ENCYCLOPEDIA OF

Natural Medicine

· ·

REVISED 2ND EDITION

ENCYCLOPEDIA OF

Natural Medicine

· ·

REVISED 2ND EDITION

Michael T. Murray, N.D.

Joseph E. Pizzorno, N.D.

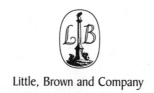

Little, Brown and Company

A *Little, Brown* Book

First published in the USA in 1998
by Prima Publishing

First published in Great Britain in 1998
by Little, Brown and Company

A CIP catalogue record for this book
is available from the British Library

ISBN 0 316 64678 4

Printed and bound in Great Britain by MPG Books Ltd Bodmin Cornwall

Little, Brown and Company (UK)
Brettanham House
Lancaster Place
London WC2E 7EN

To the Beauty, Truth, and Wisdom of Naturopathic Medicine

This book is dedicated to Dr. John Bastyr and all the natural healers of the past and the future who bring the virtues of the "healing power of nature" to all the people of the world. Dr. Bastyr, the namesake for Bastyr University, exemplified the ideal physician/healer/teacher we endeavor to become in our professional lives. We pass on a few of his words to all who strive to provide the best of health care and healing: "Always touch your patients—let them know you care" and "Always read at least one research article or learn a new remedy before you retire at night."

CONTENTS

Preface ix

Acknowledgments x

What Is Natural Medicine? 1

PART I

THE FOUR CORNERSTONES OF GOOD HEALTH 17

A Positive Mental Attitude 19

A Healthy Lifestyle 33

A Health-Promoting Diet 44

Supplementary Measures 71

PART II

ENHANCING KEY BODY SYSTEMS 81

Heart and Cardiovascular Health 83

Detoxification 104

Digestion and Elimination 126

Immune Support 145

Longevity and Life Extension 162

Stress Management 175

PART III

SPECIFIC HEALTH PROBLEMS 189

Acne 191

AIDS and HIV Infection 199

Alcoholism 211

Alzheimer's Disease 221

Anemia 233

Angina 242

Anxiety 252

Asthma and Hay Fever 260

Attention Deficit Disorders 273

Bipolar (Manic) Depression 282

Bladder Infection (Cystitis) 285

Boils 292

Bronchitis and Pneumonia 295

Candidiasis, Chronic 300

Canker Sores 313

Carpal Tunnel Syndrome 316

Cataracts 319

Celiac Disease 325

Cellulite 329

Cerebral Vascular Insufficiency 335

Cervical Dysplasia 341

Cholesterol 347

Chronic Fatigue Syndrome   359
Common Cold   371
Depression   377
Diabetes Mellitus   401
Diarrhea   431
Ear Infection (Otitis Media)   440
Eczema (Atopic Dermatitis)   448
Fibrocystic Breast Disease   455
Fibromyalgia   459
Food Allergies   464
Gallstones   476
Glaucoma   485
Gout   489
Headache   497
Heart Disease   500
Hemorrhoids   507
Hepatitis   512
Herpes   520
High Blood Pressure   524
Hives   536
Hypoglycemia   548
Hypothyroidism   558
Impotence   564
Infertility, Male   575
Inflammatory Bowel Disease   587
Insomnia   602
Irritable Bowel Syndrome   609
Kidney Stones   614
Leukoplakia   620

Macular Degeneration · 622
Menopause   628
Menstrual Blood Loss, Excessive   645
Migraine Headache   648
Multiple Sclerosis   666
Nausea and Vomiting of Pregnancy   677
Obesity   680
Osteoarthritis   695
Osteoporosis   706
Periodontal Disease   722
Premenstrual Syndrome   730
Prostate Enlargement   753
Psoriasis   763
Rheumatoid Arthritis   770
Rosacea   790
Seasonal Affective Disorder   792
Seborrheic Dermatitis   794
Sinusitis   797
Sore Throat   801
Sports Injuries, Tendinitis, and
   Bursitis   805
Ulcers   810
Vaginitis   818
Varicose Veins   826

Glossary   831
References   839
Index   923

PREFACE

This book was written in an effort to update the public's knowledge on the use of "natural" medicines in the maintenance of health and treatment of disease. It dispels a common myth that natural medicine is "unscientific." This book contains information based on firm scientific inquiry and represents countless hours of research. We believe it continues to be the most thoroughly researched and referenced book on the use of natural medicines ever written for the public.

The book must not be used in place of a physician or qualified health care practitioner. It is designed for use in conjunction with the services provided by physicians practicing, or receptive to, natural medicine. Readers are strongly urged to develop a good relationship with a physician knowledgeable in the art and science of natural and preventive medicine, such as a naturopathic physician. Unfortunately, there are not many of us, so you may need to reeducate your family physician. In all cases involving physical complaints, ailments, or therapies, please consult a physician. Proper medical care and advice can significantly improve the quality and duration of your life.

With this in mind, it can be stated that the information in this book is meant to be used, not simply read. Commit yourself to following the guidelines of natural health care as outlined in this book and you will be rewarded immensely. Your reward will be a life full of health, vitality, and vigor.

Michael T. Murray, N.D.
Joseph E. Pizzorno, N.D.

ACKNOWLEDGMENTS

MICHAEL T. MURRAY, N.D.

Most of all I would like to acknowledge that inner voice that has guided me in my life, providing me with inspiration, strength, and humility at the most appropriate times.

This work represents a great deal of things to me, including commitment and dedication. My motivation was to share the good that I know can come from using natural medicine appropriately. It can literally change people's lives. I know it changed mine.

There are many things that I am thankful for. I am especially thankful for my wife and best friend, Gina. I have also been blessed by having wonderful parents whose support and faith have never waned. If every child were loved as much as I was, it would truly be a wonderful world. Thank you Mom and Dad. I now have the opportunity to carry on their legacy of love with my own children, Alexa and Zachary.

In addition to my family, those people who have truly inspired me include Dr. Ralph Weiss, Dr. Ed Madison, Dr. Bill Mitchell, my classmates and the entire Bastyr University community, Terry Lemerond, Anthony Robbins, Dr. Gaetano Morello, and all of the special people I am lucky enough to call friends who have helped me on my life's journey.

And finally, I am deeply honored to have Dr. Joe Pizzorno, not only as my co-author, but also as a truly valued friend and inspiration. The world is truly a better place because of the vision, commitment, and qualities of this man.

JOSEPH E. PIZZORNO, N.D.

Many people have helped me throughout my life to be a better human being, healer, and educator. I hope this work will help repay all the care I have received.

In particular, I would like to thank my parents, Joe and Mary Pizzorno, for their love and support, Mary Ann Feller for seeing and nurturing the human within, Madison for her spiritual guidance, John Bastyr, N.D., for the inspiration, Jeff Bland, Ph.D., for helping me see how to bring science into natural medicine, Michael Murray, N.D., for so effectively bringing natural medicine to the public, Sheila Quinn for her friendship and help creating Bastyr College, and John Daley, Ph.D., for helping me mature the College into a University.

Finally, and most important, my appreciation and love for my dear wife, Lara, and wonderful children, Raven and Galen, for their inexhaustible love and patience. They mean the world to me.

FROM BOTH MICHAEL T. MURRAY, N.D., AND JOSEPH E. PIZZORNO, N.D.

We would also like to acknowledge the tremendous support and encouragement from Ben Dominitz and everyone at Prima. We are especially grateful to Leslie Yarborough Eschen, the editor on this project, for the huge effort she put forth coordinating the enormous task of getting this book revised (and significantly improved). We would also like to acknowledge the copy editor on this project, Carol Venolia, for helping put this book into a language and format that is "reader friendly." Thank you to everyone at Prima involved in this project.

What Is Natural Medicine?

Naturopathic medicine is a system of medicine that focuses on prevention and the use of non-toxic, natural therapies.

Naturopathic medicine is based on seven principles:
1. **First, do no harm** (*primum no nocere*)
2. **Nature has healing powers** (*vis medicatrix naturae*)
3. **Identify and treat the cause** (*tolle causam*)
4. **Treat the whole person**
5. **The physician is a teacher**
6. **Prevention is the best cure**
7. **Establish health and wellness**

As health care costs skyrocket, there is a tremendous need for naturopathic medicine.

Nature is doing her best each moment to make us well. She exists for no other end. Do not resist. With the least inclination to be well, we should not be sick.

HENRY DAVID THOREAU

A revolution is occurring in health care. At the forefront of this revolution is naturopathic medicine, a system that focuses on promoting health and on treating disease with natural, nontoxic therapies.

Before defining naturopathic medicine more fully, let's take a look at the emerging paradigm in medicine. A paradigm is a model that is used to explain events. As our understanding of the environment and the human body evolves, new paradigms (explanations) are developed.

This situation is most evident in the realm of physics. The classical cause-and-effect views of Descartes and Newton have been replaced by quantum mechanics, Einstein's theory of relativity, and the theoretical physics of Stephen Hawking. In classical physics, every action was viewed as having an equal and opposite reaction. The new paradigm incorporates possibilities instead of certainties and takes into consideration the tremendous interconnectedness of the universe. In other words, it takes a holistic view rather than breaking complex phenomena down into simplified terms.

Historically, paradigm shifts in medicine have lagged behind those in physics, but the medical paradigm shift is now in progress. The old paradigm was that the human body functions like a machine. The new paradigm focuses on the interconnectedness of body, mind, emotions, social factors, and the environment in determining the status of health. Rather than relying on drugs and surgery, the emerging model utilizes natural, noninvasive techniques to promote health and healing.

The relationship between the physician and patient is also evolving. The era of the physician as a demigod is over. The era of self-empowerment is beginning.

A Brief History of Naturopathy

Naturopathy, or "nature cure," is a method of healing that employs various natural means to empower an individual to achieve the highest possible level of health. Although the term "naturopathic medicine" was not used until the late nineteenth century, its philosophical roots go back thousands of years. Naturopathy draws on the healing wisdom of many countries, including India (Ayurveda), China (Taoism), and Greece (Hippocrates).

The European tradition of "taking the cure" at natural springs or spas gained a foothold in America by the middle of the eighteenth century, making the United States receptive to the ideas of naturopathy. Among the movement's earliest promoters were Father Sebastian Kneipp, a priest who credited his recovery from tuberculosis to bathing in the Danube, and Benedict Lust, a physician who trained at the water-cure clinic that Kneipp founded in Europe. Lust arrived in the United States in the 1890s and began using the term "naturopathy" to describe an eclectic combination of natural healing doctrines.[1]

In 1902, Lust founded the first U.S. college of naturopathic medicine in New York City. It taught a system of medicine that included the best of what was then known about nutritional therapy, natural diet, herbal medicine, homeopathy, spinal manipulation, exercise therapy, hydrotherapy, electrotherapy, stress reduction, and other natural therapies. The basic

Old Paradigm	New Paradigm
The body is a machine	Address the whole patient
The body and mind are separate	The body and mind are interconnected
Emphasize the elimination of disease	Emphasize achieving good health
Treat symptoms	Treat underlying causes
Specialize (with the risk of tunnel-vision)	Take an integrated approach
Use high-technology, heroic measures	Focus on diet, lifestyle, and preventive measures
Focus on objective information (how the patient is doing based on charts, statistics, test results, etc.)	Focus on subjective information (how the patient is feeling)
The physician should be emotionally neutral and detached	The physician's caring and empathy are critical to healing
The physician is the all-knowing authority	The physician is a partner in the healing process
The physician is in control of the patient's health decisions	The patient is in charge of health care choices

tenets of Lust's view of naturopathy are summarized in his book, *The Principles, Aim, and Program of the Nature Cure:*[2]

The natural system for curing disease is based on a return to nature in regulating the diet, breathing, exercising, bathing, and the employment of various forces to eliminate the poisonous products in the system, and so raise the vitality of the patient to a proper standard of health . . .

THE PROGRAM OF NATUROPATHIC CURE

1. ELIMINATION OF EVIL HABITS, or the weeds of life, such as overeating, alcoholic drinks, drugs, the use of tea, coffee, and cocoa that contain poisons, meat eating, improper hours of living, waste of vital forces, lowered vitality, sexual and social aberrations, worry, etc.

2. CORRECTIVE HABITS. Correct breathing, correct exercise, right mental attitude. Moderation in the pursuit of health and wealth.

3. NEW PRINCIPLES OF LIVING. Proper fasting, selection of food, hydropathy, light and air baths, mud baths, osteopathy, chiropractic and other forms of mechano-therapy, mineral salts obtained in organic form, electropathy, heliopathy, steam or Turkish baths, sitz baths, etc. . . .

There is really but one healing force in existence and that is Nature herself, which means the inherent restorative power of the organism to overcome disease. Now the question is, can this power be appropriated and guided more readily by extrinsic or intrinsic methods? That is to say, is it more amenable to combat disease by irritating drugs, vaccines, and serums employed by superstitious moderns, or by the bland intrinsic congenial forces of Natural Therapeutics, that are employed by this new school of medicine, that is Naturopathy, which is the only orthodox school of medicine? Are not these natural forces much more orthodox than the artificial resources of the druggist? The practical application of these natural agencies, duly suited to the individual case, are true signs that the art of healing has been elaborated by the aid of absolutely harmless, congenial treatments.

The early naturopaths and their contemporaries attached great importance to a natural, healthful diet. John Kellogg was a physician, Seventh-Day Adventist, and vegetarian who ran the Adventist Battle Creek Sanitarium, which utilized natural therapies. His brother, Will, built and ran a factory in Battle Creek, Michigan, to produce health foods such as shredded wheat and granola biscuits. Driven both by personal convictions about the benefits of cereal fibers and by commercial interests, the Kellogg brothers helped popularize naturopathic ideas about food, as did their former employee C. W. Post.

Naturopathic medicine grew and flourished from the early 1900s until the mid-1930s. At that point, several factors allowed the conventional medical profession to initiate its virtual monopoly of health care:

- The medical profession finally stopped using such "heroic" therapies as bloodletting and mercury dosing and replaced them with new therapies that were more effective and much less toxic
- Foundations supported by the drug industry began heavily subsidizing medical schools
- The medical profession became much more of a political force, and legislation was passed that severely restricted the use of other health care systems[1,3]

However, in the last two decades naturopathy has experienced a tremendous resurgence, largely as a result of two factors: increased public awareness of the role of diet and lifestyle in chronic disease, and the failure of modern medicine to deal effectively with these disorders. In addition, the emergence of Bastyr University (founded in 1978) and its focus on teaching science-based natural medicine has played a major role.

The Philosophy of Naturopathic Medicine

Let's take a closer look now at the seven time-tested medical principles on which naturopathic medicine is based:

1. First, do no harm *(primum no nocere)*.

Naturopathic physicians seek to do no harm with medical treatment by employing safe and effective natural therapies.

2. Nature has healing powers *(vis medicatrix naturae)*.

Naturopathic physicians believe that the body has considerable power to heal itself. It is the role of the physician to facilitate and enhance this process with the aid of natural, nontoxic therapies.

3. Identify and treat the cause *(tolle causam)*.

Naturopathic physicians are trained to seek the underlying causes of a disease rather than to simply suppress the symptoms. Symptoms are viewed as expressions of the body's attempt to heal, while the causes can spring from the physical, mental-emotional, and spiritual levels.

4. Treat the whole person.

Naturopathic physicians are trained to view an individual as a whole, composed of a complex set of physical, mental-emotional, spiritual, social, and other factors.

5. The physician is a teacher.

Naturopathic physicians are primarily teachers, educating, empowering, and motivating patients to assume more personal responsibility for their health by adopting a healthy attitude, lifestyle, and diet.

6. Prevention is the best cure.

Naturopathic physicians are preventive medicine specialists. Prevention of disease is accomplished through education and encouraging life habits that support health and prevent disease.

7. Establish health and wellness.

The primary goals of the naturopathic physician are to establish and maintain optimum health and to promote wellness. While "health" is defined as the state of optimal physical, mental, emotional, and spiritual well-being, "wellness" is defined as a state of health, characterized by a positive emotional state. The naturopathic physician strives to increase the patient's level of wellness, regardless of the level of health or disease. Even in cases of severe disease, a high level of wellness can often be achieved.

Naturopathic Therapies

In addition to providing recommendations on lifestyle, diet, and exercise, naturopathic physicians may utilize a variety of therapeutic modalities to promote health. Some naturopathic physicians emphasize a particular therapeutic modality, while others utilize a number of modalities. Furthermore, some naturopaths focus in particular medical fields such as pediatrics, natural childbirth, or physical medicine (including massage and therapeutic manipulation).

The current range of therapies in which naturopathic physicians are trained includes clinical nutrition, botanical medicine, homeopathy, Traditional Chinese Medicine and acupuncture, hydrotherapy, physical medicine, counseling and other psychotherapies, and minor surgery (i.e., suturing wounds, removing warts or moles, and other minor office procedures). In addition, in certain states (notably Oregon and Washington), licensed naturopathic physicians are granted prescription privileges for naturally derived prescription items, including vitamins, minerals, hormones (corticosteroids, estrogen, thyroxine, etc.), pancreatin, bile acids, antibiotics, and plant-based drugs such as belladonna and scopolamine.

Clinical Nutrition

Clinical nutrition—the use of diet as a therapy—serves as the foundation of naturopathic medicine. There is a growing body of knowledge that supports the use of whole foods and nutritional supplements in the maintenance of health and the treatment of disease.

Botanical Medicine

Plants have been used as medicines since antiquity. Naturopathic physicians are professionally trained herbalists; they know both the historical uses of plants and their modern pharmacological mechanisms.

Homeopathy

The term "homeopathy" is derived from the Greek words *homeos,* meaning similar, and *pathos,* meaning disease. Homeopathy is a system of medicine that treats a disease with very minute quantities of an agent, or drug, that will produce the same symptoms as the disease when given to a healthy individual; the fundamental principle is that "like cures like." Homeopathic medicines are derived from a variety of plant, mineral, and chemical substances.

Traditional Chinese Medicine and Acupuncture

Traditional Chinese Medicine and acupuncture are part of an ancient system of techniques used to enhance the flow of vital energy *(chi).* Acupuncture involves the stimulation of certain specific points on the body along *chi* pathways called "meridians." Acupuncture points can be stimulated by inserting and withdrawing needles, applying heat ("moxibustion"), massage, a laser beam, electricity, or a combination of these methods.

Hydrotherapy

Hydrotherapy may be defined as the use of water in any of its forms (hot water, cold water, ice, steam, etc.) and methods of application (sitz bath, douche, spa or hot tub, whirlpool, sauna, shower, immersion bath, pack, poultice, foot bath, fomentation, wrap, colonic irrigation, etc.) in the maintenance of health or treatment of disease. It is one of the most ancient methods of treatment. Hydrotherapy was used to treat disease and injury in many different cultures, including Egyptian, Assyrian, Persian, Greek, Hebrew, Hindu, and Chinese.

Physical Medicine

"Physical medicine" refers to the use of physical measures in the treatment of an individual. This includes physiotherapy, such as ultrasound, diathermy, and other electromagnetic energy agents; therapeutic exercise; massage; joint mobilization (manipulative) and immobilization techniques; and hydrotherapy.

Counseling and Lifestyle Modification

Counseling and lifestyle modification techniques are essential to the naturopathic practice. A naturopath is formally trained in the following counseling areas:

- Interviewing and responding skills, active listening, assessing body language, and other contact skills necessary for the therapeutic relationship
- Recognizing and understanding prevalent psychological issues, including developmental problems, abnormal behavior, addictions, stress, sexual problems, etc.
- Various treatment measures, including hypnosis and guided imagery, counseling techniques, correcting underlying organic factors, and family therapy

The Naturopathic Medical Practice

The modern naturopathic physician provides all phases of primary health care. In other words, a naturopathic physician is trained to be the first doctor seen by a patient for general (non-emergency) health care. Naturopathic clinical assessment generally follows the conventional medical model, with a reliance on medical history, a physical exam, laboratory evaluation, and other well-accepted diagnostic procedures. In addition, the clinical assessment may be influenced by nonconventional diagnostic techniques, depending upon the orientation of the naturopathic physician. For example, a naturopathic physician who has been trained in Traditional Chinese Medicine or Ayurvedic medicine will probably also utilize diagnostic techniques based on these systems of medicine.

A typical first office visit with a naturopathic doctor takes one hour. Since teaching the patient how to live healthfully is a primary goal of naturopathy, the time devoted to discussing and explaining principles of health maintenance sets naturopaths apart from many other health care providers.

The patient-physician relationship begins with a thorough medical history and an interview designed to cover all aspects of a patient's lifestyle. Making a diagnosis of a disease is only one part of this process. If needed, the physician will perform standard diagnostic procedures, including a physical exam and a blood and urine analysis. Once a good understanding of the patient's health and disease status is established, the doctor and patient will work together to establish a treatment and a health-promoting program.

Because many naturopathic physicians function as primary health care providers, standard medical monitoring, follow-up, and exams are critical to good patient care. Patients are encouraged to receive yearly checkups, including a full physical.

When therapies are used, conventional tools are used to assess the outcomes. These tools may include a patient interview, a physical exam, laboratory tests, radiological imaging, or other diagnostic techniques.

Contrasting Naturopathy with Allopathy

You may be wondering how a naturopathic physician views health differently than a conventional medical doctor. Conventional medicine is also referred to as *allopathic* medicine. The definition of allopathy is "a term that describes conventional medicine as practiced by a graduate of a medical school or college granting the M.D. degree." Allopathy is a system of medicine that focuses primarily on treating disease rather than on promoting health.

The biggest difference between naturopathy and allopathy is that the allopathic physician tends to view good health as a physical state in which there is no obvious disease present. In contrast, naturopathic physicians recognize true health as an optimal state of physical, mental, emotional, and spiritual well-being. The key differences between a naturopathic and an allopathic physician are apparent if we look at how each doctor views both health and disease.

To illustrate the differences, let's take a look how each views and addresses the infection equation. The infection equation is like a mathematical equation, such as $1 + 2 = 3$. In the infection equation, the outcome is determined by the interaction of a person's immune system with the infecting organism. In other words, immunity plus infection equals state of health. A naturopathic doctor tends to use treatments designed to enhance the immune system, while most allopathic doctors tend to use treatments designed to kill the infecting organism.

Allopathic physicians have long been obsessed with the agent that causes infection rather than with the immune system of the patient. This obsession began with Louis Pasteur, the nineteenth-century physician and researcher who discovered the antibiotic effects of penicillin. Pasteur played a major role in the development of the germ theory. This theory holds that different diseases are caused by different infectious organisms. Much of Pasteur's life was dedicated to finding substances that would kill the infecting organisms. Pasteur—and others who pioneered effective treatments for infectious diseases—gave us a great deal for which we can be thankful. However, there is more to the infection equation than the virility of the infecting organism.

Another nineteenth-century French scientist, Claude Bernard, also made major contributions to medical understanding. But Bernard had a different view of health and disease. Bernard believed that the state of a person's internal environment was more important in determining disease than the infecting organism or pathogen itself. In other words, Bernard believed that the internal "terrain," or the susceptibility of an individual to infection, was more important than the germ. Physicians, he believed, should focus more of their attention on making this internal terrain an inhospitable place for disease to flourish.

Bernard's theory led to some interesting studies. In fact, a firm advocate of the germ theory would find some of these studies to be absolutely crazy. One of the most interesting studies was conducted by a Russian scientist named Elie Metchnikoff, who discovered white blood cells. He and his research associates consumed cultures that contained millions of cholera bacteria, yet none of them developed cholera. The reason: their immune systems were not compromised. Metchnikoff believed, like Bernard, that the correct way to deal with infectious disease was to focus on enhancing the body's own defenses.

During the last part of their lives, Pasteur and Bernard engaged in scientific discussions on the virtues of the germ theory and Bernard's perspective on the internal terrain. On his death bed, Pasteur said: "Bernard was right. The pathogen is nothing. The terrain is everything." Unfortunately, Pasteur's legacy is the obsession with the pathogen; modern medicine has largely forgotten the importance of the "terrain."

The Role of Antibiotics

Now, I want to make it clear that antibiotics have their place in modern medicine. In fact, I am extremely grateful that we have these wondrous agents. When my daughter Alexa was eleven months old, she developed a kidney infection that she probably would not have recovered from without the help of antibiotics.

There is little argument that, when used appropriately, antibiotics can save lives. However, there is also little argument that antibiotics are grossly overused. While the appropriate use of antibiotics makes good medical sense, what does not make sense is the reliance on antibiotics for such conditions as acne, recurrent bladder infections, chronic ear infections, chronic sinusitis, chronic bronchitis, and nonbacterial sore throats. Relying on antibiotics in the treatment of these conditions does not make sense; the antibiotics rarely provide benefit, and these conditions are effectively treated with natural measures.

The widespread use and abuse of antibiotics is increasingly alarming for many reasons, including the near-epidemic growth of chronic candidiasis and the development of "superbugs" that are resistant to currently available antibiotics. According to many experts, including the World Health Organization, we are coming dangerously close to arriving at a "post-antibiotic era," in which many infectious diseases will once again become almost impossible to treat.[4-6]

Since there is evidence that resistance to antibiotics is less of a problem when antibiotics are used sparingly, reduction in antibiotic prescriptions may be the only significant way to address the problem. According to several authorities, antibiotic use must be restricted if the growing trend toward bacterial resistance to antibiotics is to be stopped.

As we naturopathic doctors see it, this challenge will force conventional medical practitioners to look at ways of enhancing resistance to infection. Our belief is that, as they do so, they will discover the healing power of nature. There is a growing body of knowledge that supports the use of whole foods and nutritional supplements in maintaining health and treating disease.

Treatment with Naturopathic Medicines

In addition to promoting good health, herbal products and nutritional supplements are often used as direct substitutes for conventional drugs. However, an important distinction must be made: in most cases, these natural medicines promote the healing process, rather than suppressing symptoms. To illustrate this point, let's compare the natural approach with the drug approach to osteoarthritis—the most common form of arthritis.

Osteoarthritis is characterized by a breakdown of cartilage. Cartilage plays an important role in joint function. Its gel-like nature protects the ends of joints by acting as a shock absorber. When this cartilage degenerates, it causes inflammation, pain, deformity, and limitation of motion in the joint.

The primary drugs used to treat osteoarthritis are the "nonsteroidal anti-inflammatory drugs," or NSAIDs, including aspirin, ibuprofen, Aleve, Feldene, and Voltaren. These drugs are used extensively in the United States, but research indicates that, while they may produce short-term benefit in the treatment of osteoarthritis, they actually accelerate the progression of joint destruction and cause more problems down the road.[7-13]

NSAIDs hinder cartilage repair by inhibiting the formation of compounds known as glycosaminoglycans (GAGs). These compounds are responsible for maintaining the proper water content in the cartilage matrix, thereby helping cartilage keep its gel-like nature and shock-absorbing qualities. NSAIDs are also associated with side effects—including gastrointestinal upset, headaches, and dizziness—and are therefore recommended for only short periods of time.

Simply stated, aspirin and other NSAIDs appear to suppress the symptoms but accelerate the progression of osteoarthritis. They are designed to fight disease rather than promote health.

The use of glucosamine sulfate in the treatment of osteoarthritis is consistent with the philosophy and practice of naturopathic medicine because of its action in facilitating the body's natural healing process. The clinical benefits of treating osteoarthritis with glucosamine sulfate are impressive.[14–22] In head-to-head comparison studies, glucosamine sulfate has been shown to provide greater benefit than ibuprofen and piroxicam (Feldene). While side effects are common—even expected—when using NSAIDs, glucosamine sulfate does not cause side effects.

In the most recent study, 329 patients were given one of the following for ninety days: 1,500 mg of glucosamine sulfate; 20 mg of piroxicam (Feldene); both compounds; or a placebo.[22] The results of the study were strikingly in favor of glucosamine sulfate alone. Not only was glucosamine sulfate more effective, but it was without significant side effects. In fact, patients who took glucosamine sulfate had fewer side effects than the placebo group, and no dropouts occurred in the glucosamine sulfate group. In contrast, over forty percent of the subjects taking Feldene experienced side effects, and twenty patients taking Feldene had to drop out of the study because the side effects were so severe.

While NSAIDs offer purely symptomatic relief from osteoarthritis—and may actually promote the disease process—glucosamine sulfate appears to address one of the underlying causes of osteoarthritis: reduced manufacture of GAGs. By getting at the root of the problem, glucosamine sulfate not only reduces the symptoms, but also helps the body repair damaged joints. This effect is outstanding, especially considering glucosamine's safety and lack of side effects.

The treatment of osteoarthritis is just one example in which a more natural approach produces better results and does so without side effects.

Complementary Aspects of Naturopathic Medicine

In addition to being used as primary therapy, naturopathic medicine is useful as a complementary approach to conventional medicine. This is especially true with more severe illnesses that require pharmacological and/or surgical intervention, such as cancer, angina, congestive heart failure, Parkinson's disease, and trauma. For example, a patient who has severe congestive heart failure that requires such drugs as digoxin and furosemide can benefit from the appropriate use of thiamin, carnitine, and coenzyme Q_{10} supplementation. Although there are double-blind studies demonstrating the value of these agents as complementary therapies in congestive heart failure, they are rarely prescribed by conventional medical doctors in the United States.[23–29]

Naturopathic Medicine as Prevention

Ultimately, naturopathic medicine may prove most useful in the prevention of disease.

Naturopathic physicians are trained to spend considerable time and effort in teaching patients the importance of a health-promoting lifestyle, diet, and attitude. True primary prevention involves addressing a patient's risk for disease (especially for heart disease, cancer, stroke, diabetes, or osteoporosis) and instituting a course of action designed to reduce controllable risk factors.

The health benefits and cost-effectiveness of disease-prevention programs have been clearly demonstrated. Studies have consistently found that participants in wellness-oriented programs reduced their number of days of disability (by forty-three percent in one study), number of days spent in a hospital (by fifty-four percent in one study), and amount of money spent on health care (by a remarkable seventy-six percent in one study).[30]

The Need for Naturopathic Medicine

There is a tremendous need for naturopathic medicine to become the dominant method of medicine in practice. In the United States,

we spend over one trillion dollars each year on health care—or, more accurately, on "disease care." Health care costs now consume fifteen percent of the gross national product (GNP), with the percentage of GNP spent on health care increasing at twice the rate of inflation. If the rate of increase continues, health care costs will consume the entire GNP by the year 2040! We cannot afford to continue going in this direction.

Why have health care costs skyrocketed? There are three primary reasons:

1. We have too many doctors. The number of practicing medical doctors went from 151 doctors per 100,000 people in 1970 to 245 per 100,000 in 1992—an increase of sixty-two percent.

2. We have too many medical specialists. From 1950 to 1990, specialists went from comprising thirty percent of the physician workforce to accounting for seventy to eighty percent.[31]

3. There are too many medical procedures, surgeries, unnecessary visits to doctors, and drugs being administered by doctors. Currently, medical analysts estimate that thirty-six percent of visits to physicians are unnecessary, fifty-six percent of surgeries are unnecessary, fifteen percent of hospital out-

TABLE 1	Definitions of Prevention	
Primary prevention	Lifestyle modification, decreased dietary fat, increased fiber intake, increased intake of plant foods, nutritional supplementation, smoking cessation, alcohol abuse cessation, counseling, immunization
Secondary prevention	Early detection of subclinical disease to prevent further disability; screening for hypertension, hearing impairment, visual acuity, osteoporosis, high cholesterol, malignant diseases (e.g., regular gynecological exams, mammograms, prostate-specific antigen testing)
Tertiary prevention	Minimizing disability and handicap from established disease

patient visits are unnecessary, and half of all the time spent in hospitals is not medically indicated.

One of the most disturbing findings is that the rate of surgeries performed in a given area has more to do with the number of surgeons in the area than with the size of the population. One study showed that an area with 4.5 surgeons per 10,000 people experienced 940 operations per 10,000, while an area with 2.5 surgeons per 10,000 people experienced 590 operations per 10,000.[32] In other words, when the concentration of surgeons doubles, so does the rate of surgeries. After all, these surgeons need to perform surgeries to cover overhead and maintain their desired income.

The problem is apparently worse for the especially expensive surgeries. For example, it has been clearly demonstrated that eighty percent of scheduled coronary artery bypass surgeries are inappropriate.[33] This surgical procedure carries an average price tag of $40,000. The increase in expensive hospital-based procedures, such as coronary artery bypass operations prescribed by highly specialized physicians, is considered by health economists to be the primary cause of our escalating health care costs.

If naturopathic medicine, with its focus on promoting health and preventing disease, became the dominant medical model, not only would health care costs be drastically reduced, but the health of Americans would improve dramatically. It is a sad fact that while we are grossly outspending the rest of the world in health care, as a nation we are not composed of healthy individuals.

Table 2 shows the appalling statistics: almost half of all working Americans have either a serious chronic disease (arthritis, heart disease, high blood pressure, cancer, gall bladder disease, diabetes, rheumatism, emphysema, serious arteriosclerosis, and so on) or are in poor health. But the health of their nonworking dependents is even worse. As shown in Table 3, half to two-thirds of these adults suffer from chronic disease (such as cancer, diabetes, and heart disease) and poor

TABLE 2   Health Status of Working Americans Aged Eighteen to Sixty-Five

INSURANCE STATUS	POOR HEALTH	CHRONIC HEALTH PROBLEMS
Uninsured	17%	23%
Insured	12%	29%
Federal/state employee	21%	37%

TABLE 3   Health Status of Nonworking Dependents of Americans Aged Eighteen to Sixty-Five

INSURANCE STATUS	POOR HEALTH	CHRONIC HEALTH PROBLEMS
Uninsured	23%	27%
Insured	17%	32%
Dependent of federal/state employee	30%	33%

TABLE 4	The Percentage of Adult Americans Suffering from the Ten Most Common Chronic Diseases[35]						
	MEN			WOMEN			
CONDITION	18–44	45–64	65+	18–44	45–64	65+	UNDERLYING DISORDER
Arthritis	4.1%	21.4%	38.3%	6.4%	33.9%	54.4%	Inflammation, toxicity, degeneration
Asthma, emphysema, and chronic bronchitis	5.5%	8.8%	16.7%	9.3%	11.4%	12.6%	Inflammation, toxicity
Cancer	0.2%	2.3%	5.2%	0.5%	2.2%	3.8%	Toxicity, immune dysfunction
Chronic sinusitis	13.6%	16.3%	14.1%	18.3%	19.9%	17.0%	Immune dysfunction
Diabetes	0.8%	5.1%	9.1%	1.0%	5.7%	9.9%	Metabolic dysfunction, toxicity
Hay fever	10.3%	7.9%	na*	12.1%	9.8%	na*	Inflammation
Hearing impairment	6.3%	19.6%	36.2%	4.0%	10.6%	26.8%	Degeneration
High blood pressure	6.6%	25.4%	32.7%	5.7%	27.4%	45.6%	Metabolic dysfunction
Ischemic heart disease	0.3%	8.7%	17.9%	0.3%	4.3%	12.1%	Metabolic dysfunction
Visual impairment	4.3%	6.2%	10.4%	1.7%	3.2%	18.8%	Degeneration

*na = data not available

health. What's especially alarming about these statistics is that these are adults supposedly in their prime. It gets worse for the elderly, virtually all of whom suffer from one or more chronic degenerative diseases. Table 4 lists alphabetically how shockingly common many diseases related to diet and lifestyle choices are in America.

Patient Satisfaction with Naturopathic Medicine

Equally important as naturopathic medicine's clinical efficacy and cost-effectiveness is its high rate of patient satisfaction. Studies have shown that patients who utilize natural medicine and a health-promotion approach are more satisfied with the results of their treatment than are patients who receive conventional treatments such as drugs and surgeries.

A few studies have directly compared patient satisfaction using natural medicine to patient satisfaction using conventional medicine. The largest study was done in the Netherlands, where natural medicine practitioners are an integral part of the health care system.[36] This extensive study compared satisfaction in 3,782 patients who were seeing either a conventional physician or a "complementary practitioner." The patients seeing the natural medicine practitioner reported better results for almost every condition (see Table 5). Of particular interest was the observation that the patients seeing the complementary practitioners were somewhat sicker at the start of therapy, and that in only four of the twenty-three conditions did the conventional medical patients report better results. What

TABLE 5 Patient Satisfaction with Complementary Practitioners Compared to Medical Specialists[36]

SYMPTOM	COMPLEMENTARY PRACTITIONER PATIENTS % IMPROVED	MEDICAL PATIENTS % IMPROVED
Palpitations	63	59
Stiffness	67	54
Feeling very ill	75	78
Itching or burning	71	50
Tiredness or lethargy	70	60
Fever	86	100
Pain	70	58
Tension or depression	69	65
Coughing	76	50
Blood loss	100	100
Tingling, numbness	59	40
Shortness of breath	77	53
Nausea and vomiting	71	67
Diarrhea and constipation	67	50
Poor vision or hearing	31	47
Paralysis	80	67
Insomnia	58	45
Dizziness and fainting	80	53
Anxiety	65	64
Skin rash	58	50
Emotional instability	56	63
Sexual problems	57	57
Other	75	56

can be concluded from this study is that for most common health problems, alternative therapies provide better success rates in treatment than conventional medicine!

Training in Naturopathic Medicine

There are currently three accredited schools that train naturopathic physicians. Bastyr University in Seattle, Washington, founded in 1978, is accredited by the Commission on Colleges of the Northwest Association of Schools and Colleges (an institutional accrediting body recognized by the U.S. Department of Education) and the Council of Naturopathic Medical Education (CNME). The National College of Naturopathic Medicine in Portland, Oregon, founded in 1956, is accredited by the CNME. And the Southwest College of Naturopathic Medicine & Health Sciences in Tempe, Arizona, founded in 1992, is also accredited by the CNME. All three colleges offer a four-year program leading to the Doctor of Naturopathic Medicine (N.D.) degree.

Undergraduate premedical coursework is required for admission to a college of naturopathy. This includes classes in general chemistry, organic chemistry, physics, algebra, general biology, psychology, and English composition.

Curriculum

The curriculum is divided into two primary categories: academic and clinical. The first academic year primarily covers the normal structure and function of the human body (anatomy, physiology, biochemistry, histology, embryology, etc.). The second year focuses on the pathological transitions through disease, along with clinical recognition of these processes using physical, clinical, radiological, and laboratory diagnostics.

The third and fourth academic years focus on the conventional and naturopathic perspectives on clinical aspects of pediatrics, gynecology, obstetrics, dermatology, neurology, endocrinology, cardiology, gastroenterology, and geriatrics. During the third and fourth years, there is also a focus on naturopathic therapies.

Students are required to take core classes (usually two or three quarters) in botanical medicine, homeopathy, counseling, therapeutic nutrition, and physical medicine. They are then able to choose which modality to focus on in elective advanced courses, or they may choose courses in other areas such as acupuncture and Ayurvedic medicine to meet elective requirements.

The clinical curriculum begins in the first year, with students assisting in patient care and/or in the pharmacy and laboratory. Although no naturopathic medical school currently has inpatient facilities, all three schools have extensive clinical facilities where stu-

dents work under the direction of supervising naturopathic physicians, conduct complete patient evaluation, treatment, and monitoring, and perform other aspects of patient care. Students are also required to fulfill preceptorship requirements by observing or working under the direction of licensed primary care physicians.

For more information, contact

Bastyr University
14500 Juanita Drive NE
Bothell, WA 98011-4995
206-823-1300

National College of
Naturopathic Medicine
11231 Southeast Market Street
Portland, OR 97216
503-255-4860

Southwest College of Naturopathic
Medicine & Health Sciences
2140 East Broadway Road
Tempe, AZ 85282
602-858-9100

Professional Licensing

Naturopathic physicians are currently licensed as primary health care providers in Alaska, Arizona, Connecticut, Hawaii, Maine, Montana, New Hampshire, Oregon, Utah, Vermont, and Washington. In the District of Columbia, naturopathic physicians must register in order to practice. Legal provisions allow the practice of naturopathic medicine in several other states. Efforts to gain licensure elsewhere are currently underway. Naturopathic physicians are also recognized throughout all provinces in Canada.

Professional Licensing Requirements

All states and provinces with licensure laws require a resident course of at least four years and 4,100 hours of study from a college or university recognized by the State Examining Board. To qualify for a license, the applicant must satisfactorily pass the Naturopathic Physicians Licensing Exam (NPLEX), which includes basic sciences, diagnostic and therapeutic subjects, and clinical sciences. An applicant must also satisfy all licensing requirements for the individual state or province to which they have applied. In states that license naturopathic physicians, this requirement is a comprehensive written state board exam divided into main areas of focus and given over a two- to three-day period.

Professional Organizations

The American Association of Naturopathic Physicians (AANP) is the national professional organization of licensed naturopathic physicians. The organization also seeks to differentiate the professionally trained naturopath from unscrupulous individuals claiming to be naturopaths because they received a "mail-order" degree. In states that license naturopaths, it is apparent who is a qualified naturopathic physician. In other states, since there is no licensing board overseeing the profession, many people who receive mail-order diplomas from non-accredited correspondence schools call themselves naturopaths. In such states, the best criterion of legitimacy is whether a person graduated from one of the three schools listed above or is a member of the AANP. For more information, contact

The American Association of
Naturopathic Physicians
P.O. Box 20386
Seattle, WA 98102
206-323-7610

The Future of Naturopathic Medicine

To many people, naturopathic medicine and the entire concept of natural medicine appears to be a fad that will soon pass away. However, when viewed with an open mind it is clear that naturopathic medicine points the way to the future. There is a revolution occurring in health care, resulting in more natural therapies gaining acceptance even in mainstream medical circles.

One of the great myths about naturopathic medicine has been that there is no firm scientific evidence of the efficacy of natural therapies. However, as this book chronicles, scientific studies and observations have validated not only the use of diet, nutritional supplements, and herbal medicines, but also some of the more esoteric natural healing treatments, including acupuncture, biofeedback, meditation, and homeopathy.

In many instances, scientific investigation has not only validated the natural treatment measure (such as diet therapy, nutritional supplementation, or herbal medicine), but also led to significant improvements and greater understanding. In the past thirty or so years, there have been tremendous advances in the understanding of how many natural therapies and compounds work to promote health or treat disease.

Even in mainstream medicine, there is a growing trend toward using substances found in nature—including compounds found in the human body, such as interferon, interleukin, insulin, and human growth hormone—over synthetic drugs. Add to this the growing popularity of nutritional supplements and herbal products, and it becomes obvious that there is an emerging trend toward the use of natural medicine. It appears that the concepts and philosophy of naturopathic medicine will persist and be a major part of medicine in the future.

The doctor of the future will give no medicine, but will interest his patient in the care of the human frame, in diet, and in the cause and prevention of disease.

THOMAS EDISON

PART ONE

THE FOUR CORNERSTONES OF GOOD HEALTH

· ·

T he World Health Organization defines health as "a state of complete physical, mental, and social well-being, not merely the absence of disease or infirmity." This definition includes a positive range of health, well beyond the absence of sickness.

The issue of health and disease often comes down to individual responsibility. In this context, responsibility means choosing a healthy alternative over a less healthy one. If you want to be healthy, simply make healthy choices.

Many of our health practices and lifestyle factors are based on habit and marketing hype. The health practices and lifestyles of our parents usually become intricately woven into the fabric of our own lifestyles. Meanwhile, a great deal of time, energy, and money is spent to market bad health practices. The mass media constantly bombard us with messages affecting health, diet, and lifestyle.

The first step in achieving and maintaining health is taking personal responsibility. The second step is taking the appropriate action to achieve the results you desire.

If you have a strong foundation, achieving and maintaining health is usually quite easy when you focus on strengthening the "four cornerstones of good health." You can liken these cornerstones to the four legs on a chair or table. If you want that chair or table to remain upright when stress is placed upon it, the four legs must be intact and strong. Likewise, if you want to have good, or better yet, ideal health it is essential that the following four areas be strong

- A Positive Mental Attitude
- A Healthy Lifestyle: Exercise, Sleep, and Health Habits
- A Health-Promoting Diet
- Supplementary Measures

If you desire ideal health, it is essential that you incorporate the principles and recommendations given in Part I into your life.

A Positive Mental Attitude

. . . .

A positive mental attitude is the real foundation for optimal health.

There is an innate drive in all living things to be the best that they can be.

Achieving self-actualization begins by taking personal responsibility for your own positive mental state, your life, your current situation, and your health.

The seven key steps to developing and maintaining a positive mental attitude are
1. **Become an optimist**
2. **Become aware of self-talk**
3. **Ask better questions**
4. **Employ positive affirmations**
5. **Set positive goals**
6. **Practice positive visualizations**
7. **Laugh long and often**

Read or listen to inspiring messages.

Although all four cornerstones of good health are equally important, just as all four legs on a chair or table are essential, the cornerstone that we feel acts as the real foundation for optimal health is a positive mental attitude. There is a growing body of evidence that your habitual thoughts and emotions largely determine your level of health and the quality of your life.

Life is full of events that are beyond our control. However, we do have control over our response to these events. Our attitude goes a long way in determining how we view and respond to all of the challenges of life. You will be much happier, healthier, and more successful if you adopt a positive mental attitude than if you have a pessimistic view.

Maslow's Theory of Self-Actualization

A positive mental attitude is absolutely essential if we want to live life to the fullest. It is also essential to propel us to be the best that we can be. There appears to be an innate drive within each of us to achieve the experience of *self-actualization* in our lives. Self-actualization is a concept developed by Abraham Maslow, the founding father of humanistic psychology. His work and theories were the result of intense research on psychologically healthy people over a period of more than thirty years. Maslow was really the first psychologist to study healthy people. He strongly believed the study of healthy people would create a firm foundation for the theories and values of a new psychotherapy.

Maslow discovered that healthy individuals are motivated toward self-actualization, a process of "ongoing actualization of potentials, capacities, talents, as fulfillment of a mission (or call, fate, destiny, or vocation), as a fuller knowledge of, and acceptance of, the person's own intrinsic nature, as an increasing trend toward unity, integration, or synergy within the person." In other words, healthy people are driven to be all that they can be.

Maslow developed a five-step pyramid of human needs, in which personality development progresses from one step to the next. The needs of the lower levels must be satisfied before the next level can be achieved. When needs are met, the individual moves toward well-being and health. Figure 1 displays Maslow's hierarchy of needs.

The primary needs that form the base of the pyramid are basic survival or physiological needs: the satisfaction of hunger, thirst, sexuality, and shelter. These are essential biological needs. The next step consists of needs for safety: security, order, and stability. These

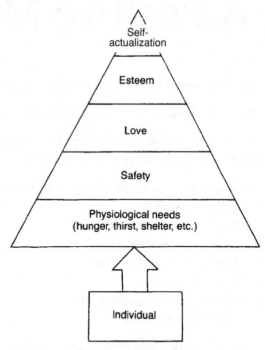

FIGURE 1 Maslow's Hierarchy of Needs

feelings are essential in dealing with the world. If these needs are satisfied, the individual can progress to the next step: love. This level refers to the ability to love and be

QUICK REVIEW

Our attitude is just like our physical body, in that it requires constant conditioning to stay fit. Just as you do not find yourself in excellent physical condition after one exercise session, you may not find yourself with a positive mental attitude after reading this chapter. We encourage you to really work at staying positive and optimistic through life. We all have our

feel unfair and undeserved; bad things do happen to good people. But it is not what happens in our lives that determines our direction; it is our response to the challenges that shapes the quality of our life. Hardship, heartbreak, disappointments, and failures are often the fuel for joy, ecstasy, compassion, and success. By conditioning your attitude to be positive, our hope is that you will experience a higher level of health and happiness in your life.

loved. The next step involves self-esteem: approval, recognition, and acceptance. These elements contribute strongly to high self-esteem and self-respect. The final step is self-actualization: the utilization of one's creative potential for self-fulfillment.

Maslow studied self-actualized people and noted that they had strikingly similar characteristics. Here, in an abbreviated form, are some of Maslow's findings:

- Self-actualized people perceive reality more effectively than others and are more comfortable with it. They have an unusual ability to detect the spurious, the fake, and the dishonest in personality. They judge experiences, people, and things correctly and efficiently. They possess an ability to be objective about their own strengths, possibilities, and limitations. This self-awareness enables them to clearly define values, goals, desires, and feelings. They are not frightened by uncertainty.
- Self-actualized people have an acceptance of self, others, and nature. They can accept their own human shortcomings without condemnation. They do not have an absolute lack of guilt, shame, sadness, anxiety, and defensiveness, but they do not experience these feelings to unnecessary or unrealistic degrees. When they do feel guilty or regretful, they do something about it. Generally, they will feel bad about discrepancies between what is and what ought to be.
- Self-actualized people are relatively spontaneous in their behavior, and even more spontaneous in their inner life, thoughts, and impulses. They are unconventional in their impulses, thoughts, and consciousness. They are rarely nonconformists, but they seldom allow convention to keep them from doing anything they consider important or basic.
- Self-actualized people have a problem-solving orientation toward life instead of an orientation centered on self. They commonly have a mission in life—some problem outside themselves that enlists much of their energies. In general, this mission is unselfish and is involved with the philosophical and the ethical.
- Self-actualized people have a quality of detachment and a need for privacy. It is often possible for them to remain above the battle, to be undisturbed by that which upsets others. They are self-governing people who find meaning in being active, responsible, self-disciplined, and decisive rather than being a pawn or a person helplessly ruled by others.
- Self-actualized people have a wonderful capacity to appreciate again and again the basic pleasures of life, such as nature, children, music, and sexual experience. They approach these basic experiences with awe, pleasure, wonder, and even ecstasy.
- Self-actualized people commonly have mystical or "peak" experiences—times of intense emotions in which they transcend the self. During a peak experience, they experience feelings of limitless horizons and unlimited power while simultaneously feeling more helpless than ever before. There is a loss of place and time, and feelings of great ecstasy, wonder, and awe. The peak experience ends with the conviction that something extremely important and valuable has happened, so that the person is to some extent transformed and strengthened by the experience.
- Self-actualized people have deep feelings of identification, sympathy, and affection for other people in spite of occasional anger, impatience, or disgust.
- Self-actualized people have deeper and more profound interpersonal relationships than most other adults, but not necessarily deeper than children's. They are capable of more closeness, greater love, more perfect identification, and more erasing of ego

boundaries than other people would consider possible. One consequence is that self-actualized people have especially deep ties with rather few individuals, and their circle of friends is small. They tend to be kind or at least patient with almost everyone, yet they do speak realistically and harshly of those who they feel deserve it, especially the hypocritical, pretentious, pompous, or self-inflated individual.

- Self-actualized people are democratic in the deepest possible sense. They are friendly toward everyone, regardless of class, education, political beliefs, race, or color. They believe it is possible to learn something from everyone. They are humble, in the sense of being aware of how little they know in comparison with what could be known and what is known by others.

- Self-actualized people are strongly ethical and moral. However, their notions of right and wrong and of good and evil are often not conventional ones. For example, a self-actualized person would have never thought segregation, apartheid, or racism to be morally right even though it may have been legal.

- Self-actualized people have a keen, unhostile sense of humor. They don't laugh at jokes that hurt other people or are aimed at others' inferiority. They can make fun of others in general, or of themselves, when they are foolish or when they try to be big when they are small. They are inclined toward thoughtful humor that elicits a smile, is intrinsic to the situation, and is spontaneous.

- Self-actualized people are highly imaginative and creative. The creativeness of a self-actualized individual is not of the special-talent type, such as Mozart's, but rather is similar to the naive and universal creativeness of unspoiled children.

The Road to Self-Actualization

Self-actualization doesn't happen all at once. It happens by degrees—subtle changes accumulating one by one. Self-actualization begins by taking personal responsibility for your own positive mental state, your life, your current situation, and your health. Once you take on this responsibility, it is up to you to direct your life. You must commit yourself to being the best you can be at whatever you do in life. For motivation, here is an all-time favorite quote from Goethe:

Until one is committed there is hesitancy, the chance to draw back, always ineffectiveness. Concerning all acts of initiative (and creation), there is one elementary truth, the ignorance of which kills countless ideas and splendid plans: that the moment one definitely commits oneself, then Providence moves too. All sorts of things occur to help one that would never have otherwise occurred. A whole stream of events issues from the decision raising in one's favor all manner of unforeseen incidents and meeting and material assistance which no man could have dreamed would have come his way. Whatever you can do, or dream you can, begin it. Boldness has genius, power and magic in it. Begin it now!

The Seven Steps to a Positive Mental Attitude

To provide some guidance toward your goal of self-actualization, we offer the following seven key steps.

Step 1: Become an Optimist

The first step in developing a positive mental attitude is to become an optimist rather than a pessimist. Fortunately, according to Martin Seligman, Ph.D. (author of *Learned Optimism*[1] and one of the world's leading authorities on optimism), we are optimists by nature. Optimism is a necessary step toward achieving self-actualization as well as our goal of ideal health. Not only does optimism help prevent disease, but science is discovering that it's a vital ally in the healing process. Conversely, a pessimistic attitude can seriously erode our health. Detailed evidence supports the contention that optimists live longer, suffer from fewer and less severe diseases, and are much healthier than pessimists.[2,3]

What distinguishes an optimist from a pessimist is the way in which they explain both good and bad events. Dr. Seligman has developed a simple test to determine your level of optimism. Take the test to determine your own level.

Are You an Optimist?

To determine whether you are an optimist, answer the following questions. Take as much time as you need. There are no right or wrong answers. It is important that you take the test before you read the interpretation. Read the description of each situation and vividly imagine it happening to you. Choose the response that most applies to you by circling either A or B. Ignore the letter and number codes for now; they will be explained later.

1. The project you are in charge of is a great success. **PsG**

   A. *I kept a close watch over everyone's work.* 1
   B. *Everyone devoted a lot of time and energy to it.* 0

2. You and your spouse (boyfriend/girlfriend) make up after a fight. **PmG**

   A. *I forgave him/her.* 0
   B. *I'm usually forgiving.* 1

3. You get lost driving to a friend's house. **PsB**

   A. *I missed a turn.* 1
   B. *My friend gave me bad directions.* 0

4. Your spouse (boyfriend/girlfriend) surprises you with a gift. **PsG**

   A. *He/she just got a raise at work.* 0
   B. *I took him/her out to a special dinner the night before.* 1

5. You forget your spouse's (boyfriend's/girlfriend's) birthday. **PmB**

   A. *I'm not good at remembering birthdays.* 1
   B. *I was preoccupied with other things.* 0

6. You get a flower from a secret admirer. **PvG**

   A. *I am attractive to him/her.* 0
   B. *I am a popular person.* 1

7. You run for a community office position and you win. **PvG**

   A. *I devote a lot of time and energy to campaigning.* 0
   B. *I work very hard at everything I do.* 1

8. You miss an important engagement. **PvB**

   A. *Sometimes my memory fails me.* 1
   B. *I sometimes forget to check my appointment book.* 0

9. You run for a community office position and you lose. **PsB**

   A. *I didn't campaign hard enough.* 1
   B. *The person who won knew more people.* 0

10. You host a successful dinner. **PmG**

    A. *I was particularly charming that night.* 0
    B. *I am a good host.* 1

(continues)

11. You stop a crime by calling the police. — PsG

    A. *A strange noise caught my attention.* — 0
    B. *I was alert that day.* — 1

12. You were extremely healthy all year. — PsG

    A. *Few people around me were sick, so I wasn't exposed.* — 0
    B. *I made sure I ate well and got enough rest.* — 1

13. You owe the library ten dollars for an overdue book. — PmB

    A. *When I am really involved in what I am reading, I often forget when it's due.* — 1
    B. *I was so involved in writing the report that I forgot to return the book.* — 0

14. Your stocks make you a lot of money. — PmG

    A. *My broker decided to take on something new.* — 0
    B. *My broker is a top-notch investor.* — 1

15. You win an athletic contest. — PmG

    A. *I was feeling unbeatable.* — 0
    B. *I train hard.* — 1

16. You fail an important examination. — PsB

    A. *I wasn't as smart as the other people taking the exam.* — 1
    B. *I didn't prepare for it well.* — 0

17. You prepared a special meal for a friend and he/she barely touched the food. — PvB

    A. *I wasn't a good cook.* — 1
    B. *I made the meal in a rush.* — 0

18. You lose a sporting event for which you have been training for a long time. — PvB

    A. *I'm not very athletic.* — 1
    B. *I'm not good at that sport.* — 0

19. Your car runs out of gas on a dark street late at night. — PsB

    A. *I didn't check to see how much gas was in the tank.* — 1
    B. *The gas guage was broken.* — 0

20. You lose your temper with a friend. — PmB

    A. *He/she is always nagging me.* — 1
    B. *He/she was in a hostile mood.* — 0

21. You are penalized for not returning your income-tax forms on time. — PmB

    A. *I always put off doing my taxes.* — 1
    B. *I was lazy about getting my taxes done this year.* — 0

22. You ask a person out on a date and he/she says no. — PvB

    A. *I was a wreck that day.* — 1
    B. *I got tongue-tied when I asked him/her on the date.* — 0

23. A game-show host picks you out of the audience to participate in the show. — PsG

    A. *I was sitting in the right seat.* — 0
    B. *I looked the most enthusiastic.* — 1

24. You are frequently asked to dance at a party. — PmG

    A. *I am outgoing at parties.* — 1
    B. *I was in perfect form that night.* — 0

25. You buy your spouse (boyfriend/girlfriend) a gift he/she doesn't like. — PsB

    A. *I don't put enough thought into things like that.* — 1
    B. *He/she has very picky tastes.* — 0

26. You do exceptionally well in a job interview. — PmG

    A. *I felt extremely confident during the interview.* — 0
    B. *I interview well.* — 1

27. You tell a joke and everyone laughs. — PsG

    A. *The joke was funny.* — 0
    B. *My timing was perfect.* — 1

28. Your boss gives you too little time in which to finish a project, but you get it finished anyway. — PvG

    A. *I am good at my job.* — 0
    B. *I am an efficient person.* — 1

29. You've been feeling run-down lately. — PmB

    A. *I never get a chance to relax.* — 1
    B. *I was exceptionally busy this week.* — 0

30. You ask someone to dance and he/she says no. — PsB

    A. *I am not a good enough dancer.* — 1
    B. *He/she doesn't like to dance.* — 0

31. You save a person from choking to death. PvG

    A. I know a technique to stop someone from choking. 0
    B. I know what to do in crisis situations. 1

32. Your romantic partner wants to cool things off for a while. PvB

    A. I'm too self-centered. 1
    B. I don't spend enough time with him/her. 0

33. A friend says something that hurts your feelings. PmB

    A. She always blurts things out without thinking of others. 1
    B. My friend was in a bad mood and took it out on me. 0

34. Your employer comes to you for advice. PvG

    A. I am an expert in the area about which I was asked. 0
    B. I'm good at giving useful advice. 1

35. A friend thanks you for helping him/her get through a bad time. PvG

    A. I enjoy helping him/her through tough times. 0
    B. I care about people. 1

36. You have a wonderful time at a party. PsG

    A. Everyone was friendly. 0
    B. I was friendly. 1

37. Your doctor tells you that you are in good physical shape. PvG

    A. I make sure I exercise frequently. 0
    B. I am very health-conscious. 1

38. Your spouse (boyfriend/girlfriend) takes you away for a romantic weekend. PmG

    A. He/she needed to get away for a few days. 0
    B. He/she likes to explore new areas. 1

39. Your doctor tells you that you eat too much sugar. PsB

    A. I don't pay much attention to my diet. 1
    B. You can't avoid sugar, it's in everything. 0

40. You are asked to head an important project. PmG

    A. I just successfully completed a similar project. 0
    B. I am a good supervisor. 1

41. You and your spouse (boyfriend/girlfriend) have been fighting a great deal. PsB

    A. I have been feeling cranky and pressured lately. 1
    B. He/she has been hostile lately. 0

42. You fall down a great deal while skiing. PmB

    A. Skiing is difficult. 1
    B. The trails were icy. 0

43. You win a prestigious award. PvG

    A. I solved an important problem. 0
    B. I was the best employee. 1

44. Your stocks are at an all-time low. PvB

    A. I didn't know much about the business climate at the time. 1
    B. I made a poor choice of stocks. 0

45. You win the lottery. PsG

    A. It was pure chance. 0
    B. I picked the right numbers. 1

46. You gain weight over the holidays and you can't lose it. PmB

    A. Diets don't work in the long run. 1
    B. The diet I tried didn't work. 0

47. You are in the hospital and few people come to visit. PsB

    A. I'm irritable when I am sick. 1
    B. My friends are negligent about things like that. 0

48. They won't honor your credit card at a store. PvB

    A. I sometimes overestimate how much money I have. 1
    B. I sometimes forget to pay my credit-card bill. 0

Scoring Key

PmB ____		PmG ____
PvB ____		PvG ____
	HoB ____	
PsB ____		PsG ____
Total B ____		Total G ____
	G–B ____	

Interpreting Your Test Results The test results will give you a clue as to your explanatory style. In other words, the results will tell you about the way in which you explain things to yourself. It tells you your habit of thought. Again, remember that there are no right or wrong answers.

There are three crucial dimensions to your explanatory style: permanence, pervasiveness, and personalization. Each dimension, plus a couple of others, will be scored from your test.

Permanence When pessimists are faced with challenges or bad events, they view these events as being permanent. In contrast, people who are optimists tend to view the challenges or bad events as temporary. Here are some statements that reflect the subtle differences:

PERMANENT (PESSIMISTIC)	TEMPORARY (OPTIMISTIC)
"My boss is always a jerk."	"My boss is in a bad mood today."
"You never listen."	"You are not listening."
"This bad luck will never stop.	"My luck has got to turn."

To determine how you view bad events, look at the eight items coded PmB (for Permanent Bad): 5, 13, 20, 21, 29, 33, 42, and 46. Each one with a "0" after it is optimistic; each one followed by a "1" is pessimistic. Total the numbers at the right-hand margin of the questions coded PmB, and write the total on the PmB line on the scoring key.

If you totaled 0 or 1, you are very optimistic on this dimension; 2 or 3 is a moderately optimistic score; 4 is average; 5 or 6 is quite pessimistic; and 7 or 8 is extremely pessimistic.

Now let's take a look at the difference in explanatory style between pessimists and optimists when there is a positive event in their lives. It's just the opposite of what happened with a bad event. Pessimists view positive events as temporary, while optimists view

them as permanent. Here again are some subtle differences in how pessimists and optimists might communicate their good fortune:

TEMPORARY (PESSIMISTIC)	PERMANENT (OPTIMISTIC)
"It's my lucky day."	"I am always lucky."
"My opponent was off today."	"I am getting better every day."
"I tried hard today."	"I always give my best."

Now total all the questions coded PmG (for Permanent Good): 2, 10, 14, 15, 24, 26, 38, and 40. Write the total on the line in the scoring key marked PmG.

If you totaled 7 or 8, you are very optimistic on this dimension; 6 is a moderately optimistic score; 4 or 5 is average; 3 is pessimistic; and 0, 1, or 2 is extremely pessimistic.

Are you starting to see a pattern? If you are scoring as a pessimist, you may want to learn how to be more optimistic. Your anxiety may be due to your belief that bad things are always going to happen, while good things are only a fluke.

Pervasiveness Pervasiveness refers to the tendency to describe things either in universals (everyone, always, never, etc.) versus specifics (a specific individual, a specific time, etc.). Pessimists tend to describe things in universals, while optimists describe things in specifics.

UNIVERSAL (PESSIMISTIC)	SPECIFIC (OPTIMISTIC)
"All lawyers are jerks."	"My attorney was a jerk."
"Instruction manuals are worthless."	"This instruction manual is worthless."
"He is repulsive."	"He is repulsive to me."

Total your score for the questions coded PvB (for Pervasive Bad): 8, 17, 18, 22, 32, 44, and 48. Write the total on the PvB line.

If you totaled 0 or 1, you are very optimistic on this dimension; 2 or 3 is a moderately optimistic score; 4 is average; 5 or 6 is quite pessimistic; and 7 or 8 is extremely pessimistic.

Now let's look at the level of pervasiveness of good events. Optimists tend to view good events as universal, while pessimists view them as specific. Again, it's just the opposite of how each views a bad event.

Total your score for the questions coded PvG (for Pervasive Good): 6, 7, 28, 31, 34, 35, 37, and 43. And write the total on the line labeled PvG.

If you totaled 7 or 8, you are very optimistic on this dimension; 6 is a moderately optimistic score; 4 or 5 is average; 3 is pessimistic; and 0, 1, or 2 is extremely pessimistic.

Hope Our level of hope or hopelessness is determined by our combined level of permanence and pervasiveness. Your level of hope may be the most significant score for this test. Take your PvB and add it to your PmB score. This is your hope score.

If it is 0, 1, or 2, you are extraordinarily hopeful; 3, 4, 5, or 6 is a moderately hopeful score; 7 or 8 is average; 9, 10, or 11 is moderately hopeless; and 12, 13, 14, 15, or 16 is severely hopeless.

People who make permanent and universal explanations for their troubles tend to suffer from stress, anxiety, and depression; they tend to collapse when things go wrong. According to Dr. Seligman, no other score is as important as your hope score.

Personalization The final aspect of explanatory style is personalization. When bad things happen, we can either blame ourselves (internalize) and lower our self-esteem as a consequence, or we can blame things beyond our control (externalize). Although it may not be right to deny personal responsibility, people who tend to externalize blame in relation to bad events have higher self-esteem and are more optimistic.

Total your score for those questions coded PsB (for Personalization Bad): 3, 9, 16, 19, 25, 30, 39, 41, and 47.

A score of 0 or 1 indicates very high self-esteem and optimism; 2 or 3 indicates moderate self-esteem; 4 is average; 5 or 6 indicates moderately low self-esteem; and 7 or 8 indicates very low self-esteem.

Now let's take a look at personalization and good events. Again, just the exact opposite occurs compared to bad events. When good things happen, the person with high self-esteem internalizes while the person with low self-esteem externalizes.

Total your score for those questions coded PsG (for Personalization Good): 1, 4, 11, 12, 23, 27, 36, and 45. Write your score on the line marked PsG on your scoring key.

If you totaled 7 or 8, you are very optimistic on this dimension; 6 is a moderately optimistic score; 4 or 5 is average; 3 is pessimistic; and 0, 1, or 2 is extremely pessimistic.

Your Overall Scores To compute your overall scores, first add the three B's (PmB + PvB + PsB). This is your B (bad event) score. Do the same for all of the G's (PmG + PvG + PsG). This is your G score. Subtract B from G; this is your overall score.

If your B score is from 3 to 6, you are marvelously optimistic when bad events occur; 10 or 11 is average; 12 to 14 is pessimistic; anything above 14 is extremely pessimistic.

If your G score is 19 or above, you think about good events extremely optimistically; 14 to 16 is average; 11 to 13 indicates pessimism; and a score of 10 or less indicates great pessimism.

If your overall score (G minus B) is above 8, you are very optimistic across the board; if it's from 6 to 8, you are moderately optimistic; 3 to 5 is average; 1 or 2 is pessimistic; and a score of 0 or below is very pessimistic.

Learning Optimism

If you are a pessimist, it is important to learn how to be optimistic. Why? Studies have shown that optimists are healthier and happier; they enjoy life at a much higher level than pessimists do. Learning to be optimistic means getting in the habit of thinking with a positive attitude. If you are pessimistic, it is only because you have gotten into the habit of thinking in a negative framework. The remaining six steps will help condition your attitude to become positive.

Step 2: Become Aware of Self-Talk

We all talk to ourselves. There is a constant dialog taking place in our heads. Our self-talk makes an impression on our subconscious mind. In order to develop or maintain a positive mental attitude, you must guard against negative self-talk. Become aware of your self-talk, and then consciously work to imprint positive self-talk on your subconscious mind. Two powerful tools in creating positive self-talk are questions and affirmations, Steps 3 and 4.

Step 3: Ask Better Questions

One of the most powerful tools that we have found for improving the quality of self-talk—and, hence, the quality of our lives—is a series of questions originally given to us by Anthony Robbins, author of the bestsellers *Unlimited Power* and *Awaken the Giant Within*. According to Tony, the quality of your life is equal to the quality of the questions you habitually ask yourself. Tony believes that whatever question you ask your brain, your brain will answer.

Let's look at the following example: A man is met with a particular challenge or problem. He can ask himself a number of questions when in this situation. Questions many people might ask include: "Why does this always happen to me?" or "Why am I always so stupid?" Do they get answers to these ques-

tions? Do the answers build self-esteem? Does the problem keep reappearing? What would be a higher-quality question? How about: "This is a very interesting situation; what do I need to learn from this situation so that it never happens again?" Or how about: "What can I do to make this situation better?"

In another example, let's look at an individual who suffers from depression. What are some questions they might ask themselves that may not be helping their situation? How about: "Why am I always so depressed? Why do things always seem to go wrong for me? Why am I so unhappy?"

What are some better questions they may want to ask themselves? How about: "What do I need to do to gain more enjoyment and happiness in my life? What do I need to commit to doing in order to have more happiness and energy in my life?" After they have answered these questions, we have depressed patients ask themselves this one: "If I had happiness and high energy levels right now, what would it feel like?" You will be amazed at how powerful questions can be in your life.

When the mind is searching for answers to these questions, it is reprogramming your subconscious into believing that you have an abundance of happiness. Unless there is a physiological reason for the depression, it won't take long before your subconscious believes it.

Regardless of the situation, asking better questions is bound to improve your attitude. If you want to have a better life, simply ask better questions. It sounds simple because it is. If you want more energy, excitement, and/or happiness in your life, simply ask yourself the following questions on a consistent basis:

1. What am I most happy about in my life right now?
   Why does that make me happy?
   How does that make me feel?

2. What am I most excited about in my life right now?

   Why does that make me excited?

   How does that make me feel?

3. What am I most grateful about in my life right now?

   Why does that make me grateful?

   How does that make me feel?

4. What am I enjoying most in my life right now?

   What about that do I enjoy?

   How does that make me feel?

5. What am I committed to in my life right now?

   Why am I committed to that?

   How does that make me feel?

6. Who do I love? (Starting close and moving out)

   Who loves me?

7. What must I do today to achieve my long-term goal?

Step 4: Employ Positive Affirmations

An affirmation is a statement with some emotional intensity behind it. Positive affirmations can make imprints on the subconscious mind to create a healthy, positive self-image. In addition, affirmations can actually fuel the changes you desire. I use certain phrases and sentences as affirmations each day. I have these affirmations in plain sight on my desk:

I am blessed with an abundance of energy!

Love, joy, and happiness flow through me with every heartbeat.

I am thankful to God for all of my good fortune!

YES I CAN!

Here are some simple guidelines for creating your own affirmations. Have fun with it! Positive affirmations can make you feel really good if you follow these guidelines:

- Always phrase an affirmation in the present tense. Imagine that it has already come to pass.
- Always phrase the affirmation as a positive statement. Do not use the words "not" or "never."
- Do your best to totally associate (link up emotionally) with the positive feelings that are generated by the affirmation.
- Keep the affirmation short and simple, but full of feeling.
- Be creative.
- Imagine yourself really experiencing what you are affirming.
- Make the affirmation personal to you and full of meaning.

Using these guidelines and examples, write down five affirmations that apply to you. State these affirmations aloud while you are taking your shower, driving, or praying.

Step 5: Set Positive Goals

Learning to set goals in a way that results in a positive experience is another powerful method for building a positive attitude and raising self-esteem. Goals can be used to create a "success cycle." Achieving goals helps you feel better about yourself, and the better you feel about yourself the more likely you are to achieve your goals. Here are some guidelines to use when setting goals:

- State the goal in positive terms; do not use any negative words in your goal statement. For example it is better to say, "I enjoy eating healthy, low-calorie, nutritious foods," than, "I will not eat sugar, candy, ice cream, and other fattening foods." Remember, always state the goal in positive terms, and do not use any negative words in the goal statement.
- Make your goal attainable and realistic. For example, if you are fully grown and 5

feet tall it isn't very realistic to set the goal of becoming a professional basketball player. If you are not used to setting goals, start out with ones that are easily attainable, like getting up in the morning at a specific time or being punctual. Again, goals can be used to create a success cycle and a positive self-image. Little things add up to make a major difference in the way you feel about yourself.

- Be specific. The more clearly your goal is defined, the more likely you are to reach it. For example, if you want to lose weight, what is the weight you desire? What body fat percentage or measurements do you desire? Clearly define what it is you want to achieve.
- State the goal in the present tense, not the future tense. In order to reach your goal, you have to believe that you have already attained it. You must literally program yourself to achieve the goal. See and feel yourself having already achieved the goal, and success will be yours.

Any voyage begins with one step and is followed by many other steps. Remember to set short-term goals that can be used to help you achieve your long-term goals. Get in the habit of asking yourself the following question each morning and evening: "What must I do today to achieve my long-term goal?"

Step 6. Practice Positive Visualizations

Positive visualization or imagery is another powerful tool in creating health, happiness, or success. We believe that we have to be able to see our lives the way we want them to be before it happens. In terms of ideal health, you must picture yourself in ideal health if you truly want to experience this state. You can use visualization in all areas of your life, but especially in your health. In fact, some of the most promising research on the power of visualization involves enhancing the immune system in the treatment of cancer. Be creative and have fun with positive visualizations, and you will soon find yourself living your dreams. It is our dreams that propel us as we roll through this life. They are powerful and inspirational. In fact, the famous author Anatole France said something about dreams and life that we think really hits home: "Existence would be intolerable if we were never to dream."

Step 7. Laugh Long and Often

By laughing frequently and taking a lighter view of life, you will find that life is much more enjoyable and fun. Researchers are discovering that laughter enhances the immune system and promotes improved physiology. Recent medical research has also confirmed that laughter

- Enhances the blood flow to the body's extremities and improves cardiovascular function.
- Plays an active part in the body's release of endorphins and other natural mood-elevating and pain-killing chemicals.
- Improves the transfer of oxygen and nutrients to internal organs.

Here are eight tips to help you have more laughter in your life

1. Learn to laugh at yourself.

Recognize how funny some of your behavior really is—especially your shortcomings or mistakes. We all have little idiosyncrasies or behaviors that are unique to us that we can recognize and enjoy. Do not take yourself too seriously.

2. Inject humor any time it is appropriate.

People love to laugh. Get a joke book and learn how to tell a good joke. Humor and laughter really make life enjoyable.

3. Read the comics to find one that you find funny and follow it.

Humor is very individual. What I may find funny, you may not, but the comics or "funny papers" have something for everybody. Read them thoroughly to find a comic strip that you find particularly funny and look for it every day or week.

4. Watch comedies on television.

With modern cable systems, I am amazed at how easy it is to find something funny on television. When I am in need of a good laugh, I try to find something I can laugh at on TV. Some of my favorites are the classics, like *Andy Griffith, Gilligan's Island,* and *Mary Tyler Moore.*

5. Go see a funny movie with a friend.

My wife and I love to go to the movies, especially a comedy. If we see a funny movie together, I find myself laughing harder and longer than if I had seen the same scene by myself. We feed off each other's laughter during and after the movie. Laughing together helps build good relationships.

6. Listen to comedy audiotapes in your car while driving.

Check your local record store, bookstore, video store, or library for recorded comedy routines of your favorite comic. If you haven't heard or seen many comics, go to your library first. You'll find an abundance of tapes to investigate, and you can check them out for free.

7. Play with kids.

Kids really know how to laugh and play. If you do not have kids of your own, spend time with your nieces, nephews, or neighborhood children with whose families you are friendly. Become a Big Brother or Sister. Investigate local Little Leagues. Help out at your church's Sunday School and children's events.

8. Ask yourself, "What is funny about this situation?"

Many times we find ourselves in seemingly impossible situations, but if we can laugh about them, somehow they become enjoyable or at least tolerable. Many times people say, "This is something that you will look back on and laugh about." Well, why wait? Find the humor in the situation and enjoy a good laugh immediately.

Recommended Reading

We recommend regular reading or listening to inspiring books. Here are some of the authors and books (in alphabetical order by author) that have inspired us the most. Most of these authors also have cassette tapes available. A good resource for tapes is Nightingale-Conant (800-525-9000).

Leo Buscaglia
  Living, Loving, and Learning
  Loving Each Other
Jack Canfield and Mark Victor Hansen
  Chicken Soup for the Soul
  All of the other "Chicken Soup" books
Dale Carnegie
  How to Win Friends & Influence People
Stephen R. Covey
  The 7 Habits of Highly Effective People
Victor Frankl
  Man's Search for Meaning
Herman Hesse
  Siddhartha
Gerald Jampolsky
  Love Is Letting Go of Fear
Og Mandino
  Mission Success
  The Greatest Salesman in the World
  The Greatest Success in the World
Alan Loy McGinnis
  The Friendship Factor
  Bringing Out the Best in People
Norman Vincent Peale
  The Power of Positive Thinking

Ken Pelletier
 Sound Mind, Sound Body
 Mind as Healer, Mind as Slayer
Anthony Robbins
 Unlimited Power
 Awaken the Giant Within
Martin Seligman
 Learned Optimism
 What You Can Change and
  What You Can't

Bernie Siegel
 Love, Medicine, and Miracles
Andrew Weil
 Spontaneous Healing
Zig Ziglar
 See You at the Top

A Healthy Lifestyle

. . . .

If you smoke, take steps to stop.

Physical inactivity is a major reason why so many Americans are overweight.

Tensions, depressions, feelings of inadequacy, and worries diminish greatly with regular exercise.

Following these seven steps will help you add regular exercise to your routine:
1. **Recognize the importance of physical exercise**
2. **Consult your physician**
3. **Select an activity you enjoy**
4. **Monitor exercise intensity**
5. **Do it often**
6. **Make it fun**
7. **Stay motivated**

Many health conditions, particularly depression, chronic fatigue syndrome, and fibromyalgia, are either entirely or partially related to sleep deprivation or disturbed sleep.

Dreams are important to mental and physical health.

Without question, a healthy lifestyle improves the quality and length of a person's life. The key components of a healthy lifestyle discussed in this chapter are avoiding cigarette smoke, following a regular exercise program, and practicing good sleep habits.

Smoking Is America's Number-One Killer

According to a report from the U.S. Surgeon General, cigarette smoking is the most important risk factor for cancer and heart disease.[1] Since these are the leading causes of death, it is quite clear that cigarette smoking is in fact America's number-one killer. There is substantial evidence to back up this statement. Detailed calculations reveal that smokers have at least three to five times as much risk of getting cancer and heart disease as nonsmokers. The more cigarettes smoked and the longer a person has smoked, the greater the risk of dying from cancer, a heart attack, or a stroke. Overall, the average smoker dies seven to eight years sooner than the nonsmoker.

Cigarette smoking is the single greatest cause of cancer death in the United States. Tobacco smoke contains more than four thousand chemicals, of which more than fifty have been identified as carcinogens. Cigarette smokers have overall cancer death rates twice those of nonsmokers. The greater the number of cigarettes smoked, the greater the risk.

Smoking is also a major factor in heart disease. For more information on smoking and cardiovascular health, refer to the section on smoking in the chapter HEART AND CARDIOVASCULAR HEALTH. If you want good health, you absolutely must not smoke!

Various measures, including acupuncture, hypnosis, and nicotine-containing skin patches or chewing gum, have all been shown to provide some benefit, but not much. In a systematic review of the efficacy of interventions intended to help people stop smoking, data were analyzed from 188 randomized controlled trials.[2] Encouragement to stop smoking given by physicians during a routine office call resulted in a two-percent cessation rate after one year. Supplementary measures such as follow-up letters or visits had an additional effect, but only slightly better than two percent. Behavioral modification techniques, such as relaxation, reward-and-punishment, and avoiding trigger situations, in group or individual sessions led by a psychologist had no greater effect than the two-percent rate achieved by simple advice from a physician. Eight studies using acupuncture have produced an overall effectiveness rate of roughly three percent. Hypnosis was judged ineffective, even though trials have shown a success rate of twenty-three percent. The reason hypnosis was judged to be ineffective was because no biochemical marker was used to accurately determine effectiveness in those particular trials. Nicotine replacement therapy (gum or patch) is effective in about thirteen percent of smokers who seek help in quitting. All together, these results are not very encouraging. It appears the best results occur when people quit "cold turkey." If you smoke, we strongly encourage you to quit now! You have got to make the commitment. It is something that only you can do.

Here are eleven tips to help:

1. List all the reasons why you want to quit smoking and review them daily.
2. Set a specific day to quit, tell at least ten friends that you are going to quit smoking, and then DO IT!
3. Throw away all cigarettes, butts, matches, and ashtrays.
4. Use substitutes. Instead of smoking, chew on raw vegetables, fruits, or gum. If your fingers seem empty, play with a pencil.
5. Take one day at a time.
6. Realize that forty million Americans have quit. If they can do it, so can you!
7. Visualize yourself as a nonsmoker with more available money, pleasant breath,

. . . .

QUICK REVIEW

Just like the other three cornerstones of good health, the importance of a health-promoting lifestyle cannot be overstated. Lifestyle definitely comes down to choices. If you want to be healthy, simply make healthy choices. Choose to not smoke. Choose to find physical activities that you enjoy, and do them often. Make getting a good night's sleep a priority, and have fun with your dreams. These simple lifestyle choices will have a profound effect on your health and the quality of your life.

unstained teeth, and the satisfaction that comes from being in control of your life.

8. Join a support group. Call the local American Cancer Society and ask for referrals. You are not alone.

9. When you need to relax, perform deep breathing exercises rather than reaching for a cigarette.

10. Avoid situations that you associate with smoking.

11. Each day, reward yourself in a positive way. Buy yourself something with the money you've saved, or plan a special reward as a celebration for quitting.

The Importance of Regular Exercise

Regular physical exercise is obviously a major key to good health. We all know this, yet only a small fraction (fewer than twenty percent) of Americans exercise on a regular basis. Why? Well, I imagine that excuses like lack of time, energy, or motivation could be given. Are these excuses valid? How important is your health? How important is regular exercise to your overall health?

Exercise is absolutely vital. While the immediate effect of exercise is stress on the body, with regular exercise the body adapts; it becomes stronger, functions more efficiently, and has greater endurance. The entire body benefits from regular exercise, largely as a result of improved cardiovascular and respiratory function. Simply stated, exercise enhances the transport of oxygen and nutrients into cells. At the same time, exercise enhances the transport of carbon dioxide and waste products from the tissues of the body to the bloodstream and ultimately to the eliminative organs. As a result, regular exercise increases stamina and energy levels.

Physical inactivity is a major reason why so many Americans are overweight.[3] This is especially true of children, as studies have demonstrated that childhood obesity is associated more with inactivity than overeating.[4] Since strong evidence suggests that eighty to eighty-six percent of adult obesity begins in childhood, it could be concluded that lack of physical activity is the major cause of obesity. If you have kids, get them active. If you are not active yourself, make a change; get active, especially if you have weight to lose. Adults who are physically active tend to have less of a problem losing weight.

Regular exercise is a necessary component of weight-loss programs due to the following factors:

- When weight loss is achieved by dieting without exercise, a substantial portion of the total weight lost comes from the lean tissue, primarily as water loss.[5]
- When exercise is included in a weight-loss program, there is usually an improvement in body composition due to a gain in lean body weight because of an increase in muscle mass and a decrease in body fat.
- Exercise helps counter the reduction in basal metabolic rate (BMR) that usually accompanies dieting alone.
- Exercise increases the BMR for an extended period of time following the exercise session.
- Moderate to intense exercise may have a suppressing effect on the appetite.
- People who exercise during and after weight reduction are better able to maintain their weight loss than those who do not exercise

Exercise promotes the development of an efficient method to burn fat. Muscle tissue is the primary user of fat calories in the body; the greater your muscle mass, the greater your fat-burning capacity. If you want to be healthy and achieve your ideal body weight, you must exercise.

Exercise and Mood

Regular exercise also exerts a powerful positive effect on mood. Tensions, depressions, feelings of inadequacy, and worries diminish greatly with regular exercise. Exercise alone has been demonstrated to have a tremendous impact on improving mood and the ability to handle stressful life situations.

In a study published in the *American Journal of Epidemiology*, increased participation in exercise, sports, and physical activities was strongly associated with decreased symptoms of anxiety (restlessness, tension, etc.), depression (feelings that life is not worthwhile, low spirits, etc.), and malaise (run-down feeling, insomnia, etc.).[5] Simply stated, people who participate in regular exercise have higher self-esteem and are happier.

Regular exercise has been shown to enhance powerful mood-elevating substances in the brain known as *endorphins*. These compounds exert effects similar to those of morphine, although much milder. In fact, their name (endo = endogenous, -rphins = morphines) was given to them because of their morphine-like effects. There is a clear association between exercise and endorphin elevation, and when endorphin levels go up, mood follows.[6]

Dennis Lobstein, Ph.D., a professor of exercise psychobiology at the University of New Mexico, compared the beta-endorphin levels and depression profiles of ten joggers to those of ten sedentary men of the same age.[7] The ten sedentary men tested out more depressed, perceived greater stress in their lives, and had more stress-circulating hormones and lower levels of beta-endorphins. As Dr. Lobstein stated, this "reaffirms that depression is very sensitive to exercise and

helps firm up a biochemical link between physical activity and depression."

If the benefits of exercise could be put in a pill, you would have the most powerful health-promoting medication available. Take a look at this long list of health benefits produced by regular exercise.

BENEFITS OF EXERCISE

Musculoskeletal System

Increases muscle strength
Increases flexibility of muscles and range of joint motion
Produces stronger bones, ligaments, and tendons
Lessens chance of injury
Enhances posture, poise, and physique

Heart and Blood Vessels

Lowers resting heart rate
Strengthens heart function
Lowers blood pressure
Improves oxygen delivery throughout the body
Increases blood supply to muscles
Enlarges the arteries to the heart

Bodily Processes

Improves the way the body handles dietary fat
Reduces heart disease risk
Helps lower blood cholesterol and triglyceride levels
Raises levels of HDL, the "good" cholesterol
Helps improve calcium deposition in bones
Prevents osteoporosis
Improves immune function
Aids digestion and elimination
Increases endurance and energy levels
Promotes lean body mass; burns fat

Mental Processes

Provides a natural release from pent-up feelings
Helps reduce tension and anxiety
Improves mental outlook and self-esteem
Helps relieve moderate depression

Improves the ability to handle stress

Stimulates improved mental function

Induces relaxation and improves sleep

Increases self-esteem

Longevity

For every hour of exercise, there is a two-hour increase in longevity

Physical Fitness and Longevity

The better shape you are in physically, the greater your odds of enjoying a healthier and longer life. Most studies have shown that an unfit individual has an eight times greater risk of having a heart attack or stroke than a physically fit individual. Researchers have estimated that for every hour of exercise, there is a two-hour increase in longevity. That is quite a return on investment.

Studies on physical fitness and mortality rate have historically relied on a single initial assessment of fitness, with subsequent follow-up for mortality. Unfortunately, with such single-exposure assessments there is no clear indication of change in fitness or activity level. To counteract this deficiency in the medical research, there are several long-term studies in progress. Recent results from two of these studies, The Aerobics Center Longitudinal Study and The Harvard Alumni Health Study, provide further documentation of the benefits of being physically fit in improving cardiovascular health and reducing mortality from all causes.

The following information on The Aerobics Center Longitudinal Study may be a bit technical, but it is worth taking a look at because of the findings. Participants were 9,777 men, ranging in age from twenty to eighty-two, who completed at least two preventive medical examinations at the Cooper Clinic in Dallas, Texas, from December

1970 through December 1989. All study subjects achieved at least eighty-five percent of their age-predicted maximal heart rate (220 minus their age) during the treadmill tests at both exams. The average interval between the two exams was 4.9 years. Men were considered healthy if, in addition to normal resting and exercise electrocardiogram (EKG), they had no history or evidence of heart attack, stroke, diabetes, or high blood pressure at both exams. Men were considered unhealthy if they had one or more of these conditions, even though they had a normal resting and exercising EKG. A total of 6,819 men were classified as healthy, and 2,958 as unhealthy.[8]

Even though, by a standard definition, all men in the study could be classified as fit, for the purpose of analyzing the effect of different levels of exercise the men were further divided into groups by their level of fitness based on their exercise tolerance to a standard treadmill test. This measure is a very sound indicator of physical fitness, as the amount of time a person can stay on the treadmill reflects their level of cardiovascular fitness. Based on the results of the treadmill test, the men were divided into five groups, with the first group labeled as "unfit" and groups two through five categorized as "fit." The higher the group number, the higher the level of fitness.

The highest death rate (from all causes) was observed in men who were unfit at both exams (122.0 deaths per 10,000 man-years); the lowest death rate was in men who were physically fit at both examinations (39.6 deaths per 10,000 man-years). Furthermore, men who progressed from "unfit" to "fit" between the first and subsequent examination had an age-adjusted death rate of 67.7 per 10,000 man-years, representing a reduction in mortality of forty-four percent relative to men who remained unfit at both exams.

Improvement in fitness was associated with lower death rates after adjusting for age, health status, and other risk factors for premature mortality. For each minute of increase in maximal treadmill time between examinations, there was a corresponding 7.9 percent decrease in the risk of dying.

The Harvard Alumni Health Study also demonstrated a strong inverse relationship between total physical activity and mortality from all causes.[9] The study was conducted in healthy, middle-aged, inactive men who were divided into two groups—those who began a regular exercise program and those who remained inactive. The exercise group had a twenty-three-percent lower risk of dying than the sedentary men. And, as in the Aerobics Center Study, the higher the activity level, the lower the death rate.

Creating an Effective Exercise Routine

Exercise is clearly one of the most powerful medicines available. The time you spend exercising is a valuable investment in your good health. To help you develop a successful exercise program, here are seven steps to follow:

Step 1. Recognize the Importance of Physical Exercise

The first step is realizing just how important it is to get regular exercise. We cannot stress enough just how vital regular exercise is to your health. But as much as we stress this fact, it means nothing unless it really sinks in and you accept it, too. You must make regular exercise a top priority in your life.

Step 2. Consult Your Physician

If you are not currently on a regular exercise program, get medical clearance if you have health problems or if you are over forty years of age. The main concern is the functioning of your heart. Exercise can be quite harmful

(and even fatal) if your heart is not able to meet the increased demands placed on it.

It is especially important to see a physician if any of the following applies to you:

- Heart disease
- Smoking
- High blood pressure
- Extreme breathlessness with physical exertion
- Pain or pressure in chest, arm, teeth, jaw, or neck with exercise
- Dizziness or fainting
- Abnormal heart action (palpitations or irregular beat)

Step 3. Select an Activity You Enjoy

If you are fit enough to begin, the next thing to do is select an activity that you will enjoy. Using the list below, choose from one to five of the activities that you think you may enjoy—or fill in a choice or two of your own. Make a commitment to do one activity a day for at least twenty minutes, and preferably an hour. Make your goal be to enjoy the activity. The important thing is to move your body enough to raise your pulse a bit above its resting rate.

Bicycling
Bowling
Cross-country skiing
Dancing
Gardening
Golfing
Heavy housecleaning
Jazzercise
Jogging
Stair climbing
Stationary bicycling
Swimming
Tennis
Treadmill
Walking
Weight lifting

The best exercises are the ones that get your heart moving. Aerobic activities such as walking briskly, jogging, bicycling, cross-country skiing, swimming, aerobic dance, and racquet sports are good examples. Brisk walking (5 miles per hour) for approximately thirty minutes may be the very best form of exercise for weight loss. Walking can be done anywhere, and the risk of injury is extremely low. It doesn't require any expensive equipment—just comfortable clothing and well-fitting shoes. If you are going to walk on a regular basis, we strongly urge you to first purchase a pair of high-quality walking or jogging shoes. They will not only make walking more enjoyable and comfortable, but they can also reduce the risk of injury.

Step 4. Monitor Exercise Intensity

Exercise intensity is determined by measuring your heart rate (the number of times your heart beats per minute). This determination can quickly be made by placing the index and middle finger of one hand on your opposite wrist, or on the side of your neck just below the angle of your jaw. Beginning with zero, count the number of heartbeats for six seconds. Simply add a zero to this number, and you have your pulse rate. For example, if you counted fourteen beats, your heart rate would be 140. Would this be a good number? It depends upon your "training zone," which is defined in the following paragraph.

A quick and easy way to determine your maximum training heart rate is to simply subtract your age from 185. For example, if you are forty years old your maximum heart rate would be 145. To determine the bottom of the training zone, simply subtract 20 from this number. In the case of a forty-year-old, this would be 125. So the training range for a forty-year-old would be between 125 and 145 beats per minute. For maximum health benefits, you must stay within your training zone or range and never exceed it.

Step 5. Do It Often

You don't get in good physical condition by exercising once; it must be done on a regular basis. A minimum of fifteen to twenty minutes of exercising at your training heart rate at least three times a week is necessary to gain any significant cardiovascular benefits from exercise. It is better to exercise at the lower end of your training zone for longer periods of time than it is to exercise at a higher intensity for a shorter period of time. It is also better if you can make exercise a part of your daily routine.

Step 6. Make It Fun

The key to getting the maximum benefit from exercise is to make it enjoyable. Choose an activity that you enjoy and have fun with. If you can find enjoyment in exercise, you are much more likely to exercise regularly. One way to make it fun is to get a workout partner. For example, if you choose walking as your activity, here is a great way to make it fun:

Find one or two people in your neighborhood whom you would enjoy walking with. If you are meeting others, you will certainly be more regular than if you depend solely on your own intentions. Commit to walking three to five mornings or afternoons each week, and increase the exercise duration from an initial ten minutes to at least thirty minutes.

Step 7. Stay Motivated

No matter how committed you are to regular exercise, at some point in time you are going to be faced with a loss of enthusiasm for working out. Here is a suggestion: take a break. Not a long break; just skip one or two workouts. It gives your enthusiasm and motivation a chance to recoup so that you can come back with an even stronger commitment.

Here are some other things to help you to stay motivated:

- Read or thumb through fitness magazines like *Shape, Men's Fitness, Muscle & Fitness,* and *Muscular Development.* Looking at pictures of people in fantastic shape really inspires me. In addition, these magazines typically feature articles on new exercise routines that interest me.
- Set exercise goals. Being a goal-oriented individual, goals really help keep me motivated. Success breeds success, so set a lot of small goals that can easily be achieved. Write down your daily exercise goal and check it off when you have it completed.
- Vary your routine. Variety is important to help you stay interested in exercise. Doing the same thing every day becomes monotonous and drains motivation. Continually find new ways to enjoy working out.
- Keep a record of your activities and progress. Sometimes it is hard to see the progress you are making, but if you write in a journal you'll have a permanent record of your progress. Keeping track of your progress will motivate you to continued improvement.

The Importance of Sleep

Human sleep is perhaps one of the least understood physiological processes. Its value to human health and proper functioning is without question. Sleep is absolutely essential to both the body and mind. Impaired sleep, altered sleep patterns, and sleep deprivation impair mental and physical function. Many health conditions, particularly depression, chronic fatigue syndrome, and fibromyalgia, are either entirely or partially related to sleep deprivation or disturbed sleep.

Over the course of a year, over one-half of Americans will have difficulty falling asleep. About thirty-three percent of the population experiences insomnia on a regular basis, with seventeen percent claiming that insomnia is a major problem in their lives. Many use over-the-counter sedative medications to combat insomnia, while others seek stronger prescription medications from their physicians. Each year up to ten million people in the United States receive prescriptions for drugs to help them go to sleep. The natural treatment of insomnia is described in Part III, INSOMNIA.

As with other health conditions, the most effective treatment for insomnia is based on identifying and addressing causative factors. The most common causes of insomnia are psychological: depression, anxiety, and tension. If psychological factors do not seem to be the cause, various foods, drinks, and medications may be responsible. There are numerous compounds in food, drink, and well over three hundred drugs that can interfere with normal sleep.

How Much Sleep Do You Need?

Exactly how much sleep an individual requires varies from one person to the next. Sleep needs tend to decrease with age. A one-year-old baby requires about fourteen hours of sleep a day, a five-year-old about twelve hours, and adults about seven to eight. In addition, women tend to require more sleep than men. As people age their sleep needs may decline, but so does their ability to sustain sleep, probably as a result of decreased levels of important brain chemicals such as *serotonin* and *melatonin.* The elderly tend to sleep less at night than younger adults, but they also doze more during the day.

Based on observation of eye movement and brain wave, or electroencephalographic (EEG), recordings, sleep is divided into two distinct types: REM (rapid eye movement) and non-REM (non-rapid eye movement) sleep. During REM sleep, the eyes move rapidly and dreaming takes place. When people are awakened during non-REM sleep, they will report that they were thinking about everyday matters but rarely report dreams.

Non-REM sleep, also known as *slow-wave sleep*, is divided into four stages based upon the level of EEG activity and ease of arousal. As sleep progresses, there is a deepening of sleep from Stage 1 to Stage 4, with progressively slower brain wave activity until REM sleep, when suddenly the brain becomes much more active. In adults, the first REM sleep cycle is usually triggered ninety minutes after going to sleep and lasts about five to ten minutes. After the flurry of activity, brain wave patterns will return to non-REM sleep for another ninety-minute sleep cycle.

Each night, most adults experience five sleep cycles. REM sleep periods grow progressively longer as sleep continues, and the last sleep cycle may produce a REM sleep period that can last about an hour. Non-REM sleep lasts for approximately fifty percent of this ninety-minute sleep cycle in infants, and about eighty percent in adults. As people age, in addition to needing less REM sleep, they tend to awaken at the transition from non-REM to REM sleep.

The Importance of Dreams

Dreams are very important to our physical and mental well-being. The primary definition of a dream refers to a sequence of sensations, images, and thoughts passing through a sleeping person's mind. A dream can also refer to a wish, fantasy, desire, or fanciful vision. It is our dreams that propel us as we roll through life. They are powerful, inspirational, and potentially healing.

The importance of dreams to mental health is obvious if we examine what happens to people who are deprived of REM sleep. In the early 1960s, the pioneering dream researcher William C. Dement conducted several interesting studies at Mount Sinai Hospital in New York. In one of these studies, subjects sleeping in a laboratory setting were awakened the moment REM began to occur and then allowed to go back to sleep. The experiment continued for one week. During this time the test group reported increased irritability, anxiety, and appetite. In other studies, people deprived of REM sleep exhibited profound personality changes—extreme irritability, depression, anxiety, etc.—that disappeared when they were allowed to dream again.[10]

A Contemporary View of Dreams

People have attempted to answer the question "Where do dreams come from and what do they mean?" since the dawn of time. While many ancient cultures actually considered their dream lives to be more significant than their waking lives, the modern view of dreams was initially swayed a bit by fears that dreams undermine moral conduct and are meaningless symbols that result from random nerve firings or physical discomfort. The emerging view is a more holistic one that recognizes that dreams have both physiological and psychological causes.

Modern psychology's fascination with dreams began with the work of Sigmund Freud. It was Freud who stated that dreams were the "window to the soul." Freud viewed dreams as expressions of the subconscious mind—safe expressions of buried impulses and desires.

Other psychologists in the early 1900s also began looking into dreams. Carl Jung, Alfred

Adler, William Stekel, and many others developed their own theories about the meanings and interpretations of dreams.

Dreams can sometimes aid us in working out the issues of our waking lives. Dreams allow us to view what is being imprinted on our subconscious mind. They are often symbolic attempts to sort among our choices in life.

The Talmud, which serves as a foundation of the Jewish religion, extensively discusses the purpose of dreams. The authors of the Talmud clearly recognized the importance of dreams in spiritual and personal development. To dream, however, is not enough. The dreams must be interpreted. The Talmud states: "An uninterpreted dream is like an unopened letter from God."

Obviously, there are times when dreams are not psychologically meaningful. For example, if you are suffering from indigestion or a peptic ulcer and experience a violent dream in which you are being stabbed in the stomach, there is no need to uncover a deep psychological issue. The problem with trying to interpret every dream is that not every dream will be meaningful. Nonetheless, it is important to examine every dream for possible clues to personal growth.

The Interpretation of Dreams

There are many theories on how to interpret dreams. Our advice is to focus on how the dream relates to what is going on in your waking life. Often dreams speak to us in symbols, so it may not be clear at first. Examine each person or item in the dream from a simplistic view: what does it mean to you? Describe it as if you were talking to someone from another planet who has no idea of what anything means here on Earth. To help you with interpreting dreams, here are some important questions to ask:

- What are you doing in the dream?
- What is the story line?
- What were the feelings you experienced in this dream?
- What was your mood upon waking?
- How does this dream relate to what is going on in your waking life?
- What are the issues, conflicts, and unresolved situations in the dream, and how might these relate to your waking life? Is there a parallel?
- What are the insights you have gained from this dream?

Techniques to Help in Recalling Dreams

It can be frustrating to try to recall dreams. Not only do we not remember most of them, but the ones we do recall can easily slip away and evaporate as well. But with a little guidance and effort, you will soon have more dream recall than you know what to do with! Here is a quick five-step process for dream recall:

1. Before Going to Bed: Keep a pad of paper and a pen or pencil beside your bed. Date the paper. If you are keeping a dream journal, read the last dream you had.

2. When you go to bed, relax your body and review the day in reverse. How did I get ready for bed? What was I doing just before going to bed? What did I do this evening? What was it like coming home from work, what did I do at the office, what did I have for lunch? And so on, all the way back to how you got up the previous morning and either recalled your last dream or wrote down "I recall nothing this morning." This exercise is very relaxing and helps us learn to reflect back and focus, the same way we need to focus to recall dreams.

3. As you are getting close to falling asleep, repeat over and over, "When I wake up, I will remember my dreams."

4. When you wake up in the morning, don't move! Stay in the same position, relax your body, and let your mind drift closer to your dream. Remind yourself that you want to remember your dream. When you begin to recall your dream, rewind it and play back what you remember. Shutting your eyes may help. Thinking about what you are going to do in the future, like take a shower or go to work, is the best way to miss a dream.

5. Once you begin to recall a dream, start writing! Write down whatever you remember right away so that you're not trying to remember that material while trying to recall new material. If after a minute you don't have any recall, write down "I don't recall anything." Even better, write a short fantasy about what you would have liked to dream. If you have other dreams in the journal, read one of them.

Dream Resources

If you are interested in learning more about dreams, there are several excellent books on the subject. The books that we found the most interesting and useful are

Breakthrough Dreaming: How to Tap the Power of Your 24-Hour Mind, by Gayle Delaney (Bantam Books, 1991)

The Natural Artistry of Dreams, by Jill Mellick (Conari Press, 1996)

The Dream Sourcebook, by Phyllis R. Koch-Sheras, Ph.D., and Amy Lemley (Lowell House, 1996)

The Internet has many interesting sites regarding dreams, such as *dreamtree.com* and *dreamgate.com.*

There is also a nonprofit organization, the Association for the Study of Dreams, dedicated to the pure and applied investigation of dreams and dreaming. Its purposes are to promote an awareness and appreciation of dreams in both professional and public arenas; to encourage research into the nature, function, and significance of dreaming; to advance the application of the study of dreams; and to provide a forum for the exchange of ideas and information on dreams. You can contact them at

Association for the Study of Dreams
P.O. Box 1600
Vienna, VA 22183
703-242-0062
Fax: 703-242-8888

A Health-Promoting Diet

. . . .

Eat a plant-based, predominantly vegetarian diet.

Reduce the intake of fat.

Eliminate the intake of refined sugar.

Reduce exposure to pesticides and herbicides.

Eliminate the intake of food additives and coloring agents.

Keep salt intake low and potassium intake high.

Drink 32 to 48 ounces of water daily.

Identify and address food allergies.

Determine caloric needs to achieve or maintain ideal body weight.

Use the Healthy Exchange System to construct a health-promoting diet.

Let your food be your medicine and let your medicine be your food.

HIPPOCRATES

Eat a Plant-Based, Predominantly Vegetarian Diet

There is a growing appreciation of the role of diet in determining our level of health. It is now established that certain dietary practices can cause or prevent a wide range of diseases. In addition, research increasingly indicates that certain diets and foods offer immediate therapeutic benefit. The purpose of this chapter is to introduce you to the growing field of nutritional medicine by focusing on ten key recommendations for a health-promoting diet. These ten principles are utilized by most naturopathic physicians to educate and inspire their patients to attain a higher level of wellness.

Based on detailed anatomical and historical evidence, it is thought that humans evolved as "hunter-gatherers." That is, humans appear to be *omnivores*—capable of surviving on both gathered (plant) and hunted (animal) foods.[1] However, while the human gastrointestinal tract is able to digest both animal and plant foods, there are indications that it can accommodate plant foods much more easily than the harder-to-digest animal foods.[2]

Specifically, our teeth are composed of twenty molars, which are perfect for crushing and grinding plant foods, along with eight front incisors, which are well suited for biting into fruits and vegetables. Only our front four canine teeth are designed for meat eating. Our jaws swing both vertically to tear and laterally to crush, while a carnivore's jaws only swing vertically.

In addition, the long human intestinal tract appears to favor plant foods. Carnivores typically have a short bowel, while herbivores have a bowel length proportionally comparable to that of humans.

To further examine what humans should eat, many researchers look to other primates, such as chimpanzees, monkeys, and gorillas. Nonhuman primates are also omnivores—or, as they are often described, "herbivores and opportunistic carnivores." They mainly eat fruits and vegetables but may also eat small animals, lizards, and eggs if given the opportunity. In primates, animal food consumption is inversely related to body weight. In other words, the smaller primates eat more animal food while the larger primates eat less animal food. The gorilla consumes only one percent of its total calories as animal foods, and the orangutan consumes two percent animal foods. The remainder of their diet comes from plants. Since humans are between the weight of the gorilla and the orangutan, it has been suggested that humans are designed to eat around one-and-one-half percent of their diet as animal foods.[2] Most Americans currently derive well over fifty percent of their calories from animal foods.[3]

It should also be pointed out that the meat our ancestors consumed was different from the meat we find in supermarkets today. Domesticated animals generally have higher fat levels than their wild counterparts, but the desire for tender meat has produced beef with a fat content of twenty-five to thirty percent or higher, compared to a fat content of lower than four percent for free-living animals or wild game.

In addition, the type of fat is considerably different. Domestic beef contains primarily saturated fats and virtually undetectable amounts of omega-3 fatty acids. In contrast, the fat of wild animals contains over five times more polyunsaturated fat per gram, and approximately four percent of the fat is beneficial omega-3 fatty acids.[1] While a diet high in saturated fat is associated with an increase in blood cholesterol levels and the risk of heart disease, a diet rich in omega-3 fatty acids exerts a protective effect against both.

Basically, humans appear to be best suited to a diet composed primarily of plant foods. This contention is supported not only by the information summarized above, but also by the tremendous amount of evidence showing that deviating from a predominantly plant-based diet is a major factor in the development of heart disease, cancer, strokes, arthritis, and many other chronic degenerative diseases. It is now the recommendation of many health and medical organizations that the human diet should focus primarily on plant-based foods, such as vegetables, fruits, grains, legumes, nuts, and seeds. Such a diet is thought to offer significant protection against the development of chronic degenerative disease.[3–5]

The Health-Promoting Components of a Plant-Based Diet

One of the key aspects of a predominantly plant-based diet is its high content of dietary fiber. Generally, the term "dietary fiber" refers to plant cell walls and non-nutritive residues. In addition, a plant-based diet is low in saturated fat, high in essential fatty acids, and high in antioxidant nutrients and phytochemicals. These important plant compounds offer significant protection against diseases like heart disease, cancer, and arthritis. They will be discussed in more detail following.

BENEFICIAL EFFECTS OF DIETARY FIBER

Decreased intestinal transit time

Delayed gastric emptying, resulting in reduced postprandial (after-meal) hyperglycemia

Increased satiety

Increased pancreatic secretion

Increased stool weight

More advantageous intestinal microflora

Increased production of short-chain fatty acids

Decreased serum lipid levels

More soluble bile

A good goal for dietary fiber intake is 25 to 35 grams daily. This can be easily achieved if the dietary focus is on whole, unprocessed plant foods. Vegetables are excellent sources of fiber. In fact, 1 cup of cooked carrots has almost the same amount of fiber as 3 slices of whole wheat bread or 2 cups of oatmeal.

A diet high in fiber is important in the prevention and treatment of a number of diseases. Table 2 lists diseases linked to a low-fiber diet.

Naturopathic physicians are not alone in the recommendation to eat more plant foods. Many medical experts, as well as the National Academy of Science, the U.S. Department of Agriculture, the U.S. Department of Health and Human Services, the National Research Council, and the National Cancer Institute, recommend that Americans consume two to three servings of fruit and three to five servings of vegetables per day to reduce the risk of developing heart disease, cancer, and other chronic degenerative diseases. Unfortunately, less than ten percent of the population meets even the lowest recommendation of five servings of a combination of fruits and vegetables.

Numerous population studies have repeatedly demonstrated that a high intake of *carotene*-rich fruits and vegetables reduces the risk of cancer, heart disease, and strokes.[3,5] Carotenes represent the most widespread group of naturally occurring pigments in nature. They are a highly colored (red and yellow) group of fat-soluble compounds. Over six hundred carotenoids have been characterized, including thirty to fifty

. . . .

QUICK REVIEW

The human body is truly one of the universe's major wonders. It deserves to be fed a high-quality diet, but most Americans are not giving their bodies the nutrition it needs or deserves. When a machine does not receive the proper fuel or maintenance, how long can it be expected to run in an efficient manner? If your body is not fed the full range of nutrients it needs, how can it be expected to stay in a state of good health? The health-promoting diet featured in this chapter goes a long way in preventing disease and maintaining or achieving good health.

Good health often comes down to the sum of the habitual choices we make on a day-to-day basis. Make a commitment to following the guidelines in this chapter, and you will be building a strong foundation for optimal health.

TABLE 1   Dietary Fiber Content of Selected Foods

FOOD	SERVING SIZE	CALORIES	GRAMS OF FIBER
Fruits			
Apple (with skin)	1 medium	81	3.5
Banana	1 medium	105	2.4
Cantaloupe	1/4 melon	30	1.0
Cherries, sweet	10 cherries	49	1.2
Grapefruit	1/2 medium	38	1.6
Orange	1 medium	62	2.6
Peach (with skin)	1	37	1.9
Pear (with skin)	1/2 large	61	3.1
Prunes	3	60	3.0
Raisins	1/4 cup	106	3.1
Raspberries	1/2 cup	35	3.1
Strawberries	1 cup	45	3.0
Vegetables, Raw			
Bean sprouts	1/2 cup	13	1.5
Celery, diced	1/2 cup	10	1.1
Cucumber	1/2 cup	8	0.4
Lettuce	1 cup	10	0.9
Mushrooms	1/2 cup	10	1.5
Pepper, green	1/2 cup	9	0.5
Spinach	1 cup	8	1.2
Tomato	1 medium	20	1.5
Vegetables, Cooked			
Asparagus, cut	1 cup	30	2.0
Beans, green	1 cup	32	3.2
Broccoli	1 cup	40	4.4
Brussels sprouts	1 cup	56	4.6
Cabbage, red	1 cup	30	2.8
Carrots	1 cup	48	4.6
Cauliflower	1 cup	28	2.2
Corn	1/2 cup	87	2.9
Kale	1 cup	44	2.8
Parsnip	1 cup	102	5.4
Potato (with skin)	1 medium	106	2.5
Potato (without skin)	1 medium	97	1.4
Spinach	1 cup	42	4.2
Sweet potato	1 medium	160	3.4
Zucchini	1 cup	22	3.6
Legumes			
Baked beans	1/2 cup	155	8.8
Dried peas, cooked	1/2 cup	115	4.7

(continues)

TABLE 1	Continued		
FOOD	**SERVING SIZE**	**CALORIES**	**GRAMS OF FIBER**
Kidney beans, cooked	1/2 cup	110	7.3
Lima beans, cooked	1/2 cup	64	4.5
Lentils, cooked	1/2 cup	97	3.7
Navy beans, cooked	1/2 cup	112	6.0
Rice, Breads, Pastas, and Flour			
Bran muffins	1 muffin	104	2.5
Bread, white	1 slice	78	0.4
Bread, whole wheat	1 slice	61	1.4
Crisp bread, rye	2 crackers	50	2.0
Rice, brown, cooked	1/2 cup	97	1.0
Rice, white, cooked	1/2 cup	82	0.2
Spaghetti, reg., cooked	1/2 cup	155	1.1
Spaghetti, whole wheat, cooked	1/2 cup	155	3.9
Breakfast Cereals			
All-Bran	1/3 cup	71	8.5
Bran Chex	2/3 cup	91	4.6
Corn Bran	2/3 cup	98	5.4
Cornflakes	1 1/4 cup	110	0.3
Grape-Nuts	1/4 cup	101	1.4
Oatmeal	3/4 cup	108	1.6
Raisin Bran	2/3 cup	115	4.0
Shredded Wheat	2/3 cup	102	2.6
Nuts			
Almonds	10 nuts	79	1.1
Filberts	10 nuts	54	0.8
Peanuts	10 nuts	105	1.4

that the body can transform into vitamin A. Beta-carotene has been termed the most active of the carotenoids, due to its higher provitamin A activity (the ability to be converted into vitamin A), but several other carotenes exert greater antioxidant effects.

The best dietary sources of carotenes are green leafy vegetables and yellow-orange fruits and vegetables such as carrots, apricots, mangoes, yams, and squash. Legumes, grains, and seeds are also significant sources of carotenoids.

The *flavonoids* are another group of plant pigments that provide remarkable protection against cancer, heart disease, and strokes. These compounds are largely responsible for the colors of fruits and flowers. Flavonoids act as powerful antioxidants in providing protection against oxidative and free-radical damage (cellular damage caused by highly reactive toxic molecules). Good dietary sources of flavonoids include citrus fruits, berries, onions, parsley, legumes, green tea, and red wine. The average daily intake of flavonoids

TABLE 2	Diseases Highly Associated with a Low-Fiber Diet
Metabolic	Obesity, gout, diabetes, kidney stones, gallstones
Cardiovascular	Hypertension, cerebrovascular disease, ischemic heart disease, varicose veins, deep vein thrombosis, pulmonary embolism
Colonic	Constipation, appendicitis, diverticulitis, diverticulosis, hemorrhoids, colon cancer, irritable bowel syndrome, ulcerative colitis, Crohn's disease
Other	Dental caries, autoimmune disorders, pernicious anemia, multiple sclerosis, thyrotoxicosis, dermatological conditions

in the United States is estimated to be somewhere between 150 and 200 mg.

Reduce the Intake of Fat

There is a great deal of research linking a diet high in fat—particularly a diet high in saturated fat (fats that are solid at room temperature and contain saturated carbon bonds) and cholesterol—to numerous cancers, heart disease, and strokes. Both the American Cancer Society and the American Heart Association recommend a diet in which less than thirty percent of the calories are derived from fat.[3] The easiest way for most people to achieve this goal is to eat fewer animal products and more plant foods. Most plant foods are very low in fat. Nuts and seeds contain high levels of fat calories; their calories are derived largely from polyunsaturated essential fatty acids.

Linoleic and linolenic acid are the essential fatty acids provided by plant foods. In addition to providing the body with energy, they protect against heart disease, cancer, autoimmune diseases (multiple sclerosis, rheumatoid arthritis, and others), skin diseases, and many others. These essential polyunsaturated fats function in our bodies as components of nerve cells, cellular membranes, and *prostaglandins*.

Much of the therapeutic benefit of essential fatty acids is related to altering prostaglandin metabolism. Prostaglandins and related compounds (thromboxanes and leukotrienes) are hormone-like molecules derived from 20-carbon-chain fatty acids that contain three, four, or five double bonds. Linoleic and linolenic acids can be converted to prostaglandins by adding two carbon molecules and removing hydrogen molecules if necessary. There are several types of prostaglandins, and some are considered to be more healthful than others. The number of double bonds in the fatty acid determines the classification of the prostaglandin.

Prostaglandins of the 1 and 3 Series are generally viewed as "good" prostaglandins, while prostaglandins of the 2 Series are viewed as "bad." This is most evident by looking at their effects on blood platelets. Prostaglandins of the 2 Series promote platelet stickiness, a factor that leads to hardening of the arteries, heart disease, and strokes. In contrast, the 1 and 3 Series prostaglandins prevent platelet adhesiveness, improve blood flow, and reduce inflammation. Although the

TABLE 3	Fat Content (as a Percentage of Calories) of Selected Foods		
Meats		Mackerel, Pacific	50%
Sirloin steak, hipbone, lean w/fat	83%	Sardines, Atlantic, in oil, drained	49%
Pork sausage	83%	Salmon, sockeye (red)	49%
T-bone steak, lean w/fat	82%		
Porterhouse steak, lean w/fat	82%	*Vegetables*	
Bacon, lean	82%	Mustard greens	13%
Rib roast, lean w/fat	81%	Kale	13%
Bologna	81%	Beet greens	12%
Country-style sausage	81%	Lettuce	12%
Spareribs	80%	Turnip greens	11%
Frankfurters	80%	Mushrooms	8%
Lamb rib chops, lean w/fat	79%	Cabbage	7%
Duck meat, w/skin	76%	Cauliflower	7%
Salami	76%	Eggplant	7%
Liverwurst	75%	Asparagus	6%
Rump roast, lean w/fat	71%	Green beans	6%
Ham, lean w/fat	69%	Celery	6%
Stewing beef, lean w/fat	66%	Cucumber	6%
Goose meat, w/skin	65%	Turnip	6%
Ground beef, fairly lean	64%	Zucchini	6%
Veal breast, lean w/fat	64%	Carrots	4%
Leg of lamb, lean w/fat	61%	Green peas	4%
Chicken, dark meat w/skin, roasted	56%	Artichokes	3%
Round steak, lean w/fat	53%	Onions	3%
Chuck rib roast, lean only	50%	Beets	2%
Chuck steak, lean only	50%	Chives	1%
Sirloin steak, hipbone, lean only	47%	Potatoes	1%
Turkey, dark meat w/skin	47%		
Lamb rib chops, lean only	45%	*Legumes*	
Chicken, light meat w/skin, roasted	44%	Tofu	49%
		Soybean	37%
		Soybean sprouts	28%
Fish		Garbanzo bean	11%
Tuna, chunk, oil-packed	63%	Kidney bean	4%
Herring, Pacific	59%	Lima bean	4%
Anchovies	54%	Mung bean sprouts	4%
Bass, black sea	53%	Lentil	3%
Perch, ocean	53%	Broad bean	3%
Caviar, sturgeon	52%	Mung bean	3%

precursor to 2 Series prostaglandins can be derived from linoleic acid, in humans the greatest source is directly from the diet in the form of arachidonic acid. This omega-6 fatty acid is found only in animal foods.

Series 1 and 2 prostaglandins come from the omega-6 fatty acids (unsaturated fatty acids where the first double bond is at the sixth carbon), with linoleic acid serving as the starting point. Linoleic acid is changed to gamma-linolenic acid, and then to dihomo-gamma-linolenic acid (DHGLA), which contains three double bonds and is the precursor to prostaglandin of the 1 Series. DHGLA can also be converted to arachidonic acid, which contains four double bonds and is the precursor to the 2 Series of prostaglandins. However, because the enzyme (delta-5 desaturase) responsible for the conversion of DHGLA to arachidonic acid prefers the omega-3 oils, the greatest source of arachidonic acid for humans is in their diet. Arachidonic acid is found almost entirely in animal foods, accompanied by saturated fats. Therefore, by restricting the amount of arachidonic acid in the diet and increasing the intake of omega-3 fatty acids there are more prostaglandins of the 1 and 3 Series being formed and lower levels of the 2 Series.

The 3 Series prostaglandins are particularly beneficial. These prostaglandins are produced from the omega-3 prostaglandin pathway. This pathway can begin with linolenic acid, which can be eventually converted to eicosapentaenoic acid (EPA), which is the precursor to the 3 Series prostaglandins.

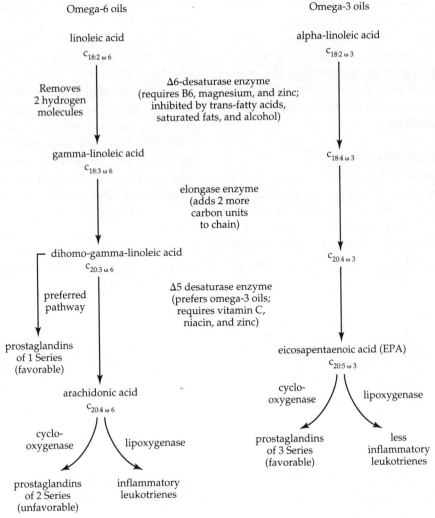

FIGURE 1 Prostaglandin Metabolism

Although EPA is found preformed in cold-water such fish as salmon, mackerel, and herring, certain vegetable oils, such as flaxseed and canola, provide linolenic acid and can thereby increase the level of EPA and 3 Series prostaglandins in the human body.

Prostaglandin metabolism can be manipulated for better health by restricting the intake of saturated fat and arachidonic acid while increasing the intake of the other precursors, such as linolenic acid, gamma-linolenic acid, and EPA. This manipulation can improve such conditions as atherosclerosis, multiple sclerosis, psoriasis, eczema, menstrual cramps, rheumatoid arthritis, and many other allergic or inflammatory conditions.

Prostaglandin metabolism can be greatly inhibited by *trans-fatty acids,* which are found primarily in margarines and shortenings, as well as by alcohol, saturated fats, and deficiencies of vitamin C, niacin, B6, zinc, and magnesium.

Avoid Trans-Fatty Acids

For optimal health, it appears important to eliminate the intake of margarine and other foods that contain trans-fatty acids and partially *hydrogenated* oils (basically most processed foods). Hydrogenation—the addition of hydrogen molecules—changes the structure of natural essential fatty acids from their original *cis-* configuration to an unnatural *trans-* configuration.

Margarine and shortening are made by hydrogenating vegetable oils. In other words, a hydrogen molecule is added to the natural unsaturated fatty acid molecules of the vegetable oil to make it more saturated. These trans-fatty acids interfere with the body's ability to utilize essential fatty acids.

Many researchers and nutritionists have been concerned about the health effects of margarine since it was first introduced. Although many Americans assume that they do their bodies good by consuming margarine instead of butter and saturated fats, in truth they are doing more harm. Margarine and other hydrogenated vegetable oils not only raise LDL cholesterol (the "bad" form of cholesterol linked to heart disease); they also lower the protective HDL ("good") cholesterol level, interfere with essential fatty acid metabolism, and are suspected of causing certain cancers, including breast cancer.[6-9]

At the very least, we encourage you to consume less saturated fat and cholesterol by reducing or eliminating the amount of animal products in your diet and increasing your consumption of fiber-rich plant foods such as fruits, vegetables, grains, and

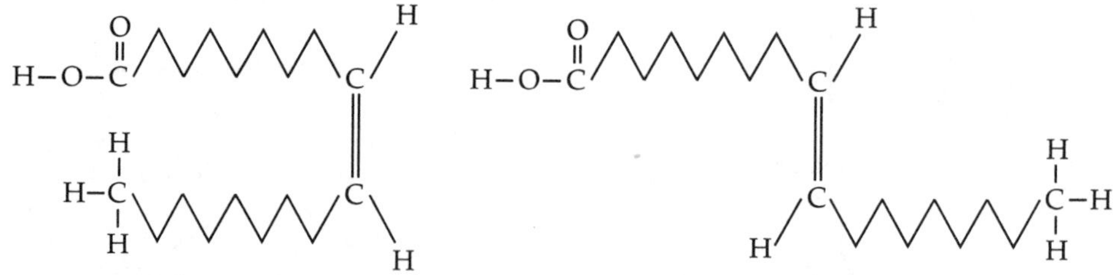

cis fatty acid

The H's are on the same side of the double bond, forcing the molecule to assume a horseshoe shape.

trans fatty acid

The H's are on opposite sides of the double bond, forcing the molecule into an extended position.

FIGURE 2 *Cis vs. Trans Fatty Acid Configuration*

legumes. Limit your intake of animal protein to 4 to 6 ounces per day, and choose fish, skinless poultry, and lean cuts rather than fat-laden types of meat.

Eliminate the Intake of Refined Sugar

Refined sugar, and simple sugars (corn syrup, honey, maple syrup, white grape juice concentrate, etc.) in general, place stress on our blood sugar control and other body control mechanisms. When high-sugar foods are eaten alone, blood sugar levels rise quickly, producing a heightened release of insulin. Eating foods high in simple sugars is usually harmful to blood sugar control—especially in hypoglycemics and diabetics. Sugar also has a detrimental effect on mood, premenstrual syndrome, and many other health conditions, especially when combined with caffeine.

Currently, more than half of the carbohydrates being consumed by most Americans are in the form of sugars that are added to foods as sweetening agents.[3] Read food labels carefully for clues to sugar content. If the words "sucrose," "glucose," "maltose," "lactose," "fructose," "corn syrup," or "white grape juice concentrate" appear on the label, extra sugar has been added. For more information on the negative effects of sugar, see the chapter HYPOGLYCEMIA.

Reduce Exposure to Pesticides and Herbicides

In the United States each year, over 1.2 billion pounds of pesticides and herbicides are sprayed or added to our crops. That is roughly 10 pounds of pesticides for each man, woman, and child. Although the pesticides are designed to kill insects and other organisms, experts estimate that only two percent of the pesticide actually serves its purpose, while over ninety-eight percent of the pesticide is absorbed into the air, water, soil, or food supply. Most pesticides in use are synthetic chemicals of questionable safety. Over the long term, exposure to pesticides can cause cancer and birth defects. In the short term, the major health risks of acute pesticide intoxication include vomiting, diarrhea, blurred vision, tremors, convulsions, and nerve damage.[10–12]

To get a glimpse of the scope of the problem, let's examine the case of the farmer. The lifestyle of a farmer is generally a healthy one in that a farmer eats fresh food, breathes clean air, works hard, and avoids such unhealthy habits as cigarette smoking and alcohol use. Despite this lifestyle, it has been shown in several studies that farmers are at greater risk for certain cancers, including lymphomas, leukemias, and cancers of the stomach, prostate, brain, and skin.[13]

This leads to a question: Are pesticides, herbicides, and other synthetic chemicals responsible for this increased risk for certain cancers? The answer appears to be "yes." Large studies of farmers in Canada, Australia, Europe, New Zealand, and the United States have demonstrated that the greater the exposure to these chemicals, the greater the risk for non-Hodgkin's lymphoma.[11,12]

Because the evidence for the cancer-causing capabilities of pesticides in animals is inadequate, the formal opinion of many "experts" is that these products pose no significant risk to the public or the farmer. This opinion reflects a major dilemma among scientists. What is more valid, studies in laboratory animals or population studies in humans? But more and more human evidence is accumulating. Increased cancer and birth defect rates after pesticide exposure seem to indicate that pesticides are not as safe as the "experts" would like us to believe.

The history of pesticide use in this country is riddled with episodes in which particular pesticides were once extensively used, then later banned due to health risks. Perhaps the best-known example of this is DDT. Widely used from the early 1940s until 1973, DDT was largely responsible for increasing farm productivity in this country—but at what cost? In 1962, Rachel Carson's classic book, *Silent Spring,* detailed the full range of DDT's hazards, including its persistence in the food chain and its deadly effects. But it was another ten years before the U.S. government banned the use of this deadly compound. Unfortunately, although DDT has been banned for nearly twenty years, it is still found in the soil and in root vegetables such as carrots and potatoes. In studies performed by the National Resources Defense Council, a public-interest environmental group, seventeen percent of the carrots analyzed contained detectable levels of DDT.[14]

A group of compounds known as *halogenated hydrocarbons* have also caused widespread environmental contamination. Included in this group are the toxic pesticides DDT, DDE, PCB, PCP, dieldrin, and chlordane. These molecules are stored in fat cells and are difficult to break down. They mimic estrogen in the body and are thought to be a major factor in the growing epidemic of estrogen-related health problems such as PMS, breast cancer, and low sperm counts.[15,16]

Pesticides in Use Today

The majority of pesticides currently used in the United States are probably less toxic than DDT and other banned pesticides (aldrin, dieldrin, endrin, and heptachlor). However,

many pesticides banned from use here are shipped to other countries such as Mexico, which in turn sends it back to the United States on agricultural products. Although over six hundred pesticides are currently used in the United States, most experts are highly concerned about a relative few. The Environmental Protection Agency (EPA) has identified sixty-four pesticides as potential cancer-causing compounds, while the National Research Council found that eighty percent of our cancer risk from pesticides is due to thirteen pesticides used widely on fifteen important food crops.[11,14] The thirteen pesticides are linuron, permethrin, chlordimeform, zineb, captafol, captan, maneb, mancozeb, folpet, chlorothalonil, metiram, benomyl, and o-phenylphenol. These pesticides are found in many crops, but those of greatest concern, in descending order, are tomatoes, beef, potatoes, oranges, lettuce, apples, peaches, pork, wheat, soybeans, beans, carrots, chicken, corn, and grapes.

Pesticide residue levels in food are monitored by both state and federal regulatory agencies. Such monitoring is used to enforce legal tolerance levels. However, there has been increasing public and governmental concern about the adequacy of the residue monitoring programs.

In theory, here is how the monitoring system is designed to work. The EPA establishes tolerance levels for pesticides in raw or unprocessed foods. The Food and Drug Agency (FDA) is then responsible for enforcing the EPA limits. Individual state organizations, such as the departments of health and agriculture, may also be involved in monitoring food safety. This system falls short in several ways: the EPA's tolerance levels may not reflect actual safe levels; probably less than one percent of our domestic food supply is screened by the FDA; the FDA does not test for all pesticides; and the FDA does not prevent the marketing of foods that it finds to contain illegal residues.

A number of pesticide poisoning epidemics have been reported over the years. The largest one to date occurred in 1985 and involved the illegal use of aldicarb—an extremely toxic pesticide—on watermelons. Aldicarb is a *systemic pesticide,* which means that it permeates the entire fruit. Over one thousand people in the western United States and Canada were poisoned in this incident. Illness ranged from mild gastrointestinal upset to severe vomiting, diarrhea, blurred vision, tremors, convulsions, and nerve damage.[11]

While the EPA and FDA estimate that excessive pesticide residues are found on about three percent of domestic and six percent of foreign produce, and acceptable pesticide levels are found in thirteen percent of domestic produce, other organizations report much higher numbers. For example, the National Resources Defense Council conducted a survey of pesticide residues on fresh produce sold in San Francisco markets. They found that forty-four percent of seventy-one fruits and vegetables had detectable levels of nineteen different pesticides, and forty-two percent of produce with detectable pesticide residues contained more than one pesticide.[14] The sheer number and quantity of pesticides showered on certain foods is astounding. For example, over 50 different pesticides are used on broccoli, 110 on apples, and 70 on bell peppers.[10] As many of the pesticides penetrate the entire fruit or vegetable and cannot be washed off, it is obviously best to buy organically grown produce. Crop-yield studies support the use of organic farming if the risk of human health·is added to the equation.

Many supermarket chains and produce suppliers are employing their own testing measures for determining the pesticide content of produce and are refusing to stock foods treated with the more toxic pesticides such as alachlor, captan, or EBDCs (ethylenebisdithiocarbamates). In addition, many stores are asking growers to disclose all pesticides used on foods and to phase out the use of the sixty-four pesticides suspected of causing cancers. Ultimately, pressure from consumers will influence food suppliers the most.

Waxes

In addition to pesticides, consumers must be aware of the waxes applied to many fruits and vegetables. These waxes seal in the water contained in the produce, thereby keeping it looking fresh. According to FDA law, grocery stores must display a sign noting that waxes or post-harvest pesticides have been applied. Unfortunately, most stores do not comply with the law and the FDA lacks the personnel to enforce it.

Currently, the FDA has approved six types of wax for use on produce, including shellac, paraffin, palm oil derivatives, and synthetic resins. These are the same items used in furniture, floor, and car waxes. Foods to which these compounds can be applied include apples, avocados, bell peppers, cantaloupes, cucumbers, eggplants, grapefruits, lemons, limes, melons, oranges, parsnips, passion fruits, peaches, pineapples, pumpkins, rutabagas, squashes, sweet potatoes, tomatoes, and turnips.[10]

The waxes are added primarily to keep produce from spoiling during the often long period of time between harvest and arrival on grocery store shelves. If grocery store chains bought more local produce, chemicals would not be required to keep it looking fresh. But instead, the large chain stores sign contracts with large produce suppliers regardless of their location. This is why, for example, a grocery store in New York is stocked with Washington state apples and California broccoli.

The waxes themselves probably pose little health risk, but most waxes have powerful pesticides or fungicides added to them. Since the waxes cannot be washed off with water, the fungicide or pesticide literally becomes cemented to the produce.

How to Reduce Pesticide Exposure

Here are some ways to reduce your exposure to pesticides:

1. Since pesticide residues are concentrated in animal fat, meat, eggs, cheese, and milk, avoid these foods.

2. Buy organically grown produce. In the context of food and farming, the term "organic" means that the produce was grown without the aid of synthetic chemicals, including pesticides and fertilizers. In 1973, Oregon became the first state to pass labeling laws for organic produce. By 1989, sixteen other states (California, Colorado, Iowa, Maine, Massachusetts, Minnesota, Montana, Nebraska, New Hampshire, North Dakota, Ohio, South Dakota, Texas, Vermont, Washington, and Wisconsin), had also adopted state laws governing organic agriculture. Consumers should ask if produce is "certified organic," and, if so, by whom. Highly reputable certification organizations include California Certified Organic Farmers, Demeter, Farm Verified Organic, Natural Organic Farmers Association, and the Organic Crop Improvement Association. Although under three percent of the total produce grown in the United States is grown without the aid of pesticides, organic produce is widely available.

3. If organic produce is not readily available, develop a good relationship with your local grocery store produce manager. Explain your desire to reduce your exposure to pesticides and waxes. Ask what measures the store takes to assure that pesticide residues are within the tolerance limits. Ask where the store buys produce from, since foreign produce is more likely to contain excessive levels of pesticides, including pesticides banned in the United States. Try to buy local produce that is in season. It increases the likelihood of the produce being produced domestically rather than from countries that have poor control over the amount of pesticides farmers use.

4. To remove surface pesticide residues, waxes, fungicides, and fertilizers, soak produce in a mild solution of additive-free soap, such as Ivory or pure castile soap from the health food store. There are also all-natural, biodegradable cleansers available at most health food stores. Simply spray the produce with the cleanser, gently scrub, then rinse off. Alternatively, you can peel off the skin or remove the outer layer of leaves. The downside of peeling is that many of the nutritional benefits are concentrated in the skin and outer layers.

The presence of pesticides in fruits and vegetables should not deter you from eating a diet high in these foods. The concentration of pesticides in fruits and vegetables is much lower than the levels found in animal fats, meat, cheese, whole milk, and eggs. Furthermore, the various antioxidant components in fruits and vegetables help the body deal with the pesticides.

Eliminate the Intake of Food Additives and Coloring Agents

Food additives are used to prevent spoiling or to enhance flavor. They include such substances as preservatives, artificial colors, artificial flavorings, and acidifiers. Although the government has banned many synthetic food additives, it should not be assumed that all the additives currently used in our food supply are safe. There are still a great number of synthetic food additives in use that are being linked to such diseases as depression, asthma or other allergy, hyperactivity or learning disabilities in children, and migraine headaches.

The FDA has approved the use of over 2,800 different food additives. In 1985, the per capita daily consumption of these food additives was approximately 13 to 15 grams.[17] This is astounding and leads to many questions. Which food additives are safe? Which should be avoided? An extremist might argue that no food additive is safe. However, many food additives fulfill important functions in our modern food supply. Many compounds approved as additives are natural in origin and possess health-promoting properties, while others are synthetic compounds with known cancer-causing effects. Obviously, the most sensible approach is to focus on whole, natural foods and to avoid foods that are highly processed.

Food Coloring

The total annual consumption of food coloring in the United States is approximately 100 million pounds for the entire population. Food color additives are officially designated as either certified or exempt from certification.[18] The food color additives that are exempt from certification are primarily natural in origin. This reflects the popular belief that natural compounds are safer. This contention appears to hold up to scientific scrutiny.

One of the most widely used food colors is FD&C Yellow Dye #5, or *tartrazine*. Tartrazine is added to almost every packaged food and to many drugs, including some antihistamines, antibiotics, steroids, and sedatives.[19] In the United States, the average daily per capita consumption of certified dyes is 15 mg, of which eighty-five percent is tartrazine. Among children, consumption is usually much higher.

Although the overall rate of allergic reactions to tartrazine is quite low in the general population, allergic reactions due to tartrazine are extremely common. In fact, twenty to fifty percent of allergic individuals, especially those who are sensitive to aspirin, will react in an allergic manner to tartrazine.[20,21] Like aspirin, tartrazine is a known inducer of asthma, hives, and other allergic conditions, particularly in children.[21] In addition, tartrazine, as well as benzoates and aspirin, increases the production of a compound that increases the number of *mast cells* in the body.[22] Mast cells are involved in producing *histamine* and other allergic compounds that are responsible for producing the signs and symptoms of allergies. A person with more mast cells in the body will typically be more prone to allergies. For example, examination of patients with hives shows that greater than ninety-five percent have a high number of mast cells.[23]

Several studies have been performed on patients with hives to determine their sensitivity to tartrazine and other food additives. Using provocation testing (a method of testing designed to provoke the allergic syndrome), allergic reactions have been noted in from five percent to forty-six percent of these subjects.[24–37] Diets that eliminate tartrazine and other food additives have been shown to be of great benefit to many patients who have hives and other allergic conditions, such as asthma and eczema.[24–32] Obviously, people who suffer from allergic conditions should eliminate artificial food colors from their diets.

Antioxidants

The two most widely used antioxidants are butylated hydroxyanisole (BHA) and butylated hydroxytoluene (BHT). These food additives have caused cancers in rats. However, there are other studies showing that these antioxidants actually protect against the development of cancers. In fact, many so-called experts in life-extension have recommended that these substances be taken as a food supplement at very high doses (2 g/day). Based on extensive research, this recommendation appears extremely unwise. Two grams per day is 100 times the estimated acceptable intake of BHA, BHT, or the sum of both as set by the Joint Food and Agriculture Organization of the United Nations/World Health Organization Expert Committee on Food Additives.[38] It is also over 100 times the estimated inhibitory activity against cancer and may actually promote cancer at high dosages. While BHA and BHT may be safe at low levels in foods, in the future they will probably be replaced by naturally occurring antioxidants.

Preservatives

Preservatives such as sodium benzoate, nitrates, nitrites, and sulfites work to prevent spoilage primarily by checking the growth of microorganisms. All of these preservatives have come under attack recently. In the case of nitrates and nitrites, these compounds are known carcinogens. Sulfites and benzoates, on the other hand, are capable of producing allergic reactions.[17,39] Clearly, preservatives should be avoided, especially by people prone to allergies. The best way of doing this is by consuming fresh, whole foods.

Benzoic acid and benzoates are the most commonly used food preservatives.[17] Although the rate of allergic response for the general population is thought to be less than one percent, the frequency of allergic responses among patients with chronic hives or asthma ranges from four to forty-four percent.[24–32]

Sulfites pose an even greater problem. Sulfites were once widely used on produce at restaurant salad bars. Since most people were not aware that sulfites were being added, and because most people were unaware that they had a sensitivity to sulfites, many unsuspecting people experienced severe allergic or asthmatic reactions. For years, the FDA refused to even consider a ban on sulfites, even while admitting that these agents provoked attacks in an unknown number of people and in five to ten percent of asthma sufferers. It was not until 1985, after sulfite sensitivity was linked to fifteen deaths between 1983 and 1985, that the FDA agreed to review the matter. In 1986, the FDA finally banned sulfite use on produce and required labeling of other foods such as wine, beer, and dried fruit that contain added sulfites. The average person consumes about 2 to 3 mg of sulfites per day, while wine and beer drinkers typically consume up to 10 mg per day.[39]

The Feingold Hypothesis

The hypothesis that food additives can cause hyperactivity in children stemmed from the research of Benjamin Feingold, M.D., and is commonly referred to as the "Feingold hypothesis." According to Feingold, perhaps forty to fifty percent of hyperactive children are sensitive to artificial food colors, flavors, and preservatives as well as to naturally occurring *salicylates* (aspirin-like compounds) and *phenolic compounds* (compounds with a phenol ring).[40] For more information on the Feingold hypothesis, see ATTENTION DEFICIT DISORDER in Part III.

Keep Salt Intake Low and Potassium Intake High

Excessive consumption of salt (sodium chloride), coupled with low levels of dietary

TABLE 4 Potassium/Sodium Content of Selected Foods, in Milligrams per Serving

FOOD	PORTION SIZE	POTASSIUM	SODIUM
Fresh Vegetables			
Asparagus	1/2 cup	165	1
Avocado	1/2	680	5
Carrot, raw	1	225	38
Corn	1/2 cup	136	trace
Lima beans, cooked	1/2 cup	581	1
Potato	1 medium	782	6
Spinach, cooked	1/2 cup	292	45
Tomato, raw	1 medium	444	5
Fresh Fruits			
Apple	1 medium	182	2
Apricots, dried	1/4 cup	318	9
Banana	1 medium	440	1
Cantaloupe	1/4 melon	341	17
Orange	1 medium	263	1
Peach	1 medium	308	2
Plums	5	150	1
Strawberries	1/2 cup	122	trace
Unprocessed Meats			
Chicken, light meat	3 ounces	350	54
Lamb, leg	3 ounces	241	53
Roast beef	3 ounces	224	49
Pork	3 ounces	219	48
Fish			
Cod	3 ounces	345	93
Flounder	3 ounces	498	201
Haddock	3 ounces	297	150

potassium, greatly stresses the kidneys' ability to maintain proper fluid volume. As a result, some people become "salt-sensitive." For them, high salt intake causes high blood pressure or water retention. In order to avoid becoming salt-sensitive, you must not only reduce salt intake, but simultaneously increase your intake of potassium. This is easily done by increasing your intake of high-potassium foods and avoiding high-sodium foods (most processed foods). Read labels carefully to keep your total daily sodium intake below 1,800 mg.

Most Americans have a potassium-to-sodium (K:Na) ratio of less than 1:2 in their diets. This means that most people ingest twice as much sodium as potassium. Researchers recommend a dietary potassium-to-sodium ratio of greater than 5:1 for health maintenance. This is ten times higher than the average intake of potassium. However, even this may not be optimal. A natural diet rich in fruits and vegetables can produce a K:Na ratio greater than 100:1, as most fruits and vegetables have a K:Na ratio of at least 50:1.

If you really must have the taste of salt, use the so-called salt substitutes, such as the popular brands NoSalt and Nu-Salt. These products are composed of potassium chloride, which tastes very similar to sodium chloride.

Drink 32 to 48 Ounces of Water Daily

Water is vital to our health. In fact, water is the most plentiful substance in our body, as it constitutes over sixty percent of our body weight. Each day our body requires an intake of over two quarts of water to function optimally. About one quart each day is provided in the foods that we eat. This means that we need to drink at least one quart of liquids each day to maintain good water balance. More liquids are needed in warmer climates or for physically active people.

Not drinking enough liquids puts a great deal of stress on the body. Kidney function is likely to be affected, gallstones and kidney stones are likely to form, and immune function will be impaired. It is clear that water is one of our most critical nutrients.

There is currently a great concern over our water supply. It is becoming increasingly difficult to find pure water. Most of our water supply is full of chemicals, including not only chlorine and fluoride, which are routinely added, but a wide range of toxic organic compounds and chemicals such as PCBs, pesticide residues, nitrates, and heavy metals such as lead, mercury, and cadmium.[41] It is estimated that lead alone may contaminate the water of more than forty million Americans.

In an effort to reduce exposure to these toxic compounds, roughly two million home water-filtration units are purchased annually. What is the best home filtration unit? It depends on the predominant toxic substance. For example, if the primary toxic is lead, a carbon filter provides very little benefit. This fact is significant, since carbon filters are the most popular water purification units sold. To determine the safety of tap or well water, contact your local water company; most cities have quality assurance programs that perform routine analyses. Simply ask for the most recent water analysis. In addition, look in the Yellow Pages of your telephone book under "Water Purification & Filtration Equipment" for a list of local companies that sell water purification units. Many of their ads will mention free water testing. Make sure that the company you call is certified as a water treatment specialist (certified by the Water Quality Association or some other third-party organization). The water treatment specialist can determine which contaminants are an issue and can recommend the appropriate filtration method for your needs.

Identify and Address Food Allergies

The importance of identifying and addressing food allergies and sensitivities is fully discussed in the chapter FOOD ALLERGY. Food allergies are an underlying feature in many health conditions, especially allergic and inflammatory conditions like asthma, eczema, chronic hives, rheumatoid arthritis, Crohn's disease, and ulcerative colitis. Food allergies can develop when foods are introduced at too early an age or when food is not being properly digested.

Determine Caloric Needs to Achieve or Maintain Ideal Body Weight

In determining caloric needs, it is necessary to first determine ideal body weight. The most popular height and weight charts are the tables of "desirable weight" provided by the Metropolitan Life Insurance Company. The most recent edition of these tables, published in 1983, gives weight ranges for men and women at 1-inch increments of height for three body frame sizes.

Determine Your Frame Size

The following technique will allow you to make a simple determination of your frame

TABLE 5	1983 Metropolitan Life Height and Weight Table*		
HEIGHT	**SMALL FRAME**	**MEDIUM FRAME**	**LARGE FRAME**
Men			
5'2"	128–134	131–141	138–150
5'3"	130–136	133–143	140–153
5'4"	132–138	135–145	142–156
5'5"	134–140	137–148	144–160
5'6"	136–142	139–151	146–164
5'7"	138–145	142–154	149–168
5'8"	140–148	145–157	152–172
5'9"	142–151	148–160	155–176
5'10"	144–154	151–163	158–180
5'11"	146–157	154–166	161–184
6'0"	149–160	157–170	164–188
6'1"	152–164	160–174	168–192
6'2"	155–168	164–178	172–197
6'3"	158–172	167–182	176–202
6'4"	162–176	171–187	181–207
Women			
4'10"	102–111	109–121	118–131
4'11"	103–113	111–123	120–134
5'0"	104–115	113–126	122–137
5'1"	106–118	115–129	125–140
5'2"	108–121	118–132	128–143
5'3"	111–124	121–135	131–147
5'4"	114–127	124–138	134–151
5'5"	117–130	127–141	137–155
5'6"	120–133	130–144	140–159
5'7"	123–136	133–147	143–163
5'8"	126–139	136–150	146–167
5'9"	129–142	139–153	149–170
5'10"	132–145	142–156	152–173
5'11"	135–148	145–159	155–176
6'0"	138–151	148–162	158–179

*Weights for adults aged twenty-five to fifty-nine years, based on lowest mortality. Weight in pounds according to frame size in indoor clothing (5 pounds for men and 3 pounds for women), wearing shoes with 1-inch heels.

size. Extend your arm and bend your forearm upward at a ninety-degree angle. Keep your fingers straight and turn the inside of your wrist away from your body. Place the thumb and index finger of your other hand on the two prominent bones on either side of your elbow. Measure the space between your fingers with a tape measurer. Compare the measurement with the measurements in Table 6 for medium-framed individuals. A lower reading indicates a small frame; higher readings indicate a large frame.

After determining your desirable weight in pounds, convert it to kilograms by dividing it by 2.2. Next, take this number and multiply it by the following number of calories, depending upon your general activity level:

Little physical activity:	30 calories
Light physical activity:	35 calories
Moderate physical activity:	40 calories
Heavy physical activity:	45 calories

Weight (in kg) multiplied by activity level equals approximate daily caloric requirement.

The Healthy Exchange System described next will provide you with a simple way to consume the appropriate number of calories

for your frame, while assuring appropriate proportions of fats, carbohydrates, proteins, and fiber. In order to lose weight you must either consume fewer calories or burn more than what your body requires to maintain its current weight.

Use the Healthy Exchange System to Construct a Health-Promoting Diet

The American Dietetic Association (ADA), in conjunction with the American Diabetes Association and other groups, has developed the Exchange System, a convenient tool for rapidly estimating the calorie, protein, fat, and carbohydrate content of a diet. Originally created for designing dietary recommendations for diabetics, the exchange method is now used in virtually all therapeutic diets. Unfortunately, the ADA exchange plan does not place a strong enough focus on the quality of food choices.

The Healthy Exchange System presented here is a healthier version because it emphasizes healthier food choices and focuses on unprocessed, whole foods. The diet is prescribed by recommending a particular number of exchanges per list for each day. There are seven exchange lists, but the milk and meat lists should be considered optional.

TABLE 6 Determining Frame Size	
HEIGHT IN 1" HEELS	**ELBOW BREADTH**
Men	
5'2" to 5'3"	$2^1/2"$ to $2^7/8"$
5'4" to 5'7"	$2^5/8"$ to $2^7/8"$
5'8" to 5'11"	$2^3/4"$ to 3"
6'0" to 6'3"	$2^3/4"$ to $3^1/8"$
6'4"	$2^7/8"$ to $3^1/4"$
Women	
4'10" to 5'3"	$2^1/4"$ to $2^1/2"$
5'4" to 5'11"	$2^3/8"$ to $2^5/8"$
6'0"	$2^1/2"$ to $2^3/4"$

THE HEALTHY EXCHANGE SYSTEM
List 1: Vegetables
List 2: Fruits
List 3: Breads, Cereals, and Starchy Vegetables
List 4: Legumes
List 5: Fats
List 6: Milk
List 7: Meats, Fish, Cheese, and Eggs

Because the food portions within each exchange list provide approximately the same amount of calories, proteins, fats, and carbohydrates per serving, it is easy to construct a diet consisting of the recommended percentages of these items.

RECOMMENDED DIETARY PERCENTAGES

Carbohydrates:	60–70% of total calories
Fats:	15–25% of total calories
Proteins:	15–20% of total calories
Dietary fiber:	at least 50 grams

Of the carbohydrates ingested, ninety percent should be complex carbohydrates or naturally occurring sugars. Intake of refined carbohydrates and concentrated sugars (including honey, pasteurized fruit juices, and dried fruit, as well as sugar and white flour) should be limited to less than ten percent of the total calorie intake.

Constructing a diet that meets these recommendations is simple using the exchange lists. In addition, the recommendations ensure a high intake of vital whole foods, particularly vegetables, that are rich in nutritional value.

Examples of Exchange Recommendations

The following diets are examples of exchange recommendations for different calorie needs.

1,500-Calorie Vegan Diet

List 1: Vegetables	5 servings
List 2: Fruits	2 servings
List 3: Breads, Cereals, and Starchy Vegetables	9 servings
List 4: Legumes	2.5 servings
List 5: Fats	4 servings

This recommendation would result in an intake of approximately 1,500 calories, of which sixty-seven percent are derived from complex carbohydrates and naturally occurring sugars, eighteen percent from fat, and fifteen percent from protein. The protein intake is entirely from plant sources, but this diet still provides approximately 55 grams of protein—well above the recommended daily allowance for someone requiring 1,500 calories. At least one-half of the fat servings should be from nuts, seeds, and other whole foods from the Fat Exchange List. The dietary fiber intake would be approximately 31 to 74.5 grams.

Carbohydrate calories: 67%
Fat calories: 18%
Protein calories: 15%
Protein content: 55 g
Dietary fiber content: 31–74.5 g

1,500-Calorie Omnivore Diet

List 1: Vegetables	5 servings
List 2: Fruits	2.5 servings
List 3: Breads, Cereals, and Starchy Vegetables	6 servings
List 4: Legumes	1 serving
List 5: Fats	5 servings
List 6: Milk	1 serving
List 7: Meats, Fish, Cheese, and Eggs	2 servings

Carbohydrate calories: 67%
Fat calories: 18%
Protein calories: 15%
Protein content: 61 g (75% from plant sources)
Dietary fiber content: 19.5–53.5 g

2,000-Calorie Vegan Diet

List 1: Vegetables	5.5 servings
List 2: Fruits	2 servings
List 3: Breads, Cereals, and Starchy Vegetables	11 servings
List 4: Legumes	5 servings
List 5: Fats	8 servings

Carbohydrate calories: 67%
Fat calories: 18%
Protein calories: 15%

Protein content: 79 g
Dietary fiber content: 48.5–101.5 g

2,000-Calorie Omnivore Diet

List 1: Vegetables	5 servings
List 2: Fruits	2.5 servings
List 3: Breads, Cereals, and Starchy Vegetables	13 servings
List 4: Legumes	2 servings
List 5: Fats	7 servings
List 6: Milk	1 serving
List 7: Meats, Fish, Cheese, and Eggs	2 servings

Carbohydrate calories: 66%
Fat calories: 19%
Protein calories: 15%
Protein content: 78 g (72% from plant sources)
Dietary fiber content: 32.5–88.5 g

2,500-Calorie Vegan Diet

List 1: Vegetables	8 servings
List 2: Fruits	3 servings
List 3: Breads, Cereals, and Starchy Vegetables	17 servings
List 4: Beans	5 servings
List 5: Fats	8 servings

Carbohydrate calories: 69%
Fat calories: 15%
Protein calories: 16%
Protein content: 101 g
Dietary fiber content: 33–121 g

2,500-Calorie Omnivore Diet

List 1: Vegetables	8 servings
List 2: Fruits	3.5 servings
List 3: Breads, Cereals, and Starchy Vegetables	17 servings
List 4: Legumes	2 servings
List 5: Fats	8 servings
List 6: Milk	1 serving
List 7: Meats, Fish, Cheese, and Eggs	3 servings

Carbohydrate calories: 66%
Fat calories: 18%
Protein calories: 16%
Protein content: 102 g (80% from plant sources)
Dietary fiber content: 40.5–116.5 g

3,000-Calorie Vegan Diet

List 1: Vegetables	10 servings
List 2: Fruits	4 servings
List 3: Breads, Cereals, and Starchy Vegetables	17 servings
List 4: Legumes	6 servings
List 5: Fats	10 servings

Carbohydrate calories: 70%
Fat calories: 16%
Protein calories: 14%
Protein content: 116 g
Dietary fiber content: 50–84 g

3,000-Calorie Omnivore Diet

List 1: Vegetables	10 servings
List 2: Fruits	3 servings
List 3: Breads, Cereals, and Starchy Vegetables	20 servings
List 4: Legumes	2 servings
List 5: Fats	10 servings
List 6: Milk	1 serving
List 7: Meats, Fish, Cheese, and Eggs	3 servings

Carbohydrate calories: 67%
Fat calories: 18%
Protein calories: 15%
Protein content: 116 g (81% from plant sources)
Dietary fiber content: 45–133 g

You can use the above recommendations as the basis for calculating diets with other calorie contents. For example, for a 4,000-calorie diet add the 2,500-calorie diet to the 1,500-calorie diet. For a 1,000-calorie diet, divide the 2,000-calorie diet in half.

Menu Planning

The Healthy Exchange System was created by us to help ensure that people will consume a health-promoting diet. After you determine your daily caloric needs and calculate the number of servings required from each Healthy Exchange List, you can construct a daily menu. Please take into account the following suggestions.

Breakfast

Eating breakfast is an absolute must. Healthy breakfast choices include whole grain cereals, muffins, and breads along with fresh whole fruit or fresh fruit juice. Both hot and cold cereals, preferably from whole grains, may be the best food choices for breakfast. The complex carbohydrates in the grains provide sustained energy. Furthermore, an evaluation of data provided by the National Health and Nutrition Examination Survey II (a survey of the nutritional and health practices of Americans) showed that serum cholesterol levels are lowest among adults who eat whole grain cereal for breakfast.[42] Interestingly, levels were highest among those who typically skipped breakfast.

Lunch

Lunch is a great time to enjoy a healthy bowl of soup, a large salad, and some whole grain bread. Bean soups and other legume dishes are especially good lunch selections for people with diabetes and blood sugar problems due to their ability to improve blood sugar regulation. Legumes are filling, yet low in calories.

Dinner

For dinner, the healthiest meals contain a fresh vegetable salad, a cooked vegetable side dish or a bowl of soup, whole grains, and legumes. The whole grains may be provided in bread, pasta, or pizza, or as a side dish or part of a recipe for an entrée. The legumes can be utilized in soups, salads, and main dishes.

Although a varied diet rich in whole grains, vegetables, and legumes provides optimal levels of protein, some people like to eat meat. The important thing is not to overconsume animal products. Limit your intake to 4 to 6 ounces per day, and choose fish, skinless poultry, and lean cuts rather than fat-laden meats.

The Healthy Exchange Lists

List 1: Vegetables

Vegetables provide the broadest range of nutrients of any food class. They are rich sources of vitamins, minerals, carbohydrates, and protein. The little fat they contain is in the form of essential fatty acids. Vegetables provide high quantities of other valuable health-promoting substances, especially fiber and carotenes. In Latin, the word "vegetable" means "to enliven or animate." Vegetables give us life. More and more evidence is accumulating that vegetables can prevent as well as treat many diseases.

The best way to consume many vegetables is in their fresh, raw form. In their fresh form, many of the nutrients and health-promoting compounds of vegetables are provided in much higher concentrations. Drinking fresh vegetable juices is an excellent way to make sure that you are achieving your daily quota of vegetables.

When cooking vegetables, it is important that they not be overcooked. Over-cooking will not only result in loss of important nutrients, but it will alter the flavor of the vegetable. Light steaming, baking, and quick stir-frying are the best ways to cook vegetables. Do not boil vegetables unless you are making soup, because many of the nutrients will be left in the cooking water. If fresh vegetables are not available, frozen vegetables are preferred over their canned counterparts.

Vegetables are fantastic "diet" foods because they are very high in nutritional value but low in calories. In the list below, you will notice that there is also a list of "free" vegetables. These vegetables can be eaten in any desired amount because the calories they contain are offset by the calories your body burns in the process of digesting them. If you are trying to lose weight, these foods are especially valuable because they can help keep you feeling satisfied between meals.

The list below shows the vegetables to use for List 1: Vegetables. One cup of cooked vegetables or fresh vegetable juice, or 2 cups of raw vegetables, equals one exchange. Please notice that starchy vegetables such as potatoes and yams are included in List 3: Breads, Cereals, and Starchy Vegetables.

Artichoke (1 medium)
Asparagus
Bean sprouts
Beets
Broccoli
Brussels sprouts
Carrots
Cauliflower
Eggplant
Greens:
    Beet
    Chard
    Collard
    Dandelion
    Kale
    Mustard
    Spinach
    Turnip
Mushrooms
Okra
Onions

Rhubarb
Rutabaga
Sauerkraut
String beans, green or yellow
Summer squash
Tomatoes, tomato juice, vegetable juice cocktail
Zucchini

The following vegetables are "free" vegetables; they may be used as often as desired, especially in their raw form:

Alfalfa sprouts
Bell peppers
Bok choy
Cabbage
Celery
Chicory
Chinese cabbage
Cucumber
Endive
Escarole
Lettuce
Parsley
Radishes
Spinach
Turnips
Watercress

List 2: Fruits

Fruits are a rich source of many beneficial compounds. Regular fruit consumption has been shown to offer significant protection against many chronic degenerative diseases, including cancer, heart disease, cataracts, and strokes. Fruits make excellent snacks because they contain fructose (fruit sugar). This sugar is absorbed slowly into the bloodstream, thereby allowing the body time to utilize it.

Fruits are also excellent sources of vitamins and minerals as well as health-promoting fiber compounds. However, fruits are not as dense with nutrients as vegetables because they are typically higher in calories. That is why vegetables are favored over fruits in weight-loss plans and overall healthy diets.

Each of the following equals one exchange:

Apple	1 large
Applesauce (unsweetened)	1 cup
Apricots, fresh	4 medium
Apricots, dried	8 halves
Banana	1 medium
Berries	
Blackberries	1 cup
Blueberries	1 cup
Cranberries	1 cup
Raspberries	1 cup
Strawberries	1 1/2 cups
Cherries	20 large
Dates	4
Figs, fresh	2
Figs, dried	2
Grapefruit	1
Grapes	20
Juice	
Fresh	1 cup (8 oz.)
Pasteurized	2/3 cup
Mango	1 small
Melons	
Cantaloupe	1/2 small
Honeydew	1/4 medium
Watermelon	2 cups
Nectarine	2 small
Orange	1 large
Papaya	1 1/2 cups
Peach	2 medium
Persimmon	2 medium
Pineapple	1 cup
Plums	4 medium
Prunes	4 medium
Prune juice	1/2 cup
Raisins	4 tbsp
Tangerine	2 medium

Additional fruit exchanges (no more than one per day):

Honey	1 tbsp
Jams, jellies, preserves	1 tbsp
Sugar	1 tbsp

List 3: Breads, Cereals, and Starchy Vegetables

Breads, cereals, and starchy vegetables are classified as complex carbohydrates. Chemically, complex carbohydrates are made up of long chains of simple carbohydrates or sugars. This means that the body has to digest or break down the large sugar chains into simple sugars. Therefore, the sugar from complex carbohydrates enters the bloodstream more slowly than refined sugars do, keeping blood sugar levels and appetite better controlled.

Complex carbohydrate foods, such as breads, cereals, and starchy vegetables, are higher in fiber and nutrients but lower in calories than foods high in simple sugars, such as cakes and candies. Choose whole grain products (whole grain breads, whole grain flour products, brown rice, etc.) over their processed counterparts (white bread, white flour products, white rice, etc.).

Whole grains provide substantially more nutrients and health-promoting properties than refined grains. Whole grains are a major source of complex carbohydrates, dietary fiber, minerals, and B-vitamins. The quality and content of protein in whole grains is greater than that in refined grains. Diets rich in whole grains have been shown to protect against the development of chronic degenerative diseases, especially cancer, heart disease, diabetes, varicose veins, and diseases of the colon, including colon cancer, inflammatory bowel disease, hemorrhoids, and diverticulitis. Whole grains can be used as breakfast cereals, side dishes, casseroles, or part of the entrée.

Each of the following equals one exchange:

Breads

Bagel, small	1/2
Dinner roll	1
Dried bread crumbs	3 tbsp
English muffin, small	1/2

| Tortilla (6-inch) | 1 |
| Whole wheat, rye, or pumpernickel bread | 1 slice |

Cereals

Bran flakes	1/2 cup
Cooked cereal	1/2 cup
Cornmeal (dry)	2 tbsp
Flour	2 1/2 tbsp
Grits (cooked)	1/2 cup
Pasta (cooked)	1/2 cup
Puffed cereal (unsweetened)	1 cup
Rice or barley (cooked)	1/2 cup
Wheat germ	1/4 cup
Other unsweetened cereal	3/4 cup

Crackers

Arrowroot	3
Graham (2 1/2" square)	2
Matzo (4" × 6")	1/2
Rye wafers (2" × 3 1/2")	3
Saltines	6

Starchy vegetables

Corn	1/3 cup
Corn on cob	1 small
Parsnips	2/3 cup
Potato, mashed	1/2 cup
Potato, white	1 small
Squash (winter, acorn, or butternut)	1/2 cup
Yam or sweet potato	1/4 cup

Prepared foods

Biscuit, 2" diameter (omit 1 fat exchange)	1
Corn bread, 2" × 2" × 1" (omit 1 fat exchange)	1
French fries, 2–3" long (omit 1 fat exchange)	8
Muffin, small (omit 1 fat exchange)	1
Pancake, 5" × 1/2" (omit 1 fat exchange)	1
Potato or corn chips (omit 2 fat exchanges)	15
Waffle, 5" × 1/2" (omit 1 fat exchange)	1

List 4: Legumes

Legumes (beans) are among the oldest cultivated plants. Fossil records indicate that even prehistoric people domesticated and cultivated certain legumes for food. Today, legumes are a mainstay of most diets around the world; they are second only to grains in supplying calories and protein to the world's population. Compared with grains, legumes supply about the same number of total calories per serving, but they usually provide two to four times as much protein.

One-half cup of the following cooked or sprouted beans equals one exchange:

Black-eyed peas
Garbanzo beans (chickpeas)
Kidney beans
Lentils
Lima beans
Pinto beans
Soybeans, including tofu (omit 1 fat exchange)
Split peas
Other dried beans and peas

List 5: Fats

As mentioned earlier in this chapter, the human body needs the fatty acids linoleic and linolenic acids. They function in our bodies as components of nerve cells, cellular membranes, and the hormone-like substances known as prostaglandins. While essential fatty acids fats are critical to human health, too much fat—especially saturated fat—in the diet is linked to numerous cancers, heart disease, and strokes. It is strongly recommended by most nutritional experts that the total fat intake be kept below thirty percent of a person's total caloric intake. It is also recommended that the ratio of unsaturated fat to saturated fat in the diet be at least two to one. This recommendation is easy to follow by simply reducing the amount of animal products in the diet, increasing the amount of nuts and seeds consumed, and using natural polyunsaturated oils such as canola, safflower, soy, and flaxseed oils for salad dressings.

Each of the following equals one fat exchange:

Polyunsaturated oils

Vegetable Oils	1 tsp
Canola	
Corn	
Flaxseed	
Safflower	
Soy	
Sunflower	
Almonds	10 whole
Avocado (4" diameter)	1/8
Pecans	2 large
Peanuts	
Spanish	20 whole
Virginia	10 whole
Peanut butter	1 tbsp
Seeds	1 tbsp
Flaxseed	
Pumpkin	
Sesame	
Sunflower	
Walnuts	6 small

Monounsaturated oils

Olive oil	1 tsp
Olives	5 small

Saturated oils (use sparingly)

Bacon	1 slice
Butter	1 tsp
Cream, light or sour	2 tbsp
Cream, heavy	1 tbsp
Cream cheese	1 tbsp
Mayonnaise	1 tsp
Salad dressings	2 tsp

List 6: Milk

Drinking cow's milk is a relatively new dietary practice for humans. Many people are allergic to milk or lack the necessary enzymes to digest it. Milk consumption should be limited to one or two servings per day.

One cup of the following equals one milk exchange:

Nonfat milk or yogurt
Nonfat soy milk

2% milk (omit 1 fat exchange)
Cottage cheese, lowfat (omit 1 fat exchange)
Lowfat yogurt (omit 1 fat exchange)
Whole milk (omit 2 fat exchanges)
Yogurt (omit 2 fat exchanges)

One ounce of cheese equals one milk exchange and one fat exchange.

List 7: Meats, Fish, Cheese, and Eggs

When choosing from this list, it is important to choose primarily from the lowfat group and remove the skin from poultry. This will keep the amount of saturated fat low. Although many people advocate vegetarianism, the exchange list below provides high concentrations of certain nutrients that are difficult to get in an entirely vegetarian diet, such as the full range of amino acids, vitamin B12, and iron. It may be best to use these animal foods in small amounts as "condiments," rather than as a mainstay of a diet. Stay away from cured meats such as bacon, pastrami, and some types of sausages; these foods are rich in compounds that can lead to the formation of cancer-causing compounds known as *nitrosamines*.

As mentioned earlier in this chapter, there is a possible exception to the recommendation to reduce animal food intake: cold-water fish such as salmon, mackerel, and herring provide oils known as omega-3 fatty acids. In hundreds of studies, these beneficial oils have been shown to lower cholesterol and triglyceride levels, thereby reducing the risk of heart disease and strokes. The omega-3 fatty acids are also recommended for treating or preventing high blood pressure, other cardiovascular diseases, cancer, autoimmune diseases (multiple sclerosis, rheumatoid arthritis, and others), allergies and inflammation, eczema, psoriasis, and many other conditions.

Each of the following equals one exchange:

Lowfat (less than 15% fat content)

Beef (baby beef, chipped beef, chuck steak, flank, tenderloin, round, rump, plate, spareribs, tripe)	1 oz
Fish	1 oz
Lamb (leg, rib, sirloin, loin roast or chops, shank, shoulder)	1 oz
Poultry (chicken or turkey, without skin)	1 oz
Veal (leg, loin, rib, shank, shoulder, cutlet)	1 oz

Medium fat (for each, omit 1/2 fat exchange)

Beef (canned corned beef, rib eye, commercial ground round, ground with 15% fat)	1 oz

Cheese (mozzarella, ricotta, farmer's, Parmesan)	1 oz
Eggs	1
Organ meats	1 oz
Pork (all tenderloin loin, picnic & boiled ham, shoulder, Boston butt, Canadian bacon)	1 oz

High fat (for each exchange, omit 1 fat exchange)

Beef (brisket, corned beef, ground beef with more than 20% fat, hamburger, rib roasts, club and rib steaks)	1 oz
Duck or goose	1 oz
Lamb breast	1 oz
Pork (spareribs, loin, ground pork, country-style ham, deviled ham)	1 oz

Supplementary Measures

Supplementary measures are divided into two categories: essential and adjunctive to good health.

Two supplementary measures that could be viewed as essential, based on their tremendous health impact, are nutritional supplementation and physical care.

A tremendous amount of scientific research indicates that the optimal level for many nutrients—especially the antioxidant nutrients, such as vitamins C and E, beta-carotene, and selenium—may be much higher than their current RDA.

We recommend three primary elements for a basic nutritional supplement program:
1. Take a high-quality multiple-vitamin-and-mineral supplement
2. Take extra antioxidants
3. Take 1 tablespoon of flaxseed oil daily

The physical care of the human body involves the following four areas:
1. Breathing
2. Posture
3. Bodywork
4. Exercise

Breathing with the diaphragm promotes good health, higher energy levels, and decreased feelings of stress.

Posture is extremely important to the physical care of the body.

There are many types of bodywork to choose from that can provide benefit, including various massage techniques, chiropractic spinal adjustment and manipulation, Rolfing, reflexology, shiatsu, and many more.

This chapter will explore the use of supplementary measures to support and achieve good health. What do we mean by supplementary measures? Well, in this day and age everyone can use a little more support to supplement a health-promoting attitude, diet, and lifestyle. Examples of supplementary measures include medication; surgery; nutritional supplements; herbal medicines; physical therapies such as chiropractic care, massage, and other bodywork; acupuncture; homeopathy; glandular therapy; and any other treatment designed to support or improve health. We will divide supplementary measures into two categories: essential and adjunctive.

An example of an essential supplementary measure is the use of insulin in the treatment of insulin-dependent diabetes. At this time, insulin is absolutely essential to these individuals; without it, they would either die or suffer greatly. There are numerous other examples in which an appropriately used medication or surgical procedure is absolutely essential to good health.

Very few natural approaches are considered essential in a strict sense. Most would be classified as adjunctive. What this means is that they complement, complete, or support other therapies. For example, St. John's wort extract has shown very good results in the treatment of depression. However, it is not an "essential" medication; it is an important adjunctive tool that supports psychological therapies, lifestyle modification, and dietary recommendations used to treat depression. You can liken these adjunctive therapies to temporary crutches that can be discarded when and if function is restored.

Although in the strict sense very few natural measures are essential, there are two supplementary measures that could be viewed as essential based on their tremendous impact on health: nutritional supplementation and physical care. Both will be defined and discussed in this chapter.

Nutritional Supplementation

The term "nutritional supplementation" refers to the use of vitamins, minerals, and other food factors to support good health and to prevent or treat illness. Nutritional supplements are just that: supplementary. A person cannot make up for poor dietary habits, a negative attitude, and a lack of exercise by taking pills, whether the pills are drugs or nutritional supplements. Although many nutritional supplements are effective in improving health, for the long term it is absolutely essential that attention be devoted to developing a positive mental attitude, a regular exercise program, and a healthful diet.

The key functions of nutrients such as vitamins and minerals in the human body revolve around their role as essential components in enzymes and coenzymes. *Enzymes* are molecules involved in speeding up chemical reactions necessary for human bodily function. *Coenzymes* are molecules that help the enzymes in their chemical reactions.

Enzymes and coenzymes work to either join molecules together or split them apart by making or breaking the chemical bonds between them. One of the key concepts in nutritional medicine is to supply the necessary support or nutrients to allow the enzymes of a particular tissue to work at their optimum levels.

Most enzymes are composed of a protein along with an essential mineral and possibly a vitamin. If an enzyme is lacking the essential mineral or vitamin, it cannot function properly. If provided the necessary mineral

QUICK REVIEW

Supplementary measures can make a dramatic impact on a person's quality of health and quality of life. In some cases, a supplementary measure is a primary therapy; in other situations it may be simply supporting or promoting good health. We highly recommend incorporating nutritional supplementation and physical care as essential supplementary measures in your program of good health.

through diet or a nutritional formula, the enzyme is then able to perform its vital function. For example, zinc is necessary for the enzyme that activates vitamin A in the visual process. Without zinc in the enzyme, the vitamin A cannot be converted to the active form. This deficiency can result in what is known as "night blindness." By supplying the enzyme with zinc, we are performing "enzymatic therapy" and allowing the enzyme to perform its vital function.

Many enzymes require additional support in order to perform their function. The support is in the form of a coenzyme—a molecule that functions along with the enzyme. Most coenzymes are composed of vitamins and/or minerals. Without the coenzyme, the enzyme is powerless. For example, vitamin C functions as a coenzyme to the enzyme *proline hydroxylase,* which is involved in collagen synthesis. Without vitamin C, collagen synthesis is impaired, resulting in bleeding gums, easy bruising, and failure of wounds to heal. There may be plenty of proline hydroxylase (the enzyme), but in order for it to function it needs vitamin C.

The Growing Popularity of Nutritional Supplementation

In the last few years, more Americans than ever are taking nutritional supplements. It is estimated that over 100 million Americans take dietary supplements on a regular basis.[1] Despite the fact that there is tremendous scientific evidence to support the use of nutritional supplementation, many medical experts and researchers have not wholeheartedly endorsed nutritional supplementation—even though ninety-eight percent of them take supplements!

Why are so many Americans taking supplements? They know that they are not getting all they need from their diets, and they realize that supplements can make them feel healthier. Numerous studies have demonstrated that most Americans consume a diet inadequate in nutritional value. Comprehensive studies sponsored by the U.S. government (HANES I and II, Ten State Nutrition Survey, USDA nationwide food consumption studies, etc.) have revealed that marginal nutrient deficiencies exist in a substantial portion of the U.S. population (approximately fifty percent) and that for selected nutrients in certain age groups more than eighty percent of study participants consume less than the recommended dietary allowance (RDA).[2,3]

These studies indicate that the chances of consuming a diet that meets the RDA for all nutrients is extremely unlikely for most Americans. In other words, while it is theoretically possible that healthy individuals can get all the nutrition they need from foods, the fact is that most Americans do not even come close to meeting all their nutritional needs through diet alone. In an effort to increase their intake of essential nutrients, many Americans look to vitamin-and-mineral supplements.

While most Americans are deficient in many vitamins and minerals, the level of deficiency is usually not such that obvious nutrient deficiencies are apparent. A severe deficiency disease like scurvy (caused by lack of vitamin C) is extremely rare, but marginal vitamin C deficiency is thought to be relatively common. The phrase "subclinical deficiency" is often used to describe marginal nutrient deficiencies. A subclinical or marginal deficiency indicates a deficiency of a particular vitamin or mineral that is not severe enough to produce a classic deficiency sign or symptom. In many instances, the only clue of a subclinical nutrient deficiency may be fatigue, lethargy, difficulty in concentrating, a lack of well-being, or some other vague symptom. Diagnosis of subclinical deficiencies is an extremely difficult process that involves detailed dietary or laboratory analysis. It's not worth the cost to perform these tests, because they are usually far more expensive than taking a year's supply of the vitamin being tested for.

The RDA Is Not Enough

Recommended dietary allowances (RDAs) for vitamins and minerals have been prepared by the Food and Nutrition Board of the National Research Council since 1941. These guidelines were originally developed to reduce the rates of severe nutritional deficiency diseases such as scurvy (deficiency of vitamin C), pellagra (deficiency of niacin), and beriberi (deficiency of vitamin B1). Another critical point is that the RDAs were designed to serve as the basis for evaluating the adequacy of diets of groups of people, not individuals. Individuals simply vary too widely in their nutritional requirements. As stated by the Food and Nutrition Board, "Individuals with special nutritional needs are not covered by the RDAs."[3]

A tremendous amount of scientific research indicates that the optimal level for many nutrients, especially the antioxidant nutrients, such as vitamins C and E, beta-carotene, and selenium, may be much higher than their current RDAs. The RDAs focus only on the prevention of nutritional deficiencies in population groups; they do not define optimal intake for an individual.

The RDAs also do not adequately take into consideration environmental and lifestyle factors that can destroy vitamins and bind minerals. For example, even the Food and Nutrition Board acknowledges that smokers require at least twice as much vitamin C as nonsmokers. But what about other nutrients and smoking? And what about the effects of alcohol consumption, food additives, heavy metals (lead, mercury, etc.), carbon monoxide, and other chemicals associated with our modern society that are known to interfere with nutrient function? Dealing with hazards of modern living is another reason why many people take supplements.

While the RDAs have done a good job of defining nutrient intake levels to prevent nutritional deficiencies, there is still much to be learned regarding the optimum intake of nutrients.

Accessory Nutrients

In addition to essential nutrients, there are a number of food components and natural physiological agents discussed in this book that have demonstrated impressive health-promoting effects. Examples include flavonoids, probiotics, carnitine, and coenzyme Q_{10}. These compounds exert significant therapeutic effects with little, if any, toxicity. More and more research indicates that these accessory nutrients, although not considered "essential" in the classical sense, play a major role in preventing illness.

Some Practical Recommendations

There are three primary recommendations to help people design a basic nutritional supplement program:

1. Take a high-quality multiple-vitamin-and-mineral supplement
2. Take extra antioxidants
3. Take 1 tablespoon of flaxseed oil daily

Recommendation 1: Take a High-Quality Multiple-Vitamin-and-Mineral Formula

Taking a high-quality multiple-vitamin-and-mineral supplement that provides all of the known vitamins and minerals serves as a foundation upon which to build. Dr. Roger

Williams, one of the premier biochemists of our time, states that healthy people should use multiple-vitamin-and-mineral supplements as an "insurance formula" against possible deficiency. This does not mean that a deficiency will occur in the absence of the vitamin-and-mineral supplement, any more than not having fire insurance means that your house is going to burn down. But given the enormous potential for individual differences from person to person, and the varied mechanisms of vitamin and mineral actions, supplementation with a multiple formula seems to make sense. The recommendations in Table 1 provide an optimum intake range in selecting a high-quality multiple.

Recommendation 2:
Take Extra Antioxidants
The terms "antioxidants" and "free radicals" are becoming familiar to most health-minded individuals. Loosely defined, a *free radical* is a highly reactive molecule that can bind to and destroy body components. Free-radical, or "oxidative," damage is what makes us age. Free radicals have also been shown to be responsible for the initiation of many diseases, including the two biggest killers of Americans: heart disease and cancer.

Antioxidants, in contrast, are compounds that help protect against free-radical damage. Antioxidant nutrients such as beta-carotene, selenium, vitamin E, and vitamin C have been shown to be very important in protecting against the development of heart disease, cancer, and other chronic degenerative diseases. In addition, antioxidants are also thought to slow the aging process.

Based on extensive data, it appears that a combination of antioxidants will provide greater antioxidant protection than any single nutritional antioxidant. Therefore, in addition to consuming a diet rich in plant foods—especially fruits and vegetables—we recommend using a combination of antioxidant nutrients rather than high doses of any single antioxidant. Mixtures of antioxidant nutrients appear to work together harmoniously to produce the phenomenon of synergy. In other words, 1 + 1 = 3.

The two primary antioxidants in the human body are vitamin C and vitamin E. Vitamin C is an "aqueous phase" antioxidant. This means that it is found in body compartments composed of water. In contrast, vitamin E is a "lipid phase" antioxidant because it is found in lipid-soluble (fat-soluble) body compartments such as cell membranes and fatty molecules. If you are taking a high-potency multiple-vitamin-and-mineral formula, many of the supportive antioxidant nutrients, such as selenium, zinc, and beta-carotene, are provided for. Therefore, your primary concern may be simply to ensure beneficial levels of vitamin C and vitamin E.

Here is a daily supplementation guideline for these key nutritional antioxidants for supporting general health. Be sure to recognize how much your multiple-vitamin-and-mineral formula is providing.

Vitamin E (d-alpha tocopherol)	400–800 IU
Vitamin C (ascorbic acid)	500–1,500 mg

Recommendation 3:
Take One Tablespoon of Flaxseed Oil Daily
In this age of concern over fat in our foods, a recommendation to supplement an individual's daily diet with one tablespoon of flaxseed oil may be puzzling. However, this recommendation makes perfectly good sense. While it is true that Americans should not consume more than thirty percent of their daily calories as fats, a lack of the dietary essential fatty acids has been suggested to play a significant role in the development of many chronic degenerative diseases such as heart disease, cancer, and stroke.

TABLE 1   Optimal Intake Range for Vitamins and Minerals

VITAMIN	RANGE FOR ADULTS
Vitamin A (retinol)	5,000 IU*
Vitamin A (from beta-carotene)	5,000–25,000 IU
Vitamin D	100–400 IU†
Vitamin E (d-alpha tocopherol)	100–800 IU‡
Vitamin K (phytonadione)	60–300 mcg
Vitamin C (ascorbic acid)	100–1,000 mg§
Vitamin B1 (thiamin)	10–100 mg
Vitamin B2 (riboflavin)	10–50 mg
Niacin	10–100 mg
Niacinamide	10–30 mg
Vitamin B6 (pyridoxine)	25–100 mg
Biotin	100–300 mcg
Pantothenic acid	25–100 mg
Folic acid	400 mcg
Vitamin B12	400 mcg
Choline	10–100 mg
Inositol	10–100 mg
MINERALS	
Boron	1–6 mg
Calcium	250–1,500 mg‖
Chromium	200–400 mcg#
Copper	1–2 mg
Iodine	50–150 mcg
Iron	15–30 mg**
Magnesium	250–500 mg††
Manganese	10–15 mg
Molybdenum	10–25 mcg
Potassium	200–500 mg
Selenium	100–200 mcg
Silica	1–25 mg
Vanadium	50–100 mcg
Zinc	15–45 mg

*Women of childbearing age should not take more than 2,500 IU of retinol daily if becoming pregnant is a possibility, due to the risk of birth defects.

†Elderly people in nursing homes who live in northern latitudes should supplement at the high end of the range.

‡It may be more cost-effective to take vitamin E separately.

§It may be easier to take vitamin C separately.

‖Taking a separate calcium supplement may be necessary in women at risk or suffering from osteoporosis.

#For diabetes and weight loss, dosages of 600 mcg can be used.

**Men and postmenopausal women rarely need supplemental iron.

††When magnesium therapy is indicated, take a separate magnesium supplement.

Many experts estimate that approximately eighty percent of our population consumes an insufficient quantity of essential fatty acids. This dietary insufficiency presents a serious health threat to Americans. In addition to providing the body with energy, the essential fatty acids linoleic and linolenic acid, provided by plant foods, function in our bodies as components of nerve cells, cellular membranes, and hormone-like substances known as *prostaglandins*.

In addition to playing a critical role in normal physiology, essential fatty acids are being shown to actually be protective and therapeutic against heart disease, cancer, autoimmune diseases like multiple sclerosis and rheumatoid arthritis, skin diseases, and many others. Over sixty health conditions have now been shown to benefit from essential fatty-acid supplementation.

Organic, unrefined flaxseed oil is considered by many to be the answer to restoring the proper level of essential fatty acids. Flaxseed oil is unique because it contains both essential fatty acids: alpha-linolenic (an omega-3 fatty acid) and linoleic acid (an omega-6 fatty acid) in appreciable amounts. Flaxseed oil is the world's richest source of omega-3 fatty acids. At a whopping fifty-eight percent by weight, it contains over twice the amount of omega-3 fatty acids found in fish oils. Omega-3 fatty acids have been extensively studied for their beneficial effects in cardiovascular disease, inflammation and allergy, and cancer.

The best way to take flaxseed oil is by adding it to foods. Do not cook with flaxseed oil; use mono-unsaturated oils like olive or canola oil because they are more stable. Because flaxseed oil is easily damaged by heat and light, you must add it to foods after they have been cooked or use it as a salad dressing. Taking flaxseed oil by swigging it down or by the spoonful is not very palatable. We rec-ommend trying to incorporate it into your foods as easily as possible. Here are some suggestions: use it as a salad dressing, dip your bread into it, add it to your hot or cold cereal, or spray it over your popcorn.

Here is a sample salad dressing featuring flaxseed oil:

Flaxseed Oil Basic Salad Dressing

4 tablespoons organic flaxseed oil
1 1/2 tablespoons lemon juice
1 medium garlic clove, crushed
Pinch of seasoned salt or salt-free seasoning
Fresh ground pepper to taste

Jazz up this basic recipe to your own personal taste by using your favorite herbs and spices. Place all ingredients into a salad bowl and whisk together until smooth and creamy. This recipe is quick and delicious!

Physical Care

A critical component of overall good health is the physical status of the body. The physical care of the human body involves the following four areas:

Breathing
Posture
Bodywork
Exercise

Since the importance of regular exercise was discussed in the chapter A HEALTHY LIFESTYLE, only the other three components are discussed here.

Breathing

Have you ever noticed how a baby breathes? With each breath, the baby's abdomen rises and falls because the baby is breathing with its diaphragm. If you are like most adults, you tend to fill only your upper chest because you do not utilize the diaphragm. Shallow breathing tends to produce tension and fatigue. One of the most important methods of maintaining health and producing more energy and less stress in the body is to breathe with the diaphragm. Try it. Take a deep, natural breath in by using your diaphragm, and let it out slowly. By using your diaphragm to breathe, you dramatically change your physiology. Learn what it feels like to breathe easily and naturally using your diaphragm, and you will definitely notice improved energy levels, reduced tension, and improved mental alertness.

Posture

Posture—the manner in which the body is held—is extremely important to good health. First of all, when the body is slouched, shoulders slumped, and head down, diaphragmatic breathing is more difficult. As a result, poor posture promotes shallow breathing and low energy levels, not to mention possible physical repercussions due to misalignment of vertebrae and/or muscle spasms. Have you noticed that when you breathe with the diaphragm, it changes your posture to expand your chest cavity? As a result of good diaphragmatic breathing, the spine becomes more erect, the shoulders are pushed back, and the head is pulled up. Energetic posture and good diaphragmatic breathing usually go hand in hand.

One of the keys to gaining more energy in your body is to assume more energetic postures. It sends a message to the subconscious that you are energized and ready to go. Become aware of how you are holding your body as well as how you are breathing. When you have low energy levels, you will probably notice that you tend to hold your body in a tight posture with your head slightly down

and shoulders slouched. When you find yourself in this position, just start breathing with your diaphragm and pull your head up by imagining a cord affixed at the top of your head gently pulling your spine and neck straight and into alignment.

By becoming aware of your breathing and your posture, you may notice a great deal of muscular tension or stress in certain areas of your body. That is where the next phase of physical care of the body comes into play: bodywork.

Bodywork

The need to touch and be touched is universal. Around the world, bodywork practitioners are relied upon much more than in the United States. However, there is a growing trend in America toward receiving bodywork treatments.

There are numerous types of beneficial bodywork to choose from, including various massage techniques, chiropractic spinal adjustment and manipulation, Rolfing, reflexology, shiatsu, and many more. Fortunately, all of these techniques can work, so it is really a matter of personal preference. Find a technique or practitioner that you really like and incorporate bodywork into your routine.

Both of us are fortunate to have experienced a broad range of bodywork, from Rolfing and deep-tissue massage (often referred to as a "sport massage") to more gentle techniques such as Trager massage, Feldenkrais, and craniosacral therapy. Our experience has led us to the conclusion that the therapist is more critical to the outcome than the technique. The technique is only a tool; the result is largely dependent on the person using the tool. We recommend that if your physical body and your attitude are in need of a tune-up, you begin looking for a good chiropractor or bodyworker. How do you find such a person? Word of mouth is probably the best method; ask around.

Our own personal beliefs are that techniques that teach body awareness and address underlying structural problems are most effective. We have divided these techniques into two major classifications: deep-tissue work and light-touch therapies. We have chosen techniques that require extensive education and training before practitioners can call themselves certified therapists.

Deep tissue work, such as Rolfing and Hellerwork, are probably the most powerful bodywork techniques that create change in body posture and energy levels quickly. Unlike massage and spinal adjustment, Rolfing and Hellerwork are focused not on the muscles and spine, but rather on the elastic sheathing network that helps support the body, keeping bones, muscles, and organs in place. This network is known as the *fascia*. According to Rolfers and Hellerwork practitioners, the fascia can be damaged by physical injury, emotional trauma, and bad postural habits. The result is that the body is thrown out of alignment. Rolfing, Hellerwork, and other deep-tissue treatments attempt to bring the body back into balance to restore efficiency of movement and increase mobility by stretching and lengthening the fascia to its natural form and pliability.

Rolfing or Hellerwork treatments consist of ten or eleven sessions, each lasting between sixty and ninety minutes. Treatments are sequential, beginning with more superficial treatments and ending with deeper massage. Deep-tissue treatment can be quite painful, but the rewards are worth it. Remarkable results can be achieved in the areas of breathing, posture, tolerance to stress, and, of course, energy levels. In addition,

many people going through deep-tissue therapy report resolution of emotional conflicts. It seems that many painful or traumatic experiences are stored as tension in the fascia and muscles. Releasing the tension and restoring freedom in the fascia can produce remarkable increases in energy levels. For more information on Rolfing or Hellerwork, contact

Rolf Institute
205 Canyon Boulevard
Boulder, CO 80306
800-530-8875

Hellerwork
406 Berry Street
Mt. Shasta, CA 96067
800-392-3900

If Rolfing or Hellerwork is too painful for you, there are three light-touch therapies that feel incredibly pleasurable and that can produce similar, but more gradual, results. The first technique is called Tragerwork or Trager massage. Tragerwork was the innovation of Milton Trager, M.D. According to Trager, we all develop mental and physical patterns that may limit our movements or contribute to fatigue, pain, and tension. During a typical session, the practitioner gently and rhythmically rocks, cradles, and moves the client's body to encourage the client to see that freedom of movement and relaxation are entirely possible. The aim of the treatment is not so much to massage or manipulate, but rather to promote feelings of lightness, freedom, and well-being. Clients are also taught a series of exercises to do at home. Called Mentastics, these simple, dance-like movements are designed to help clients maintain and enhance the feelings of flexibility and freedom they have experienced during the sessions.

The other light-touch therapies we recommend are two similar techniques: Alexander and Feldenkrais. These methods involve the practitioner guiding the patient to become aware of habitual and limited movement patterns and to replace them with more optimal movements. Like many bodywork techniques, these techniques are difficult to describe. Basically, they teach body awareness. The participant learns the difference between muscular tension and relaxation, and how different postures feel—restricted or free.

For information on these "gentler" therapies, or to find a practitioner near you, contact

The Trager Institute
33 Millwood
Mill Valley, CA 94941
415-388-2688

North American Society of Teachers of the Alexander Technique
P.O. Box 517
Urbana, IL 61801
800-473-0620

Feldenkrais Guild
706 SW Ellsworth Street
Albany, OR 97231
800-775-2118

PART TWO

ENHANCING KEY BODY SYSTEMS

Heart and Cardiovascular Health

Cardiovascular disease is responsible for at least forty-three percent of all deaths in the United States.

Atherosclerosis, the process of hardening of the arteries, can be stopped and even reversed through dietary and lifestyle measures.

Reducing the risk of heart disease and strokes involves eliminating as many risk factors as possible.

Cigarette smoke, even if secondhand, is bad for the heart and circulation.

Low antioxidant status has been shown to be as important as—or even more important than—high cholesterol in predicting a person's likelihood of having a stroke or heart attack.

Vitamin E supplementation has been shown to significantly reduce the risk of heart attack.

Population studies have demonstrated that people who consume a diet rich in omega-3 oils from either fish or vegetable sources have a significantly reduced risk of developing heart disease.

Type A behavior and worrying are linked to heart disease.

In many cases, EDTA chelation therapy is a suitable alternative to coronary angioplasty or by-pass surgery.

Antioxidant supplementation can prevent the harm caused by an angiogram or heart surgery.

The presence of a diagonal earlobe crease is a strong predictor of a heart attack or stroke.

The heart and vascular system is one of the largest and most important body systems. The cardiovascular system's primary functions are to deliver oxygen and vital nutrition to cells throughout the body and to aid in the removal of cellular waste products. In this goal, the human heart beats 100,000 times each day, pumping 2,500 to 5,000 gallons of blood through the 60,000 miles of blood vessels within our bodies. In an average lifetime, the heart will beat 2.5 billion times and pump 100,000 million gallons of blood!

Obviously, we need to support the heart in its tireless efforts. Unfortunately, as a nation we are doing a very poor job of keeping our hearts healthy. Heart disease and stroke are our nation's number-one and number-three killers, respectively. Altogether, these two conditions are responsible for at least forty-three percent of all deaths in the United States. Both are referred to as "silent killers" because the first symptom or sign in many cases is a fatal event. The cause of both conditions is often due to the process of *atherosclerosis*—hardening of the artery walls.

For example, "heart disease" is most often used to describe a disease of the heart's blood vessels. These blood vessels, called the *coronary arteries,* supply the heart muscle with vital oxygen and nutrients. If the blood flow through these arteries is restricted or blocked, severe damage to the heart muscle often oc-curs; this results in what is known as a "heart attack." In most cases, the condition that blocks the supply of blood and oxygen is atherosclerosis, caused by a buildup of plaque containing cholesterol, fatty material, and cellular debris. In the case of a stroke, it is an artery in the brain that is blocked instead of the artery of the heart.

The key point in regard to these two common causes of premature death is that atherosclerosis is largely a disease of diet and lifestyle. It appears that, in many cases, death could be significantly delayed by developing healthy habits.[1]

. . . .

QUICK REVIEW

There is no doubt that, in most cases, atherosclerosis is a disease directly related to diet and lifestyle. Treatment and prevention include reducing all known risk factors. For many patients, this goal requires a major change in diet and lifestyle. Since so many factors are known to be involved in atherosclerosis, any treatment plan must be individualized to assure optimal results. What follows is a general approach that needs to be tailored according to areas of concern. A complete cardiovascular assessment (as previously described) provides valuable information to differentiate which natural treatments are most appropriate. For example, here are some specific recommendations for some of the areas of concern that may arise with such a detailed evaluation:

- Elevated cholesterol, high LDL cholesterol, or low HDL cholesterol levels: please consult CHOLESTEROL (Elevated Levels) in Part III.
- Elevated lipid (cholesterol and triglycerides) and blood sugar levels (i.e., diabetes):
  Chromium (400–600 mcg per day)
  Pantethine (900 mg per day)
  Garlic (the equivalent of 4,000 mcg allicin per day)
- Elevated fibrinogen levels: exercise, omega-3 oils, niacin, and garlic.
- Elevated homocysteine: supplement with therapeutic levels of B12, folic acid, and B6 as described in SUPPLEMENTARY MEASURES.
- Elevated *ferritin* (an iron storage protein) levels: eliminate intake of meat and supplement with high doses of vitamin C (>5,000 mg per day in divided

Understanding Atherosclerosis

To fully understand the important ways in which various natural measures described in this chapter impact the health of the artery and the treatment of cardiovascular disease, it is necessary to examine closely the structure of an artery and the process of atherosclerosis.

Structure of an Artery

An artery is divided into three major layers:

1. The *intima* represents the internal lining of the artery (the medical term is *endothelium*). The intima consists of a layer of cells known as *endothelial cells*. Molecules known as *glycosaminoglycans* (GAGs) line the exposed endothelial cells to protect them from damage and to promote repair.

Beneath the surface of endothelial cells is the *internal elastic membrane*, composed of a layer of GAGs and other ground-substance compounds, which provides support to the endothelial cells and separates the intima from the smooth muscle layer.

2. The *media*, or middle layer, consists primarily of smooth muscle cells. Interposed

. . . .

doses) and grape seed extract (150 mg per day).

- Elevated lipid peroxide levels: vitamin C (1,000–3,000 mg per day), vitamin E (400–800 IU per day), and grape seed extract (150 mg per day).

General Diet and Lifestyle Recommendations

- Consume less saturated fat and cholesterol by reducing or eliminating the amounts of animal products in your diet, with the exception of cold-water fish.
- Increase your consumption of fiber-rich plant foods (fruits, vegetables, grains, legumes, and raw nuts and seeds).
- Achieve ideal body weight.

- Get regular aerobic exercise.
- Do not smoke.
- Eliminate consumption of coffee (both caffeinated and decaffeinated).
- Drink at least 48 ounces of water daily.

Nutritional Supplements

The following are basic recommendations that apply in the absence of clear-cut findings of concern:

- High-potency multiple-vitamin-and-mineral formula as recommended in the chapter SUPPLEMENTARY MEASURES
- Vitamin C: 500–1,000 mg three times per day
- Vitamin E: 400–800 IU per day
- Flaxseed oil: 1 tablespoon per day

among the cells are GAGs and other ground-substance structures that provide support and elasticity to the artery.

3. The *adventitia,* or external elastic membrane, consists primarily of connective tissue, including GAGs, providing structural support and elasticity to the artery.

The Process of Atherosclerosis

No single theory yet formulated about the development of atherosclerosis satisfies all investigators. However, the most widely accepted explanation theorizes that the lesions of atherosclerosis are initiated as a response to injury to the cells that line the inside of the artery—the arterial endothelium. Details of the progression of atherosclerosis according to this theory are illustrated in Figure 2.

1. The initial step in the development of atherosclerosis is a weakening of the GAG layer that protects the endothelial cells. As a result, the endothelial cells are exposed to damage by free radicals. Immune, physical, mechanical, viral, chemical, and drug factors have all been shown to induce damage to the endothelial cells that can lead to plaque development.

2. Once the endothelial lining has been damaged, sites of injury become more permeable to plasma constituents, especially *lipoproteins* (fat-carrying proteins). The binding of lipoproteins to GAGs leads to a breakdown in the integrity of the ground-substance matrix and causes an increased affinity for cholesterol.

Once significant damage has occurred, *monocytes* (large white blood cells) and platelets (small blood cells involved in the formation of blood clots) adhere to the damaged area, where they release growth factors that stimulate smooth muscle cells to migrate from the media into the intima and replicate.

3. The local concentration of lipoproteins, monocytes, and platelets leads to the migration of smooth muscle cells from the media into the intima, where they undergo proliferation. The smooth muscle cells dump cellular debris into the intima, leading to further development of plaque.

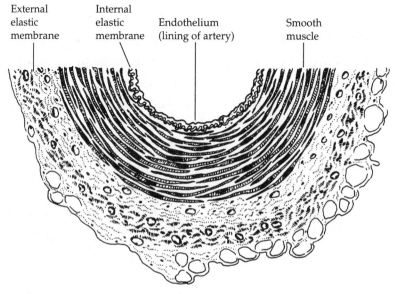

External elastic membrane | Internal elastic membrane | Endothelium (lining of artery) | Smooth muscle

FIGURE 1 Structure of an Artery

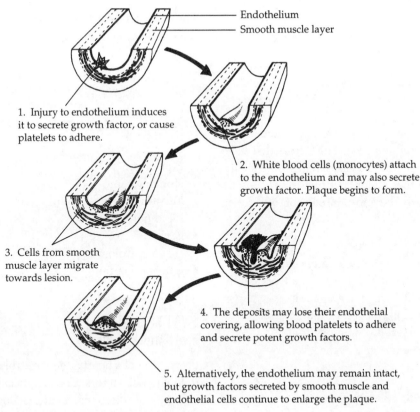

Endothelium
Smooth muscle layer

1. Injury to endothelium induces it to secrete growth factor, or cause platelets to adhere.

2. White blood cells (monocytes) attach to the endothelium and may also secrete growth factor. Plaque begins to form.

3. Cells from smooth muscle layer migrate towards lesion.

4. The deposits may lose their endothelial covering, allowing blood platelets to adhere and secrete potent growth factors.

5. Alternatively, the endothelium may remain intact, but growth factors secreted by smooth muscle and endothelial cells continue to enlarge the plaque.

FIGURE 2 Stages in the Development of Atherosclerosis

4. The formation of a *fibrous cap* (consisting of scar tissue proteins like collagen and elastin, and GAGs) over the intimal surface occurs. Fat and cholesterol deposits accumulate.

5. The plaque continues to grow, until eventually it blocks the artery. Blockage is usually around ninety percent before symptoms of atherosclerosis are apparent.

Reducing the Risk of Cardiovascular Disease

Reducing the risk of heart disease and strokes involves reducing—and when possible eliminating—various risk factors associated with premature death due to these conditions. The risk factors are divided into two primary categories: major risk factors and other risk factors.

The major risk factors are

- Smoking
- Elevated blood cholesterol levels
- High blood pressure
- Diabetes
- Physical inactivity

The risk of a heart attack increases with the presence of more than one of these major risk factors, as follows:

Presence of one of the major risk factors	30% increased risk
High cholesterol and high blood pressure	300% increased risk

High cholesterol and
    smoking   350% increased risk
High blood pressure and
    smoking   350% increased risk
Smoking, high blood cholesterol,
    and high blood pressure   720% increased risk

In addition to these well-accepted major risk factors, there are other factors that have been shown, in some cases, to be more significant than the "major" risk factors.

Here are the most important other risk factors:

- Low antioxidant status
- Low levels of essential fatty acids
- Low levels of magnesium and potassium
- Increased platelet aggregation
- Increased fibrinogen formation
- Elevated levels of homocysteine
- Type A personality

Determining Your Risk

To help you determine your overall risk for having a heart attack or stroke, we have designed a risk determinant scale (see Table 1). To determine your risk, you must obtain from your doctor your blood pressure, total cholesterol, and HDL cholesterol. All of the other items you will be able to fill in yourself. There are many important factors that this risk assessment does not take into consideration, such as the level of lipoprotein (a), *fibrinogen* (a blood protein associated with clot formation), and coping style. However, your score will give you an idea of your relative risk for a heart attack or stroke.

Clinical Evaluation

We recommend a comprehensive evaluation for people who have a significant family history of heart disease or stroke or for people who have had a prior heart attack or stroke.

The complete cardiovascular assessment we recommend should include the following tests:

- Laboratory tests
  Total cholesterol
  LDL cholesterol
  HDL cholesterol
  Lipoprotein (a)
  Fibrinogen
  Homocysteine
  Ferritin (an iron-binding protein)
  Lipid peroxides
- Exercise stress test
- Electrocardiogram (EKG)
- Echocardiogram

Primary Prevention of a Heart Attack or Stroke

Prevention of a heart attack or stroke involves reducing risk factors. The significant risk factors will be discussed in the following sections, along with natural ways to address the risk factors.

Smoking

According to a report from the U.S. Surgeon General, "Cigarette smoking should be considered the most important risk factor for coronary heart disease."[2] Statistical evidence reveals that smokers have three to five times the risk of coronary artery disease as non-smokers.

Effect on the Cardiovascular System Tobacco smoke contains more than four thousand chemicals, of which more than fifty have been identified as carcinogens. These chemicals are extremely damaging to the cardiovascular system. Specifically, they are carried in the bloodstream on LDL cholesterol molecules, where either they damage the lining of the arteries directly or they damage the

TABLE 1	Risk Determinant Scale for Heart Disease and Strokes				
SCALE OF RISK	1	2	3	4	5
			(WEIGHTING OF RISK)		
VALUES:	(LOWEST				HIGHEST)
Blood Pressure (systolic)	<125	125–134	135–149	150–164	≥165
Blood Pressure (diastolic)	<90	90–94	95–104	105–114	≥115
Smoking (cigarettes/day)	None	1–9	10–19	20–29	≥30
Heredity I[a]	None	>65	50–64	35–49	<35
Heredity II[b]	0	1	2	4	>4
Diabetes Duration (years)	0	1–5	6–10	11–15	>15
Total Cholesterol (mg/dl)	<200	200–224	225–249	250–274	≥275
HDL Cholesterol (mg/dl)	≥75	65–74	55–64	35–54	<35
Total Cholesterol/HDL Ratio[c]	<3.0	3.0–3.9	4.0–4.9	5.0–6.4	≥6.5
Exercise (hours per week)	>4	3–4	2–3	1–2	0–1
Supplemental Vitamin E Intake	>400 IU	200–399	60–199	30–59	<29
Supplemental Vitamin C Intake	>500 mg	251–499	250	125–249	0–124
Fruit and Vegetable Intake, Average Daily Servings	>5	4–5	3	1–2	0
Age	<35	36–45	46–55	56–65	>65
Subtotals					

Your risk score: _____

Your Risk

```
      15        25        35        45        55        70
  +----+----+----+----+----+----+----+----+----+----+
         Below                    Very      Extremely
  Low    Average   Average   High  High      High
  Risk   Risk      Risk      Risk  Risk      Risk
```

LDL molecule, which then damages the arteries. An elevated cholesterol level makes smoking even harder on the cardiovascular system, because more cigarette toxins will be carried through the vascular system.

Smoking also presumably contributes to an elevated cholesterol level by damaging the feedback mechanisms in the liver that control how much cholesterol is manufactured.[3] Smoking also promotes platelet aggregation and elevated fibrinogen levels, two of the other important independent risk factors for heart disease and strokes. In addition, it is well documented that cigarette smoking contributes to high blood pressure.[4]

Even Passive Exposure to Cigarette Smoke Is Damaging Convincing evidence links environmental (secondhand, or "passive") smoke to heart disease mortality and morbidity. Analysis of ten epidemiological studies indicates a consistent dose-response effect related to exposure.[5] Evidence indicates that either nonsmokers are more sensitive to smoke or secondhand smoke is more toxic, including its deleterious effects on the cardiovascular system.

Environmental tobacco smoke actually contains higher concentrations of certain smoke constituents. Pathophysiological and biochemical data after short- and long-term environmental tobacco smoke exposure show changes in the lining of the arteries and in platelet function and exercise capacity similar to those found in active smokers. In summary, passive smoking is a relevant risk factor for heart disease. In the United States, more than thirty-seven thousand coronary heart disease deaths each year are attributed to environmental smoke.

If you are regularly exposed to secondhand smoke, it is highly advised that you bolster your antioxidant nutrient intake by supplementing your diet with at least 500 mg of vitamin C and 400 IU of vitamin E each day.

If you are a smoker and you want good health, you absolutely must stop smoking! Various measures, including nicotine-containing skin patches or chewing gum, acupuncture, and hypnosis have all been shown to provide some benefit.[6] Follow the recommendations given in the chapter A HEALTHY LIFESTYLE.

Elevated Blood Cholesterol Levels

The evidence overwhelmingly demonstrates that elevated cholesterol levels greatly increase the risk of death due to heart disease. Cholesterol is transported in the blood by *lipoproteins*—carrier proteins for cholesterol. The major categories of lipoproteins are *very low-density lipoprotein* (VLDL), *low-density lipoprotein* (LDL), and *high-density lipoprotein* (HDL). VLDL and LDL are responsible for transporting fats (primarily triglycerides and cholesterol) from the liver to body cells, and elevations of either VLDL or LDL are associated with an increased risk of developing atherosclerosis, the primary cause of a heart attack or stroke. In contrast, HDL is responsible for returning fats to the liver, and elevations of HDL are associated with a low risk of heart attack.

It is currently recommended that the total blood cholesterol level be less than 200 mg/dl. In addition, it is recommended that the LDL cholesterol be less than 130 mg/dl, the HDL cholesterol be greater than 35 mg/dl, and triglyceride levels be less than 150 mg/dl.

The ratio of total cholesterol to HDL cholesterol and the ratio of LDL to HDL are referred to as the *cardiac risk factor ratios* because they reflect whether cholesterol is being deposited into tissues or being broken down and excreted. The total-cholesterol-to-HDL ratio should be no higher than 4.2, and the LDL-to-HDL ratio should be no higher than 2.5. The risk of getting heart disease can be reduced dramatically by lowering LDL cholesterol while simultaneously raising HDL cholesterol levels; for every one-percent drop in the LDL cholesterol level, the risk for a heart attack drops by two percent. Conversely, for every one-percent increase in HDL levels, the risk for a heart attack drops three to four percent.[7]

Although LDL cholesterol is referred to as "bad cholesterol," the "worst cholesterol" is *lipoprotein (a)*, or Lp(a). Lp(a) is a plasma lipoprotein with a structure and composition closely resembling that of LDL, but with an additional molecule of an adhesive protein called *apolipoprotein (a)*. Several studies have indicated that elevated plasma levels of Lp(a) constitute an independent risk factor for coronary heart disease, particularly in those patients with elevated LDL cholesterol levels.[8,9]

In fact, a high level of Lp(a) has been shown to carry a ten times greater risk of heart disease than an elevated LDL cholesterol level. That is because LDL on its own lacks the adhesive apolipoprotein (a). As a result, LDL does not easily stick to the walls of the artery. Actually, a high LDL cholesterol level carries less risk than a normal or even low LDL cholesterol with a high Lp(a) level. Levels of Lp(a) below 20 mg/dl are associated with a low risk of heart disease, levels between 20 and 40 mg/dl a moderate risk, and levels above 40 mg/dl an extremely high risk.

For information on how to lower cholesterol levels, see CHOLESTEROL in Part III.

High Blood Pressure

Elevated blood pressure is another major risk factor for a heart attack or stroke. The subject is discussed more fully in HIGH BLOOD PRESSURE, in Part III.

Diabetes

Diabetes (see DIABETES in Part III) is another major risk factor for heart disease and strokes. The diabetic has a two to three times the risk of dying prematurely from atherosclerosis as a nondiabetic individual. Because of this, diabetics must be extremely aggressive in reducing the risk factors linked to heart attacks and strokes. Foremost are the attainment of as normal a blood glucose reading as possible and the reduction of blood cholesterol levels.

Physical Inactivity

Regular exercise is extremely important in reducing the risk of heart disease and strokes. Exercise accomplishes this goal by lowering cholesterol levels, improving the supply of blood and oxygen to the heart, increasing the functional capacity of the heart, reducing blood pressure, reducing obesity, and exerting a favorable effect on blood clotting. To improve your exercise regimen, follow the recommendations given in the chapter A HEALTH-PROMOTING LIFESTYLE.

The Other Risk Factors

In addition to the major risk factors for heart disease, there are a number of other factors that have sometimes been shown to be more significant than the so-called major risk factors. These factors were listed earlier in this chapter and are discussed in the following sections.

Low Antioxidant Status

Antioxidant nutrients, such as beta-carotene, selenium, vitamin E, and vitamin C, are important in protecting against the development of heart disease, cancer, and other chronic degenerative diseases. In addition, antioxidants are also thought to slow the aging process.

Fats and cholesterol are particularly susceptible to free-radical damage—damage caused by cellular toxins like cigarette smoke. When damaged, fats and cholesterol form toxic derivatives known as *lipid peroxides* and *oxidized cholesterol,* respectively, which can then damage the artery walls and accelerate the progression of atherosclerosis. Antioxidants block the formation of these damaging compounds. Based on extensive data, it appears that a combination of antioxidants will provide greater antioxidant protection than any single nutritional antioxidant (see the chapter SUPPLEMENTARY MEASURES for a more in-depth description). In addition, extracts of grape seed or pine bark are showing antioxidant benefits beyond those of vitamin E and C. The role of grape seed and pine bark extracts in preventing heart disease is discussed following.

Vitamin E and Heart Disease   Of all the antioxidants, vitamin E may offer the greatest protection against heart disease because of its ability to be easily incorporated into the LDL-cholesterol molecule and prevent free-radical damage. There is a clear-cut dosage effect with vitamin E; the higher the dosage of vitamin E, the greater the degree of protection against oxidative damage to LDL cholesterol. Although dosages as low as 25 mg offer some protection, it appears that doses of greater than 400 IU are required to produce clinically significant effects. Dosages up to 200 IU do not provide the same degree of protection as dosages of 400 to 800 IU, especially in smokers and people exposed to greater oxidative stress.[10–12]

Vitamin E provides significant additional protection against heart disease and strokes by reducing LDL cholesterol peroxidation with an improvement in plasma LDL breakdown; inhibiting excessive platelet aggregation; increasing HDL cholesterol levels; and increasing the breakdown of fibrin (a clot-forming protein).

Vitamin E Levels Are More Significant Than Cholesterol Several large population studies have demonstrated that vitamin E levels may be more predictive of developing a heart attack or stroke than total cholesterol levels.[13–17] In one study, high blood cholesterol was predictive twenty-nine percent of the time, and high blood pressure twenty-five percent of the time, but a low level of vitamin E in the blood was shown to be predictive of a heart attack almost seventy percent of the time.[16] While the consumption of red wine has been suggested as the reason for the "French Paradox"—why the French have a lower rate of heart disease and strokes despite a higher cholesterol and fat intake—higher vitamin E levels provide at least as good an explanation.[13,16]

Vitamin E Supplementation Prevents Heart Disease and Strokes Two large-scale studies have shown relatively low-dose vitamin E supplements to be capable of significantly reducing the risk of dying from a heart attack or a stroke. One study looked at 87,245 nurses. It concluded that nurses who took 100 IU of vitamin E daily for more than two years had a forty-one-percent lower risk of heart disease than nonusers of vitamin E supplements.[17] The other study involved 39,910 male health care professionals. The results were similar: a thirty-seven-percent lower risk of heart disease with the intake of more than 30 IU of supplemental vitamin E daily.[18]

TABLE 2 Effect of Increasing Doses of Vitamin E on Oxidation Parameters		
DOSE (MG/DAY)	**LAG TIME***	**PROPAGATION RATE†**
0	94	7.8
25	99	8.0
50	100	7.9
100	106	7.7
200	111	7.5
400	116	6.8
800	120	6.5

*Lag time equals the time before oxidation occurs after the addition of an oxidizing agent. The higher the number, the greater the beneficial effect.

†Propagation rate equals the rate at which lipid peroxidation progresses. The lower the number, the greater the beneficial effect.

A recent study has demonstrated more clearly the benefits of "low-dosage" vitamin E supplementation in preventing heart disease. The study utilized the extensive dietary and nutritional supplement database collected in the Cholesterol Lowering Atherosclerosis Study. A total of 156 men aged forty to fifty-nine years who had previous coronary artery bypass graft surgery were studied. For two years, the subjects underwent randomized therapy, consisting of a cholesterol-lowering diet and either a cholesterol-lowering drug (colestipol-niacin combination) or a placebo in association with supplemental antioxidant vitamins. The main outcome was the change in the percentage of vessel diameter obstructed because of hardening of the artery, as determined by angiography.[19]

Overall, the results indicated that the subjects in the group that took 100 IU or more of vitamin E demonstrated significantly less coronary artery lesion progression than did subjects taking less than 100 IU. No benefit of vitamin E supplementation could be demonstrated in the placebo group. These results indicate that vitamin E supplementation, even at a relatively low dosage (100 IU), can reduce the progression of coronary artery disease when used in conjunction with cholesterol-lowering therapy (preferably natural).

These recent studies on vitamin E confirm what people in the health food industry and nutritionally minded physicians have known for more than fifty years: vitamin E is good for the cardiovascular system. However, based on studies on the protective effects of different dosages of vitamin E, the aforementioned studies might have had even more impressive results if dosages of at least 400 IU had been used.

In addition to offering protection against cardiovascular disease, vitamin E supplementation plays a major role in the treatment of heart disease, recovery from stroke, and peripheral vascular diseases such as intermittent claudication—a painful cramp usually occuring in the calf muscle in response to exercise or walking.

The "mecca" for vitamin E research in cardiovascular disease is the Shute Institute and Medical Clinic in London, Ontario, Canada. The Shute Institute has been active in the use of vitamin E therapy since the 1940s. The Shute brothers, Drs. Evan and Wilfred Shute, were instrumental in bringing to light many of the now substantiated cardiovascular benefits of taking vitamin E. The Shute brothers believed that vitamin E is vital to cardiovascular health and that it is important to supplement the diet with high doses of vitamin E in many health conditions, especially those involving the cardiovascular system. Once scorned in mainstream medical circles, the Shute brothers have now been vindicated. For over a half-century, the Shute Institute has successfully treated over sixty thousand patients using vitamin E and other natural therapies. Vitamin E has been at the center stage in their treatment programs.

Vitamin C as an Antioxidant   Vitamin C works as antioxidant in aqueous (water) environments in the body, both outside and inside human cells. Vitamin C is the first line of antioxidant protection in the body. In other words, it is the body's most important antioxidant. Its primary antioxidant partners are vitamin E and carotenes, as these antioxidants are fat-soluble. Vitamin C also works along with antioxidant enzymes such as glutathione peroxidase, catalase, and superoxide dismutase. Vitamin C is also responsible for regenerating oxidized vitamin E in the body, thus increasing the antioxidant benefits of vitamin E.[20]

In health food stores and health magazines, customers and readers are constantly bombarded by the word "antioxidant." Often they are pointed in the direction of some rather high-priced "super-antioxidants." But when we compare these super-antioxidants to vitamin C in terms of cost-to-benefit, vitamin C comes out far superior.

Vitamin C vs. Red Wine Another popular recommendation to improve antioxidant status and reduce the risk of heart attack is to drink red wine. This recommendation is based on several studies showing that frequent red wine ingestion offers protection against heart disease and stroke. Because the French consume more saturated fat than Americans, yet have a lower incidence of heart disease, red wine consumption has been suggested to be the key reason behind the "French Paradox." Presumably this protection is the result of flavonoids in red wine protecting against oxidative damage to LDL cholesterol.

To better determine the antioxidant capacity of red wine, a study was conducted comparing the effects of red wine, white wine, and vitamin C on the serum antioxidant capacity. The *serum antioxidant capacity* (SAOC) was determined in nine subjects after they consumed one glass (300 ml) of red wine and compared to the levels of nine subjects who consumed one glass of white wine and four subjects who consumed 1,000 mg of vitamin C.[21] The results indicated that significantly better protection is offered by consuming 1,000 mg of vitamin C than by consuming one glass of either red or white wine. Here are the results:

SUBSTANCE	% INCREASE IN SAOC	
	AT 1 HOUR	AT 2 HOURS
White wine	4%	7%
Red wine	18%	11%
Vitamin C	22%	29%

Vitamin C as Prevention against Heart Disease A high dietary vitamin C intake has been shown to significantly reduce the risk of death from heart attacks and strokes (as well as all other causes, including cancer) in numerous population studies.[22,23] One of the most detailed studies provides the most insight. The vitamin C intake of 11,348 adults was analyzed over a period of 5 years. The subjects were divided into three groups: (1) less than 50 mg daily dietary intake; (2) greater than 50 mg daily dietary intake with no vitamin C supplementation; and (3) greater than 50 mg dietary intake plus vitamin C supplementation (estimated to be 300 mg or more).[22] Analysis of the *standardized mortality ratio* (SMR), a comparison to the average death rate, showed up to forty-eight percent lower SMR in the high-vitamin-C-intake group vs. the low-intake group for cardiovascular disease and overall mortality. In practical terms, these differences correspond to an increase in longevity of five to seven years for men and one to three years for women.

So, how does vitamin C lower the risk for cardiovascular disease? It appears to act as an antioxidant, and it also strengthens the collagen structures of the arteries; lowers total cholesterol level and blood pressure; raises HDL cholesterol levels; and inhibits platelet aggregation.[22–27]

Vitamin C has been shown to be extremely effective in preventing LDL cholesterol from being oxidized, even in smokers. In addition, because vitamin C regenerates oxidized vitamin E in the body, it potentiates the antioxidant benefits of vitamin E.

Grape Seed and Pine Bark Extracts One of the most beneficial groups of plant flavonoids is the *proanthocyanidins* (also referred to as procyanidins). These flavonoids exert many health-promoting effects. The most potent proanthocyanidins are those bound to other proanthocyanidins. Collectively, mixtures of proanthocyanidin molecules are referred to as *procyanidolic oligomers,* or PCO for short. PCOs exist in many plants and are found in red wine. In addition, commercially available sources of PCO include extracts from grape seeds and the bark of the maritime (Landes) pine.

The primary uses of PCO extracts are in the treatment of venous and capillary disorders, including venous insufficiency, varicose veins, capillary fragility, and disorders of the retina such as diabetic retinopathy and macular degeneration. Good clinical studies have shown positive results in the treatment of these conditions using PCOs.[28]

Based on the relatively recent demonstration of potent antioxidant activity—effects greater than 20 to 50 times as strong as vitamin E or C—the list of clinical uses of PCO extracts will surely increase. Perhaps the most significant use will eventually be in the prevention of heart disease and strokes. Since PCOs have a greater antioxidant effect than vitamins C and E, it is only natural to assume that they could offer greater protective effects than these antioxidant vitamins.

PCO extracts have been shown in animal studies to prevent damage to the lining of the artery, to lower blood cholesterol levels, and to shrink the size of the cholesterol deposit in the artery.[29,30] Additional mechanisms of PCOs that are useful in preventing atherosclerosis include inhibition of platelet aggregation and inhibition of vascular constriction.[31,32] Presumably, PCO extracts may exert similar benefits in humans. PCO extracts in a supplement form should be thought of as a necessary food in the prevention and treatment of heart disease or strokes.

As a preventive measure and as antioxidant support, a daily dose of 50 mg of either the grape seed or pine bark extract is suitable. When being used for therapeutic purposes, the daily dosage should be increased to 150 to 300 mg.

Low Levels of Essential Fatty Acids

Population studies have demonstrated that people who consume a diet rich in omega-3 oils from either fish or vegetable sources have a significantly reduced risk of developing heart disease.[33,34] Furthermore, results from autopsy studies have shown that the highest degree of coronary artery disease is found in individuals with the lowest concentration of omega-3 oils in their fat tissues. Conversely, individuals with the lowest degree of coronary artery disease had the highest concentration of omega-3 oils.[35] Omega-3 fatty acids lower levels of LDL cholesterol and triglycerides, inhibit excessive platelet aggregation, lower fibrinogen levels, and lower blood pressure in individuals with high blood pressure.

The two populations with the lowest rate of heart attacks—the Japanese of Kohama Island and the inhabitants of Crete—have a relatively high intake of alpha-linolenic acid (the essential omega-3 fatty acid).[36,37] Typically, Cretans have a three times higher concentration of alpha-linolenic acid in their diet and body tissues compared to members of other European countries, due to their frequent consumption of walnuts and purslane.[36]

Another important dietary factor in both the Kohamans and Cretans is their use of oils that contain *oleic acid*—canola and olive oil, respectively. LDL cholesterol largely composed of oleic acid is less susceptible to becoming damaged by free radicals, a process known as peroxidation. Although the oleic acid content of the diet offers some degree of protection, the rate of heart attacks among the Kohamans and Cretans is much lower than the rate in populations that consume only oleic acid sources and little alpha-linolenic acid. The intake of alpha-linolenic acid is viewed as a more significant protective factor.[36,37]

Here are four recommendations for achieving better health and more optimal levels of essential fatty acids in body tissues:

1. Reduce your intake of saturated fat by decreasing the intake of animal foods.
2. Eliminate your intake of trans-fatty acids by avoiding margarine, shortening, and most processed foods.
3. Increase your consumption of cold-water fish such as salmon, mackerel, herring, and halibut.
4. Take 1 tablespoon of flaxseed oil daily.

Low Levels of Magnesium and Potassium

Magnesium and potassium are essential to the proper functioning of the entire cardiovascular system. Their critical roles in preventing heart disease and strokes are now widely accepted. In addition, there is a substantial body of knowledge demonstrating that magnesium and/or potassium supplementation is effective in treating a wide range of cardiovascular diseases, including angina, arrhythmia, congestive heart failure, and high blood pressure. Supplementation with magnesium and/or potassium has been used to treat many of these conditions for over fifty years.[38–40]

Since the role of potassium on the cardiovascular system is described in detail in HIGH BLOOD PRESSURE (in Part III), the focus here will be on magnesium. Most Americans simply do not get enough of this important mineral. The average intake of magnesium by healthy adults in the United States ranges between 143 and 266 mg per day. This level is well below the recommended dietary allowance (RDA) of 350 mg for men and 300 mg for women. Food choices are the main reason. Since magnesium occurs abundantly in whole foods, most nutritionists and dietitians assume that most Americans get enough magnesium in their diet. But most Americans are not eating whole, natural foods. They are consuming large quantities of processed foods. Since food processing refines out a large portion of magnesium, most Americans are not getting the RDA for magnesium.

The best dietary sources of magnesium are tofu, legumes, seeds, nuts, whole grains, and green leafy vegetables. Fish, meat, milk, and most commonly eaten fruit are low in magnesium. The diet of most Americans is low in magnesium because they eat primarily processed foods, meat, and dairy products.

Magnesium in Acute Myocardial Infarction   *Acute myocardial infarction* (MI) is the medical term for a heart attack. It is now well established that people who die from a heart attack have lower heart magnesium levels than people of the same age who die from other causes.[41] Intravenous magnesium therapy has now emerged as a valued treatment measure in acute myocardial infarction.[42–44]

The major obstacle to magnesium becoming the preferred method for saving a person's life appears to be financial interests. Magnesium is cheap compared to the new, high-tech, high-priced, genetically engineered drugs currently being promoted by the drug companies. The treatment of acute myocardial infarctions is a big business. Each year, over 1.5 million Americans will experience an acute MI. Magnesium therapy is now being used in many parts of the world to treat acute MI, due to its effectiveness, low cost, safety, and ease of administration. But in the United States it plays second fiddle to the high-tech drugs.

The fact is that, during the past decade, eight well-designed studies involving over four thousand patients have demonstrated that intravenous magnesium supplementation during the first hour of admission to a hospital for an acute MI produces a favorable effect in reducing immediate and long-term complications as well as death rates.[42-44]

The beneficial effects of magnesium in an acute MI relate to its ability to improve energy production within the heart; dilate the coronary arteries, resulting in improved delivery of oxygen to the heart; reduce peripheral vascular resistance, resulting in reduced demand on the heart; inhibit platelets from aggregating and forming blood clots; reduce the size of the *infarct* (blockage); and improve heart rate and arrhythmias.

Increased Platelet Aggregation

Excessive stickiness of blood platelets is another independent risk factor for heart disease and strokes. Once platelets adhere to each other or aggregate, they release potent compounds that dramatically promote the formation of the atherosclerotic plaque. Alternatively, they may form a clot that can get stuck in small arteries and produce a heart attack or stroke. What determines the stickiness of platelets is largely the type of fats and the level of antioxidants in the diet. While saturated fats and cholesterol increase platelet aggregation, omega-3 oils have the opposite effect.

In addition to the omega-3 fatty acids, antioxidant nutrients, and flavonoids, vitamin B6 inhibits platelet aggregation (in addition to lowering blood pressure and homocysteine levels).[45,46] In a recent study, the effect of vitamin B6 (pyridoxine HCl) supplementation on platelet aggregation, plasma lipids, and serum zinc levels was determined in twenty-four healthy male volunteers, ranging from nineteen to twenty-four years old. The volunteers were given either pyridoxine, at a dosage of 5 mg per 2.2 pounds of body weight, or a placebo for four weeks.[46] Results demonstrated that pyridoxine inhibited

platelet aggregation by forty-one to forty-eight percent, while there was no change in the control group. Pyridoxine prolonged both bleeding and coagulation time, but not over the physiological limits. It had no effect on platelet count.

In the same study, pyridoxine was also shown to lower total plasma lipid and cholesterol levels considerably from pretreatment levels. Total plasma lipid levels were reduced from 593 to 519 mg/dl, and total cholesterol level was reduced from 156 to 116 mg/dl. HDL cholesterol levels increased from 37.9 to 48.6. Serum zinc levels increased from 96 to 138 µg/dl. These results provide further evidence that vitamin B6 supplementation may reduce the risk of atherosclerotic mortality.

Garlic preparations standardized for *alliin*—the storage form of allicin, the key compound of garlic—as well as garlic oil have also demonstrated inhibition of platelet aggregation. In one study, 120 patients with increased platelet aggregation were given either 900 mg/day of a dried garlic preparation containing 1.3 percent alliin or a placebo for four weeks.[47] In the garlic group, spontaneous platelet aggregation disappeared, the microcirculation of the skin increased by 47.6 percent, plasma viscosity decreased by 3.2 percent, diastolic blood pressure dropped from an average of 74 to 67 mm Hg, and fasting blood glucose concentration dropped from an average of 89.4 to 79 mg/dl.

Increased Fibrinogen Formation

Elevated fibrinogen levels are a primary risk factor for cardiovascular disease. *Fibrinogen* is a protein involved in the clotting system. However, it plays many other important roles, including several that promote atherosclerosis, such as acting as a cofactor for platelet aggregation; determining the viscosity of blood; and stimulating the formation of the atherosclerotic plaque.

Early clinical studies stimulated detailed epidemiological investigations on the possible link between fibrinogen and cardiovascular disease.[48] The first such study was the Northwick Park Heart Study in the United Kingdom. This large study involved 1,510 men aged forty to sixty-four who were randomly recruited and tested for a range of clotting factors, including fibrinogen. At four years' follow-up, there was a stronger association between cardiovascular deaths and fibrinogen levels than that for cholesterol. This association has been confirmed in five other prospective epidemiological studies.

The clinical significance of these findings can be summarized as follows:

1. Fibrinogen levels should be determined and monitored in patients with or at high risk for coronary heart disease or stroke.

2. Natural therapies (e.g., exercise, omega-3 oils, niacin, and garlic) designed to promote fibrinolysis may offer significant benefit in the prevention of heart attacks and strokes.

Elevated Levels of Homocysteine

Homocysteine is an intermediate compound in the conversion of the amino acid methionine to cysteine. If a person is relatively deficient in folic acid, vitamin B6, or vitamin B12, there will be an increase in the level of homocysteine. This compound has been implicated in a variety of conditions, including atherosclerosis. Homocysteine is thought to promote atherosclerosis by directly damaging the artery and by reducing the integrity of the vessel wall, as well as by interfering with the formation of *collagen* (the main protein in bone).

Elevated homocysteine levels are an independent risk factor for heart attack, stroke,

or peripheral vascular disease. Elevations in homocysteine are found in approximately twenty to forty percent of patients with heart disease.[49,50] It is estimated that folic acid supplementation (400 mcg daily) alone would reduce the number of heart attacks suffered by Americans each year by ten percent. However, given the importance of vitamin B12 and B6 to proper homocysteine metabolism, it simply makes more sense to use all three together.[51–53]

In one study, the frequency of suboptimal levels of these nutrients in men with elevated homocysteine levels was found to be 56.8 percent for folic acid, 59.1 percent for vitamin B12, and 25 percent for vitamin B6. These results suggest that folic acid supplementation alone would not lower homocysteine levels in many cases since homocysteine levels would still be elevated in men with either B12 or B6 deficiency.[52] In other words, folic acid supplementation will only lower homocysteine levels if there are adequate levels of vitamin B12 and B6. Because of the interconnectedness of these three B-vitamins, the best approach to lowering homocysteine levels is to supplement all three.[53] A good multiple-vitamin-and-mineral formula (see SUPPLEMENTARY MEASURES) should provide adequate levels in most cases.

Type A Personality

Type A behavior is characterized by an extreme sense of time urgency, competitiveness, impatience, and aggressiveness. This behavior carries twice the risk of coronary heart disease, compared to non–Type A behavior.[54,55] Particularly damaging to the cardiovascular system is the regular expression of anger.

In one study, the relationship between habitual anger coping styles, especially anger expression, and serum lipid concentrations was examined in eighty-six healthy subjects.[56]

Habitual anger expression was measured on four scales: Aggression, Controlled Affect, Guilt, and Social Inhibition. A positive correlation between serum cholesterol level and Aggression was found. The higher the Aggression score, the higher the cholesterol level. A negative correlation was found between the LDL/HDL ratio and Controlled Affect score. In other words, the greater the ability to control anger, the lower the LDL/HDL ratio. Learning to control anger or express it appropriately leads to a significant reduction in the risk for heart disease, while a predominantly aggressive (hostile) anger coping style is linked to an unfavorable lipid profile. In addition to the recommendations given in the chapter A POSITIVE MENTAL ATTITUDE, here are ten tips for improving coping strategies

1. Don't starve your emotional life. Foster meaningful relationships. Make time to give and receive love in your life.

2. Learn to be a good listener. Allow the people in your life to really share their feelings and thoughts uninterrupted. Empathize with them; put yourself in their shoes.

3. Don't try to talk over somebody. If you find yourself being interrupted, relax; don't try to out-talk the other person. If you are courteous and allow other people to speak, they will eventually respond in kind (unless they are extremely rude). If they don't, point out to them that they are interrupting the communication process. You can only do this if you have been a good listener.

4. Avoid aggressive or passive behavior. Be assertive, but express your thoughts and feelings in a kind way to help improve relationships at work and at home.

5. Avoid excessive stress in your life as best you can by avoiding excessive work hours, poor nutrition, and inadequate rest. Get as much sleep as you can.

6. Avoid such stimulants as caffeine and nicotine. Stimulants promote the fight-or-flight response and tend to make people more irritable in the process.

7. Take time to build long-term health and success by performing stress-reduction techniques and deep-breathing exercises (see the chapter on STRESS).

8. Accept gracefully those things over which you have no control. Save your energy for those things that you can do something about.

9. Accept yourself. Remember that you are human and will make mistakes, from which you can learn, along the way.

10. Be patient and tolerant of other people. Follow the Golden Rule.

Worrying Is Bad for Your Heart   Recent research has suggested that anxiety and stress are associated with an increased risk of having a heart attack. Because worry is an important component of anxiety, researchers decided to assess the level of worry and how it affected the number of heart attacks in a twenty-year study.[57] In 1975, 1,759 men without apparent heart disease completed a "Worries Scale"—a scale developed to assess the extent to which the men worried about social conditions, health, finances, self-definition, and aging. During the twenty years of follow-up, 86 cases of fatal heart attack and 124 cases of angina were reported. Worry about social conditions (political, economic, and environmental factors) was the area of worry most strongly associated with heart disease. Compared with men who reported the lowest levels of worry about social conditions, men who worried about social conditions had a 241-percent increased risk of getting heart disease.

While worrying can be a positive experience if it focuses on problem solving about factors that a person can control, worrying appears to be extremely damaging when the focus is on social concerns that a person has little, if any, control over. Worry about social concerns is likely to be a more significant focus among people who are depressed or anxious.

The results of this study clearly demonstrate that comprehensive prevention of heart disease involves much more than focusing on the physical process of hardening of the arteries. A "happy heart" may prove to be the most powerful medicine against heart disease.

Preventing a Recurrent Heart Attack

People who have experienced a heart attack or stroke and lived through it are extremely likely to experience another. The primary prevention of subsequent cardiovascular events is to control the major cardiac risk factors (e.g., elevations in cholesterol, hypertension, cigarette smoking, diabetes, and physical inactivity). The most popular secondary recommendation given by physicians for reducing the risk of a subsequent heart attack is low-dose aspirin (325 mg per day). But is this recommendation the best one for survivors of heart attacks?

Aspirin and the Prevention of Subsequent Heart Attacks

There have seven prospective, randomized, placebo-controlled trials, involving almost fifteen thousand survivors of heart attacks, that have examined the use of aspirin to reduce the incidence of recurrent heart attack and death. These trials have used several dosages of aspirin, ranging from 325 mg to 1,500 mg daily, and enrolled patients at various intervals after infarction, ranging from four weeks to five years. Not a single study demonstrated a statistically significant reduc-

tion in mortality with aspirin use. If not one study demonstrated a benefit, how did aspirin become the "drug of choice" for these patients? Although not a single isolated study showed benefits, when all the results from these studies were pooled, aspirin was shown to produce a reduction in mortality rate from all causes and cardiovascular deaths. The mortality rate for all causes in the aspirin group was 5.8 percent, compared to 8.3 percent in the placebo group, indicating a reduction in mortality by thirty percent with aspirin.[58]

Although it is becoming popular to recommend dosages of aspirin lower than 325 mg (e.g., 50 mg to 150 mg daily), these lower dosages have not been tested in properly designed trials.

The Safety of Aspirin   Aspirin and other NSAIDs (nonsteroidal anti-inflammatory drugs) are associated with a significant risk of peptic ulcer. However, most studies that document the relative frequency of peptic ulcers as a consequence of aspirin and NSAID use have focused on their use in the treatment of arthritis and headaches. Recently, the risk of gastrointestinal bleeding due to peptic ulcers was evaluated for aspirin usage at daily doses of 300 mg, 150 mg, and 75 mg.

The study, conducted at five test hospitals in England, found an increased risk of gastrointestinal bleeding due to peptic ulcer at all dosage levels. However, subjects who took 75 mg per day had forty percent less gastrointestinal bleeding than those who took 300 mg per day, and those who took 150 mg per day had thirty percent less. The researchers concluded that "no conventionally used prophylactic aspirin regimen seems free of the risk of peptic ulcer complications."[59]

Given the fact that it is not known whether 75 mg of aspirin per day is at all helpful in preventing a second heart attack, most physicians recommend taking at least 300 mg—a dosage that has been shown to be effective. In the prevention of stroke, the dosage of aspirin necessary appears to be 900 mg. These dosage recommendations carry with them a significant risk for developing a peptic ulcer, but in high-risk patients unwilling to adopt the natural approach, I would certainly recommend aspirin therapy as the second choice.

Natural Alternatives to Aspirin   The best approach to preventing repeat heart attacks may not be low-dose aspirin, especially in aspirin-sensitive patients. The first alternative to aspirin is too often overlooked by many physicians: diet. As of September 1995, three studies had shown that dietary modifications are more effective in preventing heart attack recurrence than aspirin. The results of these studies clearly indicate that diet and lifestyle are not only protective against heart disease, but also can dramatically reverse the blockage of clogged arteries.

The most famous of the three studies that showed this effect is the Lifestyle Heart Trial conducted by Dr. Dean Ornish.[60] In this study, subjects with heart disease were divided into a control group and an experimental group. The control group received regular medical care, while the experimental group was asked to eat a lowfat vegetarian diet for at least one year. The diet included fruits, vegetables, grains, legumes, and soybean products. Subjects were allowed to consume as many calories as they wished. No animal products were allowed except egg whites and one cup per day of nonfat milk or yogurt. The diet contained approximately ten percent fat, fifteen to twenty percent protein, and seventy to seventy-five percent carbohydrate of total calorie intake, which was predominantly complex carbohydrate from whole grains, legumes, and vegetables.

The experimental group was also asked to perform stress-reduction techniques such as breathing exercises, stretching exercises, meditation, imagery, and other relaxation techniques for an hour each day and to exercise at least three hours each week. At the end of the year, the subjects in the experimental group showed significant overall regression of atherosclerosis of the coronary blood vessels. In contrast, subjects in the control group who were being treated with regular medical care and following the standard American Heart Association diet showed progression of their disease; the control group actually got worse. Ornish states: "This finding suggests that conventional recommendations for patients with coronary heart disease (such as a thirty-percent fat diet) are not sufficient to bring about regression in many patients."

The other two studies on diet and prevention of second heart attacks highlight the importance of omega-3 fatty acids and again show the ineffectiveness of the American Heart Association's dietary recommendations.

As stated previously, numerous population studies have demonstrated that people who consume a diet rich in omega-3 oils from either fish or vegetable sources have a significantly reduced risk of developing heart disease.[61] Furthermore, results from autopsy studies have shown that the highest degree of coronary artery disease is found in individuals with the lowest concentration of omega-3 oils in their fat tissues. Conversely, individuals with the lowest degree of coronary artery disease had the highest concentration of omega-3 oils.[62]

In the Dietary and Reinfarction Trial (DART), it was only when the intake of omega-3 fatty acids (from fish) was increased that the number of repeat heart attacks was reduced.[63] The other study, the Lyon Diet Heart Study, determined that increasing the intake of omega-3 fatty acids from plant sources (alpha-linolenic acid) offers the same degree of protection as increased fish intake.[64] The diet used in the Lyon Heart Study is often referred to as the Mediterranean or Cretan diet. Compared to the standard American diet (the SAD), the Cretan diet consists of more bread, more root vegetables, more green vegetables, more fish, less meat (beef, lamb, and pork are replaced with poultry), fruit every day, and canola and olive oil instead of butter and cream. Compared to the control group, the group that followed the Cretan diet had a sixty percent reduction in overall mortality.

Additional Measures   Several natural inhibitors of platelet aggregation were described above, notably omega-3 fatty acids, antioxidant nutrients, flavonoids, garlic, and vitamin B6. In addition to these natural compounds, a mixture of highly purified bovine-derived glycosaminoglycans (GAGs) naturally present in the human aorta (including dermatan sulfate, heparan sulfate, hyaluronic acid, chondroitin sulfate, and related hexosaminoglycans) has been shown to inhibit platelet aggregation and protect and promote normal artery and vein function.

Over fifty clinical studies have shown that an orally administered complex of aortic GAGs is effective in treating a number of vascular disorders, including cerebral and peripheral arterial insufficiency; venous insufficiency and varicose veins; hemorrhoids; vascular retinopathies, including macular degeneration; and post-surgical edema. Significant improvements in both symptoms and blood flow have been noted.[65–69]

We recommend aortic GAGs primarily to patients recovering from heart attack or stroke and to those who have had either angiograms, coronary artery bypass surgery, or angioplasty. The dosage of aortic GAGs is 100 mg daily.

Similar results, though not nearly as impressive, have been noted with the use of chondroitin sulfate at a daily dose of 3 grams (1 gram with meals, three times per day).[70]

Preventing Recurrence of Stroke

To prevent a second stroke, as well as to promote recovery from a stroke, we recommend adding *Ginkgo biloba* extract to the program given above for preventing a subsequent heart attack. The extract of *Ginkgo biloba* leaves, standardized to contain twenty-four percent ginkgo flavonglycosides and six percent terpenoids, has been the subject of over three hundred published scientific papers and over forty double-blind studies on the treatment of decreased blood supply to the brain *(cerebral vascular insufficiency)*. It is currently the third most widely prescribed drug of all kinds in Germany. *Ginkgo biloba* extract has demonstrated remarkable effects in improving many symptoms associated with aging, including short-term memory loss, depression, dizziness, ringing in the ears, and headache. *Ginkgo biloba* extract has also been shown to enhance stroke recovery.[71–74]

Considering Coronary Artery Bypass Surgery or Angioplasty

If you have had a heart attack or are experiencing *angina* (chest pain), your physician is probably urging you to have an *angiogram* (cardiac catheterization) or is recommending coronary artery bypass surgery or angioplasty. However, before electing to have these procedures performed, examine the benefits and risks carefully. Please see the chapter on ANGINA for a complete description and alternative therapies.

Earlobe Crease

The presence of a diagonal earlobe crease has been recognized as a sign of cardiovascular disease since 1973. Since then, over thirty studies have been reported in the medical literature, with the largest to date involving one thousand unselected patients. The earlobe is richly veined, and a decrease in blood flow over a period of time is believed to result in collapse of the vascular bed. This leads to a diagonal crease.[75,76]

In one study, angiograms performed on 205 consecutive patients showed an eighty-two-percent accuracy in predicting heart disease based on the earlobe crease, with a false positive rate of twelve percent and a false negative rate of eighteen percent.[76] A false positive situation exists when there is an earlobe crease and no evidence of heart disease. A false negative situation occurs when there is no earlobe crease, but there is evidence of heart disease. So you can see that the presence of an earlobe crease was quite significant in this study.

The crease is seen more commonly with advancing age until the age of eighty, when the incidence drops dramatically. However, the association with heart disease is age-independent. In other words, the presence of a diagonal earlobe crease is just as significant if you are forty years old as if you are eighty years old.

In conclusion, the earlobe crease appears to be a better predictor of heart disease than any other known risk factor, including age, smoking, sedentary lifestyle, hyperlipidemia, and others. While the presence of an earlobe crease does not prove that heart disease exists, it strongly suggests it; examination of the earlobe should be a useful screening procedure. The correlation does not hold true for Asians, Native Americans, and children with a rare condition known as Beckwith's syndrome.

Detoxification

The ability to detoxify is a major determinant of a person's level of health.

It is conservatively estimated that up to twenty-five percent of the U.S. population suffers from heavy metal poisoning to some extent.

Exposure or toxicity to food additives, solvents (cleaning materials, formaldehyde, toluene, benzene, etc.), pesticides, herbicides, and other toxic chemicals can give rise to a number of psychological and neurological symptoms.

Toxins produced by bacteria and yeast in the gut can be absorbed, causing significant disruption of body functions.

The liver is a complex organ that plays a key role in most metabolic processes, especially detoxification.

The liver's detoxification mechanisms include
- Filtration of the blood
- Formation of bile
- Phase I detoxification reactions
- Phase II detoxification reactions

Glutathione is an important detoxification compound.

Vitamin C supplementation is the most cost-effective method of raising glutathione levels.

Taking silymarin, the flavonoid complex from milk thistle, is a well-researched way to improve liver function.

Fasting is one of the fastest ways to increase elimination of wastes and enhance the healing processes of the body.

The concepts of internal cleansing and detoxification have been around for quite some time. In modern times, as society has increasingly been exposed to toxic compounds in the air, water, and food, it has become apparent that our ability to detoxify substances to which we are exposed is of critical importance in our overall health.

This chapter identifies *toxins* in the body and natural ways to support the detoxification and elimination of these harmful compounds.

Toxic substances are everywhere—in the air we breathe, the food we eat, and the water we drink. Even our bodies and the bacteria in our intestines produce toxic substances.

Toxins can damage the body in an insidious and cumulative way. Once the detoxification system becomes overloaded, toxic *metabolites* (products of metabolism) accumulate, and we become progressively more sensitive to other chemicals, some of which are not normally toxic. This accumulation of toxins can wreak havoc on our normal metabolic processes.

This chapter will focus on enhancing detoxification primarily by promoting improved liver function. Our modern environment seriously overloads our liver, resulting in increased levels of circulating toxins in the blood, which damage most of our body's systems. An overburdened liver sends out alarm signals that manifest as psoriasis, acne, chronic headaches, inflammatory and auto-immune diseases, and chronic fatigue.

Types of Toxins

You may be asking, "What exactly is a toxin?" A *toxin* is defined as any compound that has a detrimental effect on cell function or structure. Obviously, some toxins cause minimal negative effects while others can be fatal. We have organized the discussion of toxins in this chapter into the following areas

- Heavy metals
- Liver toxicants
- Microbial compounds
- Breakdown products of protein metabolism

Heavy Metals
Included in this category are the following heavy metals: lead, mercury, cadmium, arsenic, nickel, and aluminum. These metals tend to accumulate within the brain, kidneys, and immune system, where they can severely disrupt normal function.[1-6]

Most people have more lead and other heavy metals in their body than is compatible with good health. It is conservatively estimated that up to twenty-five percent of the U.S. population suffers from heavy-metal poisoning to some extent. Hair mineral analysis is a good screening test for heavy-metal toxicity.[1]

Most of the heavy metals in the body are a result of environmental contamination due to industry. For example, in the United States alone, industrial processes and leaded gasoline contribute more than 600,000 tons of lead to the atmosphere, to be inhaled or—after being deposited on food crops, in fresh water, and in soil—to be ingested.[1]

Common sources of heavy metals, in addition to industrial sources, include lead from pesticide sprays, cooking utensils, and the solder in tin cans; cadmium and lead from cigarette smoke; mercury from dental fillings, contaminated fish, and cosmetics; and aluminum from antacids and cookware.[1]

Early signs of heavy-metal poisoning are vague or attributed to other problems. Early symptoms can include headache, fatigue, muscle pains, indigestion, tremors, constipation, anemia, pallor, dizziness, and poor coordination. The person with even mild heavy-metal toxicity will experience impaired ability to think or concentrate. As toxicity increases, so does the severity of signs and symptoms.[1-6]

Numerous studies have demonstrated a strong relationship between childhood learning disabilities (and other disorders, including criminal behavior) and body stores of heavy metals, particularly lead.[7-12] (See At-TENTION DEFICIT DISORDER in Part III).

More and more information is accumulating to indicate that chronic heavy-metal toxicity is a major problem in our modern society. Every effort should be made to reduce heavy-metal levels. This is particularly true for individuals who are exposed to high levels of heavy metals. Workers with extremely high exposure include: battery makers, gasoline station attendants, printers, roofers, solderers, dentists, and jewelers.[1]

Nutritional factors that combat heavy-metal poisoning include

- A high-potency multiple-vitamin-and-mineral supplement[13-20]

- Minerals such as calcium, magnesium, zinc, iron, copper, and chromium
- Vitamin C and B-complex vitamins
- Sulfur-containing amino acids (methionine, cysteine, and taurine) and high-sulfur-content foods such as garlic, onions, and eggs[21-23]
- Water-soluble fibers such as guar gum, oat bran, pectin, and psyllium seed[1,13]

Liver Toxicants

This category of toxins is primarily dealt with by the liver and includes toxic chemicals, drugs, alcohol, solvents, formaldehyde, pesticides, herbicides, and food additives. It is staggering to contemplate the tremendous load placed on the liver as it detoxifies the incredible quantity of toxic chemicals it is constantly exposed to. Below we will discuss compounds that support the liver's detoxification mechanisms, such as methionine, antioxidants, choline, and milk thistle extract.

Exposure or sensitivity to food additives, solvents (cleaning materials, formaldehyde, toluene, benzene, etc.), pesticides, herbicides, and other toxic chemicals can give rise to a number of symptoms. Most common are psychological and neurological symptoms such as depression, headaches, mental confusion, mental illness, tingling in the hands and feet, abnormal nerve reflexes, and other signs of impaired nervous system function. The nervous system is extremely sensitive to these chemicals. Respiratory tract allergies and increased rates for many cancers are also noted in people chronically exposed to chemical toxins.[24-30]

Microbial Compounds

Toxins produced by bacteria and yeast in the gut can be absorbed, causing significant disruption of body functions. Examples of these types of toxins include toxins from bacteria (endotoxins and exotoxins), toxic amines,

QUICK REVIEW

Detoxification of harmful substances is a continual process in the body. The ability to detoxify and eliminate toxins largely determines an individual's health status. A number of toxins (heavy metals, solvents, pesticides, microbial toxins, etc.) are known to cause significant health problems.

A rational approach to aiding the body's detoxification involves

- Eating a diet that focuses on fresh fruits and vegetables, whole grains, legumes, nuts, and seeds
- Adopting a healthy lifestyle, including avoidance of alcohol and exercising regularly
- Taking a high-potency multiple-vitamin-and-mineral supplement
- Using special nutritional and herbal supplements to protect the liver and enhance liver function
- Going on a three-day fast four times per year (fasting at the change of each season is a good rule of thumb).

toxic derivatives of bile, and various carcinogenic substances.

Gut-derived microbial toxins have been implicated in a wide variety of diseases, including liver diseases, Crohn's disease, ulcerative colitis, thyroid disease, psoriasis, lupus erythematosis, pancreatitis, allergies, asthma, and immune disorders.

In addition to toxic substances being produced by microorganisms, antibodies formed against microbial molecules (antigens) can "cross-react" with the body's own tissues, thereby causing *autoimmunity*. The list of autoimmune diseases that have been linked to cross-reacting antibodies includes rheumatoid arthritis, myasthenia gravis, diabetes, and autoimmune thyroiditis.

To reduce the absorption of toxic substances, it is recommended that the diet be rich in fiber, particularly the water-soluble fibers such as those found in vegetables, guar gum, pectin, and oat bran. Fiber has an ability to bind to toxins within the gut and promote their excretion.

The immune system, in addition to the liver, is responsible for dealing with the toxic substances that are absorbed from the gut.

Breakdown Products of Protein Metabolism

The kidneys are largely responsible for the elimination of toxic waste products of protein breakdown (ammonia, urea, etc.). Drinking adequate amounts of water and avoiding excessive protein intake can support the kidneys in their important function.

The Diagnosis of Toxicity

A number of special laboratory techniques are useful in detecting toxins in the body. For heavy metals, the most reliable measure of chronic exposure is the hair mineral analysis.

Reliable results from hair analysis are dependent upon (1) a properly collected, cleaned, and prepared sample of hair and (2) the test being performed by experienced personnel using appropriate analytical methods in a qualified laboratory.

For determining exposure to toxic chemicals, a detailed medical history by a physician experienced in these matters is essential. When appropriate, the laboratory analysis for this group of toxins can involve measuring blood and fatty tissue for suspected chemicals. It is also necessary to measure the effect that these chemicals have on the liver. This goal is best accomplished by clearance tests that measure the levels of caffeine, acetaminophen, benzoic acid, and other compounds after ingestion of a specified amount. Other tests for liver function (serum bilirubin and liver enzymes) are also important but are less sensitive.

Perhaps the best recommendation to help you determine if your liver is functioning up to par is to look over the following list. If any factor applies to you, we recommend following the guidelines for improving liver function given later under Diet and Liver Function; Special Nutritional Factors; and Plant-Based Medicines and Liver Function.

- More than 20 pounds overweight
- Diabetes
- Gallstones
- History of heavy alcohol use
- Psoriasis
- Natural and synthetic steroid hormone use: anabolic steroids, estrogens and oral contraceptives
- High exposure to certain chemicals or drugs: cleaning solvents, pesticides, antibiotics, diuretics, nonsteroidal anti-inflammatory drugs, thyroid hormone
- History of viral hepatitis

To determine the presence of microbial compounds, naturopathic physicians use a number of special laboratory techniques, including tests for the presence of: (1) abnormal microbial concentrations and disease-causing organisms (stool culture), (2) microbial byproducts (urinary indican—a byproduct indicating excessive bacterial putrefaction or, breakdown of protein) and (3) endotoxins (erythrocyte sedimentation rate is a rough estimator).

To determine the presence of high levels of protein metabolism and kidney function breakdown products, both blood and urine measurements of these compounds are performed.

How the Detoxification System Works

The body eliminates toxins either by directly neutralizing them or by excreting them in the urine or feces (and to a lesser degree via the lungs and skin). Toxins that the body is unable to eliminate build up in the tissues, typically in our fat stores. The liver, intestines, and kidneys are the primary organs of detoxification.

The Liver

The liver is a complex organ that plays a key role in most metabolic processes, especially detoxification. The liver is constantly bombarded with toxic chemicals, both those produced internally and those coming from the environment. The metabolic processes that make our bodies run normally produce a wide range of toxins for which the liver has evolved efficient neutralizing mechanisms. However, the level and type of internally produced toxins increase greatly when metabolic

processes go awry, typically as a result of nutritional deficiencies.

Many of the toxic chemicals the liver must detoxify come from our environment: the content of our bowel, the food we eat, the water we drink, and the air we breathe. The polycyclic hydrocarbons (e.g., DDT; dioxin; 2,4,5-T; 2,4-D; PCB; and PCP), which are components of various herbicides and pesticides, are one example. Yet, as mentioned above, even people who eat unprocessed organic foods need an effective detoxification system because even organically grown foods have naturally occurring toxic constituents.

The liver plays several roles in detoxification: It filters the blood to remove large toxins, synthesizes and secretes bile full of cholesterol and other fat-soluble toxins, and enzymatically disassembles unwanted chemicals. This enzymatic process usually occurs in two steps, referred to as Phase I and Phase II, with Phase I chemically modifying the chemicals to make them an easier target for one or more of the several Phase II enzyme systems. These processes are summarized in Figure 1.

Proper functioning of the liver's detoxification systems is especially important for the prevention of cancer. Up to ninety percent of all cancers are thought to be due to the effects of environmental carcinogens, such as those in cigarette smoke, food, water, and air, combined with deficiencies of the nutrients the body needs for proper functioning of the detoxification and immune systems. Our levels of exposure to environmental carcinogens vary widely, as does the efficiency of our detoxification enzymes. High levels of exposure to carcinogens, coupled with sluggish detoxification enzymes, significantly increases our susceptibility to cancer.

The link between our detoxification system's effectiveness and our susceptibility to

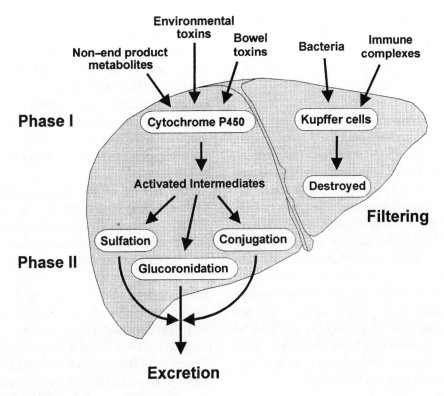

FIGURE 1 The Liver's Detoxification Pathways

environmental toxins, such as carcinogens, is exemplified in a study of chemical plant workers in Turin, Italy, who had an unusually high rate of bladder cancer. When the liver detoxification enzyme activity of all the workers was tested, it was found that those with the poorest detoxification systems were the ones who developed bladder cancer.[31] In other words, all were exposed to the same level of carcinogens, but those with poor liver function were the ones who developed the cancer.

Fortunately, the detoxification efficiency of the liver can be improved with dietary measures, special nutrients, and herbs. Ultimately, your best protection from cancer is to avoid carcinogens and to make sure your detoxification system is working well in order to eliminate those you can't avoid before they can hurt you.

Filtering the Blood

One of the liver's primary functions is filtering the blood. Almost 2 quarts of blood pass through the liver every minute for detoxification. Filtration of toxins is absolutely critical for the blood that comes from the intestines because it is loaded with bacteria, *endotoxins* (toxins released when bacteria die and are broken down), *antigen-antibody complexes* (large molecules produced when the immune system latches on to an invader to neutralize it), and various other toxic substances.

When working properly, the liver clears ninety-nine percent of the bacteria and other toxins from the blood before it is allowed to re-enter the general circulation. However, when the liver is damaged this filtration system breaks down.

The Bile

The liver's second detoxification process involves the synthesis and secretion of bile. Each day the liver manufactures approximately 1 quart of bile, which serves as a carrier in which many toxic substances are effectively eliminated from the body. Sent to the intestines, the bile and its toxic load are absorbed by fiber and excreted. However, a diet low in fiber means that these toxins are not bound in the feces very well and are reabsorbed. Even worse, bacteria in the intestine often modify these toxins so that they become even more damaging. In addition to eliminating unwanted toxins, the bile emulsifies fats and fat-soluble vitamins in the intestine, improving their absorption.

Phase I Detoxification

The liver's third role in detoxification involves a two-step enzymatic process for the neutralization of unwanted chemical compounds. These include not only drugs, pesticides, and toxins from the gut, but also normal body chemicals such as hormones and inflammatory chemicals (e.g., histamine) that would be toxic if allowed to build up. Phase I enzymes directly neutralize some chemicals, but many others are converted to intermediate forms that are then processed by Phase II enzymes. Unfortunately, these intermediate forms are often much more chemically active and therefore more toxic, so if the Phase II detoxification systems aren't working adequately, these intermediates hang around and are far more damaging.

Phase I detoxification of most chemical toxins involves a group of enzymes that collectively, have been named *cytochrome P450.* Some fifty to one hundred enzymes make up the cytochrome P450 system. Each enzyme works best in detoxifying certain types of chemicals, but with considerable overlap in activity among the enzymes. In other words, they all metabolize the same chemicals, but with differing levels of efficiency. This fail-safe system ensures maximum detoxification.

The activity of the various cytochrome P450 enzymes varies significantly from one individual to another based on genetics, the individual's level of exposure to chemical toxins, and his or her nutritional status. Since the activity of cytochrome P450 varies so much, so does an individual's risk for various diseases. For example, as highlighted in the study of chemical plant workers in Turin discussed above, those with underactive cytochrome P450 are more susceptible to cancer.[32] This variability of cytochrome P450 enzymes is also seen in the variability of people's ability to detoxify the carcinogens found in cigarette smoke and helps to explain why some people can smoke without too much damage to their lungs, while others develop lung cancer after only a few decades of smoking. Those who develop cancer are typically those who are exposed to a lot of carcinogens and/or those whose cytochrome P450 isn't working very well.

The level of activity of Phase I detoxification varies greatly, even among healthy adults. One way of determining the activity of Phase I is to measure how efficiently a person detoxifies caffeine. Using this test, researchers have found a surprising fivefold difference in the detoxification rates of apparently healthy adults.[33]

When cytochrome P450 metabolizes a toxin, it tries to either chemically transform it to a less toxic form, make it water-soluble, or convert it to a more chemically active form.

The best results come from the first option—simply neutralizing the toxin. This is what happens to caffeine. Making a toxin water-soluble is also effective because this makes it easier for the kidneys to excrete it in the urine. The final option is to transform the toxin to more chemically reactive forms, which are more easily metabolized by the Phase II enzymes. While ultimately very important for our health, this transformation of toxins into more chemically active toxins can cause several problems.

A significant side effect of all this metabolic activity is the production of free radicals as the toxins are transformed. In other words, for each toxin metabolized by Phase I, a free radical is generated. Without adequate free-radical defenses, every time the liver neutralizes a toxin, it is damaged by the free radicals produced.

The most important antioxidant for neutralizing the free radicals produced as Phase I byproducts is glutathione (a small *tripeptide* [protein] composed of three amino acids: cysteine, glutamic acid, and glycine). In the process of neutralizing free radicals, however, glutathione (GSH) is oxidized to glutathione disulfide (GSSG). Glutathione is required for one of the key Phase II detoxification processes. When high levels of toxin exposure produce so many free radicals from Phase I detoxification that all the glutathione is used up, Phase II processes dependent upon glutathione stop.

Another potential problem occurs because the toxins transformed into "activated intermediates" by Phase I are even more toxic than before. Unless quickly removed from the body by Phase II detoxification mechanisms, they can cause widespread problems. Therefore, the rate at which Phase I produces activated intermediates must be balanced by the rate at which Phase II finishes their processing. Unfortunately, some people have a very active Phase I detoxification system but very slow or inactive Phase II enzymes. The end result is that these people suffer severe toxic reactions to environmental poisons.

An imbalance between Phase I and Phase II can also occur when a person is exposed to large amounts of toxins or to lower levels of toxins for a long period of time. In these situations, so many toxins are being neutralized that the critical nutrients needed for Phase II detoxification get used up, which allows the highly toxic activated intermediates to build up.

Recent research shows that cytochrome P450 enzyme systems are found in other parts of the body, especially the brain cells. Inadequate antioxidants and nutrients in the brain result in an increased rate of neuron damage, as seen in Alzheimer's and Parkinson's disease patients.

As with all enzymes, the cytochrome P450s require several nutrients in order to function. A deficiency of any of these means more toxins floating around doing damage. The nutrients needed for Phase I detoxification are

- Copper
- Magnesium (deficiency substantially increases toxicity of many drugs)
- Zinc
- Vitamin C

A considerable amount of research has shown that various substances activate cytochrome P450, while other substances inhibit it.

Inducers of Phase I Detoxification

Cytochrome P450 is induced by some toxins and by some foods and nutrients. Obviously, it is beneficial to improve Phase I detoxification in order to get rid of the toxins as soon as possible. This is best accomplished by providing the needed nutrients and nontoxic stimulants while avoiding those substances that are toxic. However, stimulation of Phase I is not a good idea if your Phase II system is not functioning properly.

SUBSTANCES THAT ACTIVATE PHASE I DETOXIFICATION

Drugs
  Alcohol
  Nicotine in cigarette smoke
  Phenobarbital
  Sulfonamides
  Steroids
Foods
  Cabbage, broccoli, and brussels sprouts
  Charcoal-broiled meats (due to their high levels of toxic
    compounds)
  High-protein diet
  Oranges and tangerines (but not grapefruits)
Nutrients
  Niacin
  Vitamin B1 (riboflavin)
  Vitamin C
Herbs
  Caraway and dill seeds
Environmental toxins
  Carbon tetrachloride
  Exhaust fumes
  Paint fumes
  Dioxin
  Pesticides

All of the drugs and environmental toxins listed in Substances That Activate Phase I Detoxification activate P450 to combat their destructive effects. In so doing, they not only use up compounds needed for this detoxification system but contribute significantly to free-radical formation and oxidative stress.

Among foods, the Brassica family (cabbage, broccoli, and brussels sprouts) contains chemical constituents that stimulate both Phase I and Phase II detoxification enzymes. One such compound is a powerful anticancer chemical called indole-3-carbinol. It is a very active stimulant of detoxifying enzymes in the gut as well as the liver.[34] The net result is significant protection against several toxins, especially carcinogens. This helps explain why consumption of cabbage-family vegetables protects against cancer.

Oranges, tangerines, and the seeds of caraway and dill contain *limonene,* a *phytochemical* (plant chemical) that has been found to prevent and even treat cancer in tests on animals.[35] Limonene's protective effects are probably due to the fact that it is a strong inducer of both Phase I and Phase II detoxification enzymes that neutralize carcinogens.

Inhibitors of Phase I Detoxification

Many substances inhibit cytochrome P450. This situation is perilous, as it makes toxins potentially more damaging because they remain in the body longer before detoxification. For example, if you are taking drugs or are exposed to elevated levels of toxins, don't eat grapefruit or drink grapefruit juice. Grapefruit juice decreases the rate of elimination of drugs from the blood.[36] Grapefruit contains a flavonoid called *naringenin* that can decrease cytochrome P450 activity by a remarkable thirty percent.

INHIBITORS OF PHASE I DETOXIFICATION

Drugs
  Benzodiazapines (e.g., Halcion, Centrax, Librium,
    Valium, etc.)
  Antihistamines (used to treat allergies)
  Cimetidine and other stomach-acid-secretion-blocking
    drugs (used for stomach ulcers)
  Ketoconazole
  Sulfaphenazole

Foods
   Naringenin from grapefruit juice
   Curcumin from the spice turmeric
   Capsaicin from red chili pepper
   Eugenol from clove oil
Other
   Aging
   Toxins from inappropriate bacteria in the intestines

Curcumin, the compound that gives turmeric its yellow color, is interesting because it inhibits Phase I while stimulating Phase II. This effect is also very useful in preventing cancer. Curcumin has been found to inhibit carcinogens, such as benzopyrene (the carcinogen found in charcoal-broiled meat), from inducing cancer in several animal studies. It appears that the curcumin exerts its anticarcinogenic activity by lowering the activation of carcinogens while increasing the detoxification of those that are activated. Curcumin has also been shown to directly inhibit the growth of cancer cells.[37]

We recommend eating a lot of curries (turmeric is the key component of curry) to smokers and people exposed to a lot of secondhand smoke. As stated previously, most of the cancer-inducing chemicals in cigarette smoke are only carcinogenic during the period between activation by Phase I and final detoxification by Phase II. The curcumin in the turmeric can help prevent the cancer-causing effect in dramatic fashion. In one human study, sixteen chronic smokers were given 1.5 grams of turmeric daily, while six nonsmokers served as a control group for comparison.[38] At the end of the thirty-day trial, the smokers who received the turmeric demonstrated significant reduction in the level of urinary excreted mutagens comparable to the nonsmokers' levels. These results are quite significant, as the level of urinary mutagens is thought to correlate with the systemic load of carcinogens and the efficacy of detoxification mechanisms. Due to widespread exposure to smoke, aromatic hydrocarbons, and other environmental carcinogens, the frequent use of curry or turmeric as a spice appears warranted.

The Phase I detoxification enzymes are less active in old age. Aging also decreases blood flow though the liver, further aggravating the problem. Lack of the physical activity necessary for good circulation, combined with the poor nutrition commonly seen in the elderly, adds up to a significant impairment of detoxification capacity, which is typically found in aging individuals. This helps to explain why toxic reactions to drugs are seen so commonly in the elderly; they are unable to eliminate them fast enough, so toxic levels build up.

To ensure that Phase I is working well, we recommend that you eat plenty of

- Brassica-family foods (cabbage, broccoli, and brussels sprouts)
- Vitamin B–rich foods (nutritional yeast, whole grains)
- Vitamin C–rich foods (peppers, cabbage, and tomatoes)
- Citrus foods (oranges and tangerines, but not grapefruit)

Phase II Detoxification

Phase II detoxification involves a process called *conjugation*, in which various enzymes in the liver attach small chemicals to the toxin. This term will be used extensively in the next few paragraphs, so it is important to remember that conjugation is the process in which a protective compound becomes bound to a toxin. This conjugation reaction either neutralizes the toxin or makes the toxin more easily excreted through the urine or bile.

Phase II enzymes act on some toxins directly, while others must first be activated by the Phase I enzymes. There are essentially six Phase II detoxification pathways: glutathione conjugation, amino acid conjugation, methylation, sulfation, sulfoxidation, acetylation, and glucuronidation. Table 1 provides examples of toxins neutralized by each of these pathways. Some toxins are neutralized through several pathways.

In order to work, these enzyme systems need nutrients, both for their activation and to provide the small molecules they add to the toxins. In addition, they need metabolic energy to function and to synthesize some of the small conjugating molecules. If the liver cells' energy-producing plants, the *mitochondria,* are not functioning properly (which can be caused by a magnesium deficiency or lack of exercise), Phase II detoxification slows down, allowing the buildup of toxic intermediates. Table 2 lists the key nutrients needed by each of the six Phase II detoxification systems. Table 3 lists the activators, and Table 4 the inhibitors, of Phase II enzymes.

Glutathione Conjugation

A primary detoxification route is the conjugation of glutathione (a tripeptide composed of three amino acids: cysteine, glutamic acid, and glycine). Many toxic chemicals, including heavy metals, solvents, and pesticides, are fat-soluble. This makes it very difficult for the body to eliminate them. The primary way the body eliminates fat-soluble compounds is by excreting them in the bile. The problem is that ninety-nine percent of the bile, including the excreted toxins, is reabsorbed.

Fortunately, the body is able to convert the fat-soluble toxins into a water-soluble form. The body performs this feat with the help of glutathione. When glutathione binds to a fat-soluble toxin, it ultimately converts it to a water-soluble form called a *mercaptate,* allow-

ing more efficient excretion via the kidneys. The elimination of fat-soluble compounds—especially heavy metals such as mercury and lead—is dependent on adequate levels of glutathione, which in turn is dependent on adequate levels of methionine and cysteine.

When increased levels of toxic compounds are present, more methionine is converted to cysteine and glutathione. Methionine and cysteine have a protective effect on glutathione and prevent its depletion during toxic overload. This, in turn, protects the liver from the damaging effects of toxic compounds and promotes their elimination.

Glutathione is also an important antioxidant. This combination of detoxification and protection from free radicals results in glutathione being one of the most important anticarcinogens and antioxidants in our cells, which means that a deficiency is devastating.[39]

When we are exposed to high levels of toxins, glutathione is used up faster than it can be produced or absorbed from the diet. We then become much more susceptible to toxin-induced diseases, such as cancer, especially if our Phase I detoxification system is highly active.[40]

Diseases that result from glutathione deficiency are not uncommon. A deficiency can be induced either by diseases that increase the need for glutathione, deficiencies of the nutrients needed for glutathione synthesis, or diseases that inhibit the formation of glutathione. For example, people with idiopathic pulmonary fibrosis, adult respiratory distress syndrome, HIV infection, hepatic cirrhosis, cataract formation, or advanced AIDS have been found to have a deficiency of glutathione, probably due to their greatly increased need for it, both as an antioxidant and for detoxification.[41] Also, smoking increases the rate of glutathione utilization, both to

TABLE 1	Major Detoxification Systems	

ORGAN	METHOD	TYPICAL TOXIN NEUTRALIZED
Skin	Excretion through sweat	Fat-soluble toxins such as DDT, heavy metals such as lead
Liver	Filtering of the blood	Bacteria and bacterial products, immune complexes
	Bile secretion	Cholesterol, hemoglobin breakdown products, extra calcium
	Phase I detoxification	Many prescription drugs (e.g., amphetamine, digitalis, pentobarbital), many over-the-counter drugs (acetaminophen, ibuprofen), caffeine, histamine, hormones (both internally produced and externally supplied), benzopyrene (carcinogen from charcoal-broiled meat), aniline (the yellow dyes), carbon tetrachloride, insecticides (e.g., Aldrin, Heptachlor), arachidonic acid
	Phase II detoxification: Glutathione conjugation	Acetaminophen, nicotine from cigarette smoke, organophosphates (insecticides), epoxides (carcinogens)
	Phase II detoxification: Amino acid conjugation	Benzoate (a common food preservative), aspirin
	Phase II detoxification: Methylation	Dopamine (neurotransmitter), epinephrine (hormone from adrenal gland), histamine, thiouracil (cancer drug)
	Phase II detoxification: Sulfation	Estrogen, aniline dyes, coumarin (blood thinner), acetaminophen, methyl-dopa (used to treat Parkinson's disease)
	Phase II detoxification: Acetylation	Sulfonamides (antibiotics), mescaline
	Phase II detoxification: Glucuronidation	Acetaminophen, morphine, diazepam (sedative, muscle relaxant), digitalis
	Phase II detoxification: Sulfoxidation	Sulfites, garlic compounds
Intestines	Mucosal detoxification	Toxins from bowel bacteria
	Excretion through feces	Fat-soluble toxins excreted in the bile
Kidneys	Excretion through urine	Many toxins after they are made water-soluble by the liver

detoxify the nicotine and to neutralize the free radicals produced by the toxins in the smoke.

Glutathione is available through two routes: diet and synthesis. Dietary glutathione (found in fresh fruits and vegetables, cooked fish, and meat) is well absorbed by the intestines and does not appear to be affected by the digestive processes. Dietary glutathione also appears to be efficiently absorbed into the blood,[42] but the same may not be true for glutathione supplements.

TABLE 2 Nutrients Needed by Phase II Detoxification Enzymes

PHASE II SYSTEM	REQUIRED NUTRIENTS
Glutathione conjugation	Glutathione, vitamin B6
Amino acid conjugation	Glycine
Methylation	S-adenosyl-methionine
Sulfation	Cysteine, methionine, molybdenum
Acetylation	Acetyl-CoA
Glucuronidation	Glucuronic acid

TABLE 3 Inducers of Phase II Detoxification Enzymes

PHASE II SYSTEM	INDUCERS
Glutathione conjugation	Brassicas-family foods (cabbage, broccoli, and brussels sprouts), limonene-containing foods (citrus peel, dill weed oil, and caraway oil)
Amino acid conjugation	Glycine
Methylation	Lipotropic nutrients (choline, methionine, betaine, folic acid, and vitamin B12)
Sulfation	Cysteine, methionine, taurine
Acetylation	None found
Glucuronidation	Fish oils, cigarette smoking, birth-control pills, phenobarbital, limonene-containing foods

To assess the feasibility of taking supplementary oral glutathione, seven healthy subjects were given a single dose of up to 3,000 mg of glutathione. Blood values indicated that the concentration of glutathione did not increase significantly, suggesting that the systemic availability of a single dose of up to 3,000 mg of glutathione is negligible.[43]

The authors of the study concluded: "It is not feasible to increase circulating glutathione to a clinically beneficial extent by the oral administration of a single dose of 3 grams of glutathione."[43] In contrast, in healthy individuals, a daily dosage of 500 mg of vitamin C may be sufficient to elevate and maintain good tissue glutathione levels. Vitamin C raises glutathione levels by helping the body manufacture it. In one double-blind study, the average red blood cell (RBC) glutathione concentration rose nearly fifty percent with 500 mg per day of vitamin C.[44] Increasing the dosage to 2,000 mg only raised RBC glutathione levels by another five percent. In light of these findings, a person who

TABLE 4 Inhibiters of Phase II Detoxification Enzymes	
PHASE II SYSTEM	**INHIBITORS**
Glutathione conjugation	Selenium deficiency, vitamin B2 deficiency, glutathione deficiency, zinc deficiency
Amino acid conjugation	Low-protein diet
Methylation	Folic acid or vitamin B12 deficiency
Sulfation	Nonsteroidal anti-inflammatory drugs (e.g., aspirin), tartrazine (yellow food dye), molybdenum deficiency
Acetylation	Vitamin B2, B5, or C deficiency
Glucuronidation	Aspirin, probenecid

desires to increase tissue levels of glutathione may want to use vitamin C instead of glutathione supplements.

In addition to vitamin C, other compounds that encourage glutathione synthesis include N-acetylcysteine (NAC), glycine, and methionine. Once again, vitamin C appears to offer greater benefit in raising glutathione levels. In an effort to increase antioxidant status in individuals with impaired glutathione synthesis, a variety of antioxidants have been used. Of these agents, only vitamin C and NAC have been able to offer some possible benefit.

To determine the relative effectiveness of vitamin C vs. NAC, a forty-five-month-old girl with an inherited deficiency in glutathione synthesis was recently followed before and during treatment with vitamin C or NAC. High doses of vitamin C (500 mg or 3 g per day) or NAC (800 mg per day) were given for one to two weeks. Measurements of glutathione (GSH) levels indicated that 3 g per day of vitamin C increased white blood cell GSH fourfold and plasma GSH levels eightfold. NAC also increased white blood cell count (3.5-fold) and plasma (twofold to five-

fold). Based on these results, it was decided that vitamin C would be given to her for one year at the 3-grams-per-day dosage. At the end of one year, her glutathione levels remained elevated, her hematocrit (the percentage of red blood cells) increased from a baseline 25.4 percent to 32.6 percent, and the number of her immature red blood cells (*reticulocyte count*) decreased from 11 percent to 4 percent. These results indicate that vitamin C can decrease cellular damage in patients with hereditary glutathione deficiency; it is also more effective and less expensive than NAC.[45]

For the general population, the significance of these results is that vitamin C may offer the benefits being attributed to NAC at only a slightly reduced cost. To put this in perspective, a daily dosage of 3 grams of vitamin C costs about $10.00 per month, while a dosage of 1 gram of NAC would cost about $20.00 per month.

There is more to this story. Over the past five to ten years, the use of NAC and glutathione products as antioxidants has become increasingly popular among nutritionally oriented physicians and the public. But is this use valid?

There is a biochemical rationale for this practice. It is thought that NAC acts as a precursor for glutathione, and that taking extra glutathione should raise tissue glutathione levels. While supplementing the diet with high doses of NAC may be beneficial in cases of extreme oxidative stress (e.g., AIDS, cancer patients going through chemotherapy, or drug overdose), it may be an unwise practice in healthy individuals. The reason? One study indicated that when NAC was given orally to six healthy volunteers at a dosage of 1.2 grams per day for four weeks, followed by 2.4 grams per day for an additional two weeks, it actually increased oxidative damage by acting as a pro-oxidant.[46]

Compared with the control group, the concentration of glutathione in NAC-treated subjects was reduced by forty-eight percent and the concentration of oxidized (inactive) glutathione was eighty percent higher. Oxidative stress actually increased by eighty-three percent in those receiving NAC, and there was no sign of the desired antioxidant effects. From the results of this study, it can be concluded that, at high doses, NAC may act as a pro-oxidant in healthy subjects. Unfortunately, 1.2 grams per day is not an unreasonable dosage to attain from commercially available sources of NAC.

With or without supplementation, to ensure that glutathione conjugation is working well eat plenty of glutathione-rich foods (i.e., asparagus, avocado, and walnuts), Brassica-family foods (cabbage, broccoli, brussels sprouts), and limonene-rich foods, which stimulate glutathione conjugation (orange peel oil, dill and caraway seeds). In addition, we recommend taking extra vitamin C (1,000 to 3,000 mg per day in divided doses).

Amino Acid Conjugation

Several amino acids (glycine, taurine, glutamine, arginine, and ornithine) are used to combine with and neutralize toxins. Of these, glycine is the most commonly utilized in Phase II amino acid detoxification. People who suffer from hepatitis, alcoholic liver disorders, carcinomas, chronic arthritis, hypothyroidism, toxemia of pregnancy, and excessive chemical exposure are commonly found to have a poorly functioning amino acid conjugation system.

For example, using the benzoate clearance test (a measure of the rate at which the body detoxifies benzoate by conjugating it with glycine to form hippuric acid, which is excreted by the kidneys), the rate of clearance in those with liver disease is half that of healthy adults. This means that, in those with liver disease, all the toxins that require this pathway stay in the body doing damage for almost twice as long.[47]

Even in apparently normal adults, a wide variation exists in the activity of the glycine conjugation pathway. This is due not only to genetic variation, but also to the availability of glycine in the liver. Glycine and the other amino acids used for conjugation become deficient on a low-protein diet and when chronic exposure to toxins results in depletion.

To ensure that amino acid conjugation is working well, simply make sure that you are eating adequate amounts of protein-rich foods.

Methylation

Methylation involves conjugating methyl groups to toxins. Most of the methyl groups used for detoxification come from S-adenosylmethionine (SAM). SAM is synthesized from the amino acid methionine. This synthesis requires the nutrients choline, vitamin B12, and folic acid.

SAM is able to inactivate estrogens (through methylation), supporting the use of methionine in treating conditions of estrogen excess, such as PMS. Its effects in preventing estrogen-induced *cholestasis* (stagnation of bile in the gallbladder) have been demonstrated in pregnant women and those on oral contraceptives.[48] In addition to its role in promoting estrogen excretion, methionine has been shown to increase the membrane fluidity that is typically decreased by estrogens, thereby restoring several factors that promote bile flow. Methionine also promotes the flow of lipids to and from the liver in humans. Methionine is a major source of numerous sulfur-containing compounds, including the amino acids cysteine and taurine.

To ensure that methylation is working adequately, eat foods rich in folic acid (green leafy vegetables), vitamin B6 (whole grains and legumes), and vitamin B12 (animal products or supplements). Methionine deficiency is not likely to be a problem because methionine is widely available in the diet.

Sulfation

Sulfation is the conjugation of toxins with sulfur-containing compounds. The sulfation system is important for detoxifying several drugs, food additives, and, especially, toxins from intestinal bacteria and the environment.

Sulfation, like the other Phase II detoxification systems, results in decreased toxicity and increased water-solubility of toxins, making it easier for them to be excreted in the urine or sometimes the bile. Sulfation is also used to detoxify some normal body chemicals and is the main way we eliminate steroid hormones (such as estrogen) and thyroid hormones so that they don't build up to damaging levels. Since sulfation is also the primary route for the elimination of neurotransmitters, dysfunction in this system may contribute to the development of some nervous system disorders.

Many factors influence the activity of sulfate conjugation. For example, a diet low in the amino acids methionine and cysteine has been shown to reduce sulfation.[49] Sulfation is also reduced by excessive levels of molybdenum or vitamin B6 (over about 100 mg per day).[50] In some cases, sulfation can be increased by supplemental sulfate, extra amounts of sulfur-containing foods in the diet, and the amino acids taurine and glutathione.

To ensure that sulfation is working adequately, consume adequate amounts of sulfur-containing foods: egg yolks, red peppers, garlic, onions, broccoli, and brussels sprouts.

Acetylation

Conjugation of toxins with acetyl CoA is the method by which the body eliminates sulfa drugs (antibiotics commonly used to treat urinary tract infections). This system appears to be especially sensitive to genetic variation; people who have a poor acetylation system are far more susceptible to sulfa drugs and other antibiotics. While not much is known about how to directly improve the activity of this system, it is known that acetylation is dependent on thiamin (vitamin B2), pantothenic acid (B5), and vitamin C.[51]

To ensure that acetylation is working adequately, eat foods rich in B-vitamins (yeast, whole grains) and vitamin C (peppers, cabbage, citrus fruits).

Glucuronidation

Glucuronidation—the combining of glucuronic acid with toxins—requires the enzyme UDP-glucuronyl transferase (UDPGT). Many of the commonly prescribed drugs are detoxified through this important pathway. It also helps to detoxify aspirin, menthol, vanillin (synthetic vanilla), food additives such as benzoates, and some hormones.

Glucuronidation appears to work well in most of us and doesn't seem to require special attention, except for those with Gilbert's syndrome—a relatively common syndrome characterized by a chronically elevated serum bilirubin level (1.2 to 3.0 mg/dl). Previously considered rare, this disorder is now known to affect as much as five percent of the general population. The condition is usually without symptoms, although some patients do complain about loss of appetite, malaise, and fatigue (typical symptoms of impaired liver function). The main way this condition is recognized is by a slight yellowish tinge to the skin and white of the eye, due to inadequate metabolism of bilirubin, a breakdown product of hemoglobin.

The activity of UDPGT is increased by foods rich in a monoterpene called limonene (citrus peel, dill weed oil, and caraway oil). Eating these foods not only improves glucuronidation but has also been shown to protect us from chemical carcinogens.

To ensure that glucuronidation is working properly, eat sulfur-rich foods (see above) and citrus fruit (but not grapefruit). If you have Gilbert's syndrome, be sure to drink at least 48 ounces of water daily. Also, methionine administered as SAM has been shown to be quite beneficial in treating Gilbert's syndrome.[52]

Sulfoxidation

Sulfoxidation is the process by which the sulfur-containing molecules in drugs (such as chlorpromazine, a tranquilizer) and foods (such as garlic) are metabolized. It is also the process by which the body eliminates sulfite food additives used to preserve foods and drugs. Various sulfites are widely used in potato salad (as a preservative), salad bars (to keep the vegetables looking fresh), dried fruits (they keep dried apricots orange), and in some drugs (such as those used to treat asthma). Normally, the enzyme sulfite oxidase metabolizes sulfites to safer sulfates, which are then excreted in the urine. Those with a poorly functioning sulfoxidation system, however, have an increased ratio of sulfite to sulfate in their urine.

When the sulfoxidation detoxification pathway isn't working well, people become sensitive to sulfur-containing drugs and foods. This is especially important for asthmatics, who can react to these additives with life-threatening attacks.

Dr. Jonathan Wright, one of the leading holistic medical doctors in the country, discovered several years ago that providing molybdenum to asthmatics who have an elevated ratio of sulfites to sulfates in their urine resulted in a significant improvement in their condition. Molybdenum helps because sulfite oxidase is dependent upon this trace mineral. Although most nutrition textbooks believe it to be an uncommon deficiency, an Austrian study of 1,750 patients found that 41.5 percent were molybdenum-deficient.[53]

To ensure that sulfoxidation is working adequately, eat foods rich in molybdenum such as legumes (beans) and whole grains.

Practical Applications

The activity of and interplay between Phase I and Phase II reactions is probably the single most important factor that determines our biochemical individuality. Genetic factors are clearly important. To put this in a practical perspective, the strong odor in the urine after eating asparagus is an interesting phenomenon because, while it is unheard of in China, one hundred percent of the French have been estimated to experience such an odor and about fifty percent of adults in the United States notice this effect. This situation is an excellent example of genetic variability in liver detoxification function.

While sophisticated laboratory tests are necessary to prove a dysfunction of a specific liver detoxification system, several signs and symptoms can give us a good idea of when our liver's detoxification systems are not functioning well or are overloaded. In general, any time you have a bad reaction to a drug or environmental toxin, you can be pretty sure there is a detoxification problem. Table 5 lists symptoms that are directly tied to a particular dysfunction.

The Importance of Bile Flow

Once the liver has modified a toxin, it needs to be eliminated from the body as soon as possible. One of the primary routes of elimination is through the bile. However, when the excretion of bile is inhibited (a condition called cholestasis), toxins stay in the liver longer. Cholestasis has several causes, including obstruction of the bile ducts and impairment of bile flow within the liver. The most common cause of obstruction of the bile ducts is the presence of gallstones.

Currently, it is conservatively estimated that twenty million people in the United States have gallstones. Nearly twenty percent of the female and eight percent of the male population over the age of forty are found to have gallstones on biopsy, and approximately five hundred thousand gallbladders are removed because of stones each year in the United States. The prevalence of gallstones in this country has been linked to the high-

fat, low-fiber diet consumed by the majority of Americans. (For more information, see GALLSTONES in Part III.)

Impairment of bile flow within the liver can be caused by a variety of agents and conditions. These conditions are often associated with alterations of liver function in laboratory tests (serum bilirubin, alkaline phosphatase, SGOT, LDH, GGTP, etc.), signifying cellular damage. However, relying on these tests alone to evaluate liver function is not adequate since, in the initial or subclinical stages of many problems with liver function, laboratory values remain normal. Among the symptoms people with enzymatic damage may complain of are fatigue, general malaise, digestive disturbances, allergies and chemical sensitivities, premenstrual syndrome, and constipation.

CAUSES OF CHOLESTASIS

Gallstones
Alcohol
Endotoxins
Hereditary disorders such as Gilbert's syndrome
Hyperthyroidism or thyroxine supplementation
Viral hepatitis
Pregnancy
Certain chemicals or drugs:
    Natural and synthetic steroidal hormones:
        Anabolic steroids
        Estrogens
        Oral contraceptives
    Aminosalicylic acid
    Chlorothiazide
    Erythromycin estolate
    Mepazine
    Phenylbutazone
    Sulphadiazine
    Thiouracil

Perhaps the most common cause of cholestasis and impaired liver function is

TABLE 5 Dysfunctional Liver Detoxification Systems	
SYMPTOM	**SYSTEM MOST LIKELY DYSFUNCTIONAL**
Adverse reactions to sulfite food additives (such as in commercial potato salad or salad bars)	Sulfoxidation
Asthma reactions after eating at a restaurant	Sulfoxidation
Caffeine intolerance (even small amounts keep you awake at night)	Phase I
Chronic exposure to toxins	Phase II glutathione conjugation
Eating asparagus results in a strong urine odor	Sulfoxidation
Garlic makes you sick	Sulfoxidation
Gilbert's disease	Phase II glucuronidation
Intestinal toxicity	Phase II sulfation and amino acid conjugation
Liver disease	Phase I and Phase II dysfunction
Perfumes and other environmental chemicals make you feel ill	Phase I
Toxemia of pregnancy	Phase II amino acid conjugation
Yellow discoloration of eyes and skin, not due to hepatitis	Phase II glucuronidation
Rapid metabolism of caffeine (you can drink two cups of coffee and still sleep well at night)	Overactive Phase I

alcohol ingestion. In some especially sensitive individuals, as little as 1 ounce of alcohol can produce damage to the liver, which results in fat being deposited within the liver. All active alcoholics demonstrate fatty infiltration of the liver.

Methionine administered as SAM has been shown to be quite beneficial in treating two common causes of stagnation of bile in the liver: estrogen excess (due to either oral contraceptive use or pregnancy) and Gilbert's syndrome.[52,54]

Diet and Liver Function

The first step in supporting proper liver function is following the dietary recommendations given in the chapter A HEALTH-PROMOTING DIET. Such a diet will provide a wide range of essential nutrients that the liver needs to carry out its important functions. If you want to have a healthy liver, there are three things you definitely want to stay away from: saturated fats, refined sugar, and alcohol. A diet high in saturated fat increases the risk of developing fatty infiltration and/or cholestasis. In contrast, a diet rich in dietary fiber, particularly the water-soluble fibers, promotes increased bile secretion.

Special foods rich in factors that help protect the liver from damage and improve liver function include

- High-sulfur-content foods, such as garlic, legumes, onions, and eggs

- Good sources of water-soluble fibers, such as pears, oat bran, apples, and legumes
- Cabbage-family vegetables, especially broccoli, brussels sprouts, and cabbage
- Artichokes, beets, carrots, dandelion, and many herbs and spices such as turmeric, cinnamon, and licorice

Avoid alcohol if you suffer from impaired liver function, and only drink in moderation (no more than two glasses of wine or beer or 2 ounces of hard liquor per day). Alcohol stresses detoxification processes and can lead to liver damage and immune suppression.

Follow the Recommendations for Nutritional Supplementation

The recommendations given in the chapter SUPPLEMENTARY MEASURES for nutritional supplementation are quite useful in the goal of promoting detoxification. A high-potency multiple-vitamin-and-mineral is a must in trying to deal with all the toxic chemicals we are constantly exposed to. Antioxidant vitamins such as vitamin C, beta-carotene, and vitamin E are obviously quite important in protecting the liver from damage as well as helping in detoxification mechanisms, but even simple nutrients like B-vitamins, calcium, and trace minerals are critical in the elimination of heavy metals and other toxic compounds from the body.[55–57]

Special Nutritional Factors

Choline, betaine, methionine, vitamin B6, folic acid, and vitamin B12 are important. These nutrients are referred to as *lipotropic agents*. Lipotropic agents are compounds that promote the flow of fat and bile to and from the liver. In essence, they produce a "decongesting" effect on the liver and promote improved liver function and fat metabolism.

Formulas that contain lipotropic agents are useful in enhancing detoxification reactions and other liver functions. Lipotropic formulas have been used by nutrition-oriented physicians to treat a wide variety of conditions, including a number of liver disorders such as hepatitis, cirrhosis, and chemical-induced liver disease.

Most major manufacturers of nutritional supplements offer lipotropic formulas. The important thing, when taking a lipotropic formula, is to take enough of the formula to provide a daily dose of 1,000 mg of choline and 1,000 mg of either methionine and/or cysteine.

Lipotropic formulas appear to increase the levels of two important liver substances: SAM (S-adenosylmethionine), the major lipotropic compound in the liver, and glutathione, one of the major detoxifying compounds in the liver. Although SAM is not currently available in the United States, various lipotropic factors, including methionine, choline, and betaine, have been shown to increase the levels of SAM.[58–60]

Plant-Based Medicines and Liver Function

There is a long list of plants that exert beneficial effects on liver function. However, the most impressive research has been done on a special extract of milk thistle (*Silybum marianum*) known as *silymarin*, a group of flavonoid compounds. These compounds exert a tremendous effect in protecting the liver from damage and enhancing detoxification processes.

Silymarin prevents damage to the liver by acting as an antioxidant.[61–63] It is many times more potent in antioxidant activity than vitamin E and vitamin C. The protective effect of silymarin against liver damage has been demonstrated in a number of experimental studies. Experimental liver damage in animals is produced by extremely toxic chemicals such as carbon tetrachloride, amanita toxin, galactosamine, and praseodymium nitrate. Silymarin has been shown to protect against liver damage by all of these agents.[61–63]

One of the key ways in which silymarin enhances the detoxification reaction is by preventing the depletion of glutathione. As discussed above, the level of glutathione in the liver is critically linked to the liver's ability to detoxify. The higher the glutathione content, the greater the liver's capacity to detoxify harmful chemicals. Typically, when we are exposed to chemicals that can damage the liver, including alcohol, the concentration of glutathione in the liver is substantially reduced. This reduction in glutathione makes the liver cell susceptible to damage. Silymarin not only prevents the depletion of glutathione induced by alcohol and other toxic chemicals, but has been shown to increase the level of glutathione of the liver by up to thirty-five percent.[64] Since the ability of the liver to detoxify is largely related to the level of glutathione in the liver, the results of this study seem to indicate that silymarin can increase detoxification reactions by up to thirty-five percent.

In human studies, silymarin has been shown to have positive effects in treating liver diseases of various kinds, including cirrhosis, chronic hepatitis, fatty infiltration of the liver (chemical- and alcohol-induced fatty liver), and inflammation of the bile duct.[65–69] The standard dosage for silymarin is 70 to 210 mg three times per day.

Fasting

Fasting is often used as a detoxification method, as it is one of the quickest ways to increase elimination of wastes and enhance the healing processes of the body. Fasting is defined as abstinence from all food and drink except water for a specific period of time, usually for a therapeutic or religious purpose.

Although therapeutic fasting is probably one of the oldest known therapies, it has been largely ignored by the medical community despite the fact that significant scientific research on fasting exists in the medical literature. Numerous medical journals have carried articles on the use of fasting in the treatment of obesity, chemical poisoning, rheumatoid arthritis, allergies, psoriasis, eczema, thrombophlebitis, leg ulcers, the irritable bowel syndrome, impaired or deranged appetite, bronchial asthma, depression, neurosis, and schizophrenia.

One of the most significant studies regarding fasting and detoxification appeared in the *American Journal of Industrial Medicine* in 1984.[70] This study involved patients who had ingested rice oil contaminated with polychlorinated-biphenyls, or PCBs. All patients reported improvement in symptoms, and some observed "dramatic" relief, after undergoing seven-to-ten-day fasts. This research supports past studies of PCB-poisoned patients and indicates the therapeutic effects of fasting as an aid to detoxification.

Caution must be used when fasting. For example, if you are a diabetic your blood sugar levels could drop too low and produce a diabetic coma. Please consult a physician before going on any unsupervised fast.

If you elect to try a fast, it is a good idea to support detoxification reactions while fasting, especially if you are particularly overloaded with toxins or have a long history of exposure to fat-soluble toxins like pesticides. The reason is that, during a fast, stored toxins in the fat cells are released into our system. For example, the pesticide DDT has been shown to be mobilized during a fast and may reach blood levels toxic to the nervous system.[6]

The best way to support detoxification reactions during a fast is to go on a three-day fresh juice fast rather than a water fast or a longer fast. Longer fasts require strict medical supervision, while the short fast can usually be conducted at home rather than at an inpatient facility.

A three-day "juice fast" consists of three or four 8-to-12-ounce juice meals spread throughout the day. During this period, your body will begin ridding itself of stored toxins. Drinking fresh juice for cleansing reduces some of the side effects associated with a water fast, such as light-headedness, tiredness, and headaches. While on a fresh juice fast, individuals typically experience an increased sense of well-being, renewed energy, clearer thought, and a sense of purity.

To further aid in detoxification during the fast, follow the following guidelines

- Take a high-potency multiple-vitamin-and-mineral formula to provide general support
- Take a lipotropic formula according to the aforementioned guidelines
- Take 1,000 mg of vitamin C three times per day
- Take 1 to 2 tablespoons of a fiber supplement at night before retiring (the best fiber sources are the water-soluble fibers, such as powdered psyllium seed husks, guar gum, oat bran, etc.)
- If you are particularly overloaded with toxins, take silymarin at a dosage of 70 to 210 mg three times per day

Other Tips on Fasting

Although a short juice fast can be started at any time, it is best to begin on a weekend or during a time period when adequate rest can be assured. The more rest, the better results, as energy can be directed toward healing instead of other body functions.

Prepare for a fast on the day before solid food is stopped by making the last meal one of only fresh fruits and vegetables (some authorities recommend a full day of raw food to start a fast, even a juice fast).

Only fresh fruit and vegetable juices (ideally prepared from organic produce) should be consumed for the next three to five days. Four 8-to-12-ounce glasses of fresh juice should be consumed throughout the day. In addition to the fresh juice, pure water should also be consumed. The quantity of water should be dictated by thirst, but at least four 8-ounce glasses should be consumed every day during the fast.

Do not drink coffee; bottled, canned, or frozen juice; or soft drinks. Herbal teas can be quite supportive of a fast, but they should not be sweetened.

Exercise is not usually encouraged while fasting. It is a good idea to conserve energy and allow maximal healing. Short walks or light stretching are useful, but heavy workouts tax the system and inhibit repair and elimination.

Rest is one of the most important aspects of a fast. A nap or two during the day is recommended. Less sleep will usually be required at night, since daily activity is lower. Body temperature usually drops during a fast, as do blood pressure, pulse, and respiratory rate—all measures of the slowing of the body's metabolic rate. It is important, therefore, to stay warm.

When it is time to break your fast, it is important to reintroduce solid foods gradually by limiting portions. Do not overeat. It is also a good idea to eat slowly, chew thoroughly, and eat foods at room temperature.

Digestion and Elimination

. . . .

One of the most useful tools in determining the possible causes of digestive disturbance is the Comprehensive Digestive Stool Analysis.

Indigestion can be attributed to a great many causes, including not only increased secretion of acid but also decreased secretion of acid, enzymes, and other digestive factors.

Heartburn (reflux esophagitis) is usually caused by overeating.

In the person with chronic indigestion, rather than focus on blocking the digestive process with antacids, the natural approach focuses on aiding digestion.

Common symptoms of pancreatic insufficiency include abdominal bloating and discomfort, gas, indigestion, and the passing of undigested food in the stool.

Just as important as digestion is the elimination of waste from the body.

Constipation affects over four million people in the United States on a regular basis.

Maintaining and/or attaining good colon health is straightforward: eat a high-fiber diet; drink plenty of water; seed and maintain health-promoting microflora.

In order to gain nutritional benefits from foods, it is critical that they be properly digested, absorbed, and eliminated. The best nutrition in the world will go to waste if the body is unable to process it. Fortunately, the human digestive system is quite efficient in extracting the necessary nutrients from foods.

The major function of the digestive (or gastrointestinal, GI) system is to break down and absorb nutrients. The digestive system extends from the mouth to the anus. It consists of the gastrointestinal tract (the mouth, throat, esophagus, and intestines) and its related organs: the salivary glands, the liver and gallbladder, and the pancreas.

Digestion occurs as a result of both mechanical and chemical processes. The mechanical processes of digestion include grinding, crushing, and mixing of the food mass with digestive juices during propulsion through the digestive tract. The digestive juices are responsible for the chemical breakdown of food, breaking large molecules into smaller molecules by breaking chemical bonds. The active compounds in the digestive juices are primarily enzymes.

The Digestive Process

The digestive process begins in the mouth. Chewing food thoroughly is the first step toward getting the most from the food you eat. Chewing signals other components of the digestive system to get ready to go to work: it also allows food to mix with saliva. Saliva contains the enzyme *salivary amylase,* which breaks down starch molecules into smaller sugars. Once the food has been chewed, it is transported by the esophagus into the stomach.

Food is broken down in the stomach by mechanical as well as chemical means. The stomach churns and gyrates to promote the mixing of the food with its digestive secretions, including hydrochloric acid and the enzyme *pepsin.* These factors are critical to proper protein digestion and mineral absorption. If hydrochloric acid secretion is insufficient or inhibited, proper protein digestion will not occur. Food remains in the stomach until it is reduced to a semiliquid consistency. In general, this process takes anywhere from forty-five minutes to four hours. Once the food material leaves the stomach it is referred to as *chyme.*

It takes chyme approximately two to four hours to make its way through the 21-foot-long small intestine. The small intestine is divided into three segments: the *duodenum* is the first 10 to 12 inches, the *jejunum* is the middle portion and is about 8 feet long, and the *ileum* is about 12 feet long. The small intestine participates in all aspects of digestion, absorption, and transport of ingested materials. It secretes a variety of digestive and protective substances and receives the secretions of the pancreas, liver, and gallbladder.

Absorption of minerals occurs predominantly in the duodenum; absorption of water-soluble vitamins, carbohydrates, and protein occurs primarily in the jejunum; and the ileum absorbs fat-soluble vitamins, fat, cholesterol, and bile salts (compounds secreted by the gallbladder to aid in digestion).

Diseases involving the small intestine often result in malabsorption syndromes characterized by multiple nutrient deficiencies. Examples of common causes of malabsorption include *celiac disease* (gluten intolerance), food allergy or intolerance, intestinal infections, and Crohn's disease.

The Pancreas

The pancreas produces enzymes that are required for the digestion and absorption of food. Each day, the pancreas secretes about 1.5 quarts of pancreatic juice into the small intestine. Enzymes secreted include lipases, proteases, and amylases.

Lipases, along with bile, function in the digestion of fats. Deficiency of lipase results in malabsorption of fats and fat-soluble vitamins. *Amylases* break down starch molecules into smaller sugars. Amylase is secreted by the salivary glands as well as the pancreas. The *proteases* secreted by the pancreas (*trypsin, chymotrypsin,* and *carboxypeptidase*) function in digestion by breaking down protein molecules into single amino acids. Incomplete digestion of proteins creates a number of problems for the body, including the development of allergies and formation of toxic substances produced during putrefaction. *Putrefaction* refers to the breakdown of protein material by bacteria.

In addition to being necessary for protein digestion, the proteases serve several other important functions. The proteases are largely responsible for keeping the small intestine free from parasites (including bacteria, yeast, protozoa, and *helminths,* or parasitic worms). A lack of proteases or other digestive secretions greatly increases an individual's risk of having an intestinal infection, including chronic candida infections of the gastrointestinal tract. The proteases also are important in preventing the formation of fibrin clots, tissue damage during inflammation, and the depositing of immune complexes in body tissues.

The Liver and Biliary System

The liver manufactures *bile,* an extremely important substance in the absorption of fats, oils, and fat-soluble vitamins. Bile produced by the liver is either taken up by the small intestine or stored in the gallbladder. Bile also plays an important role in making the stool soft by promoting the incorporation of water into the stool. Without enough bile, the stool can become quite hard and difficult to pass.

Like pancreatic enzymes, bile also serves to keep the small intestine free from microorganisms. Each day, about 1 quart of bile is taken up by the small intestine. About ninety-nine percent of what is excreted in the bile (bile salts, cholesterol, fat-soluble toxins, etc.)

is reabsorbed back into the body at the ileum.

When additional bile acids are ingested in pill form, usually as *ursodeoxycholic acid,* or "ox bile salts," they are known to increase the output of bile and help promote a mild laxative effect. Another method of increasing the output of bile is to use nutritional formulas that contain choline and methionine. A daily dose of 1,000 mg of choline and 500 mg of methionine is sufficient in most cases to increase bile flow.

The Colon

The colon is about 5 feet long and functions in the absorption of water, *electrolytes* (salts), and, in limited amounts, some of the final products of digestion. The large intestine also provides temporary storage for waste products, which serve as a medium for bacteria.

QUICK REVIEW

This chapter highlights the importance of proper digestion for optimum health. Incomplete or disordered digestion can be a major contributor to the development of many diseases. The problem is not only that ingestion of foods and nutritional substances are of little benefit when breakdown and assimilation are inadequate, but also that incompletely digested food molecules can be inappropriately absorbed into the body. Determining digestive function and assessing the intestinal environment through proper clinical and laboratory investigation can provide valuable information as to the cause of intestinal dysfunction. This information can then be used to restore or achieve improved digestion and a more optimal intestinal environment.

In regard to indigestion, although antacids and H2-receptor antagonists may lead to relief of symptoms, they actually interfere with the digestive process and disrupt gut microbial ecology. A better approach involves enhancing digestion with the help of digestive aids such as hydrochloric acid, pancreatin, and enzyme preparations.

The health of the colon is largely determined by the types of foods that are eaten. In particular, dietary fiber is of critical importance in maintaining the health of the colon.

Equally as important as proper digestion is the proper elimination of waste products. A bowel movement every twelve to fourteen hours is critical to good health. This proper elimination requires a diet high in fiber. Such a diet is rich in fruits, vegetables, whole grains, legumes, nuts, and seeds. A high-fiber diet increases both the frequency and quantity of bowel movements, decreases the transit time (the elapsed time from when the food is ingested till it is excreted in the feces) of stools, decreases the absorption of toxins from the stool, and appears to be a preventive factor in several diseases that affect the colon, including constipation, colon cancer, diverticulitis, hemorrhoids, and irritable bowel syndrome.

Evaluating Digestive Function

The digestive system is a truly integrated system; the function of one aspect usually affects the others. This interrelationship among the components of the digestive system often makes it difficult to determine the exact cause when there is digestive disturbance. Yet proper evaluation is, in many cases, essential to developing effective treatment. One of the most useful tools in determining the possible causes of digestive disturbance is the Comprehensive Digestive Stool Analysis (CDSA). The CDSA is a battery of integrated diagnostic laboratory tests that evaluate digestion, intestinal function, intestinal environment, and absorption by carefully examining the stool.

Since most nutrients are absorbed in the small intestine, altered small intestine function and integrity have significant repercussions on nutritional status and overall health. Proper small intestine function requires effective digestive secretions coupled with a fully functional absorptive surface and barrier. Methods for improving small intestine function include addressing the underlying issues, such as food intolerance/allergy, lack of digestive secretions, low immune status, and too much sugar in the diet.

At least equally as important to good health as proper digestion of food is the elimination of waste products. An old-time naturopathic belief was "good health begins in the colon." There appears to be great wisdom in that statement. It can be definitely stated that, without proper elimination of waste products, there are serious repercussions to our health. Maintaining and/or attaining good colon health is straightforward: eat a high-fiber diet; drink plenty of water; seed and maintain health-promoting microflora; and take appropriate actions when there are problems.

Several laboratories provide this often necessary battery of tests:

Great Smokies Diagnostic Laboratory (800-522-4762)
National BioTech Laboratory (800-846-6285)
Diagnost-Techs (800-87-TESTS)
Meridian Valley Clinical Laboratory (206-859-8700)

The CDSA provides information that is useful in leading to the correct diagnosis and development of appropriate therapeutic resources. Many physicians consider it a "foundation" screening test that consistently provides valuable clinical information. The CDSA can uncover the causes of both acute and chronic illnesses.

The test involves following a special diet for at least two days. Each lab has slightly different recommendations, but basically the goal is to eat a variety of foods and avoid laxatives, iron supplements, vitamin C, multivitamin formulas, and digestive enzymes, as they may interfere with test results. Here are the individual components analyzed in a CDSA, followed by a brief discussion of their significance:

Digestion
    Triglycerides
    Chymotrypsin
    Meat fibers
    Vegetable fibers
    Valerate, iso-butyrate
Absorption
    Long-chain fatty acids
    Cholesterol
    Total fecal fat
    Total short-chain fatty acids
Colonic environment
    Beneficial bacteria
        E. coli
        Lactobacillus
        Bifidobacteria

Additional bacteria
Mycology
Metabolic markers
    pH
    Short-chain fatty acid distribution
    Butyrate
    Beta-glucuronidase
Immunology
    Fecal secretory IgA
Dysbiosis index (Great Smokies only)
Macroscopic
    Fecal color
    Mucus
    Occult blood

Triglycerides (normal range: <0.3%)

Triglycerides are the major dietary fat component. Elevated levels of triglycerides in the stool reflect incomplete fat breakdown by pancreatic lipase and suggest pancreatic insufficiency.

Chymotrypsin (normal range: 6.2–41.0 IU/g)

Fecal chymotrypsin is a measure of proteolytic enzyme activity that is both sensitive and specific. Chymotrypsin activity in the stool is closely correlated with activity in the duodenum and small intestine. Decreased quantitative fecal values reflect pancreatic insufficiency or decreased hydrochloric acid output by the stomach. As a consequence, there is potential for food allergies, incomplete digestion of proteins, bacterial and candida overgrowth in the small intestine, and an increased risk of parasitic infections. Elevated levels of chymotrypsin suggest that food is traveling too quickly through the intestines (diarrhea may be present).

Meat Fibers (normal range: 0, meaning none seen)

The presence of microscopic meat fibers indicates incomplete protein digestion. There is a correlation between presence of excessive fecal meat fibers and lack or absence of hydrochloric acid secretion (hypo- and *achlorhydria*, respectively) and/or insufficient output of pancreatic enzymes.

Vegetable Fibers
(normal range: 0–4 fibers)
The presence of an excess of vegetable fibers may be a sign of inadequate chewing more than anything else.

Valerate, Iso-Butyrate
(normal range: 0–10 mmoles/g)
These compounds are *short-chain fatty acids* (SCFAs), produced by the bacteria in the gut through breakdown of proteins. In a healthy colon, these specific SCFAs constitute less than ten percent of the total concentration of all SCFAs. Higher levels may indicate hypo- or achlorhydria, and/or insufficient output of pancreatic enzymes.

Long-Chain Fatty Acids
(normal range: <1.1%)
These free fatty acids are normally readily absorbed by healthy intestines. In cases of mucosal malabsorption, they accumulate and reach substantial fecal levels. Elevated levels of free fatty acids may reflect malabsorption. Malabsorption may be caused by parasitic infection, inflammatory bowel disease, food allergy, gluten intolerance, or small intestine bacterial overgrowth.

Cholesterol (normal range: <0.3%)
An elevated cholesterol level in feces is abnormal and usually reflects malabsorption.

Total Fecal Fat (normal range: <1.6%)
This parameter reflects the sum of all fats except the short-chain fatty acids. Elevations may reflect either malabsorption (if long-chain fatty acid levels are elevated) or impaired digestion (if triglyceride levels are elevated).

Total Short-Chain Fatty Acids
(normal range: 25–155 mmoles/g)
Short-chain fatty acids (SCFAs) are the end products of bacterial breakdown, primarily of carbohydrates. Elevated total levels of the four main SCFAs may reflect malabsorption or bacterial overgrowth. Increased levels also suggest disordered fluid, electrolyte, and acid/base balances in the body. Decreased levels reflect disruption of the normal colonic flora, usually due to antibiotic use.

Beneficial Bacteria (normal range:
2+ to 4+, within a 0- to 4+ scale)
There are several important resident bacteria that should always be present for optimal intestinal health and function. They are

Escherichia coli (nonpathogenic resident strain)
Lactobacillus species
Bifidobacteria

These three organisms are cultured, and growth is quantitatively measured.

Pathogenic Bacteria
The CDSA should also report the presence of bacterial *pathogens* (disease-causing agents), by type and amount. Some common pathogens include

Aeromonas
Campylobacter
Salmonella
Shigella
Staphylococcus aureus
Vibrio
Yersinia

There are other intestinal bacteria that, while not causing acute GI tract disturbances, may be involved in the etiology of various chronic or systemic problems and, through molecular mimicry, in several autoimmune diseases. The presence of any of the following "possible pathogens" should also be reported:

Klebsiella
Proteus
Pseudomonas
Citrobacter

The CDSA should also report organisms that are characteristic of "imbalanced flora." It is important to know if bacteria are present that are markers of an imbalanced intestinal ecology. Some bacteria reported in this category include

Enterobacter
Beta-hemolytic Streptococci
Hemolytic E. coli
Hafnia
Mucoid E. coli

Mycology (normal range: 2+ to 4+ is considered abnormal)

The identification and amount of various yeast species cultured is reported. The common species reported are

Candida albicans
C. tropicalis
Rhodotorula
Geotrichum

pH (normal range: pH 6.0–7.2)

There is considerable interest in fecal pH in relation to the risk of colon cancer, especially as affected by fiber intake and the subsequent production of short- and long-chain fatty acids. A correlation between alkaline pH and decreased short-chain fatty acid values (particularly butyrate) has been observed. Clinical studies have also shown a relationship between elevated fecal pH and hypochlorhydria. A combination of elevated pH values

and diminished SCFA levels suggests inadequate bacterial digestion of fiber and/or inadequate intake of dietary fiber.

Short-Chain Fatty Acid Distribution

The amount and proportion of the different short-chain fatty acids reflects the basic health of the intestinal metabolism. The most important SCFAs and their proper percent of the total SCFAs are

Acetate 54–67%
Proprionate 16–24%
Butyrate 14–23%

Imbalanced ratios of the SCFAs reflect disordered bowel flora (dysbiosis).

Butyrate (normal range: 10–50 m/gww)

Butyrate is the most important of the SCFAs and is the main energy source for the cells that line the colon (colonic epithelial cells). Adequate amounts of butyrate are necessary for healthy metabolism and welfare of the colonic mucosa. Butyrate has been shown to have protective effects against colorectal cancers. Elevated levels are associated with active colitis and inflammatory bowel diseases.

Beta-Glucuronidase (normal range: 70–1,000 IU/g)

One of the key ways in which the liver detoxifies cancer-causing chemicals and body hormones like estrogen is by attaching glucuronic acid to the toxin and excreting it in the bile. Beta-glucuronidase is a bacterial enzyme that breaks the bond between excreted toxins and glucuronic acid. Excess beta-glucuronidase activity is associated with an increased cancer risk, particularly estrogen-dependent breast cancer. The activity of this enzyme can be reduced by taking Lactobacilli and Bifidobacteria, reducing meat intake, and increasing dietary fiber intake.

Secretory IgA
(normal range: 22–140 mcg/g)

Secretory IgA (s-IgA) is an antibody secreted by the intestinal lining that acts as the first line of defense in the gastrointestinal tract. Reduced levels of s-IgA mean that the intestinal tract is very susceptible to infection. Reduced levels are commonly seen in food allergies, bacterial overgrowth of the small intestine, chronic candidiasis, and parasitic infections. Elevated levels may reflect an activated immune response to the same factors that can reduce s-IgA. The thought is that the initial response is an elevation in s-IgA, but then the s-IgA is depleted with continued exposure.

Dysbiosis Index
(normal range: <3)

The CDSA from Great Smokies comes with a "dysbiosis index," calculated from all the relevant digestive, metabolic, and microbiological markers. It is often helpful in analyzing the multiple data and provides a quick assessment of the microecology of the gastrointestinal tract.

Fecal Color (normal range:
light brown to brown)

The color of feces is observed, and it can be indicative of various conditions. Possible indications of abnormality are

Yellow to green	diarrhea, bowel sterilized by antibiotics
Black	usually the result of upper GI tract bleeding
Tan or gray	blockage of the common bile duct, severe pancreatic insufficiency (greasy stool), fat malabsorption
Red	possible lower GI tract bleeding
Blood mixed in stool	colonic bleeding (including hemorrhoids)

Mucus (normal range: absence of mucus)

The presence of mucus or pus can be an indication of irritable bowel syndrome, intestinal wall inflammation (caused by infection such as typhoid, shigella, or amoebas), diverticulitis, or other intestinal abscess.

Blood (normal range: negative)

The presence of fecal blood represents gastrointestinal tract bleeding. It may be due to something as benign as a hemorrhoid or something as serious as colon cancer.

Clinical Application of the CDSA

The CDSA is an integrated battery of tests that can be used to design treatment measures. Therapeutic intervention should be based not only on single test results, but also on patterns and interrelationships. That being the case, this valuable tool is best used by a knowledgeable physician. You should consult a physician if you are suffering from any chronic or acute digestive disturbance. See the INTRODUCTION for a list of referral organizations.

Stress and Digestion

When evaluating digestive disturbances, it is critical to assess your stress level. During the stress response, the sympathetic arm of the autonomic nervous system dominates over the parasympathetic. The autonomic nervous system controls all unconscious nervous activity. While the sympathetic nervous system stimulates the fight-or-flight response, it is the parasympathetic nervous system that is responsible for the processes of digestion, repair, restoration, and rejuvenation. If a person is in a stressed state, the body is programmed to shunt blood and energy away from the digestive tract in favor of the skeletal muscles and brain. Regularly achieving a relaxed state (learning to calm the mind and body) is extremely important in relieving stress and improving digestion.

Indigestion

The term "indigestion" is often used to describe a feeling of gaseousness or fullness in the abdomen. It can also be used to describe "heartburn." Indigestion can be attributed to a great many causes, including not only increased secretion of acid but also decreased secretion of acid and other digestive factors and enzymes. The dominant treatment of indigestion is the use of over-the-counter preparations. These preparations include antacids and histamine H2-receptor antagonists.

The stomach's optimal pH range is 1.5 to 2.5, with hydrochloric acid being the primary stomach acid. The use of antacids and H2-receptor antagonists will typically raise the pH above 3.5. This increase effectively inhibits the action of pepsin, an enzyme involved in protein digestion that can be irritating to the stomach. Although raising the pH can reduce symptoms, it must be pointed out that hydrochloric acid and pepsin are important factors in protein digestion. If their secretion is insufficient or inhibited, proper protein digestion and mineral dissociation will not occur. In addition, the change in pH can adversely affect gut microbial flora, including the promotion of an overgrowth of *Helicobacter pylori* (see The Cause of Hypochlorhydria in the

next section of this chapter for further discussion *of H. Pylori*). Therefore, it is important to use antacids wisely and sparingly.

In addition, many nutrition-oriented physicians believe that it is not too much acid, but rather a lack of acid, that is the problem. In addressing indigestion, naturopathic physicians typically use measures to enhance rather than inhibit digestion. Commonly used digestive aids include hydrochloric acid and pancreatic enzyme preparations. This chapter will take a critical look at the use of these agents and contrast their use with natural digestive aids.

The reason most people use antacids is to relieve symptoms of *reflux esophagitis,* the medical term for heartburn.[1] Reflux esophagitis usually results from overeating, which causes gastric juices to flow up the esophagus, leading to a burning discomfort that radiates upward and is made worse by lying down. Other common causes include obesity, cigarette smoking, and consuming chocolate, fried foods, carbonated beverages (soft drinks), alcohol, or coffee. These factors either increase intra-abdominal pressure, thereby causing the gastric contents to flow upward, or decrease the tone of the esophageal sphincter. The first step in treating reflux esophagitis is prevention. In most cases, this step simply involves eliminating or reducing the causative factor.

For occasional heartburn, antacids may well be appropriate. However, they should not be abused. If heartburn is a chronic problem, it may be a sign of a *hiatal hernia* (outpouching of the stomach above the diaphragm). However, it is interesting to note that while fifty percent of people over the age of fifty have hiatal hernias, only five percent of patients with hiatal hernias actually experience reflux esophagitis.

Perhaps the most effective treatment of chronic reflux esophagitis and symptomatic hiatal hernias is to utilize gravity. The standard recommendation is to simply place 4-inch blocks under the bedposts at the head of the bed. This elevation of the head is very effective in many cases. Another recommendation is to heal the esophagus using deglycyrrhizinated licorice (DGL). This herbal approach is discussed in The Cause of Hypochlorhydria, in the next section of this chapter.

Hypochlorhydria

In the person with chronic indigestion, rather than focus on blocking the digestive process with antacids, the natural approach focuses on aiding digestion. Although much is said about hyperacidity conditions, a more common cause of indigestion is a lack of gastric acid secretion. *Hypochlorhydria* refers to deficient gastric acid secretion, while *achlorhydria* refers to a complete absence of gastric acid secretion.

There are many symptoms and signs that suggest impaired gastric acid secretion, and a number of specific diseases have been found to be associated with insufficient gastric acid output.[2–12] These are listed in the following boxes.

COMMON SIGNS AND SYMPTOMS OF LOW GASTRIC ACIDITY

A sense of fullness after eating

Acne

Bloating, belching, burning, and flatulence immediately after meals

Chronic candida infections

Chronic intestinal parasites or abnormal flora

Dilated blood vessels in the cheeks and nose

Indigestion, diarrhea, or constipation

Iron deficiency

Itching around the rectum

Multiple food allergies

Nausea after taking supplements

Undigested food in the stool

Upper digestive tract gassiness

Weak, peeling, and cracked fingernails

DISEASES ASSOCIATED WITH LOW GASTRIC ACIDITY

Addison's disease

Asthma

Chronic autoimmune disorders

Celiac disease

Dermatitis herpetiformis

Diabetes mellitus

Eczema

Gallbladder disease

Graves disease

Hepatitis

Chronic hives

Lupus erythematosis

Myasthenia gravis

Osteoporosis

Pernicious anemia

Psoriasis

Rheumatoid arthritis

Rosacea

Sjogren's syndrome

Thyrotoxicosis

Hyper- and hypothyroidism

Vitiligo

Several studies have shown that the ability to secrete gastric acid decreases with age.[13–16] Some studies found low stomach acidity in over half of those over age sixty. The best method of diagnosing a lack of gastric acid is a special procedure known as the Heidelberg gastric analysis.[17] This technique utilizes an electronic capsule attached to a string. The capsule is swallowed and then kept in the stomach with the aid of the string. The capsule measures the pH of the stomach and sends a radio message to a receiver, which then records the pH level. It has been suggested by Jonathan Wright, M.D., that the response to a bicarbonate challenge during Heidelberg gastric analysis is the true test of the functional ability of the stomach to secrete acid.[18] After the test, the capsule is pulled up from the stomach by the string attached to it.

Since not everyone can have detailed gastric acid analysis to determine the need for gastric acid supplementation, a practical method of determination is often used. If an individual is experiencing any signs and symptoms of gastric acid insufficiency as listed or has any of the diseases listed, the method outlined below can be employed.

Protocol for Hydrochloric Acid Supplementation

1. Begin by taking one tablet or capsule, containing 10 grains (600 mg) of hydrochloric acid, at your next large meal. If this does not aggravate your symptoms, at every subsequent meal of the same size, take one more tablet or capsule. (One at the next meal, two at the meal after that, then three at the next meal.) When taking a number of tablets or capsules, it is best to take them throughout the meal.

2. Continue to increase the dose until you reach seven tablets or until you feel a warmth in your stomach, whichever occurs first. A feeling of warmth in the stomach means that you have taken too many tablets for that meal, and you need to take one less tablet for that meal size. It is a good idea to try the larger dose again at another meal to make sure that it was the HCl that caused the warmth, and not something else.

3. After you have found the largest dose you can take at your large meals without feeling any stomach warmth, maintain that dose

at all meals of a similar size. You will need to take less at smaller meals.

4. As your stomach begins to regain the ability to produce the amount of HCl needed to properly digest your food, you will notice the warm feeling again and will have to cut down the dose level.

The Cause of Hypochlorhydria

Like peptic ulcer disease, achlorhydria and hypochlorhydria have been linked to the overgrowth of the bacteria *Helicobacter pylori*. It has been shown that ninety to one hundred percent of patients with duodenal ulcers, seventy percent with gastric ulcers, and about fifty percent of people over the age of fifty test positive for *H. pylori*.[19] The presence of *H. pylori* is determined by measuring the level of antibodies to *H. pylori* in the blood or saliva or by culturing material collected during an endoscopy (a procedure where a flexible tube with a microscopic lens attached is inserted through the mouth into the stomach or small intestine) measuring the breath for urea.

Low gastric output is thought to encourage *H. pylori* colonization, and *H. pylori* colonization increases gastric pH, thereby setting up a positive feedback scenario and increasing the likelihood of the colonization of the stomach and duodenum with other organisms.[20] Interestingly, there has been scant research into the effects of antacids and H2-receptor antagonists on promoting *H. pylori* overgrowth.[21] It appears that habitual use of either could promote *H. pylori* overgrowth.

If *H. pylori* infection and stomach irritation (gastritis) lead to achlorhydria, the next obvious question is: What are the factors that lead to *H. pylori* gastritis? Consistent with history, conventional medicine is obsessed with the infective agent rather than internal defense factors. Because research focuses on eradicating the organism, there is little information on protective factors against infectivity. Proposed protective factors against *H. pylori*-induced intestinal damage are maintaining a low pH and ensuring adequate antioxidant defense mechanisms.[22-24] Low levels of vitamin C, vitamin E, and other antioxidant factors in the gastric juice appear to encourage progression of *H. pylori* colonization. Since the mechanism by which *H. pylori* damages the stomach and intestinal mucosa is oxidative damage, such a condition also contributes to the ulcer-causing potential of *H. pylori*.[25] Furthermore, antioxidant status and gastric acid output appear to explain why not everyone who is infected with *H. pylori* gets get peptic ulcer disease or gastric cancer.

Deglycyrrhizinated licorice (DGL) may also prove useful in eradicating *H. pylori* and stimulating internal defenses. DGL has shown good results in healing both duodenal ulcers and gastric ulcers (discussed more fully in ULCERS, in Part III). Rather than inhibit the release of acid, DGL stimulates the normal defense mechanisms that prevent ulcer formation. Specifically, DGL improves both the quality and quantity of the protective substances that line the intestinal tract, increases the life span of the intestinal cell, and improves blood supply to the intestinal lining.[26,27]

The active components of DGL are believed to be special flavonoid derivatives. These compounds have demonstrated impressive protection against chemically induced ulcer formation in animal studies. Several similar flavonoids have been shown to inhibit *H. pylori* in a clear-cut concentration-dependent manner.[28] In addition, unlike antibiotics, the flavonoids also were shown to augment natural defense factors that prevent ulcer formation. The activity of flavone, the most potent flavonoid in the study, was shown to be similar to that of bismuth subcitrate.

Bismuth is a naturally occurring mineral that can act as an antacid and exert activity against *H. pylori*.[29] The best known and most widely used bismuth preparation is *bismuth subsalicylate*—Pepto-Bismol. However, bismuth subcitrate has produced the best results against *H. pylori* and in the treatment of non-ulcer-related indigestion and peptic ulcers.[30,31] In the United States, bismuth subcitrate preparations are available through compounding pharmacies (pharmacies where the pharmacists still mix up preparations on the premises); contact the International Academy of Compounding Pharmacists at 800-927-4227.

One of the key advantages of bismuth preparations over standard antibiotic approaches to eradicating *H. pylori* is that, while the bacteria may develop resistance to various antibiotics, it is unlikely to develop resistance to bismuth.

The usual dosage for bismuth subcitrate is 240 mg twice daily before meals. For bismuth subsalicylate, the dosage is 500 mg (2 tablets or 30 ml of standard-strength Pepto-Bismol) four times daily.

Bismuth preparations are extremely safe when taken at prescribed dosages. Bismuth subcitrate may cause a temporary and harmless darkening of the tongue and/or stool. Bismuth subsalicylate should not be taken by children recovering from the flu, chicken pox, or another viral infection, as it may mask the nausea and vomiting associated with Reye's syndrome, a rare but serious illness.

Pancreatic Insufficiency

Both physical symptoms and laboratory tests can be used to assess pancreatic function. Common symptoms of pancreatic insufficiency include abdominal bloating and discomfort, gas, indigestion, and the passing of undigested food in the stool. For laboratory diagnosis, most nutrition-oriented physicians use the CDSA.

Pancreatic insufficiency is characterized by impaired digestion, malabsorption, nutrient deficiencies, and abdominal discomfort. The most severe level of pancreatic insufficiency is seen in cystic fibrosis. Although cystic fibrosis is rare, mild pancreatic insufficiency is thought to be a relatively common condition, especially in the elderly.

Pancreatic enzyme products are the most effective treatment for pancreatic insufficiency and are also popular digestive aids. Most commercial preparations are prepared from fresh hog pancreas *(pancreatin).*

The dosage of pancreatic enzymes is first based on the level of enzyme activity of the particular product. The United States Pharmacopoeia (USP) has set a strict definition for level of activity. A 1X pancreatic enzyme (pancreatin) product has in each milligram not less than 25 USP units of amylase activity, not less than 2 USP units of lipase activity, and not less than 25 USP units of protease activity. Pancreatin of higher potency is given a whole-number multiple, indicating its strength. For example, a full-strength undiluted pancreatic extract that is ten times stronger than the USP standard would be referred to as 10X USP. Full-strength products are preferred to lower-potency pancreatin products because lower-potency products (e.g., 4X or 1X) are often diluted with salt, lactose, or galactose to achieve the desired strength. The dosage recommendation for a 10X USP pancreatic enzyme product would be 350 to 1,000 mg three times per day immediately before meals when used as a digestive aid, and ten to twenty minutes before meals or on an empty stomach when antiinflammatory effects are desired.

Enzyme products are often *enteric*-coated. That is, they are often coated to prevent digestion in the stomach, so that the enzymes will be liberated in the small intestine. However, numerous studies have shown that non-enteric-coated enzyme preparations actually outperform enteric-coated products if they are taken prior to a meal (for digestive purposes) or on an empty stomach (for antiinflammatory effects).

For vegetarians, *bromelain* and *papain* (protein-digesting enzymes from pineapple and papaya, respectively) can substitute for pancreatic enzymes in the treatment of pancreatic insufficiency. However, in my experience, the best results are obtained if they are used in combination with pancreatin and ox bile.

Pancreatin and Food Allergies

Food allergies have been implicated as a causative factor in a wide range of conditions; no part of the human body is immune from being a target cell or organ. The actual symptoms produced during an allergic response depend on the location of the immune system activation, the allergic compounds (mediators), inflammation involved, and the sensitivity of the tissues to specific mediators. Since the gastrointestinal tract is a common site of immune system activation by a food allergy, it is not surprising that food allergies often produce gastrointestinal symptoms.

Pancreatic insufficiency and hypochlorhydria play a major role in many cases of food allergies, particularly if a patient has multiple allergies. While starch and fat digestion can be carried out satisfactorily without the help of pancreatic enzymes, the proteases are critical to proper protein digestion. Incomplete digestion of proteins creates a number of problems for the body, including the development of food allergies. Typically, individuals who do not secrete enough proteases will suffer from multiple food allergies.

In order for a food molecule to produce an allergic response, it must be a fairly large molecule. When pancreatic enzyme output is low, a person is much more likely to develop food allergies as a result of incomplete digestion. In studies performed in the 1930s and 1940s, pancreatic enzyme supplementation was shown to be effective in preventing food allergies.[31] It appears that many practitioners are not aware of—or have forgotten about—these early studies.

Small Intestine Bacterial Overgrowth

The upper portion of the human small intestine is designed to be relatively free of bacteria. The reason is simple: when bacteria are present in significant concentrations in the duodenum and jejunum, they compete with their host for nutrition. When bacteria (or yeast) get to the food first, problems can occur. The organism can ferment the carbohydrates and produce excessive gas, bloating, and abdominal distension. If this is not bad enough, the bacteria can also break down protein via the process of putrefaction to produce what are known as *vasoactive amines*.[32] For example, bacteria and yeast contain enzymes *(decarboxylases)* that can convert the amino acid *histidine* to *histamine* and *tyrosine* to *tyramine*. Even more dangerous-sounding are the compounds produced from the amino acids *ornithine* and *lysine*—namely, *putrescine* and *cadaverine*, respectively. All of these compounds are termed "vasoactive amines" because they can cause

constriction and relaxation of blood vessels by acting on the smooth muscle that surrounds the vessels. In the intestinal tract, excessive vasoactive amine synthesis can lead to increased gut permeability ("leaky gut" syndrome), abdominal pain, altered gut motility, and pain.

Diagnosis of small intestine overgrowth involves careful evaluation of the CDSA. There are also breath tests that measure the levels of hydrogen and methane after the administration of carbohydrates (lactulose and glucose). If there is bacterial overgrowth in the small intestine, there will be higher than normal amounts of hydrogen and/or methane in the breath.

Symptoms of small intestine bacterial overgrowth are similar to those generally attributed to achlorhydria and pancreatic insufficiency—namely, indigestion and a sense of fullness (bloating). They may also include arthritis, nausea, diarrhea, and symptoms generally associated with candida overgrowth (discussed later in this section). In fact, a study published in the journal *Annals of the Rheumatic Diseases* in 1993 demonstrated that many people with rheumatoid arthritis exhibit small intestine bacterial overgrowth and that the severity of symptoms is related to the level of disease activity.[33]

There are several protective measures that can prevent bacterial overgrowth in the small intestine.[34] The first area to consider is the digestive secretions. In particular, hydrochloric acid, bile, and pancreatic enzymes play a critical role in preventing significant numbers of bacteria from migrating up the small intestine.[35,36] The next area to consider is that decreased motility *(peristalsis)* in the small intestine, due to a motility disorder (e.g., systemic sclerosis) or a meal high in refined sugar, can also contribute to small intestine bacterial overgrowth.[37,38]

The third area to consider is that low immune function, food allergies, stress, and other factors associated with a reduced level of *secretory IgA*—the antibody that protects and lines mucous membranes—can also contribute to bacterial overgrowth in the small intestine. And finally, a weak *ileocecal valve* (the valve that separates the bacteria-rich colon contents from the ileum, the final segment of the small intestine) can lead to overpopulation of the small intestine tract with bacteria. A weak ileocecal valve is typically the consequence of long-term constipation or straining excessively at defecation. In both of these cases, a low-fiber diet is often responsible.

FACTORS ASSOCIATED WITH SMALL INTESTINE BACTERIAL OVERGROWTH

Decreased digestive secretions
Achlorhydria
Hypochlorhydria
Drugs that inhibit hydrochloric acid
Pancreatic insufficiency
Decreased bile output due to liver or gallbladder disease
Decreased motility
Scleroderma (progressive systemic sclerosis)
Systemic lupus erythematosus
Intestinal adhesions
Sugar-induced hypomotility
Radiation damage
Low secretory IgA
Weak ileocecal valve

Obviously, addressing the cause of the small intestine bacterial overgrowth is the first step. The subject of decreased digestive secretions was discussed previously. As for decreased motility, this usually results from a meal that is too high in sugar.[38] The mechanism is simple. When blood sugar levels rise too rapidly, a signal is sent to the gastrointestinal tract to slow down. Since glucose is primarily absorbed in the duodenum and jejunum, the message affects this portion of the gastrointestinal tract the most strongly. The result is that the duodenum and jejunum become *atonic,* meaning that they literally stop propelling chyme through the intestinal tract via peristalsis.

Restoring secretory IgA to normal levels involves eliminating food allergies (see FOOD ALLERGY in Part III) and enhancing immune function. Stress is particularly detrimental to secretory IgA. This effect offers an additional explanation as to why stressful events tend to worsen gastrointestinal function and food allergies.

Possible natural medicines to use in cases of small intestine bacterial overgrowth include pancreatic enzymes and herbs that contain *berberine*. In addition to exerting broad-spectrum antibiotic activity (including activity against the yeast *Candida albicans),* berberine has been shown to inhibit the bacterial enzyme *decarboxylase*, which converts the amino acids into vasoactive amines.[40] In regard to pancreatic enzymes, as discussed previously, the protein-digesting enzymes from the pancreas are largely responsible for keeping the small intestine free from bacterial parasites (pathogenic bacteria, yeast, protozoa, and helminths).[41] A lack of proteases or other digestive secretions greatly increases an individual's risk of having an intestinal infection, including chronic candida infections of the gastrointestinal tract.

An overgrowth in the gastrointestinal tract of the usually benign yeast *Candida albicans* is now becoming recognized as a complex medical syndrome known as "the yeast syndrome" or "chronic candidiasis" (see CHRONIC CANDIDIASIS, in Part III). The overgrowth of candida is believed to cause a wide variety of symptoms in virtually every system of the body, with the gastrointestinal, genitourinary, endocrine, nervous, and immune systems being the most susceptible. Eventually this syndrome will be replaced by a more comprehensive term to include small intestine bacterial overgrowth and leaky gut syndrome.

Elimination and Colon Function

Just as important as digestion is the elimination of waste from the body. The health and function of the *colon* (the large intestine) is very important to proper elimination. The colon is really not involved in digestion to any significant extent. It does function in the absorption of water and *electrolytes* (salts). But its primary function is to provide temporary storage for waste products and the formation of stool. The health of the colon is largely determined by the amount of fiber in the diet. Without enough dietary fiber, waste material tends to accumulate.

Constipation

Constipation affects over four million people in the United States on a regular basis.[42] This high rate of constipation translates to over $500 million in annual sales of laxatives in the United States. There are a number of possible causes of constipation, but the most common cause of constipation is a low-fiber diet.

CAUSES OF CONSTIPATION
Diet
    Highly refined and low-fiber foods
    Inadequate fluid intake
Physical inactivity
    Inadequate exercise
    Prolonged bed rest

Pregnancy
Advanced age
Drugs
    Anesthetics
    Antacids (aluminum and calcium salts)
    Anticholinergics (bethanechol, carbachol, pilocarpine, physostigmine, ambenonium)
    Anticonvulsants
    Antidepressants (tricyclics, monoamine oxidase inhibitors)
    Antihypertensives
    Anti-Parkinsonism drugs
    Antipsychotics (phenothiazines)
    Beta-adrenergic blocking agents (propranolol)
    Bismuth salts
    Diuretics
    Iron salts
    Laxatives and cathartics (chronic use)
    Muscle relaxants
    Opiates
Metabolic abnormalities
    Low potassium stores
    Diabetes
    Kidney disease
Endocrine abnormalities
    Low thyroid function
    Elevated calcium levels
    Pituitary disorders
Structural abnormalities
    Abnormalities in the structure or anatomy of the bowel
Bowel diseases
    Diverticulosis
    Irritable bowel syndrome (alternating diarrhea and constipation)
    Tumor
Neurogenic abnormalities
    Nerve disorders of the bowel (aganglionosis, autonomic neuropathy)
    Spinal cord disorders (trauma, multiple sclerosis, tabes dorsalis)

Disorders of the splanchnic nerves (tumors, trauma)
Cerebral disorders (strokes, Parkinsonism, neoplasm)
Enemas (chronic use)

While constipation usually responds to a high-fiber diet, plentiful fluid consumption, and exercise, this appears too much to ask of many sufferers of chronic constipation. Instead of following this natural approach, many people are content to become dependent upon laxatives.

It is well-accepted that increasing the level of fiber in the diet is an effective treatment for chronic constipation. High levels of dietary fiber increase both the frequency and quantity of bowel movements, decrease the transit time of stools and the absorption of toxins from the stool, and appear to be a preventive factor in several diseases. Particularly effective in relieving constipation are bran and prunes. The typical recommendation for bran is 1/2 cup of bran cereal, increasing to 1 1/2 cups over several weeks. When using bran, make sure to consume enough liquids. Drink at least six to eight glasses of water per day. Whole prunes as well as prune juice also possess good laxative effects. Eight ounces is usually an effective dose. In addition, 25 to 35 grams of fiber from food sources are recommended.

If you need additional support, consider using fiber formulas. These formulas act as bulking agents. Some are composed of natural plant fibers derived from psyllium seed, kelp, agar, pectin, and plant gums such as karaya and guar. Others are purified semisynthetic polysaccharides such as methyl-cellulose and carboxymethyl cellulose sodium. Psyllium-containing laxatives are the most popular and usually the most effective. Fiber formulas are the laxatives that approximate most closely the natural mechanism that promotes a bowel movement.

If you have been using stimulant laxatives, even natural ones like Cascara sagrada *(Rhamnus purshiana)* or senna *(Cassia senna)*, you will need to "retrain" your bowels. The recommended procedure for reestablishing bowel regularity will take four to six weeks.

RULES FOR BOWEL RETRAINING

- Find and eliminate known causes of constipation.
- Never repress an urge to defecate.
- Eat a high-fiber diet, particularly fruits and vegetables.
- Drink six to eight glasses of fluid per day.
- Sit on the toilet at the same time every day (even when the urge to defecate is not present), preferably immediately after breakfast or exercise.
- Exercise for at least twenty minutes, three times per week.
- Stop using laxatives (except as discussed below to reestablish bowel activity) and enemas.

Week one: Every night before bed, take a stimulant laxative containing either cascara or senna. Take the lowest amount necessary to reliably ensure a bowel movement every morning.

Weekly: Each week, decrease the laxative dosage by half. If constipation recurs, go back to the previous week's dosage. Decrease the dosage if diarrhea occurs.

Diverticular Disease

Diverticula are small sacs caused by the protrusion of the inner lining of the colon into areas of weakness in the colon wall. The term *diverticulosis* refers to the presence of diverticula in the colon. Typically the presence of diverticula is without symptom. However, if the diverticula become inflamed, perforated, or impacted, the condition is referred to as *diverticulitis.* Only about twenty percent of people who have diverticulosis develop diverticulitis. Symptoms of diverticulitis include episodes of lower abdominal pain and cramping, changes in bowel habits (constipation or diarrhea), and a sense of fullness in the abdomen. In more severe cases, fever may be present, along with tenderness and rigidity of the abdomen over the area of the intestine involved.

Treatment of diverticular disease involves a high-fiber diet. In severe cases of diverticulitis, an antibiotic may be warranted.

Irritable Bowel Syndrome

The irritable bowel syndrome (IBS) is a common condition in which the large intestine, or colon, fails to function properly. Estimates suggest that approximately fifteen percent of the population have suffered from IBS.

IBS has also been known as "nervous indigestion," "spastic colitis," "mucous colitis," and "intestinal neurosis." IBS has characteristic symptoms, which can include a combination of any of the following: abdominal pain and distension; more frequent bowel movements with pain, or relief of pain with bowel movements; constipation; diarrhea; excessive production of mucus in the colon; symptoms of indigestion, such as flatulence, nausea, or anorexia; and varying degrees of anxiety or depression.

The irritable bowel syndrome is usually caused by either food allergies, stress, or a lack of fiber in the diet. Simply increasing the intake of plant food in the diet is effective in most cases. IBS is discussed in more detail in IRRITABLE BOWEL SYNDROME in Part III.

Dysbiosis

The microecology of the human gastrointestinal tract is incredibly complex, as there are at least five hundred different species of microflora that are part of the normal intestinal flora.[43] There are nine times as many bacteria in the gastrointestinal tract as there are cells in the human body. The type and number of gut bacteria play an important role in determining health and disease. A state of altered bacterial flora in the gut has become popularly known as *dysbiosis*. The term was first used by noted Russian scientist Elie Metchnikoff to reflect a state of living with intestinal flora that has harmful effects. He theorized that toxic compounds produced by the bacterial breakdown of food were the cause of degenerative disease.[44] There is a growing body of evidence that is supporting and refining Metchnikoff's theory.

MAJOR CAUSES OF DYSBIOSIS

Dietary disturbances
    High protein
    High sugar
    High fat
    Low fiber
    Food allergies
Lack of digestive secretions
Stress
Antibiotic/drug therapy
Decreased immune function
Malabsorption
Intestinal infection
Altered pH

Obviously, treatment begins with addressing these major causes. In addition, it is important to "re-seed" the gastrointestinal tract with probiotics. *Probiotic*, literally translated, means "for life" and is used to signify the health-promoting effects of "friendly bacteria." The most important friendly bacteria are *Lactobacillus acidophilus* and *Bifidobacterium bifidum*.

What determines whether any of the five hundred normal microbial inhabitants of the human digestive tract become parasitic is whether they are living in harmony (*symbiosis*) or causing problems. *Candida albicans* is an example of an organism that, under normal circumstances, lives in harmony with its host. But if candida overgrows and is out of balance with other gut microbes, it can cause problems. In general, parasites cause most of their problems by interfering with digestion and/or damaging the intestinal lining, either of which can lead to diarrhea.

Diarrheal diseases caused by parasites still constitute the greatest single worldwide cause of illness and death. The problem is magnified in underdeveloped countries with poor sanitation, but even in the United States diarrheal diseases are the third major cause of sickness and death. Furthermore, the ease and frequency of worldwide travel and increased migration to the United States is resulting in growing numbers of parasitic infections. In addition to normal inhabitants of the gastrointestinal system acting as parasites, there are also significant diarrheal diseases associated with protozoa and helminths (discussed in greater detail in DIARRHEA in Part III).

While the most commonly reported symptoms of parasitic infection are diarrhea and abdominal pain, these symptoms do not occur in every case. In fact, there appears to be a growing number of individuals who experience milder-than-usual gastrointestinal symptoms from parasitic infections and/or symptoms not traditionally linked to parasitic infections. For example, many cases of irritable bowel syndrome, indigestion, and poor digestion may result from parasites. In addition, parasitic infections are often an unsuspected cause of chronic illness and fatigue.

SIGNS AND SYMPTOMS OF PARASITIC INFECTION

Abdominal pain and cramps
Constipation
Depressed secretory IgA
Diarrhea
Fatigue
Fever
Flatulence
Food allergy
Foul-smelling stools
Gastritis
Headaches
Hives
Increased intestinal permeability
Indigestion
Irregular bowel movements
Irritable bowel syndrome
Loss of appetite
Low back pain
Malabsorption
Weight loss

Detection of parasites involves taking multiple stool samples collected at two- to four-day intervals. The stool sample is analyzed by microscopy, specialized staining techniques, and fluorescent antibodies (the antibodies attach and to any parasites present and give off fluorescence).

There are a number of natural compounds that can be useful in helping the body get rid of parasites. However, before selecting a natural alternative to an antibiotic for the treatment of parasitic infections, we recommend trying to discern what factors may have been responsible for setting up the internal terrain for a parasitic infection. In other words, do you have achlorhydria, decreased pancreatic enzyme output, or one of the other conditions discussed here? Proper treatment with either an antibiotic or a natural alternative requires proper monitoring by again collecting multiple stool samples two weeks after therapy. For more information on dealing with parasites, see DIARRHEA in Part III.

Immune Support

. . . .

The immune system protects the body against infection and the development of cancer.

Recurrent or chronic infections, even very mild colds, are signs that the immune system is weakened.

Supporting immune function involves a comprehensive approach.

The immune system is one of the most complex and fascinating systems of the human body. The immune system's prime function is to protect the body against infection and the development of cancer. The importance of susceptibility to infection or disease is too often overlooked in conventional medicine. Support and enhancement of the immune system is perhaps the most important step in achieving resistance to disease and reducing susceptibility to colds, flus, and cancer.

Recurrent or chronic infections—even very mild colds—only occur when the immune system is weakened. Under such circumstances, there is a repetitive cycle that makes it difficult to overcome the tendency toward infection: a weakened immune system leads to infection, infection causes damage to the immune system, which further weakens resistance. Enhancing the immune system by following the guidelines in this chapter may provide the answer to breaking the cycle.

Determining Immune Function

If you answer "yes" to any of the following questions, your immune system would probably benefit from support:

- Do you catch colds easily?
- Do you get more than two colds a year?
- Are you suffering chronic infection?
- Do you get frequent cold sores or have genital herpes?
- Are your lymph glands sore and swollen at times?
- Do you have now or have you ever had cancer?

Components of the Immune System

The immune system is composed of the lymphatic vessels and organs (lymph nodes, thymus, spleen, and tonsils), white blood cells (neutrophils, eosinophils, basophils, lymphocytes, monocytes, etc.), specialized cells residing in various tissue (macrophages, mast cells, etc.), and specialized chemical factors.

Lymph, Lymphatic Vessels, and Lymph Nodes

Approximately one-sixth of the entire body is the space between cells. Collectively, this space is referred to as the *interstitium,* and the fluid contained within the space is referred to as the *interstitial fluid.* This fluid flows into the lymphatic vessels and becomes the *lymph*—the fluid that flows through the body in lymphatic vessels.

Lymphatic vessels, which drain waste products from the tissues, usually run parallel to arteries and veins. The lymphatic vessels transport the lymph to *lymph nodes,* which filter the lymph. The cells responsible for filtering the lymph are called *macrophages.* These large cells engulf and destroy foreign particles, including bacteria and cellular debris.

The lymph nodes also contain *B lymphocytes,* the white blood cells that are capable of initiating antibody production in response to the presence of viruses, bacteria, yeast, and other organisms.

The Thymus

The thymus is the major gland of our immune system. It is composed of two soft pinkish-gray lobes lying in a bib-like fashion just below the thyroid gland and above the heart. To a great extent, the health of the thymus determines the health of the immune system. Individuals who get frequent infections or suffer from chronic infections typically have impaired thymus activity. Also, people affected with hay fever, allergies, migraine headaches, and rheumatoid arthritis usually have altered thymus function.

The thymus is responsible for many immune system functions, including the production of *T lymphocytes,* a type of white blood cell responsible for *cell-mediated immunity.* Cell-mediated immunity refers to immune mechanisms not controlled, or mediated, by antibodies.

Cell-mediated immunity is extremely important in the resistance to infection by mold-like bacteria, yeast (including *Candida albicans*), fungi, parasites, and viruses (including Herpes simplex, Epstein-Barr, and viruses that cause hepatitis). If an individual is suffering from an infection from these organisms, it is a good indication that their cell-

QUICK REVIEW

- The mind and emotions have a tremendous impact on immune function.
- Stress depresses immune function.
- Nutrient deficiency is the most common cause of low immune function.
- Too much sugar in the diet leads to lowered white blood cell activity.
- Obesity is associated with decreased immune status.
- Alcohol consumption apparently inhibits white blood cell activity.

- Key nutrients for supplementation to support the immune system are vitamin A, carotenes, vitamin C, vitamin E, B-vitamins, iron, zinc, and selenium.
- Supporting the thymus, the major gland of the immune system, is one of the primary goals of therapy.
- The spleen is important in fighting bacterial infections.
- The herbs echinacea and astragalus exert broad-spectrum positive effects on immune function.

mediated immunity is not functioning up to par. Cell-mediated immunity is also critical in protecting against the development of cancer, autoimmune disorders such as rheumatoid arthritis, and allergies.

The thymus gland also releases several hormones, such as thymosin, thymopoietin, and serum thymic factor, which regulate many immune functions. A low level of these hormones in the blood is associated with depressed immunity and an increased susceptibility to infection. Typically, thymic hormone levels will be very low in the elderly, individuals prone to infection, cancer and AIDS patients, and individuals exposed to undue stress.

The Spleen

The spleen is the largest mass of lymphatic tissue in the body. Weighing about 7 ounces, the spleen is a fist-sized, spongy, dark purple organ that lies in the upper left abdomen behind the lower ribs. The spleen's functions include: producing white blood cells; engulfing and destroying bacteria and cellular debris; and destroying worn-out red blood cells and platelets. The spleen also serves as a blood reservoir; during times of demand, such as hemorrhage, the spleen can release its stored blood and prevent shock.

Like the thymus, the spleen releases many potent immune-system-enhancing compounds. For example, *tuftsin, splenopentin* (two small proteins secreted by the spleen), and spleen extracts have been shown to exert profound immune-enhancing activity. The benefits of spleen extracts will be discussed later in this chapter.

White Blood Cells

There are several types of white blood cells, including neutrophils, eosinophils, basophils, lymphocytes, and monocytes.

Neutrophils

These cells actively *phagocytize*—engulf and destroy—bacteria, tumor cells, and dead particulate matter. Neutrophils are especially important in preventing bacterial infection.

Eosinophils and Basophils

These cells are involved in allergic conditions. They secrete histamine and other inflammatory compounds that are designed to break down antigen-antibody complexes, but they also promote allergic mechanisms.

Lymphocytes

There are several types of lymphocytes, including T cells, B cells, and natural killer cells.

T Cells   *T cells* are thymus-derived lymphocytes. These cells orchestrate many immune functions and are the major components of cell-mediated immunity (discussed earlier in this chapter). There are different types of T cells, including helper T cells, which help other white blood cells to function; suppressor T cells, which inhibit white blood cell functions; and cytotoxic T cells, which attack and destroy foreign tissue, cancer cells, and virus-infected cells.

The ratio of helper T cells to suppressor T cells is a useful determinant of immune function. If the ratio is low, immunodeficiency is present. For example, AIDS is characterized by a very low ratio of helper T cells to suppressor T cells. If the ratio of helper T cells to suppressor T cells is too high, allergies or autoimmune disorders such as rheumatoid arthritis and lupus are often present. Both high and low T cell ratios have been found in chronic fatigue syndrome (CFS; see Part III).

B Cells   B cells are responsible for producing *antibodies*, which are large protein molecules that bind to *antigens*—molecules that the body recognizes as foreign molecules on bacteria, viruses, other organisms, and tumor cells. After the antibody binds to the antigen, it sets up a sequence of events that ultimately destroys the infectious organism or tumor cell.

Natural Killer Cells   *Natural killer cells,* or NK cells, received their name because of their ability to destroy cells that have become cancerous or infected with viruses. They are the body's first line of defense against cancer development. The level or activity of natural killer cells in chronic fatigue syndrome, cancer, and chronic viral infections is usually low.

Monocytes

Monocytes are the garbage collectors of the body. These large white blood cells are responsible for cleaning up cellular debris after an infection. Monocytes are also responsible for triggering many immune responses.

Special Tissue Cells

Macrophages

As stated earlier, the lymph is filtered by specialized cells known as macrophages. Macrophages are actually monocytes that have taken up residence in specific tissues, such as the liver, spleen, and lymph nodes. These large cells phagocytize, or engulf, foreign particles, including bacteria and cellular debris. Macrophages are essential in protecting against both invasion by microorganisms and damage to the lymphatic system.

Mast Cells

Mast cells are basophils that have taken up residence primarily along blood vessels. The mast cell, like the basophil, is responsible for releasing histamine and other compounds involved in allergic reactions.

Specialized Serum Factors

There are a number of specialized serum factors that enhance the immune system, including interferon, interleukin II, and *complement fractions.* These compounds are produced by various white blood cells. For example, interferon is produced primarily by T cells, interleukins are produced by macrophages and T cells, and complement fractions are manufactured in the liver and spleen. These specialized serum factors are extremely important in activating the white blood cells to destroy cancer cells and viruses. Complement fractions are produced by the liver and involved in the final destruction of viruses, bacteria, other organisms, immune complexes, and cancer cells.

Supporting the Immune System

Supporting the immune system is critical to good health. Conversely, good health is critical to supporting the immune system.

There isn't any single magic bullet that can immediately restore immune function. Instead, a comprehensive approach involving lifestyle, stress management, exercise, diet, nutritional supplementation, glandular therapy, and the use of plant-based medicines is used.

The immune system is a complex system of parts that are continuously under attack. The immune system is truly holistic, as evidenced by the close association of psychological, neurological, nutritional, environmental, and endocrinologic factors with immune function.

Psychoneuroimmunology

Psychoneuroimmunology is a term used to describe the interactions between the emotional state, nervous system function, and the immune system.[1] There is a growing body of knowledge documenting the mind's profound influence on health and disease. A complete and detailed account of the many facets of psychoneuroimmunology (PNI), or behavioral immunology, is beyond the scope of this chapter. Instead, we will concentrate on the effects of emotions and stress on the immune response.

Emotional State and Immune Function

Our mood and attitude have a tremendous bearing on the function of our immune system.[1] When we are happy and optimistic, our immune system functions much better. Conversely, when we are depressed, our immune system tends to be depressed. Employing measures outlined in the chapter A POSITIVE MENTAL ATTITUDE can be useful in improving the immune system.

It is not only major life stresses that can cause depressed immune function, but the more significant the stressor the greater the impact on the immune system. The loss of a spouse—perhaps the most stressful life event—was strongly associated with increased sickness and death well before a link between the mind and immune function was documented. In fact, it was not until 1977 that a study of twenty-six bereaved spouses documented a causal link between grief and a significant depression in immune function (natural killer cell activity was significantly reduced).[2] Subsequent studies have further demonstrated that bereavement, depression,

and stress significantly diminish important immune functions.[1,3]

By the end of the 1970s, several studies had shown that negative emotions suppress immune function. Conventional medical authorities have easily accepted the idea that negative emotional states adversely affect the immune system, but for some reason they initially scoffed at the notion that positive emotional states can actually enhance immune function.

Positive Emotional State and Immune Function In 1979, Norman Cousins' popular book, *Anatomy of an Illness,* caused a significant stir in the medical community. The book provided an autobiographical, anecdotal account indicating that positive emotional states can cure the body of a serious disease.[4] Cousins' healing appeared to result from watching *Candid Camera* and Marx Brothers films and reading humorous books.

Originally, physicians and researchers scoffed at Cousins' account. Now, however, it has been demonstrated in numerous studies that laughter and other positive emotional states can, in fact, enhance the immune system.[5,6] In addition, the use of guided imagery, hypnosis, and other meditative states has been shown to enhance immune system function.[1,7]

If you want to have a healthy immune system, you need to laugh often, view life with a positive eye, and put yourself in a relaxed state of mind on a regular basis.

Stress

Stress increases the levels of adrenal gland hormones, including adrenaline and corticosteroids. Among other things, these hormones inhibit white blood cell formation and function and cause the thymus gland to shrink (involute). The effects of these hormones lead to a significant suppression of immune function, leaving the individual susceptible to infections, cancer, and other illnesses. The level of immune suppression is usually proportional to the level of stress; the greater the stress, the greater the negative impact on the immune system.[8]

Stress also leads to immune suppression by stimulating the *sympathetic nervous system*. This is a part of the *autonomic nervous system*—the part of the nervous system over which we have little conscious control. The sympathetic nervous system is responsible for the fight-or-flight response. The immune system functions better under the other arm of the autonomic nervous system: the *parasympathetic nervous system*. The parasympathetic nervous system assumes control over bodily functions during periods of rest, relaxation, visualization, meditation, and sleep. During the deepest levels of sleep, potent immune-enhancing compounds are released, and many immune functions are greatly increased.[9] The value of good-quality sleep and of relaxation techniques in counteracting the effects of stress and enhancing our immune system cannot be overemphasized.

Lifestyle

A healthy lifestyle goes a long way toward establishing a healthy immune system. This benefit is perhaps most obvious when looking at the effects of lifestyle on natural killer cell activity.[10,11]

LIFESTYLE PRACTICES ASSOCIATED WITH HIGHER NATURAL KILLER CELL ACTIVITY

Not smoking
Increased intake of green vegetables
Regular meals
Proper body weight
More than 7 hours of sleep per night
Regular exercise
A vegetarian diet
Nutritional factors

The health of the immune system is greatly impacted by a person's dietary habits and nutritional status. Dietary factors that depress immune function include nutrient deficiency, excess consumption of sugar, consumption of allergenic foods, and high cholesterol levels in the blood. Dietary factors that enhance immune function include all essential nutrients, antioxidants, carotenes, and flavonoids.

Consistent with good health, optimal immune function requires a healthy diet that (1) is rich in whole, natural foods, such as fruits, vegetables, grains, beans, seeds, and nuts, (2) is low in fats and refined sugars, and (3) contains adequate, but not excessive, amounts of protein. On top of this, individuals are encouraged to drink five or six 8-ounce glasses of water per day (preferably pure water). These dietary recommendations, along with a positive mental attitude, a good high-potency multivitamin-mineral supplement, a regular exercise program, daily deep breathing and relaxation exercises (meditation, prayer, etc.), and at least seven to eight hours of sleep daily, will go a long way in helping the immune system function at an optimum level.

Nutrient Deficiency

Nutrient deficiency is, without question, the most frequent cause of a depressed immune system. Although, historically, research relating nutritional status to immune function has concerned itself with severe malnutrition states, attention is now shifting toward marginal deficiencies of single or multiple nutrients and the effects of too many calories, sugar, and fat. An overwhelming number of clinical and experimental studies lead us to the conclusion that any single nutrient deficiency can profoundly impair the immune system.

Given the widespread problem of marginal (subclinical) nutrient deficiency in Americans, it can be concluded that many are suffering from impaired immunity that will respond to nutritional supplementation. This statement is particularly true of the elderly. Numerous studies have shown that most elderly Americans are deficient in at least one nutrient.[12] Likewise, there are numerous studies that show that taking a multiple-vitamin-and-mineral supplement enhances immune function in elderly subjects, whether or not they suffer from overt nutritional deficiency.[13,14]

Protein

The importance of adequate protein intake to proper immune function has been extensively studied.[15] The most severe effects of protein deficiency are on cell-mediated immunity, although all facets of immune function are ultimately affected. Protein deficiency is not, however, usually a single-nutrient deficiency. It is normally associated with multiple nutrient deficiencies, and some immune dysfunctions attributed to severe protein deficiency are probably due to these other factors. Partial deficiencies of dietary vitamins produce a comparatively greater depression in immune function than do partial protein deficiencies. Nonetheless, adequate protein is essential for optimal immune function. Please follow the recommendations given in the chapter A HEALTH-PROMOTING DIET to attain adequate protein levels. In certain disease states, e.g., cancer and AIDS, it is appropriate to supplement the diet with a high-quality protein (e.g., whey protein, soy protein isolate, and egg pro-

tein) at a dosage of 0.8 gram per 2.2 pounds body weight. The protein will help prevent the wasting away (cachexia) associated with these conditions.

Sugar

Consuming 100 grams (roughly 4 ounces) of carbohydrate in the form of glucose, fructose, sucrose, honey, or orange juice can significantly reduce the ability of white blood cells to destroy foreign particles and microorganisms. As shown in Figure 1, the negative effects start within thirty minutes, last for over five hours, and typically include a fifty-percent reduction in the ability of white blood cells to destroy and engulf foreign particles at the peak of inhibition (usually two hours after ingestion).[16–18]

Since white blood cell function constitutes a major portion of the defense mechanism against infection, impairment of their activity obviously leads to an immune-compromised state. Ingesting increasing amounts of glucose progressively lowers white blood cell function, with maximal inhibition corresponding to maximal blood glucose levels. In other words, the more sugar you consume the greater the negative impact on immune function.

It is thought that the negative effects of high sugar levels result from the elevation of insulin levels and the competition with vitamin C for membrane transport sites.[19,20] This is based on evidence that vitamin C and blood sugar appear to have opposite effects on white blood cell function and the fact that both require insulin for membrane transport into many tissues.

Considering that the average American consumes 125 grams of sucrose each day, plus 50 grams of other refined simple sugars, the inescapable conclusion is that most Americans have chronically depressed

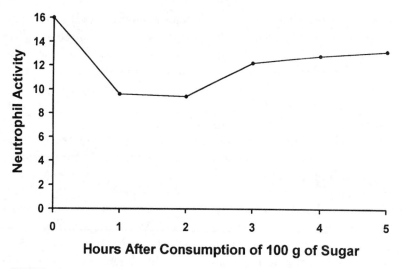

FIGURE 1 The Effects of Sugar on White Cell Phagocytic Activity

immune systems. It is clear that the consumption of simple sugars—even in the form of fruit juice—impairs immune function, particularly during an infection. To aid the immune system during an infection, it is important to stay away from sugar.

Also, short-term fasting can help improve immune function by lowering the blood sugar levels, particularly during the first twenty-four to forty-eight hours of an acute infectious illness, since this results in a significant (up to fifty percent) increase in the ability of white blood cells to destroy microorganisms.[16] The fast should not be continued for an excessive period, since eventually the leukocytes' energy sources will become depleted.

Obesity

Obesity is associated with decreased immune status. People who are overweight suffer from more infections than do people of normal weight; in experimental studies, the white blood cells of overweight individuals were less able to destroy bacteria.[21] The levels of cho-

lesterol and other fatty substances (lipids) are usually elevated in obese individuals, which may explain their impaired immune function, as described in the following section.

Lipids

Increased levels of cholesterol, free fatty acids, triglycerides, and bile acids inhibit various immune functions, including the ability of white blood cells to divide, move to areas of infection, and destroy microorganisms.[22–25] Optimal immune function is therefore dependent on control of these serum components. Interestingly, L-carnitine, a vitamin-like compound and popular nutritional supplement, has been shown to overcome the negative effects that elevated cholesterol and triglyceride levels have on immune function.[25] This is probably due to carnitine's role in the removal of fat from the blood.[26]

Alcohol

Alcohol increases susceptibility to experimental infections in animals, and alcoholics are known to be more susceptible to pneumonia. Studies of human white blood cells show a profound depression in the rate of mobilization into areas of infection after people consume alcohol.[27] The effects are somewhat dose-related; the more alcohol consumed, the greater the impairment of white blood cell mobility.

Vitamin A

Once known as the "anti-infective vitamin," vitamin A has recently regained recognition as a major determinant of immune status. Vitamin A affects the immune system in several ways. Primarily, it plays an essential role in maintaining the surfaces of the skin, respiratory tract, gastrointestinal tract, and other body tissues as well as their secretions. These surface systems constitute a primary barrier to microorganisms. In addition to this role, vitamin A has been shown to stimulate and/or enhance numerous immune processes, including induction of anti-tumor activity, enhancement of white blood cell function, and increased antibody response.[28] These effects are not due simply to a reversal of vitamin A deficiency, since many of these effects are further enhanced by large doses of vitamin A.

Vitamin A has also demonstrated significant antiviral activity and has prevented the immune suppression induced by adrenal hormones, severe burns, and surgery. Some of these effects are probably related to vitamin A's ability to prevent stress-induced shrinkage of the thymus gland and to promote thymus growth.

People who are deficient in vitamin A are more susceptible to infectious diseases in general, but especially viral infections. In addition, vitamin A stores typically plummet during the course of an infection.

Vitamin A in Children

Low vitamin A levels are a major problem in many developing countries, where five to ten million children exhibit severe vitamin A deficiency.[29] As a result, these children experience a tremendous amount of suffering and death due to impared immune function. Vitamin A deficient children are particularly susceptible to viral infections like measles.

Vitamin A supplementation in the treatment of measles is indicated in children in the United States as well as third-world countries. In a study of "well-nourished" children in Long Beach, California, who suffered from measles, it was shown that fifty percent were deficient in vitamin A.[30]

Recently, a number of well-designed studies have confirmed an effect first noted in 1932: Vitamin A supplementation can significantly reduce infant mortality among measles patients by at least fifty percent. Typically, the dosage of vitamin A in double-blind studies has been 200,000 to 400,000 IU, administered only once or twice to replenish body stores.[31]

Vitamin A therapy appears appropriate for other childhood viral illnesses as well. One of the more common viruses nowadays is the *respiratory syncytial virus* (RSV), a common cause of severe respiratory disease in young children. Studies have shown that children with RSV have low serum vitamin A levels. Furthermore, the lower the vitamin A level the greater the severity of the disease, similar to the relationship shown in measles. Because vitamin A supplementation diminishes the morbidity and death caused by measles, a group of researchers decided to determine vitamin A's safety and absorption pattern in RSV as a first step in determining the therapeutic effectiveness.[32]

Twenty-one children with a mean age of 2.3 months (range: 1 to 6 months) with mild RSV infection were treated with 12,500 to 25,000 IU of oral micellized (emulsified in water by making the fat droplets extremely small) vitamin A. Baseline vitamin A levels were shown to be low, but within six hours after receiving 25,000 IU of vitamin A, normal levels were reestablished. This did not occur with doses of 12,500 IU. Despite their young age, none of the children experienced any obvious signs or symptoms of vitamin A toxicity. Although the study was not designed as a therapeutic trial, the subjects receiving vitamin A had shorter hospital stays than did children with a similar severity of illness who were not enrolled in the study.

Placebo-controlled trials are necessary to determine the true effectiveness of vitamin A in RSV infection. Vitamin A supplementation is an attractive treatment of RSV infections for many reasons, including its low cost, wide availability, and ease of administration.

During an acute viral infection, a single oral dose of 50,000 IU for one or two days appears to be safe even for infants.

Vitamin A supplementation must be absolutely avoided during pregnancy. Women who might be pregnant may substitute beta-carotene for vitamin A. A recent study published in the prestigious *New England Journal of Medicine* demonstrated that dosages greater than 10,000 IU during pregnancy (specifically during the first seven weeks after conception) have probably been responsible for one out of each fifty-seven cases of birth defects in the United States. Women who are at risk for becoming pregnant should keep their supplemental vitamin A levels below 5,000 IU or, better yet, look to carotenes.

Carotenes

Carotenes, some of which can be converted into vitamin A, are gaining a great deal of attention as immune system enhancers. Carotenes represent the most widespread group of naturally occurring pigments in nature. They are a highly colored (red and yellow) group of fat-soluble compounds. Over six hundred carotenoids have been characterized, but only about thirty to fifty are believed to have vitamin A activity. Beta-carotene is the most widely studied and has been termed the most active of the carotenes due to its higher provitamin A activity.

However, several other carotenes exert greater antioxidant effects than beta-carotenes. Because carotenes are better antioxidants than vitamin A, they may turn out to be even better in protecting the thymus gland, since the thymus is particularly susceptible to free-radical and oxidative damage.

Carotenes have demonstrated a number of immune-enhancing effects in recent studies.[33] However, awareness of such effects goes back to 1931, when an inverse relationship was found between a diet rich in carotenes (determined by blood carotene levels) and the number of school days missed by children.[34] Originally it was thought that the immune-enhancing properties of carotenes resulted from their conversion to vitamin A. Researchers now know that carotenes exert many immune system–enhancing effects independent of any vitamin A activity.[33]

One of the most impressive studies was conducted on normal human volunteers.[35] Results indicated that oral beta-carotene (180 mg/day; approximately 300,000 IU) significantly increased the number of helper/inducer T cells by approximately thirty percent after seven days and all T cells after fourteen days.[35] Because helper T cells play a critical role in determining immune status, this study indicates that oral beta-carotene may be effective in increasing the immune function in conditions characterized by decreased T-cell count, such as AIDS and cancer.

However, rather than supplementing the diet with synthetic beta-carotene, it may be more advantageous to use natural carotene sources or increase the intake of carotene-rich foods. To support this notion, let's take a look at a comparative study. In the study, 126 healthy college students were randomly assigned to one of the following groups: Group A, the control group; Group B, which took a 15 mg (25,000 IU) beta-carotene supplement daily; and Group C, which consumed approximately 15 mg of beta-carotene per day from carrots. The group that ate carrots showed the greatest increase in white blood cell number and function.[36]

These results are baffling, because absorption studies have shown that beta-carotene in pill form is better absorbed than the carotenes from carrots and other vegetables.[37] What can be concluded from these studies is that beta-carotene is probably just one of the immune-enhancing compounds in whole, carotene-rich foods. Therefore, our recommendation is to try to focus on meeting high carotene intake through diet rather than supplementation. That being said, when immediate immune enhancement is desired, supplemental carotene may be an easier way to raise carotene intake to the 180 mg per day mark—the level which has been shown to significantly enhance thymus function. While carotenes do not possess the antiviral and tumor-killing properties of vitamin A,[38-43] carotenes are inherently safer and exert multiple beneficial effects on immune function.[44]

Vitamin C

Vitamin C (ascorbic acid) plays an important role in the natural approach to immune enhancement. Although vitamin C has been shown to be antiviral and antibacterial, its main effect is via improvement in immune function. Many different immune-enhancing effects have been demonstrated, including enhancing white blood cell response and function, increasing interferon (a special chemical factor that fights viral infection and cancer) levels, increasing the secretion of thymic hormones, and improving the integrity of the linings of mucous membranes.[45] Vitamin C has direct biochemical effects on white blood cells similar to those of the immune-enhancing compound interferon.[46]

Numerous clinical studies support the use of vitamin C in the treatment of infectious conditions, particularly the common cold. In addition to its well-known effects in reducing the frequency, duration, and severity of the common cold, vitamin C has also been shown to be useful in other infectious conditions.[45,47-51] Vitamin C levels are quickly depleted during the stress of an infection.[52]

It is useful to supplement with flavonoids —the plant pigments that give color to many fruits, vegetables, and flowers—along with vitamin C, since these compounds raise the concentration of vitamin C in some tissues and increase its effects, in addition to exerting their own effects.[53]

Vitamin E

Vitamin E exerts very good immune-enhancing activity, as it enhances both arms of immunity (antibody-related or humoral and cell-mediated immunity). A vitamin E deficiency results in significant impairment of immune function.[38,39] Even without signs of vitamin E deficiency, supplementation with vitamin E has been shown to exert a number of positive effects on immune functions.[54] The benefits of vitamin E are especially helpful in enhancing immune function in the elderly.

A recent study sought to determine the effect of vitamin E supplementation at different dosages on immune function in eighty-eight patients over the age of sixty-five years.[55] The researchers measured T-cell function as an indicator of immune system condition. Vitamin E was given at either 60 IU, 200 IU, or 800 IU for 235 days. While the placebo group only experienced an eight-percent increase in T-cell function, the 60 IU group had a twenty-percent increase; the 200 IU group had a fifty-eight-percent increase; and the 800 IU group had a sixty-five-percent increase. No adverse effects were observed at any of the three dosage schedules of vitamin E.

Vitamin B6

Vitamin B6 deficiency results in depressed immune function—both antibody-related and cell-mediated immunity are suppressed. This suppression is apparent as the number of white blood cells plummets, there is a tremendous reduction in quantity and quality of antibodies produced, and there is decreased thymic hormone activity.[38,39] Vitamin B6 deficiency may result from low dietary intake of vitamin B6, excess protein intake, consumption of yellow food dyes (hydralazine), alcohol consumption, or use of oral contraceptives.

Folic Acid and Vitamin B12

A deficiency of vitamin B12, or folic acid, results in significantly reduced white blood cell production and abnormal white blood cell responses. Folic acid deficiency—the most common vitamin deficiency in the United States—has been shown to result in *atrophy* (shrinkage) of the thymus and lymph nodes and significantly impaired white blood cell function. A B12 deficiency produces identical findings and is especially harmful to the ability of white blood cells to engulf and destroy infecting organisms.[38,39]

Other B-Vitamins

Thiamin (B1), riboflavin (B2), and pantothenic acid (B5) deficiencies lead to reduced antibody response, decreased white blood cell response, and atrophy of the thymus and lymph tissue.[38,39]

Iron

Iron deficiency is a common condition that causes immune dysfunction in large numbers of people, particularly children, menstruating women, and elderly people who take aspirin and other drugs that can cause gastrointestinal bleeding due to ulcer formation. Marginal iron deficiency—even at levels that do not lower blood values—can influence the immune system. Marginal iron deficiency can cause thymus and lymph node atrophy, decreased white blood cell response and function, and a decreased ratio of T cells to B cells.[38,39]

Iron is an important nutrient to bacteria as well as humans. During infection, one of the body's defense mechanisms to limit bacterial growth is to reduce iron levels in the blood. Laboratory studies have shown that the antibacterial effects of human serum are eliminated by the addition of iron to the serum.[56] As body temperature rises, plasma iron levels drop; when the temperature is raised to fever levels, the growth of bacteria is inhibited, but not at high iron concentrations.

These observations lead us to the conclusion that iron supplementation is probably contraindicated during acute infection. However, in patients with impaired immune function, chronic infections, and subnormal iron levels, adequate supplementation is essential.

Zinc

The hereditary zinc-deficiency disease, *acrodermatitis enteropathica* (AE), offers an excellent model for understanding the role of zinc in immunity. In AE, the number of T cells is reduced, white blood cell function is significantly impaired, and thymic hormone levels are lower. All of these effects are reversible upon adequate zinc administration and absorption.[57]

Other studies have shown that zinc serves a vital role in many immune system reactions; it promotes the destruction of foreign particles and microorganisms, acts as a protectant against free-radical damage, acts synergistically with vitamin A, is required for proper white blood cell function, and is a necessary cofactor in activating serum thymic factor—a thymus hormone with profound immune-enhancing properties.[58,59]

Zinc also inhibits the growth of several viruses, including common cold viruses and herpes simplex virus.[60] Throat lozenges containing zinc have become popular in the treatment of the common cold for good reason: they work (see COMMON COLD in Part III).

Adequate zinc levels are particularly important in the elderly, and zinc supplementation in elderly subjects results in increased numbers of T cells and enhanced cell-mediated immune responses.[61]

Selenium

Selenium plays a vital role in the functioning of the antioxidant enzyme *glutathione peroxidase*. As such, it affects all components of the immune system, including the development and activity of all white blood cells. Selenium deficiency results in depressed immune function, whereas selenium supplementation results in augmentation and/or restoration of immune functions. Selenium deficiency has been shown to inhibit resistance to infection as a result of impaired white blood cell and thymus function, while selenium supplementation (200 mcg/day) has been shown

to stimulate white blood cell and thymus function.[61,64]

The ability of selenium supplementation to enhance immune function goes well beyond simply restoring selenium levels in selenium-deficient individuals.[65,66] For example, in one study selenium supplementation (200 mcg/day) to individuals with normal selenium concentrations in their blood resulted in a 118-percent increase in the ability of lymphocytes to kill tumor cells and an 82.3-percent increase in the activity of natural killer cells.[66] These effects were apparently related to selenium's ability to enhance the expression of the immune-enhancing compound interleukin-II and, consequently, the rate of white blood cell proliferation and differentiation into forms capable of killing tumor cells and microorganisms. The results indicated that the immune-enhancing effects of selenium in humans require supplementation above the normal dietary intake.

Enhancing Thymus Function

Perhaps the most effective way to reestablish a healthy immune system is to improve the functioning of the thymus gland. Promoting optimal thymus gland activity involves

- Prevention of thymic involution or shrinkage by ensuring adequate dietary intake of antioxidant nutrients
- Using nutrients that are required in the manufacture or action of thymic hormones
- Using botanical medicines or glandular products that contain concentrates of calf thymus tissue to enhance thymus activity

The Role of Breast-Feeding

Breast-feeding is associated with giving a child a better immune function. Breast-fed infants tend to have fewer infections and allergies. One of the key benefits of breast milk may involve stimulating the thymus gland to grow. It is important for mothers to breast-feed their infants for at least the first four months of life.

In a recent study, breast-fed infants were shown to have a larger *mean thymus index* (a volume estimate based on ultrasound assessment) when compared to formula-fed infants.[67] The thymic index was assessed in healthy term infants at birth and at four months of age. While there was no significant difference in thymic index at birth, at four months of age the mean thymic index was 383 in exclusively breast-fed infants, 27.3 in partially breast-fed infants, and only 18.3 in formula-fed infants. This finding was independent of weight, length, sex, and previous or current illness. Let us put these numbers in better perspective: the thymus glands of breast-fed infants were over twenty times larger than those of formula-fed infants!

Antioxidants

The thymus gland shows maximum development in infancy; the importance of breast-feeding is clearly the determining factor in maximal development, based on the previously described study. During the aging process, the thymus gland undergoes a process of shrinkage, or involution. The reason for this involution is that the thymus gland is extremely susceptible to free-radical and oxidative damage caused by stress, radiation, infection, and chronic illness.

Many patients with impaired immune function as well as conditions associated with impaired immunity (chronic fatigue syndrome, cancer, AIDS, etc.) suffer from a state of *oxidative imbalance*. This condition is characterized by a greater number of free radicals than antioxidants in their system—a situation that is quite detrimental to thymus function. One of the primary ways in which antioxidants impact the immune system—particularly cell-

mediated immunity—may be via protecting the thymus gland from damage. The antioxidant nutrients most important for protecting the thymus include the carotenes, vitamin C, vitamin E, zinc, and selenium.

Nutrients to Enhance Thymus Function

Many nutrients function as important cofactors in the manufacture, secretion, and function of thymic hormones. Deficiencies of any one of these nutrients result in decreased thymic hormone action and impaired immune function. Zinc, vitamin B6, and vitamin C are perhaps the most critical. Supplementation with these nutrients has been shown to increase thymic hormone function and cell-mediated immunity.

Zinc is perhaps the critical mineral involved in thymus gland function and thymus hormone action. Zinc is involved in virtually every aspect of immunity. When zinc levels are low, the number of T cells is reduced; thymic hormone levels are lower, and many white blood functions critical to the immune response are severely lacking. All of these effects are reversible with zinc supplementation.[68]

Thymus Extracts

A substantial amount of clinical data now supports the effectiveness of orally administered calf thymus extracts in restoring and enhancing immune function.[69,70] The effectiveness of thymus extracts is reflective of broad-spectrum immune system enhancement, presumably mediated by improved thymus gland activity. This effect fits nicely with one of the basic concepts of glandular therapy: that the oral ingestion of glandular material of a certain animal gland will strengthen the corresponding human gland. The result is a broad general effect indicative of improved glandular function. In other words, glandular therapy is designed to increase the tone, function, and/or activity of the corresponding gland.

Thymus extracts may provide a solution to chronic viral infections and low immune function. The ability of thymus extracts to treat and then reduce the number of recurrent infections was studied in groups of children with a history of recurrent respiratory tract infections. Double-blind studies revealed not only that orally administered thymus extracts were able to effectively eliminate infection, but that treatment over the course of a year significantly reduced the number of respiratory infections and significantly improved numerous immune parameters.[71]

Thymus extract has also been shown to normalize the ratio of T helper cells to suppressor cells, whether the ratio is low (as in AIDS or cancer) or high (as in allergies or rheumatoid arthritis).[69,70]

Spleen Extracts

Like thymus extracts, pharmaceutical grade bovine spleen extracts are useful in the treatment of infectious conditions and as an immune-enhancing agent in cancer. The benefits are attributed to small-molecular-weight proteins such as tuftsin and splenopentin. Tuftsin stimulates macrophages in the liver, spleen, and lymph nodes. Remember, macrophages are large cells that engulf and destroy foreign particles, including bacteria, cancer cells, and cellular debris. Macrophages are essential in protecting against invasion by microorganisms as well as cancer. Tuftsin also helps mobilize other white blood cells to fight against infection and cancer. A deficiency of tuftsin is associated with signs and symptoms of frequent infections.[72]

Splenopentin's effects are primarily directed toward enhancing the immune system's response to regulating compounds known as *colony-stimulating factors*.[73] These compounds stimulate the production of white blood cells. Clinical studies performed during the 1930s used spleen extracts to treat depressed white blood cell counts; splenopentin is probably the factor responsible for the results.[74–76] Splenopentin has also been shown to enhance natural killer cell activity.[77]

The primary use of spleen extracts is after a *splenectomy*, or removal of the spleen. This operation is usually performed after the spleen has been seriously injured, causing severe hemorrhage. It is necessary to remove the spleen after significant trauma because it is difficult to repair. The spleen is also removed in the medical treatment of certain diseases, such as idiopathic thrombocytic purpurea (ITP), and to determine the extent of Hodgkin's disease. The removal of the spleen is associated with an increased risk for infection, particularly bacterial infection. Spleen extracts can be quite helpful in such cases.

Spleen extracts are also useful in the treatment of low white blood cell counts and bacterial infections and as an adjunct to cancer therapy.[78]

Botanicals

Many herbs have been shown to have antibacterial, antiviral, and immunostimulatory effects, and a complete discussion is outside the scope of this chapter. This chapter focuses on two of the most popular immune-enhancing botanicals: echinacea and astragalus. These two herbs were selected based on their ability to exert broad-spectrum effects on immune functions. They stimulate the body's natural defense mechanisms via slightly different mechanisms and are in many ways the prototypes of the hundreds of plants with known antimicrobial and immunological activity.

Echinacea

Perhaps the most widely used Western herb for enhancement of the immune system is echinacea. The two most widely used species are *Echinacea angustifolia* and *Echinacea purpurea*. Both have been shown to exert profound immune-enhancing effects. Several classes of constituents contribute to this action.[79]

Among the most important immune-stimulating components of Echinacea are the large polysaccharides, such as *inulin*, that activate the *alternative complement pathway* (one of the immune system's nonspecific defense mechanisms) and increase the production of immune chemicals that activate macrophages. The result is increased activity of many key immune parameters: production of T cells, macrophage phagocytosis, antibody binding, natural killer cell activity, and levels of circulating neutrophils.[79]

Echinacea strengthens the immune system even in healthy people. For example, oral administration of an *E. purpurea* root extract (a dose of thirty drops three times daily) to healthy males for five days resulted in a remarkable 120-percent increase in leukocyte phagocytosis.[80] In another study of healthy volunteers aged twenty-five to forty years, the fresh-pressed juice of *E. purpurea* extract was found to increase the phagocytosis of *Candida albicans* by thirty to forty percent; it also increased the migration of white cells to the scene of battle by thirty to forty percent.[81]

In addition to immune support, echinacea exerts direct antiviral activity and helps prevent the spread of bacteria by inhibiting a bacterial enzyme called *hyaluronidase*. This enzyme is secreted by bacteria in order to break through the body's first line of defense—the protective membranes such as the skin or mucous membranes—so that the organism can enter the body.

Echinacea's effects against the common cold are discussed in COMMON COLD in Part III.

Astragalus membranaceus

Astragalus root is a traditional Chinese medicine used to treat viral infections. Clinical studies in China have shown it to be effective when used as a preventive measure against the common cold.[82] It has also been shown to reduce the duration and severity of symptoms in acute treatment of the common cold, as well as raise white blood cell counts in chronic leukopenia (a condition characterized by low white blood cell levels).

Research in animals indicates that a stragalus apparently works by stimulating several factors of the immune system: phagocytic activity of monocytes and macrophages; interferon production and natural killercell activity; T-cell activity; and other antiviral mechanisms.[82,83] Astragalus appears particularly useful in cases where the immune system has been damaged by chemicals or radiation (e.g., in patients undergoing chemotherapy and/or radiation treatment).[84] As with echinacea, the polysaccharidescontained in the root of *Astragalus membranaceus* contribute to the immune-enhancing effects.

TREATMENT SUMMARY

The recommendations listed below are meant as a general approach to enhancing immune function during an infectious process.

General Measures

- Rest (ideally bed rest)
- Drink large amounts of fluids (preferably diluted vegetable juices, soups, and herb teas)
- Limit simple sugar consumption (including fruit sugars) to less than 50 grams per day

Nutritional Supplements

- High-potency multiple-vitamin-and-mineral formula
- Vitamin C: 500 mg every two hours
- Bioflavonoids: 1,000 mg per day
- Vitamin A: 50,000 IU per day for up to two days in infants and up to one week in adults

---

NOTE: Do not use vitamin A in sexually active women of child-bearing age unless effective birth control is being used due to possible birth defects at high dosages.)

OR beta-carotene: 200,000 IU per day

- Zinc: 30 mg per day
- If a viral infection: Thymus extract (the equivalent of 120 mg of pure polypeptides with molecular weights less than 10,000, or roughly 500 mg of the crude polypeptide fraction; read product labels to verify dosage)
- If a bacterial infection: Spleen extract (the daily dose should provide 50 mg of tuftsin and splenopentin, or roughly 1.5 g of total spleen peptides)

Botanical Medicines

All dosages are three times daily.

- *Echinacea* sp.
  Dried root (or as tea): 0.5–1 g
  Freeze-dried plant: 325–650 mg
  Juice of aerial portion of *E. purpurea* stabilized in 22% ethanol: 2–3 ml
  Tincture (1:5): 2–4 ml
  Fluid extract (1:1): 2–4 ml
  Solid (dry powdered) extract (6.5:1 or 3.5% echinacoside): 150–300 mg
- *Astragalus membranaceus*
  Dried root (or as decoction): 1–2 g
  Tincture (1:5): 2–4 ml
  Fluid extract (1:1): 2–4 ml
  Solid (dry powdered) extract (0.5% 4-hydroxy-3-methoxy isoflavone): 100–150 mg

Longevity and Life-Extension

If infant mortality is taken out of the equation, life expectancy has really only improved a maximum of 3.7 years during this century.

The longest a person ever lived, based on confirmed records, was 122 years, 188 days.

Increasing life expectancy involves reducing causes of premature death.

The latest and best theory of aging is the telomere-shortening theory; telomeres (the end caps of our DNA molecules) are the "clocks of aging."

Free-radical damage causes cellular aging, and antioxidant nutrients prevent it.

Individuals who are either severely overweight or severely underweight have the shortest life span, while individuals whose weight is just below the average weight for their height have the longest life span.

Researchers estimate that for every hour of exercise, there is a two-hour increase in longevity.

The level of antioxidant enzymes in the body, as well as the level of dietary antioxidants such as beta-carotene, determines the life span of mammals.

The *Ginkgo biloba* extract, standardized to contain twenty-four percent ginkgoflavonglycosides, has demonstrated remarkably beneficial effects in relieving many symptoms associated with aging.

Because DHEA levels tend to decline with aging, it has been postulated that DHEA supplementation may offer some protection against the effects of aging.

Melatonin is not likely to extend life in humans based solely on its antioxidant effects.

Life-extension has been a goal of humans since long before Ponce DeLeon's search for the mythical fountain of youth. In recent decades, a number of books advocating the use of vitamins, minerals, hormones, drugs, and other compounds to extend life have made the bestseller lists. Whether or not following such recommendations will have an impact on human longevity remains to be seen. Some of the recommendations to slow down the aging process do make sense and appear to be sound. This chapter will focus on such recommendations.

Current Life Expectancy and Maximum Life Span

Life expectancy refers to the average number of years that a person is expected to live in a given population, while *life span* refers to the maximum obtainable by a member of a species.

On the surface it appears that, in the United States, impressive gains in extending life have been made in this century. In 1900, the average life expectancy was forty-five years. Now it is seventy-one years for men and seventy-eight years for women. However, if we really examine what was responsible for this increase in life expectancy, it is almost entirely due to decreased infant mortality. If infant mortality is taken out of the equation, life expectancy has really only improved by a maximum of 3.7 years during this century. Life span has remained constant during this century.[1]

Increasing life expectancy involves reducing causes of premature death. Since cardiovascular disease due to hardening of the arteries (atherosclerosis) is the number-one killer of Americans, and cancer the number-

TABLE 1 Top Ten Causes of Death in 1995[2]	
Diseases of the heart	737,563
Cancer	538,455
Strokes	157,991
Lung disease	102,899
Accidents and adverse events	93,320
Pneumonia and influenza	82,923
Diabetes mellitus	59,254
AIDS	43,115
Suicide	31,284
Chronic liver disease	25,222

two killer, every effort should be made to reduce the risk of getting these diseases.

Longevity Myths and Reality

Myths still circulate about certain groups of people (the Hunzas of Pakistan, Georgian Russians, and Andean villagers in Ecuador, for example) who are reported to live to an extremely old age—between 125 and 150 years. However, detailed scientific reports have refuted these claims.[3–5]

For example, one group of investigators who studied the people of Vilcabamba, Ecuador, made a revealing discovery. Their intention was to determine whether the degree of bone loss that occurred during aging was different in that population than in the U.S. population.[4] They did an initial survey, then went back five years later for a follow-up. After this five-year interval, a number of individuals reported being ten years older than they had been during the first survey. From studying existing birth records, it became obvious that there was considerable exaggeration of age. In this society, as well as in the other societies associated with longevity, social standing increases with age.

In the Georgia region of Russia, it has been demonstrated that the majority of reported centenarians (people older than 100 years) are actually in their seventies and eighties. They just look like they are 140 years old as a result of their arduous existence.[5]

The current official world record for longevity is 122 years, reached by a French woman named Jeanne Louise Calment. Born on February 21, 1875, she lived through France's Third and Fourth Republics, and into its Fifth. She was fourteen when the Eiffel Tower was completed in 1889. She died on August 28, 1997. In her later years, she lived mostly off the income from her apartment. In 1966 she had sold her apartment to a lawyer, André-François Raffray, who had agreed to make monthly payments on the apartment in exchange for taking possession when she died but never got to do so. He died a year before Jeanne Calment at the age of seventy-seven; his family was required to keep making the payments.

What Causes Aging?

Answers to the question "What causes aging?" are coming rapidly as a result of research in *gerontology*, the science of aging. There are many interesting theories of aging, but only the most significant will be briefly discussed in this chapter.

There are basically two types of aging theories: *programmed theories* and *damage theories*. Programmed theories state that there is some sort of a genetic clock ticking away that determines when old age sets in, while damage theories hold that aging is a result of cumulative damage to cells and genetic materials. Our opinion is that both are valid. Such apparent dichotomies seem to repeat themselves in science. The nature of light is a case in point; light functions as both a particle and a wave. Well, human aging is the result of both programmed cell life and cellular damage.

The Hayflick Limit

In 1912, Dr. Alexis Carrel—one of the foremost biologists of his time—began an experiment at the Rockefeller Institute that would last for over thirty-four years. Dr. Carrel set out to find out how long he could keep chicken fibroblasts dividing. *Fibroblasts* are connective tissue cells that manufacture colla-

. . . .

QUICK REVIEW

At this time, there is no "magic bullet" to halt the aging process. However, there are steps that can be taken to slow the aging process and reduce the risk of the major causes of premature death. The best way to ensure a long, healthy, high-quality life is to adopt the guidelines described in Part I: The Four Cornerstones of Good Health. In addition, specific recommendations and dosages of supplements for slowing the aging process are given in this section. While trying to lengthen one's life span (quantity) is important, we want to encourage you to focus on improving the quality of your life as well.

Diet

A high intake of vegetables and fruits is essential to a life-extension program, due to the high content of vitamins, minerals, carotenes, flavonoids, and dietary fibers in these foods. It is especially important to follow the dietary recommendations

TABLE 2	Ten Oldest Living People, Based on Confirmed Records				
YEARS	DAYS	BORN	DIED	COUNTRY	NAME
122	188	21 Feb 1875	28 Aug 1997	France	Jeanne Louise Calment
120	237	29 Jun 1865	21 Feb 1986	Japan	Shigechiyo Izumi
115	50+	16 Aug 1882	Still alive as of 21 Oct 1997	U.S.A.	Chris Mortenson
116	88	18 Nov 1874	14 Feb 1991	U.S.A.	Carrie White (born Joyner)
114	213	1 Aug 1877	Mar 1992	U.K.	Charlotte Hughes (born Milburn)
113	124	15 Jul 1701	16 Nov 1814	Canada	Pierre Joubert
112	330	11 Dec 1874	6 Nov 1987	Australia	Caroline Maud Mockridge
112	228	14 Jul 1860	27 Feb 1973	Spain	Josefa Salas Mateo
112		1844	16 Sep 1957	Morocco	El Hadj Mohammed el Mokri
112		1868	7 Jan 1981	Poland	Roswlia Mielczarak (Mrs.)

gen. Fed with a special broth containing an extract of chick embryo, the chicken fibroblasts grew quite well in flasks. They regularly divided and formed new cells, periodically discarding excess cells. This "tissue culture" system kept dividing for thirty-four years, until two years after Dr. Carrel's death, when his coworkers discarded the culture. Dr. Carrel's work prompted the idea that cells are inherently immortal if given an ideal environment.[6]

This idea was not challenged until the early 1960s, when Dr. Leonard Hayflick observed that human fibroblasts in tissue cul-

. . . .

for reducing the risk of heart disease (atherosclerosis), such as increasing intake of cold-pressed vegetable oils, fish, and dietary fiber, especially the gel-forming or mucilaginous fibers (flaxseed, oat bran, pectin, etc.), while reducing consumption of saturated fats, cholesterol, sugar, and animal proteins.

Nutritional Supplements

- High-potency multiple-vitamin-and-mineral, as recommended in the chapter SUPPLEMENTARY MEASURES.

- Vitamin C: 500–3,000 mg per day
- Vitamin E: 400–800 IU per day
- For patients over the age of fifty: *Ginkgo biloba* extract (twenty-four percent ginkgo flavonglycosides): 40 mg three times per day in the absence of any symptoms; 80 mg three times per day if symptoms are present

DHEA: As described in this chapter

Melatonin: physiological dosages of 0.1 to 0.3 mg; for insomnia, no more than 3 mg

ture wouldn't divide more than about fifty times.[7] Why the discrepancy? It appears that Dr. Carrel had inadvertently added new fibroblasts via the embryo broth used as nutrition for the tissue culture.

Hayflick found that, if he froze cells in culture after twenty divisions, they would "remember" that they had thirty doublings left when they were thawed and refed. Fifty cell divisions or doublings became called "the Hayflick limit." As fibroblasts approach fifty divisions, they begin looking old. They become larger and accumulate an increased amount of *lipofuscin,* a yellow pigment. The brownish "age spots" that appear on the skin are the result of cellular debris and lipofuscin clumping together.

The Telomere-Shortening Theory

Based on the Hayflick limit, experts on aging theorized that there is a genetic clock ticking away within each cell that determines when old age sets in. The latest, and most creditable, program theory of aging is the *telomere-shortening theory. Telomeres* are the end-cap segments of DNA (our genetic material). The concept that shortening of the telomere with each cellular replication leads to aging was first proposed by Russian scientist Alexaie Olovnikov in 1971, and soon after by James Watson (the codiscoverer of the structure of DNA) in 1972.[8] But it really wasn't until 1990, when a seminal paper was published based on the research of Cal Harley at McMaster University in Canada and Bruce Futcher and Carol Greider at Cold Spring Harbor Laboratory in New York, that the telomere theory of aging really began to be accepted.[9] New evidence supports the notion that telomeres are, in fact, the "clocks of aging."

Each time a cell replicates, a small piece of DNA is taken off the end of each chromo-

some. At conception, each telomere is about 10,000 base-pairs long. By birth, a telomere will have already been shortened by 5,000 base-pairs. Compared with the rest of the chromosome, the telomere is small; an average chromosome is 130,000,000 base-pairs long, or about 25,000 times as long as the telomere at birth. Every time a body cell replicates, the telomere gets shorter. The shorter the telomere gets, the more it affects the way the cell expresses its genetic code. The result is cellular aging.

In addition to serving as a clock for aging, the telomere is involved in: protecting the end of the chromosome from damage; allowing for more complete replication of the chromosome; controlling gene expression; and aiding in the organization of the chromosome. In other words, the telomere determines not only the aging of the cell, but our risk for cancer, Alzheimer's disease, and other degenerative diseases.[9]

Perhaps the greatest support for the telomere theory of aging is provided by the *Hutchinsom-Gilford syndrome.* You probably have never heard of this condition, but you may have heard of its common name: *progeria.* This syndrome was first described in 1886. Children with progeria are extraordinarily rare—one in eight million births—but if you ever see one, you will never forget it. The child typically shows symptoms of aging during the first year of life and generally dies of "old age" at the age of thirteen. Another rare syndrome, known as *Werner's syndrome,* is less severe; typically symptoms begin to manifest in the early twenties, and death usually occurs by age fifty.

Much has been learned from these children with progeria. If progeria is a reflection of accelerated aging—and few would argue that it isn't—it may hold the key to understanding how to truly extend life. Researchers have been working intensely to find the mechanism responsible for the accelerated aging produced by progeria. The answer appears to be telomere shortening. Compared with normal children, the telomeres of progeria children at birth are like those of a ninety-year-old. In Werner's syndrome, telomeres are at normal length at birth but appear to shorten faster than normal telomeres.

The key to extending human life span will ultimately involve preserving or restoring telomere length to the DNA. To read more about the telomere theory of aging, we refer you to *Reversing Human Aging* by Michael Fossel, Ph.D., M.D.[9]

The Free-Radical Theory

The best damage theory is the *free-radical theory* of aging. This theory contends that damage caused by free radicals contributes to aging and age-associated disease.[10] Free radicals are highly reactive molecules that can bind to and destroy cellular compounds. Free radicals may be derived from our environment (sunlight, X rays, radiation, chemicals), ingested in our food and drinks, or produced within our bodies during chemical reactions. The majority of free radicals in the body are actually produced within the body. However, exposure to environmental and dietary free radicals greatly increases the free-radical load in the body.

Cigarette smoking is a good example of how to increase free-radical load. Many of the deleterious health effects of smoking are related to the inhalation of extremely high levels of free radicals. Other external sources of free radicals include: radiation; air pollutants; pesticides; anesthetics; aromatic hydrocarbons (petroleum-based products); fried, barbecued, and charbroiled foods; alcohol; coffee; and solvents such as formaldehyde, toluene, and benzene that are found in cleaning fluids, paints, and furniture polish. Ob-

viously, reduced exposure to these sources of free radicals is recommended in a life-extension program.

Most free radicals in the body are toxic forms of oxygen molecules. It is ironic that the oxygen molecule is the major source of free-radical damage in our bodies. In one sense, oxygen sustains our lives, yet in another it is responsible for much of the destruction and aging of our cells. Similar to the formation of rust (oxidized iron), oxygen in its toxic state is able to oxidize (damage) molecules in our bodies. As you probably already know, compounds that prevent this type of damage are referred to as *antioxidants*.

In addition to their role in aging, free radicals have been linked to a number of human diseases, including atherosclerosis, cancer, Alzheimer's disease, cataracts, osteoarthritis, and immune deficiency.[11]

Free-radical damage is not limited to our cell membranes and proteins; it extends to our DNA. DNA is responsible for transmitting the characteristics of one generation of species or cells to another. Damage to the DNA structure results in *mutations* (expression of different genetic material) or in destruction or death of the cells. DNA is constantly bombarded by free radicals and other compounds that can cause damage. However, the body has enzymes that repair damaged DNA. The differences in life spans among mammals are largely a result of an animal's or human's ability to repair damaged DNA. For example, maximum human life span (about 120 years) is more than twice as long as that of a chimpanzee (about 50 years) because human DNA repair is much more effective.[12]

Research has shown that old cells are not able to repair DNA as rapidly as young cells. It appears that nature has set the rate of DNA repair at less than the rate of damage so that animals can accumulate mutations and evolve. If repair were perfect as a result of a complete antioxidant protection, there would be no evolutionary processes.

Glycosylation and Aging

Another damage theory that deserves mentioning is the *glycosylation theory*. In a nutshell, this theory involves the continued attachment of blood sugar *(glucose)* molecules to cellular proteins until finally the protein ceases to function properly.[14] For example, cholesterol-carrying proteins that have been glycosylated do not bind to receptors on liver cells that halt the manufacture of cholesterol. As a result, too much cholesterol is manufactured. Excessive glycosylation has many adverse effects: inactivation of enzymes, damage to structural and regulatory proteins, impaired immune function, and increased likelihood of autoimmune diseases.

Obviously we want to avoid excessive glycosylation. How is this done? By keeping blood sugar levels under control and taking high doses of vitamins E and C. Glycosylation is discussed in DIABETES, in Part III.

Extending Life Span

Can life span be increased and the aging process slowed? The answer is definitely "yes." Although we can't do much about our telomere length at this time, what we can do is protect our cells and help them to be as young and vibrant as possible. Here we will discuss specific interventions that are commonly recommended for reducing the aging process. In addition, it is important to incorporate the recommendations given in the chapter HEART AND CARDIOVASCULAR HEALTH; after all, heart disease is America's number-one killer.

Caloric Restriction

Severe restriction of caloric intake is a consistent and reproducible way of increasing life span in laboratory rats and mice.[15] However, it is not known if caloric restriction has any value for humans. Based on population studies accumulated by insurance companies and others, the following conclusion can be drawn: individuals who are either severely overweight or severely underweight have the shortest life span, while those whose weight is just below the average weight for their height have the longest life span.

Exercise

As stated in the chapter A HEALTHY LIFE-STYLE, the better shape you are in physically, the greater your odds of enjoying a healthier and longer life. Most studies have shown that an unfit individual carries eight times more risk of having a heart attack or stroke than a physically fit individual. Researchers have estimated that for every hour of exercise, there is a two-hour increase in longevity. That is quite a return on an investment. For more information on the importance of exercise to longevity, see the chapter A HEALTHY LIFESTYLE.

Dietary Antioxidants

The free-radical theory of aging really lends itself to intervention. Compounds that prevent free-radical damage are known as antioxidants or "free-radical scavengers."

The body has several enzymes that prevent the damage induced by specific types of free radicals. For example, superoxide dismutase (SOD) prevents the damage caused by the toxic oxygen molecule known as *superoxide. Catalase* and *glutathione peroxidase* are two other antioxidant enzymes found in the human body.

The level of antioxidant enzymes, as well as the level of dietary antioxidants such as beta-carotene, determines the life span of mammals. Human beings live longer than chimpanzees, cats, dogs, and many other mammals because we have a greater quantity of antioxidants within our cells.[13,16] Some strains of mice live longer than other strains because they have higher levels of antioxidant enzymes. Presumably, the reason why some people outlive others is that they have higher levels of antioxidants in their cells. This line of thinking is largely the reason many progressive-minded physicians recommend increasing the level of antioxidant mechanisms within cells.[1-3]

It is unlikely that antioxidant enzyme levels within cells can be increased by taking antioxidant enzymes such as SOD and glutathione peroxidase orally. Human subjects who take a tablet containing SOD do not appear to increase the level of SOD in their blood or tissues. Enzyme levels may be increased, however, by taking other dietary antioxidants.

Several studies in animals have demonstrated that dietary antioxidants can definitely increase life expectancy. We are just beginning to see human evidence. What we do know now is that antioxidant nutrients reduce the risk of getting cancer, heart disease, and many diseases linked to aging, including cataracts, macular degeneration, and arthritis.

Dietary antioxidants of extreme significance in life-extension include vitamins C and E, selenium, beta-carotene, flavonoids, sulfur-containing amino acids, and coenzyme Q_{10}. Not surprisingly, these same nutrients are also of extreme significance in cancer prevention, as aging and cancer share many common mechanisms.

Perhaps the most important dietary antioxidants for longevity are carotene molecules. Carotenes represent the most widespread group of naturally occurring pigments in plant life. For many people (physicians included), the term "carotene" is synonymous with "provitamin A," but only thirty to fifty of the more than four hundred carotenoids that have been characterized are believed to have vitamin A activity.[17]

Considerable evidence now demonstrates that carotenes do much more than serve as a precursor to vitamin A. Included in these effects are potent antioxidant effects. It has been shown that a high intake of beta-carotene from dietary sources is associated with a reduced rate of cancers involving epithelial cells (lung, skin, uterine cervix, respiratory tract, gastrointestinal tract, etc.).[17] Although research has primarily focused on beta-carotene, other carotenes are more potent in their antioxidant activity and are deposited in tissues to a greater degree. Keep in mind that a diet rich in beta-carotene is also high in many other carotenes.

Consumption of foods rich in carotenes (green leafy vegetables, yams, sweet potatoes, carrots, etc.) and supplementation with palm-oil carotene complex or carotene complexes from algae (as opposed to isolated, synthetic beta-carotene) are the best methods of increasing tissue carotenoid levels.

High carotene intake may also offer significant benefit to the immune system, as the thymus gland is largely composed of epithelial cells. The thymus gland undergoes a process of involution (shrinking) during normal aging and stress. This is largely a result of free-radical damage. Since carotenes are concentrated in the epithelial cells of the thymus, they are able to significantly lessen thymus-gland involution. In addition, studies have shown that thymus-gland-mediated immune functions could be improved with carotene supplementation (see IMMUNE SUPPORT).

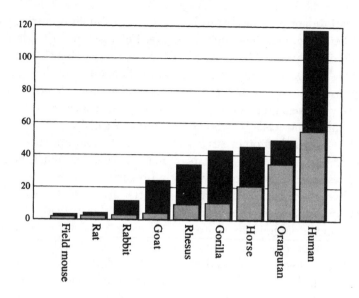

Concentration of carotenoids, in mcg/dl

Maximum life span potential, in years

FIGURE 1 Concentration of Carotenoids and Maximum Life Span Potential. Source: R. G. Cutler, Carotenoids and retinol: their possible importance in determining longevity of primate species. *Proc. Natl. Acad. Sci.* 81: 7627–31, 1984.

Flavonoids

Another group of plant pigments with remarkable protection against free-radical damage is the flavonoids. These compounds are largely responsible for the colors of fruits and flowers. However, they serve other functions in plant metabolism besides contributing to their aesthetic quality. In plants, flavonoids serve as protectors against environmental stress. In humans, flavonoids seem to function as "biological response modifiers."

Flavonoids appear to modify the body's reaction to other compounds such as allergens, viruses, and carcinogens, as evidenced by their anti-inflammatory, anti-allergic, antiviral, and anticancer properties.[18–20] Flavonoid molecules are also unique in their antioxidant and free-radical-scavenging activity, in that they are active against a wide variety of oxidants and free radicals.

The best way to assure an adequate intake of flavonoids is to eat a varied diet rich in fruits and vegetables. The best dietary sources of flavonoids include citrus fruits, berries, onions, parsley, legumes, green tea, and red wine.

Ginkgo biloba Extract

The *Ginkgo biloba* extract standardized to contain twenty-four percent ginkgoflavonglycosides has demonstrated remarkably beneficial effects in improving many symptoms associated with aging. *Ginkgo biloba* is especially useful in treating conditions linked to reduced blood flow to the brain, such as dizziness, ringing in the ears, headache, short-term memory loss, and depression.[21]

It is interesting to try to discover ginkgo's *doctrine of signature*. For centuries, it was believed that plants were "signed by the creator" with some visible or other clue that would indicate its therapeutic use. This concept is commonly referred to as "the doctrine of signatures."

Common examples of this doctrine: ginseng *(Panax ginseng)*, whose root bears strong resemblance to a human figure and whose general use is as a tonic; blue cohosh *(Caulophyllum thalictroides)*, whose branches are arranged like limbs in spasm, indicating its usefulness in the treatment of muscular spasm; bloodroot *(Sanguinaria canadensis)*, whose roots and sap are a beautiful blood color, corresponding to its traditional use as a "blood purifier"; lobelia *(Lobelia inflata)*, whose flowers are shaped like a stomach, corresponding to its emetic qualities; and goldenseal *(Hydrastis cana-densis)*, whose yellow-green root signifies its use in treating jaundice and infectious processes. All of these uses have been confirmed by recent research.

So what is ginkgo's doctrine of signature? Its long life and resistance to environmental stress. *Ginkgo biloba* is the world's oldest living tree species. The sole surviving species of the family Ginkgoaceae, the ginkgo tree can be traced back more than two hundred million years to the fossils of the Permian period. For this reason, it is often referred to as a "living fossil."

Once common in North America and Europe, the ginkgo was almost destroyed during the Ice Age in all regions of the world except China, where it is has long been cultivated as a sacred tree. The ginkgo tree was brought to America in 1784, to the garden of William Hamilton near Philadelphia. The ginkgo is now planted throughout much of the United States as an ornamental tree because it will grow where other trees are quick to die. Ginkgo is the tree most resistant to insects, disease, and pollution. As a result, it is frequently planted along streets in cities.

So ginkgo is associated with longevity and resistance to a polluted environment. It is interesting to observe it promoting longevity and helping us deal with our environment.

Key uses of *Ginkgo biloba* are in treating

Cerebral vascular insufficiency (insufficient blood flow to the brain)

Dementia

Depression

Impotence

Inner ear dysfunction (vertigo, tinnitus, etc.)

Multiple sclerosis

Neuralgia and neuropathy

Peripheral vascular insufficiency (intermittent claudication, Raynaud's syndrome, etc.)

Premenstrual syndrome

Retinopathy (macular degeneration, diabetic retinopathy, etc.)

Vascular fragility

Although the notion of a doctrine of signature is fanciful, the bottom line is this: *Ginkgo biloba* extract is extremely useful in increasing the quality of life in the elderly. Many symptoms common in the elderly are a result of insufficient blood and oxygen supply. *Ginkgo biloba* extract has demonstrated remarkable effects in improving blood and oxygen supply to tissues. Ginkgo is particularly effective in treating insufficient blood and oxygen supply to the brain, which is associated with a number of common symptoms of aging including short-term memory loss, dizziness, headache, ringing in the ears, hearing loss, lack of vigilance (get-up-and-go), and depression.[21]

Sulfur-Containing Amino Acids

The sulfur-containing amino acids methionine and cysteine are important components of a life-extension plan. Typically, as people age, the content of these amino acids in the body decreases.[22] Since supplementing the diets of mice and guinea pigs with cysteine increases life span considerably, it has been suggested that maintaining optimum levels of methionine and cysteine may promote longevity in humans.[22]

Dietary methionine and cysteine levels are a major determinant of the concentration of sulfur-containing compounds, such as glutathione, within cells. Glutathione assumes a critical role in the defense against a variety of injurious compounds by acting as part of the free-radical-scavenging enzyme glutathione peroxidase and by combining directly with these toxic substances to aid in their elimination. When increased levels of toxic compounds or free radicals are present in the body, the body needs higher levels of methionine and cysteine. For a more thorough discussion, see the section entitled Glutathione Conjugation in the chapter DETOXIFICATION.

Good dietary sources of methionine and cysteine are garlic, onions, fish, liver, eggs, Brewer's yeast, and nuts.

DHEA

The primary role of the adrenal hormone dehydroepiandrosterone (DHEA) is as a precursor for all other steroid hormones in the human body, including sex hormones and corticosteroids. Because DHEA levels tend to decline with aging, it has been postulated that raising DHEA levels through supplementation may offer some protection against the effects of aging. In fact, the benefits of DHEA supplementation may extend well beyond an anti-aging effect. Over the last decade, a number of studies have demonstrated that declining levels of DHEA are linked to such conditions as diabetes, obesity, elevated cholesterol levels, heart disease, arthritis, and autoimmune diseases. In addition, DHEA shows promise in enhancing memory and improving mental function in the elderly as well as increasing muscle strength and lean body mass, activating immune function, and enhancing the quality of life in aging men and women.[23] Further research will be required to determine whether DHEA supplementation will be a useful therapy in all of these conditions.

Although DHEA may prove useful in maintaining vim and vigor, we think it is not likely to significantly increase a person's life span. Why? For one thing, while some strains of rats live longer when taking DHEA, others do not. But probably the biggest argument against DHEA as a way to dramatically extend a healthy person's life is the observation that DHEA levels are normal in progeria. Surely if it was a significant factor in aging, levels would be low in people with progeria.

Nevertheless, although DHEA may not increase a person's quantity of life, it will often improve the quality. Our opinion is that DHEA offers significant benefits when used appropriately. One of the concerns we have about DHEA (as well as melatonin) is that so many people are using it unsupervised and with little or no respect for possible harmful effects. DHEA is not like vitamin C or many other nutrients that have virtually no toxicity. DHEA is a hormone about which we have relatively little information on long-term safety. It is safe if used appropriately, but it is a big gamble if abused.

As far as appropriate use goes, the only time we recommend DHEA to patients under the age of forty (unless they have low DHEA levels in their blood) is in women with autoimmune diseases such as lupus, rheumatoid arthritis, and multiple sclerosis. The typical dosage for these women is 50 to 100 mg per day. Dosages at this level can cause pimple formation for the first few weeks of therapy. If this occurs, try reducing the dosage. The pimples seem to be a small price to pay for significant benefits in relieving some of the symptoms of these diseases. Good results have been demonstrated in double-blind studies on women with lupus.

For men aged forty to fifty, we recommend taking DHEA if they are complaining of reduced libido or fatigue, or if they have diabetes. We recommend basing the dosage on blood levels of DHEA and testosterone. Typically, the prescribed dose ranges from 15 to 25 mg per day. For men over fifty, we recommend using blood or saliva measurements to determine the dosage. For men who desire to increase their libido and their sense of well-being, our goal has been to raise their testosterone and DHEA levels to those of a man in his early twenties. Typically, we have found the dosage required to achieve this goal is between 25 and 50 mg.

For women who have not yet passed through menopause, we do not recommend DHEA supplementation unless there is confirmation that DHEA levels are low. The reason is that, for many women approaching menopause, there is actually an increase in DHEA levels. Taking extra DHEA may lead to acne and increased facial hair. After menopause, we recommend using DHEA with caution and in low doses, ranging from 5 to 15 mg, unless the woman has an autoimmune disease or diabetes.

As men and women reach their seventies, they may require higher levels of DHEA, but until more is known we would rather err on the side of being conservative.

Melatonin

Melatonin (not to be confused with *melanin,* the compound responsible for skin pigmentation) is a hormone manufactured from *serotonin* (an important neurotransmitter; see DEPRESSION for more information) and secreted by the pineal gland. The pineal gland, a small pea-sized gland at the base of the brain, has been a source of curiosity since antiquity. The ancient Greeks considered the pineal gland to be the seat of the soul, a concept that was extended by the philosopher Descartes. In the seventeenth and eighteenth centuries, physicians associated "madness" with the pineal gland. Physicians in the early 1900s believed that the pineal gland was somehow involved with the endocrine system. The identification of melatonin in 1958 provided the first solid scientific evidence of an essential role of the pineal gland. It is now thought that the sole function of the pineal gland is to manufacture and secrete melatonin.

The exact function of melatonin is still poorly understood, but it is critically involved in the synchronization of hormone secretion. The natural daily cycle of hormone secretion is referred to as a *circadian rhythm.* The human body is governed by an internal clock that signals the secretion of various hormones at different times to regulate body functions. Melatonin plays a key role as the biological timekeeper of hormone secretion. Melatonin also helps control periods of sleepiness and wakefulness. Release of melatonin is stimulated by darkness and suppressed by light.

In addition to its role in synchronizing hormone secretion, melatonin has been shown to possess antioxidant effects.[24] This action may explain the studies in rats showing that melatonin supplementation led to longer lives (thirty-one months versus twenty-five months). However, the clinical significance of melatonin's antioxidant effects have not been fully determined. It is hard to imagine that its antioxidant effects would have greater significance than those of vitamin C, vitamin E, and a host of other antioxidants that can be delivered at much higher concentrations and, as a result, provide much greater antioxidant protection.

At this time, we believe that the same kind of precautions given in the previous section for DHEA are also appropriate for melatonin. Although there appear to be no serious side effects at recommended dosages, melatonin supplementation could conceivably disrupt normal circadian rhythms. The dosage typically recommended (3 mg per day) is much greater than the twenty-four-hour urinary excretion rate for melatonin (approximately 0.03 mg). In one study, a dosage of 8 mg per day for only four days resulted in significant alteration in circadian rhythm as noted by changes in the secretion patterns of several hormones.[25] It is not known what sort of effect would occur at commonly recommended dosages.

Melatonin has a place in the treatment of insomnia, jet lag, and possibly even some forms of cancer. Certainly, melatonin supplementation is appropriate as replacement therapy—that is, supplementing melatonin at a level that compensates for decreased synthesis (0.1 to 0.3 mg). But should higher dosages of melatonin be used as an antioxidant to promote a longer life? We think it is more important to focus on other factors.

Stress Management

. . . .

Stress produces a biological response.

Prolonged stress places a tremendous load on many organ systems, especially the heart, blood vessels, adrenals, and immune system.

Learning to calm the mind and body is extremely important in relieving stress.

One of the most powerful ways to decrease stress and increase energy in the body is by breathing with the diaphragm.

Lifestyle is a major determinant of an individual's stress levels.

In addition to addressing negative coping patterns, the two primary areas of concern are time management and relationship issues.

Key dietary recommendations:
- **Eliminate or restrict the intake of caffeine**
- **Eliminate or restrict the intake of alcohol**
- **Eliminate refined carbohydrates from the diet**
- **Increase the potassium-to-sodium ratio in the diet**
- **Eat regular planned meals in a relaxed environment**
- **Control food allergies**

Ginseng improves the ability to deal with stress.

Most Americans know something about stress. In fact, most of us have accepted the fact that everyday stress is part of modern living. Job pressures, family arguments, financial pressures, and never having enough time are just a few of the stressors most of us face daily. Although we often think of a stressor as something that causes us to feel "stressed out," technically speaking a stressor may be almost any disturbance—heat or cold, environmental toxics, toxins produced by microorganisms, physical trauma, and strong emotional reactions—that can trigger a number of biological changes to produce what is commonly known as the *stress response*.

Fortunately for us, control mechanisms known as the stress response in the body are geared toward counteracting the everyday stresses of life. Typically the stress response is so mild that it goes entirely unnoticed. However, if stress is extreme, unusual, or long-lasting, these control mechanisms can be overwhelming and quite harmful.

Recognizing Stress

Have you ever been suddenly frightened? If you have, you know what it feels like to have *adrenaline* surge through your body. Adrenaline is released from your *adrenal glands*, a pair of glands that lie on top of each kidney.

Adrenaline was designed to give the body that extra energy boost to escape from danger. Unfortunately, it can also make us feel stress, anxiety, and nervousness.

Many people are not sensitive enough to recognize what is causing them to feel stressed. What these people may notice are the physical signs of stress, such as insomnia, depression, fatigue, headache, upset stomach, digestive disturbances, and irritability. Many people going to physicians with these complaints may be suffering from unrecognized stressors.

The General Adaptation Syndrome

The stress response is actually part of a larger response known as the *general adaptation*
syndrome. To fully understand how to combat stress, it is important that we take a closer look at the general adaptation syndrome. The general adaptation syndrome is broken down into three phases: alarm, resistance, and exhaustion. These phases are largely controlled and regulated by the adrenal glands.

The initial response to stress is the *alarm reaction,* which is often referred to as the *fight-or-flight response.* The fight-or-flight response is triggered by reactions in the brain that ultimately cause the pituitary gland to release adrenocorticotropic hormone (ACTH), which causes the adrenals to secrete adrenaline and other stress-related hormones.

The fight-or-flight response is designed to counteract danger by mobilizing the body's resources for immediate physical activity. As a result, the heart rate and force of contraction of the heart increase to provide blood to areas necessary for response to the stressful

. . . .

QUICK REVIEW

Comprehensive stress management involves several approaches:

- Identify stressors
- Eliminate or reduce sources of stress
- Identify negative coping patterns and replace them with positive patterns
- Perform a relaxation/breathing exercise for a minimum of five minutes twice daily
- Manage time effectively
- Enhance relationships through better communication
- Get regular exercise

- Follow these dietary guidelines:
  Eliminate or restrict the intake of caffeine
  Eliminate or restrict the intake of alcohol
  Eliminate refined carbohydrates from the diet
  Increase the potassium-to-sodium ratio
  Eat regular planned meals in a relaxed environment
  Control food allergies
- Use adrenal supportive therapy, as described in the following section

Nutritional Supplements

Follow the recommendations given in the chapter SUPPLEMENTARY MEASURES.

situation. Blood is shunted away from the skin and internal organs, except the heart and lungs, while the amount of blood supplying needed oxygen and glucose to the muscles and brain is increased. The rate of breathing increases to supply necessary oxygen to the heart, brain, and exercising muscle. Sweat production increases to eliminate toxic compounds produced by the body and to lower body temperature. Production of digestive secretions is severely reduced since digestive activity is not critical for counteracting stress. And blood sugar levels are increased dramatically as the liver dumps stored glucose into the bloodstream.

While the alarm phase is usually short-lived, the next phase—*the resistance reaction*—allows the body to continue fighting a stressor long after the effects of the fight-or-flight response have worn off. Other hormones, such as cortisol and other cortico-steroids secreted by the adrenal cortex, are largely responsible for the resistance reaction. For example, these hormones stimulate the conversion of protein to energy so that the body has a large supply of energy long after glucose stores are depleted; they also promote the retention of sodium to keep blood pressure elevated.

In addition to providing the necessary energy and circulatory changes required to deal effectively with stress, the resistance reaction provides those changes required for meeting emotional crisis, performing strenuous tasks, and fighting infection. However, while the effects of adrenal cortex hormones are necessary when the body is faced with danger, continued stress or prolongation of the resistance reaction increases the risk of significant disease (including diabetes, high blood pressure, and cancer) and results in the final stage of the general adaptation syndrome: exhaustion.

Botanical Medicines

- *Panax ginseng*

  High-quality crude ginseng root:
    1–2 g one to three times per day
  Standardized extract (5% ginsenosides):
    100 mg one to three times per day

- *Eleutherococcus senticosus*

  (dosages are three times per day)
  Dried root: 2–4 g
  Tincture (1:5): 10–20 ml
  Fluid extract (1:1): 2–4 ml
  Solid (dry powdered) extract (20:1):
    100–200 mg

Because each individual's response to ginseng is unique, be alert for possible ginseng toxicity; irritability, nervousness, and insomnia are early manifestations. It is best to begin at lower doses and increase dosage gradually. The Russian approach for long-term administration of either Chinese or Siberian ginseng is to use ginseng cyclically for a period of fifteen to twenty days, followed by a two-week interval without any ginseng. This recommendation appears prudent to give the adrenal glands a little rest.

Exhaustion may manifest as a total collapse of body function or as a collapse of specific organs. Two of the major causes of exhaustion are losses of potassium ions and depletion of adrenal glucocorticoid hormones such as cortisone. When the cells of the body lose potassium they function less effectively and eventually die. When adrenal glucocorticoid stores become depleted, *hypoglycemia* results and cells of the body do not receive enough glucose and other nutrients.

Another cause of exhaustion is weakening of the organs. Prolonged stress places a tremendous load on many organ systems, especially the heart, blood vessels, adrenals, and immune system.

CONDITIONS LINKED TO STRESS

Angina
Asthma
Autoimmune disease
Cancer
Cardiovascular disease
Common cold
Depression
Diabetes (adult onset, Type II)
Headaches
Hypertension
Immune suppression
Irritable bowel syndrome
Menstrual irregularities
Premenstrual tension syndrome
Rheumatoid arthritis
Ulcerative colitis
Ulcers

A Healthy View of Stress

The father of modern stress research was Hans Selye, M.D. Having spent many years studying stress, Dr. Selye probably developed the best perspective on the role of stress and disease. According to Dr. Selye, stress in itself should not be viewed as a negative phenomenon. It is not the stressor that determines the response; instead it is the individual's internal reaction that triggers the response. This internal reaction is highly individualized. What one person may experience as stress, the next person may view entirely differently. Selye perhaps summarized his view best in a passage in his book, *The Stress of Life*.

No one can live without experiencing some degree of stress all the time. You may think that only serious disease or intensive physical or mental injury can cause stress. This is false. Crossing a busy intersection, exposure to a draft, or even sheer joy are enough to activate the body's stress mechanisms to some extent. Stress is not even necessarily bad for you; it is also the spice of life, for any emotion, any activity causes stress. But, of course, your system must be prepared to take it. The same stress which makes one person sick can be an invigorating experience for another.[1]

The key statement Selye made may be "your system must be prepared to take it." It is our goal to help prepare and bolster your stress-fighting system by detailing an effective comprehensive stress-management system.

Determining Stress Levels

To determine the role that stress may play in a given patient's health problems, many physicians utilize a popular method of rating stress levels—the Social Readjustment Rating Scale—developed by Holmes and Rahe.[2] The scale was originally designed to predict the likelihood of a person getting a serious

TABLE 1 The Social Readjustment Rating Scale

RANK	LIFE EVENT	MEAN VALUE
1	Death of spouse	100
2	Divorce	73
3	Marital separation	65
4	Jail term	63
5	Death of a close family member	63
6	Personal injury or illness	53
7	Marriage	50
8	Fired at work	47
9	Marital reconciliation	45
10	Retirement	45
11	Change in health of family member	44
12	Pregnancy	40
13	Sex difficulties	39
14	Gain of a new family member	39
15	Business adjustment	39
16	Change in financial state	38
17	Death of a close friend	37
18	Change to different line of work	36
19	Change in number of arguments with spouse	35
20	Large mortgage	31
21	Foreclosure of mortgage or loan	30
22	Change in responsibilities at work	29
23	Son or daughter leaving home	29
24	Trouble with in-laws	29
25	Outstanding personal achievement	28
26	Wife begins or stops work	26
27	Begin or end school	26
28	Change in living conditions	25
29	Revision of personal habits	24
30	Trouble with boss	23
31	Change in work hours or conditions	20
32	Change in residence	20
33	Change in schools	20
34	Change in recreation	19
35	Change in church activities	19
36	Change in social activities	18
37	Small mortgage	17
38	Change in sleeping habits	16
39	Change in number of family get-togethers	15
40	Change in eating habits	15
41	Vacation	13
42	Christmas	12
43	Minor violations of the law	11

disease due to stress. Various life-change events are numerically rated according to their potential for causing disease. Notice that even events commonly viewed as positive, such as an outstanding personal achievement, cause stress.

If a person is under a great deal of immediate stress or has endured a fair amount of stress over a few months' time or longer, it is appropriate to more accurately assess adrenal dysfunction by utilizing laboratory methods that measure levels of cortisol and dehydroepiandrosterone (DHEA).

Interpretation

The standard interpretation of the Social Readjustment Rating Scale is that a total of 200 or more points in one year indicates a likelihood of getting a serious disease. However, rather than using the scale solely to predict the likelihood of the patient getting a serious disease, we utilize the scale to gain insight into a person's stress level. Not everyone reacts to stressful events in the same way. The scale is a rough indicator of stress level.

Managing Stress

Whether you are aware of it or not, you have developed a pattern for coping with stress. Unfortunately, most people have found patterns and methods that ultimately do not support good health. Negative coping patterns must be identified and replaced with positive ways of coping. Use the following box to try to identify any negative or destructive coping patterns that you may have developed, and replace the pattern with more positive measures for dealing with stress described later.

NEGATIVE COPING PATTERNS
- Dependence on chemicals
  Drugs, legal and illicit
  Alcohol
  Smoking
- Overeating
- Watching too much television
- Emotional outbursts
- Feelings of helplessness
- Overspending
- Excessive behavior

In order to deal with stress effectively, it is critical that an individual concentrate on five equally important areas. The five components of an effective positive stress management program are

1. Techniques to calm the mind and promote a positive mental attitude
2. Lifestyle factors (time management, relationship issues)
3. Exercise
4. A healthful diet designed to nourish the body and support physiological processes
5. Supplementary measures designed to support the body as a whole, but especially the adrenal glands

Calming the Mind and Body

Learning to calm the mind and body is extremely important in relieving stress. When the mind and body are calm, stress seems to simply melt away. Relaxation exercises are among the easiest methods for quieting the body and mind. The goal of relaxation techniques is to produce a physiological response known as the *relaxation response*—a response that is exactly the opposite of the stress response. Although an individual may relax by simply sleeping, watching television, or reading a book, relaxation techniques are designed specifically to produce the relaxation response.

The term "relaxation response" was coined in the early 1970s by Harvard professor and cardiologist Herbert Benson, M.D., to describe a physiological response that is just the opposite of the stress response.[3] In the stress response, the sympathetic nervous system dominates. In the relaxation response, the parasympathetic nervous system dominates. The *parasympathetic nervous system* controls bodily functions such as digestion, breathing, and heart rate during periods of rest, relaxation, visualization, meditation, and sleep. While the sympathetic nervous system is designed to protect us against immediate danger, the parasympathetic nervous system is designed for repair, maintenance, and restoration of the body.

To achieve the relaxation response, a variety of techniques can be used. It really doesn't matter which technique is used; in the end they all should produce the same physiological state of deep relaxation. Some of the popular techniques are meditation, prayer, progressive relaxation, self-hypnosis, and biofeedback. The type of relaxation technique best for each person is totally individual. The important thing is that at least five to ten minutes be set aside each day for performing a relaxation technique.

TABLE 2   The Stress Response vs. the Relaxation Response

THE STRESS RESPONSE	THE RELAXATION RESPONSE
The heart rate and force of contraction of the heart increases to provide blood to areas necessary for response to the stressful situation.	The heart rate is reduced and the heart beats more effectively. Blood pressure is reduced.
Blood is shunted away from the skin and internal organs, except the heart and lungs, while at the same time the amount of blood supplying needed oxygen and glucose to the muscles and brain is increased.	Blood is shunted toward internal organs, especially those organs involved in digestion.
The rate of breathing increases to supply necessary oxygen to the heart, brain, and exercising muscle.	The rate of breathing decreases as oxygen demand is reduced during periods of rest.
Sweat production increases to eliminate toxic compounds produced by the body and to lower body temperature.	Sweat production decreases, as a person who is calm and relaxed does not experience nervous perspiration.
Production of digestive secretions is severely reduced since digestive activity is not critical for counteracting stress.	Production of digestive secretions is increased, greatly improving digestion.
Blood sugar levels are increased dramatically as the liver dumps stored glucose into the bloodstream.	Blood sugar levels are maintained in the normal physiological range.

Diaphragmatic Breathing

Producing deep relaxation with any technique requires learning how to breathe. One of the most powerful ways to decrease stress and increase energy in the body is by breathing with the diaphragm. By using the diaphragm to breathe, a person's physiology can be dramatically changed, literally activating the relaxation centers in the brain.

Here is a popular way to learn to breathe with your diaphragm:

- Find a quiet, comfortable place to sit or lie down.
- Place your feet slightly apart. Place one hand on your abdomen near your navel. Place the other hand on your chest.
- Inhale through your nose and exhale through your mouth.
- Concentrate on your breathing. Notice which hand is rising and falling with each breath.
- Gently exhale most of the air in your lungs.
- Inhale while slowly counting to four. As you inhale, slightly extend your abdomen, causing it to rise about 1 inch. Make sure that you are not moving your chest or shoulders.
- As you breathe in, imagine the warmed air flowing in. Imagine this warmth flowing to all parts of your body.
- Pause for one second, then slowly exhale to a count of four. As you exhale, your abdomen should move inward.
- As the air flows out, imagine all your tension and stress leaving your body.
- Repeat the process until you achieve a sense of deep relaxation.

Progressive Relaxation

One of the most popular techniques for producing the relaxation response is *progressive relaxation*. Many people are not aware of the sensation of relaxation. In progressive relaxation, an individual is taught what it feels like to relax by comparing relaxation to muscle tension. This technique is often used in the treatment of anxiety and insomnia.

The basic procedure is to forcefully contract a muscle for one to two seconds and then give way to a feeling of relaxation. Since the procedure goes progressively through all the muscles of the body, eventually a deep state of relaxation will result.

Begin by contracting the muscles of your face and neck, holding the contraction for a period of at least one to two seconds and then relaxing the muscles. Next, contract and relax your upper arms and chest, followed by your lower arms and hands. Repeat the process progressively down your body: abdomen, buttocks, thighs, calves, and feet. Then repeat the whole sequence two or three times.

Lifestyle Factors

Lifestyle is a major determinant of an individual's stress levels. In addition to addressing negative coping patterns, the two primary areas of concern are time management and relationship issues.

Time Management

One of the biggest stressors for most people is time; they simply feel they do not have enough of it. Here are some tips on time management:

- Set priorities. Realize that you can only accomplish so much in a day. Decide what is most important, and limit your efforts to that goal.
- Organize your day. There are always interruptions and unplanned demands on your time, but create a definite plan for the day based on your priorities. Avoid the pitfall of always letting the immediate demands control your life.

- Delegate as much authority and work as you can. You can't do everything yourself. Learn to train and depend on others.
- Tackle tough jobs first. Handle the most important tasks first, while your energy levels are high. Leave the busywork or running around for later in the day.
- Minimize meeting time. Schedule meetings to bump up against the lunch hour or quitting time; that way they can't last forever.
- Avoid putting things off. Work done under the pressure of an unreasonable deadline often has to be redone. That creates more stress than if it had been done right the first time. Plan ahead.
- Don't be a perfectionist. You can never really achieve perfection anyway. Do your best in a reasonable amount of time and then move on to other important tasks. If you find time, you can always come back later and polish the task some more.

Relationship Issues

Another major cause of stress for many people is interpersonal relationships. Relationships can be divided into three major categories: marital, family, and job-related. The quality of any relationship ultimately comes down to the quality of the communication. Learning to communicate effectively goes a long way toward reducing the stress and conflicts of interpersonal relationships. Here are some tips for effective communication, regardless of the type of relationship:

- The first key to successful communication is the most important: learn to be a good listener. Allow the people you are communicating with to really share their feelings and thoughts uninterrupted. Empathize with them; put yourself in their shoes. If you first seek to understand, you will find yourself being better understood.

- Be an active listener. This means that you must act really interested in what the other person is communicating. Listen to what is being said instead of thinking about your response. Ask questions to gain more information or clarification; good questions open lines of communication.
- Be a reflective listener. Restate or reflect back to the other person your interpretation of what he or she is telling you. This simple technique shows the other person that you are both listening and understanding. Restating what you think is being said may cause some short-term conflict in some situations, but it is certainly worth the risk.
- Wait to speak until the people you want to communicate with are listening. If they are not ready to listen, you will not be heard no matter how well you communicate.
- Don't try to talk over somebody. If you find yourself being interrupted, relax; don't try to out-talk the other person. If you are courteous and allow people to speak, all but the rudest ones will eventually respond in kind. If they don't, point out that they are interrupting the communication process. You can only do this if you have been a good listener; double standards in relationships seldom work.
- Help other people to become active listeners. This can be done by asking if they understood what you were communicating. Ask them to tell you what they heard. If they don't seem to understand what you are saying, persist until they do.
- Don't be afraid of long silences. Human communication involves much more than words; a great deal can be communicated during silences. Unfortunately, in many situations, silence can make us feel uncomfortable. Relax. Some people need silence to collect their thoughts and feel safe in communicating. The important thing to

remember during silences is to remain an active listener.

Exercise

The immediate effect of exercise is to cause stress on the body. However, with a regular exercise program the body adapts. The body's response to this regular stress is to become stronger, function more efficiently, and have greater endurance. Exercise is a vital component of a comprehensive stress management program and of overall good health.

People who exercise regularly are much less likely to suffer from fatigue and depression. Tension, depression, feelings of inadequacy, and worries diminish greatly with regular exercise. Exercise alone has been demonstrated to have a tremendous impact on improving mood and the ability to handle stressful life situations.

Healthful Diet

People who suffer from stress or anxiety need to support the biochemistry of the body by following some important dietary guidelines. Specifically

- Eliminate or restrict the intake of caffeine
- Eliminate or restrict the intake of alcohol
- Eliminate refined carbohydrates from the diet
- Increase the potassium-to-sodium ratio in the diet
- Eat regular planned meals in a relaxed environment
- Control food allergies

According to Hans Selye, M.D., the difference between stress that is harmful and stress that is not harmful depends on the strength of a person's system. From a purely physiological perspective, it can be strongly argued that delivery of high-quality nutrition to the cells of the body is the critical factor in determining the strength of the system.

When the eating habits of Americans are examined as a whole, it is little wonder that so many people are suffering from stress, anxiety, and fatigue. Most Americans are not providing the body the high-quality nutrition it deserves. Instead of eating foods rich in vital nutrients, most Americans focus on refined foods high in calories, sugar, fat, and cholesterol.

Caffeine and Stress Levels

The average American consumes 150 to 225 mg of caffeine daily, or roughly the amount of caffeine in one to two cups of coffee. Although most people can handle this amount, some people are more sensitive to the effects of caffeine than other people due to a slower elimination of these substances from the body. Even small amounts of caffeine, as found in decaffeinated coffee, are enough to affect some people adversely and produce *caffeinism*—a medical condition characterized by symptoms of depression, nervousness, irritability, recurrent headache, heart palpitations, and insomnia. People prone to feeling stress and anxiety tend to be especially sensitive to caffeine.[4,5]

Chronic caffeine intake is linked to anxiety as well as depression for the same reasons that it produces mental and physical stimulation. Caffeine produces significant alteration of brain chemistry. Long-term use of caffeine-containing beverages, especially coffee, should be avoided by people who suffer from stress, anxiety, insomnia, depression, or any other psychiatric disorder.

Alcohol Intake

Alcohol produces chemical stress on the body. It also increases adrenal hormone output, interferes with normal brain chemistry, and interferes with normal sleep cycles.

While many people believe that alcohol has a calming effect, a study in which ninety healthy male volunteers were given either a placebo or alcohol demonstrated significant increases in anxiety scores after drinking the alcohol.[5] It is our recommendation that alcohol be avoided entirely by people with symptoms of stress, anxiety, or insomnia.

Refined Carbohydrates

Refined carbohydrates (sugar and white flour) are known to contribute to problems with blood sugar control, especially hypoglycemia. The association between hypoglycemia and impaired mental function is well known. Unfortunately, most individuals who experience depression, anxiety, or other psychological conditions are rarely tested for hypoglycemia, nor are they prescribed a diet that restricts refined carbohydrates.

Numerous studies of depressed individuals have shown a high occurrence of hypoglycemia.[6,7] Because depression is one of the most frequent causes of anxiety, this provides a link between hypoglycemia and feelings of stress. Simply eliminating refined carbohydrates from the diet is sometimes all that is needed for effective therapy in patients who have depression or anxiety due to hypoglycemia.

Increased Potassium-to-Sodium Ratio

One of the key dietary recommendations to support the adrenal glands is to ensure adequate potassium levels within the body. This can best be done by consuming foods rich in potassium and avoiding foods high in sodium. Please refer to the chapter A HEALTH-PROMOTING DIET for more information on potassium and sodium in the diet.

Mealtime Atmosphere

Mealtimes should be spent in a relaxed environment. As noted above, digestion is a process largely controlled by the parasympathetic nervous system. Eating in a rushed manner or in a noisy environment is not conducive to good digestion or good health. It is important to plan meals out in advance to avoid eating on the run or under stress.

Food Allergies

People with symptoms of anxiety or chronic fatigue need to investigate possible food allergies. As far back as 1930, noted allergist Dr. Albert Rowe noticed that anxiety and fatigue were key features associated with food allergies.[8] Originally, Dr. Rowe described a syndrome he called *allergic toxemia*, with symptoms that included anxiety, fatigue, muscle and joint aches, drowsiness, difficulty in concentration, and depression. Around the 1950s, this syndrome became referred to as the *allergic tension-fatigue syndrome*. With the current focus on chronic fatigue syndrome, many physicians and other people are forgetting that food allergies can lead to chronic fatigue.

Nutritional and Herbal Support

Nutritional and herbal support for a person who has signs and symptoms of stress largely involves supporting the adrenal glands. The adrenal glands control many body functions and play a critical role in the resistance to stress. If an individual has experienced a great deal of stress or has taken corticosteroids for a long period of time, the adrenal glands will shrink and not perform properly, causing the person to experience anxiety, depression, or chronic fatigue.

An abnormal adrenal response—either deficient or excessive hormone release—

significantly alters an individual's response to stress. Often the adrenals become "exhausted" as a result of constant demands placed upon them. An individual with adrenal exhaustion will usually suffer from chronic fatigue, may complain of feeling stressed out or anxious, and will typically have a reduced resistance to allergies and infection.

Atrophy of the adrenal cortex is a common side effect of continual stress or cortisone administration. Due to the importance of the adrenal gland, optimal stress management is dependent on optimal adrenal function.

Key Nutrients

Several nutrients are especially important in supporting adrenal function: vitamin C, pantothenic acid, vitamin B6, zinc, and magnesium. All of these nutrients play a critical role in the health of the adrenal gland as well as the manufacture of adrenal hormones. Evidence indicates that the levels of these nutrients in the adrenals can plummet during times of stress.

For example, it is well known that during times of chemical, emotional, psychological, or physiological stress, the urinary excretion of vitamin C is increased, signifying an increased need for vitamin C during these times. Examples of chemical stressors include cigarette smoke, pollutants, and allergens. Extra vitamin C, in the form of supplementation along with an increased intake of vitamin C–rich foods, is often recommended to keep the immune system working properly during times of stress.

Pantothenic acid (vitamin B5) is equally important during periods of high stress or in individuals who need adrenal support. Pantothenic acid deficiency results in adrenal atrophy characterized by fatigue, headache, sleep disturbances, nausea, and abdominal discomfort. Pantothenic acid is found in whole grains, legumes, cauliflower, broccoli, salmon, liver, sweet potatoes, and tomatoes. For patients who suffer from chronic stress or who have a history of corticosteroid (prednisone) use, nutritionally oriented physicians often recommend supplementing the diet with 100 to 500 mg of pantothenic acid daily.

The other key nutrients—vitamin B6, zinc, and magnesium—should be taken in daily dosages of 50 to 100 mg, 20 to 30 mg, and 250 to 500 mg, respectively.

Ginseng and Stress

There are numerous botanical medicines that support adrenal function. Most notable are the ginsengs. Both Chinese ginseng (*Panax ginseng*) and Siberian ginseng (*Eleutherococcus senticosus*) exert beneficial effects on adrenal function and enhance resistance to stress. These ginsengs are often referred to as *general tonics* or *adaptogens*.

The term "general tonic" implies that an herb will increase the overall tone of the whole body. The ginsengs are also often referred to as *adrenal tonics* because they increase the tone and function of the adrenal glands. Both Chinese and Siberian ginseng can be used to: restore vitality in debilitated and feeble individuals; increase feelings of energy; increase mental and physical performance; prevent the negative effects of stress and enhance the body's response to stress; offset some of the negative effects of cortisone; enhance liver function; and protect against radiation damage. All of these applications are backed up by good clinical research.[9–11]

The modern term "adaptogen" is a more descriptive term applied to the general tonic effects of Chinese and Siberian ginseng. An *adaptogen* is a substance that

1. Must be innocuous and cause minimal disorders in the physiological functions of an organism

2. Must have a nonspecific action (i.e., it should increase resistance to adverse influences by a wide range of physical, chemical, and biochemical factors)

3. Usually has a normalizing action irrespective of the direction of the pathologic state

According to tradition and scientific evidence, both Chinese and Siberian ginseng possess this kind of equilibrating, tonic, antistress action, so the term "adaptogen" is appropriate in describing their general effects.

The ginsengs have been shown to enhance a person's ability to cope with various stressors, both physical and mental.[9–11] Presumably this antistress action is regulated by mechanisms that control the adrenal glands. Ginseng delays the onset and reduces the severity of the alarm phase response of the general adaptation syndrome.

People who take either of the ginsengs typically report an increased sense of well-being. Clinical studies have confirmed that both Chinese and Siberian ginseng significantly reduce feelings of stress and anxiety. For example, in one double-blind clinical study, nurses who had switched from day to night duty rated themselves for competence, mood, and general well-being. They were also given a test for mental and physical performance, along with blood cell counts and blood chemistry evaluation.[12] The group administered Chinese ginseng demonstrated higher scores in competence, mood parameters, and mental and physical performance than the placebo group. The nurses who took the ginseng felt more alert yet more tranquil and were able to perform better than the nurses who did not take the ginseng.

In addition to these human studies, several animal studies have shown the ginsengs to exert significant anti-anxiety effects. In several of these studies, the stress-relieving effects were comparable to those of diazepam (Valium). However, while diazepam causes behavior changes, sedative effects, and impaired motor activity, ginseng produces none of these negative effects.[13]

Based on the clinical studies and the animal studies, it appears that ginseng offers significant benefit to people who suffer from stress and anxiety. Chinese ginseng is generally regarded as being more potent than Siberian ginseng. If a person has been under a great deal of stress, or is recovering from a long-standing illness, or has taken corticosteroids such as prednisone for a long period of time, the best ginseng is probably Chinese (Panax) ginseng. If a person has been under mild to moderate stress and has less obvious impaired adrenal function, Siberian ginseng may be the best choice.

PART THREE

SPECIFIC HEALTH PROBLEMS

Acne

Blackheads: dilated skin follicles with central dark, horny plugs

Whiteheads: red, swollen follicles with or without white pustules

Nodules: tender collections of pus deep in the skin that discharge to the surface of the skin

Cysts: deep nodules that fail to discharge contents to surface

Large deep pustules: cysts that contain inflammatory compounds that break down adjacent skin tissue, leading to scar formation

Acne is the most common of all skin problems. There are three major forms: acne vulgaris, acne conglobata, and acne rosacea. *Acne vulgaris* is characterized as a superficial disease that affects the hair follicles and oil-secreting glands of the skin; it manifests as blackheads, whiteheads, and inflammation (redness). Acne vulgaris is the least severe form of acne. On the other hand, *acne conglobata* is a more severe form, with cyst formation and subsequent scarring. *Acne rosacea* is a chronic acne-like eruption on the face of middle-aged and older adults, associated with facial flushing. It is discussed in its own chapter, ROSACEA.

In both superficial (acne vulgaris) and cystic (acne conglobata) acne, the lesions occur predominantly on the face and, to a lesser extent, on the back, chest, and shoulders. Both forms of acne are more common among males, and onset is typically at puberty (somewhat later for the cystic form).

Causes

Acne has its origin in the skin pore or, more accurately stated, the *pilosebaceous unit* (see Figure 1). These units usually consist of a hair follicle and the associated sebaceous glands, which are connected to the skin by the follicular canal through which the hair shaft passes. The *sebaceous glands* produce *sebum,* a mixture of oils and waxes that lubricates the skin and prevents the loss of water. Sebaceous glands are most highly concentrated on the face and, to a lesser extent, on the back, chest, and shoulders.

Acne is most common among males, with the onset usually at puberty. This occurrence is due to the fact that male sex hormones, such as testosterone, stimulate the cells that line the follicular canal to produce *keratin.* Keratin is a fibrous protein that is the main component of the outermost layer of skin as well as of hair and nails. Overproduction of keratin can block skin pores. In addition, the testosterone causes the sebaceous glands to enlarge and produce more sebum. So higher testosterone levels increase the likelihood that pores will become blocked by either excessive keratin or too much sebum. While boys are at greater risk, there is an increase in testosterone level in girls during puberty, making them susceptible as well.

While the onset of acne usually reflects an increase in testosterone level, the severity and progression of acne is determined by a complex interaction among hormonal factors, keratin-producing cells, sebum, and bacteria. Here is the basic scenario: pimples begin forming near the surface of the skin pore when the cells that line the canal start producing an excess of keratin; this eventually leads to blockage of the canal, resulting in ballooning and thinning; eventually a whitehead or blackhead is formed. A blackhead will form if the blockage is incomplete—allowing the sebum to make its way to the surface, thereby avoiding the inflammation of a whitehead (discussed below)—and a whitehead will form if the blockage is complete.

With the blockage of the canal, a bacterium known as *Propionibacterium acnes* (*Corynebacterium acnes*) is allowed to overgrow and release enzymes that break down sebum and promote inflammation. The redness of pimples is a result of this inflammation. If the bacterium grows out of control or if the inflammation is severe, it can result in the rupture of the wall of the hair canal and damage to surrounding tissue. If this happens at the skin surface, it simply causes superficial redness and pustules. However, if it occurs deeper within the skin, a nodule or cyst can form, leading to more significant damage and possibly scar formation.

Acne is typically considered to be a male-hormone-dependent condition. These hormones control sebaceous gland secretion and exacerbate the development of abnormal growth of the hair-follicle cells. But excessive secretion of male hormones is not necessarily the cause, since there is only a poor correlation between blood levels of these hormones and the severity of the disease.[1–3] What may be more important is that the skin of patients with acne shows greater activity of an enzyme called 5-alpha-reductase, which converts testosterone to a more potent form known as dihydrotestosterone (DHT).[4,5] In other words, it is not necessarily an increase in testosterone level in the blood that leads to the problem of acne; it is how the skin metabolizes this hormone.

Nutritional status seems to play a major role in acne, from both a preventive and therapeutic perspective. Another contributor to acne that is seldom recognized is intestinal toxemia. One study showed that fifty percent of patients with severe acne had increased blood levels of toxins absorbed from the intestines.[6] This situation has not been fully

. . . .

QUICK REVIEW

- Acne is the most common skin problem.
- Acne is most common among males during puberty, due to hormonal changes.
- Acne is dependent upon male hormones, such as testosterone, that stimulate the manufacture of sebum.
- Long-term use of antibiotics may result in an overgrowth of the yeast *Candida albicans*.
- The key dietary recommendation is to avoid sugar, trans-fatty acids, milk, fried foods, and iodine.
- Key nutrients to aid in the treatment of acne include chromium, vitamin A, vitamin E, selenium, and zinc.
- Topical treatment with tea tree oil or azelaic acid has produced results equal to benzoyl peroxide without the side effects.

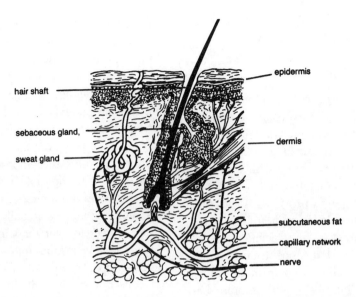

FIGURE 1 Normal Pilosebaceous Unit

evaluated at this time, but it is an interesting finding given that naturopathic physicians at the turn of the century viewed acne as largely a condition reflecting poor colon health.

If a person appears to have acne, it is important to make sure that it truly is acne. Exposure to a variety of compounds can produce the characteristic lesions of acne.

AGENTS THAT CAUSE ACNE-LIKE LESIONS

Drugs: steroids, diphenylhydantoin, and lithium carbonate

Industrial pollutants: machine oils, coal tar derivatives, and chlorinated hydrocarbons

Local actions: use of cosmetics or pomades, overwashing, or repetitive rubbing

---

Therapeutic Considerations

There are many important aspects to consider in the treatment of acne. An integrated therapeutic approach is required in order to

attain the desired results. Also, because many individuals have been treated with long-term, broad-spectrum antibiotics, they often develop intestinal overgrowth of the yeast *Candida albicans*. This chronic yeast infection may actually make acne worse and must be treated when present. (See CANDIDIASIS, CHRONIC.)

In addition to orally administered antibiotics, another popular treatment for acne is the use of over-the-counter preparations containing benzoyl peroxide (e.g., Oxy 5/Oxy 10, Clearasil, Benoxyl, etc.). Benzoyl peroxide acts as a skin antiseptic to keep the growth of bacteria down. It is most effective in superficial pimples that are inflamed. In order to be effective, benzoyl peroxide preparations must be applied on a daily basis. The primary side effect of benzoyl peroxide preparations is that they have a tendency to dry out the skin and/or cause redness and peeling.

The prescription topical medicine most often used is tretinoin (Retin-A). Side effects are more common with Retin-A than with benzoyl peroxide. The peeling and drying can be quite severe. It literally acts to improve acne by chemically burning the skin.

Dietary Considerations

Theories about direct dietary influences on acne are somewhat controversial in the medical literature. For example, theories implicating chocolate are extremely conflicting. Rather than get too caught up with specifics, we feel that it is most important to support the health of the skin by providing it with the best nutrition possible. In addition to a generally healthful diet, a few specifics are in order. All refined and/or concentrated simple sugars should be eliminated from the diet, and intake of high-fat foods should be limited. Foods containing trans-fatty acids (milk, milk products, margarine, shortening, and other synthetically hydrogenated vegetable oils) or oxidized fatty acids (fried oils) should be avoided. For those who are iodine-sensitive, foods high in iodine should be eliminated, including foods with a high salt content (most salt is "iodized"; this means that it has iodine added to it). Milk consumption should be limited due to its high hormone content in addition to its trans-fatty acid content.[7]

A high-protein diet may help. In one study, subjects fed a high-protein diet (forty-four percent protein, thirty-five percent carbohydrate, and twenty-one percent fat) showed substantially less conversion of testosterone to its more potent form (DHT).[8] A high-carbohydrate diet (ten percent protein, seventy percent carbohydrate, and twenty percent fat) had the opposite effect. These results suggest that a higher protein intake may help with acne, but this has yet to be proven.

Sugar, Insulin, and Chromium

Many dermatologists have reported that the hormone insulin is effective in the treatment of acne.[9–11] *Insulin* is the hormone that regulates blood sugar levels by promoting uptake of sugar by body cells. One study that compared the results of oral glucose tolerance tests (see the DIABETES chapter for a description) in acne patients showed no differences between those who received insulin and the control group. However, analysis of the level of glucose in the skin demonstrated that patients with acne do not metabolize sugar properly.[11] One researcher of the role of glucose tolerance in acne actually went so far as to refer to acne as "skin diabetes."[12]

The fact that insulin appears helpful also suggests impaired uptake of blood sugar by skin cells due to insensitivity to insulin. In several studies, insulin given either systemically by injection (5 to 10 units two to three times a week) or injected directly into the lesion resulted in significant improvement.[9,10] Rather than use insulin, it makes more sense to try to improve the situation by eliminating all concentrated refined sugar from the diet.

In addition, chromium supplementation is important. Chromium is known to improve glucose tolerance and enhance insulin sensitivity (see DIABETES), and has been reported in an uncontrolled study to induce rapid improvement in patients with acne.[13]

Vitamin A

Vitamin A has been shown in many studies to reduce sebum production and the buildup of keratin in the follicle. Unfortunately, the dosages that have been shown to be effective in treating acne (300 to 400,000 IU per day for five to six months) are high and potentially toxic.[14] High-dose vitamin A treatment should not be used without close supervision by a physician.

Laboratory tests appear unreliable in monitoring for vitamin A toxicity until obvious toxicity has developed. The first significant toxic symptom is usually headache, followed by fatigue, emotional instability, and muscle and joint pain. Chapped lips and dry skin are also early warning signs. Because high doses of vitamin A during pregnancy can cause birth defects, women of childbearing age should use effective birth control during vitamin A treatment and for at least one month after discontinuation.

We believe that using high dosages of vitamin A is not necessary if other nutritional factors, such as zinc and vitamin E, are included. These nutrients work with vitamin A in promoting healthy skin. A safe and effective recommendation for vitamin A in the treatment of acne is less than 25,000 IU per day. However, for sexually active women of childbearing age we do not recommend dosages of more than 5,000 IU of vitamin A per day unless an effective form of birth control is being used.

Zinc

Zinc is a very important nutrient for the health of the skin. Optimal zinc levels are a primary therapeutic goal in the natural treatment of acne. Zinc is involved in the proper metabolism of testosterone. When zinc levels are low, there is an increase in the conversion of testosterone to DHT. Remember, DHT stimulates the manufacture of sebum and keratin. Zinc is also involved in vitamin A function, wound healing, immune system activity, inflammation control, and tissue regeneration.

Low levels of zinc play a central role in many cases of adolescent acne, as zinc levels are lower in thirteen- and fourteen-year-old males than in any other age group.[15] There have been several double-blind studies on zinc supplementation in the treatment of acne, but the subject remains controversial.[16–19] The controversy stems from the fact that zinc has produced excellent results in some studies and virtually no effect in others.

The inconsistency of the results may be due to the differing rates of absorption and utilization of the forms of zinc used. For example, studies that used effervescent zinc sulfate showed effects similar to those of tetracycline (the most popular of the broad-spectrum antibiotics commonly used to treat acne), with fewer side effects from chronic use.[16] Studies that used plain zinc sulfate have shown less beneficial results.[17] The majority of patients who responded to zinc required twelve weeks of supplementation before good results were demonstrated, although some showed dramatic improvement immediately.

In the most recent study, sixty-six patients with inflammatory acne were given zinc gluconate (30 mg of elemental zinc) or a placebo for two months.[19] Based on the number and severity of lesions, an "inflammatory score" was attributed to each patient. In the placebo group, the inflammatory score dropped from fifty-eight to forty-seven during the two-month period, while in the treatment group the score dropped from forty-nine to twenty-seven. Physicians rated twenty-four of thirty-two patients in the zinc group as responding to treatment, compared to only eight of thirty-four in the placebo group.

This latest study, which produced excellent results, utilized a common form of zinc (zinc gluconate). Unfortunately, however, there have been no studies to date using zinc picolinate or zinc monomethionine, two of the better-absorbed forms of zinc.

Vitamin E and Selenium

Vitamin E is important in its own right in the treatment of acne, but it also is important for the proper functioning of vitamin A. During a vitamin E deficiency, blood levels of vitamin A stay low regardless of the amount of oral or intravenous vitamin A supplementation. Blood levels of vitamin A return to normal after vitamin E is restored to the diet.

Vitamin E is also important for its interactions with selenium. Selenium is an important antioxidant trace mineral that functions in the enzyme *glutathione peroxidase*. This enzyme is very important in preventing the inflammation of acne. Typically, acne patients have significantly decreased levels of glutathione peroxidase. After treatment with vitamin E and selenium, the level of this enzyme increases and the acne is significantly diminished.[20]

Pyridoxine

Women with premenstrual aggravation of acne are often responsive to vitamin B6 supplementation, reflecting its role in the normal metabolism of steroid hormones.[21] In rats, a vitamin B6 deficiency appears to cause both increased uptake of and sensitivity to testosterone.[22]

Pantothenic Acid

Pantothenic acid is important in fat metabolism and may be of value at high dosages in the treatment of acne. This potential benefit was evaluated in a study of 100 Chinese with acne. The study group consisted of forty-five males and fifty-five females between ten and thirty years of age; eighty percent were between the ages of thirteen and twenty-three.[23] They were given 10 grams of pantothenic acid per day, in four divided doses. They were also given a cream consisting of twenty percent pantothenic acid by weight, and were told to apply the cream to affected areas four to six times a day. Within one or two days after starting, there was a noticeable decrease in sebum secretion. Within one to two weeks, the frequency of new acne eruptions began to decline and existing lesions started to regress. No side effects were noted.

Hypothyroidism

Correcting an underlying thyroid problem can result in marked lessening of acne.[24] For more information on thyroid function, see HYPOTHYROIDISM.

Topical Treatments

A variety of topical gels, ointments, and creams containing natural products are available for use in the treatment of acne. The goal of these preparations is the same as that of the popular over-the-counter preparations containing benzoyl peroxide: reduce the bacteria level and reduce inflammation. Although there are many possibilities to choose from, the most popular formulas are those that feature either tea tree oil, azelaic acid, or sulfur.

Tea Tree Oil

Melaleuca alternifolia, or "tea tree," is a small tree native to only one area of the world: the northeast coastal region of New South Wales, Australia. The leaves—the portion of the plant that is used medicinally—are the source of a valuable therapeutic oil.

Tea tree oil possesses significant antiseptic properties and is regarded by many as the ideal skin disinfectant. This claim is supported by its efficacy against a wide range of organisms (including twenty-seven of thirty-two strains of *P. acnes*)[25] and its good penetration and lack of irritation to the skin. The therapeutic uses of tea tree oil are based largely on its antiseptic and antifungal properties.

In a study conducted at the Royal Prince Hospital in New South Wales, Australia, a five-percent tea tree oil solution was shown to demonstrate beneficial effects similar to those of five-percent benzoyl peroxide in treating acne, but with substantially fewer side effects.[26] However, this five-percent tea tree oil solution is probably not strong enough for moderate to severe acne. Stronger solutions (up to fifteen percent) should provide even better results. Numerous studies have shown that tea tree oil is extremely safe for use as a topical antiseptic, but it can occasionally produce contact dermatitis.

Azelaic Acid

This naturally occurring acid has exerted antibiotic activity against *P. acnes*. Clinical studies using twenty-percent azelaic acid creams have shown that it produces results equal to those achieved with benzoyl peroxide, Retin-A, or oral tetracycline.[27] It has been shown to be effective in treating all of the different forms of acne. In order to achieve benefits, azelaic acid must be applied to affected areas twice daily continuously for a period of at least four weeks. Treatment usually has to be continued for at least six months to maintain the benefits produced after the first month.

A recent review article found a topical cream containing twenty percent azelaic acid to be as effective as five-percent benzoyl peroxide, four-percent hydroquinone cream, 0.05-percent tretinoin, two-percent erythromycin, or oral tetracycline in relieving superficial acne, but less effective than oral Acutane (isotretinoin) in treating cystic acne.

The authors suggested that the few side effects of topical azelaic acid and its lack of overt systemic toxicity made it a better choice for chronic use. The lower incidence of side effects and allergic reactions offer a clear advantage over conventional drugs.[27]

Sulfur

Sulfur-containing products for the treatment of skin disorders have been around for thousands of years. Sulfur is a topical antiseptic, like benzoyl peroxide, but not as potent or irritating. Although sulfur-containing formulas are still around, they have been replaced by newer compounds, such as benzoyl peroxide. This doesn't mean that sulfur is not effective. In fact, preparations that contain three- to ten-percent sulfur have produced such good results, and are so widely accepted as therapeutic, that the Food and Drug Administration (FDA) has approved sulfur as a safe and effective acne treatment. Sulfur-containing products for the treatment of acne are available in health food stores as well as drugstores.

TREATMENT SUMMARY

The natural approach to acne is designed to address the underlying hormonal and local processes.

General Recommendations

- Avoid medications that may cause acne:
  Anabolic steroids, such as testosterone
  Corticosteroids
  Oral contraceptives
  Progesterone
  Drugs that contain bromides or iodides
- Avoid exposure to oils and greases.
- Avoid the use of greasy creams or cosmetics.
- Wash the pillowcase regularly in chemical-free (no added colors or fragrances) detergents.
- Remove excess sebum and oil from the face by washing thoroughly twice daily (more if necessary).

Diet

- Eliminate all refined and/or concentrated sugars from the diet.

- Do not eat foods that contain trans-fatty acids, such as milk, milk products, margarine, shortening, and other synthetically hydrogenated vegetable oils and fried foods.

Nutritional Supplements

- Chromium: 200–400 mcg per day
- Vitamin A: a dosage of 25,000 IU per day appears reasonable (higher dosages may be useful but should be monitored closely by a physician; sexually active women of childbearing age should not take vitamin A in daily dosages greater than 5,000 IU due to the link between excessive vitamin A and birth defects)

- Vitamin E: 400 IU per day
- Selenium: 200 mcg per day
- Zinc: 45–60 mg per day
- Vitamin B6: 25 mg three times per day
- Pantothenic acid: 2.5 g four times per day for up to two weeks

Physical Medicine

Acne tends to decrease with exposure to sun or ultraviolet light.

Topical Treatment

Choose one of the following:

- Tea tree oil (5–15% preparations)
- Azelaic acid (20% preparations)
- Sulfur (3–10% preparations)

AIDS and HIV Infection

. . . .

Positive test for the human immunodeficiency virus

Onset may be sudden or insidious or may present first as an opportunistic infection such as thrush (oral candidiasis) or *Pneumocystis carinii pneumonia*

Sudden onset (duration of up to fourteen days) of fevers, sweats, malaise, fatigability, joint and muscle pain, headaches, sore throat, diarrhea, generalized swelling of lymph glands, and/or rash on the trunk

Insidious onset may present as unexplained progressive fatigue, weight loss, fever, diarrhea, and/or generalized swelling of the lymph glands

Advanced stages will show neurological changes, including dementia and loss of nerve function (e.g., partial paralysis, vertigo, visual disturbances, etc.)

Acquired immunodeficiency syndrome (AIDS) is characterized by a profound defect in cell-mediated immunity. The primary cause of AIDS is infection with the human immunodeficiency virus (HIV). The spectrum of HIV infection ranges from a person with a positive test for HIV without any signs of immune deficiency to a person with full-blown AIDS, characterized by all of the now-classic components of the disease. AIDS is now viewed as a late stage of HIV infection.[1] HIV itself does not kill; what it does is cripple the immune system to such an extent that a person dies from severe infection or cancer.

Diagnosis of HIV is made by a positive blood test for HIV antigen and antibodies. Diagnosis of AIDS depends on meeting certain criteria, such as

- Presence of one of the twenty-three *opportunistic infections* (an infection that is caused by a normally noninfectious organism) and cancers linked to AIDS, or
- A positive HIV test plus a total *helper lymphocyte* (an important white blood cell)

count (CD4 count) of less than 200 cells per microliter, or
- A percentage of helper cells to total lymphocytes (CD8 count) of less than fourteen percent.

Current estimates are that over one million Americans are infected with HIV, and a little under two hundred thousand meet the requirements to be diagnosed as having AIDS. The current average time between becoming infected with HIV and developing AIDS is ten years.[1]

HIV

HIV is now regarded as the causative agent in AIDS by virtually every expert in the field. One of the exceptions is Peter Duesberg, Ph.D., of the Department of Molecular and Cell Biology at the University of California, Berkeley.[2] Dr. Duesberg contends that AIDS is caused by the long-term consumption of recreational drugs and/or the anti-HIV drug zidovudine (AZT). Before verbalizing his dissenting opinion on HIV as the causative agent (Duesberg believes that HIV is simply a "passenger" virus that causes no serious disease), Dr. Duesberg was regarded as one of the leading experts on the family of viruses (*retroviruses*), of which HIV is one. Now he is harshly criticized by many of his peers.[3]

Our perspective is that HIV plays a major role, but that other factors—particularly nutritional status, lifestyle, and mental/emotional state—play a significant role in the progression of HIV to AIDS.

Classified as a retrovirus, HIV has the ability to transform its RNA into DNA through the activity of an enzyme called *RNA-reverse transcriptase*. The virus then incorporates this piece of DNA into the infected cell's DNA, thus promoting viral replication by the cell. The cells most affected by this process are the T4 inducer/helper subset of lymphocytes. Helper T cells function in helping another type of lymphocyte multiply in response to an infection as well as help these white blood cells destroy bacteria, viruses, other organisms, and cancer cells. HIV is highly selective for and easily isolated from these white blood cells, but it is also found in other white blood cells. It actively replicates in these cells, especially when they are activated to mount a response to an infection. This infection-replication process renders the T cells nonfunctional, eventually destroying them and dramatically reducing their number, thus contributing to the profound immune suppression seen in AIDS.

QUICK REVIEW

- Primary risk factors: sexual contact with an HIV-infected person, intravenous drug use involving needle-sharing, or being born to a mother who has HIV

- HIV itself does not kill; what it does is cripple the human system to such an extent that a person dies from severe infection or cancer.

- HIV (human immunodeficiency virus) infection plays a major role in the progression to AIDS (acquired immunodeficiency syndrome), but other factors, particularly nutritional status, lifestyle, and mental/emotional state, also play a significant role.

- At this time, we recommend that conventional therapies be used in all individuals with CD4 counts below 500.

- Malnutrition and/or nutrient deficiency is too common in HIV/AIDS patients, given the very strong association between nutritional status, immune function, and the progression from HIV to AIDS.

  In general, since the immune system is dependent on many nutrients, it is vitally important to supply optimum levels of all nutrients to patients with HIV/AIDS.

- Numerous studies have shown that individuals infected with HIV have a compromised antioxidant defense system.

Therapeutic Considerations

Conventional medical management of HIV/AIDS is constantly changing but basically revolves around two treatment principles: 1) inactivation or slowing the replication of HIV, and 2) providing antibiotics to patients with abnormally low CD4 lymphocyte counts.[1] Progress is being made in the treatment of AIDS by combining some of the antiviral drugs, specifically drugs such as didanoside (nucleoside analogues), with drugs such as lamivudine (protease inhibitors). The use of these drugs appears to be appropriate in treating HIV-positive patients with CD4 counts under 500. More controversial is the use of these drugs to treat HIV-positive patients who show no signs of immune deficiency. Our current recommendation for HIV-positive individuals is to monitor their immune function by having CD4 counts determined every six months as long as levels stay above 500, and every three months if levels drop below 500. There are also specialized tests to measure the viral load and activity (such as P24 antigen levels and PCR-based HIV-RNA levels) that can be used as monitors.

In short, at this time we recommend that conventional therapies be used for all individuals with CD4 counts below 500. That isn't to say that natural measures should be abandoned at this point. Quite the contrary; it is absolutely vital to aggressively employ natural measures that promote good health

. . . .

- Of all the antioxidants that show promise in slowing the progression of HIV to AIDS, vitamin E shows the greatest and most consistent effects.
- In a few clinical studies, supplemental beta-carotene has produced positive effects on immune function, both in HIV-positive and AIDS patients.
- Several studies have shown that selenium status is a major determinant of how fast HIV will progress to AIDS.
- Vitamin B12 deficiency is seen in ten to thirty-five percent of all HIV-positive patients, presumably as a result of either decreased intake, reduced absorption, or antagonism by the drug AZT.
- Lipoic acid is demonstrating extremely encouraging results in treating HIV patients.
- Preliminary studies indicate that carnitine supplementation can improve immune function and reduce the level of HIV-induced immune suppression.
- Curcumin exhibits potent anti-HIV activity and is showing promise in clinical trials.
- Bromelain has been shown to have better activity than known anti-HIV drugs in test tube studies.
- In clinical studies in Japan, licorice components have shown tremendous benefits in treating HIV.

TABLE 1	Relationship of CD4 Count to Development of Opportunistic Infection		
>600	**400–600**	**100–400**	**<100**
No opportunistic infections	Bacterial infections	*Pneumocystis pneumonia*	*Cytomegalovirus*
Tuberculosis	Toxoplasmosis	Brain lymphoma	*retinitis*
Herpes simplex	Cryptococcosis	Severe infections of all body	
Herpes zoster	Histoplasmosis	tissues are possible	
Vaginal candidiasis	Crysposporidiosis		
Hairy leukoplakia			
Kaposi's sarcoma			

and immune function from the very start of HIV infection, and certainly when AIDS develops. It is important to remember that HIV does not kill. It is the opportunistic infections allowed by a suppressed immune system that set into motion an accelerating downward spiral that ultimately results in death.

From a natural perspective, the basic therapeutic goal is to enhance and optimize immune function, as detailed in the chapter IMMUNE SUPPORT. All of the recommendations in that chapter should be employed, with the exception of the use of *Echinacea*. It is unclear at this time if *Echinacea* should be recommended for treating AIDS. Although this condition is associated with widespread depression of the immune system, presumably due to HIV, stimulating T-cell replication and increasing levels of tumor necrosis factor (TNF) by *Echinacea* (or any other agent) may also stimulate replication of the virus. At this time, the use of *Echinacea* in treating HIV is not recommended.

Nutrition and HIV/AIDS

The immune system requires a constant supply of nutrients to function properly. Unfortunately, the AIDS patient has many obstacles to overcome in order to supply the immune system with the nutrition it needs.

Chief among these obstacles are gastrointestinal tract infection and the *wasting* (muscle breakdown) promoted by the progressing infection. It is easier to institute nutritional therapies early on than after AIDS has developed.

As mentioned above, malnutrition and/or nutrient deficiency is too common in HIV/AIDS patients, given the very strong association between nutritional status, immune function, and the progression from HIV to AIDS.[4–7] What we mean by it being "too common" is that given all of the research, why aren't more HIV/AIDS patients taking measures (such as those given here) to maximize their nutritional status and immune function?

In general, since the immune system is so dependent on so many nutrients, it is vitally important to supply optimum levels of all nutrients. There is considerable debate over what is optimal for the general population, but there is a growing consensus that HIV/AIDS patients require higher levels of virtually all known nutrients. The levels recommended are in line with the levels given in the chapter SUPPLEMENTARY MEASURES. High dosages are necessary because more than twenty-nine percent of HIV-positive individuals are deficient in one or more of the antioxidant nutrients (beta-carotene, vitamin

E, selenium, zinc, and vitamin C), including those who take nutritional supplements.[4]

In regard to basic dietary recommendations, the HIV-positive individual should consume a diet that promotes health, as defined in the chapter A HEALTH-PROMOTING DIET. The diet should

- Be rich in whole, natural foods, such as fruits, vegetables, grains, beans, seeds, and nuts
- Be low in fats and refined sugars
- Contain adequate, but not excessive, amounts of protein

On top of this, HIV-positive individuals should drink five or six 8-ounce glasses of water (preferably pure water) per day. These dietary recommendations, along with a positive mental attitude, a good high-potency multivitamin-mineral supplement, a regular exercise program, daily deep-breathing and relaxation exercises (meditation, prayer, etc.), and at least seven to eight hours of sleep daily will go a long way toward helping the immune system function at an optimum level—a critical goal in treating HIV/AIDS.

In addition to these basic recommendations, there are some important considerations for people who have HIV/AIDS. First of all, the person with HIV/AIDS has higher nutrient requirements. For example, while the typical person does quite well with 0.8 gram of protein daily per 2.2 pounds of body weight, the individual with HIV/AIDS requires at least 2.0 grams per 2.2 pounds of body weight.[5,6] Supplementing the diet with whey protein (high in the amino acid glutamine) appears particularly useful in cases of AIDS, in terms of both its potential for addressing the wasting syndrome of AIDS and its ability to heal the gastrointestinal tract. A high-quality whey protein (micro-filtered, ion-exchanged) at a dosage of 1 gram per 2

pounds of body weight should definitely be used by people who show signs of weight loss or the wasting syndrome.

The *wasting syndrome* (severe breakdown of body tissues) is a common complication of HIV infection and is marked by progressive weight loss and weakness, often associated with fever and diarrhea. The mechanisms responsible for this syndrome are not well defined, but it is clear that this is a multifactorial process. Contributors to the wasting syndrome include inadequate overall dietary intake, nutrient malabsorption, increased metabolism, and increased levels of cytokines secreted by the immune system, such as tumor-necrosis factor, interleukin-1, interleukin-6, and alpha-interferon. These cytokines stimulate the breakdown of fat and muscle.

While general broad-spectrum nutritional support is required, there are several nutrients that deserve special attention: vitamin E, vitamin C, vitamin A and beta-carotene, selenium, zinc, lipoic acid, carnitine, vitamin B6, and vitamin B12. These nutrients will be discussed following a brief discussion of the importance of antioxidant support.

Antioxidants and HIV/AIDS

Numerous studies have shown that individuals infected with HIV have a compromised antioxidant defense system.[8,9] Blood levels of antioxidants are decreased and peroxidation products of *lipids* (fats) and proteins are increased in these patients. This blood profile may contribute to the progression of AIDS, because antioxidants such as glutathione (GSH) prevent viral replication, while reactive oxidants tend to stimulate the virus.[10] Consequently, it has been suggested that HIV-infected patients may benefit from antioxidant supplementation therapy. Antioxidant therapy, especially with vitamin E and selenium, does appear to slow down the progression from HIV to AIDS.

One of the more controversial antioxidants for treating HIV infection is N-acetylcysteine (NAC). It was proposed that NAC may act as an effective antioxidant and raise tissue glutathione levels in AIDS.[10] However, supplementation at a dosage of 1.8 grams of NAC failed to increase GSH levels in white blood cells of AIDS patients.[11] Better options for raising GSH levels are vitamin E, vitamin C, beta-carotene, selenium, and lipoic acid.

Vitamin E Of all the antioxidants that show promise in slowing down the progression of HIV to AIDS, vitamin E has had the most consistent and greatest effects.[7,12,13] In one study, men with the highest levels of vitamin E in their blood showed a thirty-four-percent decrease in their risk of progression to AIDS compared with those with the lowest levels.[13] Given the importance of vitamin E as an antioxidant as well as to immune function, it is little wonder that levels of vitamin E reflect immune status in AIDS patients.

Despite the increased need for vitamin E and the tremendous potential of vitamin E in slowing down the progression to AIDS, over fifty percent of AIDS patients and thirty-eight percent of HIV-positive individuals have intakes of less than fifty percent of the RDA for vitamin E.[7] Apparently a very large number of HIV and AIDS patients do not take vitamin E supplements; this is unfortunate.

Vitamin C Vitamin C exerts some beneficial effects in test tube studies (in vitro) against HIV replication, and it has been shown that HIV-positive people with the highest levels of vitamin C intake had the slowest progression to AIDS.[7,14] However, there is some concern that high doses of vitamin C (greater than 1,000 mg three times per day) may impair lymphocyte function.[15] Based on this conflicting information, we recommend the conservative approach of keeping vitamin C dosages in the range of 500 to 1,000 mg three times per day—a dosage that has been shown to raise glutathione levels in normal subjects, and hopefully in HIV-positive and AIDS patients as well.[16]

Vitamin A and Beta-Carotene Vitamin A deficiency is quite common during HIV infection, and is clearly associated with a decreased level of circulating helper T cells—one of the hallmark features of AIDS.[17]

Analysis of vitamin A levels, helper T cell counts, and other blood parameters in HIV-positive individuals indicated that more than fifteen percent had deficient vitamin A levels in their blood. When vitamin A levels were low, helper T cell levels were much lower than the levels in HIV-infected individuals who had normal levels of vitamin A. Vitamin A deficiency was also shown to be associated with a higher rate of mortality due to HIV.[17]

Increasing beta-carotene intake may be the preferred form of vitamin A supplementation in HIV patients, as there is concern that retinoic acid, the active form of vitamin A, may actually increase HIV replication in humans. Low beta-carotene levels are common in people with HIV/AIDS (especially children), presumably as a result of fat malabsorption. Low beta-carotene levels are associated with greater impairment of immune function.[18,19]

There have been a few clinical studies using supplemental beta-carotene that produced positive effects on immune function, both in HIV-positive and AIDS patients.[20–23] For example, let's look at a clinical study of beta-carotene supplementation in AIDS. Enrollment criteria included no evidence of active opportunistic infection, greater than 1 kilogram change in weight in the month preceding enrollment, chronic diarrhea or malabsorption, or hepatic disease or significant anemia. Beta-carotene (30 mg) was given twice daily with meals for four weeks; this was followed by no therapy for six weeks. The total white blood cell, lymphocyte, and T-lymphocyte-subset counts were measured at the beginning of the study, at the end of four weeks of treatment, and six weeks after treatment had stopped. In response to beta-carotene, total lymphocyte counts rose by sixty-six percent, and CD4 cell counts rose slightly, but insignificantly, in the entire group. In all of the patients who had baseline CD4 cell counts greater than ten per microliter, however, the mean absolute increase in CD4 cell count in response to beta-carotene was fifty-three cells per microliter. Six weeks off beta-carotene treatment, the absolute CD4 cell count had returned to pretreatment levels.

We should point out that not all the studies with beta-carotene showed such impressive results. Some showed very little or no benefit.[24] However, given the lack of side effects and the possibility of benefits, supplementation surely seems appropriate.

We recommend using natural sources of beta-carotenes, such as palm oil and algae (*Dunaliella*), rather than synthetic, isolated beta-carotene. The natural forms, particularly palm oil, are better absorbed and have far greater antioxidant activity. The dosage is based upon the milligram amount (e.g., 30 mg twice per day with meals) or the vitamin A equivalence (e.g., 50,000 IU twice per day with meals).

Selenium Selenium supplementation is an absolute necessity in the treatment of HIV-positive and AIDS patients. Levels of selenium-dependent glutathione peroxidase (GSH-PX), an important antioxidant enzyme, are usually found to be quite low in HIV patients, and even lower in AIDS patients. Selenium supplementation significantly increases GSH-PX activity in HIV-positive subjects.[25]

Given the fact that lower levels of glutathione and other sulfur-containing compounds are extremely important contributing factors in the progression of AIDS, it is obvious just how essential selenium supplementation is to the HIV-infected individual.[10,26] In addition, several studies have shown selenium status is a major determinant of how fast HIV will progress to AIDS.[27]

Lipoic Acid *Lipoic acid* (also known as *thioctic acid*) is a sulfur-containing vitamin-like substance that plays an important role as the necessary cofactor in two vital energy-producing reactions involved in the production of cellular energy (ATP). Lipoic acid is not considered a vitamin because it is thought that either the body can manufacture sufficient levels or it is acquired in sufficient quantities from food. However, as with many of the other compounds described in this section, a relative deficiency can occur in certain situations, and lipoic acid supplementation exerts benefits beyond its role in normal metabolism. Lipoic acid is an effective antioxidant. It is unique in that it is effective against both water- and fat-soluble free radicals.[28]

Lipoic acid has antioxidant effects and is able to significantly inhibit the replication of HIV by reducing the activity of *reverse transcriptase*—the enzyme responsible for manufacturing the virus from the DNA of lymphocytes. Based on these actions, it was suggested that lipoic acid might be of value in treating HIV-positive patients.[29,30]

To test this hypothesis, a small pilot study was designed to determine the short-term effect of lipoic acid supplementation (150 mg three times per day) in HIV-positive patients.[31] Lipoic acid supplementation increased plasma ascorbate levels in nine of ten patients, total glutathione levels in seven of seven patients, total plasma sulfur group levels in eight of nine patients, and T-helper lymphocyte levels and T-helper/suppressor cell ratio in six of ten patients, while the level of the lipid peroxidation product malondialdehyde decreased in eight of nine patients.

The results of this pilot study indicated that lipoic acid supplementation led to significant beneficial changes in the blood of HIV-infected patients. Perhaps the most significant of these effects was the increase in the glutathione content, since the level of glutathione is directly linked to preventing the progression to AIDS. We hope that larger, double-blind studies will support these encouraging results.

Zinc

Zinc is perhaps the most important trace element for immune function. It is also one of the more common nutrient deficiencies in cases of AIDS, presumably due to the decreased intake, impaired absorption, and increased need for zinc.[4-6] Zinc supplementation has been shown to reduce the incidence of opportunistic infections in AZT-treated AIDS patients.[32] Zinc supplementation also showed an ability to increase or stabilize body weight, increase the number of CD4 cells, and increase the blood level of an important immune system regulating hormone known as *thymulin*.

Vitamin B6

Low vitamin B6 status has been noted in HIV-positive patients. The lack of vitamin B6 correlates with a decrease in immune function.[33] Vitamin B6 is required for proper immune function (see IMMUNE SUPPORT).

Vitamin B12

Vitamin B12 deficiency is seen in ten to thirty-five percent of all HIV-positive patients, presumably as a result of either decreased intake, reduced absorption, or antagonism by the drug AZT.[34,35] As serum cobalamin levels decline, progression to AIDS increases and neurological symptoms worsen.

In one study, fifty-nine HIV-positive patients without any symptoms at the beginning of the study were followed over a two-and-one-half-year period. Serum B12 levels, CD4 (helper T cell) count, and clinical progression to AIDS were measured.[36] Twelve of the fifty-nine patients progressed to AIDS. Nine of these patients had repeat serum B12 level tests prior to progression. All nine patients had or developed falling serum B12 levels without any evidence of HIV-related bowel disorder. All patients who progressed to AIDS also had falling CD4 counts. This study indicates that serum vitamin B12 levels may serve as a surrogate marker for HIV progression. It is thought that impaired absorption explains the drop in B12 levels. Of course, malabsorption of B12 would also imply that other nutrients are not being absorbed.

Given the importance to the immune system of maintaining good nutritional status, low serum vitamin B12 levels may signify that overall nutritional status is quite poor—a harbinger of further impairment of immune status and progression to AIDS. A low level of vitamin B12 is associated with faster progression from HIV to AIDS.[7,37,38]

In addition, vitamin B12 (cyanocobalamin, methylcobalamin, and adenosylcobalamin) has been shown to inhibit HIV replication *in vitro*. Given the safety of achieving high blood and tissue levels of vitamin B12 without toxicity, vitamin B12 therapy for HIV infection holds great promise.[39]

Carnitine

Several reports indicate that systemic carnitine deficiency may be a problem in patients with AIDS. Reduced levels of carnitine are often found in the blood and blood cells of AIDS patients.[40] Increasing the carnitine content of the white blood cells has strongly improved their function, highlighting the importance of carnitine to the immune system.

Carnitine has been shown to prevent the toxicity of the drug AZT on the muscle cells.[41] AZT poisons the mitochondria of the muscle, leading to abnormal energy production within the muscle, which manifests clinically as muscle fatigue and pain.

Preliminary studies indicate that carnitine supplementation can improve immune function and reduce the level of HIV-induced immune suppression. Giving AIDS patients being treated with AZT 6 grams of L-carnitine per day led to significantly increased white blood cell proliferation and levels of circulating tumor necrosis factor—a known trigger of HIV replication.[42] Given the suspected systemic carnitine deficiency, along with the tremendous safety of use, carnitine supplementation appears warranted in AIDS.

Thymus Extract

The thymus gland is the main organ of the immune system. AIDS is associated with significant loss of thymus function. Although thymus extracts have not shown any real therapeutic benefit in treating AIDS, studies have shown an ability to improve several immune parameters, including an elevation in the level of T-helper cells, a critical goal in treating AIDS.[43]

Botanicals

There are many herbs and herbal components that are showing great promise as antiviral agents that are active against HIV. In our opinion, the three that are presented here offer the greatest promise.

Turmeric (Curcuma longa)

HIV infection and its progression to AIDS are associated with activation of HIV to replicate. This activation is governed by the *long terminal repeat* (LTR) gene in the viral DNA. The virus remains in an inactive form until

LTR tells it to replicate. Whether or not LTR signals the latent provirus to become active is determined by a complex interaction of positive and negative regulators that bind to specific sequences within the LTR. There appears to be a balance that keeps the provirus inactive. When this balance is tipped toward activation, LTR activation leads to HIV replication. It is thought that if stimuli that activate LTR can be reduced, while simultaneously using compounds that block activation of LTR, the progression of HIV infection or AIDS could be halted or at least delayed.

In March 1993, researchers at Harvard Medical School published results of a study that showed that curcumin inhibits the replication of HIV by blocking LTR expression.[44] *Curcumin* is the yellow pigment and active ingredient of the spice turmeric (*Curcuma longa*), which is the key spice in curry. The research may have been performed as a follow-up to a population study in Trinidad. About forty percent of the population are of Indian descent and use curry extensively in their diet. Another forty percent of the population are of African descent and rarely use curry. The Trinidadian study indicated that persons of African descent were more than ten times likelier to have the disease than persons of Indian descent. Whether this was due to dietary factors, genetic factors, or sexual habits remains to be shown. However, given the recent antiviral studies using curcumin, a strong case could be made for the former.

Another study shed additional light on the anti-HIV activity of curcumin. Curcumin was shown to inhibit the activity of *HIV integrase*, the enzyme that integrates a double-stranded DNA copy of the RNA genome, synthesized by reverse transcriptase, into a host chromosome.[45]

Curcumin has also been shown to inhibit other factors that stimulate HIV to replicate, such as tumor necrosis factor (TNF) and NF-kappa B.[46–48] TNF, a chemical mediator of inflammation, is part of the immune system's inflammatory response, which, when working properly, is used to kill disease-causing organisms. TNF production, however, triggers the production of NF-kappa B, a chemical messenger that plays a critical role in initiating HIV replication.

Curcumin's ability to inhibit all of these aspects of HIV makes it one of the best choices for additional research. In addition, curcumin is a powerful antioxidant, showing activity as much as three hundred times greater than that of vitamin E.[49] Preliminary studies in treating HIV/AIDS with curcumin are encouraging. For example, in a controlled clinical study, a group of eighteen HIV-positive patients, with CD4 counts ranging from 5 to 615, took an average of 2,000 mg of curcumin daily.[50] This regimen resulted in an increase in CD4 counts, compared to control treatment. Unfortunately, the study failed to report the level of the increase. Larger trials of curcumin's effect on HIV are under way.

The curcumin content of turmeric is about one percent. To reach an effective dosage of curcumin (1.2 grams per day), a person would need to consume nearly 100 grams (roughly 3½ ounces) of turmeric. For this reason, pure curcumin preparations are preferred to crude curry when medicinal effects are desired. Although the benefit of curcumin in treating HIV and AIDS remains to be proven, given the safety of curcumin and its possible benefit, supplementing pure curcumin as well as increasing the dietary intake of curry makes sense. Pure curcumin products are available commercially. Because there is some debate over the oral absorption of curcumin, it is often recommended that products containing bromelain and curcumin be used, as bromelain has been shown to enhance the absorption of medicinal compounds in the treatment of AIDS.

Bromelain and Other Naturally Occurring Protease Inhibitors

Active *proteases* (protein-digesting enzymes) in the human immunodeficiency virus (HIV) are required to condense a viral protein core in subsequent viral replications. Drugs that inhibit this action—the protease inhibitors—are showing tremendous benefit in the treatment of HIV infection and AIDS, but they are expensive and associated with many side effects. The goal of one investigation was to identify natural products that inhibit HIV proteases.[51] Researchers focused on naturally occurring enzymes with low toxicity and high oral bioavailability. Compared to known HIV protease-inhibiting drugs, nineteen natural products demonstrated better activity. Among the best candidates was bromelain, which is also the most readily available. We hope that there is research underway to determine the clinical usefulness of bromelain as a naturally occurring protease inhibitor. On the surface it appears to be safer and have fewer side effects compared to the currently used protease inhibitor drugs.

Licorice (Glycyrrhiza glabra)

Licorice root's primary active component is *glycyrrhizin,* and its backbone structure is *glycyrrhetinic acid* (glycyrrhizin minus a small sugar molecule). Preparations that contain glycyrrhizin are showing promise in the treatment of HIV-related diseases, including AIDS, as well as chronic hepatitis (see HEPATITIS). Although much of the research has featured intravenous administration, this may not be necessary as glycyrrhizin and glycyrrhetinic acid are well tolerated and easily absorbed orally.

The benefit of oral administration was most evident in a recent double-blind study. The study focused on the clinical effectiveness of long-term glycyrrhizin treatment, administered orally to sixteen HIV-positive hemophilia patients.[52] The patients received daily doses of glycyrrhizin (150 to 225 mg) for three to seven years. Helper and total T lymphocyte counts, other immune system parameters, and glycyrrhizin and glycyrrhetinic acid levels in the blood were monitored. The results indicated that orally administered glycyrrhizin was converted into glycyrrhetinic acid, which was detected in the blood, without producing any side effect. None of the patients who took the glycyrrhizin progressed to AIDS or had deterioration of immune function. In contrast, the group that did not receive glycyrrhetinic acid showed decreases in helper and total T-cell counts and antibody levels. Two of the sixteen patients in the control group developed AIDS.

In another study, ten HIV-positive patients without AIDS took 150 to 225 mg of glycyrrhizin daily.[53] After two years, none had progressed to AIDS, while in a control group of HIV-positive patients three had developed AIDS (two subsequently died during the study).

The result of treating HIV-positive and AIDS patients with glycyrrhizin is an almost immediate improvement in immune function. In one study, nine symptom-free HIV-positive patients received 200 to 800 mg of glycyrrhizin intravenously each day. After eight weeks, all groups had increased helper T cell levels, improved helper/suppressor cell ratios, and improved liver function.[54]

In another study, six AIDS patients received 400 to 1,600 mg of glycyrrhizin intravenously each day.[55] After thirty days, five of the six showed a reduction or disappearance of the P24 antigen (an indicator of viral load and severity of active disease).

The results of these studies and others involving HIV-positive and AIDS patients are encouraging. The big concern is that if licorice root is ingested regularly at a dosage of more than 3 grams per day for more than six weeks, or if glycyrrhizin is taken at a dosage of more than 100 mg per day, it may cause sodium and water retention, leading to high blood pressure. Monitoring of blood pressure and increasing dietary potassium intake are suggested.

TREATMENT SUMMARY

The goal of treatment for HIV-positive individuals is to slow the progression of HIV to AIDS. This is accomplished by optimizing nutritional status, following a health-promoting lifestyle, and employing measures to enhance immune function. Particularly important are antioxidants such as vitamin E, beta-carotene, zinc, selenium, vitamin C, lipoic acid, and curcumin. In addition, vitamin B12, carnitine, licorice, and bromelain appear to offer some benefit.

In cases of AIDS the treatment goal shifts to supporting conventional therapies. It is particularly important to strive to maintain high nutritional and antioxidant status.

General Recommendations for Prevention

- Do not have sexual intercourse with persons known to have or suspected of having HIV or who use intravenous drugs

- Practice safe sex—use a condom and avoid exchange of bodily fluids
- Do not share a toothbrush, razor, or other implement that could become contaminated with blood from someone with an HIV infection

Lifestyle

- Perform a relaxation exercise (deep breathing, meditation, prayer, visualization, etc.) for ten to fifteen minutes each day
- Get regular exercise (nonstrenuous walking, Tai Chi, stretching, etc.)

Diet

- Consume a diet that focuses on whole, unprocessed foods (whole grains, legumes, vegetables, fruits, nuts, and seeds)
- Consume adequate protein (consider supplementation with a high-quality whey protein at a dosage of 1 gram per 2 pounds of body weight)
- Eliminate the intake of alcohol, caffeine, and sugar
- Identify and control food allergies
- Drink at least 48 ounces of water per day

Nutritional Supplements

- High-potency multiple-vitamin-and-mineral according to guidelines given in the chapter SUPPLEMENTARY MEASURES

- Flaxseed oil: 1 tbsp per day
- Vitamin C: 500–1,000 mg three times per day
- Vitamin E: 400–800 IU per day
- Carotene complex: 50,000–100,000 per day
- Methylcobalamin (active vitamin B12): 2 mg twice per day
- Lipoic acid: 150 mg three times per day
- Thymus extract: 750 mg of the crude polypeptide fraction per day

Botanical Medicines

- Curcumin (from *Curcuma longa*): 2,000 mg per day in divided doses (e.g., 400 mg five times per day) with an equal amount of bromelain (1,200–1,800 mcu [milk-clotting units]), preferably on an empty stomach
- *Glycyrrhiza glabra* (licorice): Powdered root: 1–2 g three times per day
  Fluid extract (1:1): 2–4 ml three times per day
  Solid (dry powdered) extract (5% glcyrrhetinic acid content): 250–500 mg three times per day
  (NOTE: If licorice is to be used over a long period of time, it is necessary to increase intake of potassium-rich foods.)

Alcoholism

Psychological/social signs of excess alcohol consumption: depression, loss of friends, arrest for driving while intoxicated, excessive drinking, drinking before breakfast, frequent accidents, unexplained work absences

Alcohol dependence as manifested when alcohol is withdrawn: tremulousness, convulsions, hallucinations, delirium

Alcoholic binges, benders (forty-eight hours or more of drinking associated with failure to meet usual obligations), or blackouts

Physical signs of excess alcohol consumption: alcohol odor on breath, flushed face, tremor, unexplained bruises

Alcoholism has been defined by the World Health Organization as "alcohol consumption by an individual that exceeds the limits accepted by the culture or injures health or social relationships." The health, social, and economic consequences of alcoholism are alarming (see box).

Current estimates indicate that over eighteen million people in the United States (roughly 10% of the adult population) are alcoholics, making alcoholism one of the most serious health problems facing the physician today. The total number of Americans affected, either directly or indirectly, is much greater when one considers disruption of family life, automobile accidents, crime, decreased productivity, and mental and physical disease.

CONSEQUENCES OF ALCOHOLISM[1]
Increased Mortality:
- Double the usual death rate in men, triple in women
- Major factor in the four leading causes of death in men between the ages of twenty-five and forty-four: accidents, homicides, suicides, cirrhosis
- Six times greater suicide rate
- Ten-year decrease in life expectancy

Economic Toll (yearly):
- Lost production: $14.9 billion
- Health care costs: $8.3 billion
- Accident and fire losses: $5.0 billion
- Cost of violent crime: $1.5 billion
- Total cost to society: $136 billion

Health Effects:
- Abstinence and withdrawal syndromes
- Acne rosacea
- Angina
- Brain degeneration
- Decreased protein synthesis
- Decreased serum testosterone levels
- Esophagitis, gastritis, ulcer
- Fetal alcohol syndrome
- Heart disease
- Hypertension
- Hypoglycemia
- Increased cancer of the mouth, pharynx, larynx, esophagus
- Increased serum and liver triglyceride levels
- Intoxication
- Fatty liver degeneration and cirrhosis

- Metabolic damage to every cell
- Muscle wasting
- Nutritional diseases
- Osteoporosis
- Pancreatitis
- Psoriasis
- Psychiatric disorders

Causes

The cause of alcoholism remains obscure. It represents a multifactorial condition with genetic, physiological, psychological, and social factors, all seemingly equally important. However, recent research indicates that genetic factors may be most important.[2] The finding of a genetic marker for alcoholism could result in the diagnosis of the disease in its initial and more reversible stage.

A number of studies have shown that alcoholism is four to five times more common in the biological children of alcoholic parents than in those of nonalcoholic parents.[2] This suggests that a biological marker may not be necessary for the implementation of a relatively innocuous primary prevention program. The genetic basis of alcoholism has been supported by (1) genealogical studies showing that alcoholism is a family condition, (2) studies of adopted children of alcoholic parents raised by foster parents, demonstrating continued higher risk of alcoholism, (3) twin studies showing differences between identical and nonidentical twins, (4) association with genetic markers, and (5) biochemical studies showing that the levels of enzymes required to detoxify alcohol are lower in people prone to alcoholism.[2–4]

Therapeutic Considerations

The primary therapeutic goal from a natural medicine perspective involves supporting the alcoholic with better nutrition, counseling, and psychological support and specific herbal medicines to deal with any alcohol-related health problem (e.g., liver damage).

QUICK REVIEW

- Genetic factors play a big role in the cause of alcoholism.
- All active alcoholics display signs of injury to the liver.
- Hypoglycemia aggravates the mental and emotional problems of the alcoholic.
- Zinc is one of the key nutrients involved in the breakdown of alcohol.
- Vitamin A deficiency is also common in alcoholics and appears to work together with the zinc deficiency to produce the major complications of alcoholism.
- Antioxidants taken either prior to or along with alcohol inhibit free-radical damage and the development of a fatty liver.
- Carnitine inhibits alcohol-induced fatty liver.

While many of the nutritional problems of alcoholics relate directly to the effects of alcohol, a major contributing factor is that alcoholics tend not to eat; they substitute alcohol for food. As a result, the alcoholic not only has to deal with secondary nutritional deficiencies caused by excessive alcohol consumption, but also primary nutritional deficiencies due to inadequate intake.

Psychosocial Aspects of Recovery

Psychological and social measures are critical in the treatment of the alcoholism. Social support for both patient and family is very important, and success often appears proportional to involvement with Alcoholics Anonymous (AA), counselors, and church.

Successful initiation of treatment requires

- The alcoholic's agreement that he or she has an alcohol problem
- Education of the alcoholic and the family about the physical and psychosocial effects of alcoholism
- Immediate involvement in a treatment program

Successful programs (such as AA) usually include strict control of drinking and replacement of the alcohol addiction with another addiction (going to meetings) that is nonchemical, time-consuming, and heavily supported by family, friends, and peers. Although strict abstinence may not be absolutely necessary, at this time it appears to be the safest and most effective choice.[1]

Fatty Liver

All active alcoholics display signs of injury to the liver. Specifically, the active alcoholic shows fatty infiltration of the liver as a sign of liver damage, with the severity roughly proportional to the duration and degree of alcohol excess. Even moderate doses of ethanol may produce fatty liver in nonalcoholics. Development of a fatty liver is a response to liver injury that is directly related to the nutritional status of the liver, the level of antioxidants in the liver, and other nutritional factors.[3,4] The fatty liver is made worse by a high-fat diet.[5]

It is very important for the alcoholic or anyone who has suffered continual assault to

- There is a direct link between the level of vitamin C in white blood cells and the rate of clearance of alcohol from the blood.
- A thiamin (vitamin B1) deficiency is both the most common and the most serious of the B-vitamin deficiencies in the alcoholic.
- Low magnesium levels are present in as many as sixty percent of alcoholics

and is strongly linked to *delirium tremens*—a state of confusion and trembling during alcohol withdrawal.
- Glutamine supplementation (1 gram per day) has been shown to reduce voluntary alcohol consumption in uncontrolled human studies.

TABLE 1   Alcohol Use Disorder Inventory Test

	0	1	2	3	4	TOTAL
1. How often do you have a drink containing alcohol? (one drink is a beer, glass of wine, or mixed drink)	Never	Monthly or less	2–4 times a month	2–3 times a week	4 or more times a week	
2. How many drinks containing alcohol do you have on a typical day when you are drinking?	1 or 2	3 or 4	5 or 6	7 to 9	10 or more	
3. How often do you have six or more drinks on one occasion?	Never	Less than monthly	Monthly	Weekly	Daily or almost daily	
4. How often during the past year have you been unable to stop drinking once you started?	Never	Less than monthly	Monthly	Weekly	Daily or almost daily	
5. How often during the past year have you failed to do what was normally expected of you because of drinking?	Never	Less than monthly	Monthly	Weekly	Daily or almost daily	
6. How often during the past year have you needed a drink in the morning to get going after a heavy drinking session?	Never	Less than monthly	Monthly	Weekly	Daily or almost daily	
7. How often during the past year have you had a feeling of guilt or remorse after drinking?	Never	Less than monthly	Monthly	Weekly	Daily or almost daily	
8. How often during the past year have you been unable to remember what happened the night before because of drinking?	Never	Less than monthly	Monthly	Weekly	Daily or almost daily	
9. Have you or someone else been injured as a result of your drinking?	No		Yes, but not in the past year		Yes, during the past year	
10. Has a relative, friend, doctor, or other health worker been concerned about your drinking or suggested you cut down?	No		Yes, but not in the past year		Yes, during the past year	

Scoring: A total score of 8–15 may indicate a problem with alcohol abuse. You may want to ask your physician about cutting down or becoming abstinent. A total score of 16 or more suggests a more serious problem. You should contact your physician or an alcohol-treatment program for help.

TOTAL

the liver to follow the recommendations given in the chapter DETOXIFICATION.

Hypoglycemia

Alcohol consumption often results in *reactive hypoglycemia*—a rapid increase in blood sugar levels, followed by a drop in blood sugar levels. The resultant drop in blood sugar pro- duces a craving for food, particularly foods that quickly elevate blood sugar, such as sugar and alcohol. Increased sugar consumption aggravates the reactive hypoglycemia, particularly in the presence of alcohol.[3] Hypoglycemia aggravates the mental and emotional problems of the alcoholic and the withdrawing alcoholic, with such symptoms as sweating, tremor, tachycardia, anxiety, hunger, dizziness, headache, visual disturbance, decreased mental acuity, confusion, and depression.[1]

Depression

Depression is common among alcoholics and is known to lead to the high suicide rate. Many alcoholics are depressed first and later become alcoholic *(primary depressives),* while others become alcoholic first and later develop a depressive condition in the context of their alcoholism *(secondary depressives).* As discussed above, alcoholics tend to have severely depleted levels of tryptophan, which may explain both the depression and the sleep disturbances common to alcoholics. Brain serotonin levels are dependent on levels of circulating tryptophan and the other amino acids, which compete with tryptophan for transport into the brain.

Intestinal Flora

The intestinal microflora are severely deranged in alcoholics.[36] Colonization of the small intestine by toxin-producing bacteria may lead to malabsorption of fats, carbohydrates, protein, folic acid, and vitamin B12. This disturbance in gut flora is probably the cause of the abnormalities of the small intestine commonly found in alcoholics. Supplementing with *Lactobacillus acidophilus* appears a worthwhile goal to try to correct the altered gut flora (see DIGESTION for further information).

Alcohol ingestion also increases intestinal permeability to toxins and macromolecules.[37] The ensuing allergic reactions and absorption of gut-derived toxins probably contribute to the many complications of alcoholism and, considering the addictive tendency of food allergies, may also contribute to alcoholic cravings.

Nutrient Support

Zinc

One of the key nutrients involved in the breakdown of alcohol is zinc.[6] Acute and chronic alcohol consumption result in zinc deficiency.[6,7] Several factors contribute to the development of zinc deficiency in alcoholics: (1) decreased dietary intake, (2) decreased absorption, and (3) increased excretion of zinc in the urine.

Low body levels of zinc are associated with impaired alcohol metabolism, a predisposition to *cirrhosis* (severe damage to the liver), impaired testicular function, and other complications of alcohol abuse.[6,8] Zinc supplementation, particularly when combined with vitamin C, greatly increases alcohol detoxification and survival in rats.[9] It may produce a similar effect in humans.

Vitamin A

Vitamin A deficiency is also common in alcoholics and appears to work with the zinc deficiency to produce the major complications of alcoholism (night blindness, hormonal disturbances, poor immune function, etc.).[5,8] The mechanism has been suggested to be as follows: reduced intestinal absorption of zinc and vitamin A, along with impaired liver function, results in reduced blood levels of zinc, vitamin A, and their transport proteins. In body tissues, these reduced concentrations of zinc and vitamin A cause abnormal enzyme activities, abnormal protein synthesis, and impaired cellular function. In the kidney, they increase the loss of zinc. These metabolic abnormalities then lead to the common disorders of alcoholism: night blindness, skin disorders, cirrhosis of the liver, reduced skin healing, decreased testicular function, and impaired immune function.[8]

Vitamin A supplementation inhibits alcohol consumption in female, but not male, rats. The effect of the vitamin A is inhibited by testosterone administration.[10] Other research on rats further highlights the impact of the endocrine system on alcohol preference. Removal of the ovaries and adrenal glands in female rats decreased their preference for alcohol, while cortisone injections increased their alcohol preference.[11]

Vitamin A supplementation in the alcoholic has produced correction of vitamin A deficiency, as noted by improvements in night blindness and sexual function.[5] Despite the importance and benefits of vitamin A to the alcoholic, great care must be employed with vitamin A supplementation. A liver that has been damaged by excessive alcohol consumption significantly loses its ability to store vitamin A. As a result, an alcoholic who continues to drink or who shows evidence of impaired liver function is at great risk for developing vitamin A toxicity when the vitamin is given at dosages above the recommended dietary allowance of 5,000 IU.

Antioxidants

Alcohol consumption causes an increase in *free-radical* (highly reactive toxins) levels and free-radical damage. Matters are made even worse by the fact that alcoholics are typically deficient in key antioxidant nutrients, particularly vitamin E, selenium, and vitamin C.[12] There is a significant link between the levels of free radicals and antioxidants and the degree of liver damage in alcoholism.[13] Antioxidants taken either prior to or along with alcohol inhibit free-radical damage and the development of a fatty liver.[14] Effective antioxidants include vitamins C and E, zinc, selenium, and cysteine.

Carnitine

Although the use of *lipotropic agents* (nutritional compounds that promote the flow of fat to and from the liver) appears warranted in treating alcoholic fatty liver disease, many commonly used lipotropic agents, including choline, niacin, and cysteine, appear to have little value.[15,16] One lipotropic agent, carnitine, does significantly inhibit alcohol-induced fatty liver disease. It has been suggested that chronic alcohol consumption results in a functional deficiency of carnitine.[17–19]

Normally the body is able to manufacture sufficient levels of carnitine. However, in order to make carnitine, the body must have adequate levels of vitamin B6, vitamin C, and several other nutrients. Since the alcoholic is often deficient in these nutrients, carnitine levels are also affected. Carnitine normally facilitates fatty acid transport and breakdown. When levels are low, fat tends to accumulate in the liver—exactly what is seen in alcohol-induced fatty liver. An even higher carnitine level than normal may be needed to handle the increased fatty acid load produced by alcohol consumption. Carnitine (300 mg three times per day) promotes fat breakdown (as evident by its ability to lower triglyceride levels) and improves liver function.[17]

Amino Acids

Blood levels of the various amino acids (building blocks of protein molecules) are disturbed in alcoholics.[20–22] Correction of this disturbance greatly aids the alcoholic patient.[20–23] Since the liver is the primary site for amino acid metabolism, it is not surprising that alcoholics develop abnormal amino acid patterns. Normalization of plasma amino acids is particularly important for patients who show signs or symptoms of hepatic cirrhosis (severe fluid retention in the abdomen, extreme weakness and fatigue, and weight loss) or depression (see DEPRESSION). Supplementation with the branched-chain amino acids (BCAA) valine, isoleucine, and leucine greatly aids the alcoholic with cirrhosis.[23]

One of the typical findings in alcoholics is a very low level of tryptophan—the amino acid that is converted to serotonin. Low serotonin levels are a hallmark of depression. Raising serotonin levels greatly helps the recovering alcoholic. Following the recommendations in the DEPRESSION chapter would definitely be appropriate to aid in recovery. Using 5-hydroxytryptophan (5-HTP) to raise brain serotonin levels may be particularly helpful.

Vitamin C

In one study, a deficiency of vitamin C was found in ninety-one percent of patients who had alcohol-related diseases.[24] Supplemental vitamin C helped reduce the effects of acute and chronic alcohol toxicity in experimental studies involving humans and guinea pigs— two species unable to synthesize their own vitamin C.[9,25] There is a direct link between the level of vitamin C in white blood cells and the rate of clearance of alcohol from the blood;[9] higher levels of vitamin C are associated with a faster rate of detoxification of alcohol from the blood.

B-Vitamins

Alcoholics are almost always deficient in at least one of the B-vitamins.[1,5,24] These deficiencies result from a variety of mechanisms: low dietary intake, impaired conversion or increased deactivation of the active form of the B-vitamin, impaired absorption, and decreased storage capacity. A thiamin (vitamin B1) deficiency is both the most common (fifty-five percent in one study[24]) and the most serious of the B-vitamin deficiencies in the alcoholic. In addition, recent evidence indicates that a thiamin deficiency results in greater intake of alcohol, suggesting that thiamin deficiency is a predisposing factor for alcoholism.[26]

A functional vitamin B6 deficiency is also common among alcoholics, due not so much to inadequate intake as to impaired conversion to its active form (pyridoxal-5-phosphate) and enhanced degradation.[27] In addition to inhibiting conversion to more active forms, alcohol also decreases the absorption and utilization of many B-vitamins by the liver—especially folic acid—and/or increases their urinary excretion.[5,28]

Magnesium

A magnesium deficiency is common among alcoholics. In fact, low magnesium levels are present in as many as sixty percent of alcoholics and are strongly linked to delirium tremens.[29] Low levels of magnesium are thought to be the major reason for the increase of cardiovascular disease noted in alcoholics.[30] This deficiency is due primarily to a reduced magnesium intake, coupled with alcohol-induced increased loss of magnesium in the urine.[1,29] The increased excretion of magnesium tends to continue during withdrawal despite low serum magnesium levels.

Essential Fatty Acids

Alcohol has been shown to interfere with essential fatty acid (EFA) metabolism and, as a result, may produce symptoms of EFA deficiency if consumed in excess.[31] Supplementing with essential fatty acids in an active alcoholic is not the answer. The answer is getting the alcoholic to stop drinking.

Glutamine

Glutamine supplementation (1 gram per day) has been shown to reduce voluntary alcohol consumption in uncontrolled human studies and experimental animal studies.[32–35] Despite the fact that this research is over forty years old now, there has never been any follow-up to these preliminary studies. This is unfortunate, as the results were quite promising and glutamine is safe and relatively inexpensive.

Other Therapies

Exercise

The involvement of the alcoholic patient in a graded, individually tailored fitness program has been shown to improve the likelihood of maintaining abstinence.[38] Research has shown that regular exercise is effective in alleviating anxiety and depression and enables individuals to respond better to stress. Improved fitness may allow more effective responses to emotional upset, thereby reducing the likelihood of resorting to alcohol when involved in conflict.

Silymarin

The flavonoid complex of milk thistle (*Silybum marianum*) appears to be of value for the alcoholic, especially in the presence of considerable liver involvement or cirrhosis. Silymarin has been shown to be effective in the treatment of the full spectrum of alcohol-related liver disease, from relatively mild to serious cirrhosis. Perhaps the most significant benefit is extending the life span of these patients.

In one study, eighty-seven cirrhotics (forty-six with alcoholic cirrhosis) received silymarin, while eighty-three cirrhotics (forty-five with alcoholic cirrhosis) received a placebo.[39] The average observation period was forty-one months. In the treatment group, there were twenty-four deaths, with eighteen related to liver disease. In the control group, there were thirty-seven deaths, with thirty-one related to liver disease. The four-year survival rate was fifty-eight percent in the treatment group, compared to thirty-nine percent in the control group.

Silymarin can also improve immune function in patients with cirrhosis.[40] Whether this effect is responsible for any direct benefit to the cirrhosis has yet to be determined.

TREATMENT SUMMARY

Alcoholism is a difficult disease to treat. Although many different strategies are promoted, there has been little documented long-term success, except for that of Alcoholics Anonymous (and even the overall success rate of this program is highly controversial). The approach presented here is unique in that we have attempted to develop an integrated, whole-person, stage-oriented program.

The treatment of the alcoholic patient must be optimized for the four stages of alcoholism: active alcohol consumption, withdrawal, recovering, and recovered.

The "recovering" stage is defined here as the period between withdrawal and full reestablishment of normal metabolic function. All alcoholics, at whatever stage, need a number of counseling, lifestyle, and metabolic-balancing therapies. Following are the recommended therapies, with additional recommendations for each stage.

Diet

Stabilization of blood sugar levels is critical to successful treatment. Although a strict hypoglycemic diet may not be necessary, most of the dietary guidelines for hypoglycemia must be followed. These include

- Elimination of all simple sugars (foods that contain added sucrose, fructose, or glucose), fruit juice, dried fruit, and low-fiber fruits (such as grapes and citrus fruits)
- Limitation of processed carbohydrates (white flour, instant potatoes, white rice, etc.)
- Increased consumption of complex carbohydrates (whole grains, vegetables, beans, etc.)

Nutritional Supplements

- Vitamin A: 25,000 IU per day (only if the person is not drinking and has normal liver function; vitamin A supplementation should not be used if there is evidence of liver damage)
- High-potency multiple-vitamin-and-mineral formula, as described in the chapter SUPPLEMENTARY MEASURES
- Vitamin C: 1,000 mg three times per day
- Vitamin E: 400–800 IU per day
- Magnesium: 200–300 mg three times per day
- Zinc: 30 mg per day
- Carnitine: 300 mg three times per day
- Glutamine: 1 g per day
- *Lactobacillus acidophilus:* one to two billion live bacteria per day
- Milk thistle extract (70–80% silymarin): 70–210 mg three times per day is a typical dosage (the dosage is based on the level of silymarin); higher

dosages should be used if there is significant liver involvement

Exercise

Establish a regular exercise program as detailed in the chapter A HEALTHY LIFESTYLE.

Counseling

Establish a good working relationship with AA and/or an experienced counselor who has particular expertise in working with alcoholics.

Additional Recommendations for the Four Stages

Active Alcohol Consumption

Seek immediate professional help or contact AA.

Withdrawal

Severity of withdrawal symptoms varies widely, although it is usually proportional to the degree of alcohol dependence and the duration of the disease. Milder cases usually start within a few hours after cessation of drinking and typically resolve within forty-eight hours. More severe cases usually occur only in patients over thirty years of age and usually develop after about forty-eight hours of abstinence. These people should be admitted to an inpatient facility.

Additional Supplement

- 5-HTP: 50–100 mg three times per day

Recovering

Establish a strong network of caring family, friends, and peers for regular support. Recognize that alcohol is no answer to the stresses of life; it is important to develop more effective ways of handling the challenges of life.

Recovered

The support group must be maintained. Continued total abstinence is the best policy.

Alzheimer's Disease

. . . .

Progressive mental deterioration, loss of memory and cognitive functions, inability to carry out activities of daily life

Characteristic symmetrical, usually diffuse, EEG pattern

Diagnosis usually made by exclusion

Definitive diagnosis can be made only by postmortem biopsy of brain, demonstrating atrophy, senile plaques, and neurofibrillary tangles

Alzheimer's disease (AD) is a degenerative brain disorder that manifests as a progressive deterioration of memory and mental function, a state of mind commonly referred to as *dementia*. In the United States, five percent of the population over sixty-five suffer from severe dementia, while another ten percent suffer from mild to moderate dementia. With increasing age, there is a rise in frequency. For example, in people over age eighty, the frequency rate for dementia is over twenty-five percent.

Autopsy studies have shown that fifty to sixty percent of all cases of dementia are the result of Alzheimer's disease. The tremendous increase (tenfold) of AD in this century in the U.S. population over the age of sixty-five is one reason why AD is referred to as "the disease of the twentieth century." AD has reached epidemic proportions.

Alzheimer's disease is characterized by distinctive changes in the brain. The primary feature is the formation of what are referred to as *neurofibrillary tangles* and *plaques*. Simplistically speaking, these neurofibrillary tangles and plaques are "scars," composed of deposits of various proteins and cellular debris. The result is massive loss of brain cells, especially in key areas of the brain that control mental function.[1]

The symptoms of AD are believed to be related to a reduced level of *acetylcholine*, a key neurotransmitter in the brain that is especially important for memory.

Causes

The cause of AD is being extensively researched. Genetic factors play a major role, with several genes being linked to AD. However, although genes probably play a significant role in determining who is going to develop AD, like most chronic degenerative diseases, environmental factors also play a significant role. Traumatic injury to the head, chronic exposure to aluminum and/or silicon, exposure to toxins from environmental sources, and free-radical damage have all been implicated as causative factors.

Fortunately, as with other chronic degenerative diseases, there is considerable evidence that increased oxidative damage plays a central role in the development of Alzheimer's disease. Therapies designed to support antioxidant mechanisms (discussed in the Therapeutic Considerations section of this chapter) may be quite helpful in the prevention of AD.[2]

Considerable attention has been given to the aluminum concentration in the neurofibrillary tangle. Whether the aluminum concentration develops in response to AD or initiates the lesions has not yet been determined, but significant evidence shows that it contributes, possibly very significantly, to the disease.

There is a great deal of circumstantial evidence linking chronic aluminum exposure to AD.[3] Greater aluminum concentrations in the brain could explain why AD symptoms worsen with increasing age. A study of 356 healthy people has shown that serum aluminum concentration increases as people age.[4] Those with Alzheimer's disease have significantly higher aluminum levels in their brains than either normal people or patients with other types of dementia, such as from alcohol, atherosclerosis, or stroke. Trying to remove the aluminum appears to help some people with AD. For example, intramuscular injections of *desferrioxamine* (a chelating agent that binds to aluminum and promotes its excretion in the urine) over a two-year period produced a significant slowing of the rate of decline of forty-eight Alzheimer's disease patients.[5] However, it's probably too late to use this type of treatment after the disease is well established.

The aluminum appears to come from the water supply, food, antacids, and deodorants. The most significant source is probably drinking water, as the aluminum in water is in a more bioavailable and thus potentially toxic form. Researchers measured the aluminum absorption of tap water by adding a small amount of soluble aluminum in a radioactive form to the stomach of animals. They discovered that the trace amounts of aluminum from this single exposure immediately entered the animal's brain tissue. The frightening news is that aluminum in water not only occurs naturally, but is also added (in the form of alum) to treat some water supplies.[6] You may want to contact your local water company and ask what the level of aluminum is in the drinking water.

Diagnostic Considerations

The process for diagnosing AD is one of exclusion. The first step is to determine if the

QUICK REVIEW

- Aluminum accumulation in the brain greatly contributes to the development of Alzheimer's disease.
- Abnormal fingerprint patterns are associated with both Alzheimer's Disease and Down's syndrome.
- From the perspective of natural medicine, the primary goals of intervention involve prevention by addressing suspected disease processes (e.g., aluminum and free-radical damage) and using natural measures to improve mental function in the early stages of the disease.
- There is evidence to suggest that antioxidant nutrients offer significant protection against Alzheimer's disease as well as therapeutic benefits.
- Aluminum absorption can be decreased by magnesium, as magnesium competes

person has true dementia as opposed to depression. Error rates of ten to fifty percent have been reported when the diagnosis of dementia is based only on the first evaluation.[7,8] Most of these misdiagnosed patients are found, on further evaluation, to have a pseudodementing functional illness.[7] Depression, which can mimic dementia in the elderly, is common. Possible causes of dementia are listed in Table 1.

The diagnosis of AD depends chiefly on clinical judgment. Complete evaluation by a competent physician includes

1. A detailed history
2. Neurological and physical examination
3. Psychological evaluation, with emphasis on the detection of subtle metabolic, toxic, or other disorders that can precipitate confusion
4. A series of tests to document the type and severity of mental impairment
5. Appropriate laboratory studies (listed in Table 1), including an electrocardiogram (EKG), electroencephalogram (EEG), and computerized tomography (CT scan)

The electroencephalogram (EEG) is an important tool in diagnosing dementia. Although a normal EEG reading does not rule out the diagnosis of dementia, particularly in its early stages, it does provide valuable information. AD is associated with a characteristic symmetrical, usually diffuse, slowing of the EEG. More importantly, the EEG differentiates focal brain dysfunction (e.g., tumor or vascular disease) from diffuse brain dysfunction (e.g., metabolic disorders).

The CT scan is a necessary part of the diagnostic protocol due to the high incidence (four to five percent) of brain tumors or other masses in patients who are examined for the diagnosis of dementia. The CT scan is of limited usefulness in diagnosing AD, since atrophy of the brain is part of the "normal" aging process. Its use is limited primarily to ruling out other causes of dementia.

Fingerprint Patterns

Abnormal fingerprint patterns are associated with both Alzheimer's disease and Down's syndrome.[9] Compared to the normal popula-

. . . .

with aluminum for absorption, not only in the intestines but also at the blood/brain barrier.

- A significant percentage of the geriatric population are deficient in one or more of the B-vitamins where low levels are linked to Alzheimer's disease.
- Zinc supplementation is demonstrating good results in the treatment of Alzheimer's disease.

- The results of using L-acetyl-carnitine to delay the progression of Alzheimer's disease have been outstanding.
- DHEA shows promise in enhancing memory and improving mental function in the elderly.
- Although preliminary studies involving established Alzheimer's patients are quite promising, at this time it appears that GBE only helps reverse or delay mental deterioration during the early stages of Alzheimer's disease.

TABLE 1 Recommended Laboratory Tests for Diagnosing Dementia	
TEST	**RATIONALE**
CBC	Anemia, infection
VDRL	Syphilis
Electrolytes	Metabolic dysfunction
Liver function tests	Hepatic dysfunction
Blood urea nitrogen (BUN)	Renal dysfunction
TSH, T4, T3, T3U	Thyroid dysfunction
Serum B12 and RBC folate	Vitamin B12 or folic acid deficiency
Urinalysis	Renal/hepatic dysfunction
Hair mineral analysis	Heavy metal intoxication
EKG	Heart function
EEG	Focal vs. diffuse brain dysfunction
CT scan	Atrophy, intracranial mass

tion, Alzheimer's and Down's patients show an increased number of ulnar loops on the fingertips, with a concomitant decrease in whorls, radial loops, and arches. *Ulnar loops* (loops that point toward the ulnar bone, away from the thumb) are frequently found on all ten fingertips. *Radial loops* (loops that point toward the thumb), when they do appear, tend to be shifted away from the index and middle fingers—where they most commonly occur—to the ring and little fingers. In patients with this fingerprint pattern characteristic of Alzheimer's disease, it is recommended that an aggressive preventive approach be instituted immediately.

Therapeutic Considerations

From the perspective of natural medicine, the primary goals of intervention involve prevention by addressing suspected disease processes (e.g., aluminum and free-radical damage) and using natural measures to im-

prove mental function in the early stages of the disease. In the advanced stages of AD, these natural measures will be unfruitful.

The Preventive Role of Antioxidants

There is considerable evidence that oxidative damage plays a major role in the development and progression of AD.[2,10,11] There is also evidence to suggest that antioxidant nutrients offer significant protection against AD.[12]

There is a tremendous need for good studies evaluating the role of antioxidant nutrients in preventing AD.[13] However, we believe that researchers will find that antioxidant nutrients, especially vitamin E, can help prevent AD in the same way they help protect against heart disease, cancer, Parkinson's disease, and other diseases linked to excessive oxidation.

Parkinson's disease is another degenerative brain disease that is caused by nerve damage to areas of the brain that control muscle tension and movement. It usually begins as a slight tremor of one hand, arm, or

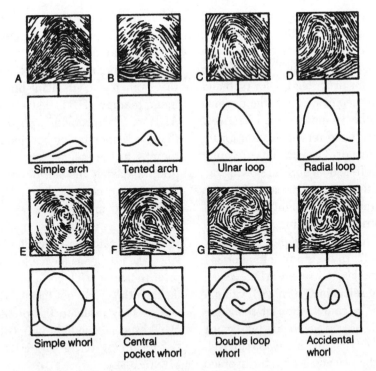

A — Simple arch
B — Tented arch
C — Ulnar loop
D — Radial loop
E — Simple whorl
F — Central pocket whorl
G — Double loop whorl
H — Accidental whorl

FIGURE 1 Fingerprint Patterns in Alzheimer's Disease

leg. In the early stages of the disease, the tremors are much worse at rest. In other words, the symptoms are most visible when a person is just sitting or standing and less visible when the hand or limb is used. One of the usual early symptoms of Parkinson's disease is called "pill-rolling." Patients move their fingers as if rolling a pill. As Parkinson's disease progresses, symptoms get much worse. It is heartbreaking to watch these people, as they are unable to control their movements.

Antioxidant nutrients, such as vitamins C and E, have been shown to be quite effective in slowing the progression of Parkinson's disease in patients who are not yet on medication. These results led to a pilot trial of high doses of vitamins C and E in treating early Parkinson's disease, as well as a large study of high-dose vitamin E and the drug Deprenyl.[14] High dosages are required because it is more difficult to increase antioxidant levels in brain tissue than in other parts of the body.

In the pilot study on vitamins C and E that began in 1979, twenty-one patients with early Parkinson's disease were given 3,000 mg of vitamin C and 3,200 IU of vitamin E each day.[14] The patients were followed closely for a period of seven years. Although all patients eventually required drug treatment (Sinemet or Deprenyl), the progression of the disease, as determined by need for medication, was considerably delayed in those who received the nutritional antioxidants compared to the rates in those not receiving the antioxidants. Dividing the patients in both groups into younger-onset and older-onset patients, those who did not receive antioxidants required medication 40 and 24 months, respectively, after the onset of the disease. In contrast, the two age groups in the pilot study were able to delay the need for drug therapy for 65.3 and 59.2 months, respectively. Thus, the patients who received the vitamins were effectively able to delay the need for medication for up to three years longer. These results are quite promising and offer some hope in slowing the progression of this dreaded disease.

The only intervention trial on the effect of antioxidant nutrients in treating AD is a study published in the *New England Journal of Medicine* in 1997. In the study, a total of 341 patients with moderately severe AD received either the drug selegiline (10 mg/d), vitamin E (2,000 IU/d), a combination of selegiline and vitamin E, or a placebo for two years. One of the key parameters was survival. Compared to the placebo group, the average survival was 230 days for vitamin E, 215 for the selegiline, and 145 days for the combination. The percentages of participants who had to be institutionalized among the four groups are as follows: vitamin E twenty-six percent; selegiline thirty-three percent; combination thirty-five percent, and placebo thirty-nine percent. These results are not outstanding, but keep in mind that these patients had moderately severe dementia. Better results are likely to be obtained if antioxidant therapy is started earlier in the disease process.

Estrogen

Estrogen is being promoted to offer protective and possibly therapeutic benefits in relation to AD. However, the epidemiological and clinical evidence to support the potential benefits of estrogen treatment is very weak because there is little evidence of major sex differences in the rate or severity of AD. In other words, men and women get AD at about the same level and frequency.[15]

Twelve population-based studies indicate that women who are taking hormone replacement therapy (HRT) have a lower rate of AD.[15-18] The problem with these studies is that the women taking hormone replacement therapy in the studies were much healthier prior to taking the hormones compared to those in the control group.[19] This situation has clouded much of the research on HRT, not only in its role in treating AD, but also in relation to cardiovascular disease. If women who take estrogens have a lower risk for AD prior to taking HRT because they are healthier than the group not taking HRT, it is difficult to fully evaluate the protective role of HRT, especially in light of possible increased risk for breast cancer with HRT therapy (see MENOPAUSE).

Some clinical trials have indicated that estrogen therapy improves mental function, but other studies have not supported those results.[15-18] It is likely that estrogen produces some benefits, but several natural products discussed in this chapter exert greater benefit without the risk of breast cancer.

The benefits of estrogen in AD could be related to many factors, but the one that appears most likely is its antioxidant effect.[19] However, a safer and probably better recommendation for these effects is vitamin E. The protective role of vitamin E against heart disease, for example, is greater than that offered by hormone replacement therapy (see HEART AND CARDIOVASCULAR HEALTH).

Aluminum

It certainly seems appropriate to encourage the avoidance of all known sources of aluminum: antacids and antiperspirants that contain aluminum; aluminum pots and pans; aluminum foil as food wrapping; and nondairy creamers. Aluminum is also found in baking powder and table salt, as it is added to keep them from becoming lumpy. In addition, citric acid and calcium citrate supplements appear to increase the efficiency of aluminum absorption (but not lead absorption) from water and food.[20]

Aluminum absorption can be decreased by magnesium, as magnesium competes with aluminum for absorption, not only in the intestines but also at the blood/brain barrier.[21] A diet rich in magnesium is recommended. Avoid processed foods, milk, and dairy products; increase the consumption of vegetables, whole grains, nuts, and seeds—all good sources of magnesium; and take a magnesium supplement or a formula that contains magnesium.

Nutritional Status, Thiamin, and Brain Function

In the elderly, cognitive function is directly related to nutritional status.[22] High nutritional status equals higher mental function. Given the frequency of nutrient deficiency in the elderly population, it is likely that many cases of impaired mental function may have a nutritional cause.

To illustrate this possibility, let's examine the role of thiamin. Although severe thiamin deficiency is relatively uncommon (except in alcoholics), many Americans do not consume the RDA of 1.5 mg, especially the elderly. In an attempt to gauge the prevalence of thiamin deficiency in the geriatric population, thirty consecutive subjects visiting a university outpatient clinic in Tampa, Florida, were tested for thiamin levels. Depending upon the thiamin measurement technique (plasma vs. red blood cell thiamin), low levels (defined as a level below the lowest level of normal) were found in fifty-seven percent and thirty-three percent, respectively.[23] In other words, somewhere between thirty-three percent and fifty-seven percent (depending upon the measurement) of the test subjects were suffering from thiamin deficiency.

These results highlight the growing body of evidence that a significant percentage of the geriatric population are deficient in one or more of the B-vitamins. Given the essential role of thiamin and other B-vitamins in normal human physiology, especially cardiovascular and brain function, routine B-vitamin supplementation appears to be worthwhile in this age group. Alzheimer's disease may simply be the result of chronic low intake of essential nutrients; key among these nutrients are the B-vitamins.

In addition to its role as a nutrient, thiamin demonstrates some pharmacological effects on the brain. Specifically, it mimics *acetylcholine*, the important neurotransmitter involved in memory and in Alzheimer's disease. Thiamin has been shown to potentiate and mimic the effects of acetylcholine in the brain.[24] This effect explains the positive clinical results that have been noted for thiamin (3 to 8 grams per day) in improving mental function in patients with Alzheimer's disease and age-related impaired mental function (senility).[25,26] High-dose thiamin supplementation exerts its benefits without side effects.

Vitamin B12

Another key B-vitamin linked to Alzheimer's disease is vitamin B12. A vitamin B12 deficiency will result in impaired nerve function, which can cause numbness, pins-and-needles sensations, or a burning feeling in the feet, as well as impaired mental function, which, in the elderly, can mimic Alzheimer's disease.

Vitamin B12 deficiency is thought to be quite common in the elderly and is a major cause of depression in this age group.

Several investigators have found that the level of vitamin B12 declines with age and that vitamin B12 deficiency is found in three to forty-two percent of persons aged sixty-five and over. It is important to diagnose B12 deficiency early in the elderly, because it is easily treatable and, if left untreated, can lead to impaired neurological and cognitive function.[27,28]

It is also crucial to measure vitamin B12 levels or activity in anyone who is experiencing dementia—especially an elderly person.[29–32] Supplementation with vitamin B12 has shown tremendous benefit in reversing impaired mental function that results from low levels of vitamin B12.[27] In one of the larger studies, a complete recovery was observed in sixty-one percent of cases of mental impairment due to low levels of vitamin B12.[33] The thirty-nine percent who did not respond probably had long-term low levels of vitamin B12.

Several studies have indicated that the best clinical responders are those who have been showing signs of impaired mental function for less than six months.[27] In one study, eighteen subjects with low serum cobalamin levels and evidence of mental impairment were given vitamin B12. Only those patients who had had symptoms for less than one year showed improvement.[34] Again, the importance of diagnosing and correcting low vitamin B12 levels in the elderly cannot be overstated.

In Alzheimer's disease patients, serum vitamin B12 levels are significantly low, and vitamin B12 deficiency is significantly common.[27,35–37] Supplementation of B12 and/or folic acid may result in complete reversal in some patients, but there is generally little improvement in patients who have had

Alzheimer's symptoms for longer than six months. It has been hypothesized that prolonged low levels of vitamin B12 may lead to irreversible changes that will not respond to supplementation.

Vitamin B12 is available in several forms. The most common form is cyanocobalamin. However, vitamin B12 is active in the human body in only two forms: methylcobalamin and adenosylcobalamin. While methylcobalamin and adenosylcobalamin are active immediately upon absorption, cyanocobalamin must be converted to either methylcobalamin or adenosylcobalamin. This occurs when the body removes the cyanide molecule from cyanocobalamin and adds either a methyl or an adenosyl group (the amount of cyanide produced in this process is extremely small). The rate at which this conversion occurs may be reduced with aging, which could contribute to the vitamin B12 disturbances noted in the elderly population.

Zinc

Zinc deficiency is one of the most common nutrient deficiencies in the elderly and has been suggested to be a major factor in the development of Alzheimer's disease.[38] The list of zinc-containing enzymes includes most of the enzymes involved in DNA replication, repair, and transcription. DNA is the genetic core that serves as the blueprint for cellular functions and cell replication. It has been suggested that dementia (possibly caused by a long-term zinc deficiency) may represent the long-term cascading effects of error-prone or ineffective activity of important enzymes that support proper DNA function.[39] In addition, zinc is required by many antioxidant enzymes, including superoxide dismutase. The end result could be the destruction of nerve cells and the formation of neurofibrillary tangles and plaques. The level of zinc in the brain and cerebrospinal fluid of Alzheimer's disease patients is markedly decreased.

Zinc supplementation is demonstrating good results in the treatment of Alzheimer's disease. In one study, ten patients with Alzheimer's disease were given 27 mg of zinc (as zinc aspartate) daily. Only two patients failed to show improvement in memory, understanding, communication, and social contact. In one seventy-nine-year-old patient, the response was labeled "unbelievable" by both medical staff and family.[40] Unfortunately, the scientific community doesn't seem very interested in following up these impressive zinc-therapy results.

Phosphatidylcholine

Since *phosphatidylcholine* (the key component of lecithin) can increase acetylcholine levels in the brain in normal patients, and since Alzheimer's disease is characterized by a decrease in acetylcholine levels, it would seem reasonable to assume that phosphatidylcholine supplementation would be of benefit to Alzheimer patients. However, the basic defect in Alzheimer's disease relates to impaired activity of the enzyme *acetylcholine transferase*. This enzyme combines choline (as provided by phosphatidylcholine) with an acetyl molecule to form the neurotransmitter *acetylcholine*. Since providing more choline will not necessarily increase the activity of this key enzyme, phosphatidylcholine supplementation would not be very beneficial.

Not surprisingly, clinical trials using phosphatidylcholine have largely been disappointing. Studies have shown inconsistent improvements in memory from phosphatidylcholine supplementation in both normal and Alzheimer's patients.[41–43] The studies have been criticized for small sample size, low dosage of phosphatidylcholine, and poor design. The lack of high-quality studies makes it difficult to assess just how helpful phosphatidylcholine might be.

In a patient with mild to moderate dementia, the use of a high-quality phosphatidylcholine preparation may be worth a try. A dosage of 15 to 25 grams of phosphatidylcholine daily is required. If there is no noticeable improvement within two weeks, supplementation should be halted since phosphatidylcholine at this dosage is expensive as well as being associated with some side effects such as nausea.

Phosphatidylserine

Phosphatidylserine plays a major role in determining the integrity and fluidity of brain cell membranes. Normally, the brain can manufacture sufficient levels of phosphatidylserine, but if there is a deficiency of folic acid and vitamin B12, or of essential fatty acids, the brain may not be able to make sufficient phosphatidylserine. Low levels of phosphatidylserine in the brain are associated with impaired mental function and depression in the elderly.

The primary use of phosphatidylserine is in the treatment of depression and/or impaired mental function in the elderly, including Alzheimer's disease patients. To date, eleven double-blind studies have been completed using phosphatidylserine in the treatment of age-related cognitive decline, Alzheimer's disease, or depression. Good results have been obtained in these studies.[44–53] In the largest study, a total of 494 elderly patients (aged between sixty-five and ninety-three years) with moderate to severe senility were given either phosphatidylserine (100 mg three times daily) or a placebo for six months.[44] The patients were assessed for mental performance, behavior, and mood at the beginning and end of the study. Statistically significant (p<0.01) improvements were noted in mental function, mood, and behavior in the phosphatidylserine-treated group.

L-Acetylcarnitine

Carnitine is a vitamin-like compound that is responsible for the transport of long-chain fatty acids into the energy-producing units in cells: the *mitochondria*. In the 1980s and 1990s, a special form of carnitine—L-acetylcarnitine (LAC)—has been the subject of numerous studies on the treatment of Alzheimer's disease, senile depression, and age-related memory defects. LAC is a molecule composed of acetic acid and carnitine bound together. The manufacture of LAC occurs naturally in the human brain, so it is not exactly known how much greater of an effect is noted with LAC vs. carnitine. However, LAC is thought to be substantially more effective than carnitine in conditions that involve the brain.[54,55]

The close structural similarity between LAC and acetylcholine led researchers to begin testing LAC as a treatment for Alzheimer's disease. Researchers have now shown that LAC does indeed mimic acetylcholine and is of benefit not only in treating patients with early-stage Alzheimer's disease, but also for elderly patients who are depressed or who have impaired memory.[55] LAC has also been shown to stabilize cell membranes, to act as a powerful antioxidant within brain cells, to improve energy production within brain cells, and to enhance or mimic the function of acetylcholine.[56]

The results of using LAC to delay the progression of Alzheimer's disease have been outstanding. The studies have been well controlled and extremely thorough.[54,57-59] For example, in one study LAC (2 grams twice daily) or a placebo was given to 130 patients with Alzheimer's disease over the course of one year.[59] The patients were evaluated by fourteen different outcome measures, such as assessment scales, cognitive function tests, memory tests, and physician evaluations. The group that received the LAC ranked better on all outcome scores.

Memory impairment need not be as severe as that found in Alzheimer's disease in order for LAC to demonstrate benefit.[60-62] In one double-blind study of 236 elderly subjects with mild mental deterioration (as evident by detailed clinical assessment), the group that received 1,500 mg of LAC daily demonstrated significant improvement in mental function, particularly in memory and constructional thinking.[62]

DHEA

DHEA (dehydroepiandrosterone) is the most abundant hormone in the bloodstream and is found in extremely high concentrations in the brain. As DHEA levels decline dramatically with aging, low levels of DHEA in the blood and brain are thought to contribute to many symptoms associated with aging, including impaired mental function.

DHEA itself has no known function other than to serve as the source for all other steroid hormones in the body, including sex hormones and corticosteroids. Therefore, the function of DHEA seems to be to supply the body with what it needs to maintain optimum levels and balance of all the steroid hormones that regulate the body's activities.

Over the last decade, it has been demonstrated that declining levels of DHEA are linked to such conditions as diabetes, obesity, elevated cholesterol levels, heart disease, arthritis, and other age-related conditions. In addition, DHEA shows promise in enhancing memory and improving cognitive function.[63,64]

The level of DHEA necessary to improve brain power in men over age fifty appears to be 25 to 50 mg per day. For women, a dosage of 15 to 25 mg appears to be sufficient in most cases. As men and women reach their seventies, they may require higher levels (50 to 100 mg). Taking too much DHEA can cause acne. If this occurs, reduce the dosage.

Ginkgo biloba Extract

The *Ginkgo biloba* extract (GBE) standardized to contain twenty-four percent ginkgo flavonglycosides is showing great benefit in treating many cases of senility, including Alzheimer's disease. In addition to GBE's ability to increase the functional capacity of the brain, it also has been shown to normalize the acetylcholine receptors in the hippocampus (the area of the brain most affected by Alzheimer's disease) of aged animals, to increase cholinergic transmission, and to address many of the other major elements of Alzheimer's disease.[65-68]

Although preliminary studies involving established Alzheimer's patients are quite promising, at this time it appears that GBE only helps reverse or delay mental deterioration during the early stages of Alzheimer's disease.[69-71] This improvement may help to enable the patient to maintain a normal life and to avoid being put in a nursing home.

The benefits of GBE in early-stage Alzheimer's disease are quite evident when looking at the results from two recent double-blind studies. In the first study, 216 patients with Alzheimer's disease or multi-infarct dementia (dementia caused by multiple "mini strokes") were given either 240 mg of GBE daily or placebo for 24 weeks.[70] The data from the 156 patients who completed the study in-

TABLE 2 Clinical Global Impression Ratings: GBE vs. Placebo		
	GBE	**PLACEBO**
Very much improved	3%	1%
Much improved	29%	16%
Slightly improved	41%	38%
Unchanged	28%	30%
Moderately worse	0	14%
Much worse	0	1%

dicated quite clearly that GBE was very useful in the treatment of both types of dementia. Improvements were noted in the same clinical parameters as the first study described above as well as a Clinical Global Impressions (CGI) scale. The results from the CGI illustrate the superiority of GBE over placebo.

The second study, published in the JAMA (*Journal of the American Medical Association*), was the first clinical study on GBE conducted in the United States.[71] The study was conducted at six research centers with the design of the study being approved by the Harvard Medical School and the New York Institute for Medical Research. In the study, 202 patients with Alzheimer's disease were given either GBE (120 mg per day) or a placebo for one year. The study provided tremendous evidence on the value of GBE in Alzheimer's disease. GBE not only stabilized Alzheimer's disease but led to significant improvements in mental function in sixty-four percent of the patients. There were no side effects with GBE.

In addition to offering benefit in early-stage Alzheimer's disease, if the mental deficit is due to vascular insufficiency or depression and not Alzheimer's disease, GBE will usually be effective in reversing the deficit.

It must be pointed out that GBE should be taken consistently for at least twelve weeks in order to determine effectiveness. Although some people with AD report benefits within a two- to three-week period, most will need to take GBE for a longer period of time (e.g., six months) before seeing results, and will need to take GBE indefinitely to maintain the improvement.

TREATMENT SUMMARY

The primary therapeutic goal is either prevention or to begin therapy as soon as any dementia is noted.

Diet and Lifestyle

- Avoid aluminum (found in many anti-perspirants, antacids, and cookware).
- Follow a general healthful dietary and lifestyle plan as detailed in Part I.

Nutritional Supplements

- High-potency multiple-vitamin-and-mineral supplement, according to guidelines given in the chapter SUP-PLEMENTARY MEASURES.

- Vitamin C: 500–1,000 mg three times per day
- Vitamin E: 400–800 IU per day
- Flaxseed oil: One tbsp per day
- Thiamin: 3–8 g per day
- Phosphatidylserine: 100 mg three times per day
- L-acetyl-carnitine: 500 mg three times per day
- Methylcobalamin: 1,000 mcg twice per day

Botanical Medicine

- *Ginkgo biloba* extract (24% ginkgo flavonglycosides): 80 mg three times per day

Anemia

. . . .

Pallor, weakness, and a tendency to become fatigued easily

Low volume of blood, low level of total red blood cells, or abnormal size or shape of red blood cells

Anemia refers to a condition in which the blood is deficient in red blood cells or the *hemoglobin* (iron-containing) portion of red blood cells. The primary function of the red blood cell (RBC) is to transport oxygen from the lungs to the tissues of the body in exchange for carbon dioxide. The symptoms of anemia, such as extreme fatigue, reflect a lack of oxygen being delivered to tissues and a buildup of carbon dioxide.

There are three major classifications of anemia. Each classification is subdivided and briefly described in the following text.

1. Anemia due to excessive blood loss
2. Anemia due to excessive RBC destruction
3. Anemia due to deficient RBC production

Excessive Blood Loss

Anemia can be produced during *acute* (rapid) or *chronic* (slow but constant) blood loss. Acute blood loss can be fatal if more than one-third of total blood volume is lost (roughly 1.5 liters). Since acute blood loss is usually quite apparent, there is little difficulty in diagnosis. Often blood transfusion is required.

Chronic blood loss from a slow-bleeding peptic ulcer, hemorrhoids, or menstruation can also produce anemia. This highlights the importance of identifying the cause through a complete diagnostic workup by a qualified health care professional.

Excessive Red Blood Cell Destruction

Old RBCs, as well as abnormal RBCs, are removed from the circulation primarily by the spleen. If destruction of old or abnormal RBCs exceeds the body's ability to manufacture new RBCs, anemia can result. The most common cause of excessive destruction of RBCs is abnormal RBC shape.

A number of things can lead to abnormal RBC shape, including: defective hemoglobin synthesis, as seen in hereditary conditions like sickle-cell anemia; mechanical injury due to trauma or turbulence within arteries; hereditary RBC enzyme defects; and vitamin or mineral deficiency.

Deficient Red Blood Cell Production

This is the most common category of anemia. The most common cause of deficient RBC production is nutritional deficiency. Although

233

deficiency of any of several vitamins and minerals can produce anemia, only the most common—iron, vitamin B12, and folic acid—will be discussed here. Iron-deficiency anemia is characterized as a *microcytic anemia* because the RBCs become very small, while folic acid and B12 deficiency anemias are classified as *macrocytic anemias* because the RBCs become quite large.

Iron-Deficiency Anemia

Iron deficiency is the most common cause of anemia. However, it must be pointed out that anemia is the last stage of iron deficiency. Iron-dependent enzymes involved in energy production and metabolism are the first to be affected by low iron levels. *Serum ferritin* is the best laboratory test for determining body iron stores.[1]

The groups at highest risk for iron deficiency are infants under two years of age, teenage girls, pregnant women, and the elderly. Studies have found evidence of iron deficiency in as many as thirty to fifty percent of people in these groups. For example, some degree of iron deficiency occurs in thirty-five to fifty-eight percent of young, healthy women. For pregnant women, the number is even higher.[1]

Iron deficiency may be caused by an increased iron requirement, decreased dietary intake, diminished iron absorption or utilization, blood loss, or a combination of factors. Increased requirements for iron occur during the growth spurts of infancy and adolescence and during pregnancy and lactation. Currently, the vast majority of pregnant women are routinely given iron supplements during their pregnancy, as the dramatically increased need for iron during pregnancy cannot usually be met through diet alone. Inadequate intake of iron is common in many parts of the world, especially areas where people consume primarily a vegetarian diet.

Typical infant diets in developed countries (high in milk and cereals) are also low in iron. The adolescent who consumes a "junk food" diet is at high risk for iron deficiency. However, the population at greatest risk for a diet deficient in iron is the low-income elderly population.[2] This situation is complicated by the fact that decreased absorption of iron is extremely common in the elderly. Decreased absorption of iron is often caused by a lack of hydrochloric acid secretion in the stomach—

QUICK REVIEW

- Identifying the cause of anemia through a complete diagnostic workup by a qualified health care professional is essential.

- Anemia caused by deficient red blood cell (RBC) production is almost always due to nutrient deficiency. The three most common are due to deficiencies of either iron, vitamin B12, or folic acid.

- Iron deficiency is the most common cause of anemia.

- Perhaps the best food for an individual with any kind of anemia is calf liver.

- Although it is popular to inject vitamin B12 in the treatment of vitamin B12 deficiency, injection is not necessary as the oral administration of an appropriate dosage has been shown to produce excellent results.

an extremely common condition in the elderly.[3,4]

Other causes of decreased absorption include chronic diarrhea or malabsorption, the surgical removal of the stomach, and antacid use. Blood loss is the most common cause of iron deficiency in women of childbearing age. This blood loss is most often due to excessive menstrual bleeding. Interestingly enough, iron deficiency is a common cause of excessive menstrual blood loss. Other common causes of blood loss include bleeding from peptic ulcers, and hemorrhoids and donating blood.

The negative effects of iron deficiency are due largely to the impaired delivery of oxygen to the tissues and the impaired activity of iron-containing enzymes in various tissues. Iron deficiency can lead to anemia, excessive menstrual blood loss, learning disabilities, impaired immune function, and decreased energy levels and physical performance.[1]

Several researchers have clearly demonstrated that even slight iron-deficiency anemia leads to a reduction in physical work capacity and productivity.[5–8] Supplementation with iron has produced rapid improvements in work capacity among iron-deficient individuals. Impaired physical performance due to iron deficiency is not dependent on anemia. Again, the iron-dependent enzymes involved in energy production and metabolism will be impaired long before anemia occurs.[1]

Vitamin B12–Deficiency Anemia

Vitamin B12 deficiency is most often due to a defect in absorption, not a dietary lack. In order for vitamin B12 from food to be absorbed, it must be liberated from food by hydrochloric acid and bond to a substance known as *intrinsic factor* within the small intestine. Intrinsic factor is secreted by the *parietal cells* of the stomach. These same cells are responsible for the secretion of hydrochloric acid. Hence, the secretion of intrinsic factor parallels that of hydrochloric acid. The B12-intrinsic factor complex is absorbed in the small intestine with the aid of the pancreatic enzyme *trypsin*.

In order for vitamin B12 to be absorbed, an individual must secrete enough hydrochloric acid and intrinsic factor and adequate pancreatic enzymes, including trypsin, and have a healthy and intact *ileum* (the end portion of the small intestine, where the vitamin B12-intrinsic factor complex is absorbed).

Lack of intrinsic factor results in a condition known as *pernicious anemia*. The defect is rare before the age of thirty-five, and it is more common in individuals of Scandinavian, English, and Irish descent. It is much less common in southern Europeans, Asians, and Blacks. Pernicious anemia is frequently associated with iron deficiency as well.[6]

A dietary lack of vitamin B12 is most often associated with a strict vegetarian diet. Unlike other water-soluble nutrients, vitamin B12 is stored in the liver, kidney, and other body tissues. As a result, signs and symptoms of vitamin B12 deficiency may not show themselves until after five to six years of poor dietary intake or inadequate secretion of intrinsic factor. Since normal body stores of vitamin B12 may last an individual three to six years, deficiency of vitamin B12 is usually not apparent in a vegetarian until after many years. The classic symptom of vitamin B12 deficiency is pernicious anemia. However, it appears that a deficiency of vitamin B12 will actually affect the brain and nervous system first.

The diagnosis of vitamin B12 deficiency is best made by measuring the vitamin B12 level in the blood. Most physicians, however, simply rely on the presence of large red blood cells and characteristic symptoms. Symptoms of severe B12 deficiency can include: paleness; easy fatigability; shortness of breath; a sore, beefy red, and swollen tongue; diarrhea; and heart and nervous system disturbances.

The nervous system disturbances of a vitamin B12 deficiency can be quite serious. Common nervous system symptoms include numbness and tingling of the arms or legs, depression, mental confusion, loss of vibration sense, and loss of deep tendon reflexes. In the elderly, a vitamin B12 deficiency can mimic Alzheimer's disease.

Folic Acid Deficiency

Folic acid deficiency is the most common vitamin deficiency in the world. Unlike vitamin B12, the body does not store a large surplus of folic acid. Folic acid stores in the body are only sufficient to sustain the body for one to two months.

Folic acid deficiency is extremely common among alcoholics, as alcohol consumption impairs folic acid absorption, disrupts folic acid metabolism, and causes the body to excrete folic acid.

Folic acid deficiency is also common among pregnant women. This is due to an increased demand for folic acid. Folic acid is vital to cell reproduction within the fetus. If the fetus does not have a constant source of folic acid, birth defects such as neural tube defects will result. Pregnant women may become deficient in folic acid because of the high demand of the developing fetus. If alcohol is consumed during pregnancy, the lowering of folic acid levels by the alcohol may lead to fetal alcohol syndrome or neural tube defects.[9]

In addition to alcohol, there are a number of drugs that can induce a folic acid deficiency, including anticancer drugs, drugs for epilepsy, and oral contraceptives.

Folic acid deficiency is quite common among patients who have chronic diarrhea or malabsorption states such as celiac disease,

Crohn's disease, or tropical sprue. Since a deficiency of folic acid will result in diarrhea and malabsorption, often a vicious circle ensues. The administration of folic acid as a preventive measure is warranted in anyone experiencing chronic diarrhea. Often this has a therapeutic effect as well.

Folic acid deficiency will result in the same type of anemia as is caused by a vitamin B12 deficiency: an anemia characterized by enlarged RBCs (macrocytic anemia). The most sensitive test to assess folic acid deficiency is determining the folic acid content of the serum and RBC. In addition to anemia, other symptoms of folic acid deficiency include diarrhea, depression, and a swollen, red tongue.

NOTE: It is always necessary to supplement vitamin B12 with folic acid to prevent the folic acid supplement from masking a vitamin B12 deficiency. Supplementing with folic acid will correct the anemia of a vitamin B12 deficiency, but it cannot overcome the problems that vitamin B12 deficiency causes in the brain.

Therapeutic Considerations

The treatment of anemia is dependent on proper clinical evaluation by a physician. It is imperative that a comprehensive laboratory analysis of the blood be performed. Do not be satisfied with the diagnosis of "anemia." It is critical that the underlying cause for the anemia be uncovered if appropriate therapy is to be employed.

Recommended therapy in this chapter will be divided into four categories: general nutritional support, iron-deficiency anemia, vitamin B12 deficiency anemia, and folic acid-deficiency anemia.

General Nutritional Support for All Types

Perhaps the best food for an individual with any kind of anemia is calf liver. It is rich not only in iron, but also in all B-vitamins. *Hydrolyzed* (liquefied) liver extracts are perhaps an even better source of highly bioavailable nutrients than regular liver. These extracts have the benefits of liver but are free of fats, cholesterol, and fat-soluble vitamins.

The use of liver or liver extracts has fallen out of favor in mainstream medicine. Instead, isolated vitamin B12, folic acid, or iron is used. The use of liver therapy in the treatment of anemia was viewed as a "shotgun" approach since liver contains such a large number of factors that can stimulate normal RBC production in addition to vitamins and minerals. In the authors' opinion, liver or hydrolyzed liver extracts still represent an effective natural treatment for all types of anemia. Contrary to popular opinion, toxins are not stored in the liver. The liver quickly processes toxins. Because it is such a vital organ, the body takes great strides to protect it. When the healthy liver cannot handle the toxin load, the toxins are quickly delivered to fatty tissues for storage. The liver itself is actually quite low in toxins compared to fatty tissue.

Green leafy vegetables are also of great benefit to individuals with any kind of anemia. These vegetables contain natural fat-soluble chlorophyll as well as other impor-tant nutrients, including iron and folic acid. The chlorophyll molecule is similar to the hemoglobin molecule. Fat-soluble (but not water-soluble) chlorophyll products may be taken by an anemic individual. Water-soluble chlorophyll is not absorbed from the gastrointestinal tract and therefore has no use in the treatment of anemia.

Since a large percentage of individuals with anemia do not secrete enough hydrochloric acid, it is often appropriate to take hydrochloric acid supplements with meals. See the chapter DIGESTION AND ELIMINATION for more information and dosage instructions.

Iron-Deficiency Anemia

Again, treatment of any type of anemia should focus on underlying causes. For iron-deficiency anemia, this typically involves finding a reason for chronic blood loss or for why an individual is not absorbing sufficient amounts of dietary iron. Lack of hydrochloric acid is a common reason for impaired iron absorption, especially among the elderly.

Increasing iron levels in the food may help partially or completely overcome poor iron absorption. In addition to liver and green leafy vegetables, foods rich in iron include: dried beans, blackstrap molasses, lean meat, organ meats, dried apricots and other dried fruits, almonds, and shellfish. Vitamin C supplementation has been shown to greatly enhance the absorption of dietary iron.[1] Vitamin C alone will often increase body iron stores. Five hundred milligrams of vitamin C with each meal is a suitable dose for this effect.

Several foods and beverages contain substances that inhibit iron absorption, including tea, coffee, wheat bran, and egg yolk. Antacids and overuse of calcium supplements also decrease iron absorption. These items should be restricted from the diet in individuals who have iron deficiency.[1]

Available Forms of Iron

There are two forms of dietary iron: *heme iron* and *non-heme iron*. Heme iron is iron bound to the oxygen-binding proteins *hemoglobin* and *myoglobin*. It is the most efficiently absorbed form of iron. The absorption rate of non-heme iron supplements, such as ferrous sulfate and ferrous fumarate, is 2.9 percent on an empty stomach and 0.9 percent with food, much less than the absorption rate of heme iron, as found in liver, which is as high as 35 percent.[1] In addition, heme iron is without the side effects associated with non-heme sources of iron, such as nausea, flatulence, and diarrhea.

Unbound non-heme iron is also more likely to spin off pro-oxidants and lead to the formation of free radicals than heme iron. For this reason, many practitioners are electing to use heme iron over non-heme iron sources when iron supplementation is necessary.

Despite the superiority of heme iron, non-heme iron salts are the most popular iron supplements. One reason is that even though heme-iron is better absorbed, it is easy to take higher quantities of non-heme iron salts so that the net amount of iron absorbed is about equal. In other words, if you take 3 mg of heme iron and 50 mg of non-heme iron the net absorption for each will be about the same. The best form of non-heme iron is ferrous succinate.

Vitamin B12 Deficiency Anemia

In 1926, it was shown that injectable liver extracts were effective in the treatment of pernicious anemia. Soon after, active concentrates of liver were available for intra-muscular as well as oral administration. As mentioned earlier, the use of liver and liver extracts has fallen out of favor in mainstream medicine. In regard to pernicious anemia, standard medical treatment involves injecting vitamin B12 at a dose of 1 mg daily for one week, but oral therapy has shown equal effectiveness (discussed in the section Oral vs. Injectable B12 later in this chapter).

Vitamin B12 is found in significant quantities only in animal foods. The richest sources are liver and kidney, followed by eggs, fish, cheese, and meat. Strict vegetarians (vegans) are often told that fermented foods such as tempeh and miso are excellent sources of vitamin B12. However, in addition to tremendous variation of B12 content in fermented foods, there is some evidence that the form of B12 in these foods is not the form that meets our body's requirements and is therefore useless. The same holds true for certain cooked sea vegetables. Although the vitamin B12 content of these foods is in the same range as beef, it is not known how well this form is utilized. Therefore, at this time it appears that it is an extremely good idea that vegetarians supplement their diets with vitamin B12.

Available Forms of Vitamin B12

Vitamin B12 is available in several forms. The most common form is *cyanocobalamin*. However, vitamin B12 is active in only two forms: *methylcobalamin* and *adenosylcobalamin*. Methylcobalamin is the only active form of vitamin B12 that is available commercially in tablet form in the United States. While methylcobalamin is active immediately upon absorption, cyanocobalamin must be converted by the body to either methylcobalamin or adenosylcobalamin by removing the cyanide molecule (the amount of cyanide produced in this process is extremely small) and adding either a methyl or adenosyl group. Cyanocobalamin is not active in many experimental models, while both methylcobalamin and adenosylcobalamin demonstrate exceptional activity. For example, in a model examining the ability of vitamin B12 to extend life in mice with cancer, methylcobalamin and adenosylcobalamin led to significant increases in survival time while cyanocobalamin had no effect.[10] Methylcobalamin has also produced better results in clinical trials than cyanocobalamin, and should therefore be considered the best available form.

Oral vs. Injectable B12

Although it is popular to inject vitamin B12, injection is not necessary; the oral administration of an appropriate dosage, even in the absence of intrinsic factor, can result in effective elevations of vitamin B12 levels in the blood. This fact has gone relatively ignored among most physicians. An editorial entitled "Oral Cobalamin for Pernicious Anemia: Medicine's Best-Kept Secret," which appeared in the January 2, 1991, edition of *JAMA* (the *Journal of the American Medical Association*), attests to the fact that oral therapy produces reliable and effective treatment even in severe cases of pernicious anemia.[11]

In the United States, oral vitamin B12 therapy is rarely used despite the fact that it has been shown to be fully (100 percent) effective in the long-term treatment of pernicious anemia. Let's first discuss the data showing effectiveness with oral administration before discussing the dogma cited for injectable administration.

Almost as soon as vitamin B12 was isolated in 1948, it was introduced in an injectable form and researchers busily sought an oral alternative. Oral preparations containing intrinsic factor were tried, but some patients developed antibodies against intrinsic factor and therefore would not respond.[12] Other studies soon documented that a small but constant proportion of an oral dose of cyanocobalamin was absorbed without intrinsic factor through the process of diffusion, so that by sufficiently increasing the dose, adequate absorption could be attained.[13,14]

In early studies, it was shown that pernicious anemia could be completely controlled with doses of cyanocobalamin in the range of 300 to 1,000 mcg daily.[15–18] The largest of these studies described sixty-four Swedish patients with pernicious anemia and other vitamin B12–deficiency states who were treated with 1,000 mcg of oral cyanocobalamin daily.[17,18] Complete normalization of serum levels and liver stores for vitamin B12,

as well as full clinical remission, was observed in all patients studied over a three-year period.

Despite the research, oral vitamin B12 therapy is not used in the United States. Why? Education and bias. Physicians have erroneously been educated by medical texts that first state that oral vitamin B12 therapy for pernicious anemia is "unpredictable," has poor patient compliance, and is more costly. These same texts then state that oral cobalamin is effective and can be used when injection therapy is problematic, but the bias against oral treatment has already been established. In a survey of internists, ninety-one percent erroneously believed that vitamin B12 could not be absorbed in sufficient quantities without intrinsic factor. Interestingly, eighty-eight percent of these doctors also stated that an effective oral vitamin B12 therapy would be useful in their practice and further stated that it would be their preferred method of delivery if it was effective. Let's reassure these doctors by answering the concerns regarding oral therapy.[11]

Is Oral Vitamin B12 Therapy Unpredictable? No, not at an effective dosage. Some of the early studies with oral B12 therapy used only 100 to 250 mcg daily. These reports led the U.S. Pharmacopoeia Anti-Anemia Preparations Advisory Board in 1959 to caution against oral therapy for pernicious anemia as being "at best, unpredictably effective."[19] However, based on what is now known about oral vitamin B12 pharmacokinetics, the response to these low doses must now be considered predictable. It has now been established that the mean absorption rate of oral cyanocobalamin by patients with pernicious anemia is 1.2 percent across a wide range of dosages.[17] Since the daily turnover rate is about 2 mcg, an oral dosage of 100 to 250 mcg daily results in a mean absorption of 1.2 to 3 mcg, respectively—a dosage that is sufficient for many, but not all, patients. Higher dosages are necessary in order for most patients to benefit from oral therapy.

How High Must the Dosage Be to Produce Predictable Improvements? In a study of sixty-four patients taking 500 mcg of oral cyanocobalamin daily, the lowest absorption rate was determined to be 1.8 mcg.[17] Since this level is slightly less than the 2 mcg daily turnover rate, it is an insufficient dosage in some cases. Therefore, the dosage of 1,000 mcg daily has become the most popular recommendation. However, even though 1,000 mcg daily has been shown to be effective, to rapidly replenish stores in the first month of treatment a dosage of 2,000 mcg is recommended.

Does Oral Vitamin B12 Lead to Poor Patient Compliance? No. The concern about patient compliance cited by the medical texts is irrational. Why is vitamin B12 singled out from any other oral therapy? It simply does not make any sense, especially since studies with oral cobalamin have shown excellent compliance. In many cases, the compliance is higher with an oral preparation since many patients prefer taking a pill over getting a shot.[14,17]

Does Oral Vitamin B12 Cost More Than Injectable? No way! The facts are that the two forms—injectable and oral—do not differ much in price for the vitamin B12 itself. The difference is in the cost charged to administer the vitamin B12 injection—anywhere from twenty dollars in a private practice to one hundred dollars in a nursing home. This results in the injectable form being considerably more expensive.

Conclusions: Oral vs. Injectable It should be obvious that there is no basis for the dogmatic belief that vitamin B12 must be administered by injection in order to produce clinical benefit. In the treatment of pernicious anemia, the usual dosage recommended by most medical texts is 1,000 mg weekly for eight weeks, then once a month for life. For oral vitamin B12, the recommended dosage is 2,000 mcg daily (14,000 mcg weekly) for at least one month, followed by a daily intake of 1,000 mg of vitamin B12. Methylcobalamin is preferred over cyanocobalamin.

Folic Acid–Deficiency Anemia

The diet should focus on foods high in folic acid: liver, asparagus, dried beans, brewer's yeast, dark green leafy vegetables, and grains. Since folic acid is destroyed by heat and light, fruits and vegetables should be eaten fresh or with very little cooking. Poor sources of folic acid include most meats, milk, eggs, and root vegetables.

To replenish folic acid stores, 1,000 mcg (1 mg) of folic acid should be taken every day for up to one month. Folic acid is available as folic acid (folate) and folinic acid (5-methyl-tetra-hydrofolate). In order to utilize folic acid, the body must first convert it to tetra-hydrofolate and then add a methyl group to form 5-methyl-tetra-hydrofolate (folinic acid). Therefore, supplying the body with folinic acid bypasses these steps. Folinic acid is the most active form of folic acid and has been shown to be more efficient at raising body stores than folic acid.[20]

TREATMENT SUMMARY

Effective therapy for anemia is dependent on proper classification as to its cause. The following recommendations are given with this in mind. Blood tests should be performed monthly to determine when the blood count returns to normal.

Diet

The ingestion of 4 to 6 oz of calf liver per day is recommended, along with the liberal consumption of green leafy vegetables.

Nutritional Supplements

Iron-Deficiency Anemia

- Iron: 30 mg, bound to either succinate or fumarate, twice per day between meals (if this recommendation results in abdominal discomfort, take 30 mg with meals three times per day)
- An alternative recommendation is to take a high-quality aqueous (hydrolyzed) liver extract at a level that provides a daily intake of 4 to 6 mg of heme iron
- Vitamin C: 1 gram three times per day with meals

B12-Deficiency Anemia

- Oral vitamin B12: 2,000 mcg per day for at least one month, followed by 1,000 mcg per day (methylcobalamin, the active form of vitamin B12, supplied in sublingual tablets, is preferred over cyanocobalamin)
- Folic acid: 800–1,200 mcg three times per day

Folic Acid–Deficiency Anemia

- Folic acid: 800–1,200 mcg three times per day
- Vitamin B12: 1,000 mcg per day (it is always necessary to supplement vitamin B12 with folic acid to prevent the folic acid supplement from masking a vitamin B12 deficiency)

Angina

Squeezing or pressure-like pain in the chest occurring immediately after exertion. Other precipitating factors include emotional tension, cold weather, or large meals. Pain may radiate to the left shoulder blade, left arm, or jaw. The pain typically lasts for only one to twenty minutes.

Stress, anxiety, and high blood pressure typically present.

An abnormal electrocardiographic reading (transient ST segment depression) in response to light exercise (stress test).

Angina pectoris is caused by an insufficient supply of oxygen to the heart muscle, which produces a squeezing or pressure-like pain in the chest. Angina usually precedes a heart attack. Since physical exertion and stress increase the heart's need for oxygen, they are often the triggering factors. The pain may radiate to the left shoulder blade, left arm, or jaw. The pain typically lasts for only one to twenty minutes.

Angina is almost always due to *atherosclerosis*—the buildup of cholesterol-containing plaque that progressively narrows and ultimately blocks the blood vessels supplying the heart (the coronary arteries). This blockage results in a decreased supply of blood and oxygen to the heart tissue. When the flow of oxygen to the heart muscle is substantially reduced, or when there is an increased need by the heart, it results in angina. Hypoglycemia (low blood sugar) can also cause angina.[1]

There is another type of angina that is not related to a buildup of plaque on the coronary arteries. It is known as *Prinzmetal's variant angina* and is caused by spasm of a coronary artery. This form of angina is more apt to occur at rest, may occur at odd times during the day or night, and is more common in women under age fifty. It usually responds to magnesium supplementation.

Therapeutic Considerations

Angina is a serious condition that requires careful treatment and monitoring. Prescription medications may be necessary in severe cases, as well as in the initial stages of mild to moderate angina. Eventually, it should be possible to control the condition with the help of natural measures. If there is significant blockage of the coronary artery, angioplasty, coronary artery bypass, or intravenous EDTA chelation therapy (discussed in the next section) may be appropriate.

Coronary Angiogram, Angioplasty, and Artery Bypass Surgery

An *angiogram* (cardiac catheterization) is an X-ray procedure in which dye is injected into the coronary arteries to locate blockages. These blockages are then most often opened with *balloon angioplasty* (a surgical procedure where the diameter of the blocked artery is increased with the aid of a very small balloon attached to a flexible tube) and/or coronary artery bypass surgery (a procedure where the coronary artery is bypassed by constructing an alternate route using a portion of a vein from the patient's leg).

Angiograms, bypass surgery, and angioplasty are a big business. Over one million heart angiograms are performed each year, for a total annual cost of over ten billion dollars. But based upon extensive analysis, it appears that most of this money is wasted.

Several studies have now challenged the widespread recommendation of angiograms made by most cardiologists.[2] One study evaluated 168 patients who were told they needed to have an angiogram to determine the degree of blockage, followed by bypass surgery or angioplasty. Using noninvasive tests, such as the exercise stress test, the echocardiogram (an ultrasound exam that measures the size and functional status of the heart), and the Holter heart monitor (a portable heart monitor that measures the pulse and characterizes beats as normal or abnormal) that is worn for twenty-four hours, the researcher determined that 134, or eighty percent, did not need the catheterization.

Over a five-year period, this group of 168 patients had only a 1.1 percent rate of fatal heart attacks annually. This rate is much lower than the mortality rates associated with either coronary artery bypass surgery (5 to 10 percent) or angioplasty (1 to 2 percent). The researcher concluded that "in a large fraction of medically stable patients with coronary disease who are urged to undergo coronary angiography (heart catheterization), the procedure can be safely deferred." Noninvasive testing to determine the functional state of the heart is far more important in determining the type of therapy that is needed than the dangerous search for blocked arteries. If the heart is not functioning well, *then* the angiogram may be needed to see if surgery should be done.

Furthermore, the blockages found by the angiogram are usually not relevant to the patient's risk of heart attack. For instance, in the most sophisticated study of bypass surgery, the Coronary Artery Surgery Study (CASS), it was demonstrated that heart patients with healthy hearts but with one, two, or all three of the major heart vessels blocked did surprisingly well without surgery.[3–5] Regardless of the number or severity of the blockages, each group had the same low death rate of 1 percent per year.

That same year, the average death rate from bypass surgery was 10.1 percent, or about one death per ten operations. In other words, the operation being recommended supposedly to save lives was five to ten times more deadly than the disease. The best that can be said about bypass surgery and balloon angioplasty is that they are irrelevant to the course of the disease in all but the most serious cases. Patients who elect not to have the surgery live just as long as or longer than those who have the surgery.[6]

The severity of blockage does not necessarily correlate with reduction in blood flow in the artery. In one study, Iowa researchers measured blood flow in over forty-four blockages demonstrated by angiogram.[7] Much to their surprise, they found no correlation between blood flow and the severity of the heart artery blockage. In other words, the angiogram did not provide clinically relevant information.

The researchers found that "the coronary artery with a ninety-six-percent blockage had one of the most brisk blood flows, while a similar artery, with only forty-percent blockage, had severe blood-flow restriction." The authors concluded that the blockages found by the heart catheterization simply do not correlate with blood-flow restriction. The researchers also commented that "the results of these studies should be profoundly disturbing . . . Information cannot be determined accurately by conventional angiographic approaches."

The bottom line is this: when patients are advised to have a coronary angiogram, chances are eight out of ten that they do not need it. The critical factor in whether a patient needs coronary artery bypass surgery or angioplasty is how well the left ventricular pump is working, not the degree of blockage or the number of arteries affected. The left ventricle (chamber) of the heart is responsible for pumping oxygenated blood through the aorta (the large artery emanating from the heart) and to the rest of the body. Bypass surgery is only helpful when the *ejection fraction* (the amount of blood pumped by the left ventricle) is less than forty percent of capacity.[8] Up to ninety percent of all bypass procedures are done when the ejection fraction is greater than fifty percent, which is adequate for circulatory needs. In other words, as many as ninety percent of all bypass procedures may be unnecessary.

When coronary artery bypass surgery and/or angioplasty is necessary, based on these accepted criteria, they definitely increase long-term survival and give relief of symptoms for eighty-five percent of patients. However, the surgery is not without risk. Complications arising from coronary bypass operations are common, as this surgery represents one of the most technically difficult procedures in modern medicine. In one study, sixty-one percent of the patients who had coronary artery bypass surgery suffered nervous-system disorders as a result.[9] Another study found that two to five percent of individuals who have coronary bypass surgery die during or soon after the operation, and ten percent have heart attacks *(myocardial infarctions)*.[10]

Considering the cost of the procedure, the lack of long-term survival benefit, and the high level of complications, it appears that

· ·

QUICK REVIEW

- Angina is a serious condition that requires careful treatment and monitoring.
- As many as ninety percent of all bypass procedures may be unnecessary.
- The two primary therapeutic goals in the natural treatment of angina are:
  1. Improving energy metabolism within the heart
  2. Improving the blood supply to the heart
- Carnitine and coenzyme Q_{10} (CoQ_{10}) have been shown to improve angina in well-designed double-blind clinical trials.

- Magnesium deficiency plays a major role in angina.
- Hawthorn extracts improve the supply of blood and oxygen to the heart.
- Since the late 1940s, there have been numerous scientific studies that demonstrate the clinical effectiveness of khella extracts in the treatment of angina.
- EDTA chelation therapy is an alternative to coronary artery bypass surgery and angioplasty; it may prove to be more effective, and it is definitely safer and less expensive.

electing to have this surgery is unwise for the majority of patients.

This is particularly true in light of the availability of effective natural alternatives to coronary bypass surgery. Numerous studies have shown that dietary and lifestyle changes can significantly reduce the risk of heart attack and other causes of death due to atherosclerosis (see the chapter HEART AND CARDIOVASCULAR HEALTH). Simple dietary changes —decreasing the amount of saturated fat and cholesterol in the diet; increasing the consumption of dietary fiber, complex carbohydrates, fish oils, and magnesium; eliminating alcohol consumption and cigarette smoking; and reducing high blood pressure—would greatly reduce the number of coronary bypass operations performed in Westernized countries. In addition, clinical studies have shown that several nutritional supplements and botanical medicines improve heart function in even the most severe angina cases. Another important alternative is intravenous EDTA chelation therapy. Although this therapy is controversial, considerable clinical research has proven its efficacy (EDTA chelation therapy is discussed later in this chapter).

When an Angiogram Is Unavoidable

When an angiogram is deemed necessary, the goal is then to prevent the damaging effects produced by this procedure. This can be accomplished by prescribing a high-potency multiple-vitamin-and-mineral formula, along with additional vitamin C (minimum 500 mg three times daily) and CoQ_{10} (300 mg daily two weeks prior to surgery and for three months afterward). Note: it is generally recommended that garlic supplementation and high dosages of vitamin E (greater than 200 IU) be avoided prior to any surgery, due to their ability to possibly promote excessive bleeding by inhibiting platelet aggregation— a key aspect of blood clot formation.

Vitamin C supplementation is rarely employed in hospitals, despite the fact that it may provide significant benefits; low vitamin C status is quite common in hospitalized patients. In a study analyzing the vitamin C status of patients undergoing coronary artery bypass, the plasma concentration of vitamin C was shown to plummet by seventy percent twenty-four hours after coronary artery bypass surgery; this level persisted in most patients for up to two weeks after surgery.[11] In contrast, vitamin E and carotene levels did not change to any significant degree, presumably because they are fat-soluble and are therefore retained in the body for longer periods of time. Given the importance of vitamin C, the serious depletion of vitamin C may deteriorate defense mechanisms against free radicals, infection, and wound repair in these patients. Supplementation appears to be essential in patients recovering from heart surgery, or any surgery for that matter.

Return of blood flow (*reperfusion*) after coronary artery bypass surgery results in oxidative damage to the vascular endothelium and myocardium and thus greatly increases the risk of subsequent coronary artery disease. Coenzyme Q_{10} is recommended in an attempt to prevent such oxidative damage after bypass surgery or angioplasty. In one study, forty patients undergoing elective surgery either served in the control group or received 150 mg of CoQ_{10} each day for seven days before the surgery.[12] The concentrations of lipid peroxides and the enzyme creatine kinase, which indicate myocardial damage, were significantly lower in patients who received CoQ_{10} than in the control group. The treatment group also showed a statistically significant lower incidence of ventricular arrhythmias during the recovery period. These results clearly demonstrate that pretreatment with CoQ_{10} can play a protective role during routine bypass surgery by reducing oxidative damage.

In addition to vitamin C and CoQ_{10}, a mixture of highly purified bovine-derived glycosaminoglycans (GAGS) naturally present in the aorta of the human heart is beneficial in preventing reperfusion injury and in restoring the proper structure, integrity, and function of the coronary vascular endothelium.[13] These GAGs include dermatan sulfate, heparan sulfate, hyaluronic acid, chondroitin sulfate, and related hexosaminoglycans. The dosage of purified aortic GAGs is 100 mg daily.

Goals of Therapy

From a natural perspective, there are two primary therapeutic goals in the treatment of angina:

- Improving energy metabolism within the heart
- Improving the blood supply to the heart

These goals are interrelated, because increased blood flow means improved energy metabolism and vice versa. The treatment goals are best achieved by a combination of important nutrient factors (e.g., carnitine, pantethine, CoQ_{10}, and magnesium) and herbs like hawthorn and khella which improve the delivery and utilization of oxygen to the heart muscle. In severe cases, EDTA chelation therapy may be a suitable alternative to angioplasty or coronary bypass.

Carnitine, CoQ$_{10}$, and Pantethine

The heart utilizes fats as its major metabolic fuel. It converts free fatty acids into energy,

much as an automobile uses gasoline. Defects in the utilization of fats by the heart greatly increase the risk of atherosclerosis, heart attacks, and angina pains. Specifically, impaired utilization of fatty acids by the heart results in accumulation of high concentrations of fatty acids within the heart muscle. This then makes the heart extremely susceptible to cellular damage, which ultimately leads to a heart attack.

Carnitine, pantethine, and coenzyme Q_{10} are essential compounds in the normal metabolism of fat and energy; they are of extreme benefit to sufferers of angina. These nutrients prevent the accumulation of fatty acids within the heart muscle by improving the conversion of fatty acids and other compounds into energy.

Carnitine

Carnitine is a vitamin-like compound that stimulates the breakdown of fats by the *mitochondria*—the energy-producing units in cells. Carnitine is essential in the transport of fatty acids into the mitochondria. A deficiency of carnitine results in a decrease in fatty acid concentrations in the mitochondria, thereby reducing energy production.

Normal heart function is critically dependent on adequate concentrations of carnitine. While the normal heart stores more carnitine than it needs, if the heart does not have a good supply of oxygen, carnitine levels quickly decrease. This leads to decreased energy production in the heart and increased risk of angina and heart disease. Since angina patients have a decreased supply of oxygen, carnitine supplementation makes good sense.

Several clinical trials have demonstrated that carnitine relieves angina and heart disease.[14–18] Supplementation with carnitine normalizes heart carnitine levels and allows the heart muscle to utilize its limited oxygen supply more efficiently. In cases of angina treated with carnitine, improvements have been noted in exercise tolerance and heart function. The results indicate that carnitine is an effective alternative to drugs in the treatment of angina.

In one study of patients with angina, oral administration of 900 mg of L-carnitine increased mean exercise time and the time necessary for abnormalities to occur during a stress test (6.4 minutes in the placebo group, compared to 8.8 minutes in the carnitine-treated group).[18]

These results indicate that carnitine may be an effective alternative to other anti-anginal agents, such as beta-blockers, calcium-channel antagonists, and nitrates, especially in patients with chronic angina.

Carnitine, by improving fat metabolism and thereby increasing energy production in the heart muscle, may also prevent the production of toxic fatty acid *metabolites* (products of metabolism). These compounds are extremely harmful to the heart and are thought to contribute to impaired heart muscle contractility, increased susceptibility to irregular beats, and eventual death of heart tissue. Supplemental carnitine increases heart carnitine levels and prevents the production of toxic fatty acid metabolites. In a clinical trial, early administration of L-carnitine (40 mg/kg/d) in heart attack patients was found to considerably reduce heart damage.[19]

Pantethine

Pantethine is the stable form of pantetheine, the active form of pantothenic acid, which is the fundamental component of coenzyme A (CoA). CoA is involved in the transport of fatty acids to the mitochondria and to and from cells. The pathway of synthesis from pantethine to CoA is much shorter than that from pantothenic acid to CoA, making pantethine the preferred therapeutic substance. In addition, pantethine has significant lipid-lowering activity, while pantothenic acid has very little (if any) effect in lowering cholesterol and triglyceride levels.

Pantethine acts by inhibiting cholesterol synthesis and accelerating fatty acid breakdown in the mitochondria. The standard dose of pantethine is 900 mg per day. Like carnitine, it has been shown in clinical trials to significantly reduce serum triglyceride and cholesterol levels, while increasing HDL-cholesterol levels.[20–22] Its lipid-lowering effects are most impressive when its toxicity (virtually none) is compared to that of conventional lipid-lowering drugs.

Pantethine is well indicated for treating angina. Like carnitine, heart pantethine levels decrease during times of reduced oxygen supply. Demonstrated effects in animals further indicate that pantethine would greatly benefit individuals with angina.[23]

Coenzyme Q$_{10}$

Coenzyme Q$_{10}$ (CoQ$_{10}$), also known as *ubiquinone,* is an essential component of the mitochondria, where it plays a major role in energy production. Like carnitine and pantethine, CoQ$_{10}$ can be synthesized within the body. Nonetheless, deficiency states have been reported. Deficiency can result from impaired CoQ$_{10}$ synthesis due to nutritional deficiencies, from a genetic or acquired defect in CoQ$_{10}$ synthesis, or from increased tissue needs.[24] In addition, many of the elderly may have increased CoQ$_{10}$ requirements; the decline of CoQ$_{10}$ levels that occurs with age may be partly responsible for the age-related deterioration of the immune system.

One of the most metabolically active tissues in the body, the heart may be unusually susceptible to the effects of CoQ$_{10}$ deficiency.

Accordingly, CoQ_{10} has shown great promise in the treatment of heart disease.

CoQ_{10} deficiency is common among individuals with heart disease. Heart tissue biopsies in patients with various heart diseases show a CoQ_{10} deficiency in fifty to seventy-five percent of cases.[24] Furthermore, cardiovascular diseases, including angina, hypertension, mitral valve prolapse, and congestive heart failure, require increased tissue levels of CoQ_{10}.[24] In one study, twelve patients with stable angina pectoris were treated with CoQ_{10} (150 mg/day for four weeks). The frequency of anginal attacks was reduced by fifty-three percent compared to a placebo group.[25] In addition, there was a significant increase in treadmill exercise tolerance (time to onset of chest pain and time to development of electrocardiogram abnormalities) during CoQ_{10} treatment. The results of this study and others suggest that CoQ_{10} is a safe and effective treatment for angina pectoris.

Carnitine, pantethine, and coenzyme Q_{10} should be considered in all heart disorders, not just angina (see also HEART DISEASE).

Magnesium

Magnesium deficiency plays a major role in angina, especially in Prinzmetal's variant. A magnesium deficiency has been shown to produce spasms of the coronary arteries, and is thought to be a cause of nonocclusive heart attacks.[26] Furthermore, it has been observed that men who die suddenly of heart attacks have significantly lower levels of heart magnesium, as well as potassium, than matched controls.[27]

It has been suggested that magnesium should become the treatment of choice for angina caused by coronary artery spasm.[27–29] Magnesium administration has also been found to be helpful in the management of arrhythmias and in angina due to atherosclero-

sis. Its benefit in all of these situations is presumably via the same mechanisms responsible for its effects in an acute heart attack (myocardial infarction). It improves the delivery of oxygen to the heart muscle by relaxing the coronary artery as well as improving the production of energy within the heart muscle.

Since the mid-1980s, over four thousand patients have been involved in eight well-designed studies that demonstrated the effectiveness of intravenous (IV) magnesium supplementation. During the first hour of admission to a hospital for an acute heart attack, administering IV magnesium reduced both immediate and long-term complications as well as death rates.[30–32]

The beneficial effects of magnesium in an acute heart attack relate to its ability to: improve energy production within the heart; dilate the coronary arteries, resulting in improved delivery of oxygen to the heart; reduce peripheral vascular resistance, resulting in reduced demand on the heart; inhibit platelets from aggregating and forming blood clots; reduce the size of the *infarct* (blockage); and improve heart rate and arrhythmias.

Hawthorn

Hawthorn (*Crataegus* sp.) berry and extracts of its flowering tops are widely used in Europe for their cardiovascular activity. They exhibit a combination of effects that are of great value to patients with angina and other heart problems. Studies have demonstrated that hawthorn extracts are effective in reducing angina attacks as well as in lowering blood pressure and serum cholesterol levels.[33–35]

The beneficial effects of hawthorn in the treatment of angina are due to improvement in the blood and oxygen supply of the heart, resulting from dilation of the coronary vessels, as well as improvement of the metabolic processes in the heart.[33–36]

Hawthorn's ability to dilate coronary blood vessels has been repeatedly demonstrated in experimental studies.[33–35] In addition, hawthorn extracts have been shown to improve cardiac energy metabolism in human and experimental studies. This combined effect is extremely important in the treatment of angina, as it results in improved myocardial function with more efficient use of oxygen. The improvement results not only from increased blood and oxygen supply to the heart muscle, but is also due to the interaction of hawthorn flavonoids with key enzymes to enhance the heart muscle's ability to contract.

Khella

Khella (Ammi visnaga) is an ancient medicinal plant native to the Mediterranean region, where it has been used in the treatment of angina and other heart ailments since the time of the pharaohs. Several of its components have demonstrated effects in dilating the coronary arteries. Its mechanism of action appears to be very similar to the calcium-channel-blocking drugs—it relaxes the blood vessels by blocking the entry of calcium through small channels. Calcium influx into the blood vessel cells leads to constriction. By inhibiting this influx, the vessel relaxes and the diameter of the vessel increases.

Since the late 1940s, there have been numerous scientific studies on the clinical effectiveness of khella extracts in the treatment of angina. More specifically, *khellin*—a derivative of the plant—was shown to be extremely effective in relieving angina symptoms, improving exercise tolerance, and normalizing electrocardiographic tests. This is evident by the concluding statements in a study published in the *New England Journal of Medicine* in 1951:

The high proportion of favorable results, together with the striking degree of improvement

frequently observed, has led us to the conclusion that khellin, properly used, is a safe and effective drug for the treatment of angina pectoris.[36]

At higher doses (120 to 150 mg per day) pure khellin was associated with mild side effects such as anorexia, nausea, and dizziness. Although most clinical studies used high dosages, several studies show that as little as 30 mg of khellin per day appears to offer equally good results with fewer side effects.[37,38]

Rather than using the isolated compound khellin, khella extracts standardized for khellin content (typically twelve percent) are the preferred form as they can deliver a consistent dosage of these keys compounds. A daily dose of such an extract would be 250 to 300 mg. Khella appears to work very well with hawthorn extracts.

Intravenous EDTA Chelation Therapy

EDTA chelation therapy is an alternative to coronary artery bypass surgery and angioplasty that may prove to be more effective; it is definitely safer and less expensive. While coronary artery bypass surgery or angioplasty usually costs $40,000 to $100,000, EDTA chelation therapy is an in-office procedure that usually costs less than $2,500 for a full set of treatments.

EDTA (ethylenediaminetetraacetic acid) is an amino-acid-like molecule that, when slowly infused into the bloodstream, chelates (binds) with minerals such as calcium, iron, copper, and lead and carries them to the kidneys, where they are excreted. EDTA chelation has been commonly used for lead poisoning, but in the late fifties and early sixties it was found to help patients with atherosclerosis.

The discovery that EDTA chelation therapy can be used in the treatment of angina and other conditions associated with atherosclerosis happened accidentally. In 1956, while Dr.

Norman Clarke was treating a battery worker for lead poisoning using EDTA, the patient noticed that his symptoms of angina disappeared. Dr. Clarke and others began using EDTA chelation therapy in patients with angina, cerebral vascular insufficiency, and occlusive peripheral vascular disease.

Between 1956 and 1960, Dr. Clarke and his colleagues treated 283 patients with EDTA chelation therapy; eighty-seven percent showed improvements in their symptoms. Heart patients got better, angina disappeared or was significantly improved, and patients with blocked leg arteries—particularly those with diabetes—avoided amputation.[39,40]

It was originally thought that EDTA opened blocked arteries by chelating out the calcium deposits in the cholesterol plaque. However, it now seems that the therapeutic effect results from chelating out excess iron and copper—minerals that, in the presence of oxygen, stimulate free radicals. Free radicals damage the cells in the artery and are a primary cause of atherosclerosis. The authors of a review of the progression and regression of atherosclerosis wrote that the process of "atherosclerosis is dependent on the presence of some metals (copper and iron) and can be completely inhibited by chelating agents such as EDTA."[41]

In spite of obvious benefits to heart patients, EDTA fell into disfavor in the mid-sixties. Advocates of EDTA use believe that this occurred for two reasons: the lucrative surgical approach to heart and vessel disease was on the rise, and the patent on EDTA that was held by Abbott Laboratories expired, so there was no financial motivation for drug companies to fund any research. Fortunately, a small group of practicing physicians who use EDTA chelation therapy banded together. In 1972, they founded an organization that is now called the American College for the Advancement of Medicine to continue education and research in this important area.

In the early days of EDTA chelation therapy, several serious problems were discovered. Giving too much of the EDTA or giving it too fast was soon found to be dangerous. In fact, there were several deaths attributed to kidney failure caused by toxic reactions to EDTA. Fortunately, additional research resulted in more appropriate protocols, and EDTA chelation therapy as used now is very safe. There have not been any deaths or significant adverse reactions in over 500,000 patients who have undergone EDTA chelation therapy. Because EDTA chelation improves blood flow throughout the body, the "side effects" are usually beneficial, and only a few adverse effects are noticed (most often the only side effect is irritation at the site of injection).

There now exists a substantial body of scientific evidence on the use of EDTA chelation therapy in the treatment of angina, peripheral vascular disease, and cerebral vascular disease.[42] Since 1987, numerous FDA-approved studies have demonstrated some impressive results.[42–46] Again, patients with angina have had symptoms improve or disappear and patients with blockages in their legs have had blood flow restored or significantly improved.

For more information, contact

American College for the Advancement in Medicine (ACAM)
23121 Verdugo Drive, Suite 204
Laguna Hills, CA 92653
800-532-3688 (outside California)
800-435-6199 (inside California)

TREATMENT SUMMARY

The primary therapy is prevention, since angina is usually the result of hardening of the arteries (atherosclerosis). Follow the general guidelines given in HEART AND CARDIOVASCULAR HEALTH and, if cholesterol levels are elevated, CHOLESTEROL.

Once angina has developed, restoring proper blood supply to the heart and enhancing energy production within the heart are the primary goals. In mild to moderate cases, the natural approach is usually sufficient. But in more serious cases, the natural approach should be used in conjunction with the use of conventional prescription drugs. Patients with unstable angina pectoris (characterized by progressive increase in the frequency and severity of pain, increased sensitivity to precipitating factors, progression of symptoms over several days, and prolonged coronary pain) should be hospitalized.

Diet

Increase dietary fiber especially the gel-forming or mucilaginous fibers (flaxseed, oat bran, pectin, etc.). Onions and garlic, vegetables, and fish should also be increased, while saturated fats, cholesterol, sugar, and animal proteins should be reduced. Avoid fried foods and food allergens. Patients with reactive hypoglycemia should eat regular meals and avoid all simple carbohydrates (sugar, honey, dried fruit, fruit juice, etc.).

Lifestyle

Stop smoking and drinking alcohol and coffee. Use stress-management techniques such as progressive relaxation, meditation, or guided imagery. A carefully graded, progressive aerobic exercise program (thirty minutes three times per week) is a necessity. Walking is a good exercise with which to start.

Nutritional Supplements

- Coenzyme Q_{10}: 150–300 mg per day
- L-carnitine: 500 mg three times per day
- Pantethine: 300 mg three times per day
- Magnesium (preferably bound to aspartate, citrate, or other Kreb's cycle intermediate): 200–400 mg three times per day

Botanical Medicines

- Hawthorn (*Crataegus sp.*) three times per day
  Berries or flowers (dried): 3–5 grams or as a tea
  Tincture (1:5): 4–6 ml (1–1.5 tsp)
  Fluid extract (1:1): 1–2 ml (0.25–0.5 tsp)
  Solid extract (10% procyanidins or 1.8% vitexin-4'-rhamnoside): 100–250 mg
- Khella (*Ammi visnaga*) three times per day
- Dried powdered extract (12% khellin content): 100 mg

Anxiety

. . . .

Nervousness, anxiety, or sense of inappropriate fear

Shortness of breath, heart palpitations, and tingling sensations in the extremities

Over fourteen million Americans suffer from anxiety—"an unpleasant emotional state ranging from mild unease to intense fear." Anxiety differs from fear in that, while fear is a rational response to a real danger, anxiety usually lacks a clear or realistic cause. Though some anxiety is normal and even healthy, higher levels of anxiety are not only uncomfortable but can lead to significant problems.

Anxiety is often accompanied by a variety of symptoms. The most common symptoms relate to the chest, such as *heart palpitations* (awareness of a more forceful or faster heart beat), throbbing or stabbing pains, a feeling of tightness and inability to take in enough air, and a tendency to sigh or hyperventilate. Tension in the muscles of the back and neck often leads to headaches, back pains, and muscle spasms. Other symptoms can include excessive sweating, dryness of the mouth, dizziness, digestive disturbances, and the constant need to urinate or defecate.

Anxious individuals usually have a constant feeling that something bad is going to happen. They may fear that they have a chronic or dangerous illness—a belief that is reinforced by the symptoms of anxiety. Inability to relax may lead to difficulty in getting to sleep and constant waking through the night.

Panic Attacks

Severe anxiety will often produce what are known as "panic attacks"—intense feelings of fear. Panic attacks may occur independent from anxiety but are most often associated with generalized anxiety or agoraphobia. *Agoraphobia* is defined as an intense fear of being alone or being in public places. As a result, most people with agoraphobia become housebound.

Panic attacks are very common; about fifteen percent of the United States population experience a panic attack in their lifetime. Among adults aged twenty-five to fifty-four, about 1.5 percent to 3 percent experience frequent panic attacks.

Causes of Anxiety and Panic Attacks

Clinical anxiety, including panic attacks, can be produced by caffeine, certain other drugs, and the infusion of lactate into the blood. The fact that these compounds can produce anxiety and panic attacks can be put to good use in understanding the underlying biochemical features of anxiety.

Perhaps the most significant biochemical disturbance noted in people with anxiety and

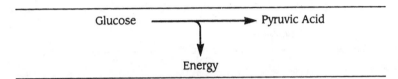

FIGURE 1 Glucose Breakdown to Pyruvic Acid

panic attacks is an elevated blood lactic acid level and an increased lactic acid to pyruvic acid ratio. *Lactate* (the soluble form of lactic acid) is the final product in the breakdown of blood sugar (glucose) when there is a lack of oxygen.

To illustrate how lactic acid is produced, let's take the classic example of the exercising muscle. Muscles prefer to use fat as their energy source, but when you exercise vigorously there isn't enough oxygen, so the muscle must burn glucose. Without oxygen, there is a buildup of lactic acid within the muscle; this is what causes muscle fatigue and soreness after exercise. Let's look more closely at this process.

The first few steps of normal glucose breakdown can occur without oxygen, until pyruvic acid is produced (see Figure 1).

The next steps require oxygen and end in the complete breakdown of pyruvic acid to carbon dioxide and water (see Figure 2).

But what happens if there is not enough oxygen? Because the exercising muscle will need energy, the muscle cell converts as much glucose as possible to pyruvic acid. This process is referred to as *anaerobic metabolism*. The pyruvic acid is converted into a temporary waste product: lactic acid (see Figure 3).

With good circulation, the lactic acid is removed from the muscle and transported to

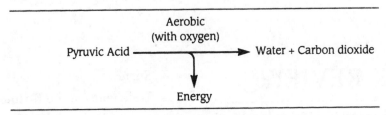

FIGURE 2 Breakdown of Pyruvic Acid to CO_2 and H_2O

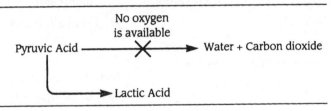

FIGURE 3 Pyruvic Acid Conversion to Lactic Acid

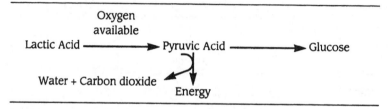

FIGURE 4 Lactic Acid Conversion to Pyruvic Acid or Glucose

the liver, where it can be turned back into pyruvic acid or even glucose if needed (see Figure 4).

All of this biochemistry plays a role in anxiety, because individuals with anxiety have elevated blood levels of lactate and a higher ratio of lactic acid to pyruvic acid when compared to normal controls. Furthermore, if people who get panic attacks are injected with lactate, severe panic attacks are produced. In normal individuals nothing happens. So it appears that individuals with anxiety may be sensitive to lactate. In other words, lactate may be causing their anxiety. Reducing the level of lactate is a critical goal in the treatment of anxiety and panic attacks.

Therapeutic Considerations

The natural approach to anxiety builds upon the recommendations given for stress in the chapter STRESS MANAGEMENT. After all, anxiety is usually a symptom of severe stress. If you suffer from mild anxiety, follow all of the recommendations given in that chapter for diet, exercise, nutritional supplementation, calming the mind and body, and taking *Panax ginseng*. If you suffer from moderate to severe anxiety, follow all of the recommendations in that chapter, but instead of taking *Panax ginseng*, try taking kava *(Piper methysticum)* (for information on kava, see Kava later in this chapter).

QUICK REVIEW

- Perhaps the most significant biochemical disturbance noted in people with anxiety and panic attacks is an elevated blood lactate level.

- There are at least six nutritional factors that may be responsible for elevated lactic acid to pyruvic acid ratio:

  1. Alcohol
  2. Caffeine
  3. Sugar
  4. Deficiency of the B-vitamins niacin, pyridoxine, and thiamin
  5. Deficiency of calcium or magnesium
  6. Food allergens

- Kava extract has produced relief from anxiety comparable to drugs like Valium but without the side effects.

Reducing Lactate Levels

As pointed out previously, increased lactic acid levels may be an underlying factor in panic attacks and anxiety. Our goal is to prevent the conversion of pyruvic acid to lactic acid and to improve the conversion of lactic acid back to pyruvic acid. Nutrition appears to play a key role in achieving this goal. According to Melvyn Werbach, M.D., author of *Nutritional Influences of Mental Illness*,[1] there are at least six nutritional factors that may be responsible for elevated lactate levels or lactic acid to pyruvic acid ratios:

1. Alcohol
2. Caffeine
3. Sugar
4. Deficiency of the B-vitamins niacin, pyridoxine, and thiamin
5. Deficiency of calcium or magnesium
6. Food allergens

By avoiding alcohol, caffeine, sugar, and food allergens, people with anxiety can go a long way toward relieving their symptoms.[1] Simply eliminating coffee can result in complete relief from symptoms. This recommendation may seem too simple to be valid, but substantial clinical evidence indicates that in many cases it is all that is necessary. For example, one study dealt with four men and two women who had generalized anxiety or panic disorder. Their caffeine consumption ranged from $1^1/2$ to $3^1/2$ cups of coffee per day. Avoiding caffeine for one week brought about significant relief of symptoms.[2] The degree of improvement was so noticeable that all patients volunteered to continue abstaining from caffeine. Previously, these patients had been only minimally helped by drug therapy. Follow-up exams six to eighteen months afterward indicated that five out of the six patients were completely without symptoms; the sixth patient became asymptomatic with a very low dose of Valium.

By following the dietary guidelines given in the chapter A HEALTH-PROMOTING DIET, as well as the recommendations for nutritional supplementation given in the chapter SUPPLEMENTARY MEASURES, you will provide your body with the kind of nutritional support it needs to counteract the biochemical derangements found in patients with anxiety and panic attacks.

Flaxseed Oil and Agoraphobia

It has been suggested that patients who get panic attacks may suffer from a deficiency of alpha-linolenic acid, the essential omega-3 fatty acid found in high concentrations in flaxseed oil. In one study, three out of four patients with a history of agoraphobia for ten or more years improved within two to three months after taking flaxseed oil at a dosage of 2 to 6 tablespoons daily, in divided doses depending upon response.[3] All patients had signs of essential fatty acid deficiency, such as dry skin, dandruff, brittle fingernails that grow slowly, and nerve disorders.

Kava *(Piper methysticum)*

The area of Oceania—the island communities of the Pacific including Micronesia, Melanesia, and Polynesia—is one of the few geographic areas in the world that did not have alcoholic beverages before European contact in the eighteenth century. However, these islanders did possess a magical drink that was used in ceremonies and celebrations because of its calming effect and ability to promote sociability. The drink, called *kava*, is still used today in this region, where the people are often referred to as the happiest and friendliest in the world. Preparations of kava root *(Piper methysticum)* are now gaining popularity in Europe and the United States as mild sedatives and anxiolytics.[4]

Several European countries have approved kava preparations for the treatment of nervous anxiety, insomnia, and restlessness on the basis of detailed pharmacological data and favorable clinical studies.

Earlier clinical trials used D,L-kavain, a purified kavalactone (the key group of compounds in kava), at a dose of 400 mg per day. For example, in one double-blind placebo-controlled study of eighty-four patients with anxiety symptoms, kavain was shown to improve vigilance, memory, and reaction time.[5] In another double-blind study, kavain was compared to the drug oxazepam (a drug similar to diazepam or Valium) in thirty-eight patients.[6] Both substances caused progressive improvements in two different anxiety scores (Anxiety Status Inventory and the Self-Rating Anxiety Scale) over a four-week period. However, while oxazepam and similar drugs are associated with side effects and with being addictive, kavain appeared to be free of these complications.

More recent studies have featured well-defined kava extracts. As mentioned earlier, evidence suggests that the whole complex of kavalactones and other compounds naturally found in kava produce greater pharmacological activity than pure kavalactone preparations. In addition, studies have shown that kavalactones are more rapidly absorbed when given orally as an extract of the root rather than as the isolated kavalactones. The bioavailability of kavalactones, as measured by peak plasma concentrations, is up to three to five times higher from the extract than when given as isolated substances.[7] Further evidence that kava root extracts are superior to isolated kavalactones is offered by an animal study showing that, while isolated kavalactones are taken up into brain tissue at a good level, when a crude kava preparation was given, the concentration of kavalactones was two to twenty times higher.[8] Based on

this evidence, it appears that crude extracts standardized for kavalactone content may offer the greatest therapeutic benefit.

Several clinical trials have featured a special kava extract standardized to contain seventy percent kavalactones. However, this high percentage of kavalactones may be sacrificing some of the other constituents that may contribute to the pharmacology of kava. Therefore, preparations around thirty percent may prove to be the most effective. More important than the actual percentage of kavalactones is the total dosage of the kavalactones and the assurance that the full range of kavalactones is present.

In perhaps the most significant study, a seventy-percent kavalactone extract was shown to exhibit significant therapeutic benefit in patients suffering from anxiety.[9] The study was double-blind; twenty-nine patients were assigned to receive 100 mg of the kava extract three times daily, while another twenty-nine patients received a placebo. Therapeutic effectiveness was evaluated using several standard psychological assessments, including the Hamilton Anxiety Scale. The results of this four-week study indicated that individuals who took the kava extract had a statistically significant reduction in symptoms of anxiety, including feelings of nervousness and somatic complaints such as heart palpitations, chest pains, headache, dizziness, and feelings of gastric irritation. No side effects were reported with the kava extract.

In another double-blind study, two groups of twenty women with menopause-related symptoms were treated for a period of eight weeks with the seventy-percent kavalactone extract (100 mg three times daily) or a placebo.[10] The target variable was once again the Hamilton Anxiety Scale. The group that received the kava extract demonstrated significant improvement at the end of the very first week of treatment. Scores continued to improve over the course of the eight-week study. In addition to reduction in symptoms of stress and anxiety, a number of other symptoms were relieved. Most notably there was an overall improvement in subjective well-being, mood, and general symptoms of menopause, including hot flashes. Again, no side effects were noted.

Two additional studies have shown that, unlike benzodiazepines, alcohol, and other drugs, kava extract is not associated with depressed mental function or impairment in driving or the operation of heavy equipment.[11,12] In one of these studies, twelve healthy volunteers were tested in a double-blind crossover manner. The first group received oxazepam (placebo on days one through three, 15 mg on the day before testing, 75 mg on the morning of the experiment); the second group received an extract of kava standardized at seventy percent kavalactones (200 mg three times daily for five days), and the third group received a placebo. The subjects were tested on behavior and event-related potentials (ERPs) in electroencephalograph (EEG) readings in a recognition memory task. Their task was to identify, within a list of visually presented words, those words that were shown for the first time and those that were being repeated. Consistent with other benzodiazepines, oxazepam inhibited the recognition of both new and old words as noted by ERP. In contrast, kava showed a slightly increased recognition rate and a larger ERP difference between old and new words. The results of this study once again demonstrate the uncharacteristic effects of kava; in this case, it relieves anxiety, but unlike standard anxiolytics, kava actually improves mental function and at the recommended levels does not promote sedation.

The dosage of kava preparations is based on their level of kavalactones. As a result of clinical studies using pure kavalactones or kava extracts standardized for kavalactones, the recommendation for anxiety-relieving effects is 45 to 70 mg of kavalactones three times per day. For sedative effects, the same daily quantity (135 to 210 mg) can be taken as a single dose one hour before retiring.

To put the therapeutic dosage in perspective it is important to point out that a standard bowl of traditionally prepared kava drink contains approximately 250 mg of kavalactones, and several bowls may be consumed at one sitting.

Side Effects of Kava

Although no side effects have been reported using standardized kava extracts at recommended levels in the clinical studies, several case reports have been presented indicating that kava may interfere with dopamine-production or binding to receptor sites and worsen Parkinson's disease, exert an additive effect when combined with benzodiazepines, and produce impaired driving ability when consumed in very large doses, sixteen cups of kava beverage as described below.[13,14] Until these issues are cleared up, kava extract should not be used in treating Parkinson's patients and should be used with extreme caution and close monitoring in patients taking benzodiazepines. In addition, patients should be instructed not to overdose on kava. In Utah, a man was charged with "driving under the influence" after he was stopped for swerving in and out of traffic lanes; he admitted to having consumed sixteen cups of kava. A cup of kava may contain an entire daily dosage of kavalactones as used in clinical studies (210 mg).

High quantities of kava beverage consumed daily over a prolonged period (a few months to a year or more) are associated with *kava dermopathy*, a condition of the skin characterized by a peculiar generalized scaly eruption known as *kani*.[15] The skin becomes dry and covered with scales, especially the palms of the hands, soles of the feet, forearms, back, and shins. It was thought at one time that kava dermopathy might be due to interference with niacin. However, in a double-blind placebo-controlled study, no therapeutic effect from niacinamide supplementation (100 mg daily) could be demonstrated.[16] It appears that the only effective treatment for kava dermopathy is reduction or cessation of kava consumption. Again, no reported cases of kava dermopathy have been noted in individuals taking standardized kava extracts at recommended levels.

Other adverse effects of extremely high doses of kava (greater than 310 grams per week) for prolonged periods include: biochemical abnormalities (low levels of serum albumin, protein, urea, and bilirubin), presence of blood in the urine, increased red blood cell volume, decreased platelet and lymphocyte counts, and shortness of breath.[17] The correlation of these adverse effects with kava is questionable because the subjects also reported heavy alcohol and cigarette usage. Nevertheless, high doses of kava are unnecessary and should not be encouraged.

TREATMENT SUMMARY

The primary treatment methods are to

- Reduce or eliminate the use of stimulants
- Follow the dietary and lifestyle recommendations given in the chapter STRESS MANAGEMENT
- Use kava when appropriate

NOTE: If you are currently taking a tranquilizer or antidepressant, you will need to work with a physician to get off the drug. Stopping the drug on your own can be dangerous; you absolutely must have proper medical supervision.

Diet

- Eliminate or restrict your intake of caffeine
- Eliminate or restrict your intake of alcohol
- Eliminate refined carbohydrates from your diet
- Design a healthful diet
- Increase the potassium-to-sodium ratio in your diet
- Eat regular planned meals in a relaxed environment
- Control food allergies

Lifestyle

- Identify stressors
- Eliminate or reduce sources of stress
- Identify negative coping patterns and replace them with positive patterns
- Perform a relaxation/breathing exercise for a minimum of five minutes twice daily
- Manage your time effectively
- Enhance your relationships through better communication

- Get regular exercise

Nutritional Supplements

- Take a high-potency multiple-vitamin-and-mineral formula, according to guidelines given in the chapter SUPPLEMENTARY MEASURES
- Flaxseed oil: 1 tablespoon daily

Botanical Medicines

- Kava *(Piper methysticum)*: 45 to 70 mg of kavalactones three times daily (the dosage of kava preparations is based on the level of kavalactones)

Asthma and Hay Fever

. . . .

Asthma:

> Recurrent attacks of shortness of breath, cough, and expectoration of tenacious mucoid sputum
>
> Prolonged expiration phase with generalized wheezing and abnormal breath sounds
>
> Laboratory signs of allergy (increased levels of eosinophils in blood, increased serum IgE levels, positive food and/or inhalant allergy tests)

Hay Fever:

> Watery nasal discharge, sneezing, itchy eyes and nose
>
> Usually associated with a particular season

Asthma and hay fever are discussed together since the mechanisms responsible for the development, as well as treatment, are similar in both. Asthma is an allergic disorder characterized by spasm of the *bronchi* (the airway tubes), swelling of the mucous lining of the lungs, and excessive production of a thick, viscous mucus. The major concern with asthma is that it can lead to respiratory failure—the inability to breathe.

WARNING: An acute asthma attack can be a medical emergency. If you are suffering from an acute attack, consult your physician or an emergency room immediately.

Asthma affects approximately three percent of the U.S. population and, although it occurs at all ages, it is most common in children under ten. Among children, there is a two-to-one male-to-female ratio of asthma sufferers, which equalizes by the age of thirty.

The rate of asthma in the United States is rising rapidly, especially among children. Reasons often given to explain the rise in asthma include: increased stress on the immune system due to greater chemical pollution in the air, water, and food; earlier weaning and earlier introduction of solid foods to infants; food additives; and genetic manipulation of plants, resulting in food components with greater allergenic tendencies. In addition, there is concern that exposure to the *pertussis* (whooping cough) vaccine may trigger asthma. A British study evaluated the health of 448 children and adolescents who had received only breast milk for the first six months of life, and in particular on the first day after birth; the study turned up some interesting findings.[1] All of the children were weaned after one year of age and were older than four years at the time their parents participated in the study. The mean age was 7.87 years.

To the question "Has your child ever been diagnosed as asthmatic?" there were thirty positive answers (6.72 percent). The surprise came when the researchers classified the respondents according to whether or not they received the pertussis vaccine.

Among the 243 immunized children, twenty-six were diagnosed as having asthma (10.69 percent). In contrast, of the 203 children who had not been immunized, only four had asthma (1.97 percent). The relative risk of developing asthma from the pertussis vaccine was 5.43 in this study.

Even though all of the children who received the pertussis vaccine received other vaccinations, the researchers felt that the statistical evidence focused on pertussis. Among the children who did not receive the pertussis vaccine, most had received some other vaccination. Of the ninety-one subjects who received no vaccines, only one had asthma, compared to three with asthma in the 112 who had other vaccinations. Therefore, based on this study, the relative risk of developing asthma is about one percent in children who receive no immunizations, three percent in those who receive vaccinations other than pertussis, and eleven percent for those who receive pertussis. Another finding to weigh: in the group not immunized to pertussis, sixteen developed whooping cough, compared to only one in the immunized group. It appears to be a trade off, a greater risk for asthma with vaccination and a greater risk for whooping cough without.

Major Categories

Asthma has typically been divided into two major categories: extrinsic and intrinsic. *Extrinsic,* or *atopic, asthma* is generally considered an allergic condition, with a characteristic increase in levels of serum IgE—the allergic antibody (see the chapter IMMUNE SUPPORT for more information). *Intrinsic asthma* is associated with a bronchial reaction that is due not to allergy, but rather to such factors as toxic chemicals, cold air, exercise, infection, and emotional upset (see Figure 1).

Both extrinsic and intrinsic factors trigger the release of chemicals that mediate (produce or control) inflammation from *mast cells*—specialized white blood cells that reside in various body tissues, including the lining of the respiratory passages. The inflammatory mediators are responsible for the signs and symptoms of asthma. They are either preformed in little packets *(granules)* within mast cells or generated from fatty acids that reside in cell membranes.

The preformed mediators include *histamine* and compounds known as leukotrienes. These compounds are responsible for producing much of the allergic reaction seen in asthma.

The most potent chemical mediators in asthma are the leukotrienes. Some leukotrienes are one thousand times more potent than histamine as stimulators of bronchial constriction and allergy. It has been observed that asthmatics have a tendency to form higher levels of leukotrienes.[2] This abnormality is further aggravated in patients with "aspirin-induced asthma." Aspirin and other nonsteroidal anti-inflammatory drugs (NSAIDs), e.g., indomethacin and ibuprofen, result in the production of excessive levels of leukotrienes in sensitive individuals.[3,4] Tartrazine (yellow dye #5) produces similar effects on leukotriene levels and is often a cause of asthma, particularly in children.[3] Tartrazine is added to most processed foods and can even be found in vitamin preparations and anti-asthma prescription drugs (e.g., aminophylline). Tartrazine may also indirectly support the asthmatic process via its role as an antimetabolite of vitamin B6 (see the discussion in Tryptophan Metabolism, later in this chapter).

Causes of Hay Fever

Ragweed pollen accounts for about seventy-five percent of the hay fever in the United States. Other significant pollens inducing hay fever include various grass and tree pollens. If the hay fever develops in the spring it is usually due to tree pollens, if it develops in the summer grass and weed pollens are usually the culprits. If hay fever symptoms persist year-round, this is known as perennial allergic rhinitis. This form of hay fever may or may not be due to pollens.

All of the discussions and therapeutic recommendations given in this chapter are appropriate for hayfever as well as asthma.

The Role of the Adrenal Gland

The activity of the adrenal gland is important in asthma due to its hormones *cortisol* and *epinephrine*. These compounds activate receptors (beta-2 receptors) on bronchial muscle, which leads to relaxation of bronchial muscle and opening of the airways. It is thought that during asthmatic attacks there is a relative deficiency of cortisol and epinephrine. The lack of stimulation of beta-2 receptors results in bronchial constriction.

Therapeutic Considerations

The first step in the natural approach to asthma is to reduce the allergic threshold. Allergens can be viewed as straws on a camel's back. Adding enough straws to the camel's back will ultimately cause the camel's back to break. Similarly, increasing the exposure to allergens will ultimately cause symptoms. By reducing the allergic threshold, as well as the offending allergen in many cases, the allergic process can be prevented. There are two

QUICK REVIEW

- Asthma occurrence is growing in number and severity.
- Hay fever (seasonal allergic rhinitis) is an allergic reaction of the nasal passages and airways to wind-borne pollens that shares many common features with asthma.
- The first step in the natural approach to asthma is to reduce the allergic threshold by avoiding airborne and food allergens.
- Elimination diets have been successful in identifying allergens and treating asthma.
- A vegan diet can be very effective in reducing asthma symptoms.
- Omega-3 fatty acids relieve asthma.
- Food additives can trigger allergic reactions and asthma.
- Vitamin B6 supplementation is recommended for the treatment of asthma, especially if the asthmatic has to take the drug theophyliine.
- Antioxidants, especially high doses of vitamin C, are highly recommended for the treatment of asthma.
- Magnesium can help open the airways and relieve asthma.
- Asthmatics should avoid salt.
- DHEA levels are typically low in asthmatics.

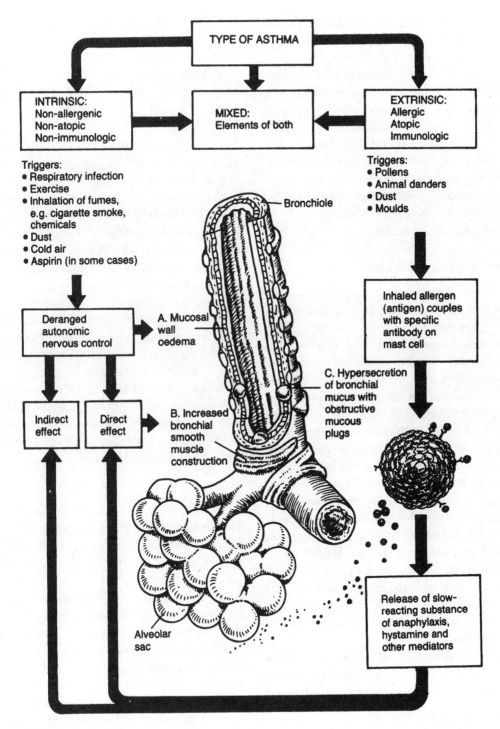

TYPE OF ASTHMA

INTRINSIC:
Non-allergenic
Non-atopic
Non-immunologic

MIXED:
Elements of both

EXTRINSIC:
Allergic
Atopic
Immunologic

Triggers:
- Respiratory infection
- Exercise
- Inhalation of fumes,
  e.g. cigarette smoke,
  chemicals
- Dust
- Cold air
- Aspirin (in some cases)

Triggers:
- Pollens
- Animal danders
- Dust
- Moulds

Bronchiole

Deranged
autonomic
nervous control

A. Mucosal
wall
oedema

Inhaled allergen
(antigen) couples
with specific
antibody on
mast cell

C. Hypersecretion
of bronchial
mucus with
obstructive
mucous
plugs

Indirect
effect

Direct
effect

B. Increased
bronchial
smooth
muscle
construction

Alveolar
sac

Release of slow-
reacting substance
of anaphylaxis,
hystamine and
other mediators

FIGURE 1 Mechanisms of Asthma

primary ways to reduce the allergic threshold: reduce exposure to airborne allergens, and reduce intake of food allergens.

Along with these recommendations, adopting a healthy lifestyle can significantly reduce allergies. In a recent study of 706 Japanese factory workers, it was demonstrated that a healthy lifestyle reduced IgE levels, while an unhealthy lifestyle increased IgE levels.[5] Lifestyle factors that tended to increase IgE levels included poor dietary habits, alcohol consumption, cigarette smoking, and increased feelings of stress.

Avoiding Airborne Allergens

Airborne allergens, such as pollen, dander, and dust mites, are often difficult to avoid entirely, but measures can be taken to reduce exposure. Removing dogs, cats, carpets, rugs, upholstered furniture, and other surfaces where allergens can collect is a great first step. If this can't be done entirely, make sure that the bedroom is as allergy-proof as possible. Encase the mattress in an allergen-proof plastic; wash sheets, blankets, pillowcases, and mattress pads every week in hot water with additive- and fragrance-free detergent; consider using bedding material made from Ventflex, a special hypoallergenic synthetic material; and install an air purifier. The best mechanical air purifiers are HEPA (high-efficiency particulate arresting) filters, which can be attached to central heating and air-conditioning systems. These units are available from suppliers of heating and air-conditioning units.

For a complete listing of special products to reduce the allergic load in the environment, contact either of the following two companies:

Allergy Control Products
89 Danbury Road
Ridgefield, CT 06877
800-422-DUST

National Allergy Supply
4579 Georgia Highway 120
Duluth, GA 30136
800-522-1448

Food Allergy

Many studies have indicated that food allergies play an important role in asthma (see FOOD ALLERGY).[6–10] Adverse reactions to food may be immediate or delayed. Double-blind food challenges in children have shown that immediate-onset sensitivities are usually due to (in order of frequency) eggs, fish, shellfish, nuts, and peanuts. Foods most commonly associated with delayed-onset sensitivities include (in order of frequency) milk, chocolate, wheat, citrus, and food colorings.[8]

Elimination diets have been successful in identifying allergens and treating asthma and are a particularly valuable diagnostic and therapeutic tool in infants.[11] Elimination of common allergens during infancy (the first two years) has been shown to reduce allergic tendencies in high-risk children (children with a strong familial history).[12]

Hypochlorhydria

Detailed analysis of gastric acid output of two hundred asthmatic children in 1931 showed that eighty percent of them had gastric acid secretions below normal levels.[13] This high occurrence suggests that decreased gastric acid output may predispose these children to food allergies. It may also have a major impact on the success of rotation and/or elimination diets and, if not corrected, on the development of additional food allergies.

The presence of food allergies is thought to be responsible for *leaky gut syndrome* in asthmatics.[14] As a result of this increased gut permeability, there is increased antigen load on the immune system. In other words, the intestinal barrier becomes too leaky and very large molecules that normally are not absorbed find their way into the body. This increased antigenic load overwhelms the immune system and increases the likelihood of developing additional allergies; it also increases the level of allergic compounds in the circulatory system that can trigger asthma. It is essential to identify offending foods as soon as possible to avoid the development of further allergies.

Candida albicans

An overgrowth of the common yeast *Candida albicans* in the gastrointestinal tract has been implicated as a causative factor in allergic conditions, including asthma. Apparently, the acid *protease,* produced by *C. albicans,* is the responsible allergen.[15] Appropriate anticandida therapy (see CANDIDIASIS, CHRONIC) may result in significant clinical improvement of asthma in many cases.

Vegan Diet

A long-term trial of a *vegan diet* (elimination of all animal products) provided significant improvement in ninety-two percent of the twenty-five patients who completed a study in 1985 (nine dropped out).[16] Improvement was determined by a number of clinical variables, including: lung capacity; the maximum amount of air expired in one second (FEV_1); physical working capacity; and laboratory assessment of IgM, IgE, cholesterol, and triglyceride levels in the blood. The researchers also found a reduction in the tendency to contract infectious disease. It is important to recognize, however, that while seventy-one percent of the patients responded (asthma significantly improved or entirely relieved) within four months, one year of diet therapy was required before the ninety-two-percent level was reached.

The vegan diet excluded all meat, fish, eggs, and dairy products. The only drinking water allowed was spring water (chlorinated tap water was specifically prohibited), and coffee, ordinary tea, chocolate, sugar, and salt were excluded. Herbal spices were allowed, and up to 1.5 liters per day of water and herbal teas were allowed. Vegetables used freely were lettuce, carrots, beets, onions, celery, cabbage, cauliflower, broccoli, nettles, cucumber, radishes, Jerusalem artichokes, and all beans except soy and green peas. Potatoes were allowed in restricted amounts. A number of fruits were also used freely: blueberries, cloudberries, raspberries, strawberries, black currants, gooseberries, plums, and pears. Apples and citrus fruits were not allowed, and grains were either highly restricted or eliminated.

The beneficial effects of this dietary regime are probably related to three areas: (1) elimination of food allergens, (2) altered prostaglandin metabolism, and (3) increased intake of antioxidant nutrients and magnesium. The importance of avoiding food allergens was discussed earlier. In regard to altered prostaglandin metabolism, the avoidance of dietary sources of arachidonic acid (derived from animal products) appears to be quite significant. The prostaglandins and leukotrienes derived from arachidonic acid contribute significantly to the allergic reaction in asthma. Decreasing the availability of arachidonic acid as the starting point of these inflammatory compounds appears to explain some aspects of the efficacy of the vegan diet. The beneficial effects of altering prostaglandin metabolism are further discussed (see Omega-3 Essential Fatty Acids), as is the role of increased dietary antioxidants in preventing asthma.

In addition to the patients' improvement in health, two significant effects were noted in the trial of the vegan diet. First, there was a great reduction in health care costs; the patients had been receiving corticosteroids and other drugs and therapies for an average of twelve years. Second, according to the authors, the patients gained a greater sense of responsibility for their own health.

Omega-3 Essential Fatty Acids

Population studies have shown that children who eat fish more than once a week have one-third the risk of getting asthma as children who do not eat fish regularly.[17] Several clinical studies have shown that increasing the intake of omega-3 fatty acids (through supplementation with fish oils that contain eicosapentaenoic acid [EPA] and docosahexanoic acid [DHA]) offers significant benefits in treating asthma. In particular, improvements in airway responsiveness to allergens have been noted, as well as improvements in respiratory function.[18,19]

These benefits are related to increasing the ratio of omega-3 to omega-6 fatty acids in cell membranes, thereby reducing the availability of arachidonic acid. In particular, omega-3 fatty acid ingestion leads to a significant shift in leukotriene synthesis from the extremely inflammatory 4-series leukotrienes to the less inflammatory 5-series leukotrienes. This shift is directly related to relief from asthma symptoms.[20] It may take as long as one year before the benefits are apparent, as it appears to take time to turn over cellular membranes in favor of the omega-3 fatty acids.

Food Additives

The elimination of synthetic food additives is vitally important in the control of asthma.[21] Artificial dyes and preservatives are widely used in foods, beverages, and drugs. The most common coloring agents are the azo dyes tartrazine (orange), sunset yellow, amaranth (red), and the new coccine (red) and the non-azo dye pate blue. The most commonly used preservatives in food are sodium benzoate, 4-hydroxybenzoate esters, and sulfur dioxide. Various sulfites are commonly used in prepared foods.

Tartrazine, benzoates, sulfur dioxide, and, in particular, sulfites have been reported to cause asthma attacks in susceptible individuals.[21,22] It is estimated that 2 to 3 mg of sulfites are consumed each day by the average U.S. citizen, while an additional 5 to 10 mg are ingested by wine and beer drinkers.[22]

It has been postulated that a molybdenum deficiency may be responsible for sulfite sensitivity.[23] Sulfite oxidase, the enzyme responsible for neutralizing sulfites, requires molybdenum to work properly.

Tryptophan Metabolism and Pyridoxine Supplementation

Children with asthma have been shown to have a defect in their metabolism of the amino acid *tryptophan* (a building block of protein).[24,25] Tryptophan is converted to *serotonin*, a compound that, among other things, can cause the airways of asthmatics to constrict. High serotonin levels in the blood and sputum are common findings in asthmatics and are reflected by an elevated urinary level of 5-hydroxyindole acetic acid (5-HIAA), the breakdown product of serotonin. The levels of 5-HIAA in the urine correlate well with the severity of asthmatic symptoms. Double-blind clinical studies have shown that patients benefit from either a tryptophan-restricted diet[24] or vitamin B6 supplementation[25,26] to correct the blocked tryptophan metabolism. Vitamin B6 is required for the proper metabolism of tryptophan.

Vitamin B6 may also be of direct benefit to asthmatic patients. In one study, blood levels of the active form of vitamin B6 in fifteen adult patients with asthma were found to be significantly lower than in sixteen controls, but still above the level found in vitamin B6 deficiency.[25] Oral supplementation with 50 mg of vitamin B6 twice per day to seven of the patients failed to produce a substantial elevation of these low levels. However, all seven patients reported a dramatic decrease in frequency and severity of wheezing and asthmatic attacks while taking the supplements. This result means that vitamin B6 produces beneficial effects in asthma even when deficiency is not apparent.

In a study of seventy-six asthmatic children, pyridoxine at a dosage of 200 mg per day produced significant reductions in symptoms and in the dosages of drugs required (bronchodilators and corticosteroids). However, a double-blind study failed to demonstrate any significant improvement with B6 supplementation in patients who were dependent upon steroids for control of symptoms.[27]

While vitamin B6 supplementation may not help patients who are taking steroids, it is definitely recommended for asthmatics who are being treated with the drug theophylline. Theophylline significantly depresses levels of the active form of vitamin B6.[28] In addition, another study has shown that vitamin B6 supplementation can significantly reduce the typical side effects of theophylline (headaches, nausea, irritability, sleep disorders, etc.).[29]

Antioxidants

The substantial increase in the rate of asthma over the past twenty years can be partially explained by the reduced dietary intake of antioxidant nutrients. These include beta-carotene and vitamins A, C, and E, as well as the mineral cofactors essential for antioxidant defense mechanisms, such as zinc, selenium, and copper.[30] Antioxidants are thought to pro-vide important defense mechanisms for the lung. Antioxidant protection is significant because free radicals and other oxidizing agents can both stimulate bronchial constriction and increase reactivity to other agents. Asthma appears to be yet another inflammatory/allergic disease process that is influenced greatly by antioxidant mechanisms.

Vitamin C

Vitamin C is especially important to the health of the lungs, as it is the major antioxidant present in the lining of the airway surfaces.[31] Vitamin C intake in the general population appears to correlate inversely with occurrence of asthma. In other words, when vitamin C intake is low, the rate of asthma is high. This association indicates that low levels of vitamin C (in the diet and the blood) are an independent risk factor for asthma. Additional support for this theory is offered by two findings: that children of smokers have a higher rate of asthma (cigarette smoke is known to deplete respiratory vitamin C and E levels), and that symptoms of ongoing asthma in adults appear to be increased by exposure to environmental free radicals and decreased by vitamin C supplementation.[32]

Both treated and untreated asthmatic patients have been shown to have significantly lower levels of vitamin C in their blood.[32] From a clinical perspective, it appears that asthmatics have a higher need for vitamin C. Since 1973, there have been eleven clinical studies of vitamin C supplementation in asthma patients.[33] Seven of these studies showed significant improvements in respiratory measures and asthma symptoms as a result of supplementing the diet with 1 to 2 grams of vitamin C per day. This dosage recommendation appears extremely wise based on the increasing exposure to inhaled oxidants and the growing appreciation of the antioxidant function of vitamin C in the respiratory system. High-dose vitamin C therapy may also help asthma patients by lowering their histamine levels.[34]

Vitamin C exerts a number of effects against histamine. Specifically, it prevents the secretion of histamine by white blood cells and increases the detoxification of histamine. A recent study examined the antihistamine effect of acute and chronic vitamin C administration and its effect on white blood cell function in healthy men and women. In the study of chronic asthma, ten subjects ingested a placebo during weeks one, two, five, and six and 2 grams of vitamin C per day during weeks three and four. Fasting blood samples were collected after the initial two-week period (baseline) and at the end of weeks four and six.

Blood vitamin C levels rose significantly following vitamin C administration, while blood histamine levels fell by thirty-eight percent during those same weeks. The ability of white blood cells to respond to an infection (*chemotaxis*) increased by nineteen percent during vitamin C administration and fell thirty percent after vitamin C withdrawal.

In the study of acute asthma and vitamin C, blood histamine concentrations and chemotaxis did not change during the four hours following a single dose of vitamin C. This result suggests that vitamin C will only lower blood histamine levels if taken over time. Individuals who are prone to allergy or inflammation are encouraged to increase their consumption of vitamin C through supplementation.[34]

Flavonoids

Flavonoids appear to be key antioxidants in the treatment of asthma. Various flavonoids —quercetin in particular—have also been shown to inhibit histamine release from mast cells and the manufacture of allergy-related compounds, including leukotrienes.[35–38] In addition, quercetin has both a vitamin C–sparing effect and a direct stabilizing effect on membranes, including mast cells.

To increase flavonoid consumption, take quercetin or flavonoid-rich extracts. The extracts—from grape seed, pine bark, green tea, or *Ginkgo biloba*—may prove even more helpful in the treatment of asthma due to their better absorption of flavonoids than quercetin.

Carotenes

Carotenes are powerful antioxidants that may increase the integrity of the epithelial lining of the respiratory tract and also decrease leukotriene formation.[39] These effects suggest that a carotene-rich diet or carotene supplementation may be helpful.

Vitamin E

Vitamin E's activity as an antioxidant and an inhibitor of leukotriene formation also suggests that vitamin E supplementation may be helpful in asthma.[40]

Selenium

Reduced selenium levels have been found in asthma patients.[41–43] Glutathione peroxidase, the selenium-dependent antioxidant enzyme, is very important for breaking down allergic leukotrienes. Reduced levels of glutathione peroxidase have also been reported in asthmatics.[41] Supplemental selenium appears warranted to address any deficiency of glutathione peroxidase. In addition, supplemental selenium may reduce the production of leukotrienes by ensuring optimal activity of glutathione peroxidase.

Vitamin B12

Jonathan Wright, M.D., believes that "B12 therapy is the mainstay in childhood asthma."[44] In one clinical trial, weekly

1,000-mcg intramuscular injections produced definite improvement in asthmatic patients.[45] Of twenty patients, eighteen showed less shortness of breath with exertion, as well as improved appetite, sleep, and general condition. Vitamin B12 appears to be especially effective in treating sulfite-sensitive individuals. It offers the best protection when given orally (1 to 4 mcg) prior to challenge, compared to other pharmacological agents (e.g., cromolyn sodium, atropine, and doxepin).[46] The mode of action is the formation of a sulfite-cobalamin complex, which blocks sulfite's allergic effect.

Magnesium

In 1912, it was demonstrated that magnesium relaxed bovine bronchial smooth muscle.[47] Later, uncontrolled clinical studies with injectable forms of magnesium revealed magnesium's beneficial effect in the treatment of patients with acute attacks of asthma.[48]

Unfortunately, this promising line of research was dropped when antihistamines and bronchodilators became available. However, recently there has been renewed interest in the therapeutic use of magnesium for treating asthma. In fact, intravenous magnesium (2 grams of magnesium sulfate every hour, up to a total of 24.6 grams) is now a well-proven and clinically accepted measure to halt an acute asthma attack.[49–53]

These studies have utilized injectable magnesium therapy, but it has been demonstrated that injectable magnesium is not necessary for restoring magnesium status (except in the case of an emergency situation, such as an acute heart attack or acute asthma attack).[54] Oral magnesium therapy can raise body magnesium stores, but it will usually take six weeks to achieve significant elevations in tissue magnesium concentrations. Supplementation appears warranted, as dietary magnesium intake is directly related to lung function and asthma severity.[55]

Salt

There is strong evidence that increased salt intake increases bronchial reactivity and mortality from asthma.[56,57] The degree of bronchial reactivity to histamine has been positively linked with increased dietary sodium and with twenty-four-hour urinary sodium excretion. Since the severity of asthma correlates with the degree of bronchial reactivity, it is clear that the severity of asthma can be influenced by alterations in dietary sodium consumption.

DHEA

Decreased levels of the adrenal hormone DHEA (dehydroepiandrosterone) have been shown to be common among postmenopausal women with asthma, compared to matched controls.[58] Whether DHEA produces any therapeutic benefit in asthma patients remains to be demonstrated. However, given its importance to proper immune function, an ability to produce positive effects is certainly possible.

Botanicals

The most popular historical herbal treatment of asthma involved the use of *Ephedra sinica* (Ma huang), in combination with herbal expectorants. Examples of commonly used expectorants include: *Glycyrrhiza glabra* (licorice), *Grindelia camporum* (grindelia), *Euphorbia hirta* (euphorbia), *Drosera rotundifolia* (sundew), and *Polygala senega* (senega). This approach appears to have considerable merit, as ephedra and its alkaloids have proven effective as bronchodilators for the treatment of mild to moderate asthma and hay fever.[59,60] The peak bronchodilation effect occurs in one hour and lasts about five hours after administration. In addition to this approach, several other botanical medicines deserve mention.

Glycyrrhiza glabra

Licorice root has a long history of use as an anti-inflammatory and anti-allergic agent—actions that have now been documented in the scientific literature. The primary active component of licorice root in this application is glycyrrhetinic acid, a compound that has shown cortisol-like activity. In particular, glycyrrhetinic acid has been shown to inhibit prostaglandin and leukotriene manufacture, in a similar manner to corticosteroids such as prednisone.[61] Licorice is also an expectorant—a useful action in treating asthma.

Lobelia inflata

Lobelia (Indian tobacco) contains the alkaloid lobeline, an efficient expectorant. It has a long history of use in treating asthma.[62] Its mechanism of action may involve stimulating the release of epinephrine by the adrenal glands, resulting in binding to beta-2 receptors, and thereby relaxing the airways.[63] Although effective when used alone, lobelia has traditionally been used in combination with other botanical agents, such as cayenne pepper (Capsicum frutescens) and lungwort (Pulmonaria officinalis).

Allium Family

Onions and garlic, both members of the Allium family, inhibit lipoxygenase and cyclooxygenases, which generate inflammatory prostaglandins and thromboxanes.[65] Oral pretreatment of guinea pigs with 1 ml of an alcohol/onion extract markedly reduced their asthmatic response to allergen-inhalation challenges.

Onion contains quercetin, which may account for some of its pharmacological effect,[66]

but the major protective actions appear to be related to its content isothiocyanates (mustard oils).[67] Although the mechanism of action is unknown, it has been suggested that it is due to inhibition of the biosynthesis of arachidonic acid metabolites.

Tylophora asthmatica

The leaves of Tylophora asthmatica have been used extensively in Ayurvedic medicine for treating asthma and other respiratory tract disorders. The mode of action of tylophora is unknown but is thought to be due to its alkaloids, especially tylophorine. These alkoloids have been reported to possess antihistamine and antispasmodic activity as well as inhibition of mast cell release of histamine and other inflammatory compounds.[68,69] However, a more central mechanism may be responsible for the clinical effects in asthma therapy.

Several double-blind clinical studies have shown tylophora to produce good results.[70–73] In one study of 135 patients, those who were given 200 mg of tylophora leaves twice daily for six days demonstrated improvements in symptoms and respiratory function during the treatment period and for up to two weeks after treatment[70]. Symptom score, FEV_1, and other respiratory function tests were used as parameters. Side effects, such as nausea and vomiting, occurred in 9.8 percent of the tylophora group and 14 percent of the placebo group.

In another double-blind study, of 103 patients, those who received 40 mg of a dry alcoholic extract of tylophora daily for only six days demonstrated significant relief from symptoms of asthma compared to a placebo group.[72] At the end of the first week, 56 percent of the tylophora group had complete-to-moderate improvement, as compared to 31.6 percent of the patients who received the placebo. At the end of four weeks, the respective figures were 32 and 23.8 percent; at eight weeks, 23.8 and 8.4 percent; and at twelve weeks, 14.8 and 7.2 percent. The incidence of side effects, such as nausea, partial diminution of taste for salt, and slight mouth soreness, was 16.3 percent in the tylophora group and 6.6 percent in the placebo group. These results, as well as the results from an additional study, indicate that the benefits of tylophora are short-lived.[73]

Ginkgo biloba

Ginkgo biloba contains several unique terpene molecules, known collectively as ginkgolides, that antagonize platelet activating factor (PAF), a key chemical mediator in asthma, inflammation, and allergies. Ginkgolides compete with PAF for binding sites and inhibit the various events induced by PAF. In several double-blind studies, the anti-asthmatic effects of orally administered or inhaled ginkgolides have been shown to produce improvements in respiratory function and to reduce bronchial reactivity.[74,75] Treatment consisted of 120 mg of the pure ginkgolides daily—a dosage that is currently expensive to achieve using Ginkgo biloba extract, which contains twenty-four percent ginkgo flavonglycosides and six percent total terpenoids. Nevertheless, ginkgo extracts provide good antioxidant support and may also prove useful in the treatment of asthma.

TREATMENT SUMMARY

The effective treatment of asthma requires the consideration and control of many aspects. The following seven recommendations are given in order of priority.

1. Avoid airborne allergens, and allergy-proof the house.
2. Eliminate food allergens and food additives from the diet.
3. Follow a vegan diet with the possible exception of cold-water fish (salmon, mackerel, herring, halibut, etc.) for their omega-3 fatty acids.
4. Support the body's anti-allergy mechanisms with vitamin C, other antioxidants, quercetin, vitamin B12, and vitamin B6.
5. Use grape seed extract, green tea extract, or Ginkgo biloba extract.
6. Use ephedra- or tylophora-based herbal products in conjunction with licorice.
7. Use asthma medications as prescribed.

NOTE: In severe cases of asthma, the best treatment is a combined approach, using natural measures to reduce the allergic threshold and prevent acute attacks, along with proper drug treatment of acute attacks.

Diet

Eliminate all food allergens and food additives. If you have multiple food allergies, utilize a four-day rotation diet as described in FOOD ALLERGY. Consider trying a vegan diet for a minimum of four months to judge if it will help. If you are not allergic to garlic and onions, consume them liberally.

Nutritional Supplements

The following doses are for adults; for children, divide the dosage in half if they weigh between 50 and 100 pounds. For children under 50 pounds, use one-third the adult dosage. Be sure to determine the contents and source of all supplements to assure avoidance of any allergens.

- Vitamin B6: 25–50 mg twice per day
- Vitamin B12: 1,000 mcg/day (oral) or weekly injection; evaluate for efficacy after six weeks
- Vitamin C: 10–30 mg per day for every 2 pounds of body weight, in divided doses
- Vitamin E: 200–400 IU per day
- Magnesium: 200–400 mg three times per day
- Flavonoids(choose one):
  Quercetin: 400 mg twenty minutes before each meal
  Grape seed extract (95% PCO content): 50–100 mg three times per day
  Green tea extract (50% polyphenol content): 200–300 mg three times per day (or drink green tea liberally)

Gingko biloba extract: 80 mg three times per day
- Carotenes: 25,000–50,000 IU per day
- Selenium: 200–400 mcg per day
- DHEA: follow recommendations given in LONGEVITY AND LIFE EXTENSION

Botanical Medicines

Use ephedra or tylophora preparations. In either case, licorice can be used in conjunction.

- *Ephedra sinica*: The optimum dosage of ephedra depends on the alkaloid content of the form used. Each dose should have an ephedrine content of 12.5 to 25.0 mg and be taken two to three times per day. For the crude herb, this dosage would most likely be 500 to 1,000 mg three times per day. Standardized preparations are often preferred, as they have more dependable therapeutic activity. Ephedra can be combined with herbal expectorants as described in this chapter.
- *Tylophora asthmatica*: 200 mg of tylophora leaves or 40 mg of the dry alcoholic extract twice per day
- Licorice (*Glycyrrhiza glabra*): (all dosages three times per day)
  Powdered root: 1–2 g
  Fluid extract (1:1): 2–4 ml
  Solid (dry powdered) extract (4:1): 250–500 mg

Attention Deficit Disorders

Hyperactivity (attention deficit disorder with hyperactivity): Signs of inattention, impulsiveness, and hyperactivity inappropriate for the child's age

Learning disability (attention deficit disorder without hyperactivity): Developmentally inappropriate brief attention span and poor concentration for the child's age

Attention deficit disorder" (ADD) is the current phrase that encompasses a wide variety of terms used in the past to describe similar disorders: "hyperkinetic reaction of childhood," "hyperkinetic syndrome," "hyperactive child syndrome," "minimal brain damage," "minimal brain dysfunction," "minimal cerebral dysfunction," and "minor cerebral dysfunction." Three separate ADD disorders exist

1. ADD without hyperactivity
2. ADD with hyperactivity
3. ADD, residual type

The first two disorders will be discussed separately in the following sections. The discussion of hyperactivity is concerned largely with the role of food additives, food allergies, and sucrose, while the discussion of attention deficit disorder without hyperactivity focuses on heavy metals. Residual attention deficit disorder (individuals are eighteen years or older) is viewed primarily as a continuation of the process of ADD into adulthood. Although the first two syndromes will be discussed separately, it is important to recognize that the factors discussed under one may be equally relevant to the other.

Ear infections are another important consideration, given the fact that frequent ear infections and antibiotic use are associated with a greater likelihood of developing ADD. This situation highlights the importance of following the recommendations given in the chapter EAR INFECTIONS in the treatment of frequent ear infections.

Hyperactivity (ADD with Hyperactivity)

The frequency of ADD with hyperactivity has been reported to be from four to twenty percent of school-age children. A more conservative figure of three to five is probably more accurate, due to improved diagnostic criteria.[1] Clinical observation and population-based surveys report a substantially greater incidence in boys than girls (10:1). Over two million American school-aged boys take the drug *methylphenidate* (Ritalin). Onset is usually by the age of three, although diagnosis is not generally made until later when the child is in school.

273

The characteristics of this disorder, cited in order of frequency, are

1. Hyperactivity
2. Perceptual motor impairment
3. Emotional instability
4. General coordination deficit
5. Disorders of attention (short attention span, distractibility, lack of perseverance, failure to finish things, not listening, poor concentration)
6. Impulsiveness (action before thought, abrupt shifts in activity, poor organizing, jumping up in class)
7. Disorders of memory and thinking
8. Specific learning disabilities
9. Disorders of speech and hearing
10. Equivocal neurological signs and electroencephalographic irregularities

These characteristics are frequently associated with difficulties in school, both in learning and behavior. Although other factors may be involved in the *etiology* (cause), considerable evidence points toward food additives, food sensitivities, and sucrose (sugar) consumption as being responsible for the majority of hyperactivity in this country.

Food Additives

The term "food additives" covers a wide range of chemicals. Five thousand additives are used in the United States, including: anti-caking agents (e.g., calcium silicate); antioxidants (e.g., BHT, BHA); bleaching agents (e.g., benzoyl peroxide); colorings (e.g., artificial azo dye derivatives); flavorings; emulsifiers; mineral salts; preservatives (e.g., benzoates, nitrates, sulfites); thickeners; and vegetable gums. It is now estimated that each person in the United States is consuming eight to ten pounds of food additives each year.[2] The 1985 per capita daily consumption of food additives is approximately 13 to 15 grams. The total annual consumption of food colors alone is approximately 100 million pounds for the entire population. The theory that food additives induce hyperactivity is commonly referred to as the "Feingold hypothesis," stemming from the research of Benjamin Feingold, M.D.

According to Feingold, many hyperactive children—perhaps forty to fifty percent—are sensitive to artificial food colors, flavors, and preservatives and to naturally occurring salicylates and phenolic compounds.[3] Feingold's

---

QUICK REVIEW

- Over two million American school-aged boys take the drug methylphenidate (Ritalin).
- Food additives and food allergies are the major factors in ADD with hyperactivity.
- Three factors appear to be particularly relevant to learning disabilities:

1. Otitis media
2. Nutrient deficiency
3. Heavy metals

- Several clinical studies have shown that nutritional supplementation can improve mental function in school-aged children.

claims were based on his experience with over 1,200 cases in which food additives were linked to learning and behavior disorders. Since Feingold's presentation to the American Medical Association in 1973, the role of food additives as the causative factor in hyperactivity has been hotly debated in the scientific literature.[4-16] However, researchers have focused on only ten food dyes, versus the three thousand food additives with which Feingold was concerned.

At first glance, it appears that the majority of the double-blind studies designed to test the Feingold hypothesis have shown essentially negative results.[4-9] That is, they found no link between food additives and hyperactivity. However, upon closer examination of these studies and further investigation into the literature, it becomes evident that food additives do, in fact, play a major role in hyperactivity.[10-16] This is somewhat in opposition to the final report filed by the National Advisory Committee on Hyperkinesis and Food Additives to the U.S.A. Nutrition Foundation in 1980.

However, the U.S. National Institutes of Health, Consensus Conference on Defined Diets and Childhood Hyperactivity, agreed to reconsider the Feingold diet in the amelioration of hyperkinesis.[17,18] The reason for this reconsideration is largely due to the overwhelming evidence produced in several studies[8-10,13,14] and the fact that, despite major inadequacies in the negative studies, about fifty percent of those who tried the Feingold diet in these studies displayed a decrease in symptoms of hyperactivity.[4,7] In other words, even though the studies seemed to be designed to disprove the Feingold diet, about half of the children still showed benefit. The studies were still viewed as "negative" because more children were not helped.

Schauss[11] and Rippere[12] have reviewed much of the literature concerning food addi-

tives and hyperactive children and have formulated guidelines and recommendations for future research designs that we hope will be utilized. Rippere's review is primarily a critique of C. Keith Conners' studies and book, *Food Additives and Hyperactive Children.* Conners has been the primary researcher refuting the Feingold hypothesis.[3-5] Rippere's major criticisms of Conners' work focused on six areas:

1. *Type of placebo:* In Conners' studies, the placebo used was a chocolate cookie—hardly an appropriate choice, to say the least. In Table 1 it can be seen that, in double-blind studies of reactions to foods in hyperkinetic children, chocolate produced a reaction in thirty-three percent in one study and sixty-four percent in another. Conners himself acknowledges that reaction to the placebo was not uncommon. Furthermore, Conners reports that, at a two-year follow-up, twenty-one percent of the mothers whose children took part in the diet trials mentioned that chocolate appeared to affect their children's behavior adversely. When the other constituents of the cookie are also taken into consideration (cow's milk, sugar, wheat, corn, yeast, and other additives, in addition to artificial colors), this placebo can hardly be termed inert.

2. *Adequacy of challenge dosages:* The dose of mixed food dyes in these challenge trials was based on erroneous information, being far below the average daily intake according to FDA data. The dose given in Conners' studies was 13 mg twice daily, compared with a daily dose of 150 mg estimated to be at the ninetieth percentile for children from five to twelve years of age (the average daily dose for children between five and twelve years of age is estimated at 76.5 mg). Swanson and Kinsbourne confirmed the Conners results when a daily dose of 26 mg of mixed food dyes was given; however, they demonstrated that doses of 75, 100 and 150 mg produced significant impairment of learning performance in seventeen of the twenty subjects.[13] These results were consistent with other researchers' demonstrations of severe behavioral effects provoked by administration of mixed dyes, even at the low concentrations used by Conners.[14]

3. *Length of dose interval:* The doses of food dyes were given at relatively long intervals. This, combined with the inadequate dosage, indicates that the model fell far short of real-life exposure experienced by these victims of the technicolor breakfast cereal generation.

4. *Type of blood test for allergy determination:* Conners used a highly unreliable blood test for food allergies (the cytotoxic test). The test is considered unreliable because it has a high rate of false positives and negatives. In other words, the test will register an allergy when it really isn't there (a false positive) and ignore an allergy when it really is there (a false negative). Conners use of an allergy test is irrelevant anyway because Feingold's hypothesis does not require an allergic reaction of the immune system as the basis for the reactions to the various additives.

5. *Outcome measures:* Conners' main outcome measure, a rating scale that he designed himself, was extremely imprecise. Behavioral changes were not adequately detected, due to inappropriateness of the rating scales being used.

6. *Bias in the presentation of other investigators' data:* Conners consistently minimized and discounted findings that support Feingold's hypothesis, including his own findings. In the two major double-blind studies assessing the Feingold diet (Conners' and Harley's), parental scores revealed positive behavioral changes for the Feingold diet.[3,6] The fact that

teacher ratings failed to improve may indicate that other environmental factors were having an effect. In particular, it has been demonstrated that standard cool-white fluorescent lighting increases hyperactive behavior, while full-spectrum light with radiation shields decreases hyperactivity presumably by somehow affecting the pineal gland—a small pea-sized gland in the center of the brain that secretes melatonin and regulates the release of many other hormones.[19]

It is interesting to note that, while the U.S. studies have been largely negative, the reports from Australia and Canada have been more supportive of the Feingold hypothesis.[8,10,14,21–30] Feingold has contended that there is a conflict of interest on the part of the Nutrition Foundation, an organization supported by the major food manufacturers—Coca Cola, Nabisco, General Foods, etc. It appears significant that the Nutrition Foundation has financed most of the negative studies.[19,20] Feingold contends that the conflict of interest arises because these companies would suffer economically if food additives were found to be harmful. Other countries have significantly restricted the use of artificial food additives because of the possible harmful effects.[22]

Several more recent studies have been designed to determine the effect of the common yellow dye tartrazine on behavior in hyperactive children. In the largest study, 200 children were included in a six-week open trial of a diet free of synthetic food coloring.[30] The parents of 150 children reported behavioral improvement with the diet and subsequent deterioration of behavior upon introduction of foods containing artificial colors. Thirty-four children (twenty-three suspected reactors, eleven uncertain reactors) and twenty control subjects, aged two to fourteen years, were studied in the double-blind, placebo-controlled portion of the study.

Either a placebo or one of six dose levels of tartrazine (1, 2, 5, 10, 20, and 50 mg) was administered randomly each morning, and behavioral ratings were recorded by parents at the end of each day.

The study identified twenty-four children as clear reactors (nineteen of the twenty-three "suspected reactors," three of the eleven "uncertain reactors," and two of the twenty "control subjects"). Reactors displayed irritability, restlessness, and sleep disturbances. A clear dose-response effect was obtained. With doses greater than 10 mg, the duration of effect was prolonged.

These results once again support the Feingold hypothesis. Not surprisingly, the study was not performed in the United States. The study was conducted at the Royal Children's Hospital, University of Melbourne, Australia.

The other two recent studies also found that food additives and food allergens are common causes of ADD. In one study, nineteen out of twenty-six children with ADD with hyperactivity responded favorably to an elimination diet.[31] In the other study, fifty-nine out of seventy-eight children responded to an elimination diet.[32] In both studies, double-blind, placebo-controlled food challenges confirmed the negative effects of food additives and food allergies on behavior and mental performance.

Sucrose

There appears to be a relationship between sucrose consumption and artificial food dyes.[23] It has been demonstrated that destructive-aggressive and restless behavior significantly correlates with the amount of sucrose consumed. In addition, Langseth and Dowd performed five-hour oral glucose tolerance tests on 261 hyperactive children, with the result that seventy-four percent displayed abnormal glucose tolerance curves.[24] The predominant

abnormality was a low, flat curve (see the chapter HYPOGLYCEMIA for further discussion). Hypoglycemia would obviously promote hyperactivity via increased adrenalin secretion. Refined carbohydrate consumption appears to be the major factor in promoting reactive hypoglycemia (i.e., hypoglycemia that is the result of a quick elevation in blood sugar for one to two hours followed by a severe drop in blood sugar levels).[33]

Food Allergies (Sensitivities)

The contention that food allergies provoke hyperactivity in children is another popular notion in lay publications. There are, however, much more consistent results from double-blind studies that examined the relationship between behavior and allergies to food and food additives.[25–28] While artificial colorings and preservatives were the most common substances that caused hyperactivity in two of these studies, no child was sensitive to these alone.[25,26] This situation suggests that, since food allergies or sensitivities can cause psychological symptoms, elimination of just food additives from the diet is inadequate. The diet must also be free of any food allergen. In other words, if a child has an allergy to milk, it is necessary to eliminate not only sources of food additives from the diet, but also milk.

In one large controlled trial, seventy-six severely hyperactive children were treated with a low-allergen diet (the *oligoantigenic* diet is described in the chapter FOOD ALLERGY) consisting of lamb, chicken, potatoes, rice, banana, apple, cabbage-family vegetable, a multiple vitamin, and 3 grams per day of calcium gluconate.[25] After a four-week trial, sixty-two children (eighty-two percent) improved, and a normal range of behavior was achieved in twenty-one of these. Other symptoms, such as headaches, abdominal

ITEM	% REACTING[26]	% REACTING (NUMBER OF PATIENTS)[25]
Red dye	88	NT*
Yellow dye	80	NT
Blue dye	80	NT
Coloring and preservatives	NT	79 (34
Cow's milk	73	64 (55)
Soya	NT	73 (15)
Chocolate	33	64 (34)
Grape	40	50 (18)
Orange	40	45 (49)
Peanuts	47	32 (32)
Wheat	30	49 (53)
Corn	40	29 (38)
Tomato	47	20 (35)
Egg	20	40 (50)
Cane sugar	40	16 (55)
Apple	40	13 (53)
Fish	NT	23 (48)
Oats	NT	23 (43)

TABLE 1   Food Allergy Reactions in Hyperactive Children

*NT=Not tested

pains, and fits, were also relieved.[25] Reintroduction of the foods to which the child was sensitive led to reappearance of symptoms and hyperactive behavior. No mention was made of the possibility that nonresponders were reacting to foods in the oligoantigenic diet or perhaps the vitamins, although it was noted that physical complaints were reduced in the non-responders as well.

It is also significant that, in a retrospective study, eighty-six percent of hyperactive children had elevated levels of white blood cells that are linked to allergies (eosinophils).[24]

Table 1 summarizes the results of two studies on food sensitivities and hyperactivity. In the study by O'Shea et al.[26] fifteen patients were tested for each food item. In the study by Egger et al.[25] the number of patients tested is given in parentheses after the percent reacting.

These results were reproduced in a larger study of 185 children with established hyperkinetic syndrome. The children were put on a low-allergen diet treatment for four weeks. The diet consisted of two meats (lamb and chicken), two carbohydrates (potatoes and rice), two fruits (bananas and pears), vegetables (cabbage, sprouts, cauliflower, broccoli, cucumber, celery, and carrots), and water. They were supplemented with calcium, magnesium, zinc, and some basic vitamins. Behavior in 116 of these children improved, and foods that provoked hyperactivity were identified by sequential reintroduction.[27] Other researchers have found similar improvements. For example, one double-blind study of twenty-six children who met the criteria for attention deficit hyperactivity disorder found that nineteen responded favorably to an oligoantigenic diet that also eliminated food additives.[28]

Learning Disability (Attention Deficit Disorder without Hyperactivity)

Three factors appear to be particularly relevant to learning disabilities:

1. Otitis media
2. Nutrient deficiency
3. Heavy metals

Otitis Media

Children with moderate to severe hearing loss tend to have impaired speech and language development, lowered general intelligence scores, and learning difficulties.[34,35] Current and frequent ear infections (otitis media) have been reported to be twice as common in learning-disabled children as non-learning-disabled children.[34] This reconfirms the necessity of dealing with otitis media from a preventive standpoint (see EAR INFECTION), since many of the factors associated with hyperactivity are also associated with otitis media.

Nutrient Deficiency

Virtually any nutrient deficiency can result in impaired brain function.[36,37] Iron deficiency is the most common nutrient deficiency in American children.[36] Iron deficiency is associated with: markedly decreased attentiveness; less complex or purposeful, narrower attention span; decreased persistence; and decreased voluntary activity that is usually responsive to supplementation.[36–39] Several investigators have demonstrated that correction of even subtle nutritional deficiencies exerts a substantial influence on learning and behavior.[40–42]

Heavy Metals

Numerous studies have demonstrated a strong relationship between childhood learning disabilities (and other disorders, including criminal behavior) and body stores of heavy metals, particularly lead.[43–49] Learning disabilities seem to be characterized by a general pattern of high levels of mercury, cadmium, lead, copper, and manganese, as determined by hair analysis.[43,44] Poor nutrition and elevation of heavy metal levels usually go hand in hand, due to decreased consumption of food factors known to chelate these heavy metals or decrease their absorption. Table 2 summarizes the results of several studies that examine hair heavy-metal levels in learning-disabled (LD) subjects.

Screening for lead toxicity is an essential process when evaluating a child with symptoms of ADD or developmental delay (DD). However, a recent study did not find significantly higher lead levels in children with ADD and DD than in normal controls.[50] This study seems to refute the need for lead-status evaluation in ADD and DD; however, the study used blood lead levels as an indicator of body lead burden. The problem with blood lead measurements is that they reflect recent exposure and do not accurately evaluate lead concentration in the brain. Hair mineral analysis and EDTA challenge have provided entirely different results.

Nutritional Supplements

Several clinical studies have shown that nutritional supplementation can improve mental function in school-aged children. For example, let's take a look at a study published in the medical journal *The Lancet*, that demonstrated that supplementing the diet with a multiple-vitamin-mineral formula can increase nonverbal intelligence in children.[52] This study demonstrates the essential role of many vitamins and minerals in brain function. Nutrients especially important to proper brain and nervous system function include thiamin, niacin, vitamin B6, vitamin B12, copper, iodine, iron, magnesium, manganese, potassium, and zinc. A deficiency of any of these essential nutrients will result in impaired brain and nervous system function.

The study was performed on ninety children between the ages of twelve and thirteen. The children were divided into three groups of thirty. One group took no tablet,

TABLE 2	Summary of Literature on Heavy Metals and Learning Disability				
STUDY	**CADMIUM**	**LEAD**	**MERCURY**	**COPPER**	**SUBJECTS**
Cameron et al. (1980)	+	++	++	++	66 LD
Colgan (1983)	++	++	+	0	16 LD
Ely et al. (1981)	+	NT	+	NT	77 LD males
Hansen et al. (1980)	NT	+	NT	NT	20 LD vs controls
Moore et al. (1975)	NT	++	NT	NT	45 LD
Pihl et al. (1977)	++	++	0	0	35 LD vs 22 controls
Rasmussen (1976)	NT	+	NT	+	200 LD
Thatcher et al. (1982)	++	++	NT	NT	141 children
Rudolph (1977)	0	+	NT	++	53 LD vs 1,347 controls
Tuthill (1996)	NT	++	NT	NT	277 first-graders

Key:

++   Significant positive relationship

+   Weak positive relationship

0   No relationship

NT   Not tested

one group took a typical multiple-vitamin-and-mineral tablet, and the last group took a tablet that looked and tasted just like the multiple-vitamin-and-mineral, yet contained no vitamins or minerals.

The results of this well-controlled study demonstrated that the group that took the supplement had a significant increase in non-verbal intelligence, while the placebo group and the remaining thirty who took no tablet showed no such improvement. It is a well-accepted fact that a deficiency of a number of vitamins and minerals will result in impaired mental performance. Apparently, many of the children were suffering from "subclini-cal" vitamin and mineral deficiencies to an extent that hampered their nerve cell function and impaired their mental performance. In other words, low levels of nutrients in the diet will not allow the brain to function properly. Providing the brain with the nutrients that it requires to function at its optimal level, through either diet or supplementation, can prevent or reverse these nutritional deficiencies.

Many cases of ADD may simply be reflecting poor nutritional status. High-quality nutrition is important throughout one's life, but it is probably most important earlier in life, during physical, mental, and social development.

TREATMENT SUMMARY

ADD with Hyperactivity

Despite the controversy about the significance of food additives in hyperactivity, careful reading of the published studies yields some clear conclusions:

- Virtually every study, both negative and positive, demonstrated that some hyperactive children consistently react with behavioral problems when challenged by specific food additives
- Virtually every study, whether supportive or critical of the Feingold hypothesis, is marred by significant experimental design defects
- Critics of the Feingold hypothesis are misusing the apparently inconsistent statistical group results to ignore the significance of the clear individual results, which are reproducible under double-blind conditions

Although the best approach would be to eliminate all food additives, practical realities make this difficult. Ultimately, the best results will depend upon accurate identification of the offending agents, preferably with behavioral, rather than laboratory, measurements.

Considering the importance of food allergy, recognition and control of the offending allergens is critical. The most sensible and economical approach is to follow the oligoantigenic diet for a period of four weeks, then reintroduce suspected foods (full servings at least once a day, one food introduced per week). If symptoms recur or worsen upon reintroduction/challenge, the food should be withdrawn. If there is no improvement when on the oligoantigenic diet, it is possible that the child is reacting to something else in the diet or environment. Further testing may be indicated in these cases.

All refined sugars should be eliminated from the diet, and a general multivitamin-and-mineral supplement should be used (with special care to ensure that the child is not allergic to the product used).

Also, the factors discussed in LEARNING DISABILITIES, should be considered. For example, hyperactive children have been shown to have increased lead levels in their blood.[51,52]

ADD Without Hyperactivity

The treatment plan for ADD without hyperactivity involves the elimination of any underlying otitis media, detection and elimination of any heavy-metal toxicity, and establishment of optimum nutrition for these children, including the use of a high-potency multiple-vitamin-and-mineral formula. Counseling is also indicated in most cases and, for the best results, should involve the whole family.

Bipolar (Manic) Depression

To be diagnosed as a bipolar depressive, an individual would be expected to have at least three of the following symptoms:

Excessive self-esteem or grandiosity

Reduced need for sleep

Extreme talkativeness, excessive telephoning

Extremely rapid flight of thoughts, along with the feeling that the mind is racing

Inability to concentrate; easily distracted

Increase in social or work-oriented activities, often with a sixty- to eighty-hour work week

Poor judgment, as indicated by sprees of uncontrolled spending, increased sexual indiscretions, and misguided financial decisions

In order to distinguish states of depression that alternate with mania from the more common types of depression, the terms *unipolar* and *bipolar* are commonly used. A unipolar depressive suffers from depression alone, while the bipolar depressive suffers from either mania alone or mania alternating with depression. Bipolar depression is often referred to as *manic depression.*

For a complete discussion of depression and to provide a better understanding of the natural approach discussed below, please consult the chapter DEPRESSION.

Therapeutic Considerations

Patients experiencing a manic syndrome usually require hospitalization to prevent impulsive and aggressive behavior from ruining their careers or causing injury to themselves or others. The mineral lithium has become the drug of choice for these patients. Typically, manic patients are hospitalized for two weeks and kept under heavy sedation with drugs until lithium levels reach acceptable blood levels.

Many of the principles outlined in the DEPRESSION chapter are applicable to bipolar depression. However, while the lifestyle and dietary recommendations can be employed without physician supervision, due to the seriousness of this condition we do not encourage anyone with bipolar depression to self-medicate with 5-HTP, St. John's wort extract, or any other herbal medicines. Find a qualified psychiatrist or physician to supervise you if you wish to employ any of these natural supportive therapies.

That being said, serotonin reuptake inhibitors such as Prozac, Zoloft, and Paxil are often helpful when used in combination with lithium. 5-hydroxytryptophan (5-HTP) and/or botanical medicines such as St. John's wort extract may prove to be useful adjuncts to lithium as well, but without the side effects (see DEPRESSION).

Tryptophan

Tryptophan is the amino acid that is converted to the important neurotransmitter serotonin. Although patients have responded to tryptophan supplementation, the effective doses were generally quite large (12 grams of L-tryptophan per day).[1,2] A better choice appears to be 5-HTP. 5-HTP has been shown to be helpful in the treatment of bipolar depression when used in combination with lithium at a much lower dosage (200 mg, three times per day) than L-tryptophan.[3,4]

For more information on 5-HTP, see the DEPRESSION chapter.

Phosphatidylcholine

Phosphatidylcholine is the major fat in our cell membranes, as well as in soy lecithin. Supplementation with large amounts of phosphatidylcholine (15 to 30 grams per day in both the pure form and as lecithin) has shown better results than tryptophan in the treatment of mania because of its ability to raise levels of the important neurotransmitter acetylcholine.[5-7] One of the ways in which lithium is thought to relieve bipolar depression is by promoting increased brain activity of acetylcholine.[8,9] The use of phosphatidylcholine to increase brain acetylcholine activity has been shown to produce significant improvement in symptoms in some patients.[5-7]

Vanadium

The role of vanadium in mania has been researched primarily by G. Naylor at the University of Surrey in the United Kingdom.[10-12] Increased levels of vanadium are found in hair samples from manic patients, and these values fall toward normal levels upon recovery.[10] In contrast, depressed patients typically have normal hair concentrations of vanadium, while whole blood and serum vanadium levels are elevated.[10] Their levels also return to normal upon recovery. These findings suggest that vanadium plays a major role in determining mood. Therapies designed to change the chemical structure of vanadate to the less inhibitory vanadyl form have used

. . . .

QUICK REVIEW

- Patients experiencing a manic syndrome usually require hospitalization to prevent impulsive and aggressive behavior from ruining their careers or injuring themselves or others.
- There is a link between high vanadium levels and mania.
- Vitamin C (3 grams per day) has been shown in a double-blind crossover study to result in significant clinical improvement.
- The use of phosphatidylcholine to increase brain acetylcholine activity has been shown to produce significant improvement in symptoms in some patients.

vitamin C and EDTA, separately and in combination.[11,12] Vitamin C (3 grams per day) has been shown in a double-blind crossover study to result in significant clinical improvement.[11]

The use of a "low-vanadium diet" has also been advocated by Naylor. However, his dietary suggestions for low vanadium intake are not consistent with the vanadium content of foods.[13] Low-vanadium-content foods (1 to 5 ng/g) include fats, oils, fresh fruits, and vegetables. Whole grains, seafood, meat, and dairy products are in the range of 5 to 30 ng/g, while prepared foods—such as peanut butter, white bread, and breakfast cereals—range from 11 to 93 ng/g. We recommend following this low-vanadium diet versus the diet that Naylor advocated. The benefit of the "low-vanadium diet" used in Naylor's study was probably due to his simultaneous administration of EDTA, a *chelating* (binding) agent that binds to the vanadium and other heavy metals and promotes their excretion.

Circadian Rhythms

Manic-depressive patients have a disturbed natural daily rhythm of hormonal release (the circadian rhythm), tend to be worse in the winter, and are sensitive to bright light (it's hard on their eyes). All of these findings suggest light therapy may be of value. See the chapter SEASONAL AFFECTIVE DISORDER).[14]

TREATMENT SUMMARY

In general, the same dietary and lifestyle guidelines given in the DEPRESSION are appropriate here.

Diet

A low-vanadium diet is recommended. This involves eliminating all refined and processed foods and promoting the consumption of fresh fruits and vegetables.

Nutritional Supplements

- High-potency multiple-vitamin-and-mineral formula
- Phosphatidylcholine: 10–25 g/day

NOTE: Phosphatidylcholine may induce depression in some patients.[15] If this occurs, discontinue immediately.

- Vitamin C: 3–5 grams per day in divided doses
- Vitamin E: 400–800 IU per day

Bladder Infection (Cystitis)

Burning pain on urination

Increased urinary frequency, especially at night (*nocturia*)

Cloudy, foul-smelling, or dark urine

Lower abdominal pain

Urinalysis shows significant number of bacteria and white blood cells

Bladder infections in women are surprisingly common: ten to twenty percent of all women have urinary tract discomfort at least once a year; thirty-seven percent of women with no history of urinary tract infection will have one within ten years; and two to four percent of apparently healthy women have elevated levels of bacteria in their urine, indicative of an unrecognized urinary tract infection.

Women with a history of recurrent urinary tract infections will typically have an episode at least once every year.[1] Recurrent bladder infections can be a significant problem for some women since fifty-five percent of the infections will eventually involve the upper urinary tract—the kidneys. Recurrent kidney infection can cause progressive damage, resulting in scarring and, for some, kidney failure. Kidney failure comes with a high price: lifelong dialysis or kidney transplant.

Urinary tract infections are much less common in males than in females, except in infants. In general, urinary tract infections in males indicate an anatomical abnormality, a prostate infection, or rectal intercourse.[2]

Most bladder infections are caused by bacteria. However, the diagnosis of bladder infection by culturing the urine for bacteria is imprecise since clinical symptoms and the presence of significant amounts of bacteria in the urine do not always correlate well. Only sixty percent of women with the typical symptoms of urinary tract infection actually have significant levels of bacteria in their urine.

In general, diagnosis is made according to signs and symptoms and urinary findings. Microscopic examination of the infected urine will show high levels of white blood cells and bacteria. Culturing the urine will indicate the quantity and type of bacteria involved. The *Escherichia coli*, or *E. coli*, bacteria is responsible for about ninety percent of bladder infections when bacteria can be identified.

Urine, as it is secreted by the kidneys, is sterile until it reaches the urethra, which transports it from the bladder to the urethral opening. Bacteria can reach the urinary tract by ascending from the urethra or, much less commonly, through the bloodstream. The body has several defenses against bacterial growth in the urinary tract: urine flow tends to wash away bacteria; the surface of the bladder has antimicrobial properties; the pH of the urine inhibits the growth of many bacteria; in men the prostatic fluid has many antimicrobial substances; and the body quickly secretes white cells to control the bacteria.[4]

Many factors are associated with increased

risk of bladder infection: pregnancy (twice as frequent), sexual intercourse (nuns have one-tenth the incidence), homosexual activity (in males), mechanical trauma or irritation, and, perhaps most important, structural abnormalities of the urinary tract that block the free flow of urine.

Therapeutic Considerations

Although most bladder infections are not serious, it is important that you be properly diagnosed, treated, and monitored. If you have symptoms suggestive of a bladder infection, consult a physician. If an original urine culture indicates the presence of bacteria, it is appropriate to follow up with another culture seven to fourteen days after treatment is started. Most physicians will want to prescribe antibiotics. However, please discuss with your doctor the hazards of antibiotic use

(discussed in the next paragraph) and your desire to utilize a more natural approach. Notify your physician if any change occurs in your condition (fever, more painful urination, low back pain, etc.).

For most bladder infections, the best treatment appears to be the natural approach. There is a growing concern that antibiotic therapy actually promotes recurrent bladder infection by disturbing the bacterial flora of the vagina and by giving rise to antibiotic-resistant strains of *E. coli*.[3,4] One of the body's most important defenses against bacterial colonization of the bladder is a protective shield of bacteria that line and protect the external portion of the urethra. When antibiotics are used, this normal protective shield is usually stripped away or is replaced by less effective organisms.

If a woman tends to suffer from recurrent bladder infections, or if antibiotics have been used, it is appropriate to reintroduce friendly bacteria into the vagina. The best way to do this is to use commercially available *Lacto-*

· ·

QUICK REVIEW

- If you have symptoms suggestive of a bladder infection, consult a physician.
- There is a growing concern that antibiotic therapy actually promotes recurrent bladder infections.
- The primary goal in the natural approach to treating bladder infections is to enhance the immune system and other protective factors against infection.
- Drinking at least 64 ounces of water daily increases urine flow to combat cystitis.
- Alkalinizing the urine with citrate salts relieves cystitis.
- Cranberry juice has been shown to be quite effective in several clinical studies.
- Uva ursi is effective in the treatment of acute bladder infections and is also a preventive measure.

bacillus acidophilus products. Use a product that is a capsule or tablet, and simply place one or two in the vagina before going to bed at night every other night for two weeks.

Chronic Interstitial Cystitis

Chronic interstitial cystitis is a persistent form of bladder irritation not due to infection. In addition to the general measures given below, the therapeutic focus is on enhancing the integrity of the tissue (interstitium) along with the lining of the bladder wall. Eliminating food allergens appears to be a valid goal, as food allergies have been shown to produce cystitis in some patients.[5–7] Repeated ingestion of a food allergen could easily explain the chronic nature of interstitial cystitis.

The herb gotu kola (*Centella asiatica*) appears to address some of the other features of chronic interstitial cystitis. Specifically, centella extracts have been shown to heal ulcerations of the bladder and to improve the integrity of the connective tissue that lines the bladder wall.[8,9]

Goals of Therapy

The primary goal in the natural approach to treating infectious cystitis is enhancing an individual's internal defenses against urinary tract infection. Specifically, this refers to enhancing the flow of urine by drinking at least 64 ounces of water daily; promoting a pH that will inhibit the growth of the organism; preventing bacteria from attaching to the lining of the bladder; and enhancing the immune system. The recommendations given in the chapter IMMUNE SUPPORT are appropriate to employ during a bladder or lower urinary tract infection. In addition, the herb uva ursi (*Arctostaphylos uva ursi*) can be used as an antimicrobial agent.

Increasing Urine Flow

Increasing urine flow can be easily achieved by increasing the quantity of liquids consumed. Ideally, the liquids should be in the form of pure water, herbal teas, and fresh fruit and vegetable juices diluted with at least an equal amount of water. If you have a bladder infection, you should drink at least 64 ounces of liquids from this group, with at least half of this amount being water. You should also avoid such liquids as soft drinks, concentrated fruit drinks, coffee, and alcoholic beverages.

Cranberry Juice

Cranberries and cranberry juice are particularly beneficial in the treatment of urinary tract infections; several clinical studies have shown them to be quite effective.[10–12] In one study, 16 ounces of cranberry juice per day produced beneficial effects in seventy-three percent of the subjects (forty-four females and sixteen males) with active urinary tract infections.[10] Furthermore, withdrawal of the cranberry juice in the people who benefited resulted in recurrence of bladder infection in sixty-one percent.

Many believe that the action of cranberry juice is due to acidifying the urine and to the antibacterial effects of *hippuric acid*, a component of cranberries.[13,14] However, these are probably not the major mechanisms of action. In order to acidify the urine, at least 1 quart of cranberry juice would have to be consumed at one sitting.[13] In addition, the concentration of hippuric acid in the urine as a result of drinking cranberry juice is insufficient to inhibit bacteria.[13,14] As 16 ounces of cranberry juice per day have been shown to be effective in the treatment of bladder infection, another mechanism is more likely.

Recent studies have shown that components of cranberry juice reduce the ability of *E. coli* to adhere to the lining of the bladder and urethra.[15,16] In order for bacteria to infect, they must first adhere to this mucosal lining. By interfering with adherence, cranberry juice greatly reduces the likelihood of infection and helps the body fight off infection. This is the most likely explanation of cranberry juice's positive effects in bladder infections.

In one study of seven juices (cranberry, blueberry, grapefruit, guava, mango, orange, and pineapple), only cranberry and blueberry contained this inhibitor.[16] Blueberry juice is a suitable alternative to cranberry juice in treating bladder infections.

It must be pointed out that most cranberry juices on the market contain one-third cranberry juice, mixed with water and sugar. Since sugar has such a detrimental effect on the immune system,[17–19] use of sweetened cranberry juice cannot be recommended. Fresh cranberry (sweetened with apple or grape juice) or blueberry juice is preferred. Cranberry extracts are also available commercially in pill form.

Acidify or Alkalinize?

Although many practitioners believe that acidifying the urine is the best approach in addressing cystitis, several arguments can be made for alkalinizing the urine. First, it is often difficult to acidify the urine. Many popular methods of attempting to acidify the urine, such as ascorbic acid supplementation and the drinking of cranberry juice, have very little effect on pH at commonly prescribed doses.

The best argument for alkalinizing the urine is that it appears to be more effective, especially in women without pathogenic bacteria in their urine. The best method for alkalinizing the urine appears to be the use of potassium citrate or sodium citrate. These salts are rapidly absorbed and metabolized without affecting gastric pH or producing a laxative effect. They are excreted partly as carbonate, thus raising the pH of the urine.

Potassium citrate and/or sodium citrate have long been employed in the treatment of lower urinary tract infections. They are often used as a treatment until the results of a urine culture are available because they will often provide complete relief from symptoms. There are some clinical studies to support the use of citrate salt treatment. For example, in one study, women who had symptoms of a urinary tract infection were given a 4-gram dose of sodium citrate every eight hours for forty-eight hours.[20] Of the sixty-four women evaluated, eighty percent had relief of symptoms, twelve percent had deterioration of symptoms, and ninety-two percent rated the treatment as acceptable. Of the sixty-four women, nineteen were shown to have positive bacterial cultures before treatment. There was more variation in response to treatment in the group of women with proven bacterial infection. In those with symptoms of urethral pain, seven out of ten improved. In those with dysuria (increased urinary frequency or urgency) thirteen out of eighteen improved. These results were similar to those of a previous study that demonstrated significant symptomatic relief in eighty percent of the 159 women studied who had negative urine cultures for bacteria.[21]

Because of these positive results, it has been suggested that urine culture as a diagnostic tool could be restricted to those women who fail to respond to alkalinization therapy.

Restricting urine cultures to nonresponders would lower health care costs.

There is one more possible advantage to alkalinizing rather than acidifying the urine. Many of the herbs used to treat urinary tract infections, such as goldenseal (*Hydrastis canadensis*) and uva ursi (*Arctostaphylos uva ursi*) contain antibacterial components that work most effectively in an alkaline environment.

The best way to take citrate is in the form of mineral supplements (potassium, magnesium, or calcium) in which the mineral is bound to the citrate. The dosage can be based on the appropriate level of elemental mineral. The dosage recommendation is 125 to 250 mg three to four times daily. For example, if calcium citrate is being used as the source of citrate, the dosage would be based on the level of calcium (125 to 250 mg of calcium three to four times daily).

Uva Ursi

Many herbs have been used through the centuries in the treatment of urinary tract infections. The most useful herb in most cases of bladder infection is uva ursi (*Arctostaphylos uva ursi*: bearberry or upland cranberry). Most research has focused on uva ursi's urinary antiseptic component, *arbutin*, which typically comprises seven to nine percent of the leaves. Arbutin is converted to hydroquinone (a related compound with urinary tract antiseptic properties) and glucose in the body (hydroquinone is most effective in an alkaline urine). However, crude plant extracts are more effective medicinally than isolated arbutin.[22] Uva ursi is reported to be especially active against *E. coli* and also has diuretic properties.[23]

The preventive effect of a standardized uva ursi extract on recurrent bladder infections was evaluated in a double-blind study of fifty-seven women.[24] At the end of one year, five of the twenty-seven women in the placebo group had a recurrence, while none of the thirty women receiving uva ursi extract had a recurrence. No side effects were reported in either group. These impressive results indicate that regular use of uva ursi, like cranberry, may prevent bladder infections. In fact, uva ursi appears to be more effective than cranberry.[25]

Care must be taken to avoid excessive dosages of uva ursi; as little as 15 grams ($^1/_2$ ounce) of the dried leaves has been shown to produce side effects (usually nausea) in susceptible individuals. Signs of extreme toxicity include: ringing in the ears, nausea, vomiting, sense of suffocation, and shortness of breath.[22]

Goldenseal

Goldenseal (*Hydrastis canadensis*) is another useful herb in the treatment of bladder infections, due to its antimicrobial properties. Its long history of use by herbalists and naturopathic physicians for the treatment of infections is well documented in the scientific literature. Of particular importance here is its activity against many common bacterial causes of bladder infections, including *E. coli* and *Proteus species*.[26,27] The chief antibiotic substance, *berberine*, works better in an alkaline urine, as does the hydroquinone from uva ursi.

TREATMENT SUMMARY

While the occasional acute bladder infection is easily treated, treating chronic bladder infections requires determining the underlying cause. Structural abnormalities, excessive sugar consumption, food allergies, nutritional deficiencies, chronic vaginitis, local foci of infection (e.g., prostate, kidneys), and current or childhood sexual abuse are all potential causes that must be evaluated and resolved.

General Measures

- Drink large quantities of fluids (at least 2 quarts per day), including at least 16 ounces of unsweetened cranberry or 8 ounces of blueberry juice per day.
- Urinate after intercourse. Women who develop bladder infections after intercourse should wash their labia and urethra with a strong tea of *Hydrastis canadensis* (2 tsp per cup) both before and after. If this is inadequate, a dilute solution of providone-iodine will usually prove effective.

Diet

Avoid all simple sugars, refined carbohydrates, full-strength fruit juice (diluted fruit juice is acceptable), and food allergens.

Nutritional Supplements

- Citrate: dosage can be based on the level of elemental mineral such as potassium, magnesium, or calcium. The dosage recommendation is 125 to 250 mg three to four times daily.
- Vitamin C: 500 mg every two hours
- Bioflavonoids: 1,000 mg per day
- Vitamin A: 50,000 IU per day for up to two days in infants and up to one week in adults, or beta-carotene: 200,000 IU/day

WARNING: Do not use vitamin A in sexually active women of childbearing age without effective birth control due to the link with birth defects at high dosages.

- Zinc: 30 mg per day

Botanical Medicines

Choose one; dosages can be taken three times daily with a large glass of water.

NOTE: Neither uva ursi nor goldenseal is recommended during pregnancy.

- Uva ursi (*Arctostaphylos uva ursi*)
  Dried leaves or as a tea: 1.5–4.0 g (1–2 tsp)
  Freeze-dried leaves: 500–1,000 mg
  Tincture (1:5): 4–6 ml (1–1.5 tsp)
  Fluid extract (1:1): 0.5–2.0 ml ($^1/_4$–$^1/_2$ tsp)

Powdered solid extract (10% arbutin): 250–500 mg

- Goldenseal *(Hydrastis canadensis)*
  Dried root (or as tea): 1–2 g
  Freeze-dried root: 500–1,000 mg
  Tincture (1:5): 4–6 ml (1–1$^{1}/_{2}$ tsp)

Fluid extract (1:1): 0.5–2.0 ml ($^{1}/_{4}$–$^{1}/_{2}$ tsp)

Powdered solid extract (8% alkaloid): 250–500 mg

Boils

. . . .

Painful inflammatory swelling of a hair follicle that forms an abscess; typically appears as a small rounded or conical nodule surrounded by redness, progressing to a localized pus pocket with a white center.

There is tenderness and pain and, if severe, mild fever.

***Staphylococcus aureus* is cultured from the abscess.**

A boil *(furuncle)* is a deep-seated infection *(abscess)* involving the entire hair follicle and adjacent tissue. The most commonly involved sites are the hairy parts of the body that are exposed to friction, pressure, or moisture, such as the neck, armpits, and buttocks. Plugging the hair follicles with petroleum-based products also increases the risk of boil formation. Since the boil can spread, several boils are often found at one location.[1] When several furuncles join together, they are called a *carbuncle*.

There is no particular cause of boils, although occasionally they may indicate an underlying disease that is associated with poor immune function, such as diabetes, AIDS, or cancer. Most lesions will resolve within one to two weeks. Recurrent boils can indicate a highly infective form of bacteria, poor hygiene, industrial exposure to chemicals, or depression of the immune system.

Therapeutic Considerations

Recurrent attacks of boils can also indicate a depressed immune system caused by nutritional deficiencies, food allergies, and/or excessive consumption of sugar and other concentrated refined carbohydrates (see the chapter IMMUNE SUPPORT for further discussion). Zinc and vitamin A are especially important in the treatment of boils.

Goals of Therapy

The therapeutic goals are to address any underlying immune disorder; achieve higher skin levels of vitamin A and zinc; and disinfect the area with the topical application of herbal antiseptics. However, in severe cases consult a physician immediately.

Botanical Medicines

The best herbal treatment for boils is the topical application of tea tree oil. The tea tree *(Melaleuca alternifolia)* is a small tree native to only one area of the world: the northeast coastal region of New South Wales, Australia. Tea tree oil possesses significant antiseptic properties and is regarded by many as the ideal skin disinfectant. This claim is supported by its efficacy against a wide range of organisms and by its good penetration and lack of irritation to the skin.[2] Organisms inhibited by tea tree oil include:

Candida albicans
Propionibacterium acnes
Pseudomonas aeruginosa
Staphylococcus aureus
Streptococcus pyrogenes
Trichomonas vaginalis
Trichophyton mentagrophytes

A clinical trial in patients with boils demonstrated that tea tree oil encouraged more rapid healing without scarring, compared to matched controls.[3] Presumably the positive clinical effects were due to the oil's antibiotic activity against *Staphylococcus aureus*. The method of application included cleaning the site, followed by painting the surface of the boil freely with tea tree oil two or three times a day.

For boils and most skin infections, the most effective treatment appears to be direct application of full-strength, undiluted oil at the site of infection. If irritation occurs, diluted preparations may be tried.

Poultices

Various herbal poultices are commonly used in the treatment of abscesses. Folk healers have used burdock root, castor oil, chervil, licorice root, and others. Poultices, although quite simple, appear to be highly effective. Naturopathic physicians commonly use a poultice made from a paste of goldenseal root powder. Its efficacy is probably due to the properties of *berberine*, the most active alkaloid in goldenseal. Berberine is well-documented as an antimicrobial agent.[4] It is toxic to the bacteria commonly associated with boils, particularly *Staphylococcus aureus*.[5] It has also been found to stimulate immune system function and decrease inflammatory processes.[6,7] An advantage of goldenseal poultices, as compared to hot packs and other types of poultices, is that they usually will not cause the boil to rupture.

QUICK REVIEW

- Recurrent attacks of boils can indicate a depressed immune system.
- Tea tree oil is an effective topical treatment of boils.
- If the boil is severe or does not resolve within two to three days, a physician should be consulted immediately.

TREATMENT SUMMARY

Eliminate from the diet any foods that may suppress immune function (sugar, refined simple carbohydrates, and food allergens). If the boil is severe or does not resolve within two to three days, a physician should be consulted immediately since the infection can spread through the *subcutaneous* (under the skin) tissues (causing *cellulitis*—inflammation of the connective tissue) or into the bloodstream (causing *bacteremia*—bacteria in the blood). Cleanliness should be rigorously maintained.

Nutritional Supplements

- Vitamin C: 500–1,000 mg three times per day
- Vitamin A: 50,000 IU per day for up to two days in infants and up to one week in adults (NOTE: Do not use vitamin A in sexually active women of childbearing age without effective birth control due to the link to birth defects at high dosages.)
- Zinc: 30 mg per day

Botanical Medicines

- Tea tree oil *(Melaleuca alternifolia)*: apply undiluted oil to affected area two to three times daily
- Goldenseal *(Hydrastis canadensis)* poultice: 1 tablespoon of the root powder mixed with water or egg white to form a paste; apply to abscess and cover with an absorbent bandage twice daily.

Other Recommendations

The infected area should be immobilized and not handled, except when necessary to change the poultice. If tea tree oil or goldenseal poultices are not available or if localization, rupture, and drainage are preferred, hot Epsom salts packs will bring an abscess to a head (soak a washcloth in 2 tablespoons of Epsom salts per cup of hot water).

Bronchitis and Pneumonia

. . . .

Usually preceded by upper respiratory tract infection

Sudden onset of shaking, chills, fever, and chest pain

Pneumonia shows classic signs of lung involvement (shallow breathing, cough, abnormal breath sounds, etc.)

In pneumonia, an X ray shows infiltration of fluid and lymph into the lungs

B*ronchitis* refers to an infection or irritation of the bronchi—the passageway from the windpipe (trachea) to the lungs while *pneumonia* refers to infection or irritation of the lungs. Both of these conditions are much more common in the winter, as they usually follow an upper respiratory infection (cold).

Acute pneumonia is the fifth leading cause of death in the United States; it is particularly dangerous in the elderly. Although pneumonia may appear in healthy individuals, it is usually seen in individuals with low immune function, particularly drug and alcohol abusers. The growing population of individuals with chronic lung diseases, caused primarily by smoking, has contributed to a further increase in the number of cases of chronic bronchitis and serious pneumonia, both of which have high mortality rates.

In healthy individuals, pneumonia and bronchitis most often follow an insult to the immune system: viral infection (especially influenza or the common cold), cigarette smoke and other noxious fumes, loss of consciousness (which depresses the gag reflex, allowing the breathing in of fluids [aspiration]), cancer, or hospitalization (due to increased exposure to organisms that can cuase pneumonia).

Therapeutic Considerations

Most cases of bronchitis and/or pneumonia do not require antibiotics because they are due to viral infection (antibiotics are only useful in bacterial causes), yet most physicians prescribe antibiotics for these conditions in an attempt to relieve symptoms and reduce the likelihood of secondary bacterial infection. However, there is little support for this common practice. As an example, let's look at the use of antibiotics to treat acute bronchitis.

Over the past twenty years, there have been several randomized controlled trials designed to assess the benefit of antibiotics in treating acute bronchitis.[1,2] *Acute bronchitis* refers to the acute onset of productive cough in a patient with no history of asthma, no chronic obstructive pulmonary disease, and no evidence of pneumonia. Seven double-blind studies have now shown no clinical benefit from antibiotic treatment of acute bronchitis. Nevertheless, roughly seventy percent of doctors regularly prescribe an antibiotic for acute bronchitis even though it provides no benefit and significant risk. The risks include overgrowth of *Candida albicans,* disruption of normal gut microflora, and the development of antibiotic-resistant strains of bacteria.

Why do physicians prescribe antibiotics for acute bronchitis in light of the scientific facts? There are several misconceptions, according to an editorial in the medical journal *Lancet* titled: What Will It Take to Stop Physicians from Prescribing Antibiotics in Acute Bronchitis?[2] There are no data to support the use of antibiotics when a patient says, "I've had a cough for a week, and now my phlegm has turned green." There are also no data to support the use of antibiotics in response to fever in acute bronchitis or in the hope of preventing progression to pneumonia.

Often doctors prescribe antibiotics for acute bronchitis because many patients believe that only an antibiotic can cure acute bronchitis. This belief is perhaps best exemplified by the fact that sixty percent of eligible patients refused to enter one double-blind study because they felt that antibiotics were absolutely necessary. Given the doctors' and patients' beliefs and expectations, it is little wonder that antibiotics continue to be prescribed for a condition in which they will not alter the course and are never warranted.

The bottom line is that, while antibiotics definitely have their place in the treatment of severe bacterial pneumonia, they offer no benefit in cases of bronchitis or viral pneumonia. Since bacterial pneumonia can be quite serious, it is necessary that any individual with symptoms suggestive of pneumonia consult a physician immediately.

The Natural Approach

The natural approach to bronchitis and pneumonia involves two primary goals:

1. Stimulation of normal processes that promote the *expectoration* (removal) of mucus
2. Enhancement of immune function

. . . .

QUICK REVIEW

- Most cases of bronchitis and/or pneumonia do not require antibiotics.
- The natural approach to bronchitis and pneumonia involves two primary goals: (1) stimulation of normal processes that promote the expectoration (removal) of mucus and (2) enhancement of immune function.
- Vitamin C supplementation is warranted in all elderly patients with acute respiratory infection, especially those who are severely ill.

- The application of local heat followed by postural draining can help get rid of excessive mucus.
- Bromelain (the protein-digesting enzyme complex from pineapple) has shown good results in the treatment of upper respiratory tract infections.
- Botanical expectorants act to increase the quantity, decrease the viscosity, and promote the expulsion of the secretions of the respiratory tract.

In regard to the latter goal, we recommend following the guidelines given in the chapter IMMUNE SUPPORT.

Vitamin C Therapy
Particularly helpful is high-dosage vitamin C therapy. In the early part of this century, before the advent of effective antibiotics, many controlled and uncontrolled studies demonstrated the efficacy of large doses of vitamin C, but only when started on the first or second day of infection. If administered later, vitamin C tended only to lessen the severity of the disease. Researchers also demonstrated that, in cases of pneumonia, white cells took up large amounts of vitamin C in an attempt to have the necessary ammunition they need to fight the infection.[3]

The value of vitamin C supplementation in elderly patients with pneumonia was demonstrated clearly in a more recent double-blind study. This study involved fifty-seven elderly patients who were admitted to St. Luke's Hospital in Huddersfield, England, for severe acute bronchitis or pneumonia.[4] The patients were given either 200 mg of vitamin C per day or a placebo. Patients were assessed by clinical and laboratory methods (vitamin C levels in the plasma, white blood cells, and platelets; sedimentation rates; and white blood cell counts and differential). Patients who received the modest dosage of vitamin C demonstrated substantially increased vitamin C levels in all tissues, even in the presence of an acute respiratory infection.

Using a clinical scoring system based on major symptoms of respiratory infection, results indicated that patients who received the vitamin C fared significantly better than those who took the placebo. The benefit of vitamin C was most obvious in patients with the most severe illness, many of whom had low plasma and white blood cell vitamin C levels on admission.

These results indicate that even relatively small doses of vitamin C in a hospital setting can produce significant clinical improvement. Vitamin C supplementation is warranted in all elderly patients with acute respiratory infection, especially those who are severely ill. Remember, pneumonia is still a major killer of the elderly.

Postural Draining
One of the main treatment goals in cases of bronchitis, sinusitis, and pneumonia is to help the lungs and air passages get rid of excessive mucus. In an effort to assist this process, we recommend applying heat and performing *postural drainage* twice daily, as described in the following paragraph.

Apply a heating pad, hot water bottle, or mustard poultice to the chest for up to twenty minutes. To make a mustard poultice, mix one part of dry mustard with three parts of flour, then add enough water to make a paste. Spread the paste on thin cotton (an old pillowcase works well) or cheesecloth, fold it, and place it on the chest. Check often, as the mustard can cause blisters if left on too long. After the hot pack, perform postural drainage by lying face down with the top half of the body off the bed, using the forearms as support. The position should be maintained for five to fifteen minutes, while you try to cough and expectorate into a basin or newspaper on the floor.

Bromelain
Bromelain is the protein-digesting enzyme complex from pineapple. It has shown good results in the treatment of upper respiratory tract infections. For example, in the treatment of chronic bronchitis, bromelain was shown to have an *antitussive* effect (suppression of cough) and to reduce the viscosity of sputum *(mucolytic activity)*. Examination of patients, using a specialized apparatus for

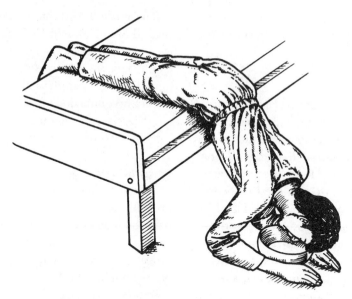

FIGURE 1 Postural Draining

determining respiratory function (a *spirometer*) before and after treatment, indicated increased lung capacity and function. These favorable effects were attributed to enhanced resolution of respiratory congestion, due to bromelain's ability to fluidify and decrease bronchial secretions. It appears that bromelain's mucolytic activity is responsible for its effectiveness in treating respiratory tract diseases.[5]

Acute sinusitis has also responded to bromelain therapy. Good-to-excellent results were obtained in eighty-seven percent of bromelain-treated patients, compared with sixty-eight percent of the placebo group.[6]

Herbal Expectorants

Botanical expectorants have a long history of use in treating bronchitis and pneumonia. Expectorants increase the quantity, decrease the viscosity, and promote the expulsion of the secretions of the mucous membranes that line the respiratory tract. Many botanical expectorants also have antibacterial and antiviral activity. It is important to note that these are not cough suppressants; suppression of coughs is contraindicated in pneumonia. Many commonly used herbal expectorants actually promote the cough reflex.

Commonly used herbal expectorants include lobelia (*Lobelia inflata*), licorice (*Glycyrrhiza glabra*), gumweed (*Grindelia camporum*), wild cherry bark (*Prunus sp.*), horehound (*Marrubium vulgare*), coltsfoot (*Tussilago farfara*), and sundew (*Drosera rotundifolia*). Another herbal expectorant is glycerol guaiacolate (also referred to as *guaifenesin*). In fact, it is probably the most popular and most effective. It is found in many over-the-counter cough formulas.

TREATMENT SUMMARY

The general approach to all infectious bronchial conditions and pneumonias includes stimulation of the immune system and support of respiratory tract drainage (for a full discussion of immune system stimulation see IMMUNE SUPPORT). Drainage is encouraged by the use of postural drainage, local heat, bromelain, and herbal expectorants.

Persistent cough may indicate a serious condition. Consult your physician if your cough persists for more than one week, if it recurs, or if it is accompanied by high fever, rash, or persistent headache.

General Measures

- Rest (bed rest is preferred)
- Drink large amount of fluids (preferably diluted vegetable juices, soups, and herb teas)
- Limit simple sugar consumption (including fruit sugars) to less than 50 grams per day

Nutritional Supplements

In general, those supplements see recommendations in IMMUNE SUPPORT. Especially important are

- Vitamin C: 500 mg every two hours
- Bioflavonoids: 1,000 mg per day
- Vitamin A: 25,000 IU per day
- Beta-carotene: 200,000 IU per day
- Zinc lozenges: One lozenge containing 23 mg elemental zinc every two waking hours for one week

NOTE: Prolonged supplementation at this dose is not recommended, as it may suppress immune function.

Herbal Expectorants

Herbal expectorants are available over the counter, or you can make your own. Follow the dosage on the product label. For glycerol guaiacolate, the dosage is 200 to 400 mg three times per day for adults and 200 mg three times per day for children ages six to twelve.

Here is an expectorant mixture you can make yourself:

> 2 oz licorice root
> 1 oz wild cherry bark
> 1 oz coltsfoot
> 1 oz lobelia
> 1 oz horehound

Mix the ingredients together. Boil the mixture slowly in 4 cups of water for 2 minutes; let it steep for 10 minutes more. Strain the mixture, and take 1 cup every 2 hours if an adult ($1/2$ cup for children). Sweeten with honey if necessary.

Drainage Techniques

Apply local heat, followed by postural drainage, as described in Postural Drainage in this chapter.

Candidiasis, Chronic

Positive demonstration of yeast overgrowth on stool culture

Higher than normal levels of candida antibodies or antigens in the blood

An overgrowth in the gastrointestinal tract of the usually benign yeast (or fungus) *Candida albicans* is now becoming recognized as a complex medical syndrome called *chronic candidiasis,* or the *yeast syndrome.*[1,2] Specifically, the overgrowth of candida is believed to cause a wide variety of symptoms in virtually every system of the body, with the gastrointestinal, genitourinary, endocrine, nervous, and immune systems being the most susceptible.[3]

Although chronic candidiasis has been clinically defined for a long time, it was not until Orion Truss published *The Missing Diagnosis* and William Crook published *The Yeast Connection* that the public and many physicians became aware of the magnitude of the problem.[1,2]

Normally, *Candida albicans* lives harmoniously in the inner warm creases and crevices of the digestive tract and in the vaginal tract in women. However, when this yeast overgrows, or when immune system mechanisms are depleted, or when the normal lining of the intestinal tract is damaged, the body can absorb yeast cells, particles of yeast cells, and various toxins.[3] As a result, there may be significant disruption of body processes resulting in the development of the yeast syndrome.

This syndrome is characterized by patients saying they "feel sick all over." Fatigue, allergies, immune system malfunction, depression, chemical sensitivities, and digestive disturbances are just some of the symptoms patients with the yeast syndrome may experience.[3]

The typical patient with the yeast syndrome is female; women are eight times more likely to experience the yeast syndrome than men, due to the effects of estrogen, birth-control pills, and the higher number of prescriptions for antibiotics.[4]

TYPICAL CHRONIC CANDIDIASIS PATIENT PROFILE

Sex: Female
Age: 15–50
General symptoms:
    Chronic fatigue
    Loss of energy
    General malaise
    Decreased libido

Gastrointestinal symptoms:
    Thrush
    Bloating, gas
    Intestinal cramps
    Rectal itching
    Altered bowel function

Genitourinary system complaints:
    Vaginal yeast infection
    Frequent bladder infections

Endocrine system complaints:
    Primarily menstrual complaints

Nervous system complaints:
    Depression

Irritability
Inability to concentrate

Immune system complaints:
   Allergies
   Chemical sensitivities
   Low immune function

Past history:
   Chronic vaginal yeast infections
   Chronic antibiotic use for infections or acne
   Oral birth control usage
   Oral steroid hormone usage

Associated conditions:
   Premenstrual syndrome
   Sensitivity to foods, chemicals, and other allergens
   Endocrine disturbances
   Eczema
   Psoriasis
   Irritable bowel syndrome

Other:
   Craving for foods rich in carbohydrates or yeast

Causes

Chronic candidiasis is a classic example of a "multifactorial" condition, as indicated by the following list. Therefore, the most effective treatment involves addressing and correcting the factors that predispose an individual to candida overgrowth; there is much more to it than killing the yeast with antifungal agents, whether synthetic or natural.

PREDISPOSING FACTORS TO CANDIDA OVERGROWTH
Altered bowel flora
Decreased digestive secretions
Dietary factors
Drugs (particularly antibiotics)
Impaired immunity
Impaired liver function
Nutrient deficiency
Prolonged antibiotic use
Underlying disease states

Prolonged antibiotic use is believed to be the most important factor in the development of chronic candidiasis. Antibiotics suppress the immune system and the normal intestinal bacteria that prevent yeast overgrowth, strongly promoting the proliferation of candida.

There is little argument that, when used appropriately, antibiotics save lives. However, there is also little argument that antibiotics are seriously overused. While the appropriate use of antibiotics makes good medical sense, using them for such conditions as acne, recurrent bladder infections, chronic ear infections, chronic sinusitis, chronic bronchitis, and nonbacterial sore throats does not. The antibiotics rarely provide benefit, and these conditions can be effectively treated with natural measures.

The widespread use and abuse of antibiotics is becoming increasingly alarming, not only because of the chronic candidiasis epidemic, but also due to the development of "superbugs" that are resistant to currently available antibiotics. According to many experts, as well as the World Health Organization, we are coming dangerously close to arriving at a "postantibiotic era," in which many infectious diseases will once again become almost impossible to treat.[6–8]

Inappropriate use of antibiotics greatly increases the risk of developing complications, such as overgrowth of *Candida albicans* and other organisms, as well as the risk of developing a bacterial infection that is resistant to antibiotics.

In addition, it may be several decades before it is truly known what role the widespread use of antibiotics plays in many health conditions. For example, antibiotic exposure is now being linked to Crohn's disease.[9]

Syndromes Related to the Yeast Syndrome

Eventually, "yeast syndrome" will probably be replaced by a more comprehensive term that includes small intestine bacterial overgrowth and the *leaky gut syndrome*. Both of these conditions are often associated with *Candida albicans* overgrowth and may produce symptoms identical to those of the yeast syndrome.

Diagnosis

One of the most useful screening methods for determining the likelihood of yeast-related illness is a comprehensive questionnaire. Here is the questionnaire that we use (adapted from W. G. Crook, *The Yeast Connection*):[2]

CANDIDA QUESTIONNAIRE

History	Point Score
1. Have you taken tetracycline or other antibiotics for acne for one month or longer?	25
2. Have you at any time in your life taken other "broad-spectrum" antibiotics for respiratory, urinary, or other infections for two months or longer, or in short courses four or more times in a one-year period?	20
3. Have you ever taken a broad-spectrum antibiotic (even a single course)?	6
4. Have you at any time in your life been bothered by persistent prostatitis, vaginitis, or other problems affecting your reproductive organs?	25
5. Have you been pregnant . . .	
One time?	3
Two or more times?	5

- -

QUICK REVIEW

- Prolonged antibiotic use is believed to be the most important factor in the development of chronic candidiasis.
- A physician knowledgeable about yeast-related illness can help in diagnosing, treating, and monitoring chronic candidiasis.
- A comprehensive approach is more effective in treating chronic candidiasis than simply trying to kill the candida with a drug or a natural anticandida agent.
- Recurrent or chronic infections, including chronic candidiasis, are characterized by a depressed immune system.
- Restoring proper immune function is one of the key goals in the treatment of chronic candidiasis.
- The most effective natural anticandida compounds are enteric-coated volatile oil preparations.

6. Have you taken birth-control pills . . .
   For six months to two years?   8
   For more than two years?   15

7. Have you taken prednisone or other cortisone-type drugs . . .
   For two weeks or less?   6
   For more than two weeks?   15

8. Does exposure to perfumes, insecticides, fabric shop odors, and other chemicals provoke . . .
   Mild symptoms?   5
   Moderate to severe symptoms?   20

9. Are your symptoms worse on damp, muggy days or in moldy places?   20

10. Have you had athlete's foot, ringworm, "jock itch," or other chronic infections of the skin or nails?
    Mild to moderate?   10
    Severe or persistent?   20

11. Do you crave sugar?   10

12. Do you crave breads?   10

13. Do you crave alcoholic beverages?   10

14. Does tobacco smoke really bother you?   10

Total Score for This Section   _____

Major Symptoms

For each of your symptoms, enter the appropriate figure in the Point Score column.

If a symptom is occasional or mild	score 3 points
If a symptom is frequent and/or moderately severe	score 6 points
If a symptom is severe and/or disabling	score 9 points

1. Fatigue or lethargy   ___
2. Feeling of being "drained"   ___
3. Poor memory   ___
4. Feeling "spacey" or "unreal"   ___
5. Depression   ___
6. Numbness, burning, or tingling   ___

7. Muscle aches   ___
8. Muscle weakness or paralysis   ___
9. Pain and/or swelling in joints   ___
10. Abdominal pain   ___
11. Constipation   ___
12. Diarrhea   ___
13. Bloating   ___
14. Persistent vaginal itch   ___
15. Persistent vaginal burning   ___
16. Prostatitis   ___
17. Impotence   ___
18. Loss of sexual desire   ___
19. Endometriosis   ___
20. Cramps and/or other menstrual irregularities   ___
21. Premenstrual tension   ___
22. Spots in front of eyes   ___
23. Erratic vision   ___

Total Score for This Section   _____

Other Symptoms

For each of your symptoms, enter the appropriate figure in the Point Score column.

If a symptom is occasional or mild	score 1 point
If a symptom is frequent and/or moderately severe	score 2 points
If a symptom is severe and/or disabling	score 3 points

1. Drowsiness   ___
2. Irritability   ___
3. Lack of coordination   ___
4. Inability to concentrate   ___
5. Frequent mood swings   ___
6. Headache   ___
7. Dizziness/loss of balance   ___

8. Pressure above ears, feeling of head swelling and tingling   ___

9. Itching   ___

10. Other rashes   ___

11. Heartburn   ___

12. Indigestion   ___

13. Belching and intestinal gas   ___

14. Mucus in stools   ___

15. Hemorrhoids   ___

16. Dry mouth   ___

17. Rash or blisters in mouth   ___

18. Bad breath   ___

19. Joint swelling or arthritis   ___

20. Nasal congestion or discharge   ___

21. Postnasal drip   ___

22. Nasal itching   ___

23. Sore or dry throat   ___

24. Cough   ___

25. Pain or tightness in chest   ___

26. Wheezing or shortness of breath   ___

27. Urinary urgency or frequency   ___

28. Burning on urination   ___

29. Failing vision   ___

30. Burning or tearing of eyes   ___

31. Recurrent infections or fluid in ears   ___

32. Ear pain or deafness   ___

Total Score for This Section   ___

Total Score for All Three Sections   ___

Interpretation

	Women	Men
Yeast-connected health problems are almost certainly present	>180	>140
Yeast-connected health problems are probably present	120–180	90–140
Yeast-connected health problems are possibly present	60–119	40–89
Yeast-connected health problems are less likely to be present	<60	<40

Although the candida questionnaire can help, ultimately the best method for diagnosing chronic candidiasis is clinical evaluation by a physician knowledgeable about yeast-related illness. The manner in which the doctor will diagnose the yeast syndrome will probably be based on clinical judgment from a detailed medical history and patient questionnaire. The doctor may also employ laboratory techniques, such as stool cultures for candida, and measurement of antibody levels to candida or candida antigens in the blood.[3,5] However, while these laboratory exams are useful diagnostic aids, they should be used to confirm the diagnosis. In other words, the diagnosis is best made by evaluation of a patient's history and clinical picture.

Therapeutic Considerations

In treating chronic candidiasis, a comprehensive approach is more effective than simply trying to kill the candida with a drug or a natural anticandida agent. Drugs such as nystatin, ketoconazol, and diflucan, as well as various natural anticandida agents, rarely produce significant long-term results because they fail to address the underlying factors that promote candida overgrowth. It is kind of like trying to weed your garden by simply cutting the weeds instead of pulling them out by the roots.

Nonetheless, in many cases it is useful to try to eradicate *Candida albicans* from the system, preferably with the help of natural anticandida therapies such as timed-release caprylic acid preparations, enteric-coated (defined below) volatile oil preparations, or fresh garlic preparations. A follow-up stool culture and candida antigen determination will confirm whether the candida has been eliminated. If it has been eliminated and symptoms are still apparent, it is likely that the symptoms are unrelated to an overgrowth of *Candida albicans*. Similar symptoms to those attributed to chronic candidiasis can be caused by small intestine bacterial overgrowth. In this scenario, pancreatic enzymes and berberine-containing plants such as goldenseal can be helpful.

In addition to using natural agents to eradicate *Candida albicans*, it is important to address predisposing factors, follow a candida-control diet, and support various body systems according to individual needs.

Diet

A number of dietary factors appear to promote the overgrowth of candida. The most important factors are high intakes of sugar, milk and other dairy products, foods with a high content of yeast or mold, and food allergens.

Sugar

Sugar is the chief nutrient for *Candida albicans*. It is well accepted that restriction of sugar intake is an absolute necessity in the treatment of chronic candidiasis. Most people do well by simply avoiding refined sugar and large amounts of honey, maple syrup, and fruit juice.[1–4]

Milk and Dairy Products

There are several reasons to restrict or eliminate the intake of milk in chronic candidiasis:

- Milk's high lactose content promotes the overgrowth of candida

- Milk is one of the most common food allergens
- Milk may contain trace levels of antibiotics, which can further disrupt the gastrointestinal bacterial flora and promote candida overgrowth[1–4]

Mold- and Yeast-Containing Foods

It is generally recommended by many experts that individuals with chronic candidiasis avoid foods with a high content of yeast or mold, including alcoholic beverages, cheeses, dried fruits, and peanuts. Even though many patients with chronic candidiasis may be able to tolerate these foods, it is still a good idea to eliminate them from the diet. At the very least, they should be avoided until the situation is under control.[1–4]

Food Allergens

Food allergies are another common finding in patients with the yeast syndrome.[3] ELISA tests, which determine both IgE- and IgG-mediated food allergies, are often helpful in identifying food allergies. See the chapter FOOD ALLERGY for more information on these tests.

Increasing Digestive Secretions

In many cases, an important step in treating chronic candidiasis is improving digestive secretions. Gastric hydrochloric acid, pancreatic enzymes, and bile all inhibit the overgrowth of candida and prevent its penetration into the absorptive surfaces of the small intestine. Decreased secretion of any of these important digestive components can lead to overgrowth of *Candida albicans* in the gastrointestinal tract. Therefore, restoration of normal digestive secretions through the use of supplemental hydrochloric acid, pancreatic enzymes, and substances that promote bile flow is critical in the treatment of chronic candidiasis.

Patients on anti-ulcer drugs such as Tagamet (cimetidine) and Zantac (ranitidine) actually develop candida overgrowth in the stomach.[10] This occurrence highlights the importance of hydrochloric acid in the prevention of candida overgrowth. Restoring proper levels of gastric acid by supplemental hydrochloric acid is often quite useful in chronic candidiasis.

Pancreatic enzymes can also be useful in the treatment of chronic candidiasis. As well as being necessary for protein digestion, the *proteases* (enzymes that break down protein) serve several other important functions. The proteases are largely responsible for keeping the small intestine free from parasites (including bacteria, yeast, protozoa, and intestinal worms).[11,12] A lack of proteases or other digestive secretions greatly increases an individual's risk of having an intestinal infection, including chronic candida infections of the gastrointestinal tract.

Please read the chapter DIGESTION to identify which of these digestive factors is most important in your particular case.

Enhancing Immunity

Recurrent or chronic infections, including chronic candidiasis, are characterized by a depressed immune system. A repetitive cycle makes it difficult to overcome chronic candidiasis: a compromised immune system leads to infection, and infection leads to damage to the immune system, further weakening resistance.

The importance of a healthy immune function to protect against candida overgrowth is well known by any physician who has seen a patient suffering from AIDS or taking drugs that suppress the immune system. In either case, severe overgrowth of *Candida albicans* is a hallmark feature. The occurrence of candida overgrowth in these conditions provides

considerable evidence that attaining better immune function is essential for the patient with chronic candidiasis.

In addition, patients with chronic candidiasis often suffer from other chronic infections, presumably due to a depressed immune system. Typically, this depression of immune function is related to decreased thymus function, which manifests as depressed cell-mediated immunity. Although expensive laboratory tests can document this depression, it is better to rely on the history of repeated viral infections (including the common cold), outbreaks of cold sores or genital herpes, and prostatic (men) or vaginal (women) infections.

Causes of Depressed Immune Function in Candidiasis

The patient with chronic candidiasis is typically stuck in a vicious cycle. In regard to the immune system, a triggering event such as antibiotic use or nutrient deficiency can lead to immune suppression, allowing *Candida albicans* to overgrow and become more firmly entrenched in the lining of the gastrointestinal tract. Once the organism attaches itself to the intestinal cells, it competes with the cell and ultimately the entire body for nutrition, potentially robbing the body of vital nutrients.

In addition, *Candida albicans* secretes a large number of toxins and antigens (compounds that the body recognizes as foreign and develops antibodies to).[13,14] *Candida albicans* is referred to as a "polyantigenic" organism because over seventy-nine distinct antigens have been identified. As a result of this tremendous number of antigens, an overgrowth of *Candida albicans* greatly taxes the immune system. The immune system is directing many of its resources to *Candida albicans*.

TRIGGERS THAT IMPAIR IMMUNITY TO CANDIDIASIS

Antibiotic use
Corticosteroid use
Food allergies
High-sugar diet
Nutrient deficiency
Other drugs that suppress the immune system
Stress

Goals of Therapy

Restoring proper immune function is one of the key goals in the treatment of chronic candidiasis. There isn't any single magic bullet that can immediately restore immune function in patients with chronic candidiasis. Instead, a comprehensive approach involving lifestyle, stress management, exercise, diet, nutritional supplementation, glandular therapy, and plant-based medicines is used.

Perhaps the most effective intervention in reestablishing a healthy immune system is employing measures designed to improve thymus function. Promoting optimal thymus gland activity involves

- Prevention of thymic involution or shrinkage by ensuring adequate dietary intake of antioxidant nutrients such as carotenes, vitamin C, vitamin E, zinc, and selenium
- Use of nutrients that are required in the manufacture or action of thymic hormones
- Use of products that contain concentrates of calf thymus tissue

The promotion of optimal thymus gland function is discussed fully in the chapter IMMUNE FUNCTION. A good high-quality multiple-vitamin-and-mineral formula and extra vitamin C and vitamin E are the most important recommendations. When thymus function is very depressed, orally administered calf thymus extracts can be quite helpful in restoring and enhancing immune function.[15,16] The effectiveness of thymus extract is reflective of broad-spectrum immune system enhancement, presumably the result of improved thymus gland activity.

The dosage will vary from one manufacturer to another, as there are no quality control procedures or standards enforced in the glandular industry. It is left up to the individual company to adopt quality control and good manufacturing procedures.

From a practical view, products concentrated and standardized for polypeptide content are preferable to crude preparations. Based on current clinical research, the daily dose should be equivalent to 120 mg of pure polypeptides with molecular weights less than 10,000, or roughly 750 mg of the crude polypeptide fraction. No side effects or adverse effects have been reported with the use of thymus preparations.

Promoting Detoxification

Candida patients usually exhibit multiple chemical sensitivities and allergies, an indicator that detoxification reactions are stressed. Therefore, the liver function of the candida patient needs to be supported. In fact, improving the health of the liver and promoting detoxification may be one of the most critical factors in the successful treatment of candidiasis.

Damage to the liver is often an underlying factor in chronic candidiasis as well as chronic fatigue. When the liver is even slightly damaged by a toxic chemical, immune function is severely compromised.

The immune-system-suppressing effect of liver damage has been repeatedly demonstrated in experimental animal studies and human studies. For example, when the liver of a rat is damaged by a toxic chemical, immune function is severely hindered.[17] Liver injury is also linked to candida overgrowth, as evident in studies of mice demonstrating that when the liver is even slightly damaged, candida runs rampant through the body.[18]

INDICATIONS OF THE NEED FOR DETOXIFICATION

More than twenty pounds overweight

Diabetes

Gallstones

History of heavy alcohol use

Psoriasis

Natural and synthetic steroid hormone use

    Anabolic steroids

    Estrogens

    Oral contraceptives

High exposure to certain chemicals or drugs

    Cleaning solvents

    Pesticides

    Antibiotics

    Diuretics

    Nonsteroidal anti-inflammatory drugs

    Thyroid hormone

History of viral hepatitis

A rational approach to aiding the body's detoxification involves

- A diet based on fresh fruits and vegetables, whole grains, legumes, nuts, and seeds
- A healthy lifestyle, including regular exercise and avoidance of alcohol
- A high-potency multiple-vitamin-and-mineral supplement

- Lipotropic formulas and silymarin (see explanation following) to protect the liver and enhance liver function
- A three-day fast at the change of each season

If any of the following factors are present, enhancing detoxification is a major therapeutic goal.

Lipotropic Factors

The nutrients choline, betaine, and methionine are often beneficial in enhancing liver function and detoxification reactions. These nutrients are referred to as *lipotropic agents*—compounds that promote the flow of fat and bile to and from the liver. In essence, they produce a "decongesting" effect on the liver and promote improved liver function and fat metabolism.

Formulas containing lipotropic agents are very useful in enhancing detoxification reactions and other liver functions. Lipotropic formulas have been used by nutrition-oriented physicians for a wide variety of conditions, including a number of liver disorders (hepatitis, cirrhosis, and chemical-induced liver disease). The dosage should provide 1,000 mg of choline and 1,000 mg of either methionine and/or cysteine daily.

Lipotropic formulas appear to increase the levels of two important liver substances: SAM (S-adenosylmethionine), the major lipotropic compound in the liver, and glutathione, one of the major detoxifying compounds in the liver.[19,20]

Silymarin

There is a long list of plants that exert beneficial effects on liver function. However, the most impressive research has been done on a special extract of milk thistle (*Silybum marianum*) known as *silymarin*. Silymarin refers to a group of flavonoid (plant pigments with impressive antioxidant effects) compounds.

These compounds protect the liver from damage and enhance its detoxification processes. Silymarin has shown impressive results in improving liver function and detoxification processes in double-blind studies.[21-23] The standard dosage for silymarin is 70 to 210 mg three times daily.

Promoting Elimination

In addition to directly supporting liver function, proper detoxification involves promoting proper elimination. A diet that focuses on high-fiber plant foods should be sufficient to promote proper elimination by supplying an ample amount of dietary fiber. If additional support is needed, fiber formulas can be taken. These formulas are composed of natural plant fibers derived from psyllium seed, kelp, agar, pectin, and plant gums such as karaya and guar. Alternatively, the formulas may contain purified semisynthetic polysaccharides such as methyl-cellulose and carboxymethyl cellulose sodium. Psyllium-containing laxatives are the most popular and usually the most effective. Fiber formulas are the laxatives that approximate most closely the natural mechanism that promotes a bowel movement. In the treatment of candidiasis, 3 to 5 grams of soluble fiber are recommended at bedtime, especially if antiyeast therapies are employed, to ensure that dead yeast cells are excreted and not absorbed.

Probiotics

Intestinal flora play a major role in a person's health and nutritional status.[24,25] The intestinal flora affect immune system function, cholesterol metabolism, carcinogenesis, and aging. Due to the importance of *Lactobacillus acidophilus* and *Bactobacillus bifidum* (see the chapter DIGESTION AND ELIMINATION for a complete discussion) to human health, supplements containing these organisms can be used to promote overall good health.

There are several specific uses for probiotics, however. The four primary areas of use related to chronic candidiasis are

- Promotion of proper intestinal environment
- Postantibiotic therapy
- Vaginal yeast infections
- Urinary tract infections

The dosage of a commercial probiotic supplement is based upon the number of live organisms it contains. The ingestion of one to ten billion viable *L. acidophilus* or *B. bifidum* cells daily is a sufficient dosage for most people. Amounts exceeding this may induce mild gastrointestinal disturbances, while smaller amounts may not be able to colonize the gastrointestinal tract.

Natural Antiyeast Compounds

There are a number of natural agents with proven activity against *Candida albicans*. Rather than relying on these agents as a primary therapy, however, it is still important to address the factors that predispose a person to chronic candidiasis, especially a lack of either hydrochloric acid or pancreatic enzymes.

The four natural agents recommended to treat *Candida albicans* are

- Caprylic acid
- Berberine-containing plants
- Garlic
- Enteric-coated volatile oil preparations

Most patients (but not all) can achieve benefits from the natural agents described here rather than the drug approach. Use of any effective antiyeast therapy alone will probably result in the *Herxheimer* ("die-off") reaction due to the rapid killing of the organism and subsequent absorption of large quantities of yeast toxins, cell particles, and antigens. The Herxheimer reaction refers to a worsening of symptoms as a result of this die-off. This reaction can be minimized by

- Following the dietary recommendations for a minimum of two weeks before taking an antiyeast agent
- Supporting the liver by following the recommendations given previously
- Starting any of the above-described antiyeast medications in low doses and gradually increasing dosage over one month to achieve full therapeutic dosage

Caprylic Acid

Caprylic acid, a naturally occurring fatty acid, has been reported to be an effective antifungal compound in the treatment of candidiasis.[26,27] Since caprylic acid is readily absorbed in the intestines, it is necessary to take timed-release or enteric-coated caprylic acid formulas to allow for gradual release throughout the entire intestinal tract.[28] The standard dosage for these delayed-release preparations is 1,000 to 2,000 mg with meals.

Berberine-Containing Plants

Berberine-containing plants include goldenseal (*Hydrastis canadensis*), barberry (*Berberis vulgaris*), Oregon grape (*Berberis aquifolium*), and goldthread (*Coptis chinensis*). Berberine, an alkaloid, has been extensively studied in both experimental and clinical settings for its antibiotic activity. Berberine exhibits a broad spectrum of antibiotic activity, including activity against bacteria, protozoa, and fungi, particularly *Candida albicans*.[30–35] Berberine's action in inhibiting both *Candida* and disease-causing bacteria prevents the overgrowth of yeast that is a common side effect of antibiotic use.

Diarrhea is a common symptom in patients with chronic candidiasis. Berberine has shown remarkable antidiarrheal activity in even the most severe cases. Positive clinical results have been shown with berberine in relieving diarrhea in cases of cholera, amebiasis, giardiasis, and other causes of acute gastrointestinal infection (e.g., *E. coli*, shigella, salmonella, and klebsiella) and may also relieve the diarrhea seen in patients with chronic candidiasis.[36–44]

The dosage of any berberine-containing plant should be based on berberine content. As there is a wide range of quality in preparations, standardized extracts are preferred. Three times a day, dosages as follows:

Dried root or as infusion (tea): 2–4 grams
Tincture (1:5): 6–12 ml (1½–3 tsp)
Fluid extract (1:1): 2–4 ml (½–1 tsp)
Solid (powdered dry) extract (4:1 or 8–12% alkaloid content): 250–500 mg

Berberine and berberine-containing plants are generally nontoxic at the recommended dosages; however, berberine-containing plants are not recommended for use during pregnancy, and higher dosages may interfere with B-vitamin metabolism.[45]

Garlic

Garlic (*Allium sativum*) has demonstrated significant antifungal activity. In fact, its inhibition of *Candida albicans* in both animal and test tube (*in vitro*) studies has shown it to be more potent than nystatin, gentian violet, and six other reputed antifungal agents.[46–48] The active component is *allicin*— the pungent and odorous principle of garlic.

The modern clinical use of garlic involves commercial preparations designed to offer the benefits of garlic without the odor. These preparations are made in such a way that the allicin is not formed until the enteric-coated tablet is delivered to the small and large intestine.

Treatment of chronic candidiasis requires a daily dose of at least 10 mg of allicin or a total allicin potential of 4,000 mcg. This amount is equal to approximately one clove (4 grams) of fresh garlic. Going beyond this dosage with these preparations usually results in the odor of garlic being detectable.

Enteric-Coated Volatile Oils

The most recent "new wave" natural anticandida formulas are enteric-coated volatile oil preparations. Volatile oils from oregano, thyme, peppermint, and rosemary are all ef-fective antifungal agents. A recent study compared the anticandida effect of oregano oil to that of caprylic acid.[49] The results indicated that oregano oil is over 100 times more potent than caprylic acid against candida. Since the volatile oils are quickly absorbed and associated with inducing heartburn, enteric-coating is recommended to ensure delivery to the small and large intestine.

An effective dosage for an enteric-coated volatile oil preparation is 0.2 to 0.4 ml twice daily between meals.

TREATMENT SUMMARY

Following is a comprehensive step-by-step approach to the successful elimination of chronic candidiasis.

Step 1: Identify and Address Predisposing Factors

- Eliminate the use of antibiotics, steroids, immune-suppressing drugs, and birth control pills (unless there is absolute medical necessity)
- Identify any lack of digestive secretions
- Follow the specific recommendations if the identifiable predisposing factor is dietary factors, impaired immunity, impaired liver function, or an underlying disease state

Step 2: Follow the Candida-Control Diet

- Eliminate refined and simple sugars
- Eliminate milk and other dairy products
- Eliminate foods with a high content of yeast or mold, including alcoholic beverages, cheeses, dried fruits, melons, and peanuts
- Eliminate all known or suspected food allergens

Step 3: Provide Nutritional Support

- Take a high-potency multiple-vitamin-and-mineral formula
- Take additional antioxidants
- Take 1 tablespoon of flaxseed oil daily

Step 4: Support Immune Function

- Promote a positive mental attitude
- Deal with stress by using positive coping techniques (see the chapter STRESS MANAGEMENT)
- Avoid alcohol, sugar, smoking, and elevated cholesterol levels, which can impair immune function
- Get plenty of rest and good sleep
- Support thymus gland function (take thymus extract: 750 mg of crude polypeptide fractions daily)

Step 5: Promote Detoxification and Elimination

- Take 3–5 grams of water-soluble fiber, such as guar gum, psyllium seed, or pectin, at night
- If necessary, take lipotropic factors and silymarin to enhance liver function

Step 6: Take Probiotics

- Dosage: 1–10 billion viable *Lactobacillus acidophilus* and *Bactobacillus bifidum* cells per day

Step 7: Use Appropriate Antiyeast Therapy

- Ideally, use the recommended nutritional and/or herbal supplements to help control against yeast overgrowth and promote a healthy bacterial flora
- If necessary, use a prescription antiyeast drug appropriately

These simple steps should take care of chronic candidiasis in most cases. If you follow these guidelines and don't have significant improvement or complete resolution, further evaluation is necessary to determine if chronic candidiasis is the underlying factor. Repeat stool cultures and antigen level tests are often helpful in this goal. If the organism has not been eradicated, stronger prescription antibiotics can be used along with the other general recommendations.

Canker Sores

. . . .

Single or clustered shallow, painful ulcers found anywhere in the oral cavity

Ulcerations usually resolve in seven to twenty-one days but are recurrent in many people

Recurrent canker sores (*aphthous stomatitis* is the medical term) are a common condition estimated to affect about twenty percent of the U.S. population. Although not a serious medical condition, recurrent canker sores are quite bothersome.

Therapeutic Considerations

Based on studies of initiating factors, recurrent canker sores appear to be related to food sensitivities (especially milk and gluten sensitivity), stress, and/or nutrient deficiency.

Food and Environmental Allergens

The mouth is, obviously, the first site of contact for ingested—and many inhaled—allergens. The association of recurrent canker sores with increased antibodies to food antigens strongly suggests that an allergic reaction is involved.[1] Furthermore, the appearance of the lesions under a microscope and elevated levels of allergic white blood cells and antibodies confirm the association.[2] It has been clearly demonstrated that allergic mechanisms are responsible for producing canker sores in many cases.[3] An elimination diet (see FOOD ALLERGY) has been shown to have good therapeutic results.[4]

The allergen doesn't have to be a food. Allergens that commonly induce canker sores include preservatives such as benzoic acid, methylparaben, dichromate, and sorbic acid.[5] Elimination of allergens usually brings complete resolution or significant improvement in people with recurrent canker sores. Follow the guidelines in the FOOD ALLERGY section of Part III.

Gluten Sensitivity

There is considerable evidence that sensitivity to *gluten* (a protein found in grains) is the primary cause of recurrent canker sores in many cases. The frequency of recurrent canker sores is increased in patients with celiac disease, a condition characterized by diarrhea and malabsorption due to a sensitivity to gluten (see CELIAC DISEASE).[6–9]

Biopsy of the small intestine of thirty-three patients with recurrent canker sores showed eight to have the type of changes (villous atrophy) typical of celiac disease along with signs of food allergy.[6] The remaining patients also exhibited these types of signs, but to a lesser degree.

If a patient with recurrent canker sores has food allergies or a sensitivity to gluten, it increases the likelihood of having a vitamin or mineral deficiency. Withdrawing gluten from the diet results in complete remission of recurrent canker sores in patients with celiac disease and some improvement in the rest of the patients.[6–10]

The best method of diagnosing sensitivity to gluten is to measure the level of antibodies against gluten in the blood. This test is called the *alpha-1-gliadin antibody assay*. This test is strongly recommended for a person who has recurrent canker sores.

Stress

Stress is often a precipitating factor in recurrent aphthous stomatitis, suggesting a breakdown in normal immune function and/or integrity of the mucosal lining.[11]

Nutrient Deficiency

The lining of the mouth and throat is often the first place where nutritional deficiency becomes visible because of the high turnover rate of the cells that line the surface. Although a number of nutrient deficiencies can lead to canker sores, thiamine deficiency appears to be the most significant. In one study seeking to examine whether thiamine deficiency is associated with recurrent canker sores, the levels of *transketolase* (a thiamine-dependent enzyme) were determined in seventy patients with recurrent canker sores and fifty patients from a control group.[12] Low levels of transketolase were found in forty-nine of the seventy patients with recurrent aphthous stomatitis, compared to only two among the fifty people in the control group. These results clearly demonstrate an associa-

tion between low thiamine levels and recurrent aphthous stomatitis.

There are several other studies that show nutrient deficiencies to be much more common among recurrent canker sore sufferers than in the general population. For example, a study of 330 patients with recurrent canker sores showed that forty-seven (14.2 percent) were deficient in iron, folate, vitamin B12, or a combination of these nutrients.[13] In another study of sixty patients, 28.2 percent were deficient in either thiamine, riboflavin, or pyridoxine.[14] When these patients' deficiencies were corrected, the majority had complete remission. Other studies have shown similar deficiency rates for the same nutrients and equally good response to supplementation.[15]

Quercetin

The bioflavonoid *quercetin* is known to inhibit mast cells from releasing inflammatory compounds and causing symptoms of allergy.[16] The anti-allergy drug *disodium cromoglycate*—a compound very similar in structure and function to quercetin—has been shown to be effective in the treatment of recurrent canker sores, resulting in an increase in the number of ulcer-free days and

QUICK REVIEW

- Recurrent canker sores can be caused by trauma, food sensitivities (especially milk and gluten sensitivities), stress, and/or nutrient deficiency.

- Eliminating food allergens, sources of gluten, and nutritional deficiencies results in complete cure in most cases.

in mild symptomatic relief.[17] Quercetin may demonstrate similar benefits.

Deglycyrrhizinated Licorice (DGL)

A special licorice extract known as DGL may be effective in promoting healing of recurrent canker sores. In one study, twenty patients were instructed to use a solution of DGL as a mouthwash (200 mg powdered DGL dissolved in 200 ml warm water) four times daily.[18] Fifteen of the twenty (seventy-five percent) experienced fifty- to seventy-five-percent improvement within one day, followed by complete healing of the ulcers by the third day. DGL in tablet form may produce even better results.

TREATMENT SUMMARY

The data presented suggest that numerous factors can lead to recurrent canker sores. Considerable evidence suggests that the underlying problem may be a gluten sensitivity and/or food allergy. In addition, nutrient deficiencies need to be corrected. DGL can be used to help heal the ulcers.

Diet

The diet should be free of known allergens and all gluten sources (i.e., grains).

Nutritional Supplements

- Vitamin C: 1,000 mg per day
- High-potency multiple-vitamin-and-mineral supplement, according to guidelines given in the chapter SUPPLEMENTARY MEASURES.
- DGL: One to two 380-mg chewable tablets twenty minutes before meals.

Carpal Tunnel Syndrome

· ·

Numbness, tingling, and/or burning pain in the first three fingers of the hand, particularly at night

Appearance or worsening of symptoms caused by flexing of the wrist for sixty seconds and relieved by extending the wrist

Carpal tunnel syndrome (CTS) is a common, painful disorder caused by compression of the nerve that passes between the bones and ligaments of the wrist. Compression of this nerve—the *median* nerve—causes weakness, pain when gripping, and burning, tingling, or aching that may radiate to the forearm and shoulder. Symptoms may be occasional or constant and usually occur most at night. Carpal tunnel syndrome is found most commonly in people who perform repetitive, strenuous work with their hands (e.g., carpenters), but may also occur in people who do light work (e.g., typists and keyboard operators). It may also follow injuries of the wrist. More frequently, however, there is no history of significant trauma.

CTS is more prevalent among women and occurs frequently between the ages of forty and sixty years. It occurs most often in pregnant women, women taking oral contraceptives, menopausal women, or patients on hemodialysis due to kidney failure. These patients tend to have a greater need for vitamin B6.

Therapeutic Considerations

Vitamin B6 (pyridoxine) supplementation appears to be quite helpful in many cases.[1-9]

John Ellis, M.D., Karl Folkers, Ph.D., and their coworkers at the University of Texas have conducted double-blind studies and have successfully treated hundreds of patients suffering from carpal tunnel syndrome with vitamin B6.[7-9] It may take as long as three months to produce a benefit, but vitamin B6 is effective in many cases.

The increased frequency of CTS since its initial description by George Phalen, M.D., in 1950 parallels the increased presence of compounds that interfere with vitamin B6 in the body. Particularly incriminating is tartrazine (FD&C yellow dye #5). A high protein intake can also lead to a relative shortage of B6. Dr. Phalen agrees that pyridoxine (in doses of 100 to 200 mg/day) may become the treatment of choice.[10]

The effectiveness of vitamin B6 may be enhanced by taking it along with other B-vitamins, especially vitamin B2. In one study, vitamin B2 was shown to be useful in the treatment of CTS; an even greater effect was seen when it was combined with vitamin B6.[7] Vitamin B2 functions in converting vitamin B6 into its more active form, pyridoxal 5'-phosphate.

Vitamin B6 can help even when there is no apparent vitamin B6 deficiency. A recent study led to much confusion about the role of vitamin B6 in CTS. In an attempt to determine whether there is a relationship between vitamin B6 status and symptoms of carpal tunnel syndrome, researchers randomly selected 125 employees at an auto parts plant and measured their vitamin B6 levels, assessed median nerve function in their wrists and hands, and noted any CTS symptoms.[11] About one-third of the employees reported CTS, one-fourth had median nerve dysfunction, and less than one-tenth had vitamin B6 deficiency. After statistical analysis, researchers found no correlation between employees' blood levels of vitamin B6 and the presence of or improvement in CTS symptoms.

Despite the lack of clinical evaluation, the authors of the study concluded that "empiric treatment for CTS with vitamin B6 supplementation is not warranted." The study did not analyze the effectiveness of vitamin B6 therapy, yet several reports in the popular press and *JAMA* (the *Journal of the American Medical Association*) advised people to "forget the vitamin B6" in the treatment of CTS. However, vitamin B6 therapy may prove to be effective in some cases of CTS regardless of the patients' vitamin B6 status. Given its safety and the positive clinical studies with vitamin B6 in reasonable doses (25 to 50 mg three times daily), treatment with vitamin B6 should still be considered, especially before opting for surgery.

Alternating Hot and Cold Water Treatment

Inflammation and swelling are present in many cases of CTS.[11] Alternating hot and cold water treatment (contrast hydrotherapy) provides a simple, efficient way to increase circulation to the area and reduce swelling. Immersion in hot water for three minutes, followed by immersion in cold water for thirty seconds, repeated three to five times, will increase local circulation, thereby increasing local nutrition, eliminating waste, and decreasing pain.

Acupuncture

Acupuncture may be helpful. In a study of the acupuncture treatment of CTS, a positive response was demonstrated in thirty-five of thirty-six patients, fourteen of whom were previously treated unsuccessfully with surgery.[12]

Stretching

Researchers have suggested that stretching exercises might reduce the need for surgery by fifty percent.[13] Stretching exercise involves flexing the wrists and fists, with the arms extended, for five minutes. This sustained movement helps prepare the carpal

. . . .

QUICK REVIEW

- Vitamin B6 supplementation appears to be quite helpful in many cases.
- Alternating hot and cold water treatment ("contrast hydrotherapy") provides a simple, efficient way to increase circulation to the area and reduce swelling.

- Additional natural measures that may be helpful include acupuncture, bromelain, and physical therapy.

tunnel nerve for repetitive actions. This exercise should be done before work starts and during every break.

Bromelain

When the carpal tunnel syndrome is due to injury or inflammation, *bromelain* (an enzyme found in pineapple) may be of benefit. Bromelain has well-documented effects in virtually all inflammatory conditions, regardless of cause. The effect of orally administered bromelain on the reduction of swelling, bruising, healing time, and pain following various injuries and surgical procedures has been demonstrated in several clinical studies.[14,15]

If surgery is absolutely necessary, bromelain should definitely be employed. In studies of patients undergoing oral surgery it was concluded that, while postsurgical medication alone is effective, a regimen of pre- and postsurgical medication with bromelain is recommended.[15–17] Start taking the bromelain three days prior to surgery and for at least two weeks after surgery for maximum benefit.

TREATMENT SUMMARY

Whenever possible, prevention is obviously best. Avoid activities that cause trauma to the median nerve through repeated flexing and extending of the wrist.

Diet

Avoid foods containing yellow dyes, and limit daily protein intake to a maximum of 1.65 g/lb of body weight.

Nutritional Supplements

- Pyridoxine: 25 mg three to four times per day
- Riboflavin: 10 mg daily

Botanical Medicine

Bromelain (1,200–1,800 mcu/gdu [milk-clotting units or gelatin-digesting units]): 250–750 mg twice daily between meals

Physical Medicine

- Hot and cold therapy: immersion for three minutes in hot water followed by a thirty-second immersion in cold water. Repeat this three to five times; perform daily.
- Regular wrist exercises

Cataracts

. . . .

Clouding or opacity in the crystalline lens of the eye

Gradual loss of vision

Cataracts are white, opaque blemishes on the normally transparent lens of the eye. They occur as a result of damage to the protein structure of the lens, similar to the damage that occurs to the protein of eggs when they are boiled or fried. Cataracts are the leading cause of impaired vision and blindness in the United States. Approximately four million people have some degree of vision-impairing cataract, and at least forty thousand people in the United States are blind due to cataracts.

Cataracts create a tremendous financial burden on our society. Among U.S. Medicare recipients, cataract surgery is the most common major surgical procedure, costing $600,000 each year.

Cataracts can be classified by location and appearance of the lens opacities, by cause or significant contributing factor, and by age of onset. Many factors may cause or contribute to the progression of lens opacity, including: ocular disease, injury, or surgery; systemic diseases (e.g., diabetes mellitus, galactosemia); exposure to toxics, radiation, or ultraviolet and near-ultraviolet light; and hereditary disease. Aging-related (or "senile") cataracts are discussed in this chapter, and diabetic and galactose-induced cataracts (*sugar cataracts*) are discussed in the DIABETES section.

The lens of the eye is, obviously, a vital component of the visual system due to its ability to focus light (via changes in shape) while maintaining transparency. Unfortunately, this transparency decreases with age.

The majority of people over sixty years of age display some degree of cataract formation. With normal aging there is a progressive increase in size, weight, and density of the lens, but although cataracts are common they should not be considered normal.

Therapeutic Considerations

In cataract formation, the normal protective mechanisms are unable to prevent free-radical damage. The lens, like many other tissues of the body, is dependent on adequate levels and activities of the antioxidant enzymes superoxide dismutase (SOD), catalase, and glutathione (GSH) and adequate levels of the accessory antioxidants vitamins E and C and selenium to aid in preventing free-radical damage. Individuals with higher dietary intakes of vitamins C and E, selenium, and carotenes have a much lower risk of developing cataracts.[1] These compounds are discussed individually below.

Can nutritional or herbal supplements reverse cataracts? In advanced cases, probably not. But in the early stages there are several possibilities.

Vitamin C

Several clinical studies have demonstrated that vitamin C supplementation can halt cataract progression and, in some cases, significantly improve vision. For example, in one study conducted in 1939, 450 patients with cataracts were placed on a nutritional program that included 1 gram of vitamin C per day, which resulted in a significant reduction in cataract development.[2] Though similar patients had previously required surgery within four years, among the vitamin-C-treated patients only a small number required surgery. During the eleven-year period of the study, most of the vitamin-C-treated patients showed no evidence that the cataract progressed.

In another study, 450 patients with incipient cataract where placed on a nutritional program that included 1 gram of vitamin C per day, which resulted in a significant reduction in cataract development.[3]

It appears that the dosage of vitamin C necessary to increase the vitamin C content of the lens is equal to or greater than 1,000 mg.[4] The active tissue of the body and the lens of the eye require higher concentrations of vitamin C. The level of vitamin C in the blood is about 0.5 mg/dl, while in the lens of the eye vitamin C is concentrated by at least a factor of twenty. In order for this concentra-tion to be maintained in these tissues, the body has to generate enormous amounts of energy to pull vitamin C out of the blood against this tremendous gradient. By keeping blood vitamin C levels elevated, you are helping the body to concentrate vitamin C into active tissue by reducing the gradient. That is probably why dosages of at least 1,000 mg are required to increase the vitamin C content of the lens.

Glutathione

Glutathione is a small protein (*peptide*) composed of the three amino acids *glycine, glutamic acid,* and *cysteine.* Glutathione is found at high concentrations in the lens and plays a vital role in maintaining a healthy lens and preventing cataract formation.[5] Glutathione levels are diminished in virtually all forms of cataracts. Glutathione works very closely with vitamin C.

Selenium and Vitamin E

These antioxidants are known to function synergistically and are therefore discussed together. Maintaining proper selenium levels

QUICK REVIEW

- In cataract formation, the normal protective mechanisms are unable to prevent free-radical damage.
- Individuals with higher dietary intakes of antioxidants have a much lower risk for developing cataracts.
- Several clinical studies have demonstrated that vitamin C supplementa-tion can halt cataract progression and, in some cases, significantly improve vision.
- Bilberry extract plus vitamin E stopped progression of cataract formation in forty-eight of fifty patients.
- An ancient Chinese formula, *Hachimijiogan,* has been shown to increase the antioxidant level of the lens of the eye.

appears to be especially important, as the antioxidant enzyme glutathione peroxidase requires selenium in order to neutralize free radicals. Low selenium levels would greatly promote cataract formation. Early studies have shown that the selenium content in a human lens with a cataract is only fifteen percent of normal levels.[6] A more recent study was conducted to better examine the role of selenium in cataract formation.[7]

Selenium levels in the serum, lens, and fluid (*aqueous humor*) of the eye were determined in forty-eight patients with cataracts and compared to matched controls. The selenium levels of the serum and aqueous humor were found to be significantly less in the patients with cataracts (serum: 0.28 vs. 0.32 mcg/ml; aqueous humor: 0.19 vs. 0.31 mcg/ml). However, the selenium levels in the lens itself did not significantly differ between patients with cataracts and normal controls.

The most important finding of the study was the decreased level of selenium in the aqueous humor of patients with cataracts. Among cataract patients, hydrogen peroxide levels in the aqueous humor are found to be up to twenty-five times the normal levels. An excess of hydrogen peroxide is associated with increased free-radical damage and damage to the lens. As a result, a cataract is formed. Since selenium-dependent glutathione peroxidase is responsible for the breakdown of hydrogen peroxide, low selenium levels appear to be a major factor in the development of a cataract.

Superoxide Dismutase

The activity of the antioxidant enzyme superoxide dismutase (SOD) in the human lens is lower than it is in other tissues. Presumably this lower level is because of the increased vitamin C and glutathione levels in the lens. However, as a cataract progresses SOD levels decrease even further. Taking oral forms of SOD is probably of little value, as it has been demonstrated that they do not affect tissue SOD activity.[8] Of greater value is supplementation with the trace mineral components of SOD, such as zinc, copper, and manganese. Levels of these cofactors (necessary components) are greatly reduced in lenses with cataracts; copper and zinc levels are reduced by over ninety percent, and manganese by fifty percent.[9]

Tetrahydrobiopterin

Tetrahydrobiopterin is believed to play a protective role against cataract formation via prevention of damage caused by ultraviolet light. Studies of human senile cataracts have demonstrated decreased levels of tetrahydrobiopterin.[10] Although tetrahydrobiopterin is not currently available as a nutritional supplement, taking extra folic acid may help compensate for this deficiency by increasing the body's ability to manufacture tetrahydrobiopterin.

Other Nutritional Factors

Riboflavin

The regeneration of active glutathione in the lens requires the vitamin riboflavin.[11,12] As a result, deficiency of riboflavin is believed to lead to cataract formation. Riboflavin deficiency is fairly common in the geriatric population (thirty-three percent of people over the age of 65 show evidence of low levels of riboflavin). Although correction of the deficiency is warranted, cataract patients should not take more than 10 mg of riboflavin per day since it is a *photosensitizing* substance. (It reacts with sunlight to produce free radicals.) Riboflavin and light exposure have been used experimentally to induce cataracts.

The evidence appears to suggest that excess riboflavin does more harm than good in the cataract patient. We need riboflavin to protect against cataract formation, but taking too much also may lead to cataract formation. Keep supplementary intake below 10 mg.

Amino Acids

Methionine is a component of *methionine sulfoxide reductase,* an important antioxidant enzyme in the lens. Methionine can also be converted to cysteine, a component of glutathione. Cysteine, along with the other amino acid precursors of glutathione, has been shown to be of some aid in cataract treatment.[13]

Zinc, Vitamin A, and Beta-Carotenes

These nutrients are known antioxidants and vital for normal integrity of eye structures. In particular, beta-carotene may act as a filter, protecting against light-induced damage to the fiber portion of the lens.[14] Low levels of these nutrients leave the lens of the eye very susceptible to free-radical damage and cataract formation. In addition to eating a diet rich in high-carotene-content vegetables like leafy greens, yams, carrots, broccoli, and other highly colored vegetables, we recommend supplementation. Dosages are given below in the Treatment Summary section.

Melatonin

Melatonin, the hormone produced by the human pineal gland in the brain, is an efficient free-radical scavenger and antioxidant. In studies on animals, melatonin has been an effective inhibitor of cataract formation.[15]

Diet

Evaluation of 207 patients with cataracts, compared to 706 controls, found a protective action from some vegetables, fruit, calcium, folic acid, and vitamin E. The study also found an increased risk for cataract formation with elevated salt and fat intake.[16]

Dairy Products

Cataracts often develop in infants who are deficient in the enzymes required to break down *galactose,* a milk sugar. However, even with normal levels of these enzymes, it has been suggested that an inability to properly break down galactose is an important factor in approximately thirty percent of cataract patients.[12] However, this factor appears to be significant only in diabetic cataract formation and is probably not relevant to senile cataract formation (for further discussion, see the section on DIABETES MELLITUS).

Heavy Metals

A number of heavy metals have been shown to have increased concentrations in both the aging lens and the lens with a cataract.[9] For example, the cadmium concentration in the lens with a cataract is two to three times higher than normal. Since cadmium prevents zinc from binding in important antioxidant enzymatic proteins, it may contribute to deactivation of free-radical quenching and other protective/repair mechanisms. Cigarette smoke is a leading source of cadmium from the environment. Other elevated elements of unknown significance include bromine, cobalt, iridium, and nickel.[9]

Botanical Medicines

There are a number of excellent choices from the botanical world to help with antioxidant mechanisms.

Flavonoid-Rich Extracts

Among the best may be flavonoid-rich extracts from *Vaccinium myrtillus* (bilberry),

Vitis vinifera (grape seed), and *Pinus maritima* (pine bark), as well as curcumin from *Curcuma longa.* The occurrence of cataracts in rats can be retarded by changing their diet from a commercial "lab chow" to a "well-defined diet."[17] Preliminary research suggests that flavonoid components in the well-defined diets may be responsible for the protective effects.[18]

Of the flavonoid-rich extracts, bilberry (*Vaccinium myrtillus*) extracts may offer the greatest protection. In one human study, bilberry extract plus vitamin E stopped progression of cataract formation in forty-eight of fifty patients with cataracts.[19]

Hachimijiogan

An ancient Chinese formula, *Hachimijiogan,* has been shown to increase the antioxidant level of the lens of the eye.[20,21] This activity may explain its use in treating cataracts for hundreds of years. According to clinical research, its therapeutic effect is quite impressive in the early stages of cataract formation. In one study, sixty percent of the subjects on *Hachimijiogan* noted significant improvement, twenty percent of the group showed no progression, and only the remaining twenty percent of the group displayed progression of the cataract. *Hachimijiogan* contains the following eight herbs per 22 grams:

Rehmania glutinosa	6,000 mg
Poria cocos sclerotium	3,000 mg
Dioscorea opposita	3,000 mg
Cormus officinalis	3,000 mg
Epimedium grandiflorum	3,000 mg
Alisma plantago	3,000 mg
Astragalus membranaceus	2,500 mg
Cinnamonum cassia	1,000 mg

TREATMENT SUMMARY

Progression of cataract formation can be stopped, and early cataracts can be reversed. However, significant reversal of well-developed cataracts does not appear possible at this time. In cases of marked vision impairment, cataract removal and lens implant may be the only alternative. As with most diseases, prevention or treatment at an early stage is most effective.

Since free-radical damage appears to be the primary factor in the induction of senile cataracts, avoidance of oxidizing agents and promotion of free-radical scavenging are critically important to successful treatment. The individual with cataracts should: avoid direct sunlight and bright light in general; wear sunglasses with UV protection when outdoors; and greatly increase intake of antioxidant nutrients.

Diet

Avoid fried foods, rancid foods, and other sources of free radicals. Increase consumption of legumes (high in sulfur-containing amino acids), yellow-orange vegetables (high in carotenes), and fresh fruits and vegetables (high in vitamins E and C).

Nutritional Supplements

- Vitamin C: 1 g three times per day
- Vitamin E: 400–800 IU per day
- Selenium: 400 mcg per day
- Beta-carotene: 200,000 IU per day
- Quercetin: 500 mg three times per day
- L-cysteine: 400 mg per day
- L-glutamine: 200 mg per day
- L-glycine: 200 mg per day

Botanical Medicines

- Bilberry extract (25% anthocyanidin content): 40 to 80 mg three times per day
- *Hachimijiogan* formula: 150 mg three times per day

Celiac Disease

. . . .

Bulky, pale, frothy, foul-smelling, greasy stools with increased fecal fat

Weight loss and signs of multiple vitamin and mineral deficiencies

Increased blood levels of antibodies for gliadin

Diagnosis confirmed by biopsy of the small intestine

Celiac disease, also known as *nontropical sprue, gluten-sensitive enteropathy,* or *celiac sprue,* is characterized by diarrhea and an abnormal small intestine structure caused by the immune system's response to a protein known as gluten. Gluten and its smaller derivative, gliadin, are found primarily in wheat, barley, and rye grains. Symptoms typically appear during the first three years of life, after cereals are introduced into the diet. A second peak occurrence rate occurs during the third decade of life. Breast-feeding appears to have a preventive effect, as breast-fed babies have a decreased risk of developing celiac disease.[1-3] The early introduction of cow's milk is also believed to be a major causative factor.[1-4] Research in the past few years has clearly indicated that breast-feeding and delayed administration of cow's milk and cereal grains are the primary preventive steps that can greatly reduce the risk of developing celiac disease.

Genetic Factors

Celiac disease appears to have a strong genetic component. There is an increased frequency of celiac disease in people with some specific genetic markers known as HLA-B_8 and DR_{w3} that appear on the surface of cells similar to the genetic markers of blood type. [3,5] For example, the HLA-B_8 marker has been found in eighty-five to ninety percent of celiac patients, as compared with twenty to twenty-five percent of normal subjects. There is a low frequency of HLA-B_8 within long-standing agrarian (farming) populations, as in Asia, while the frequency in northern and central Europe and the northwest Indian subcontinent is much higher.[3,6] Wheat cultivation in these high HLA-B_8 areas is a relatively recent development (1000 B.C.). The prevalence of celiac disease is much higher in these areas than in other parts of the world. For example, celiac disease is estimated to occur in one in every three hundred people in southwest Ireland while it is virtually unknown in Asia. In the United States, with its diverse genetic background, the frequency rate is roughly one in 2,500.

Chemistry of Grain Proteins

Gluten is the major protein component of wheat and is composed of *gliadins* and *glutenins*. Only the gliadin portion has been demonstrated to activate celiac disease. In rye, barley, and oats, the proteins that appear to activate the disease are termed *secalins, hordeins,* and *avenins,* respectively, and *prolamines* collectively. Cereal grains belong to the family Gramineae. The closer a grain is related to wheat, the greater its ability to activate celiac disease. Rice and corn, two grains that do not appear to activate celiac disease, are farther removed from wheat.[3,7]

Gliadins are single chains of amino acids that range in molecular weight from 30,000 to 75,000. Gliadins have been divided into four major fractions: alpha-, beta-, gamma-, and omega-gliadin. Alpha-gliadin is believed to be the fraction most capable of activating celiac disease, although beta- and gamma-gliadin are also capable. Gliadin that has been completely broken down by digestion does not activate celiac disease in susceptible individuals. This suggests that celiac disease may arise from a deficiency of enzymes that break down gliadin or some other factor involved with protein digestion.[3]

Opioid Activity

Partially digested wheat gluten has demonstrated opiate-like activity.[8,9] This activity is believed to be the factor responsible for the association between wheat consumption and schizophrenia.[10–12] The hypothesis that gluten is a pathogenic factor in the development of schizophrenia is substantiated by epidemiological, clinical, and experimental studies.[10]

Causes of the Intestinal Damage

Various theories have been proposed to explain what causes the damage to the intestinal tract in celiac disease. Currently, the most likely model relates to abnormalities in the immune response rather than some "toxic" property of gliadin.[13] Defects in the immune system appear to be responsible for most of the damage.[14] The damage is the result of the immune system trying to neutralize gliadin and, in the process, destroying surrounding intestinal tissue.

The intestinal damage of celiac disease is often indistinguishable from changes caused by intestinal infection, food allergy, and certain cancers (e.g., diffuse intestinal lymphoma). Furthermore, celiac disease often leads to a lactose deficiency, causing lactose intolerance, and the increased intestinal permeability usually results in multiple food allergies. As stated earlier, cow's milk intolerance may precede celiac disease.[1–4]

Associated Conditions

Conditions such as thyroid abnormalities, insulin-dependent diabetes mellitus, psychiatric disturbances (including schizophrenia), and hives have also been linked to gluten intolerance.[3] A more ominous association is the increased risk for malignant cancers seen in celiac patients.[3,15,16] This may be a result of decreased vitamin and mineral absorption, particularly of vitamin A and carotenoids. However, it may also be a result of gliadin-

QUICK REVIEW

- Celiac disease is characterized by diarrhea and an abnormal small intestine structure caused by the immune system's response to a protein known as gluten.

- A gluten-free diet is curative.
- Pancreatic enzyme supplementation enhances the benefit of a gluten-free diet during the first thirty days after the initial diagnosis.

activated suppression of immune function.[17] Alpha-gliadin has demonstrated suppressing effects on immune function in celiac patients but has no effect on the immune function of healthy controls or patients with Crohn's disease. Two other dietary proteins found in milk—*casein* and *beta-lactoglobulin*—have failed to produce suppressing effects on the immune system in similar experimental settings. This suppression in the immune response makes people with celiac disease who continue to eat gliadin more susceptible to infection and neoplasm.

Diagnosis of Celiac Disease

The definitive diagnostic procedure for celiac disease is intestinal biopsy. However, the presence of the characteristic symptoms along with a positive blood test for antibodies against gliadin (anti-alpha-gliadin antibodies) spares the patient the rigor of a small intestine biopsy. These blood tests for alpha-gliadin antibodies have a diagnostic sensitivity of one hundred percent.[18–20]

Therapeutic Considerations

Once the diagnosis has been established, the treatment is very straightforward: gluten-free diet. This diet does not contain any wheat, rye, barley, triticale, or oats. Buckwheat and millet are often excluded as well. Although buckwheat is not in the grass family, and millet appears to be more closely related to rice and corn, they do contain proteins that are similar to alpha-gliadin. A recent study of fifty-two adults with celiac disease suggests that modest amounts of oats my be tolerated without adverse side effects.[21]

In addition, other foods should be rotated (see FOOD ALLERGY), and milk and milk products should be eliminated until intestinal structure and function return to normal.

Usually, significant improvement will be apparent within a few days or weeks; thirty percent respond within three days, another fifty percent within one month, and ten percent within another month. However, ten percent of people with celiac disease only respond after twenty-four to thirty-six months of gluten avoidance.[22]

If you have celiac disease and you do not appear to be responding to a gluten-free diet after two months, the following should be considered:

1. You may have an incorrect diagnosis
2. You may be being exposed to hidden sources of gliadin
3. You may be suffering from some complications of celiac disease, such as zinc deficiency[3,23]

The latter possibility highlights the importance of multivitamin and mineral supplementation for anyone with an intestinal disorder. In addition to treating any underlying deficiency, supplementation provides the necessary cofactors for growth and repair. Celiac disease will often not clear up if there is an underlying nutrient (e.g., zinc) deficiency.[3,23]

Pancreatic Enzymes

The effect of pancreatic enzyme substitution therapy during the two months following initial diagnosis of celiac disease was investigated in a double-blind study. The study sought to clarify the benefit of pancreatic enzyme therapy because previous studies had shown that deficiency of pancreatic enzymes is found in eight to thirty percent of celiac patients.

In the study, patients followed a gluten-free diet and received either two capsules of pancreatic enzymes or two placebo capsules with each meal. The patients who received pancreatic enzymes took six to ten capsules per day depending upon the number of meals they consumed, with each capsule containing 5,000 IU of lipase, 2,900 IU of amylase, and 330 IU of protease. Complete nutritional evaluations were conducted at day zero, thirty, and sixty.

Results indicated that pancreatic enzyme supplementation enhanced the clinical benefit of a gluten-free diet during the first thirty days but did not provide any greater benefit than the placebo after sixty days.[24]

TREATMENT SUMMARY

The treatment of celiac disease is clear: eliminate all sources of gliadin, eliminate dairy products initially, correct underlying nutritional deficiencies by taking a high-potency multiple-vitamin-and-mineral formula, and identify and eliminate all food allergens. In the first two months after diagnosis, pancreatic enzymes at dosages described should be used to speed up the healing process. If you do not respond within two months, consult with your doctor again to reconsider the diagnosis.

Maintenance of a strict gluten-free diet is difficult in the United States. We encourage you to read labels carefully in order to avoid hidden sources of gliadin, such as are found in some brands of soy sauce, modified food starch, ice cream, soup, beer, wine, vodka, whisky, malt, and other foods. We also encourage you to consult resources for education and information on gluten-free recipes, such as:

American Celiac Society
45 Gifford Avenue
Jersey City, NJ 07304

American Digestive Disease Society
7720 Wisconsin Avenue
Bethesda, MD 20014

Gluten Tolerance Group of
    North America
P.O. Box 23053
Seattle, WA 98102

National Digestive Disease Education
    and Information Clearing House
1555 Wilson Boulevard, Suite 600
Rosslyn, VA 22209

Cellulite

Demonstration of the "mattress phenomenon" (pitting, bulging, and deformation of the skin)

Possible feelings of tightness and heaviness in affected areas (particularly the legs)

Tenderness of the skin when pinched, pressed upon, or vigorously massaged

The term *cellulite* is used to describe a cosmetic defect that is cause for great distress among millions of European and American women. This French word was adopted by the lay public in the United States before American physicians were educated about a condition that European physicians had been dealing with for over 150 years.[1]

The correct English translation of the French word *cellulite* would be "cellulitis." However, in the United States, "cellulitis" is used solely to describe a serious inflammatory or infectious process involving the connective tissue of the skin. In cellulite, there is no inflammatory or infectious process occurring. This difference in meaning of the translated term was just one source of confusion for American physicians.

Researchers have suggested that the technical terms *dermo-panniculosis deformans* and *adiposis edematosa* be used to designate the clinical condition.[2] In this chapter, however, the term "cellulite" will be used.

Structural Features of Cellulite

The tissue just below the surface of the skin that binds the skin loosely to underlying tissue or bones is termed the *subcutaneous tissue*. It is the subcutaneous tissue that is disturbed in cellulite. The subcutaneous tissue contains fat cells that vary in size and number from individual to individual. Since the thighs are the prime area of involvement in cellulite, the structure of the subcutaneous tissue of the thighs will be discussed in greatest detail.

The subcutaneous tissue of the thighs is composed of three layers of fat, with two planes of connective tissue (ground substance) between them. The basic construction of the subcutaneous tissue of the thigh differs in men and women, as shown in Figure 1.

In women, the uppermost subcutaneous layer consists of what are termed large *standing fat cell chambers*, which are separated by radial and arching dividing walls of connective tissue anchored to the overlying connective tissue of the skin. In contrast, the uppermost part of the subcutaneous tissue of men is thinner and has a network of crisscrossing connective tissue walls. In addition, the connective tissue structure (the *corium*) between the *dermis* and subcutaneous tissue is stronger in men than in women.[1,2]

These basic differences in subcutaneous tissue structure are the reason cellulite is seen almost exclusively in women. A simple test to illustrate these differences is the "pinch test." Pinching the skin and subcutaneous tissue of the thighs of women will result in the "mattress phenomenon"—pitting, bulging, and deformation of the skin—while in most men the skin will fold or furrow, but will not bulge or pit. These structural

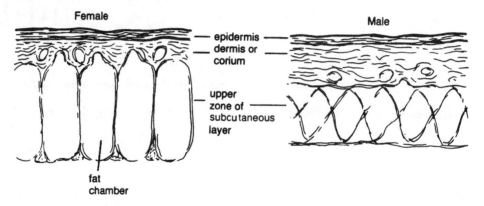

FIGURE 1 Anatomical Basis of Cellulite

differences between men and women are responsible for the fact that most women produce the mattress phenomenon in response to the pinch test, as illustrated in Figure 2.[1,2]

As women age, the corium (see Figure1), which is already thinner in women than in men, becomes progressively thinner and looser.[3] This allows fat cells to migrate into this layer. In addition, the connective tissue walls between the fat cell chambers also become thinner, allowing the fat-cell chambers to enlarge excessively *(hypertrophy)*. The breaking down or thinning of connective tis-

sue structures is a major contributor to the development of cellulite and is responsible for the granular "buckshot" feel of cellulite.[1,2]

The "mattress phenomenon" is brought about by alternating depressions and protrusions in the upper compartment systems of fat tissue. The vertical orientation of women's fat cell compartments, in conjunction with the weakening of the tissues noted above, is apparently what allows the protrusion of the fat cells into the lower corium.[2] The anatomical differences between men and women are summarized in Table 1.

QUICK REVIEW

- Cellulite is a "cosmetic" condition that results from weakened connective tissue structures just below the surface of the skin.
- Women are affected by cellulite at least nine times more often than men

due to structural differences just below the surface of the skin.
- Slim women and female athletes usually have little or no cellulite.
- An extract of gotu kola *(Centella asiatica)* has demonstrated impressive clinical results in the treatment of cellulite when given orally.

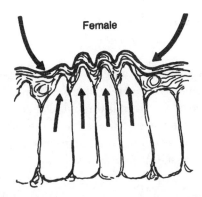
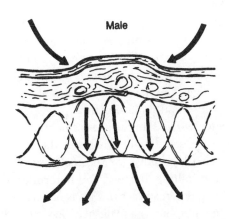

Female   Male

FIGURE 2 The Pinch Test

Examination of the tissue affected with cellulite under a microscope reveals distension of the lymphatic vessels and a decrease in the number of important elastic fibers that support the skin. This situation implies that there is congestion of lymphatic fluid and great stress on the skin in cases of cellulite.

Clinical Features

The basic appearance of cellulite is well known and described above as the "mattress phenomenon." Women comprise ninety to ninety-eight percent of the cases, reflecting differences in tissue structure between men and women. Symptoms of cellulite include feelings of tightness and heaviness in areas affected, particularly the legs. Tenderness of the skin is quite apparent when the skin is pinched, pressed upon, or vigorously massaged.[1,2]

The areas of the body involved are typically the buttocks and thigh regions, and, to a lesser extent, the lower part of the abdomen, the nape of the neck, and the upper parts of the arms. These are the areas of the body usually affected in female obesity.

Cellulite is classified in four major stages:

TABLE 1 Sex-Typical Differences in the Skin of the Lateral Thighs of Men and Women (16–50 years old)[2]		
STRUCTURE	**OF MEN**	**OF WOMEN**
Epidermis	Thicker	Thinner
Corium	Thicker	Thinner
Border zone of corium	Fewer fat cells	More fat cells and subcutaneous tissue
Subcutaneous tissue	Thinner	Thicker
	Small polygonal fat cell chambers with criss-crossing connective tissue	Large, standing fat cell with radially running connective tissue
Status protrusis cutis ("mattress phenomenon")	Does not develop	Develops

Stage 0: The skin on the thighs and buttocks has a smooth surface when the subject is standing or lying. When the skin is pinched (pinch test), it folds and furrows but does not pit or bulge. This stage is the "normal" state of most men and slim women.

Stage 1: The skin surface is smooth while a subject is standing or lying, but the pinch test is clearly positive for the mattress phenomenon (pitting, bulging, and deformity of the affected skin surfaces). This is normal for most females, but in a male may be a sign of deficiency of testosterone.

Stage 2: The skin surface is smooth while a subject is lying, but when standing there is pitting, bulging, and deformity of the affected skin surfaces. This stage is common in women who are obese or past thirty-five to forty years of age.

Stage 3: The mattress phenomenon is apparent when a subject is lying or standing. This stage is very common after menopause and in obesity.

Although most women consider Stage 0 the cosmetic ideal, Stage 1 is the best classification most can expect, due to their structural predisposition.

Therapeutic Considerations

As usual, the best approach is prevention. However, since the number and size of fat cells an individual has are largely determined by maternal prenatal nutritional status, many people have a significant predisposition to cellulite.

The next step is maintaining a slim subcutaneous fat layer. This is best done by exercising and maintaining a normal body weight throughout life. Slim women and female athletes have little or no cellulite.[1,2]

Treatment Goals

Therapeutic goals are to reduce the stress on the connective tissue structures by reducing the size of the fat cells through diet and exercise; improving the circulation to the affected area; and increasing the integrity of the connective tissue structures.

Weight Reduction and Exercise

Weight reduction and exercise can also be employed in the treatment of cellulite, and they should always be the primary method of treatment. However, weight reduction should be gradual, especially in women over the age of forty. A rapid loss of weight in individuals whose skin and connective tissues are already undergoing changes from aging will often make the mattress phenomenon more apparent.

Massage

Massage is very beneficial, particularly self-administered massage with the hand or brush. The physical and mechanical effects of massage improve circulation of blood and lymph. The direction of the massage should always be toward the heart.

Botanical Medicines

There are many cosmetic formulas and herbal preparations on the market that claim to be effective in "curing" cellulite. However, there is no scientific basis for the claims made about the majority of these formulas. In addition, long-term double-blind studies of some of the more popular cellulite treatments (e.g., Thiomucase, Nemectron, and Alec Eden-Slendertone) demonstrated that they were no more effective than a placebo.[3,4] However, several botanical compounds do have confirmed effects in the treatment of cellulite.

The comprehensive herbal treatment of cellulite involves both the oral and topical administration of botanical medicines that enhance connective tissue structures. As stated earlier, the breaking down or thinning of connective tissue structures is a major contributor to the development of cellulite.

Centella asiatica (Gotu kola)

An extract of centella containing seventy percent triterpenic acids (asiatic acid and asiaticoside) has demonstrated impressive clinical results when given orally in the treatment of cellulite and varicose veins.[5-9] In one study of cellulite in sixty-five patients who had undergone other therapies without success over a period of three months, very good results were produced in fifty-eight percent of the patients, and satisfactory results in twenty percent.[5] Other investigations have shown a similar success rate (approximately eighty percent).[6,7]

Several experimental studies have demonstrated that centella exerts a normalizing action on the metabolism of connective tissue. Specifically, it enhances connective tissue integrity by stimulating the manufacture of important structural components known as glycosaminoglycans (GAGs).[5] GAGs are the major components of the ground substance in which collagen (the main protein of connective tissue and bone) fibers are embedded. The net outcome is the development of connective tissue that is much stronger.

The effect of centella in the treatment of cellulite appears to be related to its ability to enhance connective tissue structure and reduce the formation of hardened connective tissue.

Aesculus hippocastanum (Horse Chestnut)

Horse chestnut extracts, and their key compound, *escin*, have anti-inflammatory and antiswelling properties that appear to be useful in the treatment of cellulite. One of escin's key effects is that it decreases capillary permeability by reducing the number and size of the small pores of the capillary walls.[10-12] Like centella extracts, horse chestnut extracts are very effective in the treatment of varicose veins (see VARICOSE VEINS).

In the treatment of cellulite, escin can be given orally, or an escin/cholesterol complex can be applied topically. The topical application of escin is also of benefit in the treatment of bruises, due to escin's ability to decrease capillary fragility and swelling.

Fucus vesiculosus (Bladderwrack)

Bladderwrack is a seaweed that has been used in the treatment of obesity since the seventeenth century. Its high iodine content is thought to stimulate thyroid function. Bladderwrack has also been used in toiletries and cosmetics for its soothing, softening, and toning effects.[13]

Another major topical application of bladderwrack has been in the treatment of cellulite. Its effects in this application have not been confirmed by careful scientific investigation, but bladderwrack does possess general actions (soothing, softening, and toning effects) that may be of benefit in the treatment of cellulite.

Cola Species

Cola is a rich source of caffeine and related compounds. These compounds potentiate the effect of fat breakdown (lipolysis). Topical administration of caffeine is preferable to oral administration in the treatment of cellulite, since its effects will be primarily local.

TREATMENT SUMMARY

It must be kept in mind that cellulite is not a "disease" per se. Instead, it is primarily a cosmetic disorder. Excessive accumulation of subcutaneous fat or degeneration of subcutaneous connective tissue leads to fat-chamber enlargement and greater visibility of the "mattress phenomenon." The basic therapeutic approach is straight forward: reduce subcutaneous fat and enhance connective tissue integrity.

Varicose veins are often found in conjunction with cellulite, and the two conditions have much in common. In particular, both appear to result largely from a loss of integrity of supporting connective tissue. (See VARICOSE VEINS for further discussion.)

It must be stated again that demonstration of the "mattress phenomenon" in men is a highly probable sign of androgen (male hormones) deficiency.[1]

Diet

A diet high in complex carbohydrates and low in refined carbohydrates and fats is very important. Weight loss should be promoted in obese individuals.

Physical Measures

- Exercise: twenty to thirty minutes of aerobic exercise a minimum of five days per week
- Massage: regular self-massage of the affected area with hand or brush

Botanical Medicines

Oral Administration

- *Centella asiatica* extract: 30 mg of triterpenes three times per day
- *Aesculus hippocastanum* extract: 10–20 mg of escin three times per day

Topical Application

Salve, ointment, etc., twice per day:

- Escin: 0.5–1.5%
- *Cola vera* extract (14% caffeine): 0.5–1.5%
- *Fucus vesiculosus:* 0.25–75%

Cerebral Vascular Insufficiency

. . . .

Presence of one or more of the following symptoms:

- **Short-term memory loss**
- **Dizziness (vertigo)**
- **Headache**
- **Ringing in the ears**
- **Depression**
- **Blurred vision**
- **Reduced blood flow to the brain based on ultrasound exam**

Cerebral vascular insufficiency—decreased blood supply to the brain—is extremely common among the elderly in developed countries due to the high prevalence of atherosclerosis (hardening of the arteries). The artery affected in most cases is the carotid artery. A pair of carotid arteries—one on each side of the neck running parallel to the jugular vein—are the main arteries that supply blood to the brain.

Typically, the problem develops at the *carotid bifurcation*—the splitting of the carotid artery into the internal (supplying the brain) and external (supplying the face and scalp) branches. This bifurcation is similar to a stream splitting into two branches. At the bifurcation, just like the splitting of the stream, debris and sediment accumulates. Significant symptoms begin to appear in most cases only when the blockage of the artery has reached ninety percent. This situation is similar to what occurs in angina (see ANGINA).

Symptoms of cerebral vascular insufficiency are caused by a reduced blood flow and oxygen supply to the brain. Severe disruption of blood and oxygen supply results in

a stroke. The official definition of a *stroke* is "loss of nerve function for at least twenty-four hours due to lack of oxygen." Some strokes are quite mild; others can leave a person paralyzed, in a coma, or unable to talk, depending on which part of the brain is affected. Smaller "mini-strokes," or *transient ischemic attacks* (TIAs), may result in loss of nerve function for an hour or more, but less than twenty-four hours. TIAs may produce transient symptoms of cerebral vascular insufficiency: dizziness, ringing in the ears, blurred vision, confusion, and so on.

Diagnostic Considerations

Anyone who experiences signs and symptoms of cerebral vascular insufficiency should consult a physician immediately for proper evaluation. In the past, evaluation of blood flow to the brain involved invasive techniques such as *cerebral angiography*. This procedure was similar to a cardiac (heart) angiogram (see

335

ANGINA) and carried a relatively high side-effect rate: it caused a stroke in roughly four percent of the subjects. The modern evaluation of blood flow to the brain involves the use of ultrasound techniques. These techniques determine the rate of blood flow and the degree of blockage by using sound waves. There are still other techniques that can be used to provide valuable information.

Therapeutic Considerations

The considerations and recommendations given in the chapter HEART AND CARDIOVASCULAR HEALTH are appropriate here, since the primary goal is to improve blood flow. In addition to those recommendations, it is important to address any other underlying factor, such as high cholesterol levels or high blood pressure. Beyond these general recom-

mendations, we will offer a discussion of two natural medicines with proven benefits in treating cerebral vascular insufficiency: aortic glycosaminoglycans (GAGs) and *Ginkgo biloba* extract.

Carotid Endarterectomy

Before discussing these natural approaches to improving cerebral vascular insufficiency, let's take a look at a controversial surgical procedure—*carotid endarterectomy*—that is often recommended for patients with cerebral vascular insufficiency. Carotid endarterectomy involves the surgical removal of the atherosclerotic plaque from the carotid artery. This surgical procedure is highly controversial, as approximately six to ten percent of the patients will either die or suffer severe neurological damage as a result of a stroke during the surgery.[1-3] All in all, approximately seven to eleven percent of the patients will die during or soon after (less than

- -

QUICK REVIEW

- **Symptoms of cerebral vascular insufficiency are associated with a reduced blood flow and oxygen supply to the brain.**

- **Anyone who experiences signs and symptoms of cerebral vascular insufficiency should consult a physician immediately.**

- **The modern evaluation of blood flow to the brain involves the use of ultrasound techniques.**

- **Carotid endarterectomy is a highly controversial surgical procedure be-**

cause approximately six to ten percent of the patients will either die or suffer severe neurological damage as a result of a stroke during the surgery.

- **Aortic glycosaminoglycan preparations have been effective in improving both cerebral (brain) and peripheral (hands and feet) vascular insufficiency.**

- **In well-designed studies, *Ginkgo biloba* extract (GBE) has produced a statistically significant regression of the major symptoms of cerebral vascular insufficiency and impaired mental performance.**

one month) carotid endarterectomy. Most of these patients are dying unnecessarily.

As with coronary bypass (see ANGINA), the majority of patients who have carotid endarterectomy do not need it. A 1988 article published in the *New England Journal of Medicine* described the conclusions of a panel of nationally known experts who rated the appropriateness of carotid endarterectomy. In a random sample of 1,302 Medicare patients, they found that only thirty-five percent had carotid endarterectomy for appropriate reasons.[3] This same study found that approximately 9.8 percent of the patients who underwent carotid endarterectomy died of a stroke within thirty days of the operation or suffered permanent neurological damage.

Carotid endarterectomies are of no value to patients with less than seventy percent blockage, as determined by angiograph.[4–6] Again, as with coronary bypass, it appears that most patients who elect not to have the surgery will outlive the patients who have the surgery. Even in patients with blockage greater than seventy percent, the benefits of carotid endarterectomy are not very significant to long-term survival rate, especially when risk is considered. It appears that carotid endarterectomy is extremely risky and provides little benefit.

Despite the lack of benefit in most cases, approximately 100,000 carotid endarterectomies are performed each year in the United States. At a cost of roughly $25,000 per procedure, that is a total of over $2.5 billion dollars each year.

If you have symptoms of severe cerebral vascular insufficiency, including frequent TIAs or a past stroke, along with severe (greater than seventy percent) blockage of the carotid artery, then carotid endarterectomy may be appropriate. However, before electing to proceed with this surgery, we recommend that you consult a qualified EDTA chelation specialist. (For a discussion of EDTA, see ANGINA.) For information on locating an EDTA chelation specialist, contact

The American College of Advancement
  in Medicine (ACAM)
23121 Verdugo Drive, Suite 204
Laguna Hills, CA 92653
800-532-3688 (outside California)
800-435-6199 (inside California)

Aortic GAGs

Glycosaminoglycans (GAGs) are structural components that are essential to maintaining the health of arteries and other blood vessels. A mixture of highly purified bovine-derived glycosaminoglycans naturally present in the human aorta, including dermatan sulfate, heparan sulfate, hyaluronic acid, chondroitin sulfate, and related hexosaminoglycans, has been shown to protect and promote normal artery and vein function.

A number of clinical studies have demonstrated that supplementing the diet with aortic GAGs remarkably improves the structure, function, and integrity of arteries, as well as improving blood flow.[7–9] Aortic GAGs have been shown to be effective in improving both cerebral (brain) and peripheral (hands and feet) vascular insufficiency; symptoms have been relieved, and blood flow has been increased. The effects of aortic GAGs in improving blood flow to the brain are similar to those of *Ginkgo biloba* extract (discussed in the next paragraph). Aortic GAGs should be used for at least six months after a stroke or TIA.

Ginkgo biloba Extract

The extract of *Ginkgo biloba* leaves standardized to contain twenty-four percent ginkgo flavonglycosides and six percent terpenoids has been the subject of over forty double-blind studies on the treatment of cerebral vascular insufficiency. In well-designed studies,

Ginkgo biloba extract (GBE) has produced a statistically significant regression of the major symptoms of cerebral vascular insufficiency and impaired mental performance. These symptoms included short-term memory loss, vertigo, headache, ringing in the ears, lack of vigilance, and depression.[10–18]

The significant regression of these symptoms by GBE suggests that vascular insufficiency, not a true degenerative process, may be the major cause of these so-called age-related cerebral disorders.

In a comprehensive review, an analysis was made of the quality of research in over forty

TABLE 1	Characteristics of Well-Conducted Controlled Trials	
TRIAL	**INDICATION** **DURATION OF SYMPTOMS** **AVERAGE AGE**	**DAILY DOSE/** **DURATION OF TREATMENT**
Schmidt,[11] 1991	Cerebral insufficiency 26 months 59 years	150 mg/12 weeks
Bruchert,[12] 1991	Cerebral insufficiency 46 months 69 years	150 mg/12 weeks
Meyer,[13] 1986	Tinnitus, dizziness, hearing impairment 4–5 months 50 years	16 mg (4 ml)/3 months
Taillandier,[14] 1986	Cerebral insufficiency 5 years 82 years	160 mg/12 months
Haguenauer,[15] 1986	Vertiginous syndrome and tinnitus, headaches, nausea, hearing loss 21 weeks 50 years	160 mg/3 months
Vorberg,[16] 1989	Cerebral insufficiency 21 months 70 years	112 mg/12 weeks
Eckmann,[17] 1990	Cerebral insufficiency 32 months 55 years	160 mg/6 weeks
Wesnes,[18] 1987	Mild idiopathic cognitive impairment 71 years	120 mg/12 weeks

clinical studies of GBE in the treatment of cerebral insufficiency.[10] The results of the analysis indicate that GBE is effective in reducing all symptoms of cerebral insufficiency, including impaired mental function (senility). GBE was found to be comparable to FDA-approved drugs used in the treatment of cerebral vascular insufficiency and Alzheimer's disease. Eight studies stood out as extremely well designed, and they are summarized in Table 1.[11–18]

It appears that by increasing blood flow to the brain, and therefore oxygen and glucose utilization, *Ginkgo biloba* extract offers relief

TABLE 1, *continued*

1. NO.* RANDOMIZED 2. NO. ANALYZED	ENDPOINTS	RESULTS
1. 50/49 2. 50/49	1. 12 symptoms; OS(4) 2. Overall assessment doctor; OS(3) 3. Overall assessment patient; OS(3)	1. Significant differences for 8 of 12 2. 72% vs. 8% improved 3. 70% vs. 14% improved
1. 156/157 2. 110/99	1. 12 symptoms; OS(4) 2. Overall assessment doctor; OS(3) 3. Overall assessment patient; OS(3)	1. Significant differences for 8 of 12 2. 71% vs. 32% improved 3. 83% vs. 53% improved

1. 58/45 (?)
 	
2. 55/45 (?)
	1. Symptoms; OS(4)
	
	2. Overall assessment; days to
	   improvement or cure
		1. Significant difference for intensity;
		   positive trend for discomfort
		2. 70 days vs. 119 days

1. 101/109
2. 80/86
	1. Scale for geriatric patients (17
	   items); change from randomization
	   after 3 months
	2. After 6 months
	3. After 9 months
	4. After 12 months
		1. 10% vs. 4%
		
		2. 15% vs. 4%
		3. 15% vs. 8%
		4. 17% vs. 8%

1. 35/35 2. 34/33	1. Symptoms; VAS and others 2. Overall assessment doctor; OS(5)	1. Vertigo: 75% vs. 18% beneficial change 2. 47% vs. 18% symptoms disappeared
1. 50/50 2. 49/47	6 symptoms; OS(4)	1. Concentration: 54% vs. 19% improved 2. Memory: 52% vs. 17% improved 3. Anxiety: 48% vs. 17% improved 4. Dizziness: 61% vs. 23% improved 5. Headache: 65% vs. 24% improved 6. Tinnitus: 37% vs. 12% improved
1. 30/30 2. 29/29	12 symptoms; OS(4)	Significant differences for 11 of 12 symptoms after 4 and 6 weeks

1. 28/30
 	
2. 27/27
	1. Cognitive test battery
	
	2. Behavioral rating scale
	3. VAS mood
	4. Overall assessment
	   doctor and patient
		1. Significant differences for combined
		   scores
		2. No differences
		3. No significant differences
		4. No differences, nearly all patients
		   improved

*Ginkgo/placebo
OS(4) = 4-point ordinal scale; VAS = visual analog scale

from these presumed "side effects" of aging and may offer significant protection against their development. Furthermore, *Ginkgo biloba*'s tendency to reduce blood viscosity offers additional protection against a stroke.

This has been indicated by a clinical study of post-stroke patients that demonstrated that GBE improved blood flow and blood viscosity.[19]

TREATMENT SUMMARY

In most cases, cerebral vascular insufficiency is a consequence of atherosclerosis. That being the case, appropriate treatment involves following the recommendations given in the chapter HEART AND CARDIOVASCULAR HEALTH. It may also be appropriate to consult the chapters on CHOLESTEROL and HIGH BLOOD PRESSURE.

The therapeutic goal in the treatment of cerebral vascular insufficiency is to en- hance the blood and oxygen supply to the brain. Aortic GAGs and *Ginkgo biloba* extract (alone or in combination) have shown excellent results in treating cerebral vascular insufficiency, as well as in promoting a speedier and more complete recovery from a stroke. Both aortic GAGs and GBE can be used with the blood-thinning agent Coumadin without side effect. Dosages are as follows:

- Aortic GAGs: 50–100 mg per day
- *Ginkgo biloba* extract (24% ginkgo flavonglycosides): 80 mg three times per day

Cervical Dysplasia

. . . .

Abnormal Pap smear (Classes II–IV)

ervical dysplasia involves the appearance of abnormal cells on the surface of the cervix. It is generally regarded as a precancerous lesion; in other words, it is not a cancerous state, but if untreated it could lead to cancer.

The cervix is a small, cylindrical organ that comprises the lower part and neck of the uterus. The cervix contains a central canal for passage of sperm and menstrual blood, and for childbirth. Both the canal and outer surface of the cervix are lined with two types of cells: mucus-producing cells and protective (*squamous*) cells.

Cancer of the cervix is one of the most common cancers affecting women. Fortunately, cervical cancer is one of the few cancers that has well-defined precancerous stages, so it is usually treated successfully as a result of early detection. However, cervical cancer is still the second most common malignant cancer found in women between the ages of fifteen and thirty-four (although it can occur at any age).[1,2]

Women routinely receive annual Pap smears in an attempt to detect cancer of the cervix. The *Pap smear* is a sampling of cells from the surface of the cervix. Before any cancer appears, abnormal changes occur in cells on the surface of the cervix. These abnormal cells are detected by a Pap smear, indicating possible cervical dysplasia.

The risk factors for cervical dysplasia are similar to those for cervical cancer.[1] These risk factors include early age at first intercourse; multiple sexual partners; *Herpes simplex* Type II and human papillomaviruses; low income; smoking; oral contraceptive (birth-control pills) use; and many nutritional factors.[1,2]

Therapeutic Considerations

The therapeutic approach depends upon the severity of the dysplasia. Most doctors use the numerical rating system in which "I" represents normal and "V" represents cancer. In addition to this rating system, there are the CIN and Bethesda scales (see Table 1). If the Pap smear indicates Class II or III, the recommendations given in this chapter can be employed with careful monitoring (which means getting a Pap smear every three months until the results are normal).

However, if the Pap smear demonstrates significant dysplasia (a Class IV score), proper treatment involves first ascertaining if there is cancer involved. Diagnosis and treatment of Class IV Pap usually includes a process known as *cone biopsy*. This surgical procedure involves removing a cone-shaped piece of the cervix where the abnormal cells are located in order to determine if localized cancer of the cervix (*carcinoma in situ*) has developed.

A Class III Pap should also be biopsied if a woman has had recurrent abnormal Pap smears, has significant risk factors for cervical cancer (discussed more fully in the following section), or does not respond to the therapy

341

TABLE 1   Classification Systems for Pap Smears

NUMERICAL CLASS	DYSPLASIA	CIN*	BETHESDA SYSTEM
I	Benign	Benign	Normal
II	Benign with inflammation	Benign with inflammation	Normal
III	Mild dysplasia	CIN I	Low-grade SIL†
III	Moderate dysplasia	CIN II	Low-grade SIL
III	Severe dysplasia	CIN III	High-grade SIL
IV	Carcinoma *in situ*	CIN III	High-grade SIL

*CIN = cervical intraepithelial neoplasia
*†SIL = squamous epithelial lesion

outlined in this chapter within a three-month period.

Risk Factors

The best approach to cervical dysplasia is prevention by avoidance of known risk fac-tors. When cervical dysplasia is present, the next step is to eliminate risk factors when possible and to optimize one's nutritional status. In particular, eliminate smoking and oral contraceptive use and supplement with folic acid, beta-carotenes, and vitamin C. Pap smears should be repeated every one to three

. . . .

QUICK REVIEW

- Cervical dysplasia reflects abnormal cell growth on the cervix and is usually a precancerous condition.
- Severe surgical dysplasia (Class IV Pap smear) requires cone biopsy or a similar procedure.
- Risk factors for cervical dysplasia include: early age at first intercourse; smoking; multiple sexual partners; exposure to viruses; low income; oral contraceptive use; and many nutritional factors.
- Women who have low vitamin C levels are 6.7 times more likely to develop

cervical cancer than women with sufficient vitamin C levels.
- The higher the intake of dietary sources of beta-carotene, the lower the rate of cervical dysplasia.
- Many abnormal Pap smears reflect folic acid deficiency rather than true dysplasia.
- In placebo-controlled studies, folic acid supplementation (10 mg per day) has resulted in improvement or normalization of Pap smears in patients with cervical dysplasia.
- Selenium levels are significantly lower in patients with cervical dysplasia.

months, according to severity, to judge effectiveness of treatment.

As previously stated, cervical dysplasia is associated with the same risk factors as cervical cancer. The risk factors that will be discussed here are sexual activity, viruses, smoking, oral contraceptive use, and nutritional factors.

To help you assess these risk factors, the *relative risk* for each one is provided in Table 2. The relative risk tells us the statistical probability of a particular factor causing cancer, compared to women who do not have that risk factor. For example, smoking carries a relative risk of 3. This number means that women who smoke are three times more likely to develop cervical cancer than women who don't smoke. For another example, women who have low vitamin C levels are 6.7 times more likely to develop cervical cancer than women with sufficient vitamin C levels.

Sexual Activity

Early age at first intercourse and/or multiple sexual contacts are associated with an increased risk of cervical dysplasia/carcinoma.[1,2] From this and other evidence, it has been suggested that cervical cancer is a venereal disease, in the sense that the implicated infectious agents appear to be sexually transmitted. The most likely candidates are viruses.

Viruses Two classes of virus are currently suspected of playing a causative role in cervical cancer as well as cervical dysplasia: *Herpes simplex* Type II (HSV-II) and the human papillomavirus (HPV). HPV is the virus that causes venereal warts (*Condyloma acuminata*) and is the most likely culprit in many cases of cervical dysplasia. There are over forty-five different strains of HPV, and one strain in particular appears to be a major cause of cervical dysplasia. HPV16 has been found in ninety percent of all cervical cancers and fifty to seventy percent of all cases of cervical dysplasia.

Although these viruses have been shown to be related to cervical dysplasia, it has not been determined whether they reflect decreased immunity or some other defense mechanism or are themselves the causative agents.[1,2]

Smoking

Cigarette smoking is a major risk factor for cervical cancer and/or cervical dysplasia. The incidence of cervical dysplasia in smokers is two to three times greater than that in nonsmokers (one study[3] showed the risk to be as much as seventeen times greater in women aged twenty to twenty-nine).[3-6]

Many hypotheses have been proposed to explain this association:

TABLE 2 Risk Factors in Cervical Dysplasia/Cancer	
RISK FACTOR	**RELATIVE RISK**
Age at first intercourse (<18)	2.76
Deficient dietary beta-carotene (<5,000 IU/day)	2.814
Smoking (10+ cigarettes/day)	3.06
Multiple sexual partners (2–5)	3.46
Oral contraceptive use (5–8 years)	3.66
Deficient dietary vitamin C (<30 mg/day)	6.717

- Smoking may depress immune functions, allowing a sexually transmitted agent to promote abnormal cellular development, leading to the onset of cervical dysplasia
- Smoking induces vitamin-C deficiency (vitamin C levels are significantly depressed in smokers)[7]
- Vaginal or endometrial cells may concentrate carcinogenic compounds from inhaled smoke and secrete these compounds
- There may be unrecognized associations between smoking and sexual behavior[3-6]

Oral Contraceptives

The long-term use of oral contraceptives (birth-control pills) is associated with increased risk of hospitalization for thromboembolic disease, gallbladder disease, myocardial infarction, mental illness, hyperthyroidism, and hypertension, as well as cancer of the cervix.[6-10] Birth-control pills are known to increase the adverse effects of cigarette smoking and to decrease numerous nutrient levels, including those of vitamins C, B6, and B12, folic acid, riboflavin, and zinc.[11]

Nutritional Considerations

Numerous nutritional factors have been implicated in the development of cervical dysplasia, cancer of the cervix, and other cancers of similar cell types to the cervix (such as the skin, cheek cavity, pharynx, esophagus, colon, rectum, or lung).[26] Although many single nutrients may play a significant role (particularly beta-carotene and vitamin A, folic acid, vitamin B6, and vitamin C), it is important to recognize that sixty-seven percent of patients with cervical cancer have nutritional deficiencies. Many other patients have marginal but "normal" nutritional status as determined by routine evaluations. These results suggest that multiple nutrient deficiencies are probably the rule rather than the exception.[12,13]

It is clear that vitamin deficiencies play a major role in the onset of cervical dysplasia/ carcinoma. General dietary factors are also important. A high fat intake has been associated with increased risk for cervical cancer, while a diet rich in fruits and vegetables is believed to offer significant protection against carcinogenesis, probably due to the higher intake of fiber, beta-carotenes, and vitamin C.[5]

Vitamin A and Beta-Carotene There appears to be a minor association between dietary vitamin A levels and cervical cancer/ dysplasia risk, and a strong inverse correlation between beta-carotene intake and the risk of cervical cancer/dysplasia.[14-16] An inverse relationship means that the higher the intake of beta-carotene, the lower the rate of cervical dysplasia.

Beta-carotene appears to be more important than vitamin A, possibly due to greater antioxidant properties. For example, one study found that only six percent of patients with untreated cervical cancer had below-normal serum vitamin A levels, while thirty-eight percent had stage-related abnormal levels of beta-carotene.[13] The greater the stage of dysplasia the lower the level of beta-carotene. Low serum beta-carotene levels are associated with a three times greater risk for severe dysplasia compared to women with normal beta-carotene levels.[16]

However, vitamin A is also important. In one study, vitamin A levels were significantly lower in patients with cervical dysplasia than in a control group (54 mg/dl versus 104 mg/ dl).[27] Several studies are currently being conducted to evaluate the clinical efficacy of vitamin A and related compounds (retinoids) in cervical dysplasia treatment.[15,16]

Vitamin C There is a significant decrease in vitamin C intake and blood vitamin C levels among patients with cervical dysplasia. It has also been documented that inadequate vitamin C intake is an independent risk factor for the development of cervical dysplasia and carcinoma *in situ*.[17,18] Vitamin C is known to act as an antioxidant, strengthen and maintain normal epithelial integrity, improve wound healing, enhance immune function, and inhibit carcinogen formation.[11]

Folic Acid Folic acid deficiency is characterized by abnormal red and white blood cells. Similar changes occur in the cells of the cervix. However, changes in the cells of the cervix due to folic acid deficiency precede changes in the blood cells by many weeks, if not months.[19,20] Since folic acid deficiency is the most common vitamin deficiency in the world, and quite common in women who are pregnant or taking birth-control pills,[11,21] it is probable that many abnormal Pap smears reflect folate deficiency rather than true dysplasia.[19,20,22,23] This is particularly applicable to cases in which women are taking birth-control pills.

It has been hypothesized that birth-control pills block the effects of folic acid within cells by stimulating a molecule that inhibits folate uptake by cells. Although serum levels of folic acid may be normal or even increased in many patients with cervical dysplasia, the level within the cells of the cervix may be lower than normal.[22,23] This hypothesis is consistent with the observation that tissue status, as measured by the level of folic acid in red blood cells, is typically decreased in women on birth-control pills (especially in those with cervical dysplasia), while serum levels are normal or even increased.[23]

Low levels of folic acid in the red blood cells have been shown to enhance the effect of the other risk factors for cervical dysplasia, especially human papillomavirus (HPV) infection. In other words, low red blood cell folate appears to be a major risk factor for HPV infection of the cervix.[23,24] Conversely, when folic acid status within the cells of the cervix is high, HPV does not infect the cells.

Folic acid supplementation (10 mg per day) has resulted in improvement or normalization of Pap smears in patients with cervical dysplasia in placebo-controlled[25] and clinical studies.[22] Regression rates of Pap smears to normal for patients with untreated cervical dysplasia are typically 1.3 percent for mild and 0 percent for moderate dysplasia. When patients were treated with folic acid, the regression-to-normal rate, as determined by colposcopy/biopsy examination, was observed to be twenty percent in one study,[26] sixty-four percent in another,[25] and one hundred percent in yet another.[22]

Furthermore, the progression rate of untreated cervical dysplasia to either more severe dysplasia or cancer is typically sixteen percent at four months, a figure matched in the placebo group in one study of women on the birth-control pill, while the folate-supplemented group had a zero-percent progression rate.[23] All these figures were observed despite the fact that the women remained on the birth-control pills.

The median time required for progression from cervical dysplasia to carcinoma *in situ* in untreated patients ranges from eighty-six months for patients with very mild dysplasia to twelve months for patients with severe dysplasia; regression is very uncommon. Consequently, it has been suggested that a trial of folate supplementation (along with other considerations discussed) be instituted in mild-to-moderate dysplasia, with a follow-up Pap smear at three months. Vitamin B12 supplementation should always accompany folate supplementation.

Vitamin B6 Vitamin B6 status is decreased in one-third of patients with cervical cancer.[27]

Decreased B6 status would have a significant effect on the metabolism of estrogens, as well as impairing immune response.

Selenium Serum, dietary, and soil selenium levels are significantly lower in patients with cervical dysplasia.[28,29] An increased glutathione peroxidase activity resulting from increased selenium intake is believed to be the factor responsible for selenium's anticarcinogenic effect, although other factors may be of equal significance. Many toxic elements, such as lead, cadmium, mercury, and gold possess selenium-antagonistic properties.[28] The role these heavy metals may play in cervical disease has not been determined.

TREATMENT SUMMARY

For the treatment of a Class II or III Pap smear, the program outlined in this chapter can be used if there are regular repeat Pap smears (every one to three months). For Class IV or Class V Pap smears or unresponsive cases, please consult a physician immediately for proper medical treatment.

Diet

Consumption of animal products should be decreased, particularly animal fats. Follow the recommendations given in PREMENSTRUAL SYNDROME for reducing estrogen levels.

Nutritional Supplements

- Folic acid: 10 mg per day for three months, then 2.5 mg per day until normalization of the Pap smear occurs
- Vitamin B6: 25 mg three times per day
- Vitamin B12: 1 mg per day
- Beta-carotene: 25,000–50,000 IU per day
- Vitamin C: 500–1,000 mg three times per day
- Vitamin E: 200–400 IU per day
- Selenium: 200–400 mcg per day

Cholesterol

. . . .

Total blood cholesterol level above 200 mg/dl

LDL cholesterol level above 130 mg/dl

HDL cholesterol level below 35 mg/dl

Lipoprotein (a) level greater than 30 mg/dl

Keeping cholesterol levels in the proper range is an important step in the prevention of a heart attack or stroke.[1] The role that cholesterol levels play in determining the risk of a heart attack or stroke was introduced in the chapter HEART AND CARDIOVASCULAR HEALTH.

Cholesterol is transported in the blood on carrier molecules known as *lipoproteins*. The major categories of lipoproteins are very-low-density lipoprotein (VLDL), low-density lipoprotein (LDL), and high-density lipoprotein (HDL). Since VLDL and LDL are responsible for transporting fats (primarily triglycerides and cholesterol) from the liver to body cells, while HDL is responsible for returning fats to the liver, elevations of either VLDL or LDL are associated with an increased risk of developing atherosclerosis, the primary cause of a heart attack or stroke. In contrast, elevations of HDL are associated with a low risk of heart attack.

It is currently recommended that the total blood cholesterol level be less than 200 mg/dl. In addition, it is recommended that the LDL cholesterol level be less than 130 mg/dl, the HDL cholesterol be greater than 35 mg/dl, and triglyceride (another type of blood fat) levels be less than 150 mg/dl.

The ratio of total cholesterol to HDL cholesterol and the ratio of LDL to HDL are referred to as the *cardiac risk factor ratios*, because they reflect whether cholesterol is being deposited into tissues or broken down and excreted. The total cholesterol-to-HDL ratio should be no higher than 4, and the LDL-to-HDL ratio should be no higher than 2.5. The risk of heart disease can be reduced dramatically by lowering LDL cholesterol levels while raising HDL cholesterol levels. It has been concluded that for every one-percent drop in the LDL cholesterol level, the risk of a heart attack drops by two percent. Conversely, for every one-percent increase in HDL levels, the risk of a heart attack drops three to four percent.[2]

Although LDL cholesterol is often referred to as "bad cholesterol," an even more damaging form is *lipoprotein (a),* or Lp(a). Lp(a) is a plasma lipoprotein with a structure and composition that closely resemble those of LDL (low-density lipoprotein), but with an additional molecule of an adhesive protein called *apolipoprotein (a).* Several studies have indicated that elevated plasma levels of Lp(a) are an independent risk factor for coronary heart disease, particularly in patients with elevated LDL cholesterol levels.[3,4] In fact, a high level of Lp(a) has been shown to carry a ten times greater risk for heart disease than an elevated LDL cholesterol level. That is because LDL on its own lacks the adhesive apolipoprotein (a). As a result, LDL does not easily stick to the walls of the artery. Actually,

347

a high LDL cholesterol level carries less risk than a normal or even low LDL cholesterol level with a high Lp(a) level. Levels of Lp(a) below 20 mg/dl are associated with a low risk for heart disease; levels between 20 and 40 mg/dl a moderate risk; and levels above 40 mg/dl an extremely high risk for heart disease.

Causes

Although, in most cases, elevations of blood cholesterol and/or triglyceride (another blood fat) levels are due to dietary and lifestyle factors, elevations can also be due to genetic factors. These conditions are referred to as *familial hypercholesterolemia* (FH), *familial combined hyperlipidemia* (FCH), and *familial hypertriglyceridemia* (FT). These disorders are among the most common inherited diseases, as they affect about one in every five hundred people.

The basic problem in FH is a defect in the receptor protein for LDL in the liver. Under normal situations, the LDL receptor is responsible for removing cholesterol from the blood. When the liver cell takes up the LDL after it has bound to the receptor, it signals the liver cell to stop making cholesterol. In FH, there is a defect in the LDL receptor; as a result, the liver does not get the message to stop making cholesterol.

Damage to the LDL receptor occurs with normal aging and in several disease states, with diabetes being the most important. As a result of LDL receptor damage, cholesterol levels tend to rise in diabetics and with aging in general. In addition, a diet high in saturated fat and cholesterol decreases the number of LDL receptors, thereby reducing the feedback mechanism that tells the liver cell that no more cholesterol is needed.

Fortunately, the steps for lowering your cholesterol levels, detailed in the Therapeutic Considerations section of this chapter, can increase the function and/or number of LDL receptors. The most dramatic effects will be in people without inherited causes of elevated cholesterol and/or triglycerides, but even people with FH can experience a benefit.

QUICK REVIEW

- Elevated cholesterol levels in the blood are linked to heart attacks and strokes.
- Although, in most cases, elevations of blood cholesterol levels are due to dietary and lifestyle factors, elevations can also result from genetic factors.
- Elevations in cholesterol levels may be the result of low thyroid function (hypothyroidism).
- The most important approach to lowering a high cholesterol level is a healthful diet and lifestyle.
- Several of the cholesterol-lowering drugs are actually associated with an increase in noncardiovascular mortality.
- Cholesterol-lowering drugs are toxic to the liver and extremely carcinogenic (cancer-causing).
- Niacin has demonstrated better overall results than cholesterol-lowering

Familial combined hyperlipidemia (FCH) and familial hypertriglyceridemias (FT) involve defects similar to those found in FH. In FCH, the basic defect appears to be an accelerated production of very-low-density lipoprotein (VLDL) in the liver. Individuals with FCH may have only a high blood triglyceride level, or only a high cholesterol level, or both.

In FT, there is only an elevation in blood triglyceride levels; HDL cholesterol levels tend to be low. The defect in FT is that the VLDL particles made by the liver are larger than normal and carry more triglycerides. FT is made worse by diabetes, gout, and obesity.

The recommendations given in the Therapeutic Considerations section will also be helpful to people with FCH and FT, although these conditions will usually require more aggressive support (discussed in the Treatment Summary section).

Low Thyroid Function

Elevations in cholesterol levels may be the result of low thyroid function (*hypothyroidism*). It is well established that patients with hypothyroidism are prone to coronary artery disease because of an increased LDL cholesterol and decreased HDL cholesterol level. A recent study indicates that the risk may be greater than previously suspected. The study demonstrated that patients with even very mild cases of hypothyroidism were shown to have not only significantly elevated levels of LDL cholesterol, but also elevated levels of lipoprotein (a).[5] It is extremely important to rule out hypothyroidism in cases of high cholesterol levels. For more information, see HYPOTHYROIDISM.

Therapeutic Considerations

The most important approach to lowering a high cholesterol level is a healthful diet and lifestyle. The dietary guidelines are straightforward:

- Eat less saturated fat and cholesterol by reducing or eliminating the amount of animal products in the diet

agents in reducing the risk of coronary heart disease.

- Niacin was the only cholesterol-lowering agent found to reduce the death rate in The Coronary Drug Project.
- Because of its low cost and proven efficacy, niacin should be considered the first cholesterol-lowering agent to try.
- The problems with niacin (e.g., skin flushing, other side effects, and patient compliance) can be avoided by using inositol hexaniacinate.
- Sustained-release niacin should not be used due to greater toxicity in the liver.
- The majority of studies that showed a positive effect of garlic and garlic preparations used forms of garlic that deliver a sufficient dosage of allicin.

- Eat more fiber-rich plant foods (fruits, vegetables, grains, and legumes)
- Lose weight if necessary

The lifestyle guidelines are

- Get regular aerobic exercise
- Don't smoke
- Reduce or eliminate consumption of coffee (both with caffeine and decaffeinated)

Basically, the dietary and lifestyle recommendations for lowering cholesterol levels are identical to those detailed in Part I of this book. Table 1 provides some simple recommendations, but please read Part I for a more complete discussion.

In many cases, dietary therapy alone is not sufficient to get lipid levels into the desired ranges. Fortunately, there are several natural compounds that can lower cholesterol levels and other significant risk factors for coronary artery disease. In fact, when all factors are considered (cost, safety, effectiveness, etc.), the natural alternatives presented here offer significant advantages over standard drug therapy. The natural products are best utilized in a comprehensive program that stresses a healthy diet and lifestyle.

Conventional Drug Therapy

Conventional drug therapy designed to lower cholesterol levels is prescribed at an alarming rate—nearly thirty million prescriptions per year—due to aggressive marketing by drug companies. The major problem is that these drugs have not yet been shown in long-term studies to extend a person's life span. Several of the drugs are actually associated with an increase in non-cardiovascular mortality. In other words, while these drugs reduced the number of deaths from heart attacks and strokes, they increased the overall death rate.

One of the reasons why cholesterol-lowering drugs may increase overall mortality is that they are toxic to the liver and extremely *carcinogenic* (cancer-causing). An article published in the *Journal of the American Medical Association* (*JAMA*) summarized the carcinogenicity studies of cholesterol-lowering drugs and clearly demonstrated that the risk of carcinogenicity for these drugs is far above recently issued FDA guidelines.[6] The article asked several questions and provided answers that were extremely interesting. Here is an example:

TABLE 1   Food Choices for Lowering Cholesterol Levels

EAT LESS OF THESE	SUBSTITUTE WITH THESE
Red meats	Fish and white meat or poultry
Hamburgers and hot dogs	Soy-based alternatives
Eggs	Egg Beaters and similar products, tofu
High-fat dairy products	Lowfat or nonfat dairy products
Butter, lard, and other saturated fats	Vegetable oils
Ice cream, pie, cake, cookies, etc.	Fruits
Refined cereals, white bread, etc.	Whole grains, whole wheat bread
Fried foods, fatty snack foods	Vegetables, fresh salads
Salt and salty foods	Low sodium, light salt
Coffee and soft drinks	Herbal teas, fresh fruit and vegetable juices

How did it happen that cholesterol-lowering drugs were approved by the FDA for long-term use in spite of their animal carcinogenicity? To address the question, we obtained minutes of the Endocrinologic and Metabolic Drugs Advisory Committee meetings (under the Freedom of Information Act) at which lovastatin and gemfibrozil—the two most popular cholesterol-lowering drugs—were discussed. . . . The only reported discussion of animal carcinogenicity studies at the FDA advisory committee meeting on lovastatin (February 19 and 20, 1987) was by a representative of Merck Sharp & Dohme (makers of the Mevacor brand of lovastatin), who downplayed the importance of the studies.

The minutes from the meeting on gemfibrozil (October 17, 1988) are extremely revealing. The committee did discuss the carcinogenicity of the drug. The minutes state:

Dr. Troendle [deputy director, Division of Metabolism and Endocrine Drug Products for the FDA] noted that gemfibrozil belongs to a class of drugs that has been shown to increase total mortality. It has been shown to have animal carcinogenicity, and she does not believe the FDA has ever approved a drug for long-term prophylactic use that was carcinogenic at such low multiples of the human dose as gemfibrozil.

When asked to vote at the end of the meeting, only three of the nine members of the advisory committee believed the potential benefit of gemfibrozil outweighed the risk. However, the FDA ignored the committee's recommendation and decided to grant gemfibrozil drug approval. Lopid (gemfibrozil) is now the second most popular lipid-lowering drug, behind Mevacor (lovastatin).

The bottom line is that these drugs have been shown to be extremely carcinogenic in animal studies. Although extrapolation of animal data to humans is an uncertain process,

there is enough evidence of carcinogenicity to warrant concern. The authors of the review advised that lipid-lowering drug treatment be avoided except in patients at high risk for an immediate heart attack or stroke. Yet the widespread use of these drugs defies this recommendation.

Niacin

Despite the fact that niacin has demonstrated better overall results than other cholesterol-lowering agents in reducing the risk of coronary heart disease, physicians are often reluctant to prescribe niacin.[7] The reason is a widespread perception that niacin is a difficult and somewhat dangerous medicine. There is much confusion about the benefits versus the risks for patients who take niacin. In contrast, most physicians are unaware of the considerable risks and limited benefits of commonly used prescription cholesterol-lowering agents.

In addition, since niacin is a widely available "generic" agent, no pharmaceutical company stands to generate the huge profits that the other cholesterol-lowering drugs have enjoyed. As a result, niacin is not intensively advertised like the other drugs. Despite the advantages of niacin over the cholesterol-lowering drugs, niacin accounts for only 7.9 percent of all lipid-lowering prescriptions.

The cholesterol-lowering activity of niacin was first described in the 1950s. It is now known that niacin does much more than lower the total cholesterol level. Specifically, niacin has been shown to lower LDL cholesterol, Lp(a), triglyceride, and *fibrinogen* (a blood protein that causes clot formation) levels, while raising HDL cholesterol levels.[8]

An extensive evaluation of cholesterol-lowering drugs (The Coronary Drug Project) demonstrated that niacin was the only cholesterol-lowering agent to actually reduce overall mortality.[7] Its effects are long lasting, as demonstrated in a fifteen-year follow-up study to the Coronary Drug Project. The follow-up study showed that the long-term death rate for patients treated with niacin was actually eleven percent lower than that of the placebo group, even though the treatment had been discontinued in most patients many years earlier. In other words, even though the patients were no longer taking the niacin, they still had a lower death rate. In contrast, patients being treated with cholesterol-lowering drugs (clofibrate and/or cholestyramine) actually experienced an increased death rate.[9] Clofibrate was associated with a thirty-six-percent higher mortality rate. Presumably both clofibrate and cholestyramine lowered cholesterol levels and reduced the mortality rate for coronary artery disease but increased the risk of dying prematurely from cancer, complications of gallbladder surgery (clofibrate causes gallstones), and other conditions.

Clofibrate and, to a lesser extent, cholestyramine have been replaced by drugs such as lovastatin (Mevacor), pravastatin (Pravochol), simvastatin (Zocor), and gemfibrozil (Lopid). Are these newer drugs effective in reducing mortality? The jury is still out. Preliminary studies are showing some benefits. For example, a five-year safety and efficacy study of lovastatin involved 745 patients with severe *hypercholesterolemia* (total cholesterol levels greater than 360 mg/dl). The study demonstrated that the effectiveness of lovastatin was maintained over time, there was no increase in mortality, and lovastatin was generally well tolerated.[10] Longer-term studies with larger patient populations are now in progress with all of the "statin" drugs, but these results will not be available for several years. In the meantime, millions of Americans are being placed on these drugs.

Comparative Studies: Lovastatin vs. Niacin

To evaluate how niacin compares in safety and efficacy to the new lipid-lowering drugs, one need only examine the results of several recent head-to-head comparison studies. In 1994, the *Annals of Internal Medicine* published the first clinical study that directly compared niacin and lovastatin.[11] The twenty-six-week study was performed at five clinics and involved 136 patients who had coronary heart disease and LDL cholesterol levels greater than 160 mg/dl, and/or more than two coronary heart disease risk factors, or an LDL cholesterol level greater than 190 mg/dl without coronary heart disease or with few coronary heart disease risk factors (see HEART and CARIOVASCULAR HEALTH for description of risk factors). Patients were first placed on a four-week diet, after which eligible patients were randomly assigned to receive treatment with either lovastatin (20 mg/day) or niacin (1.5 g/day). On the basis of the LDL cholesterol response and patient tolerance, the doses were sequentially increased after ten and eighteen weeks of treatment, to 40 and 80 mg/day of lovastatin or 3 and 4.5 g/day of niacin, respectively. In the two patient groups, sixty-six percent of patients treated with lovastatin, and fifty-four percent of patients treated with niacin. Here were the results on lipoprotein levels:

GROUP	WEEK 10	WEEK 18	WEEK 26
LDL Cholesterol Reduction			
Lovastatin	26%	28%	32%
Niacin	5%	16%	23%
HDL Cholesterol Increase			
Lovastatin	6%	8%	7%
Niacin	20%	29%	33%
Lp(a) Lipoprotein Reduction			
Lovastatin	0	0	0
Niacin	14%	30%	35%

These results indicate that, while lovastatin produced a greater reduction in LDL cholesterol levels, niacin provided better overall results despite the fact that fewer patients were able to tolerate a full dosage of niacin because of skin flushing. The percentage increase in HDL cholesterol, a more significant indicator for coronary heart disease, was dramatically in favor of niacin (thirty-three percent versus seven percent). Equally as impressive was the percentage decrease in Lp(a) level with niacin treatment. While niacin produced a thirty-five-percent reduction in Lp(a) levels, lovastatin did not produce any effect. Niacin's effect on Lp(a) in this study confirmed a previous study that showed that niacin (4 grams/day) reduced Lp(a) levels by thirty-eight percent.[12]

Another comparative study sought to determine the lipoprotein responses to niacin, gemfibrozil, and lovastatin in patients with normal total cholesterol levels but low levels of HDL cholesterol.[13] The first phase of the study compared lipoprotein responses to lovastatin and gemfibrozil in sixty-one middle-aged men with low HDL levels. In the second phase, thirty-seven patients agreed to take niacin; twenty-seven patients finished this phase at a dose of 4.5 g/day. In the first phase, gemfibrozil therapy increased HDL cholesterol levels by ten percent, and lovastatin by six percent. In the second phase, niacin therapy was shown to raise HDL cholesterol levels by thirty percent.

Dealing with the Side Effects of Niacin

The side effects of niacin are well known. The most common and bothersome side effect is the skin flushing that typically occurs twenty to thirty minutes after the niacin is taken. Other occasional side effects of niacin include gastric irritation, nausea, and liver damage. In an attempt to combat the acute reaction of skin flushing, several manufacturers began marketing "sustained-release," "timed-release," or "slow-release" niacin products. These formulations allow the niacin to be absorbed gradually, thereby reducing the flushing reaction. However, while these forms of niacin reduce skin flushing, they actually have proven to be more toxic to the liver. In a recent study published in *JAMA*, it was strongly recommended that sustained-release niacin be restricted from use because of the high percentage (seventy-eight percent) of patient withdrawal due to side effects; fifty-two percent of the patients who took the sustained-release niacin developed liver toxicity, while none of the patients who took regular niacin developed liver toxicity.[14]

Because niacin can impair blood sugar control, it should be used with close observation in patients with diabetes. Niacin should not be used by patients with preexisting liver disease or elevated levels of liver enzymes. For these patient groups, gugulipid (an extract of *Commiphora mukul*), garlic, or pantethine recommended.

The safest form of niacin at present is known as *inositol hexaniacinate*. This form of niacin has long been used in Europe to lower cholesterol levels and to improve blood flow in cases of intermittent claudication. It yields slightly better results than standard niacin but is much better tolerated, both in terms of flushing and, more important, long-term side effects.[15-17]

Niacin: Some Practical Recommendations

Regardless of the form of niacin being used, periodic checking (every three months, minimum) for cholesterol and liver enzyme levels in the blood is important. Please tell your physician that you are taking niacin and that you wish to be monitored.

Because of its low cost and proven efficacy, niacin should be considered the first cholesterol-lowering agent to try. The problems with niacin (skin flushing and other side effects) can be avoided by using inositol hexaniacinate. Sustained-release niacin should not be used. If pure crystalline niacin is being used, start with a dose of 100 mg three times per day, and carefully increase the dosage over a period of four to six weeks to the full therapeutic dose of 1.5 g to 3 g daily in divided doses. If inositol hexaniacinate is being used, begin with 500 mg three times per day for two weeks, then increase to 1,000 mg. It is best to take either crystalline niacin or inositol hexaniacinate with meals.

Pantethine

Pantethine is the stable form of pantetheine, the active form of vitamin B5, or pantothenic acid. Pantetheine is the most important component of coenzyme A (CoA). This enzyme is involved in the transport of fats to and from cells, as well as to the energy-producing compartments within the cell. Without coenzyme A, the cells of our body would not be able to utilize fats as energy.

For some reason, pantethine has significant lipid-lowering activity, while pantothenic acid has very little (if any) effect in lowering cholesterol and triglyceride levels. Pantethine administration (standard dose: 900 mg per day) has been shown to significantly reduce serum triglyceride levels (by thirty-two percent), total cholesterol levels (by nineteen percent), and LDL cholesterol levels (by twenty-one percent), while increasing HDL cholesterol levels (by twenty-three percent).[18,19] These effects are most impressive when the toxicity of pantethine (virtually none) is compared to that of conventional lipid-lowering drugs. Pantethine acts by in-

hibiting cholesterol synthesis and accelerating the utilization of fat as an energy source. There appears to be no toxicity or side effects from taking pantethine.

Of the four natural lipid-lowering agents discussed in this chapter, pantethine has the best effect on blood triglyceride levels. Therefore, it is quite useful for individuals who primarily have elevated triglyceride levels. Pantethine is also appropriate for treating diabetics, since niacin is associated with impairment of insulin action. Several clinical studies have shown that pantethine produces impressive lipid-lowering effects without side effects in diabetics.[20-22]

The dosage for pantethine is 300 mg three times per day. It has an excellent safety profile, and no significant side effects have been reported in the clinical trials.

Vitamin C and Cholesterol

Dozens of population-based and clinical studies have shown that vitamin C levels correspond with total cholesterol and HDL cholesterol levels.[23-26] In one of the best-designed studies, it was shown that the higher the vitamin C content of the blood, the lower the total cholesterol and triglyceride levels and the higher the HDL cholesterol level.[26] The beneficial effects on HDL levels were particularly impressive. For each 0.5 mg/dl increase in vitamin C content of the blood, there was an increase in HDL cholesterol of 14.9 mg/dl in women and 2.1 mg/dl in men. Remember, for every one-percent increase in HDL cholesterol level, the risk of heart disease drops four percent. This study and others demonstrate that vitamin C supplementation increases HDL levels even in well-nourished individuals with normal levels of vitamin C in their blood. The most significant effect of high-dosage vitamin C therapy in reducing the risk of heart disease may turn out to be a reduction in Lp(a) and its antioxidant activity.

Garlic

Although garlic exerts a broad spectrum of beneficial effects, the modern use of garlic has focused on its ability to lower blood pressure and cholesterol levels, in the attempt to reduce the risk of dying prematurely from a heart attack or stroke.

The volatile compounds of garlic are generally considered to be responsible for most of the pharmacological properties.[27] Fresh garlic contains 0.1 to 0.36 percent of a volatile oil composed of sulfur-containing compounds: alliin, allicin, diallyl disulfide, diallyl trisulfide, and others. *Allicin* is mainly responsible for the pungent odor of garlic, as well as its pharmacology. Allicin is formed by the action of the enzyme alliinase on the compound alliin. The essential oil of garlic yields approximately sixty percent of its weight in allicin after exposure to alliinase. The enzyme alliinase is inactivated by heat, which accounts for the fact that cooked garlic produces neither as strong an odor as raw garlic nor nearly as powerful physiological effects.[27]

Commercial Garlic Preparations

The majority of studies that showed a positive effect from administering garlic and garlic preparations used a form a garlic that delivers a sufficient dosage of allicin.[27] Since allicin is the component of garlic that is responsible for its easily identifiable odor, some manufacturers have developed highly sophisticated methods of providing the full benefits of garlic; they provide "odorless" garlic products concentrated for alliin because alliin is relatively odorless until it is converted to allicin in the body. Products concentrated for alliin and other sulfur components provide all of the benefits of fresh garlic but are more "socially acceptable." Based on a great deal of clinical research, the recommendation is that a commercial garlic product should provide a daily dose of at least 10 mg of alliin, or a total allicin potential of 4,000 mcg. The German Commission E, an expert panel that sets dosage requirements to allow for therapeutic claims in Germany, requires that products deliver the equivalent of 4,000 mg of fresh garlic—roughly one to four cloves.

Manufacturers of garlic products all tout their preparation as being the best. How do you know who to believe? First of all, preparations standardized for alliin content are viewed by most garlic experts as the most beneficial. However, there are other compounds in garlic that exert beneficial effects, including S-allylcysteines and gamma-glutamylpeptides. Therefore, the best product would be one that is rich in all garlic compounds and most resembles fresh garlic.

What about aged garlic? It is interesting that the expert panel of the German Commission E specified that the daily dose of garlic be equivalent to fresh, raw garlic. Since aged garlic preparations do not contain the beneficial compounds found in fresh garlic, they do not meet the Commission E monograph guidelines and cannot be marketed in Germany with the claims allowed for garlic. The Commission E was very specific: the daily dosage recommended to achieve the benefits linked to garlic requires the equivalent of 4,000 mg of fresh garlic.

To highlight the superiority of fresh garlic preparations over aged garlic, let's examine the results of the effects of both on blood pressure and cholesterol and triglyceride levels.

	AGED GARLIC	FRESH GARLIC PREPARATIONS
Total cholesterol	7% reduction	10–12% reduction
LDL cholesterol	4% reduction	15% reduction
HDL cholesterol	no effect	10% increase
Systolic blood pressure	5 mm Hg reduction	11 mm Hg reduction
Diastolic blood pressure	no effect	5 mm Hg reduction
Daily dosage	7.2 grams	>4,000 mcg of allicin

The data for aged garlic in the preceding table are based on a recently completed double-blind study of forty-one men with beginning cholesterol levels in the 220- to 290-mg/dl range.[28] The men received either aged garlic (7.2 grams per day!) or a placebo for six months and then were switched to the other supplement for an additional four months. The results demonstrated a reduction of total cholesterol of seven percent, and LDL cholesterol of four percent, but no changes in HDL cholesterol or triglyceride levels were noted. The systolic blood pressure dropped an average of 5.5 percent during the aged-garlic period, but there was no change in diastolic blood pressure.

Now let's take a look at the effect of fresh garlic preparations in similar patient populations. Numerous double-blind placebo-controlled studies have been performed on patients with initial cholesterol levels greater than 200 mg/dl. Supplementation with commercial preparations that provided a daily dose of at least 10 mg of alliin, or a total allicin potential of 4,000 mcg, were found to lower total serum cholesterol levels by about ten to twelve percent. LDL cholesterol levels decreased by about fifteen percent, HDL cholesterol levels usually increased by about ten percent, and triglyceride levels typically dropped fifteen percent.[29–33] These results

were generally achieved within one to three months; significantly better results are achieved in a shorter amount of time with the fresh garlic preparations compared to aged garlic.

Blood pressure reductions have also been greater when using fresh garlic preparations than when using aged garlic. With fresh garlic preparations, typical reductions of 11 mm Hg for the systolic and 5.0 in the diastolic are usually achieved within a one- to three-month period.[27,34]

It has been concluded in expert reviews that the anti-atherosclerotic effects of garlic are derived from alliin and allicin.[27,35] The bottom line is that preparations standardized for alliin content provide the greatest assurance of quality.

Garlic and Heart Disease

A garlic supplement may not be necessary if the dietary intake of garlic and onion can be increased.[36,37] In a 1979 population study, researchers studied three populations of vegetarians in the Jain community of India who consumed differing amounts of garlic and onions.[38] Numerous favorable effects on blood lipids were observed in the group that consumed the largest amounts of both, as shown in Table 2. Blood fibrinogen levels were highest in the group that ate no onions or garlic. This study is quite significant because the subjects had nearly identical diets, except in their levels of garlic and onion ingestion.

Gugulipid

Gugulipid is the standardized extract of the mukul myrrh tree (*Commiphora mukul*), native to India. The active components of gugulipid are two compounds: Z-guggulsterone and E-guggulsterone. Several clinical

TABLE 2 Effects of Garlic and Onion Consumption on Serum Lipids with Carefully Matched Diets		
GARLIC/ONION CONSUMPTION	**CHOLESTEROL**	**TRIGLYCERIDE**
Garlic 50 g/wk, onion 600 g/wk	159 mg/dl	52 mg/dl
Garlic 10 g/wk, onion 200 g/wk	172 mg/dl	75 mg/dl
No garlic or onions	208 mg/dl	109 mg/dl

studies have confirmed that gugulipid has an ability to lower both cholesterol and triglyceride levels.[39,40] Typically, total cholesterol levels dropped fourteen to twenty-seven percent in a four- to twelve-week period, while LDL cholesterol and triglyceride levels dropped from twenty-five to thirty-five percent and twenty-two to thirty percent, respectively. HDL cholesterol levels typically increased by sixteen to twenty percent.

The effect of gugulipid on cholesterol and triglyceride levels is comparable to that of lipid-lowering drugs. While those drugs are associated with some degree of toxicity, gugulipid is without side effects. Safety studies in rats, rabbits, and monkeys have demonstrated it to be nontoxic. It is also considered safe to use during pregnancy.

The mechanism of gugulipid's cholesterol-lowering action is its ability to increase the liver's metabolism of LDL cholesterol.[39]

In addition to lowering lipid levels, gugulipid has been shown in animals to prevent atherosclerosis and aid in the regression of preexisting atherosclerotic plaques. This implies that it may have a similar effect in humans. Gugulipid also has a mild effect in inhibiting platelet aggregation and promoting fibrinolysis, implying that it may also prevent the development of a stroke or embolism.[39]

The dosage of gugulipid is based on its guggulsterone content. Clinical studies have demonstrated that gugulipid extract, standardized to contain to 25 mg of guggulsterone per 500 mg tablet, given three times per day is an effective treatment for elevated cholesterol levels, elevated triglyceride levels, or both. No significant side effects have been reported with purified gugulipid preparations, but crude guggul preparations such as gum guggul are associated with side effects (skin rashes, diarrhea, etc.)

TREATMENT SUMMARY

In addition to diet and lifestyle measures, there are a number of natural compounds that can effectively improve cholesterol and triglyceride levels. Of the four described above (niacin, garlic, gugulipid, and pantethine), niacin in the form of inositol hexaniacinate produces the best overall effect.

In addition to the recommendations given in the chapter HEART DISEASE AND CARDIOVASCULAR HEALTH, we recommend beginning therapy with the following:

- Flaxseed oil: 1 tablespoon daily
- Niacin (as inositol hexaniacinate): 500 mg three times per day with meals for

two weeks, then increase dosage to 1,000 mg three times per day with meals

- Garlic: minimum of 4,000 mcg of allicin per day

Within the first two months, this program will typically produce reductions in total cholesterol level of 50 to 75 mg/dl in patients with initial total cholesterol levels above 250 mg/dl. In cases in which the initial cholesterol level is above 300 mg/dl, it may take four to six months before cholesterol levels begin to reach recommended levels. Once the cholesterol level is reduced below 200 mg/dl, reduce the dosage of niacin to 500 mg three times per day for two months. If the cholesterol levels creep up above 200 mg/dl, then raise the dosage of niacin back to 1,000 mg three times per day. If the cholesterol level remains below 200 mg/dl, then withdraw the niacin completely and check the cholesterol levels in two months. Reinstitute niacin therapy if levels creep up over 200 mg/dl. Garlic and flaxseed oil supplementation can be continued indefinitely, if desired.

Gugulipid can be added to the above protocol if, after four months, the total cholesterol level remains above 250 mg/dl. Gugulipid is also suitable for the rare patient who cannot tolerate inositol hexaniacinate.

Pantethine is recommended primarily to diabetics and patients who have elevated triglyceride levels. Although there are no data showing that inositol hexaniacinate affects blood sugar levels, niacin is known to adversely affect blood sugar control in some diabetics. As stated above, pantethine has demonstrated excellent effects in diabetics. It not only improves cholesterol and triglyceride levels; it also normalizes platelet lipid composition and function and blood viscosity.[15]

In regard to elevations in Lp(a), both niacin and vitamin C have shown an ability to drop Lp(a) levels dramatically (thirty-five- and twenty-seven-percent reductions, respectively). In addition, it is important to rule out low thyroid function (hypothyroidism) in all cases of elevated blood lipids, especially Lp(a).

TABLE 3　Comparative Effects of Natural Compounds on Cholesterol and Triglyceride Lipids				
	NIACIN	GARLIC	GUGULIPID	PANTETHINE
Total cholesterol (% decrease)	18	10	24	19
LDL cholesterol (% decrease)	23	15	30	21
HDL cholesterol (% increase)	32	31	16	23
Triglycerides (% decrease)	26	13	23	32

Chronic Fatigue Syndrome

Mild fever

Recurrent sore throat

Painful lymph nodes

Muscle weakness

Muscle pain

Prolonged fatigue after exercise

Recurrent headache

Migratory joint pain

Depression

Sleep disturbance (excessive sleep requirements or insomnia)

Chronic fatigue syndrome (CFS) is a newly defined syndrome that describes varying combinations of symptoms, including recurrent fatigue, sore throat, low-grade fever, lymph node swelling, headache, muscle and joint pain, intestinal discomfort, emotional distress and/or depression, and loss of concentration.

Although newly defined and currently receiving a great deal of attention, CFS is not a new disease at all. References to similar conditions in the medical literature go back as far as the 1860s. In the past, chronic fatigue syndrome has been known by a variety of names, including: chronic mononucleosis-like syndrome or chronic EBV syndrome, Yuppie flu, postviral fatigue syndrome, postinfectious neuromyasthenia, chronic fatigue and immune dysfunction syndrome (CFIDS), Iceland disease, Royal Free Hospital disease, and many more. In addition, symptoms of chronic fatigue syndrome mirror symptoms of neurasthenia, a condition first described in 1869.

Definition

In response to the growing interest, chronic fatigue syndrome was formally defined in 1988 by a consensus panel convened by the Centers for Disease Control (CDC). Their definition was an attempt to establish a guide for evaluating patients with chronic fatigue of unknown cause by clinical physicians and researchers.[1]

A formal (and controversial) set of diagnostic criteria was established by the CDC. These criteria are controversial for many reasons, including the fact that psychological symptoms are both a minor criterion as well as potential grounds for exclusion. One of the major complaints from physicians about the CDC definition is that it appears better suited for research than for clinical purposes. A major problem with the CDC criteria is that they ignore many of the common symptoms reported by patients with CFS (see Table 1).

CDC DIAGNOSTIC CRITERIA FOR CHRONIC FATIGUE SYNDROME

Major Criteria

New onset of fatigue causing fifty percent reduction in activity for at least six months

Exclusion of other illnesses that can cause fatigue

Minor criteria

Presence of eight of the eleven symptoms listed, or presence of six of the eleven symptoms and two of the three signs listed.

Symptoms

1. Mild fever
2. Recurrent sore throat
3. Painful lymph nodes
4. Muscle weakness
5. Muscle pain
6. Prolonged fatigue after exercise
7. Recurrent headache
8. Migratory joint pain
9. Neurological or psychological complaints
   Sensitivity to bright light
   Forgetfulness
   Confusion
   Inability to concentrate
   Excessive irritability
   Depression
10. Sleep disturbance (hypersomnia or insomnia)
11. Sudden onset of symptom complex

Signs

1. Low-grade fever
2. Nonexudative pharyngitis
3. Palpable or tender lymph nodes

The British and Australian criteria for the diagnosis of CFS are less strict than the CDC definition.[2] In particular, the minor diagnostic criteria are not required, and the major diagnostic criteria is not as strict. For example, in the Australian definition the major criterion is simply fatigue at a level that disrupts daily activities in the absence of other medical conditions associated with fatigue.

QUICK REVIEW

- A disturbed immune system plays a central role in chronic fatigue syndrome (CFS).

- Fibromyalgia and multiple chemical sensitivity disorder have symptoms similar to those of CFS.

- Chronic fatigue can be caused by a variety of physical and psychological factors other than the chronic fatigue syndrome.

- A person's energy level and emotional state are determined by interplay between two primary factors: internal focus and physiology.

- One of the most common findings in individuals with impaired immune function is gastrointestinal overgrowth of *Candida albicans*.

TABLE 1 Frequency of Symptoms in CFS	
SYMPTOM/SIGN	**FREQUENCY (%)**
Fatigue	100
Low-grade fever	60–95
Muscle pain	20–95
Sleep disorder	15–90
Impaired mental function	50–85
Depression	70–85
Headache	35–85
Allergies	55–80
Sore throat	50–75
Anxiety	50–70
Muscle weakness	40–70
After-exercise fatigue	50–60
Premenstrual syndrome (women)	50–60
Stiffness	50–60
Visual blurring	50–60
Nausea	50–60
Dizziness	30–50
Joint pain	40–50
Dry eyes and mouth	30–40
Diarrhea	30–40
Cough	30–40
Decreased appetite	30–40
Night sweats	30–40
Painful lymph nodes	30–40

Using the CDC criteria, the frequency of CFS in individuals suffering from chronic fatigue (a larger classification of all causes of chronic fatigue) in the United States is thought to be about 11.5 percent; using British criteria the frequency is about 15 percent; and according to Australian criteria, about 38 percent.[2]

Causes

Many research studies have focused on identifying an infectious agent as the cause of CFS. The Epstein-Barr virus (EBV) emerged as the leading, yet controversial, candidate.[3–7] EBV is a member of the Herpes group of viruses, which includes *Herpes simplex* Types 1 and 2, *Varicella zoster* virus, *Cytomegalovirus*, and *Pseudorabies* virus. A common aspect of these viruses is their ability to establish a lifelong latent infection after the initial infection. This latent infection is kept in check by a normal immune system. When the immune system is compromised in any way, these viruses can become active as viral

- As far back as 1930, chronic fatigue was recognized as a key feature of food allergies.
- The mind and attitude play a critical role in determining the status of the immune system and energy levels.
- A deficiency of virtually any nutrient can produce the symptoms of fatigue and render the body more susceptible to infection.

- Breathing with the diaphragm, good posture, and bodywork (massage, spinal manipulation, etc.) are all important in helping to relieve the stress that is a common contributor to fatigue.
- Siberian ginseng has been shown to exert a number of beneficial effects that may be useful in the treatment of CFS.
- Successful treatment of CFS requires a comprehensive approach.

replication and spread increased. This situation is commonly observed with Herpes virus infections, especially in immunocompromised individuals such as those with AIDS, cancer, or drug-induced suppression of immune function.

Infection with EBV is inevitable among humans. By the end of early adulthood, almost all individuals demonstrate detectable antibodies in their blood to the Epstein-Barr virus, indicating past infection. When the primary infection occurs in childhood, there are usually no symptoms, but when it occurs in adolescence or early adulthood, the clinical manifestations of infectious mononucleosis develop in approximately fifty percent of the cases.

Although reports of a prolonged or recurrent mononucleosis-like syndrome began appearing in the 1940s and 1950s, it wasn't until the 1980s that evidence implicated EBV in this broad clinical spectrum of chronic fatigue and associated symptoms. Numerous studies have now demonstrated persistently elevated *titers* (levels) of serum antibodies against the Epstein-Barr virus in a number of patients who have the symptom pattern of this syndrome (specifically, anti-EBV capsid antibody titers greater than 1:80).

A careful study of 134 patients who had undergone EBV antibody testing because of suspected chronic mononucleosis-like syndrome found mixed results about the importance of EBV infection.[8] Fifteen patients identified as having severe, persistent fatigue of unknown origin were compared with the remaining 119, who had less severe illness, and with thirty age- and race-matched controls. The more seriously ill patients generally had higher levels of EBV antibodies than did the comparison groups, and, interestingly, they also demonstrated higher antibody titers to *Cytomegalovirus*, *Herpes simplex* viruses Types 1 and 2, and measles. This led the researchers to conclude that "some patients with these illnesses (syndromes of chronic fatigue) may have an abnormality of infectious and/or immunological origin" and that there remain "questions concerning the relationship between CFS and EBV."

Current knowledge about EBV infection can be summarized as follows:

1. EBV and the Herpes group of viruses produce latent lifelong infections.

2. The host's immune system normally holds the latent infection in check.

3. Any compromise in the immune system can lead to the reactivation of the virus and recurrent infection.

4. The infection itself can compromise and/or disrupt immunity, thereby leading to other diseases.

5. Elevated EBV antibody levels are observed in a significant number of diseases characterized by disorders in immune function.

6. Elevated antibody levels to the Herpes-group viruses, measles, and other viruses have also been observed in patients suspected of having chronic fatigue and who also display elevated EBV antibody titers.

EBV antibody testing (and antibody testing for other Herpes-group viruses and measles) may be useful as a measure of immune function and overall host resistance but should not be relied upon for diagnosis of CFS.

Other Infectious Agents

In addition to EBV, a number of other viruses have been investigated as possible causes of CFS. This search for a viral agent is consistent with the mainstream medical approach of focusing on the infectious organism rather than on reducing susceptibility and supporting the individual's immune system to deal with the organism effectively.[3-5]

ORGANISMS PROPOSED AS CAUSATIVE AGENTS IN CFS

Epstein-Barr virus

Human herpes virus-6

Inoue-Melnich virus

Brucella

Borrelia bugdorferi

Giardia lamblia

Cytomegalovirus

Enterovirus

Retrovirus

Immune System Abnormalities

There is little argument that a disturbed immune system plays a central role in CFS. A variety of immune system abnormalities have been reported in CFS patients. While no specific immunological dysfunction pattern has been recognized, the most consistent abnormality is a decreased number or activity of natural killer (NK) cells.[3,4,9,10] NK cells received their name because of their ability to destroy cells that have become cancerous or infected with viruses. In fact, for a time CFS was also referred to as low natural killer cell syndrome (LNKS).

Other consistent findings include a reduced ability of lymphocytes (a type of white blood cell that is critical in the battle against viruses) to respond to stimuli.[10] One of the reasons for this lack of response may be a reduced activity or decreased production of interferon, a key compound produced by the body to fight viruses. While both low and high levels of interferon have been reported in CFS, levels are depressed in most cases. When interferon levels are low, reactivation of latent viral infection is likely. Conversely,

when interferon levels are high, (as well as other chemical mediators, such as interleukin-1), many of the symptoms may be related to the higher levels of interferon. When interferon is used as a therapy for cancer and viral hepatitis, the side effects produced are similar to the symptoms of CFS.

IMMUNOLOGICAL ABNORMALITIES REPORTED FOR CFS

Elevated levels of antibodies to viral proteins

Decreased natural killer cell activity

Low or elevated antibody levels

Decreased levels of circulating immune complexes

Increased cytokine (e.g., interleukin-2) levels

Increased or decreased interferon levels

Altered helper/suppressor T-cell ratio

Fibromyalgia and multiple chemical sensitivities

Fibromyalgia (FM) and multiple chemical sensitivities (MCS) are, like CFS, recently recognized disorders with a substantial overlap of symptomatology.[3,4,11-13] The only difference in diagnostic criteria for fibromyalgia and CFS is the requirement of musculoskeletal pain in fibromyalgia and fatigue in CFS. The likelihood of being diagnosed as having fibromyalgia or CFS is dependent upon the type of physician consulted. Specifically, if a rheumatologist or orthopedic specialist is consulted, the patient is more likely to be diagnosed with fibromyalgia (see the chapter FIBROMYALGIA for more information).

One group of researchers carefully compared the symptomatology of ninety patients who had been diagnosed as having CFS, MCS, or FM (thirty in each category).[13] Utilizing the same questionnaire for all ninety patients, seventy percent of the patients diagnosed with FM and thirty percent of those diagnosed with MCS met the Centers for Disease Control criteria for CFS. Particularly significant was the observation that eighty percent of both the FM and MCS patients met the CFS criterion of fatigue lasting more than six months with a fifty percent reduction in activity. More than fifty percent of the CFS and FM patients reported adverse reactions to various chemicals.

Other Causes of Chronic Fatigue

Chronic fatigue can be caused by a variety of physical and psychological factors other than the chronic fatigue syndrome. The accompanying box lists the major causes of chronic fatigue in decreasing order, according to how common the cause is among sufferers of chronic fatigue in the general population. The list is based on the findings of several large studies as well as the authors' clinical experience.

MAJOR CAUSES OF CHRONIC FATIGUE

Preexisting physical condition
  Diabetes
  Heart disease
  Lung disease
  Rheumatoid arthritis
  Chronic inflammation
  Chronic pain
  Cancer
  Liver disease
  Multiple sclerosis
Prescription drugs
  Antihypertensives
  Anti-inflammatory agents
  Birth control pills
  Antihistamines
  Corticosteroids
Tranquilizers and sedatives
Depression
Stress/Low adrenal function
Impaired liver function and/or environmental illness
Impaired immune function
  Chronic fatigue syndrome
  Chronic candida infection
  Other chronic infections
Food allergies
Hypothyroidism
Hypoglycemia
Anemia and nutritional deficiencies
Sleep disturbances
Unknown cause

Therapeutic Considerations

Since chronic fatigue and CFS generally involve many factors, the therapeutic approach typically involves multiple therapies that address different facets of the clinical picture. Breaking it down into simplistic terms, a person's energy level and emotional state are determined by interplay between two primary factors: internal focus and physiology. Internal focus refers to images held up before the mind's eye as well as our "self-talk"—the constant dialog our conscious mind has with our subconscious mind. Physiology refers to the functioning of the body and how it is affected by physical posture, breathing, nutrition, hormonal status, and other physical factors.

Let's take a look at the typical internal focus and physiology in the patient with CFS. Most people with chronic fatigue focus on how tired they are. They repeatedly reaffirm their fatigue to themselves and to anyone who will listen. This imprint on the subconscious mind must be reversed in order for energy levels to be significantly uplifted. The physiology of typical CFS patients includes alterations not only in the chemicals and hormones floating around in the body, but also in the way they hold their body (usually slouched) and the way they breathe (shallowly). In most patients with chronic fatigue, both the mind and the body need to be addressed. The most effective treatment is a comprehensive program that is designed to help CFS patients use their mind, attitude, and physiology to fuel higher energy.

Underlying Factors

There are a number of underlying factors that must be addressed in the effective treatment of CFS. Most notably: depression, stress, impaired detoxification, excessive gut permeability (see DIGESTION for more information), impaired immune function, chronic candidiasis, food allergies, hypothyroidism, hypoglycemia, and low adrenal function.

Depression

The first factor to address is any underlying depression. Depression is one of the major causes of chronic fatigue, and it is one of the common features of CFS. In the absence of a preexisting physical condition, depression is generally regarded as the most common cause of chronic fatigue. However, it is often difficult to determine whether the depression preceded the fatigue or vice versa. Depression is fully discussed in the DEPRESSION chapter.

Stress

Stress is another factor to consider in chronic fatigue or CFS. Stress can be the underlying factor in the patient with depression, low immune function, or other causes of chronic fatigue. Please see the chapter STRESS Management, and Adrenal Support for assessing the role of stress in chronic fatigue and CFS.

Impaired Detoxification

Exposure to food additives, solvents (cleaning materials, formaldehyde, toluene, benzene, etc.), pesticides, herbicides, heavy metals (lead, mercury, cadmium, arsenic, nickel, and aluminum), and other toxins can greatly stress liver and detoxification processes. This exposure can lead to a condition labeled by many naturopathic and nutrition-oriented physicians as the "congested liver" or "sluggish liver," or the more recently coined "impaired hepatic detoxification." These terms signify a reduced ability of the liver to detoxify.

Among the other symptoms people with a sluggish liver may complain of are depression, general malaise, headaches, digestive disturbances, allergies and chemical sensitivities, premenstrual syndrome, and constipation.

An interesting multiclinic research study of chronically ill patients, many of whom were diagnosed as suffering from CFS, evaluated the efficacy of a comprehensive detoxification program. Patients were placed on a hypoallergenic diet and provided a dietary food supplement rich in nutrients that facilitate liver detoxification. The patients reported a fifty-two-percent reduction in symptoms after ten weeks, and symptom improvement was mirrored by normalization of liver detoxification mechanisms.[14]

For more information on ways to enhance detoxification, see the chapter DETOXIFICATION.

Impaired Immune Function and/or Chronic Infection

When the immune system is impaired, infections can linger and fatigue may persist. There is a good reason for fatigue during an infection; fatigue is the body's response mechanism to infection because the immune system works best when the body is at rest.

In order to determine the role that the immune system is playing in the individual with

CFS, answer the the series of questions listed in the accompanying box.

QUESTIONNAIRE FOR RECOGNITION OF IMPAIRED IMMUNE FUNCTION

Do you get more than two colds per year?

When you catch a cold, does it take more than five to seven days to get rid of the symptoms?

Have you ever had infectious mononucleosis?

Do you have herpes?

Do you suffer from chronic infections of any kind?

Chronic Candida Infection

One of the most common findings in individuals with impaired immune function is gastrointestinal overgrowth of *Candida albicans*. Candidal overgrowth is now becoming recognized as a complex medical syndrome, also known as "the yeast syndrome" and "chronic candidiasis." This overgrowth is believed to cause a wide variety of symptoms in virtually every system of the body, with the gastrointestinal, genitourinary, endocrine, nervous, and immune systems being the most susceptible. Fill out the questionnaire in CANDIDIASIS, CHRONIC to determine if candida is a factor in your case.

Food Allergies

As far back as 1930, chronic fatigue was recognized as a key feature of food allergies.[15] Originally, Albert Rowe, M.D., one of the foremost allergists of this century, described a syndrome known as "allergic toxemia" that included the symptoms of fatigue, muscle and joint aches, drowsiness, difficulty in concentration, nervousness, and depression. Around the 1950s, this syndrome began to be referred to as the "allergic tension-fatigue syndrome."[16] With the current focus on CFS, many physicians and others are forgetting that food allergies can lead to chronic fatigue.

Furthermore, between fifty-five and eighty-five percent of individuals with CFS have allergies. For more information on food allergies, see FOOD ALLERGY.

Hypothyroidism

Hypothyroidism is a common cause of chronic fatigue. However, the condition is often overlooked. The reason may be the reliance on standard blood measurements of thyroid hormone levels as the method of diagnosis.[17–19] Undiagnosed hypothyroidism is a serious concern, as failure to treat such a critical underlying problem will reduce the effectiveness of all other measures designed to increase energy levels. For more information, see HYPOTHYROIDISM.

Hypoglycemia

The association between hypoglycemia and fatigue is well known. What is not as well known is the effect that hypoglycemia plays in contributing to depression. Numerous studies have shown that depressed individuals suffer from hypoglycemia.[20,21] Since depression is the most common cause of chronic fatigue, hypoglycemia must always be considered as an underlying factor (see HYPOGLYCEMIA).

Low Adrenal Function

The *adrenal glands* are two small glands that lie on top of the kidneys and secrete important hormones such as *adrenaline* and *cortisol*. Low adrenal function was first proposed as a cause of chronic fatigue over fifty years ago.[22] A small but growing body of evidence now supports the role of low or altered adrenal function in CFS.[23] One of the major symptoms of low or altered adrenal function is debilitating fatigue. Low adrenal function is also characterized by a stressful event, followed by feverishness, joint pain, muscle ache, swollen lymph glands, fatigue, worsening of allergic responses, and disturbances of mood and sleep. These symptoms are strikingly similar to those of CFS. Enhancing adrenal function, as detailed in the chapter STRESS MANAGEMENT, is an important goal in CFS.

Mind and Attitude

The mind and attitude play a critical role in determining the status of the immune system and energy levels. Many patients who have chronic fatigue (including CFS) are either depressed or seem to have lost a sense of enthusiasm for life. Of course, it's not easy to have a lot of enthusiasm when a person does not have much energy. But the two usually go hand in hand.

The first step in overcoming CFS is for the person with CFS to realize that it is possible to get better. Many people with CFS are told that it is "something they will have to live with" and that "there is no cure." Achieving or maintaining a positive mental attitude is critical to good health and high energy levels, especially in CFS. In order to achieve a positive state of mind, a person needs to exercise or condition the attitude, much like the way in which one would condition the body. To help in this process, practice the mental exercises—visualizations, goal setting, affirmations, and empowering questions—that are detailed in the chapter A POSITIVE MENTAL ATTITUDE.

Diet

Energy level appears to be directly related to the quality of the foods routinely ingested. Adhere to the dietary guidelines given in the chapter A Health-Promoting Diet. It is especially important to eliminate or restrict intake of refined sugar and caffeine. Sugar is a major contributor to hypoglycemia, and caffeine

stresses the adrenal glands. Although caffeine consumption provides temporary stimulation, regular caffeine intake may actually lead to chronic fatigue. While mice fed one dose of caffeine demonstrated significant increases in their swimming capacity, when the dose of caffeine was given for six weeks, a significant decrease in swimming capacity was observed.[24]

Be aware that abrupt cessation of coffee drinking will probably result in symptoms of caffeine withdrawal, including fatigue, headache, and an intense desire for coffee.[25] Fortunately, this withdrawal period doesn't last more than a few days.

Supplementation

Nutritional supplementation is essential in the treatment of chronic fatigue. A deficiency of virtually any nutrient can produce the symptoms of fatigue and render the body more susceptible to infection. Individuals with chronic fatigue require at the bare minimum: a high-potency multiple-vitamin-and-mineral formula, along with extra vitamin C (3,000 mg per day in divided doses) and magnesium (500 to 1,200 mg in divided doses).

Magnesium

An underlying magnesium deficiency, even if very mild, can result in chronic fatigue and symptoms similar to CFS. In addition, low red blood cell magnesium levels, a more accurate measure of magnesium status than routine blood analysis, have been found in many patients with chronic fatigue and CFS. Several studies have shown good results with magnesium supplementation.

For example, in one double-blind placebo-controlled trial, thirty-two CFS patients received either an intramuscular injection of magnesium sulfate (1 gram in 2 ml of injectable water) or a placebo (2 ml of injectable water) for six weeks. At the end of the study, twelve of the fifteen patients receiving magnesium reported, based on strict criteria, significantly improved energy levels, better emotional states, and less pain. In contrast, only three of seventeen placebo patients reported that they felt better, and only one reported an improved energy level.[26]

This study seems to confirm some impressive results obtained in clinical trials during the 1960s on patients suffering from chronic fatigue.[27–30] These studies utilized oral magnesium and potassium aspartate (1 gram each) rather than injectable magnesium. Between seventy-five and ninety-one percent of the nearly three thousand patients studied experienced relief of fatigue during treatment with the magnesium and potassium aspartate. In contrast, the number of patients responding to a placebo was between nine and twenty-six percent. The beneficial effect was usually noted after only four to five days, but sometimes ten days were required. Patients usually continued treatment for four to six weeks; afterward fatigue frequently did not return.

Injectable magnesium is not necessary to restore magnesium status.[31] Absorption studies indicate that magnesium is easily absorbed orally when it is bound to aspartate or citrate. In addition, both of these compounds may also help fight off fatigue. Aspartate feeds into the *Krebs cycle,* the final common pathway for the conversion of glucose, fatty acids, and amino acids to chemical energy (adenosine triphosphate, or ATP), while citrate is itself a component of the Krebs cycle. Krebs cycle components, including aspartate, citrate, fumarate, malate, and succinate, usually provide a better form of a mineral supplement; evidence suggests that minerals bound (chelated) to the Krebs cycle intermediates are better absorbed, utilized, and tolerated compared to inorganic or relatively insoluble mineral salts, including magnesium chloride, oxide, or carbonate.[31,32]

Other Therapies

Breathing, Posture, and Bodywork

Proper care of the body is critical to high energy levels. Breathing with the diaphragm, good posture, and bodywork (massage, spinal manipulation, etc.) are all important in helping to relieve the stress that is a common contributor to fatigue.

Exercise

Exercise alone has been demonstrated to have a tremendous impact on improving mood and the ability to handle stressful life situations.[33] Regular exercise has also been shown to lead to improved immune status. For CFS patients, regular exercise has been shown to lead to a significant increase (up to 100 percent) in natural killer cell activity.[34,35] Although more strenuous exercise is required to benefit the cardiovascular system, light to moderate exercise may be best for the immune system. One study found that immune function was significantly increased by the practice of Tai Chi exercises.[36] Tai Chi is a martial arts technique that features the movement from one posture to the next in a flowing motion resembling dance. The research thus far suggests that light to moderate exercise stimulates the immune system, while intense exercise (e.g., training for the Olympics) can have the opposite effect.[37]

Botanical Medicine

Siberian Ginseng (*Eleutherococcus senticosus***)** In addition to supporting adrenal function and acting to increase the resistance to stress, Siberian ginseng has been shown to exert a number of beneficial effects on immune function that may be useful in the treatment of CFS. In one double-blind study, thirty-six healthy subjects received either 10 ml of a fluid extract of Siberian ginseng or a placebo daily for four weeks.[38] The group receiving the Siberian ginseng demonstrated significant improvements in a variety of immune system parameters. Most notable were a significant increase in T-helper cells and an increase in natural killer cell activity—both of which are of value in the treatment of CFS.

Licorice *(Glycyrrhiza glabra)* Considering the possible roles of viral infection and low adrenal function in CFS, licorice root with its antiviral and adrenal supportive properties would seem to be an ideal botanical for this condition. Unfortunately, licorice therapy has not been rigorously evaluated, although an excellent response in a single patient has been reported.[39]

The main hazard of licorice use is that it may cause sodium and water retention, resulting in high blood pressure, if ingested regularly at a dosage of 3 grams of licorice root per day for more than six weeks.[40] Monitoring of blood pressure is suggested. Prevention of the blood pressure–raising effects of licorice may be possible by following a high-potassium, low-sodium diet. Although no formal trial has been performed, patients who normally consume high-potassium foods and restrict sodium intake, even those with high blood pressure and angina, have been reported to be free from the blood pressure–raising effects of licorice.[41]

TREATMENT SUMMARY

Successful treatment of CFS requires a comprehensive approach. Especially important is identifying underlying factors which may be impacting energy levels or the immune system. Special attention should be given the advice on immune support in the chapter IMMUNE SUPPORT.

Diet

Identify and control food allergies. Increase your consumption of water while eliminating consumption of caffeine containing drinks and alcohol. Adopt a diet of whole, organically grown foods. Control hypoglycemia through the elimination of sugar and other refined foods and the regular consumption of small meals and snacks. To speed the detoxification process, consider using a several-week course of a medical food-replacement product (e.g., UltraClear, a popular powdered meal-replacement formula).

Lifestyle

Follow the recommendations given in the chapter A HEALTHY LIFESTYLE. Especially important is a regular exercise program, with low-intensity activities producing the greatest benefits.

Nutritional Supplements

- High-potency multiple-vitamin-and-mineral formula, according to guidelines given in the chapter SUPPLEMENTARY MEASURES
- Vitamin C: 500–1,000 mg three times per day
- Vitamin E: 200–400 IU per day
- Thymus extract: 750 mg of the crude polypeptide fraction once or twice per day
- Magnesium bound to citrate or Krebs cycle intermediates: 200–300 mg three times per day
- Pantothenic acid: 250 mg per day

Botanical Medicines

Dosages are three times per day.
- Siberian ginseng (*Eleutherococcus senticosus*):
  Dried root: 2–4 g
  Tincture (1:5): 10–20 ml
  Fluid extract (1:1): 2.0–4.0 ml
  Solid (dry powdered) extract (20:1 or standardized to contain greater than 1% eleutheroside E): 100–200 mg
- Licorice (*Glycyrrhiza glabra*):
  Powdered root: 1–2 g
  Fluid extract (1:1): 2–4 ml
  Solid (dry powdered) extract (4:1): 250–500 mg

Counseling

Seek guidance from your physician or a professional counselor, to establish a regular pattern of mental, emotional, and spiritual affirmations.

Common Cold

. . . .

Nasal discomfort with watery discharge and sneezing

Dry, sore throat

Red, swollen nasal passages

Swollen lymph nodes on the neck

The common cold can be caused by a wide variety of viruses that are capable of infecting the *upper respiratory tract* (the nasal passages, sinuses, and throat). We are all constantly exposed to many of these viruses, yet the majority of us only experience the discomfort of a "cold" once or twice a year. This situation implies that a decrease in resistance or immune function is the major factor in "catching" a cold.

Typically, the individual with a cold will experience general malaise, fever, headache, and upper respiratory tract congestion. Initially, there is usually a watery nasal discharge and sneezing, followed by thicker secretions containing mucus, white blood cells, and dead organisms. The throat may be red, sore, and quite dry.

Usually a cold can be distinguished from other conditions with some similar symptoms (influenza and allergies, for example) by some common sense. Influenza is much more severe in symptoms and usually occurs in epidemics, so contacting the local Public Health Department is all that is needed to rule this out. Allergies may be an underlying factor in decreasing resistance and allowing a virus to infect the upper airways, but usually allergies can be differentiated from the common cold by the fact that, with allergies, no fever occurs, there is no evidence of infec-

tion, and there is usually a history of seasonal allergic episodes.

Therapeutic Considerations

Maintaining a healthy immune system is the primary way to protect yourself against getting an excessive number of colds. If you catch more than one or two colds per year, it may be indicative of a weak immune system. To strengthen your immune system, please follow the recommendations given in the chapter IMMUNE SUPPORT.

What to Do If You Catch a Cold

Once a cold develops, there are several things that can speed recovery, as will be detailed in this chapter. With a healthy, functioning immune system, a cold should not last more than three or four days at the most. Even if you utilize a wide variety of natural healing methods, once a cold is well underway, it is difficult to completely throw it off within two days. Do not expect immediate relief in most instances when using natural substances. In fact, since most natural therapies for colds involve assisting the body, as opposed to suppressing the symptoms, the symptoms of the cold may temporarily worsen.

Many of the symptoms of the cold are a result of our body's defense mechanisms. For example, the potent immune-stimulating compound *interferon,* released by our blood cells and other tissues during infections, is responsible for many flu-like symptoms. Another example is the beneficial effect of fever on the course of infection. While an elevated body temperature can be uncomfortable, suppression of fever is thought to counteract a major defense mechanism and prolong the infection. In general, fever should not be suppressed during an infection unless it is dangerously high (greater than 104 degrees Fahrenheit). For these and other reasons, it is not uncommon for individuals, treating themselves for the common cold with natural medicines to experience a greater degree of discomfort due to the immune-enhancing effects of these compounds. Of course, the illness is generally much shorter-lived as a result.

Rest

As detailed in the chapter IMMUNE SUPPORT, the immune system functions better under when we are under the control of the parasympathetic nervous system. This portion of our nervous system assumes control over bodily functions during periods of rest, relaxation, visualization, meditation, and sleep. During the deepest levels of sleep, potent immune-enhancing compounds are released, and many immune functions are greatly increased. The value of sleep and rest during a cold cannot be overemphasized.

Consume Liquids

Drink lots of fluids. Increased fluid consumption offers several benefits. A much more hospitable environment is provided for the virus when the membranes that line the respiratory tract get dehydrated. Consuming plenty of liquids and/or using a vaporizer maintains a moist respiratory tract that repels viral infection. Drinking plenty of liquids will also improve the function of white blood cells

QUICK REVIEW

- Many of the symptoms of the cold are a result of our body's defense mechanisms.
- The value of sleep and rest during a cold cannot be overemphasized.
- Consuming plenty of liquids and/or using a vaporizer maintains a moist respiratory tract that repels viral infection.
- Vitamin C at a dosage of 1 to 6 grams per day decreases the duration of the cold episodes by nearly one full day.
- The argument in the medical literature that vitamin C has no effect on the common cold seems to be based in large part on a faulty review written two decades ago.
- If they are properly prepared, zinc lozenges can be effective in reducing the duration of symptoms.
- In 1994, German physicians and pharmacists prescribed echinacea for the common cold more than 2.5 million times.

by decreasing the concentration of compounds that are in solution in the blood.

The type of liquids you consume is very important. Studies have shown that consuming concentrated sources of sugars, such as glucose, fructose, sucrose, honey, or orange juice, greatly reduces the ability of the white blood cells to kill bacteria.[1-3] Before being consumed, fruit juices should be greatly diluted. Drinking a lot of orange juice during a cold does more harm than good because of the much higher level of sugar than vitamin C. Keep daily intake to 4 to 8 ounces of undiluted fruit juices.

Avoid Sugar

As mentioned in the previous section, sugar consumption—even if derived from "natural" sources like fruit juices and honey—can impair immune functions.[1-3] This impairment appears to result from the fact that glucose (blood sugar) and vitamin C compete for transport sites into the white blood cells. Decreased vitamin C levels due to excessive sugar consumption may result in a significant reduction in white blood cell function.

Take Vitamin C

Many claims have been made about the role of vitamin C (ascorbic acid) in the prevention and treatment of the common cold. It has been over twenty years since Linus Pauling wrote the book Vitamin C and the Common Cold.[4] Pauling based his views on several studies that showed that vitamin C was very effective in reducing the severity of symptoms and the duration of the common cold. Since 1970, there have been over twenty double-blind studies designed to test Pauling's assertion.[5] Yet despite the fact that in every study, the group that received vitamin C had a decrease either in duration or in severity of symptoms, for some reason the clinical effect is still debated in the medical

community. A 1995 article that appeared in the Journal of the American College of Nutrition has shed some light on the controversy.[6]

In 1975, Thomas Chalmers analyzed the possible effect of vitamin C on the common cold by calculating the average difference in the duration of cold episodes between vitamin C groups and control groups in seven placebo-controlled studies. He found that episodes were 0.11 day shorter in the vitamin C groups and concluded that there was no valid evidence to indicate that vitamin C is beneficial in the treatment of the common cold. Chalmers's review has been extensively cited in scientific articles and monographs.

However, other reviewers have concluded that vitamin C significantly alleviates the symptoms of the common cold. A careful analysis of Chalmers's review reveals serious shortcomings. For example, Chalmers did not consider the amount of vitamin C used in the studies; he included in his meta-analysis a study in which only 25 to 50 mg/day of vitamin C was administered to the test subjects. For some studies, Chalmers used values that are inconsistent with the original published results.

Using data from the same studies, the authors of a new study calculated that vitamin C at a dosage of 1 to 6 g/day decreased the duration of the cold episodes by nearly a full day, or roughly twenty-one percent. The argument in the medical literature that vitamin C has no effect on the common cold seems to be based in large part on a faulty review written two decades ago.

Use Zinc Lozenges

One of the most popular natural approaches to the common cold is the use of zinc lozenges. There is good scientific data to support this practice, as several studies have now shown that zinc lozenges provide relief of a sore throat due to the common cold. Zinc is a critical nutrient for optimum immune system function and, like vitamin C, zinc also possesses direct antiviral activity.[7] There have been several double-blind, placebo-controlled studies showing the benefits of zinc lozenges in reducing the severity and duration of cold symptoms.[8,9] In the most recent study, 100 patients who were experiencing early signs of the common cold were provided a lozenge that contained either 13.3 mg of zinc (from zinc gluconate) or a placebo. They took the lozenges as long as they had symptoms.

The subjects kept track of symptoms such as cough, headache, hoarseness, muscle ache, nasal drainage, nasal congestion, scratchy throat, sore throat, sneezing, and fever (assessed by oral temperature). The duration of symptoms was significantly shorter in the zinc group than in the placebo group. Complete recovery was achieved in 4.4 days with zinc, compared to 7.6 days for the placebo. The zinc group also had significantly fewer days with coughing (2.0 days compared with 4.5 days), headache (2.0 days vs. 3.0 days), hoarseness (2.0 days vs. 3.0 days), nasal congestion (4.0 days vs. 6.0 days), nasal drainage (4.0 days vs. 7.0 days), and sore throat (1.0 day vs. 3.0 days).

Despite these promising results, it appears that not all zinc lozenges are effective. A few early studies did not show much benefit from zinc lozenges. This inconsistency was probably due to an ineffective lozenge formulation. The explanation for this can be found in an interesting study that evaluated the actual amount of ionized zinc released into the saliva by various lozenges. It appears that, in order for zinc to be effective, it must be ionized in saliva. The study showed that sucking on hard candy lozenges containing zinc gluconate and citric acid delivered an insignificant amount of ionized zinc.[10] It was found that, in the presence of citric acid, saliva com-

pletely suppressed the ionization of zinc. Sweetening agents such as mannitol or sorbitol also prevented the ionization of zinc. The best zinc lozenges were those that used the amino acid *glycine*. Even the presence of large excesses of glycine in contrast to citric acid, mannitol, or sorbitol, was found to not interfere with ionization of zinc. In fact, ninety percent of zinc was found to be ionized in a study that used zinc lozenges with glycine.

What does all this mean? It means that in order for a zinc lozenge to be effective it must be free of sorbitol, mannitol, and citric acid. The best lozenges are those that utilize glycine as a sweetener. Use lozenges that supply 15 to 25 mg of elemental zinc. If you feel a cold coming on, dissolve them in your mouth every two waking hours after an initial double dose. Continue for up to seven days.

Take Vitamin A or Beta-Carotene
Short-term, high doses of vitamin A (not recommended in pregnant women or sexually active women not employing birth control) or beta-carotene can enhance immune function. Vitamin A may be a bit more effective than beta-carotene during a cold because it also exerts antiviral effects. For more information, see IMMUNE SUPPORT.

Take Echinacea
There are many herbs to choose from that can enhance immune function. However, the herb with the greatest amount of scientific support is echinacea. There have been over three hundred scientific investigations on the immune-enhancing effects of echinacea.

One of the most popular uses of echinacea is in the treatment of the common cold. In 1994, German physicians and pharmacists prescribed echinacea for the common cold more than 2.5 million times.[11] Two recent studies offer considerable support for this clinical application.

In one study, 180 patients with cold symptoms were given either an extract of *Echinacea purpurea* root at a daily dose of 450 mg or 900 mg or a placebo. The 450-mg dose was found to be no more effective than a placebo. However, the group taking the 900 mg dose showed significant reduction of cold symptoms.[12]

In the other study, 108 patients with colds received either an extract of the fresh-pressed juice of *E. purpurea* (4 ml twice daily) or a placebo for eight weeks.[13] The percentage of patients that remained healthy was: 35.2 percent for echinacea, 25.9 percent for placebo. The length of time between infections was: forty days with echinacea, twenty-five days with placebo. When infections did occur in patients receiving echinacea, they were less severe and resolved more quickly. Patients who showed evidence of a weakened immune system (helper to suppressor cell ratio less than 1.5) benefited the most from echinacea.

TREATMENT SUMMARY

Although the focus of this chapter was on the use of natural methods to assist the body in recovering from the common cold, prevention is by far the best medicine. The old adage "an ounce of prevention is worth a pound of cure" is true for the common cold as well as the majority of other conditions afflicting human health. Prevention involves strengthening the immune system, as detailed in the chapter IMMUNE FUNCTION. The following are recommendations as to what to do if a cold develops.

- Rest (bed rest is best)
- Drink large amounts of fluids (preferably diluted vegetable juices, soups, and herb teas)
- Limit simple sugar consumption (including fruit sugars) to less than 50 grams a day

Nutritional Supplements

- Vitamin C: 500–1,000 mg every two hours (decrease if it produces excessive gas or diarrhea), along with 1,000 mg of mixed bioflavonoids per day
- Vitamin A: 15,000–25,000 IU per day for up to four days

WARNING: DO NOT FOLLOW THIS RECOMMENDATION FOR VITAMIN A IF YOU ARE PREGNANT OR A SEXUALLY ACTIVE WOMAN NOT EMPLOYING EFFECTVE BIRTH CONTROL.

- Beta-carotene: 50,000–100,000 IU per day
- Zinc lozenges: Use lozenges that supply 15 to 25 mg of elemental zinc with glycine as the sweetener; dissolve in the mouth every two waking hours after an initial double dose; continue for up to seven days. Prolonged supplementation (for more than one week) at this dose is not recommended, as it may lead to suppression

of the immune system.

Botanical Medicines

- *Echinacea* sp.
  All dosages are three times per day.
  Dried root (or as tea): 0.5–1 g
  Freeze-dried plant: 325–650 mg
  Juice of aerial portion of *E. purpurea* stabilized in 22% ethanol: 2–3 ml
  Tincture (1:5): 2–4 ml
  Fluid extract (1:1): 2–4 ml
  Solid (dry powdered) extract (6.5:1 or 3.5% echinacoside): 150–300 mg

Depression

The official definition of clinical depression, according to the American Psychiatric Association in its *Diagnostic and Statistical Manual of Mental Disorders (DSM-IV)*, is based on the following eight primary criteria:

1. Poor appetite accompanied by weight loss, or increased appetite accompanied by weight gain
2. Insomnia or excessive sleep habits (hypersomnia)
3. Physical hyperactivity or inactivity
4. Loss of interest or pleasure in usual activities, or decrease in sexual drive
5. Loss of energy; feelings of fatigue
6. Feelings of worthlessness, self-reproach, or inappropriate guilt
7. Diminished ability to think or concentrate
8. Recurrent thoughts of death or suicide

The presence of five of these eight symptoms definitely indicates clinical depression; an individual with four is probably depressed. According to the *DSM-IV,* the symptoms must be present for at least one month to be called depression. Clinical depression is also referred to as *major depression* or *unipolar depression.*

Depression and other affective (mood) disorders reflect disturbances in mood. Used in this context, *mood* means a prolonged emotional tone that dominates an individual's outlook. Normal moods (sadness, grief, elation, etc.), which are typically transient, are a part of everyday life, making the demarcation between "normal" and "abnormal" often difficult to determine. Depression is the most common mood disorder.

Obviously, there is a spectrum of clinical depression, ranging from mild feelings of depression to serious considerations of suicide. Mild depression is also known as *dysthymia.* "Dysthymia" is a term coined in the 1980s; it replaced the term *depressive neurosis,* which was used in the 1950s, and the term *depressive personality,* which was used in the 1970s.

Like clinical depression, dysthymia is diagnosed according to *DSM-IV* criteria. In order to be officially diagnosed as dysthymic, a patient must be depressed most of the time for at least two years (one year for children or adolescents) and have at least three of the following symptoms:

- Low self-esteem or lack of self-confidence
- Pessimism, hopelessness, or despair
- Lack of interest in ordinary pleasures and activities
- Withdrawal from social activities
- Fatigue or lethargy
- Guilt or ruminating about the past
- Irritability or excessive anger
- Lessened productivity
- Difficulty concentrating or making decisions

Theories on Depression

Depression is a major problem in the United States. Approximately seventeen million Americans suffer from true clinical depression each year, and over twenty-eight million Americans take antidepressant drugs or anxiety medications. The obvious question is: "Why are so many Americans depressed?" Five basic theoretical models of depression attempt to answer this question:

1. The "aggression turned inward" construct, which, although apparent in many clinical cases, has no substantial proof.

2. The "loss model," which postulates that depression is a reaction to the loss of a person, thing, status, self-esteem, or even a habit pattern.

3. The "interpersonal relationship" approach, which utilizes behavioral concepts, (i.e., the person who is depressed uses depression as a way of controlling other people, including doctors). It can be an extension and outgrowth of such simple behavior as pouting, silence, or ignoring something or someone. It fails to serve the need, and the problem worsens.

4. The "learned helplessness" model, which theorizes that depression is the result of habitual feelings of pessimism and hopelessness.

5. The "monoamine hypothesis," which stresses biochemical derangement characterized by imbalances of monoamines such as serotonin, epinephrine, and norepinephrine.

Although the monamine (also referred to as biogenic amine) model is the dominant medical model of depression, there is much value to counseling, especially in clear cases of psychological *etiology* (origin). Of the various psychological theories of depression, the

. . . .

QUICK REVIEW

- Approximately seventeen million Americans suffer from true clinical depression each year, and over twenty-eight million Americans take antidepressant drugs or anxiety medications.

- One of the most powerful techniques for producing the necessary biochemical changes in the brains of depressed individuals is to teach them to be more optimistic.

- Low levels of serotonin contribute to depression.

- It is important to rule out the simple organic factors that are known to contribute to depression, i.e., nutrient deficiency or excess, drugs (prescription, illicit, alcohol, caffeine, nicotine, etc.), hypoglycemia, consumption, hormonal derangement, allergy, environmental factors, and microbial factors.

- Cognitive therapy has been shown to be as effective as antidepressant drugs in treating moderate depression.

- Depression is often a first or early manifestation of thyroid disease.

- Increased cortisol levels are common in depression.

one that we feel has the most merit is the learned helplessness model, developed by Martin Seligman, Ph.D. During the 1960s, Dr. Seligman discovered that animals could be trained to be helpless. His animal model provided a valuable clue to human depression as well as serving as a model to test antidepressant drugs.[1]

The Learned Helplessness Model

Seligman's early experiments were performed on three groups of dogs. The first group was given an escapable electrical shock. The dogs could turn off the shock by simply pressing a panel with their noses. This group of dogs thus had control. The second group of dogs was "yoked" to the first group. They would get exactly the same shocks as the first group but would be unable to turn off the shock. The shock would cease only when the "yoked" dog in the first group pressed its nose to the panel. Thus, the second group had no control over the degree of shock they received. The third group of dogs received no shocks at all.

Once the dogs went through this first part of the experiment, they were placed in what is known as a "shuttle box"—a box separated in the middle by a small barrier that the dogs could jump over. The dogs would be electrically shocked, but they were able to escape the shock by simply jumping over the barrier to the other side. Seligman hypothesized that the first and third groups of dogs would quickly figure this out, but that the second group would have learned to be helpless and would believe that nothing they did mattered. Seligman thought that the dogs in the second group would simply lie down and accept the shock.

As predicted, the first and third groups of dogs learned within seconds that they could avoid the shock by jumping over the barrier,

. . . .

- Elimination of sugar and caffeine has been shown to produce significant benefits in clinical trials.
- Increased participation in exercise, sports, and physical activities is strongly associated with decreased symptoms of anxiety, depression, and malaise.
- A deficiency of any single nutrient can alter brain function and lead to depression, anxiety, and other mental disorders.
- Hypoglycemia can cause depression.
- An insufficiency of omega-3 oils in the diet has been linked to depression.

- Numerous double-blind studies have shown 5-hydroxytryptophan (5-HTP) to be as effective as antidepressant drugs, but it is better tolerated and is associated with fewer and much milder side effects.
- Extracts of St. John's wort standardized for hypericin (usually 0.3 percent) are the most thoroughly researched natural antidepressants.
- Over twenty-five double-blind studies have shown St. John's wort to produce as good or better results compared to standard antidepressant drugs, but with significantly fewer side effects.

while the dogs in the second group simply lay down and didn't even make an effort to jump over the barrier though they could see the shock-free side of the shuttle box. Seligman and his colleagues went on to show that many humans react in an identical fashion.

The adoption of Seligman's model was revolutionary, as it became an effective experiment for testing antidepressive drugs. Basically, when animals that had learned to be helpless were given antidepressant drugs, they unlearned their helplessness and started exerting control over their environment. Researchers discovered that animals learning to be helpless resulted in an alteration of brain chemistry. The drugs restored proper chemical balance and altered the animals' behavior. Furthermore, researchers discovered that when animals with learned helplessness were taught how to gain control over their environment, their brain chemistry also normalized. The alteration in brain chemistry (chiefly a reduced level of serotonin) in the animals with learned helplessness mirrors the altered monoamine content that characterizes human depression.

While most physicians quickly look to drugs to alter brain chemistry, helping patients gain more control over their lives will actually produce even greater biochemical changes. One of the most powerful techniques for producing the necessary biochemical changes in the brains of depressed individuals is to teach them to be more optimistic.

Outside the laboratory setting, Seligman discovered that the determining factor in how a person reacted to uncontrollable events, either "bad" or "good," was their explanatory style—the way in which they explained events. Optimistic people were immune to becoming helpless and depressed. However, pessimistic individuals were extremely likely to become depressed when something went wrong in their lives. Seligman and other researchers also found a direct correlation between an individual's level of optimism and the likelihood of developing not only clinical depression but other illnesses as well.[2,3] In one of the longer studies, patients were followed for a total of thirty-five years. While optimists rarely got depressed, pessimists were extremely likely to experience depression and other psychological disturbances.

Depression as a Result of Low Serotonin Levels

Serotonin is an important *neurotransmitter*—a chemical messenger responsible for transmitting information from one nerve cell to another. Serotonin has been referred to as the brain's own mood-elevating and tranquilizing drug. There is a lot of support for this description. Because the manufacture of serotonin in the brain depends upon how much tryptophan is delivered to the brain, in experimental studies researchers can feed subjects a diet that lacks tryptophan and then note the effects of such a diet. The results from these sorts of studies have contributed greatly to our understanding of just how vital proper levels of serotonin are to a positive human experience. Table 1 contrasts optimal serotonin levels with low serotonin levels.

The lower the level of serotonin, the more severe the consequences. For example, low levels of serotonin are linked to depression, with the lowest levels being observed in people who have committed or attempted suicide.

Therapeutic Considerations

Modern psychiatry focuses on manipulating neurotransmitter levels in the brain rather

TABLE 1 Effects of Low Serotonin Levels	
OPTIMAL LEVEL OF SEROTONIN	**LOW LEVEL OF SEROTONIN**
Hopeful, optimistic	Depressed
Calm	Anxious
Good-natured	Irritable
Patient	Impatient
Reflective and thoughtful	Impulsive
Loving and caring	Abusive
Able to concentrate	Has a short attention span
Creative, focused	Blocked, scattered
Able to think things through	"Flies off the handle"
Responsive	Reactive
Does not overeat carbohydrates	Craves sweets and high-carbohydrate foods
Sleeps well with good dream recall	Has insomnia and poor dream recall

than identifying and eliminating the psychological factors that are responsible for producing the imbalances in neurotransmitters like serotonin, dopamine, and gamma-aminobutyric acid (GABA).

Many of the commonly used antidepressant drugs, such as Prozac, Zoloft, and Paxil, work primarily by increasing the effects of serotonin. Once serotonin is manufactured in the brain, it is stored in nerve cells where it waits to be released. Once released, the serotonin carries a chemical message by binding to receptor sites on the neighboring nerve cell. Almost as soon as the serotonin is released, enzymes are at work to either break down the serotonin or aid its uptake back into the brain cells. Either event results in stopping the serotonin effect. It is at this point that various drugs typically work to either inhibit the reuptake of serotonin or prevent its breakdown. As a result, there is more serotonin hanging around capable of binding to receptor sites and transmitting the serotonin effect.

There are effective alternatives to antidepressant drugs. For example, there are a number of lifestyle and dietary factors that

lead to reduced serotonin levels. Chief among these factors are cigarette smoking, alcohol abuse, high sugar intake, overconsumption of protein, blood sugar disturbances (hypoglycemia and diabetes), and various nutrient deficiencies. All of these factors have one thing in common: they lower serotonin levels by impairing the conversion of tryptophan to serotonin. A health-promoting lifestyle and diet go a long way toward restoring optimal serotonin levels and relieving depression. But in the interim, such natural agents as 5-HTP and St. John's wort can provide the necessary serotonin boost to support making important changes in diet and lifestyle.

Rule Out an Underlying Cause

Depression can often be due to an underlying organic (chemical) or physiological cause. Identification and elimination of the underlying cause should be the primary therapy. Failure to address an underlying cause will make any antidepressant therapy less successful. It is important to rule out the simple organic factors that are known to contribute to the depression: nutrient deficiency or excess, drugs (prescription, illicit, alcohol, caffeine, nicotine, etc.), hypoglycemia, consumption, hormonal derangement, allergy, environmental factors, and microbial factors. Each of these is discussed later in this chapter. Regardless of whether there is an underlying organic cause, counseling is always recommended for the depressed individual.

ORGANIC AND PHYSIOLOGICAL CAUSES OF DEPRESSION

Food allergies

Heavy metals

Hypoglycemia

Hypothyroidism

Nutritional deficiencies

Preexisting physical condition

   Cancer

   Chronic inflammation

   Chronic pain

   Diabetes

   Heart disease

   Liver disease

   Lung disease

   Multiple sclerosis

   Rheumatoid arthritis

Premenstrual syndrome

Prescription drugs

   Antihistamines

   Antihypertensives

   Anti-inflammatory agents

   Birth-control pills

   Corticosteroids

   Tranquilizers and sedatives

Sleep disturbances

Stress/low adrenal function

Counseling

There are several counseling techniques that can be quite useful. Cognitive therapy has the most merit and support in the medical literature. In fact, cognitive therapy has been shown to be as effective as antidepressant drugs in treating moderate depression.[4,5] However, while there is a high rate of relapse of depression when drugs are used, the relapse rate for cognitive therapy is much lower. People who take drugs for depression tend to have to stay on them for the rest of their lives. That is not the case with cognitive therapy, because the patient is taught new skills for dealing with depression.[6]

Psychologists and other mental health specialists trained in cognitive therapy seek to change the way the depressed person consciously thinks about failure, defeat, loss, and helplessness. Cognitive therapists employ five basic tactics.

First, they help patients recognize the negative automatic thoughts that flit through their consciousness when they feel their worst. Second, they dispute the negative thoughts by focusing on contrary evidence. Third, they teach the patients different explanations to dispute the negative automatic thoughts. Fourth, they teach patients how to avoid rumination (the constant churning of a thought in one's mind) by helping them better control their thoughts. Finally, they question depression-causing negative thoughts and beliefs and replace them with empowering positive thoughts and beliefs.

Cognitive therapy does not involve the long, drawn-out process of psychoanalysis. It is a solution-oriented psychotherapy designed to help patients learn skills that will improve the quality of their lives.

Hormonal Factors

Many hormones are known to influence mood. However, it is beyond the current scope of this chapter to address all of them. Instead, the focus here will be on the effects of the thyroid and adrenal hormones.

Thyroid Function

Depression is often an early manifestation of thyroid disease, as even subtle decreases in available thyroid hormone are suspected of producing symptoms.[7,8] The link between low thyroid function (*hypothyroidism*) and depression is well known in medical circles, but whether the low thyroid function is a result of depression or the depression is a result of low thyroid function remains to be answered. It is probably a combination. Please see HYPOTHYROIDISM for more information on determining thyroid function.

Stress and Adrenal Function

As with the thyroid gland, altered function of the adrenal gland is closely associated with depression. Often this dysfunction is the result of stress—a major factor to consider in depression. The Adrenal Stress Index is a laboratory technique that many nutritionally oriented physicians use to assess a patient's level of, and response to, stress. This test measures the level of the adrenal hormones cortisol and dehydroepiandrosterone (DHEA) in the saliva. The typical pattern found in depression is an elevated morning cortisol level and a decreased DHEA level.

The elevations in cortisol levels reflect a disturbance in the control mechanisms for adrenal function that reside in the hypothalamus and pituitary gland, located at the center of the brain. Defects in adrenal regulation seen in affective (mood) disorders include: excessive cortisol secretion independent of stress responses, abnormal nighttime release of cortisol, and inadequate suppression by the drug dexamethasone during the dexamethasone suppression test.[9] Defects in control mechanisms for adrenal hormones and thyroid function are hallmark features of depression.[10,11]

When the adrenal gland releases increased amounts of natural cortisol, its effects on the brain mirror the effects of synthetic cortisones such as prednisone: depression, mania, nervousness, insomnia, and, at high levels, schizophrenia. The effects of cortisol on mood are related to its activation of tryptophan oxygenase (see Figure 1). This activation results in shunting of tryptophan to the kynurenine pathway at the expense of serotonin and melatonin synthesis.[12] The significance of this shunting is described later in this chapter, in The Tryptophan Catastrophe.

Environmental Toxins

Heavy metals (lead, mercury, cadmium, arsenic, nickel, and aluminum), solvents (cleaning materials, formaldehyde, toluene, benzene, etc.), pesticides, and herbicides have an affinity for nervous tissue. As a result, a variety of psychological and neurological symptoms can occur, including depression, headaches, mental confusion, mental illness, tingling in extremities, abnormal nerve reflexes, and other signs of impaired nervous system function.[13–15]

History of exposure and hair mineral analysis are good screening mechanisms for environmental toxicity. If the hair mineral analysis is inconclusive, a more sensitive indicator is the eight-hour lead mobilization test. This test employs the chelating agent EDTA (ethylenediaminetetra acetic acid), which binds to lead and promotes its excretion in the urine. The eight-hour mobilization test measures the level of lead excreted in the urine for a period of eight hours after the injection of EDTA.

Lifestyle Factors

A health-promoting lifestyle and diet are very important in the treatment of depression. Particularly important are the cessation of smoking, excessive alcohol consumption, and the intake of caffeine. These lifestyle changes, coupled with regular exercise and a healthful diet, will probably produce better clinical results than antidepressant drugs, with no side effects and no cost.

Smoking

Cigarette smoking is one of the major factors contributing to premature death in the United States. Cigarette smoking is also a significant factor in depression. Central to the effect of nicotine is the stimulation of adrenal hormone secretion, including cortisol. Elevated cortisol levels are a well-recognized feature of depression.[3] One of the key effects of cortisol (and stress) on mood is activation of tryptophan oxygenase, resulting in less tryptophan being delivered to the brain. Since the level of serotonin in the brain is dependent upon the amount of tryptophan delivered to the brain, cortisol dramatically reduces the level of serotonin and melatonin.[10] In addition, cortisol "down-regulates" serotonin receptors in the brain, making them less sensitive to the serotonin that is available.

Cigarette smoking also leads to a relative vitamin C deficiency, as the vitamin C is utilized to detoxify the cigarette smoke. Low levels of vitamin C in the brain can result in depression and hysteria.[16]

Alcohol

Alcohol, a brain depressant, increases adrenal hormone output, interferes with many brain cell processes, and disrupts normal sleep cycles. Alcohol ingestion also leads to hypoglycemia. The resultant drop in blood sugar produces a craving for sugar. Unfortunately, increased sugar consumption ultimately aggravates the hypoglycemia. Hypoglycemia aggravates the mental and emotional problems of the alcoholic.

Caffeine

Although caffeine is a well-known stimulant, the intensity of response to caffeine varies greatly; people prone to feeling depressed or anxious tend to be especially sensitive to caffeine. The term *caffeinism* is used to describe a clinical syndrome, similar to generalized anxiety and panic disorders, that includes such symptoms as depression, nervousness, palpitations, irritability, and recurrent headache.[17]

Several studies have looked at caffeine intake and depression. For example, one study found that, among healthy college students, moderate and high coffee drinkers scored higher on a depression scale than did low users. Interestingly, the moderate and high coffee drinkers also tended to have significantly lower academic performance.[18] Several other studies have shown that depressed patients tend to consume fairly high amounts of caffeine (more than 700 mg per day).[19,20] In addition, the intake of caffeine has been linked with the degree of mental illness in psychiatric patients; the higher the intake, the more severe the depression.[21,22]

The combination of caffeine and refined sugar seems to be even worse than either substance consumed alone. Several studies have found an association between this combination and depression. In one of the most interesting studies, twenty-one women and two men responded to an advertisement requesting volunteers "who feel depressed and don't know why, often feel tired even though they sleep a lot, are very moody, and generally seem to feel bad most of the time."[23] After baseline psychological testing, the subjects were placed on a caffeine- and sucrose-free diet for one week. The subjects who reported substantial improvement (about sixty percent) were then challenged in a double-blind fashion. The subjects took either a capsule containing caffeine and a Kool-Aid drink sweetened with sugar or a capsule containing cellulose and a Kool-Aid drink sweetened with NutraSweet. Each challenge lasted up to six days. About fifty percent of test subjects became depressed during the test period with caffeine and sucrose.

Another study using a format similar to the Kool-Aid study described above found that seven of sixteen depressed patients were found to be depressed with the caffeine and sucrose challenge, but became symptom-free during the caffeine- and sucrose-free diet and the cellulose and NutraSweet test period.[24]

The average American consumes 150 to 225 mg of caffeine daily, or roughly the amount of caffeine in one to two cups of coffee. Although most people appear to tolerate this amount, some people are more sensitive to the effects of caffeine than others. Even a small amount of caffeine, as found in decaffeinated coffee, is enough to affect some people adversely. Patients with depression or any psychological disorder should avoid caffeine completely.

Exercise

Regular exercise may be the most powerful natural antidepressant available. In fact, many of the beneficial effects of exercise noted in the prevention of heart disease may be related as much to its ability to improve mood as to its improvement of cardiovascular function.[25] Various community and clinical studies have clearly indicated that exercise has profound antidepressive effects.[26] These studies have shown that increased participation in exercise, sports, and physical activities is strongly associated with decreased symptoms of anxiety, depression, and malaise. Furthermore, people who participate in regular exercise have higher self-esteem, feel better, and are much happier than people who do not exercise.

Much of the mood-elevating effect of exercise may be attributed to the fact that regular exercise increases the level of endorphins, which are directly correlated with mood.[27] One of the most interesting studies that examined the role of exercise and endorphins in depression compared the beta-endorphin levels and depression profiles of ten joggers with those of ten sedentary men of the same age. The ten sedentary men tested out more depressed, perceived greater stress in their lives, and had a higher level of cortisol and lower levels of beta-endorphins. As the researchers stated, this "reaffirms that depression is very sensitive to exercise and helps firm up a biochemical link between physical activity and depression."[28]

At least 100 clinical studies have now evaluated the efficacy of an exercise program in the treatment of depression. In an analysis of the sixty-four studies prior to 1980, physical fitness training was shown to relieve depression and improve both self-esteem and work behavior.[29]

Unfortunately, the quality of many of the studies was less than ideal. However, because of the good results noted in the analysis of these studies, there was a flurry of well-designed studies conducted in the 1980s to better determine how effective exercise could be as a therapy. These studies utilized stricter scientific criteria than the earlier ones, yet they produced similar results. It was concluded that exercise can be as effective as other antidepressants, including drugs and psychotherapy.[30] More recently, even stricter studies have further demonstrated that regular exercise is a powerful antidepressant.[31–33]

The best exercises are either strength training (weight lifting) or aerobic activities such as walking briskly, jogging, bicycling, cross-country skiing, swimming, aerobic dance, and racquet sports.

Dietary Guidelines

Since the brain requires a constant supply of blood sugar to function properly, hypoglycemia must be avoided. Symptoms of hypoglycemia can range from mild to severe, and include depression, anxiety, irritability, and other psychological disturbances; fatigue; headache; blurred vision; excessive sweating; mental confusion; incoherent speech; bizarre behavior; and convulsions. Several studies have shown hypoglycemia to be very common in depressed individuals.[34-37] Simply eliminating refined carbohydrates from the diet is sometimes all that is needed for effective therapy in patients whose depression results from reactive hypoglycemia.

The dietary guidelines for depression are identical to the dietary guidelines for optimal health. It is now a well-established fact that certain dietary practices cause a wide range of diseases, while others prevent them. Quite simply, a health-promoting diet provides optimal levels of all known nutrients and low levels of food components that are detrimental to health, such as sugar, saturated fats, cholesterol, salt, and food additives. A health-promoting diet is rich in whole, "natural," unprocessed foods. It is especially high in plant foods, such as fruits, vegetables, grains, beans, seeds, and nuts, as these foods not only contain valuable nutrients but have additional compounds with remarkable health-promoting properties.

Nutritional Deficiency

A deficiency of any single nutrient can alter brain function and lead to depression, anxiety, and other mental disorders. However, the role of nutrient deficiency is just the tip of the iceberg in regard to the role of nutrient effects on the brain and mood. According to Melvin Werbach, M.D.:

It is clear that nutrition can powerfully influence cognition, emotion, and behavior. It is also clear that the effects of classical nutritional deficiency diseases upon mental function constitute only a small part of a rapidly expanding list of interfaces between nutrition and the mind . . . Even in the absence of laboratory validation of nutritional

deficiencies, numerous studies utilizing rigorous scientific designs have demonstrated impressive benefits from nutritional supplementation.[38]

A high-potency multiple-vitamin-and-mineral provides a good nutritional foundation upon which to build. When selecting a multiple-vitamin-and-mineral formula, it is important to make sure that it provides the full range of vitamins and minerals at high potency levels, as recommended in the chapter SUPPLEMENTARY MEASURES. Deficiencies of a number of nutrients are quite common in depressed individuals. The most common deficiencies are folic acid, vitamin B12, and vitamin B6. The significance of these deficiencies is discussed in the following sections of this chapter.

Folic Acid and Vitamin B12

Folic acid and vitamin B12 function together in many biochemical processes. Folic acid deficiency is the most common nutrient deficiency in the world. In studies of depressed patients, thirty-one to thirty-five percent have been shown to be deficient in folic acid.[39-42] In elderly patients, this percentage may be even higher. Studies have found that, among elderly patients admitted to a psychiatric ward, the number of patients with folic acid deficiency ranges from 35 percent to 92.6 percent.[43,44] Depression is the most common symptom of a folic acid deficiency. Vitamin B12 deficiency is less common than folic acid deficiency, but it can also cause depression, especially in the elderly.[45,46] Correcting the folic acid and/or vitamin B12 deficiency results in a dramatic improvement in mood.

Folic acid, vitamin B12, and a form of the amino acid methionine known as SAM (S-adenosyl-methionine) function as "methyl donors." They carry and donate methyl molecules to important brain compounds, includ-

TABLE 2   Behavioral Effects of Some Vitamin Deficiencies

DEFICIENT VITAMIN	BEHAVIORAL EFFECTS
Thiamin	Korsakoff's psychosis, mental depression, apathy, anxiety, irritability
Riboflavin	Depression, irritability
Niacin	Apathy, anxiety, depression, hyperirritability, mania, memory deficits, delirium, organic dementia, emotional lability
Biotin	Depression, extreme lassitude, somnolence
Pantothenic acid	Restlessness, irritability, depression, fatigue
B6	Depression, irritability, sensitivity to sound
Folic acid	Forgetfulness, insomnia, apathy, irritability, depression, psychosis, delirium, dementia
B12	Psychotic states, depression, irritability, confusion, memory loss, hallucinations, delusions, paranoia
Vitamin C	Lassitude, hypochondriasis, depression, hysteria

ing neurotransmitters. Without the methyl group being donated the neurotransmitter cannot perform its function. SAM is the major methyl donor in the body. The antidepressant effects of folic acid appear to be a result of raising brain SAM content.

One of the key brain compounds that depends on methylation is tetrahydrobiopterin (BH_4). This compound functions as an essential factor in the manufacture of neurotransmitters such as serotonin and dopamine from their corresponding amino acids. Patients with recurrent depression have been shown to have reduced BH_4 synthesis, probably as a result of low SAM levels. BH_4 supplementation has been shown to produce dramatic results in these patients.[47,48] Unfortunately, BH_4 is not currently available commercially. However, since BH_4 synthesis is stimulated by folic acid, vitamin B12, and vitamin C, it is possible that increasing these vitamin levels in the brain may stimulate BH_4 formation and the synthesis of serotonin.[49]

There is indeed evidence that supplementing the diet with folic acid, vitamin C, and vitamin B12 can increase BH_4 levels. In addition, folic acid supplementation and the promotion of methylation reactions have been shown to increase serotonin levels.[50–52] Elevation of serotonin levels is undoubtedly responsible for much of the antidepressive effects of folic acid and vitamin B12. Typically, the dosages of folic acid in the antidepressant clinical studies have been very high: 15 mg to 50 mg. High-dose folic acid therapy is safe (except in patients with epilepsy) and has been shown to be as effective as antidepressant drugs.[53]

A dosage of 800 mcg of folic acid and 800 mcg of vitamin B12 should be sufficient to prevent deficiencies in most circumstances. Folic acid supplementation should always be accompanied by vitamin B12 supplementation to prevent folic acid from masking a vitamin B12 deficiency.

Vitamin B6

Vitamin B6 (pyridoxine) levels are typically quite low in depressed patients, especially women taking birth-control pills or other forms of estrogens.[54-58] Considering the many functions of vitamin B6 in the brain, including the fact that vitamin B6 is essential to the manufacture of serotonin, it is likely that many of the millions of people who take Prozac are depressed simply as a result of low vitamin B6 levels. Patients with low B6 status usually respond well to supplementation. The typical effective dosage is 50 mg to 100 mg.

Omega-3 Fatty Acids

An insufficiency of omega-3 oils in the diet has been linked to depression.[59] This may be related to the impact of dietary fatty acids on the composition of nerve cell membranes. While it is thought that the cell is programmed to selectively incorporate the different fatty acids it needs to maintain optimal function, a lack of essential fatty acids (particularly the omega-3 oils) and an excess of saturated fats and animal fatty acids leads to the formation of cell membranes that are much less fluid than normal.

A relative deficiency of essential fatty acids in cellular membranes substantially impairs cell membrane function. Since the basic function of the cell membrane is to serve as a selective barrier that regulates the passage of molecules into and out of the cell, a disturbance of structure or function disrupts the cell's ability to control its internal environment. Because the brain is the richest source of fatty acids in the human body, and because proper nerve cell function is critically dependent on proper membrane fluidity, alterations in membrane fluidity impact behavior, mood, and mental function.

Studies have shown that the physical properties of brain cell membranes, including their fluidity, directly influence neurotransmitter synthesis, signal transmission, uptake of serotonin and other neurotransmitters, neurotransmitter binding, and the activity of *monoamine oxidase*—the enzyme that breaks down serotonin and other monoamine neurotransmitters such as epinephrine, dopamine, and norepinephrine. All of these factors have been implicated in depression and other psychological disturbances.

Researchers have concluded that omega-3 fatty acids may reduce the development of depression, just as they reduce the development of coronary artery disease.[59] This conclusion was based on several factors:

1. Recent studies have suggested that lowering plasma cholesterol levels by diet and medications increases suicide, homicide, and depression.

2. The quantity and type of dietary fats consumed influence serum lipid levels and alter the biophysical and biochemical properties of cell membranes.

3. Dietary advice to lower cholesterol levels tends to increase the ratio of omega-6 to omega-3 and decreases the level of the essential omega-3 fatty acid, docosahexanoic acid.

4. Population-based studies in various countries and the United States have indicated that decreased consumption of omega-3 fatty acids correlates with increased rates of depression.

5. There is a consistent association between depression and coronary artery disease.

Food Allergies

Depression and fatigue have been linked with food allergies for over sixty-five years. In 1930, Albert Rowe, M.D., one of the leading allergists of this century, coined the term *allergic toxemia* to describe a syndrome that included the symptoms of depression, fatigue, muscle and joint aches, drowsiness, difficulty in concentrating, and nervousness.[60] Although the term "allergic toxemia" is not used anymore, food allergies still play a major role in many people with depression.[61]

Monoamine Metabolism and Precursor Therapy

The monoamine neurotransmitters, such as serotonin, epinephrine, dopamine, and gamma-amino-butyric acid (GABA), are manufactured from amino acid precursors. The use of monoamine (MA) precursors, particularly tryptophan, 5-hydroxytryptophan (5-HTP), and tyrosine, has offered a more natural way of influencing monoamine metabolism than synthetic antidepressant drugs.

The Tryptophan Catastrophe

For more than thirty years, tryptophan was used safely and effectively by over thirty million people in the United States and around the world to treat insomnia and depression. But in October of 1989, some people who were taking tryptophan started reporting strange symptoms to physicians: severe muscle and joint pain, high fever, weakness, swelling of the arms and legs, and shortness of breath.[62] The syndrome was dubbed EMS (eosinophilia-myalgia syndrome).

Laboratory studies showed that the blood of subjects with EMS contained a very high level of eosinophils—white blood cells involved in allergic/inflammatory reactions. In patients with EMS, eosinophil levels rose to greater than 1,000 eosinophils per mm³— roughly double the normal level—and the percentage of eosinophils often increased to levels above thirty percent.

The problem with such severe elevations of eosinophil levels is that these white blood cells contain packets that have high levels of histamine and other allergic and inflammatory compounds. Releasing these compounds by eosinophils leads to intense symptoms of an allergic and inflammatory nature: severe muscle and joint pain, high fever, weakness, swelling of the arms and legs, skin rashes, and shortness of breath. It was suspected that one or more newly introduced contaminants in tryptophan that activated eosinophils and other white blood cells had to be the reason behind EMS.

Detailed analysis of all the evidence by the Centers for Disease Control (CDC) led to the conclusion that the cause of the EMS epidemic could be traced to one Japanese manufacturer, Showa Denko.[63,64] Of the six Japanese companies that supplied all of the tryptophan to the United States, Showa Denko was the largest, supplying fifty to sixty percent. The tryptophan was used not only as a nutritional supplement, but also in infant formulas and nutrient mixtures used for intravenous feeding.

The tryptophan produced from October 1988 to June 1989 by Showa Denko became contaminated due to changes in the filtration process and in the bacteria being used to produce the tryptophan. The change in the filtration process resulted in the tryptophan being contaminated with impurities linked to EMS. Examination of the pre-filtered material indicated that it had no detectable levels of these impurities. Some contaminants.

While the epidemic of EMS during the last half of 1989 was clearly related to the contaminated tryptophan produced by Showa Denko, there have been a handful of other reported cases of EMS in people who never took tryptophan and in people who took tryptophan before the contaminated batch manufactured by Showa Denko hit the shelves. It is likely that, in these earlier reports of EMS-like illnesses among tryptophan users, the subjects were also using contaminated tryptophan and also had a predisposition to EMS (discussed later in this section).[65,66] This conclusion is based on the fact that uncontaminated tryptophan 5-HTP has never produced EMS.

The total number of reported cases of EMS in the United States eventually reached 1,511. Included in this number were thirty-six deaths attributed to tryptophan. In Europe, the total number of cases was 171, and there were no deaths.[63–66] The difference between the U.S. experience and the European experience is that the dominant tryptophan supplement in Europe was Optimax, a product marketed by Merck, the largest pharmaceutical company in the world. The supplier of the tryptophan used in the Merck product was Ajimomato.

One of the interesting aspects of the entire tryptophan catastrophe is that it did not affect more people. Based on detailed studies, it was concluded that EMS affected 144 out of every 100,000 men and 268 out of every 100,000 women who took tryptophan.[67] If fifty percent of these tryptophan users were taking tryptophan supplied by Showa Denko, we can assume that EMS affected 144 out of every 50,000 men who took *contaminated* tryptophan and 268 out of every 50,000 women who took *contaminated* tryptophan. In other words, roughly 1 out of every 250 people who took the contaminated tryptophan developed EMS.

The obvious question is: "Why didn't everyone who took the contaminated tryptophan experience EMS?" The answer appears to be that only those with an abnormal activation of the kynurenine pathway reacted to the contaminant.[68] Kynurenine and its metabolites (especially quinolinic acid) are also linked to other EMS-related illnesses, including the toxic oil syndrome, one of the largest food-related epidemics that has occurred to date. This syndrome occurred in Spain during the month of May in 1991. It affected more than 20,000 people and caused over 12,000 hospitalizations. It was caused by the ingestion of canola oil contaminated with a compound very similar to one found in the contaminated Showa Denko tryptophan.[69]

One of the interesting findings in studies conducted by researchers from the CDC was that people who took a multiple-vitamin preparation were given some protection against EMS.[70] When regular vitamin users did develop EMS, it was less severe than the EMS experienced by non vitamin–users. A likely explanation for this occurrence is that either the vitamins (particularly vitamins B6 and niacin) shunted tryptophan metabolism away from the kynurenine pathway or the contaminants were somehow metabolized by vitamin-dependent enzymes.

Tryptophan as a Treatment for Depression
The basic theory behind tryptophan supplementation in treating depression and insomnia is that it will increase the levels of serotonin and melatonin in the brain. This theory is supported by the considerable evidence that many depressed individuals have low tryptophan and serotonin levels. Unfortunately, supplementation with tryptophan in depressed patients has produced mixed results in the published clinical trials. In only two out of eight studies that compared tryptophan to a placebo was tryptophan shown to be more effective than the placebo. But, interestingly, nine out of eleven studies that compared tryptophan to conventional antidepressant drugs showed no difference between them in effectiveness.[71–76]

There are many factors to consider when looking at these studies, such as study size, severity of depression, duration, and dosage. In addition, a number of factors, such as hormones (estrogen and cortisol) and tryptophan itself, stimulate the activity of tryptophan oxygenase, which results in tryptophan being converted to kynurenine and less tryptophan being delivered to the brain.

In summary, tryptophan is only modestly effective in the treatment of depression when used alone. In order to gain any real benefit from tryptophan, it must be used along with vitamin B6 and the niacinamide form of vitamin B3 to help block the kynurenine pathway to provide better results. Although tryptophan is once again entering the marketplace, better yet is the use of 5-HTP.

5-Hydroxytryptophan (5-HTP)

One step closer to serotonin manufacture from tryptophan is 5-HTP. This compound offers significant advantages over tryptophan. First of all, it is inherently safer because it is extracted from the seed of an African plant (*Griffonia simplicifolia*) rather than being synthesized with the help of bacteria. And, unlike tryptophan, 5-HTP cannot be converted to kynurenine and easily cross the blood brain barrier. As a result, while only three percent of an oral dose of tryptophan is converted to serotonin, over seventy percent of an oral dose of 5-HTP is converted to serotonin. In addition to increasing serotonin levels, 5-HTP causes an increase in levels of endorphin and other neurotransmitters that are often decreased in cases of depression. Numerous double-blind studies have shown

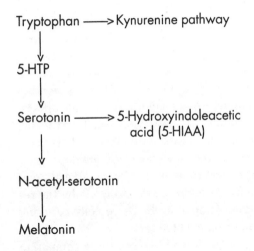

FIGURE 1 Tryptophan Metabolism

that 5-HTP has equal effectiveness compared to drugs like Prozac, Paxil, and Zoloft (the selective serotonin reuptake inhibitors, SSRIs) and tricyclic antidepressant drugs like imipramine and desipramine in terms of effectiveness, and that it offers several advantages: it is less expensive, better tolerated, and associated with fewer and much milder side effects.[77–81]

TABLE 3 5-HTP vs. Fluvoxamine: Changes in the HDS		
DECREASE IN HDS	**5-HTP (NUMBER = 34)**	**FLUVOXAMINE (NUMBER = 29)**
Mean decrease after 2 weeks (%)	23	18.9
less than 35% decrease	20	19
35–50% decrease	10	8
50–75% decrease	4	2
Mean decrease after 4 weeks (%)	46.2	46.1
less than 35% decrease	2	8
35–50% decrease	7	3
50–75% decrease	12	13
more than 75% decrease	3	5
Mean decrease after 6 weeks (%)	60.7	56.1
less than 35% decrease	4	5
35–50% decrease	8	3
50–75% decrease	12	8
more than 75% decrease	10	13

A 1987 review article on the use of 5-HTP in treating depression highlighted the need for well-designed double-blind, head-to-head studies of 5-HTP versus standard antidepressant drugs.[78] Although 5-HTP was viewed as an antidepressant agent with few side effects, the authors of this review felt that the big question to answer was how 5-HTP compared to the new breed of antidepressant drugs: SSRIs such as Prozac, Paxil, and Zoloft. These drugs selectively inhibit the reuptake of serotonin by nerve cells, resulting in an increase in the serotonin effect.

In 1991, a double-blind study comparing 5-HTP to an SSRI was conducted in Switzerland.[80] 5-HTP was compared to the SSRI fluvoxamine (Luvox). Fluvoxamine is used primarily in the United States as a treatment for obsessive-compulsive disorder (OCD), an anxiety disorder that affects an estimated five million Americans. Fluvoxamine exerts antidepressant activity comparable to (if not better than) that of other SSRIs such as Prozac, Zoloft, and Paxil.

In the study, subjects received either 5-HTP (100 mg) or fluvoxamine (50 mg) three times daily for six weeks. The assessment methods used to judge effectiveness included the Hamilton Rating Scale for Depression (HDS). As can be seen in Table 3, the percentage decrease in depression was slightly better in the 5-HTP group (60.7 percent vs. 56.1 percent). 5-HTP was faster-acting than the fluvoxamine, and a higher percentage of patients responded to 5-HTP than to fluvoxamine.

The advantages of 5-HTP over fluvoxamine are evident when looking at the subcategories of the HDS: depressed mood, anxiety, physical symptoms, and insomnia.

Perhaps more important than simply relieving insomnia is 5-HTP's ability to improve the quality of sleep. In contrast, antidepressant drugs greatly disrupt sleep processes. On the self-assessment depression scale (SADS), 5-HTP produced a 53.3-percent drop in SADS values, compared to a drop of 47.6 percent for the fluvoxamine group. Anything over a fifty-percent drop is an excellent result. In fact, a fifty-percent drop is the best that SSRIs generally produce.

5-HTP is equal to or better than standard antidepressant drugs, and its side effects are much less severe. Fourteen patients (38.9 percent) of the patients receiving 5-HTP reported side effects, compared to 18 patients (54.5 percent) in the fluvoxamine group. The most common side effects from 5-HTP were mild nausea, heartburn, and gastrointestinal problems (flatulence, feelings of fullness, and rumbling sensations). These side effects were rated as being very mild to mild. In contrast, most of the side effects experienced in the fluvoxamine group were of moderate to severe intensity. The only subject to drop out of the 5-HTP group did so after thirty-five days (five weeks), while four subjects in the fluvoxamine group dropped out after only two

TABLE 4 5-HTP vs. Fluvoxamine: Reduction in Severity for Subcategoreis of the HDS		
SUBCATEGORY	**5-HTP (%)**	**FLUVOXAMINE (%)**
Depressed mood	65.7	61.8
Anxiety	58.2	48.3
Physical symptoms	47.6	37.8
Insomnia	61.7	55.9

TABLE 5 5-HTP vs. Antidepressant Drugs: comparsion of Side Effects

	% OF PATIENTS EXPERIENCING SIDE EFFECT		
SIDE EFFECT	5-HTP	TRICYCLICS	SSRIS
Nausea	9%	15%	23%
Headache	5%	16%	20%
Nervousness	2.5%	11%	16%
Insomnia	2.5%	7%	17%
Anxiety	2.5%	9%	14%
Drowsiness	7%	23%	11%
Diarrhea	2.5%	4%	12%
Tremor	0%	18%	11%
Dry mouth	7%	64.5%	12%
Sweating	2.5%	15%	9%
Dizziness	5%	25.5%	7%
Constipation	5%	25%	5.5%
Vision changes	0%	14.5%	4%

weeks. The longer the 5-HTP was used (e.g., after four to six weeks of use), the less problem there was with any mild nausea.

In summary, 5-HTP has been shown to have equipotency with standard antidepressant drugs in terms of effectiveness, but offers several advantages in that it is better tolerated and associated with fewer and much milder side effects.

Phenylalanine and Tyrosine

Although the number of clinical studies utilizing phenylalanine or tyrosine for depression does not approach the number using tryptophan and 5-HTP, there is evidence that these monoamine precursors may be effective in some individuals.[82,83]

Phenylalanine, besides being converted to tyrosine, can be converted to phenylethylamine (PEA).[82] This biogenic amine has been suggested to be an internal stimulant and antidepressive substance in humans. It is found in high concentrations in chocolate, which might explain the latter's addictive-

ness. Low urinary PEA levels are found in depressed patients, while high levels are found in schizophrenic patients.[82,83] Phenylalanine, both D- and L- forms, has been demonstrated to increase urinary PEA output and brain PEA concentrations.

In regard to tyrosine, the activity of supplemental tyrosine in depressives may also be related to the fact that it increases PEA levels, rather than just enhancing the levels of the monoamines epinephrine, norepinephrine, and dopamine.[81] Like tryptophan, the brain tyrosine content is best determined by the ratio of serum tyrosine concentration to the sum of its brain-uptake competitors (leucine, isoleucine, valine, tryptophan, and phenylalanine). Tyrosine ratios are increased by eating high-protein meals. Table 6 summarizes clinical studies using phenylalanine and/or tyrosine to treat depression. These results indicate that phenylalanine and tyrosine supplementation offer encouraging alternatives to tricyclics and MAO inhibitors.

In the early 1970s, Herman van Praag, M.D., and colleagues discovered that about

REFERENCE	# OF PATIENTS	DOSE (MG/DAY)	DURATION (DAYS)	CLINICAL EFFECTS AND COMMENTS
Yaryura et al. (1974)	15	200–400	14	(d,l-P) 10 severely depressed patients responded
Fischer et al. (1975)	23	100	1–13	(d, or d,l-P) A complete response was observed in 17 patients previously unresponsive to tricyclics and MAO inhibitors
Beckman et al. (1977)	20	75–200	20	(d,l-P) 8 complete remissions, 4 marked improvement; used Hamilton Depression Scale and von Zerssen Self-Rating Questionnaire
Heller (1978)	55	100–400	60–180	(d-P) 73% recovered completely after 15 days, 23% had marked improvement, 4% failed to respond
Heller (1978)	60	100	30	(d-P) Complete remission and improvement 83% for the phenylalanine group compared to 73% for the imipramine group; double-blind controlled study; no diagnostic criteria or rating scales were reported
Beckman (1979)	27	200	30	(d,l-P) No significant difference between phenylalanine and imipramine groups
Gibson et al. (1983)	9	100 mg/kg	ongoing	(T) Double-blind, placebo-controlled study; tyrosine demonstrated a rate of response (60–70%) typical of most major antidepressants, without side effects

TABLE 6   Phenylalanine and Tyrosine Used in Treating Depression[82,83]

P = Phenylalanine, T = Tyrosine

one out of five patients who responded well to 5-HTP tended to relapse after one month of treatment. The antidepressant effects of 5-HTP in these subjects began to wear off gradually after the first month despite the fact that the level of 5-HTP in their blood, and presumably the level of serotonin in the brain, remained at the same level as when they were experiencing a benefit.[81] These researchers discovered that, while serotonin levels appeared to stay at the same levels after one month of treatment, the levels of the other important monoamine neurotransmitters, dopamine and norepinephrine, declined.[84] These patients responded to supplemental tyrosine.

S-Adenosyl-Methionine (SAM)

SAM was covered briefly in this chapter in the discussion of vitamin B12 and folic acid. SAM is involved in the methylation of monoamines, neurotransmitters, and phospholipids such as phosphatidylcholine and phosphatidylserine. Normally, the brain man-

TABLE 7	Double-Blind Clinical Studies with SAM vs. Placebo in Treating Depression[88]		
AUTHORS	**SAM RESPONDERS**	**PLACEBO RESPONDERS**	**CONCLUSION**
Fazio et al. (1973)	Not quantified		SAM superior to placebo based on Hamilton Depression Scale
Agnoli et al. (1976)	20/20	1/10	SAM superior to placebo
Muscettola et al. (1982)	4/10	0/10	SAM superior to placebo
Janicak (1982)	5/7	0/5	SAM superior to placebo
Caruso et al. (1984)	Not quantified		SAM superior to placebo based on Hamilton Depression Scale
Carney et al. (1986)	Not quantified		SAM superior to placebo based on Hamilton Depression Scale and Beck Scale
De Leo (1987)	Not quantified		SAM superior to placebo based on Clinical Global Impression Scale
Total	29/37 (78%)	1/25(4%)	SAM dramatically more effective than placebo

ufactures all the SAM it needs from the amino acid *methionine*. However, SAM synthesis is impaired in depressed patients. Supplementing the diet with SAM in depressed patients results in increased levels of serotonin and dopamine and improved binding of neurotransmitters to receptor sites. This causes increased serotonin and dopamine activity and improved brain cell membrane fluidity, resulting in significant clinical improvement.[85–87]

The results of a number of clinical studies suggest that SAM is one of the most effective natural antidepressants.[88–91] Unfortunately, as of this writing (October 1997) SAM is still not available in the United States. Table 7 summarizes double-blind studies that have compared SAM to either a placebo or a tricyclic drug such as imipramine.

The studies cited in Tables 7 and 8 utilized injectable SAM. However, more recent studies using a new oral preparation at a dosage of 400 mg four times daily (1,600 mg total) have demonstrated that SAM is just as effective

orally as it is when given intravenously.[92–95] SAM is also better tolerated and has a quicker onset of antidepressant action than tricyclic antidepressants.

A recent study compared SAM to the tricyclic desipramine. In addition to clinical response, the blood level of SAM was determined in both groups. At the end of the four-week trial, sixty-two percent of the patients treated with SAM and fifty percent of the patients treated with desipramine had significantly improved. Regardless of the type of treatment, patients with a fifty-percent decrease in their Hamilton Rating Scale for Depression (HDS) score showed a significant increase in plasma SAM concentration. These results suggest that one of the ways in which tricyclic drugs exert antidepressive effects is by raising SAM levels.[96]

No significant side effects have been reported from the use of oral SAM. However, because SAM can cause nausea and vomiting in some people, it is recommended that SAM be started at a dosage of 200 mg twice daily

	SAM RESPONDERS	DRUG RESPONDERS	
TABLE 8 Double-Blind Clinical Studies with SAM vs. Antidepressant Drugs in Treating Depression[88]			
AUTHORS	**SAM RESPONDERS**	**DRUG RESPONDERS**	**CONCLUSION**
Mantero et al. (1975)	11/16	9/15	SAM comparable to imipramine (75 mg/day)
Barberi et al. (1978)	10/10	8/10	SAM more effective than amitriptyline (100 mg/day)
Del Vecchio et al. (1978)	5/14	4/10	SAM comparable to clomipramine (100 mg/day)
Miccoli et al. (1978)	35/45	30/41	SAM comparable to clomipramine (100 mg/day)
Scarzella et al. [1(978)	9/10	9/10	SAM comparable to clomipramine (100 mg/day)
Scaggion et al. (1982)	18/22	10/18	SAM more effective than nomifensine (200 mg/day)
Kufferle et al. (1982)	7/9	6/9	SAM comparable to clomipramine (50 mg/day)
Plotkin (1988)	9/9	2/9	SAM more effective than imipramine (150 mg/day)
Janicak (1988)	5/7	2/3	SAM comparable to imipramine (150 mg/day)
Total	109/142 (76%)	80/124 (61%)	SAM is significantly more effective than antidepressant drugs

for the first two days, increased to 400 mg twice daily on day three, then to 400 mg three times daily on day ten, and finally to the full dosage of 400 mg four times daily after twenty days.

Individuals with bipolar (manic) depression should not take SAM. Because of SAM's antidepressant activity, individuals with bipolar depression are susceptible to experiencing hypomania or mania. This effect is exclusive to some individuals with bipolar depression.

Botanical Medicines

St. John's wort (Hypericum perforatum)

Extracts of St. John's wort standardized for hypericin content (usually 0.3 percent) are the most thoroughly researched natural antidepressants. A total of 1,592 patients have been studied in twenty-five double-blind controlled studies (fifteen compared to a placebo, ten compared to an antidepressant).[97–99] In these studies, St. John's wort extract was shown to produce improvements in many psychological symptoms, including depression, anxiety, apathy, sleep disturbances, insomnia, anorexia, and feelings of worthlessness. The main advantage of using St. John's wort extract as opposed to antidepressant drugs was found to be not so much a difference in therapeutic outcome, but rather a significant advantage in terms of side effects, cost, and patient satisfaction. The double-blind studies with the highest methodological quality rating are listed in Table 9.

In the study with the highest quality rating, 135 depressed patients were treated with

TABLE 9 Summary of Clinical Trials with St. John's wort Extract in Treating Depression

TRIAL (REF #)	# OF PATIENTS	BASELINE HDS	DOSE (HYPERICIN MG/D)	DURATION (WKS)	RESPONDER RATE* (ST. JOHN'S WORT)	RESPONDER RATE* (PLACEBO)
Trials comparing St. John's wort to a placebo						
Halama[100]	50	18.0	1.08	4	10/25	0/25
Hansgren[101]	72	20.4	2.7	4	27/34	9/38
Harrer[102]	120	20.9	0.75	6	22/58	9/58
Hubner[103]	40	12.4	2.7	4	14/20	9/20
Quandt[104]	88	17.3	0.75	4	29/44	3/44
Reh[105]	50	20.0	1.0	8	20/25	11/25
Schmidt[106]	65	16.4	1.08	6	20/32	6/33
Schmidt[107]	40	29.5	0.75	4	15/25	3/24
Sommer[108]	105	15.8	2.7	4	28/50	13/55
Totals	630				185/313 (59%)	63/322 (20%)
Trials comparing St. John's wort extract to an antidepressant drug						
Bergman[109]	80	15.4	0.75	6	32/40	28/40 (amitriptyline)
Harrer[110]	102	19.4	2.7	4	27/51	28/51 (maprotiline)
Vorbach[111]	135	9.4	2.7	4	42/67	37/68 (imipramine)
Totals	317				101/158 (64%)	93/159 (58%)

* Responder rate: a decrease in the HDS of greater than 50% or achieving a value less than 10

either St. John's wort extract (0.3 percent hypericin content, 300 mg three times per day) or imipramine (25 mg three times per day) for a period of six weeks. The main outcome criteria were the Hamilton Depression Scale (HDS) and the Depression Scale according to von Zerssen (D-S), two popular rating scales that measure severity of depression. Better overall results were seen in patients taking St. John's wort. Again, the main advantage was not so much a difference in therapeutic outcome, but a significant advantage in terms of lack of side effects and excellent patient tolerance in the St. John's wort group. The major side effect with St. John's wort is mild stomach irritation.

Kava (Piper methysticum)

Like St. John's wort, kava extracts are gaining in popularity in Europe in the treatment of anxiety and depression. Several European countries (Germany, United Kingdom, Switzerland, and Austria) have approved kava preparations for the treatment of nervous anxiety, insomnia, depression, and restlessness on the basis of detailed pharmacological data and favorable clinical studies. In fact, kava extract compares favorably to benzodiazepines in effectiveness but does not possess the major drawbacks of these drugs (impaired mental acuity, addictiveness, etc.).[112–114] These approved kava preparations are extracts standardized for kavalac-

TABLE 10 St. John's Wort Extract Compared to Imipramine		
	ST. JOHN'S WORT	IMIPRAMINE
Hamilton Depression Scale		
Initial measurement	20.2	19.4
Week 6	8.8	10.7
Depression Scale (von Zerssen)		
Initial measurement	39.6	39
Week 6	27.2	29.2

tone content (usually thirty to seventy percent). Kava appears most useful in cases of depression with severe anxiety. (For more information on kava, see ANXIETY.)

Ginkgo biloba

The extract of *Ginkgo biloba* leaves standardized to contain twenty-four percent ginkgo flavonglycosides and six percent terpenoids exerts good antidepressant effects, especially in patients over the age of fifty. Researchers became interested in the antidepressive effects of *Ginkgo biloba* extract as a result of the improvement in mood reported by patients suffering from cerebrovascular insufficiency who were treated with ginkgo in double-blind studies.[115–118] These observations led to several double-blind studies on the efficacy of ginkgo in treating depression.

In one of the more recent double-blind studies, forty older patients (ranging in age from fifty-one to seventy-eight years old) with depression who had not benefited fully from standard antidepressant drugs were given either 80 mg of *Ginkgo biloba* extract three times daily or a placebo along with their antidepressant drug.[119] By the end of the fourth week of the study, the total average score on the Hamilton Depression Scale (HDS) was reduced from 14 to 7. At the end of the eighth week, the total score in the *Ginkgo biloba* extract group had dropped to

4.5. In comparison, the placebo group only dropped from 14 to 13. This study indicates that *Ginkgo biloba* extract can be used with standard antidepressants; it may enhance their effectiveness, particularly in patients over fifty years of age.

In addition to human studies, *Ginkgo biloba* extract has demonstrated antidepressant effects in a number of animal models, including the learned helplessness model described earlier in this chapter. The most interesting of these studies demonstrated that *Ginkgo biloba* extract was able to counteract one of the major changes in brain chemistry associated with aging: the reduction in the number of serotonin receptor sites.[120] Typically, with aging there is a significant reduction in the number of serotonin receptor sites on brain cells. As a result, the elderly are more susceptible to depression, impaired mental function, insomnia, and sleep disturbances.

The study was designed to determine whether *Ginkgo biloba* extract could alter the number of serotonin receptors in aged (twenty-four-month-old) and young (four-month-old) rats. At the beginning of the study, the older rats had a twenty-two-percent lower number of serotonin binding sites compared to the younger rats. The results of ongoing treatment with *Ginkgo biloba* extract for twenty-one consecutive days demonstrated that there was no change in receptor binding in young rats, but in the aged rats there was a statistically significant increase (thirty-three percent) in the number of serotonin binding sites. These results indicate that *Ginkgo biloba* extract may counteract at least some, if not all, of the age-dependent reductions of serotonin binding sites in the human brain as well.

The exact mechanism of *Ginkgo biloba* extract's effect in increasing serotonin receptors has not yet been determined. However, *Ginkgo biloba* extract may address two major reasons why the number of serotonin receptors declines with age: (1) impaired receptor synthesis; and (2) changes in cerebral neuronal membranes or receptors as a result of free-radical damage. *Ginkgo biloba* extract has demonstrated an ability to increase protein synthesis. In addition, it is known to be a potent antioxidant. The most likely explanation is that it is the combination of these two effects (and others) rather than one single mechanism.

TREATMENT SUMMARY

Treatment is largely dependent on a few central elements: accurate determination of which factors are contributing to the depression; balancing of errant neurotransmitter levels; and optimizing nutrition, lifestyle, and psychological health.

Diet

Increase the consumption of fiber-rich plant foods (fruits, vegetables, grains, legumes, and raw nuts and seeds). Avoid the intake of caffeine, nicotine, other stimulants, and alcohol. Identify and control food allergies.

Lifestyle

Follow the recommendations given in the chapter A POSITIVE MENTAL ATTITUDE.

In addition, consult with a counselor to learn skills and tools that will help you attain a positive, optimistic mental attitude. Get regular exercise—at least thirty minutes at least three times per week—and practice a relaxation/stress reduction technique for ten to fifteen minutes each day.

Nutritional Supplements

- High-potency multiple-vitamin-and-mineral
- Vitamin C:
  500–1,000 mg three times per day
- Vitamin E:
  200–400 IU per day
- Flaxseed oil:
  1 tablespoon per day
- 5-HTP:
  100–200 mg three times per day
- Folic acid and vitamin B12:
  800 mcg of each per day

Botanical Medicines

- If under the age of fifty, St. John's wort extract (0.3% hypericin): 300 mg three times per day. In severe cases, St. John's wort extract can be used in combination with 5-HTP.
- If over the age of fifty, *Ginkgo biloba* extract (24% ginkgo flavonglycosides): 80 mg three times per day. In severe cases, can be used in combination with St. John's wort and/or 5-HTP.
- If anxiety is a significant factor, kava extract standardized for kavalactone content: 45–70 mg kavalactones three times per day.

Diabetes Mellitus

. . . .

The National Diabetes Data Group of the National Institutes of Health recommends the following criteria for diagnosing diabetes:

- Fasting (overnight): serum glucose (blood sugar) concentration greater than or equal to 140 mg/dl on at least two separate occasions
- Following ingestion of 75 g of glucose: serum glucose concentration greater than or equal to 200 mg/dl at two hours post-ingestion and at least one other sample during the two-hour test
- Classic symptoms of increased thirst, increased hunger, and increased urination

Diabetes is a chronic disorder of carbohydrate, fat, and protein metabolism characterized by fasting elevations of blood sugar (glucose) levels and a greatly increased risk of heart disease, stroke, kidney disease, and loss of nerve function. Diabetes can occur when the pancreas does not secrete enough insulin or if the cells of the body become resistant to insulin. Hence, the blood sugar cannot get into the cells, which then leads to serious complications (see Complications of Diabetes, later in this chapter).

The classic symptoms of diabetes are frequent urination, excessive thirst, and excessive appetite. Because these symptoms are not very serious, many people who have diabetes do not seek medical care. In fact, of the more than ten million Americans with diabetes, fewer than half know that they have diabetes or ever consult a physician.

Classification

Diabetes is divided into two major categories: Type I and Type II. Type I, or Insulin-Dependent Diabetes Mellitus (IDDM), occurs most often in children and adolescents. Type II, or Non-Insulin-Dependent Diabetes Mellitus (NIDDM), usually has an onset after forty years of age.

Insulin-Dependent Diabetes Mellitus

IDDM is associated with complete destruction of the beta-cells of the pancreas, which manufacture the hormone insulin. IDDM patients require lifelong insulin for the control of blood sugar levels. Type I diabetics must learn how to manage their blood sugar levels on a daily basis, modifying insulin types and dosage schedules as necessary according to the results of regular blood sugar testing. About ten percent of all diabetics are Type I.

Although the exact cause of Type I diabetes is unknown, current theory suggests that it results from injury to the insulin-producing beta-cells, coupled with some defect in tissue regeneration capacity. In Type I diabetes, the body's immune system apparently begins to attack the pancreas. Antibodies for beta-cells are present in seventy-five percent of all cases of Type I diabetes, compared to one-half percent to two percent of non-diabetics. It is probable that the antibodies to the beta-cells develop in response to cell destruction due to other mechanisms (chemical, free-radical, viral, food allergy, etc.). It appears that normal individuals either do not develop as severe an antibody reaction, or are better able to repair the damage once it occurs.

Non-Insulin-Dependent Diabetes Mellitus

About ninety percent of all diabetics are Type II. Their insulin levels are typically elevated, indicating a loss of sensitivity to insulin by the cells of the body. Obesity is a major contributing factor to this loss of insulin sensitivity; approximately ninety percent of individuals with Type II diabetes are obese. In most cases, achieving ideal body weight is associated with restoration of normal blood sugar levels in these patients.

In the treatment of Type II diabetes, diet is of primary importance and should be diligently followed before a drug is used. Most cases of Type II diabetes can be controlled by diet alone. Despite a high success rate with dietary intervention, physicians often use drugs or insulin instead.

Other Types of Diabetes

Other types of diabetes include:

- *Secondary diabetes* (a form of diabetes that is secondary to certain conditions and syndromes, such as pancreatic disease, hormone disturbances, drugs, and malnutrition)
- *Gestational diabetes* (glucose intolerance that occurs during pregnancy)
- *Impaired glucose tolerance* (a condition that includes prediabetic, chemical, latent, borderline, subclinical, and asymptomatic diabetes); individuals with impaired glucose tolerance have blood glucose levels and glucose-tolerance test (GTT) results that are intermediate between normal and clearly abnormal

In addition, many practitioners consider *reactive hypoglycemia* to be a prediabetic condition.

QUICK REVIEW

- **Diabetes is divided into two major categories: Type I and Type II.**
- **Ninety percent of diabetics are Type II and are not dependent upon insulin.**
- **Although genetic factors appear important in susceptibility to diabetes, environmental factors are required to trigger diabetes.**
- **Obesity is another significant environmental factor, as ninety percent of diabetics are obese.**
- **Exposure to a protein in cow's milk (bovine albumin peptide) in infancy**
  may trigger the autoimmune process and subsequent Type I diabetes.
- **The trace mineral chromium plays a major role in the sensitivity of cells to insulin.**
- **To reduce the risk of developing the complications of diabetes, it is important to control against elevations in blood sugar by careful monitoring.**
- **Dietary modification and treatment is fundamental to the successful treatment of diabetes, whether it be Type I or II.**
- **The treatment of diabetes requires nutritional supplementation, as diabetics**

Frequency and Epidemiology

The overall frequency of diabetes in the United States is estimated at approximately 4.5 percent, of which 90 percent are NIDDM and the rest are primarily IDDM.[1] In 1992, while diabetics accounted for only 4.5 percent of the U.S. population, diabetic care required roughly 14.6 percent of the total U.S. healthcare expenditures ($105 billion).[2]

The number of Americans with diabetes is rising. Diabetes is now the seventh leading cause of death in the United States. At the current rate of increase (six percent per year), the number of diabetics will double every fifteen years. Population studies have linked diabetes to diet and lifestyle. Diabetes is uncommon in places where people consume a more "primitive" diet.[3,4] As indigenous peoples switch from their native diets to the highly processed "foods of commerce," their rate of diabetes increases, eventually reaching the same proportions seen in Western societies.

The Hypoglycemia-Diabetes Link

Blood sugar problems are strongly associated with the so-called "Western diet."[3,4] This diet is rich in refined sugar, fat, and animal products, and low in dietary fiber. It is widely accepted that refined carbohydrates are among the most important contributing factors to diabetes and reactive hypoglycemia (as well as obesity). Refined sugars are quickly absorbed into the bloodstream, causing a rapid rise in blood sugar. The body's response is to greatly increase the secretion of insulin by the pancreas. The excessive secretion of insulin drives the blood sugar down and often causes the symptoms of hypoglycemia to appear.

In response to the rapid fall in blood glucose levels, the adrenal glands secrete *epinephrine* (adrenaline), which causes a rapid

- -

have a greatly increased need for many nutrients.

- Since the transport of vitamin C into cells is facilitated by insulin, many diabetics do not have enough intracellular vitamin C.
- Some newly diagnosed Type I diabetics have experienced complete reversal of their diabetes with niacinamide supplementation.
- Vitamin B6 supplementation appears to offer significant protection against the development of diabetic nerve disease.

- Diabetics appear to have an increased requirement for vitamin E, and benefit from high-dose supplementation.
- Onions and garlic have demonstrated blood-sugar-lowering action in several studies and help reduce the risk of cardiovascular disease.
- The oral administration of bitter melon preparations has shown good results in clinical trials in patients with both Type I and Type II diabetes.
- Recent scientific investigation has upheld the effectiveness of *Gymnema sylvestre* in treating both Type I and Type II diabetes.

TABLE 1 Comparison of Type I and Type II Diabetes		
FEATURES	**TYPE I**	**TYPE II**
Age at onset	Usually under 40	Usually over 40
% of all diabetics	Less than 10%	Greater than 90%
Seasonal trend	Fall and winter	None
Family history	Uncommon	Common
Appearance of symptoms	Rapid	Slow
Obesity at onset	Uncommon	Common
Insulin levels	Decreased	Variable
Insulin resistance	Occasional	Often
Treatment with insulin	Always	Not required
Beta-cells	Decreased	Variable
Ketoacidosis	Frequent	Rare
Complications	Frequent	Frequent

increase in the blood glucose level. In time, the adrenal glands become exhausted by the repeated stress and cannot mount an appropriate response. This lack of response leads to reactive hypoglycemia. If blood sugar control mechanisms are further stressed, the body will eventually become insensitive to insulin or the pancreas will also become exhausted, and the reactive hypoglycemia will turn into diabetes.

Diagnosis

Fasting Blood Glucose Level

The standard method of diagnosing diabetes involves the measurement of blood glucose levels. The normal fasting blood glucose level is between 70 and 105 mg/dl. A fasting blood glucose measurement greater than 140 mg/dl on two separate occasions is diagnostic of diabetes. Levels below 50 mg/dl indicate fasting hypoglycemia.[1]

The Glucose Tolerance Test

A more functional test of blood sugar control is the oral glucose tolerance test (GTT). The GTT is a very sensitive test for diabetes. However, it is also very stressful to the patient and has a relatively low specificity. The National Diabetes Data Group recommends giving a 75-gram glucose dose dissolved in 300 ml of water for adults (1.75 g per 2.2 pounds of body weight for children) after an overnight fast. Subjects are encouraged to consume at least 150 grams of carbohydrate daily for three days prior to the test. The patient is considered normal if the two-hour glucose level is less than 140 mg/dl and no value exceeds 200 mg/dl. A diagnosis of diabetes requires that levels be above 200 mg/dl both at two hours and at least once between zero time and two hours. Medications that impair glucose tolerance (diuretics, glucocorticoids, nicotinic acid, and phenytoin) may invalidate the results.

The Glucose-Insulin Tolerance Test

Relying on blood sugar levels alone is often not adequate in diagnosing blood sugar disorders. Several studies have shown that the glucose-insulin tolerance test (G-ITT) is more sensitive in the diagnosis of both hypoglycemia and diabetes than the standard GTT.

The G-ITT uses a standard six-hour glucose tolerance test coupled with measure-

TABLE 2	Glucose Tolerance Test Response Criteria
TYPE	**CRITERIA**
Normal	No elevation greater than 160 mg
	Below 150 mg at the end of first hour
	Below 120 mg at the end of second hour
	Flat
	No variation more than ± 20 mg from fasting value
Pre-diabetic	Over 120 mg at the end of second hour
Diabetic	Over 180 mg during the first hour
	200 mg or higher at the end of first hour
	150 mg or higher at the end of second hour
Reactive hypoglycemia	Normal response for the first 2 or 3 hours
	A decrease of 20 mg or more from the fasting level during the final hours
Probable reactive hypoglycemia	Normal response for the first 2 or 3 hours
	A decrease of 10 to 20 mg from the fasting level during the final hours
Flat hypoglycemia	An elevation of 20 mg or less followed by a decrease of 20 mg or more below fasting level
Pre-diabetic hypoglycemia	A 2-hour response like the pre-diabetic
	Hypoglycemic response during the final 3 hours
Hyperinsulinism	A marked hypoglycemic response, with a value of less than 50 mg during the third, fourth, or fifth hour

ments of insulin levels. The G-ITT appears to be one of the best diagnostic indicators for faulty sugar metabolism. As many as two-thirds of subjects with suspected diabetes or hypoglycemia who have normal glucose tolerance test results will demonstrate abnormal insulin tolerance tests. The downside to this test is that it is costly. For example, the glucose-insulin tolerance test (G-ITT) costs around two hundred dollars, while a standard GTT usually costs less than thirty dollars. Despite the high price, the G-ITT and other diagnostic tests are often appropriate.

Causes of Diabetes

Although genetic factors appear important in susceptibility to diabetes, environmental factors are required to trigger diabetes. Many have been identified. A diet high in refined, fiber-depleted carbohydrates is believed to induce diabetes in susceptible genetic types, while a high intake of high-fiber, complex-carbohydrate-rich foods protects against the development of diabetes.[3,4]

Obesity is another significant environmental factor, as ninety percent of NIDDM types are obese.[1] Even in normal individuals, significant weight gain results in carbohydrate intolerance, higher insulin levels, and insulin insensitivity in fat and muscle tissue. The progressive development of insulin insensitivity (which will be discussed in more detail later) is believed to be the underlying factor in the development of NIDDM. Weight loss alone can correct all of these abnormalities and either significantly improves diabetes or totally resolves it.[5]

TABLE 3	Glucose-Insulin Tolerance Test Criteria
PATTERN	**DESCRIPTION**
Pattern 1	Normal fasting insulin 0–30 units. Peak insulin at $^1/2$–1 hour. The combined insulin values for the second and third hours is less than 60 units. This pattern is considered normal.
Pattern 2	Normal fasting insulin. Peak at $^1/2$–1 hour with a delayed return to normal. Second- and third-hour levels between 60–100 units are usually associated with hypoglycemia and are considered borderline for diabetes; values greater than 100 units are considered definite diabetes.
Pattern 3	Normal fasting insulin. Peak at second or third hour instead of $^1/2$–1 hour. Definite diabetes.
Pattern 4	High fasting insulin. Definite diabetes.
Pattern 5	Low insulin response. All tested values for insulin lower than 30. When associated with elevated blood sugar levels, it indicates probable insulin-dependent diabetes (juvenile pattern).

Causative Factors in IDDM

Insulin-Dependent Diabetes Mellitus is generally recognized as due to an insulin deficiency.[1] Although the exact cause is unknown, current theory suggests a hereditary predisposition to injury to the insulin-producing beta-cells coupled with some defect in the ability of the pancreas to regenerate new beta-cells. Causes of injury are probably free radicals, viral infection, and autoimmune reactions.

Smoked or Cured Meats   Streptozotocin is a compound that is used to induce diabetes in studies with animals. It works by destroying the beta-cells.[6] It is similar in structure and function to the N-nitroso-compounds found in smoked and/or cured meats. In fact, a diet high in bacon, ham, smoked salmon, and similar products has been linked to IDDM.[7] Many other chemicals in foods and the environment have also been implicated in beta-cell damage.[6–8] These chemicals typically damage the pancreas by acting as free radicals—highly reactive molecules which destroy cellular components.

Viral Infection   Recent population-based and experimental evidence has strengthened the hypothesis that a viral infection causes IDDM in some cases.[6,8] A viral cause was initially suspected due to the seasonal variation in the onset of the disease (higher in October to March). During these months, viral diseases such as mumps, hepatitis, infectious mononucleosis, congenital rubella, and coxsackie virus infections are much more common. Viruses are capable of infecting pancreatic beta-cells and inducing antibody attack.

Autoimmunity   Developing antibodies against the pancreatic beta cells (a process known as autoimmunity) is probably the major causative factor, especially in individuals with a specific genetic makeup (the HLA-B8 genotype). Antibodies to pancreatic cells are present in seventy-five percent of all cases of IDDM, compared to one-half to two percent of people without diabetes.[6] It is probable that the antibodies to the beta-cells develop in response to cell destruction due to other mechanisms (chemical, viral, etc.)

when normally concealed cellular antigens are exposed. It appears that normal individuals either do not develop as severe an antibody reaction, or are more able to repair the damage once it occurs.

Recent studies have provided some strong evidence that exposure to a protein in cow's milk (bovine albumin peptide) in infancy may trigger the autoimmune process and subsequent Type I diabetes. Although animal and laboratory evidence exists to justify these concerns, studies involving humans have generated conflicting results.[9]

A critical review and analysis of all relevant citations in the medical literature indicated that early cow's milk exposure may, in fact, be an important determinant of subsequent Type I diabetes and may increase the risk by about 1.5 times.[9] In detailed studies, it was shown that patients with Type I diabetes were more likely to have been breast-fed for under three months and to have been exposed to cow's milk or solid foods before the age of four months. The cow's milk protein can be found in the mother's breast milk, so in cases of family history of diabetes it is recommended that the mother avoid cow's milk while breast-feeding.

Causative Factors in NIDDM

Central to the development of NIDDM is insulin insensitivity. The typical patient with NIDDM has high levels of insulin in the bloodstream. There is plenty of insulin, but it is just not performing its function because cells have become unresponsive. Measures to restore insulin sensitivity (e.g., dietary changes and/or weight loss) usually relieve NIDDM.

Obesity Obesity plays a major role as a cause of NIDDM for many patients.[1,5,10–12] As stated earlier, obesity is associated with in-

sulin insensitivity, and adipose size and distribution also seem to be important.

Weight loss, in particular a significant decrease in body-fat percentage, is a prime objective in treating the majority of NIDDM patients since it improves all aspects of diabetes and may result in cure.

Dietary Fat The percentage of calories from fat in the diet, especially saturated fat, has been shown to be associated with NIDDM as well as to predict the conversion from impaired glucose tolerance to NIDDM.[13,14] These results suggest that a high-fat, low-carbohydrate diet increases the risk of subsequently developing NIDDM. Ironically, such a diet was used in the past for the dietary management of diabetes.

Chromium Deficiency The trace mineral chromium plays a major role in the sensitivity of cells to insulin.[15–20] Chromium, as a critical component of the so-called "glucose tolerance factor" (GTF), functions as a cofactor in all insulin-regulating activities. Chromium deficiency is widespread in the United States. Supplementing the diet with chromium has been shown to significantly improve insulin action; decrease fasting glucose, cholesterol, and triglyceride levels; and increase the HDL-cholesterol level by increasing insulin sensitivity in normal, elderly, and NIDDM patients.[15–20] Chromium is not, however, a panacea for NIDDM. In other words, although chromium is important and many cases of NIDDM will be improved by chromium supplementation, it will only produce its benefits in people with low chromium levels.

Prenatal Factors Recent population-based evidence supports the concept that the nutritional status of the mother during pregnancy plays a role in determining whether the child will develop both types of diabetes later in life. Studies done in Berlin have shown that adults born during the "hypocaloric war and post-war period (1941–48)" have significantly lower rates of diabetes that those born during the years before and after this period. This is not a minor correlation; the data show a greater than fifty-percent drop in the incidence of diabetes![21] What can be gleaned from this research is that overeating (overconsumption of calories) during pregnancy may increase the risk for diabetes for the unborn fetus later in life.

Another study shows a significantly lower incidence of childhood diabetes during periods in which blood glucose level was carefully controlled.[22] Although the data in this study are based on a number of suppositions, they again indicate a greater than fifty-percent drop in the incidence of childhood diabetes when mothers avoided increases in blood sugar levels above normal.

Monitoring the Diabetic Patient

There appears to be a strong relationship between blood sugar level and the development of the complications of diabetes. Specifically, when blood sugar levels are chronically elevated, the risk for complications is very high. To reduce the risk of developing the complications of diabetes, it is important to control against elevations in blood sugar by careful monitoring. The availability of home glucose monitoring kits makes it easier now than in the past to monitor blood sugar levels, resulting in a major improvement in the care of diabetes.

Another major improvement is the measurement of the level of glycosylated hemoglobin ($HgbA_{1c}$), which allows monitoring of blood sugar levels over a long period of time. Levels of proteins that have glucose molecules attached to them (glycosylated peptides) are elevated severalfold in diabetics. Normally about five to seven percent of hemoglobin is combined with glucose. Mild elevations in blood sugar result in $HgbA_{1c}$ concentrations of eight to ten percent, while severe elevations may result in concentrations of up to twenty percent.

Since the average life span of a red blood cell is 120 days, the $HgbA_{1c}$ measurement represents the average values for blood glucose over the preceding two to four months. $HgbA_{1c}$ determination can also be used in some cases to diagnose diabetes. Although the oral glucose tolerance test is more sensitive than the $HgbA_{1c}$ assay in the diagnosis of diabetes, it is also more stressful to the patient. Because an elevated $HgbA_{1c}$ level almost always indicates diabetes, many physicians will simply measure the $HgbA_{1c}$ level rather than (or before) subjecting patients, particularly pregnant women, to the stress of a GTT.

In general, measuring glycosylated hemoglobin (and possibly other glycosylated proteins) is an important and useful test for diabetic control and the prevention of complications. We recommend periodic measurement—every three months in poorly controlled diabetes, and every year in well-controlled cases.

Conventional Medical Treatment

IDDM

There is no question that a Type I diabetic requires insulin. Insulin preparations have been used in the treatment of diabetes since

1922. Since insulin is not absorbed orally, it must be injected. Insulin preparations come in concentrations of 100 units per milliliter (U-100) and 500 units per milliliter (U-500), but can differ in their source (beef, pork, or human synthetic insulin), duration of action (rapid, intermediate, or long-acting), and solubility (crystalline versus soluble). The human synthetic insulin is gaining wider acceptance as the preferred source.

Conventional insulin therapy involves administering crystalline insulin (usually a mixture of rapid- and intermediate-acting insulin) once or twice daily. This method is being replaced by *intensified insulin therapy,* in which the insulin is given in increasingly sophisticated and complex regimens. Growing evidence is demonstrating that intensified insulin therapy significantly reduces the development of the chronic complications of diabetes (see Complications of Diabetes, later in this chapter).[23] Intensified insulin therapy is designed to mimic as closely as possible the continuous variations in plasma insulin levels produced by a healthy pancreas.

Intensified insulin therapy requires either multiple daily injections (three to five injections per day) or the use of an "insulin pump" to administer a continuous supply of insulin. The insulin pump method involves filling a syringe with soluble insulin. The syringe, which looks like a ballpoint pen, is connected via a hollow flexible hose to a needle which is inserted into a site on the abdomen. The unit must be worn twenty-four hours a day. The plunger of the syringe is pressed slowly and constantly by a small pump so that a constant trickle of soluble insulin is delivered. Fifteen minutes prior to a meal, the diabetic can press the pump manually to release a burst of insulin.

In our opinion, the insulin pump, which approximates the natural levels of insulin, is the best of the currently available techniques, but is not without drawbacks. The device must be worn constantly and can be an irritation; the patient must be highly motivated to monitor blood sugar levels quite closely; the risk for hypoglycemia is greater; and not all physicians are familiar enough with the method.

Regardless of the type of insulin therapy used, the proper care of diabetes must include appropriate diet and lifestyle (see Diet and Exercise later in this chapter).

NIDDM

When Type II diabetes cannot be controlled satisfactorily with diet therapy, drugs or insulin may be utilized for additional support. Since most Type II diabetics are obese and secrete large amounts of insulin to overcome the body's cellular resistance to insulin, additional insulin is usually of only limited value.

While healthy individuals secrete approximately 31 units of insulin daily, the obese Type II diabetic secretes an average of 114 units daily. This amount is nearly four times the normal amount. In contrast to obese Type II individuals, lean Type II individuals produce about 14 units daily and individuals with Type I diabetes secrete only 4 units of insulin daily. If a diabetic is overproducing insulin, it makes more sense to work on increasing the sensitivity to insulin by following the recommendations given in the following paragraph.

The drug treatment of Type II diabetes utilizes *oral hypoglycemic agents.* These agents are sulfa drugs (*sulfonylureas*) that appear to stimulate the secretion of additional insulin by the pancreas in addition to enhancing the sensitivity of body tissues to insulin. Some common examples of oral hypoglycemic agents are:

Chlorpropamide (Diabinese)

Glipizide (Glucotrol)
Glyburide (Diabeta, Micronase)
Tolazamide (Tolinase)
Tolbutamide (Orinase)

As a group, these drugs are not very effective. After three months of continual treatment at an adequate dosage, only about sixty percent of Type II diabetics are able to control their blood sugar levels using these drugs. Furthermore, these agents generally lose their effectiveness over time. After an initial period of success, these drugs fail to produce a positive effect in about thirty percent of cases. The overall rate of achieving adequate control by long-term use of sulfonylureas is twenty to thirty percent at best.

In addition to being of limited value, there is evidence that these drugs actually produce harmful long-term side effects. For example, in a famous study conducted by the University Group Diabetes Program (UGDP) on the long-term effects of Tolbutamide, it was shown that the rate of death due to a heart attack or stroke was two-and-one-half times greater among Tolbutamide users than in the group controlling their Type II diabetes by diet alone.[24]

The major side effect of sulfonylureas is hypoglycemia. Other possible side effects include allergic skin reactions, headache, fatigue, indigestion, nausea and vomiting, and liver damage. Due to the high risk of side effects, these drugs have to be used with caution. They should not be used in the following situations:

During infection, injury, or surgery
During long-term corticosteroid use
Known allergy to sulfa drugs
Pregnancy

In addition, oral hypoglycemics must be used with extreme caution in treating the elderly, alcoholics, those taking multiple drugs, and those with impaired liver or kidney function.

Complications of Diabetes

Diabetes can result in numerous complications due to chronic elevations in blood glucose. The likelihood of developing complications, whether acute or chronic, is ultimately a reflection of the level of blood sugar control. A large body of evidence indicates that good blood sugar control significantly reduces the development of complications. Therefore, as mentioned before, monitoring and controlling the degree of elevations in blood sugar (hyperglycemia) is critical to the prevention of the major diabetic complications. This goal cannot be stressed too much.

Acute Complications

Diabetics are susceptible to three major acute complications: hypoglycemia, diabetic ketoacidosis (primarily affects IDDM), and nonketogenic hyperosmolar syndrome (primarily affects NIDDM).

Hypoglycemia

The problem of *hypoglycemia* due to insulin or oral hypoglycemic drugs is much more common in Type I than Type II diabetes because the Type I diabetic is injecting insulin. Taking too much insulin, missing a meal, or overexercising can result in hypoglycemia. It is imperative that a good relationship exist between the patient and the physician prescribing the insulin so that dosages can be gauged correctly.

Daytime hypoglycemic episodes are usually recognized by the following symptoms: sweating, nervousness, tremor, and hunger. Nighttime hypoglycemia may be without symptoms or may manifest as night sweats, unpleasant dreams, or early morning headaches.

In response to the hypoglycemia, secretion of several hormones that raise blood glucose levels is increased: epinephrine, norepinephrine, growth hormone, and cortisol. As a result, blood sugar levels will rebound and often lead to *hyperglycemia*. This phenomenon is commonly referred to as the *Somogyi phenomenon*.

Diabetic Ketoacidosis

Another acute complication more likely to occur in IDDM is *ketoacidosis*, a condition caused by a lack of insulin leading to a buildup of ketoacids. If progressive, ketoacidosis can result in numerous metabolic problems and even coma. Since ketoacidosis is potentially a medical emergency, prompt recognition is imperative. The coma is usually preceded by a day or more of increased urination and thirst as well as marked fatigue, nausea, and vomiting. Diabetics can use a simple urine dipstick at home to measure the level of ketones (excreted ketoacids) in the urine.

Non-Ketogenic Hyperosmolar Syndrome

With a mortality rate of over fifty percent, *non-ketogenic hyperosmolar syndrome* constitutes a true medical emergency. It is usually the result of profound dehydration due to deficient fluid intake or precipitating events such as pneumonia, burns, stroke, a recent operation, or certain drugs such as phenytoin, diazoxide, glucocorticoids, or diuretics.

The onset of the syndrome may be subtle and occur over a period of days or weeks, with symptoms of weakness, increased urination and thirst, and progressively worse signs of dehydration (weight loss, loss of skin elasticity, dry mucous membranes, rapid heart beat, and low blood pressure).

Chronic Complications

Although the acute complications are more serious in the short term, the long-term consequences of diabetes are just as deadly.

Seven major long-term complications of diabetes are discussed here: atherosclerosis, diabetic retinopathy, diabetic neuropathy, diabetic nephropathy, and diabetic foot ulcers. There are two primary mechanisms behind the development of most chronic complications of diabetes: glycosylated proteins and the intracellular accumulation of sorbitol.

Glycosylated Proteins and Diabetic Complications

As described previously (Monitoring the Diabetic Patient), glycosylation—the binding of glucose to proteins—leads to changes in the structure and function of many body proteins. For example, glycosylated cholesterol-carrying LDL molecules (found in high levels in diabetics) do not bind to LDL-receptors or shut off the liver's manufacture of cholesterol. In diabetes, excessive glycosylation also occurs with the proteins of the red blood cell, lens, and myelin sheath that surrounds and insulates nerve cells. Excessive glycosylation has many adverse effects: inactivation of enzymes, inhibition of regulatory molecule binding, crosslinking of glycosylated proteins, and disruption of many cell functions.[25]

Sorbitol and Diabetic Complications

Sorbitol is a byproduct of glucose metabolism formed within the cell through the action of the enzyme *aldose reductase*. In nondiabetics, once sorbitol is formed it is broken down into fructose—another simple sugar. This conversion to fructose allows the sorbitol to be excreted from the cell. Unfortunately, in the diabetic with frequent elevations in blood sugar levels, sorbitol accumulates and plays a major role in the development of the chronic complications of diabetes.

The mechanism by which sorbitol is involved in the development of diabetic complications is best understood by considering its involvement in cataract formation.

Cataracts are opacities that occur in the lens of the eye (see CATARACTS). Although the lens does not have any blood vessels, it is an actively metabolizing tissue that continuously grows throughout life. Elevations in blood sugar level results in shunting of glucose to the sorbitol pathway. Since the lens membranes are virtually impermeable to sorbitol and lack the enzyme to convert the sorbitol into fructose, sorbitol accumulates to high concentrations that persist even if glucose levels return to normal.

This accumulation creates an osmotic gradient that draws water into the cells to maintain osmotic balance. An osmotic gradient means that there are more small molecules within the cells than outside the cells. In an effort to restore the osmotic balance the cells release small molecules such as amino acids, inositol, glutathione, niacin, vitamin C, magnesium, and potassium. Since these latter compounds function to protect the lens from damage, their loss results in increased susceptibility to damage. As a result, the delicate protein fibers within the lens become opaque and a cataract forms.

Intracellular accumulation of sorbitol is a major factor in the development of the majority of the complications of diabetes. Elevated sorbitol levels are found in high concentrations in the tissues commonly involved in the major diabetic complications: the lens, the nerve cell of the peripheral nerve, the pancreas, and the cells of the retinal blood vessels.

Measurement of the red blood cell (RBC) sorbitol concentration may become a valuable indicator of diabetic control, since RBC and nerve cell sorbitol concentrations correlate well.[28]

Atherosclerosis

The diabetic has a two to three times higher risk of dying prematurely of *atherosclerosis* (hardening of the arteries) than a nondiabetic individual. Therefore, the physician and diabetic patient must be aggressive in reducing the risk factors linked to heart attacks and strokes. Foremost is the reduction of LDL-cholesterol levels and triglycerides while increasing HDL-cholesterol levels.

The most important approach to lowering a high cholesterol level is to follow a healthy diet and lifestyle. The dietary recommendations are straightforward:

- Eat less saturated fat and cholesterol by reducing or eliminating the amount of animal products in the diet
- Increase the consumption of fiber-rich plant foods (fruits, vegetables, grains, and legumes)
- Lose weight if necessary

The lifestyle changes include getting regular aerobic exercise, quitting smoking, and reducing or eliminating the consumption of coffee (both caffeinated and decaffeinated).

Diabetic Neuropathy

Diabetic neuropathies are among the most frequent complications of long-term diabetes. Loss of peripheral nerve function, tingling sensations, numbness, loss of function, pain, and muscle weakness may occur as a result of diabetic neuropathies. Occasionally, the neuropathy can affect deeper nerves and result in impaired heart function, alternating bouts of diarrhea and constipation, inability to empty the bladder, and impotence.

TABLE 4 Recommended Blood Cholesterol and Triglyceride Levels	
Total cholesterol	Less than 200 mg/dl
LDL cholesterol	Less than 130 mg/dl
HDL cholesterol	Greater than 35 mg/dl
Triglycerides	50–150 mg/dl

There is substantial evidence that diabetic neuropathy is also due to sorbitol accumulation.[1,26] In rats, increasing the sorbitol concentration in the sciatic nerve is directly related to decreasing the rate of transmission of the impulse (the nerve conduction velocity), possibly as a result of decreased levels of a compound known as myoinositol.[27] Although some studies have shown that supplementation with inositol (a vitamin B-like substance) improves nerve conduction velocity, addressing the underlying accumulation of sorbitol is of greater importance.[28]

Diabetic Retinopathy

Diabetic retinopathy is a serious eye disease that can result in blindness. In fact, diabetic retinopathy is still the leading cause of blindness in the United States. One in twenty Type I and one in fifteen Type II diabetics develop retinopathy.[1] The development of laser therapy will probably reduce the prevalence of diabetes-induced blindness. However, laser therapy is probably not indicated in milder forms of retinopathy since the occasional side effects (hemorrhage, retinal detachment, and visual field loss) may outweigh the benefits.[1]

Diabetic Nephropathy (Kidney Disease)

Kidney disease due to diabetes is a common complication and a leading cause of death in diabetes.[1] Like the other long-term complications, good blood glucose control goes a long way in reducing the risk of diabetic nephropathy. In addition to monitoring blood sugar levels, periodic monitoring of a diabetic patient's kidney function (blood urea nitrogen, uric acid, creatinine, and creatinine clearance) is important.

Diabetic Foot Ulcers

Lack of blood supply and peripheral neuropathy are the key factors in the development of diabetic foot ulcers. The incidence of gangrene of the feet in diabetics is twenty times greater than normal.[10] Foot ulcers are largely preventable through proper foot care, the avoidance of injury and tobacco in any form, and employing methods to improve local blood circulation. Proper foot care includes keeping the feet clean, dry, and warm and wearing only well-fitted shoes. Tobacco constricts the peripheral blood vessels and can cause Buerger's disease—a severe disease where the blood vessels constrict and block blood flow that often leads to amputation of the affected limbs. Circulation can be improved by avoiding sitting with the legs crossed or in other positions that compromise circulation, and by massaging the feet lightly in an upward direction. *Ginkgo biloba* extract (see *Ginkgo biloba* in the Botanical Medicines section later in this chapter) may also be helpful in improving blood flow.

Therapeutic Considerations

Proper and effective treatment of the diabetic patient requires the careful integration of a wide range of therapies, and patients who are willing to substantially alter their diet and lifestyle. Diabetic individuals must be monitored carefully, particularly if they are on insulin or have relatively uncontrolled diabetes. Careful attention to symptoms, home glucose monitoring, and other blood tests are essential in monitoring the progress of the diabetic individual. It is important to recognize that, as the diabetic individual employs some of the suggestions described in this chapter, drug dosages will have to be altered.

Diet

Dietary modification and treatment is fundamental to the successful treatment of diabetes, whether it be Type I or II. Since diabetics have a higher incidence of death from cardiovascular disease (sixty to seventy percent, versus twenty to twenty-five percent in people without diabetes),[29] most of the dietary recommendations given in the CHOLESTEROL chapter are equally appropriate here. As stated earlier, the frequency of diabetes is highly correlated with the fiber-depleted, high-refined-carbohydrate diet of "civilization."[3] Reestablishing a traditional diet and lifestyle reverses the carbohydrate and lipid metabolism abnormalities associated with the "foods of commerce," and eventually results in a low prevalence of diabetes. The epidemiological evidence indicting the Western diet and lifestyle as the ultimate etiological factor in diabetes is overwhelming.[3,30]

Although there are several commonly recommended diets in the management of diabetes, the best one is not the one promoted by the American Diabetes Association (ADA), but rather one popularized by James Anderson, M.D.[31] The diet Dr. Anderson recommends is high in cereal grains, legumes, and root vegetables, and low in simple sugars and fats. It is called the "high-complex-carbohydrate, high-fiber diet, or "HCF diet" for short.

Clinical trials of dietary treatment with a "primitive" diet high in plant cell-wall materials and complex carbohydrates, and low in fat and animal products, have consistently demonstrated superior therapeutic effects over oral hypoglycemic agents, insulin (when less than 30 units per day), and other previously recommended dietary regimes (carbohydrate restriction, high protein, and the ADA diet).[31–36]

The ADA Diet

The diet recommended by the American Diabetes Association and the American Dietetic Association is clearly inferior to the HCF and MHCF diets (presented following). Nonetheless, it is presented here for historical purposes. The ADA's exchange system is a useful concept and, as the diet is in common use by the typical physician, familiarity is necessary. It offers some beneficial support to many, especially if supplemented with dietary fiber (guar gum at 15 to 30 g/day or pectin at 30 to 45 g/day).[4,37]

A resurgence of interest in diet therapy resulted from the Universal Group Diabetes Program (UGDP) report which, in 1970, cast serious doubt on the efficacy and safety of oral hypoglycemic drugs.[24] Prior to the report, the ADA diet consisted of high-protein, high-cholesterol, and high-fat foods. This diet obviously exacerbated the already atherosclerosis-prone state of diabetes and contributed to greater insulin insensitivity. In 1971, a revised ADA diet was developed based on the exchange system, a very useful concept for diabetic diets. A healthier version of the exchange system is presented in A HEALTH-PROMOTING DIET.

The Importance of Dietary Fiber

Population studies, as well as clinical and experimental research, show diabetes to be one of the diseases most clearly related to inadequate dietary fiber intake.[3,4] These results indicate that, while the intake of refined sugars should be curtailed, the intake of complex carbohydrate sources that are rich in fiber should be increased.

The term "dietary fiber" refers to the components of the plant cell wall as well as the indigestible residues from plant foods. Different types of fibers possess different actions. The type of fiber that exerts the most beneficial effects on blood sugar control are the water-soluble forms. Included in this class are hemicelluloses, mucilages, gums, and pectin substances. These types of fiber are capable of: slowing down the digestion and absorption of carbohydrates, thereby preventing rapid rises in blood sugar; increasing the sensitivity of tissues to insulin, thereby preventing the excessive secretion of insulin; and improving uptake of glucose by the liver and other tissues, thereby preventing a sustained elevation of blood sugar level.

Fortunately, the majority of fiber in most plant cell walls is water-soluble. Particularly good sources of water-soluble fiber are legumes (beans), oat bran, nuts, seeds, psyllium seed husks, pears, apples, and most vegetables. The optimal diet for diabetics includes a large amount of plant foods to ensure adequate levels of dietary fiber. A daily intake of 50 grams is a reasonable goal.

Frequent consumption of legumes is particularly important since a high-carbohydrate, legume-rich, high-fiber diet has been shown to improve all aspects of diabetic control.[35]

Fiber Supplementation versus a High-Fiber Diet Supplementation with the plant fibers (guar gum at a dosage of 5 g/meal orand pectin at 10 g/meal) has demonstrated a positive impact on diabetic control. These fiber supplements are now being used, along with the standard ADA diet, by many experts in diabetes.[4] For example, David Jenkins and colleagues developed a palatable crisp bread containing guar gum.[4,36] When diabetic patients ate between 14 and 26 grams of guar per day, they required less insulin and had better control of blood sugar levels.[4,36] It is interesting to note that these beneficial effects are maximized in patients whose diet includes at least forty percent complex carbohydrates.

Despite these beneficial results, fiber-supplemented diets are not as effective as the HCF diet and are reserved for the Type II patient who is unwilling to implement the more difficult dietary change and will settle

for palliative results. The insulin dosages of diabetics on fiber-supplemented diets can usually be reduced to one-third those used on control (ADA) diets, while the HCF diet has led to discontinuation of insulin therapy in approximately sixty percent of NIDDM patients and significantly reduces doses in the other forty percent.[4,32,33]

The Glycemic Index

The "glycemic index" was developed by David Jenkins in 1981 to measure the rise of blood glucose after consumption of a particular food.[40] The standard value of 100 is based on the rise seen after the ingestion of glucose. The glycemic index ranges from about 20 for fructose and whole barley to about 98 for a baked potato. The insulin response to carbohydrate-containing foods is similar to the rise in blood sugar.

The glycemic index is used as a guideline for dietary recommendations for people with either diabetes or hypoglycemia. Basically, people with blood sugar problems are advised to avoid foods with high values and choose instead carbohydrate-containing foods with lower values. However, the glycemic index, should not be the only dietary guideline. For example, while high-fat foods like ice cream and sausage may have a low glycemic index, these are not good choices for people with hypoglycemia or diabetes because a diet high in fat has been shown to impair glucose uptake.

Fruits and Fructose

Many physicians have recommended that individuals with diabetes or hypoglycemia avoid fruits and fructose (the primary form of sugar found in fruits). However, recent research challenges this approach. Fructose does not cause a rapid rise in blood sugar levels. Because fructose must be changed to glucose in the liver in order to be utilized by the

TABLE 5	Glycemic Index of Some Common Foods

FOOD	GLYCEMIC INDEX
Sugars	
Glucose	100
Maltose	105
Honey	75
Sucrose	60
Fructose	20
Fruits	
Apples	39
Bananas	62
Oranges	40
Orange juice	46
Raisins	64
Vegetables	
Beets	64
Carrot, raw	31
Carrot, cooked	36
Potato, baked	98
Potato (new), boiled	70
Grains	
Bran cereal	51
Bread, white	69
Bread, whole grain	72
Corn	59
Cornflakes	80
Oatmeal	49
Pasta	45
Rice	70
Rice, puffed	95
Wheat cereal	67
Legumes	
Beans	31
Lentils	29
Peas	39
Other foods	
Ice cream	36
Milk	34
Nuts	13
Sausages	28

body, blood glucose levels do not rise as rapidly after fructose consumption compared to other simple sugars.

While most diabetics and hypoglycemics cannot tolerate sucrose, most can tolerate moderate amounts of fruits and fructose without loss of blood sugar control. In fact, fructose and fruits are not only much better tolerated than white bread and other refined carbohydrates, they produce less sharp elevations in blood sugar levels compared to most sources of complex carbohydrates (starch).[41] As a bonus, fructose has actually been shown to enhance the sensitivity to insulin by thirty-four percent when fed to non-insulin-dependent diabetics over a period of four weeks.

Nutritional Supplements

The treatment of diabetes requires nutritional supplementation, as diabetics have a greatly increased need for many nutrients. Supplying the diabetic with additional key nutrients has been shown to improve blood sugar control and to help prevent or ameliorate many of the major complications of diabetes.

Although the following discussion of specific nutrients documents their usefulness, supplements are used as part of a comprehensive approach in which diet is the primary focus. Good blood sugar control combined with nutritional supplementation will go a long way in helping prevent many of the major complications of diabetes.

Chromium

Chromium was briefly discussed earlier in this chapter (see Causative Factors in NIDDM). Clinical studies in diabetes has shown that supplementing the diet with chromium can decrease fasting blood glucose levels, improve glucose tolerance, lower insulin levels, and decrease total cholesterol and triglyceride levels, while increasing HDL-cholesterol levels.[19,20] Although some studies have not shown chromium to exert much effect in improving glucose tolerance in diabetes, there is no doubt that it is an important mineral in blood sugar metabolism.

A recent large study clearly documented the benefit of chromium for NIDDM patients. In this study, 180 Type II diabetics were placed in one of three groups. The first group was a placebo group; the second group received 100 mcg of chromium as chromium picolinate two times per day; and the third group received 500 mcg of chromium picolinate two times per day. The patients continued their normal medication. There was a significant dose- and time-dependent decrease in glycosylated hemoglobin, fasting glucose, two-hour postprandial glucose levels, fasting and two-hour after meal (postprandial) insulin values, and total serum cholesterol.[15]

Reversing a chromium deficiency by supplementing the diet with chromium has also been demonstrated to lower body weight while increasing lean body mass. All of the effects of chromium appear to be due to increased insulin sensitivity. A chromium deficiency may be an underlying contributing factor to the large number of Americans suffering from diabetes, hypoglycemia, and obesity. There is evidence that marginal chromium deficiency is common in the United States.

Although no recommended dietary allowance (RDA) has been established for chromium, at least 200 mcg each day appears necessary for optimal sugar regulation. Chromium levels can be depleted by consuming refined sugars or white flour products, and by lack of exercise. In addition to the regular consumption of chromium-rich foods, the diabetic and hypoglycemic should supplement the diet with chromium polyni-

cotinate, chromium picolinate, or chromium-enriched yeast.

Vitamin C

A primary function of vitamin C is the manufacture of collagen, the main protein substance in the human body. Since collagen is such an important protein in connective tissue, vitamin C is vital for wound repair, healthy gums, and the prevention of excessive bruising. In scurvy or severe vitamin C deficiency, the classic symptoms are bleeding gums, poor wound healing, extensive bruising, increased susceptibility to infection, hysteria, and depression. In addition to its role in collagen metabolism, vitamin C is critical to immune function, the manufacture of certain nerve-transmitting substances and hormones, and the absorption and utilization of other nutritional factors.

Since the transport of vitamin C into cells is facilitated by insulin, many diabetics do not have enough intracellular vitamin C. Therefore, a relative vitamin C deficiency exists in many diabetics despite adequate dietary consumption.[42] A chronic, latent vitamin C deficiency will lead to a number of problems for the diabetic, including an increased tendency to bleed (increased capillary permeability), poor wound healing, vascular disease, elevations in cholesterol levels, and a depressed immune system.

Vitamin C at high doses (2,000 mg per day) has been shown to reduce the accumulation of sorbitol in the red blood cells of diabetics and to inhibit the glycosylation of proteins.[43,44] As discussed previously, sorbitol accumulation and glycosylation of proteins are linked to many complications of diabetes, especially eye and nerve diseases. The attempt to prevent sorbitol accumulation with drugs designed specifically to inhibit aldose reductase has produced equivocal results in human clinical trials along with consistent side effects. Vitamin C may be able to accomplish what these drugs could not: safe and effective inhibition of sorbitol accumulation.

A recent study provides further support for this possibility.[45] In this research, vitamin C supplements of 100 mg or 600 mg were given daily for fifty-eight days to young adults with insulin-dependent diabetes. RBC sorbitol was measured at baseline and again at thirty and fifty-eight days. The baseline results indicated that RBC sorbitol levels were nearly doubled in these patients despite "adequate" dietary intakes of vitamin C as determined by diet diaries. Vitamin C supplementation at both dosages normalized RBC sorbitol within thirty days.

This correction of sorbitol accumulation was independent of changes in diabetic control as monitored by fasting glucose, glycosylated hemoglobin, and presence of glucose in the urine. In fact, overall diabetic control during the study was moderate to poor. The researchers concluded:

Vitamin C supplementation is effective in reducing sorbitol accumulation in the erythrocytes of diabetics. Given its tissue distribution and low toxicity, we suggest a superiority for vitamin C over pharmaceutic ARIs [aldose reductase inhibitors].

Although lower levels of vitamin C achieved normal sorbitol levels, supplementation with a minimum of 2 grams of vitamin C daily in diabetics appears warranted due to its other important effects. While vitamin C supplementation will be necessary to ensure this level of intake, patients should be encouraged not to rely exclusively on supplements to meet all of their vitamin C requirements. Vitamin-C-rich foods are rich in flavonoids and carotenes, which enhance the effects of vitamin C and exert favorable effects of their own. Good dietary sources of vitamin C are broccoli, peppers, potatoes, Brussels sprouts, and citrus fruits.

Niacin and Niacinamide

Niacin-containing enzymes play an important role in energy production; fat, cholesterol, and carbohydrate metabolism; and the manufacture of many body compounds, including sex and adrenal hormones. Like chromium, niacin (vitamin B3, or *nicotinic acid*), is an essential component of the glucose tolerance factor, making it a key nutrient for treating hypoglycemia and diabetes.[46]

Supplementing the diet of diabetics with vitamin B3 in the form of *niacinamide* has been shown to exert many favorable effects. Foremost is its possible application in preventing the development of Type I diabetes.[47–50] Niacinamide, also called *nicotinamide,* has been shown to prevent the development of diabetes in experimental animals. This observation led to several pilot clinical trials which suggest that niacinamide can prevent Type I diabetes from developing, or, if given soon enough at the onset of diabetes, help restore beta-cells or at least slow their destruction.

There have been ten studies of niacinamide treatment in recent-onset IDDM or IDDM of less than five years duration. Six of these studies used a double-blind placebo-controlled format. Of these six, three studies showed a positive effect in terms of prolonged remission, lower insulin requirements, improved metabolic control, and increased beta-cell function. Some newly diagnosed Type I diabetics have experienced complete reversal of their diabetes with niacinamide supplementation.[48] The main difference between the positive and negative studies in recent-onset IDDM seems to be the older age and higher baseline fasting C-peptide (an indicator of pancreatic function) in positive studies.

In the spring of 1993, a large multi-center study involving eighteen European countries, Israel, and Canada was started to follow up these encouraging preliminary findings. Other clinical trials are also in progress or have been proposed.

The mechanism of action appears to be inhibition of damage to the beta-cells by the immune system, along with niacinamide's antioxidant role.[51] The daily dose of niacinamide is based on body weight: 25 mg per kilogram. The studies in children used 100 mg to 200 mg per day.

Niacin has also long been used to lower cholesterol levels.[52–54] Because the dose of niacin required (1 gram three times per day) to lower cholesterol levels often results in blood sugar abnormalities, flushing of the skin, stomach irritation, ulcers, liver damage, fatigue, and other side effects, many diabetics do not tolerate niacin very well. The acute reaction of skin flushing after taking niacin can be alleviated by taking "sustained-release," "timed-release," or "slow-release" niacin products. These formulations allow the niacin to be absorbed gradually, thereby reducing the flushing reaction. However, while these forms of niacin reduce skin flushing, they are more toxic to the liver.[55]

A better and safer form of niacin is *inositol hexaniacinate,* composed of one molecule of inositol (an unofficial B-vitamin) and six molecules of niacin. Inositol hexaniacinate can be used in both Type I and Type II diabetes to lower elevated blood lipid levels. This form of niacin has long been used in Europe to lower cholesterol levels and also to improve blood flow in patients with intermittent claudication (a condition characterized by severe muscle cramps in the calf produced with exercise or walking). It yields slightly better clinical results than standard niacin, including improved sugar level regulation, and is much better tolerated.[56–58] In one study of 153 patients treated with inositol hexaniacinate at dosages ranging from 600 to 1,800 mg per day, no patients reported any side effects or adverse reactions.[56]

In cases of elevated cholesterol levels, a dosage of 600 to 1,000 mg three times per day is usually sufficient to produce an eighteen-percent reduction in total cholesterol, a twenty-six-percent reduction in triglycerides, and an increase of thirty percent in HDL-cholesterol levels.

Biotin

Biotin functions in the manufacture and utilization of carbohydrates, fats, and amino acids. Since biotin is manufactured in the intestines by gut bacteria, it is not often discussed as a needed nutrient. A vegetarian diet has been shown to alter the intestinal bacterial flora so that it enhances the synthesis and promotes the absorption of biotin.

Biotin supplementation has been shown to enhance insulin sensitivity and increase the activity of *glucokinase,* the enzyme responsible for the first step in the utilization of glucose by the liver. Glucokinase concentrations in diabetics are very low. In one study, 16 mg of biotin per day resulted in significant lowering of fasting blood sugar levels and improvements in blood glucose control in IDDM.[59] In a study in NIDDM, similar effects were noted with 9 mg of biotin per day.[60]

If high-dose biotin (i.e., greater than 8 mg per day) is used in IDDM, insulin requirements must be adjusted as needed.

Vitamin B6

Vitamin B6 supplementation appears to offer significant protection against the development of diabetic nerve disease (neuropathy), as diabetics with neuropathy have been shown to be deficient in vitamin B6 and to benefit from supplementation.[61] Individuals with long-standing diabetes, or who are developing signs of peripheral nerve abnormalities, should definitely be supplemented with vitamin B6. It is interesting to note that the neuropathy of a vitamin B6 deficiency is indistinguishable from diabetic neuropathy.

Vitamin B6 may also prove to be important in preventing other diabetic complications because it inhibits glycosylation of proteins.[62] Vitamin B6 supplementation should be tried as a safe treatment for gestational diabetes. In one study of women with gestational diabetes, taking 100 mg of vitamin B6 for two weeks resulted in eliminating the diagnosis in twelve of the fourteen women.[63]

Vitamin B12

A vitamin B12 deficiency is characterized by numbness of the feet, pins-and-needles sensations, or a burning feeling—symptoms typical of diabetic neuropathy.[64,65] Vitamin B12 supplementation has been used with some success in treating diabetic neuropathy. It is not clear if this is due to the correcting of a deficiency state or to the normalization of the deranged vitamin B12 metabolism seen in diabetics.[66] Absence of anemia is not an adequate criterion for ruling out a deficiency. A deficit within the nerve cells will usually precede anemia, often by several years. Measuring blood levels of vitamin B12 is more reliable in diagnosing vitamin B12 deficiency.

Oral supplementation with 1,000 to 3,000 mcg per day is usually sufficient, but intramuscular injections of vitamin B12 may be necessary in some cases.

Vitamin E

Diabetics appear to have an increased requirement for vitamin E. High doses of vitamin E (800 to 1,200 IU) not only improves insulin action, but also exerts a number of beneficial effects that may aid in preventing the long-term complications of diabetes.

Several clinical studies have shown vitamin E supplementation to be helpful. For example, in one study examining vitamin E's role on glucose metabolism and insulin action, ten control (healthy) subjects and fifteen non-insulin-dependent diabetics underwent an oral glucose-tolerance test before and after taking 1,350 IU of vitamin E per day for four months. In the healthy subjects, vitamin E supplementation was shown to improve glucose tolerance and insulin sensitivity. In the diabetics, improvements in glucose metabolism and insulin action were even more obvious. The authors of the study concluded:

Our study demonstrates that in diabetic patients daily oral vitamin E supplements may reduce oxidative stress, thus improving membrane physical characteristics and related activities in glucose transport.[67]

Vitamin E also appears to play a significant role in the prevention of diabetes. One study followed 944 men, forty-two to sixty years of age, who did not have diabetes at the beginning of the study. Forty-five men developed diabetes during the four-year follow-up. The study indicated that a low vitamin-E concentration was associated with 3.9 times greater risk of developing diabetes.[68]

Magnesium

Magnesium is involved in several areas of glucose metabolism, and there is considerable evidence that diabetics need supplemental magnesium. The reasons: magnesium deficiency is common in diabetics, and magnesium may prevent some of the complications of diabetes, such as retinopathy and heart disease.[69] Magnesium levels are lowest in diabetics who have severe retinopathy.

The RDA for magnesium is 350 mg per day for adult males and 300 mg per day for adult females. The diabetic may need twice this amount. While the magnesium should ideally be derived from the diet, the average intake of magnesium by healthy adults in the United States ranges only between 143 and 266 mg per day. While magnesium occurs abundantly in whole foods, food processing refines out a large portion of magnesium. The best dietary sources of magnesium are tofu, legumes, seeds, nuts, whole grains, and green leafy vegetables. Fish, meat, milk, and the most commonly eaten fruits are quite low in magnesium. As most Americans consume a diet high in refined foods, meat, and dairy products, low magnesium intake is common.

In addition to eating a diet high in magnesium-rich foods, supplementation with 300 to 500 mg of magnesium as aspartate or citrate is recommended. Also, diabetics should take at least 50 mg of vitamin B6 per day; the level of intracellular vitamin B6 appears to be intricately linked to the magnesium content of the cell. In other words, without vitamin B6, magnesium will not get inside the cell.

Potassium

There are several reasons why diabetics should eat a high-potassium diet: potassium supplementation yields improved insulin sensitivity, responsiveness, and secretion; insulin administration induces a loss of potassium; and a high potassium intake reduces the risk of heart disease, atherosclerosis, and cancer.[70,71] However, there are some concerns about potassium supplementation in diabetics.

The estimated safe and adequate daily dietary intake of potassium, as set by the Committee on Recommended Daily Allowances, is 1.9 g to 5.6 g. If body potassium requirements are not being met through diet, supplementation is essential to good health. This is particularly true for the diabetic as well as athletes and the elderly. Potassium salts are commonly prescribed by physicians in the dosage range of 1.5 g to 3.0 g per day. However, potassium salts can cause nausea, vomiting, diarrhea, and ulcers. These effects are not seen when potassium levels are increased through the diet only. This highlights the advantages of using vegetable juices, foods, or food-based potassium supplements to meet the human body's potassium requirements.

While most people can handle an excess of potassium, those with diabetes and kidney disease do not handle potassium in the normal way, and are more likely to experience heart disturbances and other consequences of potassium toxicity. Individuals with kidney disorders usually need to restrict their potassium intake. Most diabetics can consume a high-potassium diet, but their kidney function should be properly evaluated before taking a potassium supplement.

Manganese

Manganese is a cofactor in many enzyme systems involved in blood sugar control, energy metabolism, and thyroid hormone function.[72,73] In guinea pigs, a deficiency of manganese results in diabetes and the frequent birth of offspring who develop pancreatic abnormalities or have no pancreas at all. Diabetics have been shown to have only one-half the manganese of normal individuals. A good daily dose of manganese for a diabetic is 30 mg.

Zinc

Zinc is involved in virtually all aspects of insulin metabolism: synthesis, secretion, and utilization. Zinc also has a protective effect against beta-cell destruction. Diabetics typically excrete excessive amounts of zinc in the urine and therefore require supplementation,[74] which has been shown to improve insulin levels in both Type I and Type II diabetes.[75] In addition, zinc helps improve the poor wound healing observed in diabetics.[76] Zinc is found in good amounts in whole grains, legumes, nuts, and seeds. The recommended level of supplementation for diabetics is at least 30 mg of zinc per day.

Flavonoids

Recent research suggests that flavonoids may be useful in treating diabetes.[77–79] Flavonoids such as *quercetin* promote insulin secretion and are potent inhibitors of sorbitol accumulation. These effects may help explain the favorable effects of many botanical medicines traditionally used in the treatment of diabetes, many of which are high in flavonoids. The nutritional effects of flavonoids include: an increase in intracellular vitamin C levels, a decrease in the leakiness and breakage of small blood vessels, the prevention of easy bruising, and immune system support, all of which are of benefit to individuals with diabetes.[79] In addition to consuming a diet rich in flavonoids, the diabetic should take an extra 1 to 2 grams of mixed flavonoids per day or a flavonoid-rich extract such as bilberry or grape seed extract.

Essential Fatty Acids

Both omega-6 and omega-3 fatty acids have shown benefit in treating various aspects of diabetes. In particular, the omega-6 fatty acid, gamma-linolenic acid, has been shown to offer significant protection against the development of diabetic neuropathy, while the omega-3 oils offer significant protection against hardening of the arteries and enhance insulin secretion in NIDDM. To sum up the following discussion, it appears that the best approach is to:

- Increase the consumption of cold-water fish such as salmon, herring, mackerel, and halibut

- Supplement the diet with 480 mg of gamma-linolenic acid from evening primrose, borage, or black currant oil
- Consume 1 tablespoon (roughly 10 grams) of flaxseed oil daily

Gamma-Linolenic Acid   Diabetes is associated with a substantial disturbance in essential fatty acid (EFA) metabolism. One of the key disturbances is the impairment in the process of converting linoleic acid to gamma-linolenic (GLA), dihomo-gamma-linolenic (DHGLA), and arachidonic acids.[80] As a result, providing GLA in the form of borage, evening primrose, or black currant oils may offer a method to bypass some of this disturbance.

To test the hypothesis, a large multicenter trial was designed. The Gamma-Linolenic Acid Multicenter Trial enrolled 111 patients with mild diabetic neuropathy from seven centers into a randomized, double-blind, placebo-controlled parallel study of GLA at a dose of 480 mg/day for one year.[81] The source of GLA used in the study was evening primrose oil. Patients in the treatment group took twelve capsules containing 40 mg of GLA per day.

Sixteen different parameters were assessed, including conduction velocities, hot and cold thresholds, sensation, tendon reflexes, and muscle strength. After one year, all sixteen parameters improved, thirteen of them to a statistically significant degree. Treatment was more effective in relatively well-controlled than in poorly controlled diabetic patients. The latter finding highlights the need for a comprehensive approach in controlling blood sugar levels rather than expecting a single physiological aid (i.e., GLA) to compensate for poor control.

Omega-3 Fatty Acids   The omega-3 fatty acids have been shown to lower cholesterol and triglyceride levels in hundreds of studies, including many studies of diabetics.[82,83] However, not all of the studies have yielded positive effects. In fact, some studies have shown deterioration of blood sugar control and elevations in blood lipid levels.[82] Although there is no obvious explanation for these contradictory findings, proper dosage and antioxidant support (especially vitamin E) appears to be critical to producing beneficial rather than deleterious effects.

The initial enthusiasm for the use of fish oils (eicosapentaenoic acid [EPA] and docosahexanoic acid [DHA]), in treating diabetes was modified by reports of potentially damaging effects, including increased levels of plasma glucose, total cholesterol, and LDL-cholesterol. The magnitude of these adverse effects was relatively small, but nonetheless their occurrence raised doubts regarding the safety of fish oil supplementation for diabetics.

These adverse effects occurred at larger doses, usually 4 to 10 grams of fish oils per day. Subsequent studies using lower doses (2.5 grams of omega-3 fatty acids) or highly purified EPA (900 mg or 1,800 mg per day) have led to a better understanding of the potential problems with fish oils.[84,85]

Specifically, dosage appears to be a critical element. At the lower dosage of 2.5 g of fish oils or 900 mg of purified EPA, supplementation appears safe.[84,85] In one study, a ninety-six-percent pure EPA product at a dose of 900 mg per day had little effect on blood sugar.[85] However, at 1,800 mg per day for eight weeks, blood sugar control deteriorated and cholesterol levels increased significantly.

Altogether, these studies seem to suggest caution when supplementing fish oils for diabetics. One reason why fish-oil products may negatively affect diabetics is the high level of lipid peroxides in these preparations, coupled with their tendency to deplete antioxidant nutrients when ingested. Diabetics might better gain the benefits of omega-3 oils by consuming fish and/or flaxseed oil, neither of which is associated with negative effects in diabetes.

Increased consumption of cold-water fish has been shown to produce effects equal or superior to fish-oil supplementation. For example, in one study, twenty-five men with high cholesterol levels were studied over a five-week period, comparing the effects of eating an equivalent amount of fish oil from whole fish versus a fish-oil supplement.[86] Although total cholesterol levels were unchanged in both groups, both fish and fish-oil supplements lowered triglycerides and raised HDL-cholesterol. However, dietary fish produced some additional benefits over the fish-oil supplements including better effects on improving blood viscosity. These findings suggest that, while both fish consumption and fish-oil supplementation produce desirable effects on lipids and lipoproteins, fish consumption is more effective in improving several other factors involved in cardiovascular disease.

Another study demonstrated an inverse correlation between fish intake and impaired glucose tolerance and diabetes. An average daily intake of 24.2 g (about one ounce) of fish was associated with a significantly lower incidence of glucose intolerance.[87] In addition, mortality was lower in fish consumers (20.6/1,000 person-years) compared to those who did not eat fish (31.2/1,000 person-years).

These studies, along with additional epidemiological studies showing a low prevalence of both IDDM and NIDDM in cultures that consume cold-water fish, indicate that omega-3 fatty acids may offer some protection against the development of diabetes.[82,83]

Although the majority of studies on omega-3 oils have utilized fish oils, flaxseed oil may offer similar benefits because it contains alpha-linolenic acid (ALA), an omega-3 oil which the body can convert to EPA. Linolenic acid exerts many of the same effects as EPA, as well as several of its own including effecting the immune system, fighting cancer, and exerting a greater positive effect on platelet function.[88]

Flaxseed oil supplementation may avoid some of the problems associated with EPA supplementation in diabetics. In the presence of omega-6 fatty acids, ALA is not as effective in increasing tissue concentrations of EPA and lowering tissue concentrations of arachidonic acid.[89] In contrast to EPA, this moderate effect of flaxseed oil in the presence of omega-6 oils may not compromise the already disturbed EFA metabolism of the diabetic. Furthermore, encapsulated fish oils have several disadvantages: they contain very high levels of lipid peroxides, they deplete body stores of antioxidant nutrients, and they are expensive to use at therapeutic dosages (1.8 g EPA/day for most clinical applications). Flaxseed oil will thus probably emerge as the preferred source of omega-3 fatty acids in the treatment of diabetes as well as in atherosclerosis, high blood pressure, and inflammatory conditions such as psoriasis, rheumatoid arthritis, eczema, multiple sclerosis, and ulcerative colitis.

In summary, diabetics can benefit from omega-3 oils. At this time the best recommendation may be to increase the amount of cold-water fish in the diet and use flaxseed oil. An average daily intake of 1 ounce of fish is appropriate. This amount works out to roughly two 3 1/2-ounce servings per week. For flaxseed oil, a daily dosage of 1 tablespoon (roughly 10 grams) is recommended for diabetics.

Carnitine

Carnitine supplementation has resulted in significantly decreased total serum lipid and increased HDL-cholesterol levels in diabetic patients.[90] In addition, carnitine increases the breakdown of fat into energy (a process known as beta-oxidation), possibly playing a role in preventing diabetic ketoacidosis.

Inositol

As mentioned above, inositol supplementation has shown some success in the treatment of experimental animal diabetic neuropathy since it helps reestablish normal levels of myoinositol in nerve cells.[6] The nerve cell myoinositol deficiency is believed to result from a combination of glucose competition with myoinositol for active transport into the cell and accumulation of sorbitol within the cell, resulting in the loss of intracellular myoinositol. Oral supplementation in human diabetics has not, however, resulted in significant clinical improvement.[28]

Botanical Medicines

Before the advent of insulin, diabetes was treated using plant medicines. In 1980, the World Health Organization urged researchers to examine whether traditional medicines produced any beneficial clinical results. In the last ten to twenty years, scientific investigation has confirmed the efficacy of many of these preparations, some of which are remarkably effective. Covered here are those plants which appear most effective, are least toxic, and have substantial documentation of efficacy.

Even though the herbs discussed possess blood-sugar-lowering effects, proper and effective natural treatment of the diabetic patient requires the careful integration of diet, nutritional supplements, lifestyle, and botanical medicine.

Onion (Allium cepa) and Garlic (Allium sativum)

Onions and garlic have demonstrated blood-sugar-lowering action in several studies.[91,92]

The active principles are believed to be sulfur-containing compounds—allyl propyl disulphide (APDS) in onions, and diallyl disulphide oxide (allicin) in garlic—although other constituents such as flavonoids may play a role as well.

Experimental and clinical evidence suggests that APDS lowers glucose levels by competing with insulin (also a disulphide) for insulin-inactivating sites in the liver.[92] This results in an increase of free insulin. APDS administered in doses of 125 mg/kg to fasting humans causes a marked fall in blood glucose levels and an increase in serum insulin. Allicin at doses of 100 mg/kg produces a similar effect.

Increasing the graded doses of onion extracts to levels sometimes found in the diet (1 to 7 ounces of onion) reduce blood sugar levels in a dose-dependent manner—the higher the intake of onion extract, the lower the level of glucose during oral or intravenous glucose tolerance tests. The effects are similar in both raw and boiled onion extracts.[92]

The cardiovascular effects of garlic and onions (lowering cholesterol and blood pressure) further substantiate the value of liberal intake of garlic and onions by the diabetic patient.

Bitter Melon (Momordica charantia)

Bitter melon—also known as balsam pear—is a tropical fruit widely cultivated in Asia, Africa, and South America. A green cucumber-shaped fruit covered with gourd-like bumps, bitter melon looks like an ugly cucumber. In addition to the unripe fruit being eaten as a vegetable, bitter melon has been used extensively in folk medicine as a remedy for diabetes. The blood-sugar-lowering action of the fresh juice or extract of the unripe fruit has been clearly established in human clinical trials as well as experimental models.[93,94]

Bitter melon is composed of several compounds with confirmed anti-diabetic properties. *Charantin*, extracted by alcohol, is a hypoglycemic agent composed of mixed steroids that is more potent than the oral hypoglycemic drug Tolbutamide. *Momordica* also contains an insulin-like polypeptide, polypeptide-P, which lowers blood sugar levels when injected like insulin into Type I diabetics.[95] Since it appears to have fewer side effects than insulin, it has been suggested as a replacement for some patients. Unfortunately, there is no further research in this area.

The oral administration of bitter melon preparations has shown good results in clinical trials in patients with Type II diabetes.[93,94] In one study, blood sugar control was improved in seventy-three percent of Type II diabetics who were given 2 ounces of the juice.[93] The total area under the glucose tolerance curves of the patients responding to the bitter melon was 187.0 cm^2, much lower than the baseline level of 243.6 cm^2. In another study, 15 grams of the aqueous extract of bitter melon produced a fifty-four-percent decrease in after-meal blood sugar level and a seventeen-percent reduction in glycosylated hemoglobin in six patients.[94]

Unripe bitter melon is available primarily at Asian grocery stores. Commercial suppliers and health food stores may have bitter melon extracts, but the fresh juice is probably the best as this traditional form was used in some of the studies. Bitter melon juice is very difficult to make palatable because, as its name implies, it is quite bitter. If you use this effective plant medicine, hold your nose and quickly drink a 2-ounce shot of the juice. The dosage of other forms should approximate this dose.

Gymnema sylvestre

Gymnema sylvestre, a plant native to the tropical forests of India, has long been used as a treatment for diabetes. Recent scientific investigation has upheld its effectiveness in both Type I and Type II diabetes.[96,97]

Gymnema sylvestre appeared on the U.S. market a few years ago, hyped as a "sugar blocker." Manufacturers erroneously claimed that *Gymnema* could allow sugar to pass through the gastrointestinal tract unabsorbed. Ridiculous advertisements contained phrases such as "how to cut down on sugar calories without cutting down on sugar."

When applied to the tongue, *Gymnema* components, such as gymnemic acid, block the sensation of sweetness. Clinically this has shown some significance. Subjects that had *Gymnema* extracts applied to their tongue have been shown to consume fewer calories at a meal, compared to controls. Consumption of capsules or tablets has not been shown to produce the same effect.

Gymnema extracts have been shown to enhance glucose control in diabetic dogs and rabbits. Interestingly, *Gymnema* has no apparent effect in animals that have had their pancreas removed, suggesting that *Gymnema* enhances the production of insulin. There is evidence in animal studies that it accomplishes this through regeneration of the insulin-producing beta-cells in the pancreas. Studies in humans with both types of diabetes also seem to support the possibility of pancreas regeneration.[96,97]

Gymnema extract has shown positive clinical results in both Type I and Type II diabetes. An extract of the leaves of *Gymnema sylvestre* given to twenty-seven patients with Type I diabetes on insulin therapy was shown to reduce insulin requirements and fasting blood sugar levels, and to improve blood sugar control.[92] In Type I diabetes, *Gymnema* appears to enhance the action of insulin. In a study of Type II diabetics, twenty-two were given *Gymnema* extract along with their oral hypoglycemic drugs. All patients demonstrated improved blood sugar control; twenty-one of the twenty-two were able to reduce their drug dosage considerably; and five sub-jects were able to discontinue their medication and maintain blood sugar control with the *Gymnema* extract alone.[97] It is interesting to note that *Gymnema* extract given to healthy volunteers does not produce any blood-sugar-lowering or hypoglycemic effects.[97]

The dosage for *Gymnema sylvestre* extract is 400 mg per day in both Type I and Type II diabetes. No side effects have been reported from *Gymnema* extract.

Fenugreek (Trigonella foenumgraecum)

Fenugreek seeds have demonstrated significant anti-diabetic effects in experimental and clinical studies. The active principle is in the defatted portion of the seed. Administration of the defatted seed (in daily doses of 1.5 to 2 g/kg) to both normal and diabetic dogs has reduced fasting and postprandial blood levels of glucose, glucagon, somatostatin, insulin, total cholesterol, and triglycerides, while increasing HDL-cholesterol levels.[99]

Human studies have confirmed these effects. Defatted fenugreek seed powder given twice daily, at a 50-gram dose, to insulin-dependent diabetics resulted in significant reduction in fasting blood sugar levels and improved glucose tolerance test results.[100] There was also a fifty-four-percent reduction in twenty-four-hour urinary glucose excretion, and significant reductions in cholesterol and triglyceride values. In non-insulin-dependent diabetics, supplementation with 15 grams of powdered fenugreek seed soaked in water significantly reduced after-meal glucose levels during the meal tolerance test.[100] These results indicate that fenugreek seeds or defatted fenugreek seed powder should be included in the diet of the diabetic.

Salt Bush (Atriplex halimu)

Salt bush is a branchy, woody shrub native to the Mediterranean, North Africa, and Southern Europe. Salt bush is especially common around the Jordan Valley in inundated saline depressions and oases. Researchers noticed that when sand rats switched from a diet rich in salt bush to standard rat chow, they would typically develop severe diabetes. Restoring *Atriplex* to the diet brought about a quick reversal of the condition.

Human studies conducted in Israel demonstrated improved blood glucose regulation and glucose tolerance in patients with Type II diabetes.[101,102] Salt bush is rich in fiber, protein, and numerous trace minerals, including chromium. The dosage used in the human studies was 3 grams per day.

Pterocarpus marsupium and Epicatechin-Containing Plants

Pterocarpus has a long history of use in India as a treatment for diabetes. The flavonoid *epicatechin*, extracted from the bark of this plant, has been shown to prevent beta-cell damage in rats. Further, both epicatechin and a crude alcohol extract of *Pterocarpus marsupium* have been shown to actually regenerate functional pancreatic beta-cells in diabetic animals.[103,104] Epicatechin and related flavonoids are very strong antioxidants.[105,106]

In addition to *Pterocarpus*, the dry-weight percentage of epicatechin is very high in a number of other plants, most notably green tea (*Camellia sinensis*; one to three percent). As commercial sources of *Pterocarpus* are lacking in the United States, green tea may be a suitable alternative. The recommended dosage is at least two cups of green tea per day, or 300 mg of green tea extract.

Bilberry (Vaccinium myrtillus)

Bilberry, or European blueberry, is a shrubby perennial plant that grows in the woods and forest meadows of Europe. The fruit is a blue-black berry that differs from an American blueberry in that its meat is also blue-black. Bilberry leaf tea has a long history of folk use in the treatment of diabetes. This use is supported by research which has shown that oral administration reduces blood sugar levels in normal and diabetic dogs, even when glucose is injected intravenously at the same time.[107,108] Although this research is interesting, it is thought that the berries or extracts of the berries offer even greater benefit.

Bilberry flavonoids (*anthocyanosides*) provide numerous benefits in diabetics. Specifically, they have been shown to increase intracellular vitamin C levels, decrease the leakiness and breakage of small blood vessels, prevent easy bruising, and exert potent antioxidant effects.

It appears that anthocyanosides have an affinity for the blood vessels of the eye and the retina, especially the macula (the area of the retina responsible for fine vision), and improve circulation to the retina.[109–111] This affinity is consistent with several of the clinical effects observed, including positive results in diabetic retinopathy, macular degeneration, cataracts, retinitis pigmentosa, and night blindness.[109,112] Bilberry extracts have been prescribed for diabetic retinopathy in France since 1945.

The standard dose for bilberry extracts is based on its anthocyanoside content, as calculated by its anthocyanidin percentage. Widely used pharmaceutical preparations in Europe are standardized for anthocyanidin content (typically twenty-five percent). These extracts are also available in the United States. The standard dose is 80 to 160 mg three times per day.

Ginkgo biloba

Although the primary clinical application of *Ginkgo biloba* extract (GBE) is cerebral vascular insufficiency,[113,114] GBE has also been shown to improve the blood flow to peripheral tissues in the arms, legs, fingers, and toes. This is an important effect, as peripheral vascular insufficiency is common in diabetics. In several double-blind trials in patients with intermittent claudication, ginkgo was shown to be quite active and superior to the placebo.[115,116] Not only were measurements of pain-free walking distance and maximum walking distance dramatically increased, but ultrasound measurements demonstrated increased blood flow through the affected limb.

The significance of demonstrating measurable improvement in blood flow through the affected areas is great. While conventional medical treatment of these patients (muscular rehabilitation and the elimination of risk factors such as smoking, excess weight, etc.) results in clinical improvement, such as increased walking tolerance, it has not shown improved blood flow of the limbs, and the results are limited over time. Therefore, the muscular rehabilitation and elimination of risk factors, while valuable therapies, are not satisfactory alone.

Ginkgo is clearly an important medicine in the treatment of peripheral vascular disease due to diabetes. *Ginkgo biloba* extract has also been shown to prevent diabetic retinopathy in diabetic rats, suggesting that it may have a protective effect in human diabetics.[117]

The dosage of the *Ginkgo biloba* extract standardized to contain twenty-four percent ginkgo flavoglycosides is 40 to 80 mg three times a day.

Ginseng

In a double-blind controlled study, thirty-six non-insulin-dependent diabetic patients were treated for eight weeks with ginseng at either 100 mg, 200 mg daily, or a placebo. Ginseng elevated mood, improved psychophysiological performance, and reduced fasting blood sugar levels and body weight. The 200-mg dose improved glycosylated hemoglobin levels and physical activity.[118]

Exercise

An appropriate exercise training program is vitally important in a diabetes treatment plan. Exercise improves many parameters and is recommended for both IDDM and NIDDM. Physically trained diabetics experience many benefits: enhanced insulin sensitivity with a consequent diminished need for exogenous insulin, improved glucose tolerance, reduced total serum cholesterol and triglycerides with increased HDL levels that result in a more anti-atherogenic state, and improved weight loss in obese diabetics.[119–121]

However, a physical fitness program does present some risk to the diabetic and must be carefully adapted to the fitness of the patient. Exercise should be avoided during periods of hypoglycemia.

In addition to its well-known and documented value, exercise may have a more specific beneficial effect for diabetics: exercise increases tissue levels of chromium in rats[122] and increases the number of insulin receptors in IDDM patients.[123] It is possible, then, that many of the beneficial effects of exercise are directly related to improved chromium metabolism.

TREATMENT SUMMARY

Effective treatment of diabetes usually requires the careful integration of a wide range of therapies and a willingness on the part of patients to substantially improve their diet lifestyles. NIDDM usually results from many years of chronic metabolic insult; although it can be treated with the natural metabolic approach presented here, its ultimate resolution will take persistence. Although much of the information presented in this chapter has focused on NIDDM, it is equally appropriate for the IDDM patient, with the exception that, according to current information, the Type I diabetic will always require insulin.

Blood sugar levels must be monitored carefully, particularly if the diabetic is on insulin or has poorly controlled diabetes. Home glucose monitoring and the $HgbA_{1c}$ test are, at this time, the best way to monitor progress. It is important to recognize that, as these natural therapies take effect, insulin requirements and drug dosages will have to be altered. It is helpful to develop a good working relationship with one's doctor.

WARNING: Under no circumstances should a patient be suddenly taken off diabetic drugs, especially insulin. According to current information, an IDDM patient will never be able to stop taking insulin.

Diet

All simple, processed, and concentrated carbohydrates must be avoided. Complex-carbohydrate, high-fiber foods, should be stressed, and fats should be kept to a minimum. Legumes, onions, and garlic are particularly useful.

Nutritional Supplements

Take a high-potency multiple-vitamin-and-mineral supplement, according to the guidelines given in SUPPLEMENTARY MEASURES.

- Vitamin C: 500–1,000 mg three times per day
- Mixed flavonoids: 1,000–2,000 mg per day
- Vitamin E: 800–1,200 IU per day
- Flaxseed oil: 1 tablespoon per day
- GLA source: 240–480 mg of GLA per day
- Magnesium: 250 mg two to three times per day
- Methylcobalamin (active vitamin B12): 1,000 mcg per day

- Fiber (guar, pectin, or oat bran): 20–30 g per day

Botanical Medicines

If diabetic retinopathy is present: Bilberry (or grape seed) extract: 40–80 mg three times per day

If diabetic neuropathy is present: *Ginkgo biloba* extract (24% ginkgo flavoglycosides): 40–80 mg three times per day

Other botanicals, listed in order of presumed effectiveness:

- *Gymnema sylvestre* extract: 200 mg twice per day
- Bitter melon *(Momordica charantia)*: 1–2 oz fresh juice three times per day
- Defatted fenugreek powder: 50 g per day
- Salt bush *(Atriplex halimus)*: 3 g per day

Exercise

Regular exercise is vitally important. Exercise at an intensity that elevates heart rate at least fifty percent for one-half hour at least three times a week.

Diarrhea

. . . .

Increase in frequency, fluidity, and volume of bowel movements

Diarrhea is a common symptom that usually indicates a mild, temporary event. However, it may also be the first suggestion of a serious underlying disease or infection. Severe bloody diarrhea, diarrhea in a child less than six years of age, or diarrhea that lasts more than three days should not be taken lightly; its cause must be determined and treated appropriately.

Diarrhea is divided into four major types: osmotic, secretory, exudative, and inadequate-contact. *Osmotic diarrhea* is caused by an excess of water-soluble molecules in the stool, which results in increased fluid retention in the bowel. *Secretory diarrhea* results from excessive secretion of ions into the bowel, with the same results of excessive water retention in the stools. *Exudative diarrhea* is usually due to infections and inflammatory bowel diseases, resulting in abnormal intestinal permeability and intestinal loss of serum proteins, blood, mucus, and pus. Frequent small, painful evacuations are usually a result of disease in the rectum or at the end of the colon. *Inadequate-contact diarrhea* is the result of inadequate contact between the intestinal contents and the absorbing surfaces, resulting in inadequate absorption.

TABLE 1   Types of Diarrhea

TYPE	CAUSES
Osmotic	Saline laxatives that contain magnesium, phosphate, or sulfate
	Carbohydrate malabsorption (e.g., lactose intolerance)
	Antacids that contain magnesium salts
	Excess consumption of nonmetabolizable low-calorie sweets, such as sorbitol
	Excessive vitamin C intake
Secretory	Toxin-producing bacteria
	Hormone-producing tumors
	Fat malabsorption (e.g., lack of bile output)
	Laxative abuse
	Surgical resection of the small intestine
Exudative	Inflammatory bowel disease (Crohn's disease or ulcerative colitis)
	Pseudomembranous colitis (a post-antibiotic diarrhea caused by an overgrowth of a bacteria [*Clostridium difficele*])
	Invasive bacteria
Inadequate-contact	Surgical removal of sections of the intestine
	Short bowel syndrome

Causes

As evident from both Tables 1 and 2, diarrhea can have many causes. Again, it is important to consult a physician for accurate determination of the cause.

Diagnostic Considerations

Diagnosis of the cause of diarrhea can be difficult for a physician. It may require microscopic examination and culturing of the stools for infectious agents, special tests such as the breath hydrogen test to discover missing enzymes, intestinal biopsy, and X rays. Acute diarrhea is usually due to benign events, such as excessive fruit consumption, eating allergenic foods, or an intestinal viral infection. Table 3 lists the key diagnostic criteria for common causes of diarrhea.

Therapeutic Considerations

Since most causes of acute diarrhea, such as mild infections due to "food poisoning," are self-limiting (they are going to resolve on their own), some general recommendations may be all that is needed. If the diarrhea is severe or bloody, or involves a child under the age of six years, a physician should be contacted immediately. A physician should also be consulted if any diarrhea lasts for more than three days.

The therapy of any chronic diarrhea requires identification of the underlying cause and then directing therapy designed to restore normal bowel function. The Comprehensive Stool and Digestive Analysis (see DIGESTION AND ELIMINATION) provides a great deal of information on the internal digestive environment and can be a valuable aid in the identification of the cause. The discussion in this chapter will focus on general support for all diarrheas, along with discus-

. . . .

QUICK REVIEW

- Severe bloody diarrhea, diarrhea in a child under six years of age, or diarrhea that lasts more than three days should not be taken lightly; its cause must be determined and treated appropriately.
- The therapy of any chronic diarrhea requires identification of the underlying cause and then directing therapy designed to restore normal bowel function.
- Replace lost water and electrolytes by drinking herbal teas, vegetable broths, fruit juices, or electrolyte-replacement drinks.
- Avoid dairy products (with the possible exception of live-cultured yogurt) while experiencing diarrhea.
- Carob powder is particularly helpful in treating diarrhea in young children.

TABLE 2 Causes of Diarrhea

CAUSE	MOST COMMON EXAMPLES
Functional disorders	Irritable bowel syndrome
Intestinal viral infections	Enterovirus, rotavirus
Intestinal bacterial infections	*Campylobacter jejuni, Shigella, Salmonella, Yersinia enterocolitica*
Intestinal bacterial toxins	*Clostridium difficele,* pathogenic *Escherichia coli, Staphylococcus, Vibrio parahaemolytica, Vibrio cholerae*
Parasitic infections	*Giardia lamblia, Entamoeba histolytica, Cryptosporium, Isospora*
Inflammatory bowel disease	Crohn's disease, ulcerative colitis, diverticulitis
Antibiotic therapy	Tetracycline
Inadequate bile secretion	Hepatitis, bile duct obstruction
Malabsorption states	Celiac sprue (severe wheat allergy), short small bowel, lactose intolerance
Pancreatic disease	Pancreatic insufficiency, pancreatic tumor
Reflex from other areas	Pelvic inflammatory disease
Neurological disease	Syphilis, diabetic neuropathy
Metabolic disease	Hyperthyroidism
Malnutrition	Severe protein and/or calorie malnutrition
	Food allergy
	Laxative abuse
	Heavy metal poisoning
Miscellaneous	Fecal impaction, cancer, etc.

- Supplementation with *Lactobacillus acidophilus* is crucial in the treatment of diarrhea of any kind, but particularly in antibiotic-associated diarrhea.
- Chronic diarrhea is one of the most common symptoms of food allergy.
- It has been estimated that seventy to ninety percent of Asian, Black, Native American, and Mediterranean adults lack the enzyme required to digest milk sugar (lactose).
- Diarrheal diseases caused by parasites still constitute the single greatest worldwide cause of illness and death.
- Popular natural treatments of parasitic infections include high dosages of pancreatic enzymes and berberine-containing plants, such as goldenseal.
- Berberine has shown significant success in the treatment of acute diarrhea in several clinical studies.

TABLE 3	Diagnostic Criteria for Common Causes of Diarrhea
CAUSE	**KEY DIAGNOSTIC CRITERIA**
Lactase deficiency	Bloated feeling, flatulence, cramps, belching, watery explosive diarrhea relieved by stopping dairy product consumption
Infectious diarrhea	Acute diarrhea in most members of the family, fever, debility
Food allergy	Eczema, asthma, chronic infections, dark circles and puffiness under the eyes
Low-calorie sweets	Explosive, watery diarrhea after consumption of large amounts of undigestible, low-calorie sweets (e.g., mannitol)

sion of diarrhea caused by food allergy, lactose intolerance, parasites, and antibiotic therapy. Treatments for some other causes of diarrhea, e.g., inflammatory bowel disease, celiac disease, and impaired digestion, can be found in their corresponding chapters.

General Support

There are several measures that can be used as general support during any case of diarrhea:

- Don't eat solid foods
- Replace water and electrolytes
- Avoid dairy products
- Use carob or pectin (alone or in combination with kaolin)
- Reestablish *Lactobacillus acidophilus*

Don't Eat Solid Foods
During the acute phase of diarrhea, no solid foods should be consumed. Instead the focus should be on liquids, as discussed in the next paragraph.

Replace Water and Electrolytes
With diarrhea, a person loses much water and a great deal of electrolytes, such as potassium, sodium, and chloride. It is important to replace these lost items. This replacement can be in the form of herbal teas, vegetable broths, fruit juices, and electrolyte-replacement drinks. An old naturopathic remedy is to sip a drink made of equal parts of sauerkraut and tomato juice.

When there are young children in the household, it is a good idea to have electrolyte replacement drinks on hand as a precautionary measure. In addition to the well-known Pedialyte and Gatorade brands, electrolyte-replacement drinks with healthier ingredients are available at health food stores. These drinks are generally marketed as "sports drinks." However, they not only provide the electrolytes and fluids lost during intense exercise, but also those lost during a bout of diarrhea.

Avoid Dairy Products
Acute intestinal illnesses, such as viral or bacterial intestinal infections, will frequently injure the cells that line the small intestine. This results in a temporary deficiency of *lactase*, the enzyme responsible for digesting milk sugar (lactose) from dairy products. Avoid dairy products (with the possible ex-

ception of live-cultured yogurt) while experiencing diarrhea.

Use Carob

Since the early 1950s, there have been several reports in the medical literature indicating that brewed teas of roasted carob powder are effective and without side effects in the treatment of acute-onset diarrhea. Carob is rich in dietary fiber (twenty-six percent) and compounds known as polyphenols (twenty-one percent). These two components are thought to be responsible for the beneficial effects.

Carob powder is particularly helpful in treating diarrhea in young children. One study involved forty-one infants, aged three to twenty-one months, with acute diarrhea of bacterial and viral origin. The infants were treated in a hospital setting with oral rehydration fluid (e.g., Pedialyte), and randomly received either carob pod powder (1.5 g/kg of body weight per day) or an equivalent placebo for up to six days.[1] The powders were either diluted in the oral rehydration solution or in milk (not recommended by us; see the previous header). The duration of diarrhea in the carob group was 2 days, compared to 3.75 days in the placebo group. Normalizations in defecation, body temperature, and weight, and cessation of vomiting, were also reached more quickly in the carob group. No side effects from carob were reported.

Use Pectin and Kaolin

An alternative approach to carob is the use of *pectin* (a fruit fiber found in citrus fruits, apples, and many other fruits and vegetables), alone or in combination with *kaolin* (clay) as a bulking agent to improve the consistency of the stool. This combination has long been used in the symptomatic treatment of diarrhea (e.g., Kaopectate, Donnagel, Kaodene,

etc.). Follow the dosage on the bottle or package insert.

Lactobacillus acidophilus

Supplementation with *Lactobacillus acidophilus* is crucial in the treatment of diarrhea of any kind, but particularly in cases of antibiotic-associated diarrhea (discussed later in this chapter). The dosage of a commercial *L. acidophilus* product is based on the number of live organisms. One to two billion viable *L. acidophilus* organisms daily is a sufficient dosage for most people. Amounts exceeding this dosage may induce mild gastrointestinal disturbances (except when taking an antibiotic), while smaller amounts may not be able to colonize the gastrointestinal tract.

Food Allergy

Chronic diarrhea is one of the most common symptoms of food allergy (see FOOD ALLERGY.) The ingestion of an allergic food can result in the release of histamine and other allergic compounds from white blood cells known as mast cells that reside in the lining of the intestines. These allergic compounds can produce a powerful laxative effect.

Lactose Intolerance

Deficiency in the enzyme lactase, responsible for digesting the lactose found in dairy products, is common worldwide. It has been estimated that seventy to ninety percent of Asian, Black, American Indian, and Mediterranean adults lack this enzyme. The frequency of deficiency is ten to fifteen percent in northern and western Europeans.

While almost all infants are able to digest milk and other dairy products, many children lose their lactase enzyme by three to seven years of age. Symptoms range from minor abdominal discomfort and bloating to severe diarrhea in response to even small amounts of lactose. The deficiency is confirmed by the lactose challenge test.

Parasites

Parasites are microorganisms that live off their host (in this case, a human being), and ultimately cause damage to the host. There are five hundred normal microbial inhabitants of the human digestive tract; whether any of them become parasitic depends on whether they are living in harmony *(symbiosis)* with the host or growing out of balance. *Candida albicans* is an example of an organism that, under normal circumstances, lives in harmony with the host. But if candida overgrows and is out of balance with other gut microbes, it can result in problems. In general, parasites cause most of their problems by interfering with digestion and/or damaging the intestinal lining, either of which can lead to diarrhea.

Diarrheal diseases caused by parasites that are not part of the normal gastrointestinal tract still constitute the greatest single worldwide cause of illness and death. The problem is magnified in underdeveloped countries that have poor sanitation, but even in the United States diarrheal diseases are the third major cause of sickness and death. Furthermore, the ease and frequency of worldwide travel and increased migration to the United States is resulting in growing numbers of parasitic infections.

There are many types of microbes that can be classified as parasites, but usually when physicians refer to parasites they mean the organisms known as *protozoa* (one-celled organisms) and *helminths* (worms).

COMMON PROTOZOA
Ameba *(primarily Entamoeba histolytica)*
Giardia
Trichomonas
Cryptosporidium
Dientamoeba fragilis
Iodamoeba butschlii
Blastocystis
Balantidium coli
Chilomastix
Helminths
Roundworm (*Ascaris lumbricoides*)
Pinworm (*Enterobius vermicularis*)
Hookworm (*Necator americanus*)
Threadworm (*Strongyloides stercoralis*)
Whipworm (*Trichuris trichiura*)
Tapeworms (various species)

Detection of parasites involves collecting multiple stool samples at two-to-four-day intervals. The stool sample is analyzed under a microscope after it has been prepared with specialized staining techniques and fluorescent antibodies (the antibodies attach to any parasites present and give off fluorescence).

There are a number of natural compounds that can be useful in helping the body get rid of parasites. However, before selecting a natural alternative to an antibiotic we recommend trying to discern what factors may have been responsible for setting up the internal terrain for a parasitic infection—decreased output of hydrochloric acid, decreased pancreatic enzyme output, and so on. Proper treatment with either an antibiotic or a natural alternative requires monitoring by repeating multiple stool samples two weeks after therapy.

Popular natural treatments for parasitic infections include high dosages of pancreatic enzymes (10X USP pancreatic enzymes, 750 to 1,000 mg ten to twenty minutes before meals) and berberine-containing plants such as goldenseal (*Hydrastis canadensis*), barberry (*Berberis vulgaris*), Oregon grape (*Berberis aquifolium*), and goldthread (*Cop-*

tis chinensis). When using these plants, the dosage should be based on berberine content. As there is a wide range of quality, standardized extracts guaranteed for their berberine content are preferred. The following dosages are to be taken three times per day:

- Dried root, or as infusion (tea): 2–4 grams
- Tincture (1:5): 6–12 ml (1 $\frac{1}{2}$ to 3 tsp)
- Fluid extract (1:1): 2–4 ml ($\frac{1}{2}$ to 1 tsp)
- Solid (dry powdered) extract (4:1 or 8–12 percent alkaloid content): 2 50–500 mg

These dosage recommendations result in a berberine dosage of 25 to 50 mg three times per day, or a daily dosage of up to 150 mg. This dosage is consistent with the dosage range in the positive clinical studies of various parasitic infections. For children, a dosage based on body weight is appropriate. The daily dosage would be the equivalent to 5 to 10 mg of berberine per kg of body weight.

Berberine in Infectious Diarrhea

Berberine has shown significant success in the treatment of acute diarrhea in several clinical studies. It has been found effective against diarrheas caused by *E. coli* (traveler's diarrhea), *Shigella dysenteriae* (shigellosis), *Salmonella paratyphi* (food poisoning), *B. Klebsiella*, *Giardia lamblia* (giardiasis), *Entamoeba histolytica* (amebiasis), and *Vibrio cholerae* (cholera).[2–12]

Berberine appears to be effective in treating the majority of common gastrointestinal infections. The clinical studies have produced results with berberine comparable to standard antibiotics in most cases. In fact, results were better in several studies.

For example, one study focused on sixty-five children below five years of age who had acute diarrhea caused by *E. coli*, *Shigella*, *Salmonella*, *Klebsiella*, or *Faecalis aerogenes*. The children who were given berberine tannate (25 mg every six hours) responded better than those who received standard antibiotic therapy.[6]

Another study involved forty children, ages one through ten years, who were infected with the parasite *Giardia*. The children received either berberine (5 mg per kg of body weight each day), the drug metronidazole (10 mg per kg of body weight each day), or a placebo of vitamin B syrup in three divided doses.[7] After six days, forty-eight percent of the children treated with berberine were symptom-free and, upon stool analysis, sixty-eight percent were found to be *Giardia*-free. In the metronidazole (Flagyl) group, thirty-three percent of the children were without symptoms and, upon stool analysis, all were found to be *Giardia*-free. In comparison, fifteen percent of the children who took the placebo were without symptoms and, upon stool analysis, twenty-five percent were found to be *Giardia*-free. These results indicate that berberine was actually more effective than metronidazole in relieving symptoms at half the dose, but was less effective than the drug in clearing the organism from the intestines.

Finally, in a study of two hundred adult patients with acute diarrhea, the subjects were given standard antibiotic treatment with or without berberine hydrochloride (150 mg per day). Results of the study indicated that the patients who received berberine recovered more quickly.[8] An additional thirty cases of acute diarrhea were treated with berberine alone. Berberine arrested diarrhea in all of these cases, with no mortality or toxicity.

Despite these results, due to the serious consequences of an ineffectively treated infectious diarrhea, the best approach may be to use berberine-containing plants along with standard antibiotic therapy.

Much of berberine's effectiveness is undoubtedly due to its direct antimicrobial activity. However, it also has an effect in blocking the action of toxins produced by certain bacteria.[13,14] This toxin-blocking effect is most evident in diarrheas caused by the enterotoxins *Vibrio cholerae* and *E. coli*), in cholera and traveler's diarrhea respectively.[10–12]

Cholera is a serious disorder that needs standard therapy. However, traveler's diarrhea is usually self-limiting. Good results have been obtained using berberine in the treatment of traveler's diarrhea. In one study, patients with traveler's diarrhea randomly served as controls or received 400 mg of berberine sulfate in a single dose.[12] In treated patients, the mean stool volumes were significantly less than those of controls during three consecutive eight-hour periods after treatment. Twenty-four hours after treatment, significantly more treated patients than controls stopped having diarrhea (forty-two percent vs. twenty percent).

If you are planning to travel to an underdeveloped country or an area where there is poor water quality or sanitation, the prophylactic use of berberine-containing herbs (and *Lactobacillus acidophilus* preparations) may be appropriate. Take them one week prior to your trip, during your stay, and one week after visiting.

Antibiotic-Associated Diarrhea

Antibiotics often cause diarrhea by altering the type of bacteria in the colon or by promoting the overgrowth of *Candida albicans*. Antibiotic use can result in a severe form of diarrhea known as *pseudomembranous enterocolitis*. This condition is attributed to an overgrowth of a bacterium *(Clostridium difficele)*, resulting from the death of the bacteria that normally keep this *Clostridium* under control.

When antibiotic use is absolutely necessary, it is important to supplement with *Lactobacillus acidophilus*. This recommendation is particularly important for preventing and treating antibiotic-induced diarrhea. *L. acidophilus* has been shown to correct diarrhea caused by antibiotics and other causes.[15–18] Although it is commonly believed that acidophilus supplements are not effective if taken during antibiotic therapy, research actually supports the use of *L. acidophilus* during antibiotic administration. Reductions of friendly bacteria and/or infection with antibiotic-resistant bacteria may be prevented by administering *L. acidophilus* products during antibiotic therapy. A dosage of at least fifteen to twenty billion organisms is required. We would still recommend taking the *L. acidophilus* supplement at a different time than the antibiotic. In fact, take it as far away from the antibiotic as possible.

TREATMENT SUMMARY

Since most acute cases of diarrhea are self-limiting, the general recommendations given are often all that is needed. If any of the following apply, a physician should be consulted:

- Diarrhea in a child under six years of age
- Severe or bloody diarrhea
- Diarrhea that lasts more than three days
- Significant signs of dehydration (sunken eyes, severe dry mouth, strong body odor, etc.)

After identification of the cause of chronic diarrhea, appropriate treatment can be determined with the help of a physician.

General Support

There are several measures that can be used as general support during any case of diarrhea:

- Don't eat solid foods
- Replace water and electrolytes
- Avoid dairy products
- Use carob or pectin (alone or in combination with kaolin)
- Reestablish *Lactobacillus acidophilus*

Ear Infection (Otitis Media)

Acute middle ear infection (*acute otitis media*):
- earache or irritability
- history of recent upper-respiratory-tract infection or allergy
- red, opaque, bulging eardrum with loss of the normal features
- fever and chills

Chronic inflammation of the middle ear (*serous otitis media*):
- painless hearing loss
- dull, immobile eardrum (*tympanic membrane*)

Infection or inflammation of the external ear canal (*otitis externa*):
- itching, discharge, or burning pain

An earache occurs as a result of inflammation, swelling, or infection of the middle ear. There are basically two types of earache: chronic and acute.

Acute otitis media is usually preceded by an upper-respiratory infection or allergy. The organisms most commonly cultured from middle-ear fluid during acute otitis media include *Streptococcus pneumoniae* (forty percent) and *Haemophilus influenzae* (twenty-five percent). *Chronic otitis media* (also known as *serous, secretory,* or *nonsuppurative otitis media; chronic otitis media with effusion;* or *glue ear*) refers to a constant swelling of the middle ear.

Acute ear infections affect two-thirds of American children by two years of age, and chronic ear infections affect two-thirds of children under the age of six.[1] Ear infections are the most common diagnosis in children, and they account for over fifty percent of all visits to pediatricians. It has been conservatively estimated that approximately eight billion dollars is spent annually on medical and surgical treatment of earache in the United States.

Standard Medical Treatment

The standard medical approach to ear infections in children is antibiotics, analgesics (e.g., acetaminophen), and/or antihistamines. If the ear infection is long-standing and unresponsive to the drugs, surgery is performed. The surgery involves the placement of a tiny plastic tube known as a *myringotomy tube* through the eardrum to assist drainage of fluid into the throat via the *eustachian tube* (the passageway that connects the middle ear with the throat). This is not a curative procedure, as children with myringotomy tubes in their ears are in fact more likely to have further problems with ear infections.

Myringotomies are currently being performed on nearly one million American children each year. It appears that the unnecessary surgery of the past, the tonsillectomy, has been replaced by this new procedure. In fact, there is a direct correlation between the decline of the tonsillectomy and the rise of the myringotomy. Over two million myringotomy tubes are inserted into children's ears each year, along with six hundred thousand tonsillectomies and adenoidectomies. Are these surgeries necessary? Are they effective? Is current standard medical treatment successful? The answer to all of these questions is a resounding "no" for most kids.

An evaluation of the appropriateness of myringotomy tubes for children under sixteen years of age in the United States was published in *JAMA (the Journal of the American Medical Association)* in 1994; it found that only forty-two percent were appropriate.[2] Since nearly one million myringotomy tubes are inserted into children's ears each year, this means that several hundred thousand children are subjected to a procedure that will do them little good and possibly significant harm.

A number of well-designed studies have demonstrated that there were no significant differences in the clinical course of acute otitis media when conventional treatments were compared with a placebo. Specifically, no differences were found between nonantibiotic treatment, ear tubes, ear tubes with antibiotics, and antibiotics alone.[3-7] Interestingly, in some studies, children who did not receive antibiotics had fewer recurrences of earache than those who received antibiotics. This reduced recurrence rate undoubtedly reflects the suppressive effects antibiotics have on the immune system, as well as their disturbance of the normal flora of the upper respiratory tract.

Although some reviews showed a slight benefit from antibiotic treatment, in the most recent analysis a group of eight international experts from the United States, Britain, and the Netherlands reported that antibiotics are not recommended for treating otitis media in most cases. The experts did an extensive review of the scientific literature on the value of antibiotics in the treatment of otitis media over the past thirty years.[7] The report was published in *BMJ (the British Medical Journal)* in 1997. The group came to the following conclusions:

We conclude that the benefit of routine antimicrobials use for otitis media, judged by either short-term or long-term outcomes, is unproven.

We conclude that existing research offers no compelling evidence that children with acute otitis media routinely given antimicrobials have a shorter duration of symptoms, fewer recurrences, or better long-term outcomes than those who do not receive them.

Although preventing mastoiditis and meningitis is a rationale for antimicrobial treatment, little evidence exists that routine treatment is effective for this purpose.

Antimicrobials did not improve outcome at two months, and no differences in rates of recovery were found for either antimicrobial type or duration.

These results are not likely to be readily accepted by most pediatricians in the United States, who heavily rely on antibiotics to treat otitis media. As an alternative they recommend the use of analgesics (e.g., acetaminophen) and close observation by the parent, as over eighty percent of the children with acute otitis media respond to a placebo within forty-eight hours.

In addition to not being very effective in treating otitis media, the widespread use and abuse of antibiotics is becoming increasingly alarming for other reasons, including the near-epidemic proportion of sufferers of chronic candidiasis and the development of "superbugs" that are resistant to currently available antibiotics. According to many experts, including the World Health Organization, we are coming dangerously close to arriving at a "post-antibiotic era," in which many infectious diseases will once again become almost impossible to treat because of an overreliance on antibiotics (see the chapter IMMUNE SUPPORT for further information).[8]

The risks and failures associated with antibiotics, when coupled with the high rate of recurrent ear infections following insertion of ear tubes, suggest that conservative (nonantibiotic, nonsurgical) treatment alone would reduce the frequency rate and decrease the yearly financial costs of otitis media.

CAVEAT

Although standard antibiotic and surgical procedures may not be statistically effective, each child must be evaluated by a physician before a decision to not use these procedures is considered. As with all potentially dangerous diseases, otitis media should be treated under the supervision of a physician.

Doctors scare parents into believing that drugs and ear tubes are necessary to reduce the risk of the infection spreading to the mastoid (the area of bone behind and under the ear) and brain. Although a major concern, there is no evidence that the rate is any different with or without antibiotics or myringotomy.[7]

Causes

The primary risk factors for otitis media are day care attendance, wood-burning stoves, parental smoking (or exposure to other second-hand smoke), and not being breast-fed.[1] Besides daycare, all of the other factors have something in common: they lead to abnormal eustachian tube function, the underlying cause in virtually all cases of otitis media. The *eustachian tube* regulates gas pressure in the middle ear, protects the middle ear from nose and throat secretions and bacteria, and clears fluids from the middle ear. Swallowing causes active opening of the eustachian tube due to the action of the surrounding muscles. Infants and small children are particularly susceptible to eustachian tube problems since theirs are smaller in diameter and more horizontal.

. . . .

QUICK REVIEW

- Since an ear infection can be quite serious, it is necessary that any individual with symptoms of acute ear infection be seen by a physician.
- Ear infections are extremely common in children under the age of six years.
- Acute otitis media is usually preceded by an upper-respiratory infection or allergy.

- Only forty-two percent of myrin–gotomy tube insertions have been judged as being appropriate.
- A number of well-designed studies have demonstrated that there are no significant differences in the clinical course of acute otitis media when conventional treatments were compared with a placebo.
- The primary risk factors for otitis

Obstruction of the eustachian tube leads first to fluid buildup and then, if bacteria start to grow, bacterial infection. Obstruction results from collapse of the tube (due to weak tissues holding the tube in place and/or an abnormal opening mechanism), blockage with mucus in response to allergy or irritation, or infection.

Therapeutic Considerations

Since an ear infection can be quite serious, it is necessary that any individual with symptoms of acute ear infection be seen by a physician. The recommendations given below are to be used along with the recommendations given in: IMMUNE SUPPORT.

Bottle Feeding

Recurrent ear infection is strongly associated with early bottle feeding, while breast-feeding (for a minimum of four months) has a protective effect.[9] Whether this is due to a cow's milk allergy or the protective effect of human milk against infection has not been conclusively determined. It is probably a combination of both.

In addition, bottle feeding while a child is lying on his or her back (bottle propping) leads to regurgitation of the bottle's contents into the middle ear and should be avoided.

Whether the causative organism in otitis media is viral (*Respiratory syncytial virus* or *Influenza A*) or bacterial (*Streptococcus pneumonia* or *Haemophilus influenza*), human milk offers protection due to its high antibody content, which helps inhibit infectious agents.[10] Breast-fed infants also have a thymus gland (the major organ of the immune system) that is roughly twenty times larger than that of formula-fed infants (see the chapter IMMUNE SUPPORT for further information).[11]

Food Allergy

The role of allergy as the major cause of chronic otitis media has been firmly established in the medical literature.[12–17] Most studies show that eighty-five to ninety-three

· ·

media are day care attendance, wood-burning stoves, parental smoking (or exposure to other second-hand smoke), and not being breast-fed.

- Recurrent ear infection is strongly associated with early bottle feeding, while breast feeding (for a minimum of four months) has a protective effect.

- The role of allergy as the major cause of chronic otitis media has been firmly established in the medical literature.

- Elimination of food allergens has been shown to produce a dramatic effect in the treatment of chronic otitis media in over ninety percent of children in some studies.

percent of children with chronic otitis media have allergies: sixteen percent to inhalants, fourteen percent to food, and seventy percent to both.

One way in which prolonged breast-feeding prevents otitis media may be by avoidance of food allergens, particularly if the mother avoids eating sensitizing foods (foods to which she is allergic) during pregnancy and lactation. In addition to breast-feeding, it is valuable to exclude the foods to which children are most commonly allergic: wheat, egg, fowl, and dairy, particularly during the first nine months.

Since a child's digestive tract is quite permeable to food antigens, especially during the first three months, careful control of eating patterns will reduce food allergies and/or prevent their development. This means no frequent repetitions of any food, avoiding the common allergenic foods, and introducing foods in a controlled manner, that is, introducing one food at a time and carefully watching for a reaction.

The allergic reaction causes blockage of the eustachian tube by two mechanisms: inflammatory swelling of the tube, and inflammatory swelling of the nose which causes the *Toynbee Phenomenon* (swallowing when both mouth and nose are closed, forcing air and secretions into the middle ear). In chronic earaches, an allergic cause should always be considered, and the offending allergens determined and avoided.

One illustrative study of 153 children with earaches demonstrated that 93.3 percent of the children were allergic to foods, inhalants, or both (using the RAST test for diagnosis; see FOOD ALLERGY for description). The twelve-month success rate for 119 of the children who were treated with allergy shots for inhalant sensitivities and an elimination diet for food allergens was ninety-two percent.

This result was much better than the surgically treated control group (ear tubes and, as indicated, removal of the tonsils and adenoids), which showed only a fifty-two percent response.[12]

In another study, a total of 104 children with recurrent otitis media, ranging in age from 1.5 to 9 years, were evaluated for food allergy by means of skin-prick testing, specific IgE tests, and food challenge.[17] Results indicated a statistically significant association between food allergy and recurrent otitis media in eighty-one of the patients (seventy-eight percent). The elimination diet led to a significant amelioration of chronic otitis media in seventy of those eighty-one patients (eighty-six percent), as assessed by detailed clinical evaluation. The challenge diet with the suspected offending food(s) provoked a recurrence of serous otitis media in sixty-six out of those seventy patients (ninety-four percent).

In this study, the frequency distribution of allergies to individual foods was found to be:

FOOD	NUMBER OF PATIENTS	% OF PATIENTS
Cow's milk	31	38
Wheat	27	33
Egg white	20	25
Peanut	16	20
Soy	14	17
Corn	12	15
Tomato	4	5
Chicken	4	5
Apple	3	4

The frequency distribution according to number of food allergens indicates that 81.5 percent of the kids were allergic to two to four foods:

# OF FOOD ALLERGENS	# OF ALLERGIC PATIENTS	TOTAL PERCENTAGE
1	11/81	13.6
2–4	66/81	81.5
5–7	3/81	3.7
8–10	1/81	1.3

Thymus Gland Extract

The thymus gland secretes a family of hormones that act on white cells to ensure their proper development and function. Studies with calf thymus extracts given orally have demonstrated impressive clinical results in a variety of clinical conditions in children.[18–20] Specifically, thymus extracts have been shown to improve immune function, decrease children's food allergies, and improve a child's resistance to chronic respiratory infections. Thymus extracts may be of particular benefit in treating chronic otitis media. For more information, see IMMUNE SUPPORT.

Humidifiers

Humidifiers are popular treatments for ear infections and upper respiratory tract infections in children. Do they work? Apparently so; results from a 1994 study highlight the possibility that low humidity may play a significant role in this disorder.[21]

The study examined the effect of low humidity on the middle ear using a rat model. Twenty-three rats were housed for five days in a low-humidity environment (ten- to twelve-percent relative humidity), and twenty-three control rats were housed at fifty- to fifty-five-percent relative humidity. Microscopic ear examinations were graded for otitis media before testing and on test days three and five. The lining of the middle ears and eustachian tubes were examined by biopsy. Significantly more *effusions* (fluid in the eustachian tubes) were observed in the low-humidity group on both days three and five, but biopsy results were similar in both groups.

This study indicated that low humidity may be a contributing factor in otitis media. Possible explanations are that low humidity may induce nasal swelling and reduced ventilation of the eustachian tube, or it may dry the eustachian tube lining, which could lead to increased secretions and an inability to clear fluid. White blood cells known as *mast cells,* which reside in the lining of the eustachian tubes, may also come into play by releasing histamine and producing swelling.

Although preliminary, this research indicates that increasing the humidity level with the help of a humidifier may be an important goal in the treatment of otitis media with effusion. That being the case, humidifiers appear to be good medicine.

TREATMENT SUMMARY

The key factor in the natural approach to chronic ear infections in children appears to be the recognition and elimination of allergies, particularly food allergies. Since it is usually not possible to determine the exact allergen during an acute attack, the most common allergenic foods should be eliminated from the diet: milk and dairy products, eggs, wheat, corn, oranges, and peanut butter. The diet should also eliminate concentrated simple carbohydrates (sugar, honey, dried fruit, concentrated fruit juice, etc.) since they inhibit the immune system. These simple dietary recommendations will bring relief to most children in a matter of days.

As detailed in the chapter IMMUNE SUPPORT, measures should also be taken to enhance the immune system. Supplementing the diet with a good children's multiple-vitamin-and-mineral formula is a good foundation. Deficiencies of any of a number of essential nutrients increases the likelihood of infection. Of particular importance appears to be the trace minerals, such as zinc, selenium, and manganese. Of course, vitamin C and the B vitamins are also critically important.

In addition to avoiding allergens and enhancing the immune system, locally applied heat is often very helpful in reducing discomfort. It can be applied as a hot pack, with warm oil (especially mullein oil), or by blowing hot air into the ear with the aid of a straw and a hair dryer. These treatments help reduce the pressure in the middle ear and promote fluid drainage.

The following dosage recommendations are given for children. Adults with otitis media should follow the dosage recommendations given in the chapter IMMUNE SUPPORT.

Nutritional Supplements

- Vitamin A: 50,000 IU per day for up to two days in children under six years of age, four days in children over six years of age
- Beta-carotene: age in years x 10,000 IU per day (up to 100,000 IU per day)
- Vitamin C: age in years x 50 mg every two hours
- Bioflavonoids: age in years x 50 mg every two hours
- Zinc: age in years x 2.5 mg per day (up to 30 mg)
- Thymus extract: the equivalent of 120 mg of pure polypeptides with molecular weights less than 10,000, or roughly 500 mg of the crude polypeptide fraction, per day

Botanical Medicines

Echinacea sp. are very safe for children. One-half the adult dosage is appropriate for children under the age of six, and the full adult dosage (given below) is appropriate for children over the age of six. All dosages listed here can be given up to three times per day.

- Dried root (or as tea): 0.5–1 g
- Freeze-dried plant: 325–650 mg
- Juice of aerial portion of *E. purpurea* stabilized in 22% ethanol: 2–3 ml
- Tincture (1:5): 2–4 ml
- Fluid extract (1:1): 2–4 ml
- Solid (dry powdered) extract (6.5:1 or 3.5% echinacoside): 150–300 mg

Eczema (Atopic Dermatitis)

. . . .

Chronic itchy, inflamed skin

Skin is very dry, red, and scaly

Scratching and rubbing lead to darkened and hardened areas of thickened skin with accentuated furrows, most commonly seen on the front of the wrist and elbows and the back of the knees

Personal or family history of allergy

Eczema *(atopic dermatitis)* is a common condition that affects approximately two to seven percent of the population. Current research indicates that eczema is, at least partially, an immediate allergic disease because:

- Serum IgE (an allergic antibody) levels are elevated in eighty percent of patients
- All eczema patients have positive allergy tests
- There is a family history of eczema in two-thirds of eczema patients
- Many eczema patients eventually develop hay fever and/or asthma
- Most eczema patients improve with a diet that eliminates common food allergens[1]

Eczema is also characterized by a variety of physiological and anatomical abnormalities of the skin. The type of abnormality determines the manner in which eczema is manifested in each patient. The major abnormalities are:

- A higher tendency to itch
- Dry, thickened skin that has decreased water-holding capacity
- An increased tendency to thickening of the skin in response to rubbing and scratching

- A tendency of the skin to be overgrown by bacteria, especially *Staphylococcus aureus*

The physiological abnormalities primarily originate in the immune system. For example, the specialized white blood cells known as *mast cells* from the skin of patients with eczema have abnormalities that cause them to release higher amounts of histamine and other allergic compounds compared to people without eczema.[1] Histamine and other allergic compounds result in the inflammation and itching of eczema.

Another key immune-system abnormality is a defect in the ability to kill bacteria.[2] The defect involves the *alternate complement pathway* (ACP), an immune mechanism that is important in destroying bacteria and foreign particles. Interestingly, the historic use of herbs such as burdock root (*Arctium lappa*) and dandelion root (*Taraxacum officinale*) appears to have some scientific validity, since the major polysaccharide in these plants (*inulin*) activates the ACP.[3] This activation could result in restoration of the ability to destroy bacteria.

These defects in immune function, coupled with scratching and the predominance of the bacteria *Staphylococcus aureus* in the skin flora in ninety percent of eczema patients, lead to the increased susceptibility to *staph infections*—potentially severe infections of the skin. There are also other immune defects in patients with eczema that lead to increased susceptibility to other infections of the skin, including infections caused by *Herpes simplex* and common wart viruses.

Therapeutic Considerations

The primary treatment consideration is identification and elimination of food allergy. Many studies have now documented the major role of food allergy in eczema (also see FOOD ALLERGY). Like other conditions associated with food allergy, the best treatment is prevention, and the best preventive measure is breast-feeding in infancy. Studies support the position that breast-feeding offers significant protection against eczema and allergies in general.[4]

If infants who are breast-fed develop eczema, it usually is the result of transfer of allergic antigens in the breast milk. If this occurs, a mother should avoid the common food allergens: milk, eggs, and peanuts, and to a lesser extent, fish, soy, wheat, citrus, and chocolate.[5] Having the mother avoid these common allergens is associated with complete cure in the majority of cases.

In older or formula-fed infants, milk, eggs, and peanuts appear to be the most common food allergens that induce eczema. In one study, these three foods accounted for roughly eighty-one percent of all cases of childhood eczema,[6] while in another study sixty percent of children with severe eczema had an allergic reaction to one or two of the following: egg, cow's milk, peanut, fish, wheat, or soybean.

However, virtually any food can be the offending agent.[7]

Diagnosis of food allergy is usually best achieved using the "elimination diet and challenge" method—eliminate suspected allergens for a period of at least ten days followed by careful reintroduction (see the chapter FOOD ALLERGY for more information). This approach is especially useful in childhood eczema. A simple elimination of milk products, eggs, peanuts, tomatoes, and artificial colors and preservatives results in significant improvement in at least seventy-five percent of cases.[6–8] If laboratory methods are used to identify food allergies in eczema, the most useful method appears to be ELISA IgE and IgG4 (see FOOD ALLERGY).[9]

The presence of food allergies is thought to be responsible for the "leaky gut" condition in children with eczema.[10] As a result of this increased gut permeability there is an added load on the immune system, which consequently overwhelms the immune system, increasing the likelihood of developing additional allergies. It is essential to identify offending foods as soon as possible to avoid the development of further allergies. Trying to deal with multiple food allergies can be a difficult task, as the diet often becomes unrealistically restrictive. But early elimination of allergenic foods appears to stop the development of new allergies.[11]

If you have allergies to a particular food, stay away from it for at least one year. Studies have shown that, if patients can avoid allergenic foods for a period of up to one year, in many cases they will "lose" or "outgrow" their allergy. One study showed that, when patients with eczema avoided the five major food allergens (egg, milk, wheat, soy, and peanut) for one year, their "loss rate" of food allergies was twenty-six percent; for other food allergies, their loss rate was sixty-six percent.[12]

Candida albicans

An overgrowth of the common yeast *Candida albicans* in the gastrointestinal tract has been implicated as a causative factor in many allergic conditions, including eczema. Elevated levels of anticandida antibodies are common in atopic individuals. Furthermore, the severity of lesions tends to correlate with the level of IgE antibodies to candida antigens. The higher the level of antibodies to candida (which usually means a greater overgrowth), the more severe the eczema. Appropriate anticandida therapy (see CHRONIC CANDIDIASIS) may result in significant clinical improvement of eczema.[13]

Essential Fatty Acids and Prostaglandin Metabolism

Patients with eczema appear to have altered essential fatty acid (EFA) and *prostaglandin* metabolism (prostaglandins are hormone-like compounds made from essential fatty acids). Analysis of fatty acids in blood, red blood cells, and white blood cells in patients with eczema demonstrates a tendency for linoleic acid levels to be increased while levels of longer-chain polyunsaturated fatty acids, such as gamma-linolenic acid, arachidonic acid, and the long-chain omega-3 oils eicosapentaenoic acid (EPA) and docosahexanoic acid (DHA), tend to be relatively low. These changes lead to a greater tendency to allergies and inflammation.[14,15]

Initially, it was thought that patients with eczema might have a decreased activity of delta-6-desaturase, the zinc-dependent enzyme that converts linoleic acid to gamma-linolenic acid. If such a defect exists, supplementing the diet with evening primrose, borage, or black currant oil (commercial sources of gamma-linolenic acid) should prove helpful. In fact, several double-blind studies using evening primrose oil have shown benefit in improving the symptoms of eczema (at dosages of at least 3,000 mg of evening primrose oil daily [providing 270 mg of GLA]).[16–18] However, the results generally appear more favorable and less expensive using omega-3 oil supplementation than with evening primrose oil; several studies using evening primrose oil failed to demonstrate any benefit over a placebo. In the largest and highest-quality of these studies, no bene-

QUICK REVIEW

- Food allergy is the major cause of eczema.
- Allergies to milk, eggs, and peanuts account for roughly eighty-one percent of all cases of childhood eczema.
- Omega-3 oils (fish oils and flaxseed oil) appear to offer greater treatment benefits than evening primrose oil.
- Effective treatment involves simultaneously reducing the load on the immune system by identifying and eliminating food allergies, while inhibiting the tendency to release histamine and other allergic factors in the skin.

fit of evening primrose oil could be demonstrated.[19]

In general, treatment with omega-3 oils appears to deal more effectively with prostaglandin abnormalities.[20] In a recent study, the ratio of omega-3 to omega-6 fatty acids was found to be significantly lower in people with eczema than in people who did not have eczema.[21] Furthermore, there was no evidence to suggest that delta-6-desaturase activity is impaired in atopic patients. Without this defect, it doesn't make sense to use high-priced GLA supplements such as evening primrose oil. This analysis seems to provide a reason why clinical studies show omega-3 fatty acids to be more effective in treating eczema than evening primrose oil.

Dietary enrichment with "fish oil" supplements that provide EPA and DHA, or simply eating more fatty fish (e.g., mackerel, herring, and salmon), results in significant incorporation of omega-3 fatty acids into the cell membranes. Flaxseed oil, which contains alpha-linolenic acid (the precursor to omega-3 fatty acid), may provide some benefit to patients with eczema. However, the degree of clinical improvement correlates with the increase in the concentration of DHA in serum phospholipids, and fish oils tend to be more effective in raising DHA levels than flaxseed oil. Therefore, either supplementation with EPA/DHA or increasing the consumption of cold-water fish is likely to produce better overall results in eczema than flaxseed oil.[22]

Inhibition of Excess Histamine Release

There are a number of natural agents that address the excessive histamine release in patients with eczema. An ancient East Indian plant, *Coleus forskolii*, may prove to be the most potent herbal antihistamine.[23] Licorice (*Glycyrrhiza glabra*) also shows very good antiallergy properties.[24] But the most useful natural antihistamines and antiallergy compounds are the flavonoids. In particular, the flavonoid *quercetin* typically shows the greatest activity in experimental studies.[25,26] It not only inhibits the release of histamine, it acts as a potent antioxidant and actually inhibits the formation of histamine and other allergic compounds.

Flavonoid-rich extracts from grape seed (*Vitis vinifera*), bilberry (*Vaccinium myrtillus*), *Ginkgo biloba,* and green tea (*Camellia sinensis*) are also capable of inhibiting allergic mechanisms and may prove helpful in the treatment of eczema.[27]

In addition to flavonoids, *Ginkgo biloba* extract contains several unique *terpene* molecules known collectively as *ginkgolides* that block the effects of *platelet activating factor* (PAF), a key chemical mediator in eczema. Preliminary studies have indicated that mixtures of ginkgolides, as well as the *Ginkgo biloba* extract standardized to contain twenty-four percent ginkgo flavonglycosides and six percent terpenoid are capable of demonstrating clinically significant antiallergy effects.[28,29]

Zinc

Zinc supplementation appears to be indicated in treating eczema, given that low zinc levels are common in eczema patients and that zinc is important to proper essential fatty acid metabolism (zinc is required to create delta-6-desaturase, the enzyme that is responsible for converting linoleic acid to gamma-linolenic acid).[30]

Licorice

The use of botanical medicines in treating eczema can be generally divided into two categories: internal and external. Licorice (*Glycyrrhiza glabra*) appears to be useful in either application. Internally, licorice preparations can exert significant anti-inflammatory and antiallergic effects. These benefits are perhaps best exemplified in several recent double-blind studies featuring a licorice-containing Chinese herbal formula.[31] In addition to licorice, the formula contained *Ledebouriealla seseloides, Potentilla chinensis, Clematis chenisis, Clematis armandi, Rehmania glutinosa, Paeonia lactiflora, Lophatherum gracile, Dictamnus dasycarpus, Tribulus terrestris,* and *Schizonepeta tenuiflora*. Interest in this formula by a group of researchers began after one of their patients with eczema experienced tremendous improvement after taking a *decoction* (tea produced by boiling the herbal material rather than steeping) prescribed by a Chinese doctor.

Several double-blind studies have confirmed this benefit. In one study, forty adult patients with long-standing eczema that resisted treatment were randomized to receive two month's treatment of either the active formula or a placebo decoction, followed by a crossover to the other treatment after a four-week "washout" period.[32] The treatment group demonstrated significant superiority over the placebo in clinical evaluation. In addition, of the thirty-one patients who completed the study, twenty preferred the active formula while only four patients preferred the placebo. There was also a decrease in itching and an improvement in sleep during the active treatment phase. No side effects were reported, although many complained about how awful the decoctions tasted.

Similar results were demonstrated in a double-blind study in children.[33] These positive preliminary studies will hopefully be followed by more extensive investigations to determine proper dosages and perhaps different forms of administration (e.g., pills, tablets, or capsules versus unpalatable decoctions).

Licorice undoubtedly plays a major role in the effectiveness of the Chinese herbal formula. At this time, until the benefits of the other components can be confirmed, it makes the most sense to base the dosage level upon the level of delivered licorice as recommended in the Treatment Summary section.

In regard to using licorice topically, the best results are likely to be obtained by using commercial preparations featuring pure glycyrrhetinic acid (e.g., Simicort from Enzymatic Therapy). Several studies have shown glycyrrhetinic acid to exert an effect similar to that of topical hydrocortisone in the treatment of eczema, contact dermatitis (e.g., poison oak), allergic dermatitis, and psoriasis. In one study, nine of twelve patients with intractable eczema noted marked improvement, and two patients noted mild improvements, when an ointment containing glycyrrhetinic acid was applied topically. In another study of patients with eczema, ninety-three percent of the patients who applied glycyrrhetinic acid demonstrated improvement, compared to eighty-three percent of the patients who used cortisone.[34]

Other popular topical treatments for eczema are creams containing chamomile extracts (e.g., CamoCare) or witch hazel. There is good evidence that this type of preparation can help reduce inflammation and itching in patients with eczema.[35,36]

Miscellaneous Factors

Hypothyroid patients with eczema respond well to thyroid treatment (see the chapter HYPOTHYROIDISM) presumably as a result of improved immune function.

Itching is extremely detrimental to eczema because it breaks the skin, which aids bacterial ingress and promotes *lichenification*—hardening of the skin. Factors that limit itching such as glycyrrhetinic acid or chamomile-containing creams, therefore, promote healing and prevent recurrence.

Emotional tension can provoke and aggravate itching in patients with eczema. Also, according to a number of studies, eczema patients show higher levels of anxiety, hostility, and neurosis than matched controls.[38] It is very important that the person with eczema learn positive coping skills (see the chapter STRESS MANAGEMENT).

TREATMENT SUMMARY

In most cases, effective treatment involves simultaneously reducing the load on the immune system and inhibiting the tendency to release histamine and other allergic factors in the skin.

Diet

Start by eliminating all major allergens (remember, milk, eggs, and peanuts account for approximately eighty-one percent of cases). Limit animal products and add fatty fish such as salmon, mackerel, herring, and halibut to the diet.

Nutritional Supplements

- Vitamin A: 5,000 IU per day
- Vitamin E (mixed tocopherols): 400 IU per day
- Zinc: 45–60 mg per day (decrease to 30 mg when condition clears)
- Flavonoids (choose one):

  Quercetin: 400 mg 20 minutes before meals

  Grape seed extract (95% procyanidolic oligomers content): 50–100 mg three times per day

  Green tea extract (50% polyphenol content): 200–300 mg three times per day (NOTE: Liberal drinking of green tea can be used instead.)
- *Gingko biloba* extract: 80 mg three times per day
- EPA and DHA: 540 and 360 mg per day (or flaxseed oil: 1 tablespoon per day). If there is no response after three months, try evening primrose oil: 3,000 mg per day

Botanical Medicines

Choose one of the following (take dosage three times per day).

- *Glycyrrhiza glabra*

  Powdered root: 1–2 g

  Fluid extract (1:1): 2–4 ml

  Solid (dry powdered) extract (4:1): 250–500 mg
- *Arctium lappa or Taraxacum officinale*

  Dried root: 2–8 g by infusion or decoction

  Fluid extract (1:1): 4–8 ml (1–2 tsp)

  Tincture: alcohol-based tinctures of dandelion are not recommended because of the extremely high dosage required

  Juice of fresh root: 4–8 ml (1–2 tsp)

Powdered solid extract (4:1):
250–500 mg
- *Coleus forskolii*
  Extract standardized to contain 18%
  forskolin: 50 mg (9 mg of forskolin)
  two to three times per day

Topical Treatment

Choose commercial preparations that contain either glycyrrhetinic acid, chamomile, or witch hazel. In addition, avoid rough-textured clothing; wash clothing with mild soaps only and rinse thoroughly; and avoid exposure to chemical irritants and any other agents that might cause skin irritation. Local application of soothing lotions ameliorates itching (zinc oxide works well), but greasy preparations should not be used for extended periods since they block the sweat ducts.

Fibrocystic Breast Disease

. . . .

Characteristically cyclic and bilateral, with multiple cysts of varying sizes giving the breast a nodular consistency

Pain or premenstrual breast pain and tenderness common, although condition often without symptoms

Occurs in twenty to forty percent of premenopausal women

Benign fibrocystic breast disease (FBD), also known as *cystic mastitis*, is usually a component of premenstrual syndrome (PMS) and is considered a risk factor for breast cancer. It is not, however, as significant a factor as the classic breast cancer risk factors, family history, early onset of menstruation (*menarche*), and late or no first pregnancy.

FBD is apparently the result of an increased estrogen-to-progesterone ratio. However, other hormones are also important. For example, the changes within the breast in FBD may be due to the hormone *prolactin.* Typically, significantly elevated levels of prolactin are found in women with FBD.[1,2] The levels are higher, but not so high has to cause loss of menstruation (*amenorrhea*). The increase in prolactin is thought to be the result of higher estrogen levels.

FBD cannot be definitively differentiated from breast cancer on clinical criteria alone. Although pain, cyclic variations in size, high mobility, and multiplicity of nodules are indicative of FBD, you should see a physician immediately if you notice a lump of any kind. Noninvasive procedures, such as ultrasound, can help to aid differentiation further, but at this time definitive diagnosis depends upon biopsy.

Therapeutic Considerations

For a more comprehensive discussion of the many factors involved in FBD, please read PREMENSTRUAL SYNDROME first. The factors discussed here were chosen because they are not covered in depth in the PMS chapter and are particularly relevant to FBD.

Caffeine and Other Methylxanthines

Population studies, experimental evidence, and clinical evaluations indicate a strong association between caffeine consumption and FBD. Caffeine, theophylline, and theobromine are known as *methylxanthines.* These compounds elevate the levels of compounds that promote overproduction within breast tissue of cellular products, such as fibrous tissue and cyst fluid, that are linked to FBD.[3–7]

In one study, limiting sources of methyl–xanthines (coffee, tea, cola, chocolate, and caffeinated medications) resulted in improvement in 97.5 percent of the forty-five women who completely abstained, and in 75 percent of the twenty-eight who limited their consumption. Those who continued with little change in their methylxanthine consumption showed little improvement.[4] According to this study, women may have varying thresholds of response to methylxanthines. Stress may also play an important role, since fibrocystic breasts appear more responsive to the changes caused by adrenaline (epinephrine).

Vitamin E

Vitamin E (*alpha-tocopherol*) has been shown to relieve many PMS symptoms, particularly FBD, as evidenced by several double-blind clinical studies.[8,9] The mode of action remains obscure, although vitamin E has been shown to normalize circulating hormones in PMS and FBD patients.[8–10] Vitamin E supplementation (600 IU/day) also normalizes the elevated levels of the pituitary hormones FSH and LH commonly seen in FBD patients.[10]

Vitamin A

After three months of high-dose (150,000 IU/day) supplementation with vitamin A, five of the nine patients who completed one study had complete or partial remission of their FBD.[11] However, some patients developed mild side effects, resulting in two of the original twelve withdrawing due to headaches and one patient having her dosage reduced. We recommend high-dosage vitamin A therapy only in cases that are unresponsive to other measures, and only under the direct supervision of a physician. Prolonged high dosages of vitamin A can lead to serious side effects and should never be used if there is a chance of pregnancy; at higher dosages (prolonged intake of as little as 10,000 IU per day), vitamin A can produce birth defects.

Thyroid and Iodine

Experimental iodine deficiency in rats results in changes very similar to human FBD.[12] Thyroid hormone replacement therapy in patients with low or even normal thyroid function may result in clinical improvement.[12,13] Research has shown that thyroid supplementation decreases breast pain, serum prolactin levels, and breast nodules in patients thought to have normal thyroid function. These results suggest that subclinical hypothyroidism and/or iodine deficiency may be a causative

QUICK REVIEW

- Fibrocystic breast disease is most often a component of premenstrual syndrome.
- Elevated estrogen-to-progesterone ratio and/or increased prolactin levels are common.
- Eliminating caffeine and similar compounds has produced improvements in

as high as ninety-seven percent of women in clinical trials.
- Hypothyroidism and/or iodine deficiency may be a causative factor in fibrocystic breast disease.
- Women who have fewer than three bowel movements per week have a 4.5 times greater rate of fibrocystic breast disease than women who have at least one bowel movement a day.

factor in FBD. Hypothyroidism and/or iodine deficiency are also associated with a higher incidence of breast cancer.

Iodine (specifically iodine caseinate) may be an effective treatment of FBD.[14] It is theorized that an absence of iodine renders the breast cells more sensitive to estrogen stimulation. Also, oral iodine supplementation is known to have significant anti-inflammatory and antifibrotic effects in both acute and chronic experimental models.[15] This hypersensitivity to estrogen in iodine deficiency leads the breast ducts to produce small cysts and later *fibrosis* (hardening of the tissue due to the deposition of fibrin similar to the formation of scar tissue).

Since 1975, three clinical trials have been performed on women with FBD:

1. A study with sodium iodide and protein-bound iodide
2. A study where subjects were switched from iodide to molecular iodine (or vice versa)
3. A double-blind study with molecular iodine[14]

Results from these studies indicate that, while treatment with iodides was effective in about seventy percent of subjects, it was associated with a high rate of side effects (altered thyroid function in four percent, iodism [iodine poisoning characterized by a watery nose, weakness, excessive salivation, and bad breath] in three percent, and acne in fifteen percent). Results with elemental iodine were about the same, but there were no significant side effects. The most significant side effect with molecular iodine was short-term increased breast pain, which seemed to correspond to a softening of the breast and disappearance of fibrous tissue plaques on physical examination. The short-term pain was viewed as a positive sign since it was followed by resolution of the fibrous tissue.

The dosage of molecular iodine was 70 to 90 mcg of iodine per kilogram of body weight. This dosage appears to be safe and effective treatment for FBD. Unfortunately, as of this writing (October, 1997) the forms of iodine supplement used in the studies (iodine caseinate and liquid iodine) were not yet available on the marketplace.

Liver Function

Since the liver is the primary site for estrogen clearance, any factor (e.g., cholestasis, "toxic liver syndrome," environmental pollution) that interferes with proper liver function may lead to estrogen excess. Adequate levels of B-vitamins are necessary for estrogen clearance from the body. It is the liver's role to detoxify estrogen by binding (conjugating) it to glucoronic acid so that it can be excreted in the bile. The liver requires vitamin B6, folic acid, and other B vitamins to accomplish this goal. A deficiency of any of these B vitamins makes it very difficult for the liver to do its job.

Colon Function

Breast disease has been linked to constipation and to a diet low in fiber.[16] Women who have fewer than three bowel movements per week have a 4.5 times greater rate of FBD than women who have at least one bowel movement a day. This association is probably due to the bacterial flora in the large intestine transforming excreted steroids into toxic derivatives or allowing these excreted steroids to be reabsorbed.[17,18]

Comparing the diet of 354 women with benign proliferative epithelial disorders of the breast to 354 matched controls and 189 unmatched controls found an inverse association between dietary fiber and the risk of benign, proliferative, epithelial disorders of the breasts. An increased intake of dietary fiber may be associated with a reduced risk of both benign breast disease and breast cancer.

These benefits may be due to an increase in the amount of estrogen being excreted. For example, it has been shown that women on a vegetarian diet excrete two to three times more estrogens than women on an omnivorous diet. This difference in excretion is responsible for vegetarian women having a fifty-percent lower level of unbound estrogen in their blood. *Lactobacillus acidophilus* supplementation may also help promote increased excretion of estrogens.[19]

. . . .

TREATMENT SUMMARY

Unless a woman has pure FBD (no other PMS symptom), the therapeutic approach outlined in PREMENSTRUAL SYNDROME will more definitively meet her individual needs, as FBD is often a component of the more encompassing PMS. The therapy recommended here includes key factors discussed in that chapter.

Diet

The diet should be primarily vegetarian, with large amounts of dietary fiber. All methylxanthines should be eliminated until symptoms are alleviated; they then can be reintroduced in small amounts. External (exogenous) estrogens should be avoided (oral contraceptives, animal products with high estrogen content such as meats raised with the help of growth stimulators, etc.). The diet should emphasize whole, unprocessed foods: whole grains, legumes, vegetables, fruits, nuts, and seeds. Drink at least 48 ounces of water daily.

Nutritional Supplements

- High potency multiple vitamin and mineral formula as described in the chapter SUPPLEMENTARY MEASURES
- Lipotropic factors
  Choline: 500–1,000 mg per day
  Methionine: 500–1,000 mg per day
- Vitamin B6: 25–50 mg three times per day
- Vitamin C: 500 mg three times per day
- Vitamin E: 400–800 IU per day of d-alpha tocopherol
- Beta-carotene: 50,000 IU per day
- Iodine (caseinate or liquid iodine): 70–90 mcg of iodine per kilogram of body weight per day (other forms of iodine 500 mcg daily)
- Zinc: 15–30 mg per day
- Flaxseed oil: 1 tablespoon per day
- *Lactobacillus acidophilus:* 1–2 billion live organisms per day

Fibromyalgia

. . . .

Diagnosis requires fulfillment of all three major criteria and four or more minor criteria

MAJOR CRITERIA:

1. Generalized aches or stiffness of at least three anatomical sites for at least three months
2. Six or more typical, reproducible tender points
3. Exclusion of other disorders that can cause similar symptoms

MINOR CRITERIA:

1. Generalized fatigue
2. Chronic headache
3. Sleep disturbance
4. Neurological and psychological complaints
5. Joint swelling
6. Numbing or tingling sensations
7. Irritable bowel syndrome
8. Variation of symptoms in relation to activity, stress, and weather changes

Fibromyalgia is a recently recognized disorder that is regarded as a common cause of chronic musculoskeletal pain and fatigue. Fibromyalgia is a relatively common condition, estimated to affect about four percent of the general population. As described in the chapter on CHRONIC FATIGUE SYNDROME, there is tremendous overlap between fibromyalgia and chronic fatigue syndrome (CFS); approximately seventy percent of patients diagnosed with fibromyalgia meet all the diagnostic criteria for CFS.[1] The only difference in diagnostic criteria for fibromyalgia and CFS is the requirement of musculoskeletal pain in fibromyalgia and fatigue in CFS.

Therapeutic Considerations

Because of the close link with CFS, we recommend taking a good look at the CHRONIC FATIGUE SYNDROME chapter to determine which recommendations given there are appropriate to your case (e.g., if you have evidence of needing liver support, as described and recommended in Chronic Fatigue Syndrome, please follow that recommendation).

Although fibromyalgia has many facets, the central cause of the pain of fibromyalgia is a low level of serotonin. Chronic low levels of serotonin cause the sensation of pain to be greatly exaggerated (see MIGRAINE).

The primary treatment goals in fibromyalgia (in addition to those named in the CHRONIC FATIGUE SYNDROME chapter) are to raise serotonin levels, improve sleep quality, and assure adequate magnesium levels.

Sleep Disturbances

One of the key findings in patients with fibromyalgia is altered sleep patterns—presumably as a result of the low serotonin levels (see INSOMNIA). Specifically, fibromyalgia patients tend to have reduced REM sleep and increased non-REM sleep.[2]

Based on observations of eye movement and brain-wave or electroencephalogram (EEG) recordings, sleep is divided into two distinct types: REM (rapid-eye-movement) and non-REM (non-rapid-eye-movement) sleep. During REM sleep, the eyes move rapidly and dreaming takes place. When people are awakened during non-REM sleep, they report that they were thinking about everyday matters but rarely report dreams.

Non-REM sleep, also known as slow-wave sleep, is divided into four stages, graded 1 to 4, based on level of EEG activity and ease of arousal. As sleep progresses, there is a deepening of sleep from Stage 1 to Stage 4, with progressively slower brain-wave activity until REM sleep, when suddenly the brain becomes much more active. In adults, the first REM sleep cycle is usually triggered ninety minutes after going to sleep and lasts about five to ten minutes. After the flurry of activity, brain-wave patterns return to non-REM sleep for another ninety-minute sleep cycle.

Most adults experience five or six sleep cycles each night. REM sleep periods grow progressively longer as sleep continues; the last sleep cycle may produce a REM sleep period that lasts about an hour. In general, non-REM sleep lasts approximately fifty percent of the ninety-minute sleep cycle in infants and about eighty percent in adults.

The sleep defects in fibromyalgia go well beyond reduced REM sleep and increased non-REM sleep. For example, the deeper levels (Stages 3 and 4) are not achieved for long enough periods. As a result, people with fibromyalgia wake up feeling tired, worn out, and in pain. The severity of the pain of fibromyalgia correlates with the rating of sleep quality; when patients with fibromyalgia get a good night's sleep, they have less pain. Conversely, when they sleep poorly, their symptoms are more severe.

This association between pain level and sleep quality in fibromyalgia patients was shown clearly in a study conducted at the

. . . .

QUICK REVIEW

- Fibromyalgia and chronic fatigue syndrome share many features.
- Although fibromyalgia is a disorder that has many facets, the central cause of the pain of fibromyalgia is a low level of serotonin.

- The primary treatment goals in fibromyalgia are to raise serotonin levels, improve sleep quality, and assure adequate magnesium levels.
- Individuals with fibromyalgia have altered sleep patterns: reduced REM sleep and increased non-REM sleep.

University of Connecticut School of Medicine.[3] Fifty women with fibromyalgia syndrome recorded their sleep quality, pain intensity, and attention to pain for thirty days, using palm-top computers programmed as electronic interviewers. They described their previous night's sleep quality within one-half hour of awakening each day. Then, at randomly selected times in the morning, afternoon, and evening, they rated their present pain. This detailed study and analysis found that poor sleep resulted in significantly more pain. However, the problems did not end there. The researchers found that a night of poor sleep was followed by a significantly more painful day, and a more painful day was followed by a night of even poorer sleep.

An analogy is that sleep is like a battery charger. If the body is not being recharged, especially the muscles, the result is pain. With a good, restful sleep, the battery becomes fully charged and functions optimally. The outcome is that the pain goes away or is significantly relieved.

5-HTP and Fibromyalgia

5-Hydroxytryptophan (5-HTP) is converted to the important neurotransmitter serotonin. The role of serotonin and the benefits of 5-HTP in raising serotonin levels are detailed in the chapter on DEPRESSION. In addition to being helpful in treating depression, 5-HTP is proving effective in the treatment of fibromyalgia—as it should be, since a deficiency of serotonin is linked to fibromyalgia.

The history of the development of 5-HTP in the treatment of fibromyalgia began with studies on a drug known as fenclonene. This drug blocks the enzyme that enables the conversion of tryptophan to 5-HTP and, as a result, it effectively blocks serotonin production.[4] When subjects took this drug, they experienced severe symptoms of fibromyalgia. This association led to the discovery of the link between low serotonin levels and fibromyalgia, as well as to the use of 5-HTP in the treatment of fibromyalgia.[5] According to one of the world's leading authorities on fibromyalgia, professor Federigo Sicuteri of the University of Florence, "In our experience, as well as in that of other pain specialists, 5-HTP can largely improve the painful picture of primary fibromyalgia."[6]

Several clinical studies confirm this opinion.[7,8] In one double-blind study, fifty patients with fibromyalgia were given either 5-HTP (100 mg) or a placebo three times per day.[7] The group that received the 5-HTP experienced significant improvements in their

. . . .

- The severity of the pain of fibromyalgia correlates with the rating of poor sleep quality.
- 5-HTP has shown considerable benefit in treating fibromyalgia in double-blind studies.
- Although 5-HTP can be effective on its own, we recommend the combination of 5-HTP (100 mg), St. John's wort extract (300 mg, 0.3-percent hypericin content), and magnesium (150 to 250 mg) three times per day.
- Magnesium supplementation has produced very good results in treating fibromyalgia.

symptoms. In contrast, the group that received the placebo did not improve much at all. As shown in Table 1, 5-HTP was rated significantly better than the placebo by subjects and evaluating physicians. Improvements were noted in all symptom categories: number of painful areas, morning stiffness, sleep patterns, anxiety, and fatigue. Although 5-HTP produces very good results within thirty days, even better results are obtained at ninety days of use.

The beneficial effects of 5-HTP are thought to be due to elevation of serotonin levels, which increases pain tolerance (see MIGRAINE) and improves sleep quality (see INSOMNIA).

Combined Therapy with 5-HTP, St. John's wort, and Magnesium

Although 5-HTP can be effective on its own, we recommend the combination of 5-HTP (100 mg), St. John's wort extract (300 mg, 0.3-percent hypericin content), and magnesium (200 to 250 mg) three times per day. This approach is likely to work better than using any of these treatments alone. We recommend St. John's wort extract (see DEPRESSION) largely because of a study in which a combination of 5-HTP and an antidepressant drug produced significantly better results than when either was used alone.[2] Even in conventional circles, combined antidepressant agents—usually Prozac (fluoxetine) and Elavil (amitriptyline)—have been shown to produce much better results than using either drug alone.[9]

The magnesium comes into play because low magnesium levels are a common finding in patients with fibromyalgia (as well as in CFS).[10,11] Magnesium is critical to many cellular functions, including energy production, protein formation, and cellular replication. Magnesium participates in more than three hundred enzymatic reactions in the body, particularly those processes that produce energy (i.e., the production of ATP). When magnesium levels are low, energy levels are low.

Magnesium supplementation has produced very good results in treating both fibromyalgia and CFS. This improvement may be due to magnesium's importance to serotonin function and the production of cellular energy.[12,13]

In addition to supplementing with magnesium, we recommend increasing dietary intake of magnesium. The best food sources of magnesium are legumes, tofu, seeds, nuts, whole grains, and green leafy vegetables. Fish, meat, milk, and most commonly eaten fruit are low in magnesium. Most Americans consume a low-magnesium diet because their diet is high in refined foods, meat, and dairy products.

TABLE 1	Patient's and Physician's Opinion on the Effectiveness of 5-HTP vs. Placebo in Fibromyalgia	
RESPONSE	**5-HTP**	**PLACEBO**
Good	11	1
Fair	8	5
Poor	4	8
None	0	9

TREATMENT SUMMARY

The primary treatment goals in fibromyalgia are to raise serotonin levels, improve sleep quality, and assure adequate magnesium levels. In addition, there may be recommendations given in the CHRONIC FATIGUE SYNDROME chapter that are appropriate in any given case. Please follow the relevant recommendations given there.

Diet

Follow the recommendations given in A HEALTH-PROMOTING DIET.

Lifestyle

Follow the recommendations given in A HEALTHY LIFESTYLE.

Nutritional Supplements

- High-potency multiple-vitamin-and-mineral formula, according to guidelines given in SUPPLEMENTARY MEASURES
- 5-HTP: 50–100 mg three times per day
- Magnesium bound to citrate or Krebs-cycle intermediates (citrate, malate, fumarate, succinate, aspartate): 150–250 mg three times per day

Botanical Medicines

- St. John's wort extract (0.3% hypericin): 300 mg three times per day

Food Allergies

. . . .

Significant improvement in symptoms and signs of a disease linked to food allergy while on an allergy-elimination diet

Positive test result from an acceptable food allergy test

Typical signs of allergy:
- Dark circles under the eyes ("allergic shiners")
- Puffiness under the eyes
- Horizontal creases in the lower eyelid
- Chronic (noncyclic) fluid retention
- Chronic swollen glands

A food allergy occurs when there is an adverse reaction to the ingestion of a food. The reaction may or may not be mediated (controlled and influenced) by the immune system. The reaction may be caused by a protein, starch, or other food component, or by a contaminant found in the food (colorings, preservatives, etc.).

A classic food allergy occurs when an ingested food molecule acts as an *antigen*—a substance that can be bound by an antibody. Antibodies are the protein molecules made by white blood cells that bind to foreign substances, in this case, antigens. The food antigen is bound by allergic antibodies known as IgE (immunoglobulin E). The IgE are specialized immunoglobulins (proteins) that bind to specialized white blood cells known as *mast cells* and *basophils*. When the IgE and food antigen bind to a mast cell or basophil, it causes the release of *histamines,* which cause swelling and inflammation. The mechanisms which lead to allergy symptoms are further discussed following in the Immune System and Allergies section.

Other terms often used to refer to food allergy include: food hypersensitivity, food anaphylaxis, food idiosyncrasy, food intolerance, pharmacological (drug-like) reaction to food, metabolic reaction to food, and food sensitivity.

The recognition of food allergy was first recorded by the famous Greek physician Hippocrates, who observed that milk could cause gastric upset and hives *(urticaria).* He wrote, "To many this has been the commencement of a serious disease when they have merely taken twice in a day the same food which they have been in the custom of taking once."[1]

Food allergies have been implicated in a wide range of medical conditions, affecting virtually every part of the body—from mildly uncomfortable symptoms, such as indigestion and gastritis, to severe illnesses, such as celiac disease, arthritis, and chronic infection. Allergies have also been linked to numerous disorders of the central nervous system, including depression, anxiety, and chronic fatigue. The actual symptoms produced during an allergic response depend on the location of the immune system activation, the mediators of inflammation involved, and the sensitivity of the tissues to specific mediators. As

TABLE 1	Symptoms and Diseases Commonly Associated with Food Allergy

SYSTEM	SYMPTOMS AND DISEASES
Gastrointestinal	Canker sores, celiac disease, chronic diarrhea, duodenal ulcer, gastritis, irritable bowel syndrome, malabsorption, ulcerative colitis
Genitourinary	Bed-wetting, chronic bladder infections, nephrosis
Immune	Chronic infections, frequent ear infections
Mental/emotional	Anxiety, depression, hyperactivity, inability to concentrate, insomnia, irritability, mental confusion, personality change, seizures
Musculoskeletal	Bursitis, joint pain, low back pain
Respiratory	Asthma, chronic bronchitis, wheezing
Skin	Acne, eczema, hives, itching, skin rash
Miscellaneous	Arrhythmia, edema, fainting, fatigue, headache, hypoglycemia, itchy nose or throat, migraines, sinusitis

evident in Table 1, food allergies have been linked to many common symptoms and health conditions.

Scope of the Problem

The frequency of food allergies and the number of individuals who have food allergies has increased dramatically in recent times. For example, it is estimated that eczema (an allergic condition of the skin that is often directly caused by food allergies) now affects between ten and fifteen percent of the population at some time during their lives.[2,3] Food allergies and other adverse reactions to food are now reported in about twenty-five percent of young children.[4] Some physicians believe that food allergies are the leading cause of undiagnosed symptoms, and that at least sixty percent of Americans suffer from symptoms associated with food reactions.

The primary causes for the increased frequency of food allergy appears to be excessive regular consumption of a limited number of foods (often hidden as ingredients in commercially-prepared foods) and the high level of preservatives, stabilizers, artificial colorings, and flavorings now added to foods.[5] Some researchers and clinicians believe that the increased chemical pollution in our air, water, and food is to blame. For example, foods can easily become contaminated following the use of pesticides in farming.

Other possible reasons for the increased occurrence of food allergy include: earlier weaning and earlier introduction of solid foods to infants; genetic manipulation of plants resulting in food components with greater allergic properties; and impaired digestion (especially lack of hydrochloric acid, see DIGESTION).

Causes and Development

It is well documented that food allergy is often inherited. When both parents have allergies, there is a sixty-seven-percent chance that the children will also have allergies. Where only one parent is allergic, the chance of a child being prone to allergies is still high, but drops from sixty-seven percent to thirty-three percent.[6]

The theory is that individuals with a tendency to develop food allergies have abnormalities in the number and ratios of special white blood cells known as *T lymphocytes* or *T cells*.[7,8] Specifically, these individuals have nearly fifty percent more helper T cells than nonallergic persons. These cells help other white blood cells make antibodies.

Individuals prone to food allergies have a lower allergic set point because they have more helper T cells in circulation. Therefore, the level of insult required to trigger an allergic response is lowered. The actual expression of an allergy can be triggered by a variety of stressors which can disrupt the immune system, such as physical or emotional trauma, excessive use of drugs, immunization reactions, excessive frequency of consumption of a specific food, and/or environmental toxins.

Other Factors

Repetitious exposure to a food, improper digestion, and poor integrity of the intestinal barrier are additional factors that can lead to the development and maintenance of food allergy. When properly chewed and digested, ninety percent of ingested proteins are absorbed as amino acids and small peptides. However, it has been well documented that partially digested dietary protein can cross the intestinal barrier and be absorbed into the bloodstream. These larger molecules can cause an allergic response that can occur either directly at the intestinal barrier, at distant sites, or throughout the body.[9]

It is often necessary to support the individual who has food allergies with supplemental levels of hydrochloric acid and/or pancreatic enzymes (see DIGESTION). Research has shown that incompletely digested proteins can impair the immune system, leading to long-term allergies and frequent infections.[10]

Stress

During stressful times, food allergies tend to develop or become worse. This situation probably results from a stress-induced decrease in secretory IgA levels.[11,12] IgA plays an important role in the lining of the mucosal membrane of the intestinal tract, where it helps protect against the entrance of foreign substances into the body. In other words, IgA

. . . .

QUICK REVIEW

- Food allergies have been linked to many common symptoms and health conditions.
- Some physicians believe that at least sixty percent of the American population suffers from symptoms associated with food reactions.

- When both parents have allergies, there is a sixty-seven-percent chance that the children will also have allergies.
- It is often necessary to support the individual who has food allergies with supplemental levels of hydrochloric acid and/or pancreatic enzymes.

acts as a barricade against the entry of food antigens. When there is a lack of IgA lining the intestines, the absorption of food allergens and microbial antigens increases dramatically. Even a relative short-term IgA deficiency predisposes a person to the development of food allergy. People with food allergies have unusually low levels of IgA, making them particularly susceptible.[13]

The Immune System and Food Allergies

Most food allergies are mediated by the immune system as a result of interactions between ingested food, the digestive tract, white blood cells, and food-specific antibodies (immunoglobulins), such as IgE and IgG. Food represents the largest antigenic challenge that confronts the human immune system whether a person suffers from food allergies or not.[14] When the immune system is activated by food antigens, white blood cells and antibodies cooperate in an immune response which, under certain circumstances, can have negative effects.

There are five major families of antibodies: IgE, IgD, IgG, IgM, and IgA. IgE is involved primarily in the classic immediate reaction, while the others seem to be involved in delayed reactions, such as those seen in the cyclical type of food allergy (one that comes and goes). Although the function of the immune system is to protect a person from infections and cancer, abnormal immune responses can lead to tissue injury and disease (food allergy reactions being one expression).

There are four distinct types of immune-mediated reactions: Type I, immediate hypersensitivity; Type II, cytotoxic; Type III, immune-complex-mediated; and Type IV, T-cell dependent.

Type I: Immediate Hypersensitivity Reactions

Type I reactions occur less than two hours after consumption of an allergenic food. Antigens bind to preformed IgE antibodies, which are attached to the surface of the mast cell or the basophil, and cause the release of mediators such as histamines and leukotrienes. A variety of allergic symptoms may result, depending on the location of the mast cell: in the nasal passages, this causes sinus congestion; in the bronchioles, constriction

- During stressful times, food allergies tend to develop or become worse.
- Many physicians believe that oral food challenge is the best way to diagnose food sensitivities.
- The skin-prick test or skin-scratch test commonly employed by many allergists is of little value in diagnosing most food allergies.

- There are now effective blood tests to identify food allergies.
- The simplest and most effective method of treating food allergies is through avoidance of allergenic foods.
- Many experts believe that the key to the dietary control of food allergies is the "Rotary Diversified Diet."

(asthma); in the skin, hives and eczema; in the synovial cells that line the joints, arthritis; in the intestinal mucosa, inflammation with resulting malabsorption; and in the brain, headaches, loss of memory, and "spaciness." It has been estimated that Type I reactions account for only ten to fifteen percent of food-allergy reactions.[14,15]

Type II: Cytotoxic Reactions

Cytotoxic reactions involve the binding of either IgG or IgM antibodies to cell-bound antigens. Antigen-antibody binding activates factors that cause the destruction of the cell to which the antigen is bound. Immune hemolytic anemia is one example of such tissue injury. The antigen-antibody complex binds to the red blood cell and ultimately causes its destruction. The destruction of the red blood cell is referred to as "hemolysis," since it is caused by immune mechanisms and can lead to anemia (lack of red blood cells); that is why it is called immune hemolytic anemia.

It has been estimated that at least seventy-five percent of all food allergy reactions are accompanied by cell destruction.[14] Normally the cells that are destroyed are intestinal since that is where the immune system and the food antigen meet.

Type III: Immune-Complex-Mediated Reactions

Immune complexes are formed when antigens bind to antibodies. They are usually cleared from the circulation by the white blood cells located in the liver (macrophages) and the spleen. However, if these complexes are deposited in tissues, they can produce tissue injury. Two factors that promote tissue injury are: (1) increased quantities of circulating complexes and (2) the presence of histamines and other amines that increase

vascular permeability and favor the deposition of immune complexes in tissues.

These responses are of the delayed type, often occurring two hours after exposure. This type of allergy has been shown to involve IgG and IgG4 immune complexes. It is estimated that eighty percent of food allergy reactions involve IgG and IgG4.[14]

Type IV: T-Cell-Dependent Reactions

This delayed reaction is mediated primarily by white blood cells known as T lymphocytes. It results when an allergen contacts the skin, respiratory tract, gastrointestinal tract, or other body surface. Within thirty-six to seventy-two hours of contact, this can cause inflammation by stimulating sensitized T cells. Type IV reactions do not involve any antibodies. Examples include poison ivy (contact dermatitis), allergic colitis, and regional ileitis.

Other Mechanisms That Trigger Food Allergies

Many adverse reactions to foods are not triggered by the immune system. Instead, the reaction is caused by inflammatory mediators (histamine, prostaglandins, leukotrienes, SRS-A, serotonin, platelet-activating factor, kinins, etc.) released by mast cells and other white blood cells. In addition, foods themselves may also produce allergy-like reactions due to a high histamine content or to histamine-releasing effects.

Cyclical vs. Fixed Food Allergies

From a clinical perspective, naturopathic and other nutrition-oriented physicians recognize two basic types of food allergies: cyclic and fixed.

Cyclic allergies are slowly developed by repetitive eating of a food. If the allergenic food is avoided for a period of time (typically over four months), it may be reintroduced and tolerated unless it is again eaten too frequently. Cyclic allergies account for eighty to ninety percent of food allergies.

Fixed allergies occur whenever a food is eaten, no matter what the time span between episodes of ingestion. In other words, in fixed allergies the person remains allergic to the food throughout life.

Diagnostic Considerations

There are two basic categories of tests commonly used: (1) food challenge and (2) laboratory methods. Each has its advantages. Food-challenge methods require no additional expense, but they do require a great deal of motivation. Laboratory procedures, such as blood tests, can provide immediate identification of suspected allergens, but they are more expensive.

Elimination Diet and Food Challenge

Many physicians believe that oral food challenge is the best way to diagnose food sensitivities. There are two broad categories of food challenge testing: (1) elimination (also known as *oligoantigenic*) diet, followed by food reintroduction, and (2) pure water fast, followed by food challenge.

A NOTE OF CAUTION: Food challenge testing should NOT be used by people who have potentially life-threatening symptoms, such as airway constriction or severe allergic reactions.

In the elimination diet method, the patient is put on a limited diet. Commonly eaten foods are eliminated and replaced with either hypoallergenic foods and foods that are rarely eaten, or special hypoallergenic formulas.[16,17] The fewer allergenic foods eaten, the greater the ease of establishing a diagnosis using an elimination diet.

The standard elimination diet consists of lamb, chicken, potatoes, rice, banana, apple, and a cabbage-family vegetable (cabbage, brussels sprouts, broccoli, etc.). There are variations of the elimination diet that are suitable. However, it is extremely important that no allergenic foods be consumed.

The individual stays on this limited diet for at least one week, and up to one month. If the symptoms are related to food sensitivity, they will typically disappear by the fifth or sixth day of the diet. If the symptoms do not disappear, it is possible that a reaction to a food in the elimination diet is responsible. In that case, an even more restricted diet must be utilized.

After the elimination-diet period, individual foods are reintroduced every two days. Methods range from reintroducing only a single food every two days, to reintroducing a food every one or two meals. Usually, after the one-week "cleansing" period, the patient will develop an increased sensitivity to offending foods.

Reintroduction of allergenic foods will typically produce a more severe or recognizable symptom than before. A careful, detailed record must be maintained, describing when foods were reintroduced and what symptoms appeared upon reintroduction.[18] It can be very useful to track the wrist pulse during reintroduction, as pulse changes may occur when an allergenic food is consumed.[19]

For many people, elimination diets offer the most viable means of detection. Because one sometimes dramatically experiences the effects of food reactions, motivation to eliminate the food can become high. The downside of this procedure is that it is time-consuming and requires discipline and motivation.

A refinement that often yields better results than the simple elimination diet is the five-day water fast with subsequent food challenge. Proponents of this approach believe that it is necessary for the patient to fast for at least five days in order to "clear" the body of allergic responses.[20] During the fast, "withdrawal" symptoms will probably be experienced. These symptoms usually subside by the fourth day. As with the elimination diet, symptoms caused by food allergy will diminish or be eliminated after the fourth day.

After the five-day fast, individual foods are singly reintroduced, with the monitoring of symptoms and pulse. Due to the person's hyperreactive state as a result of giving the immune system a bit of a rest, symptoms tend to be more acute and pronounced than before the fast. This method can produce dramatic results, greatly motivating avoidance of the offending foods.

This method is only advisable for people who are physically and mentally capable of a five-day water fast. Close monitoring by a physician with experience in fasting is highly recommended. At times, careful interpretation of results is needed, due to the occurrence of delayed reactions.

Laboratory Methods

There are two popular types of laboratory test used to diagnose food allergies: the skin-prick test, and blood tests that measure the levels of antibodies relative to food antigens.

The Skin-Prick Test

The skin-prick test or skin-scratch test commonly employed by many allergists only tests for IgE-mediated allergies. Since only about ten to fifteen percent of all food allergies are mediated by IgE, this test is of little value in diagnosing most food allergies. Nevertheless, skin tests are often performed and can provide good information if the food allergy is mediated by IgE.

In this type of test, food extracts are placed on the patient's skin using a scratch or prick method. If the patient is allergic to the food, a welt will form immediately as the allergen reacts with IgE-sensitized cells in the patient's skin.

Blood Tests

Most nutritionally oriented physicians now employ blood tests to diagnose food allergies. Despite a tremendous amount of scientific support, for some reason the diagnosis of food allergy by blood testing is still somewhat controversial in conventional medical settings. These tests are convenient, but they can range in cost from a modest $130 to an extravagant $1,200. A variety of blood tests is available to physicians, with the ELISA (enzyme-linked immunosorbent assay) test appearing to be the best and most popular laboratory method currently available (and most reasonably priced). This test can measure IgE, IgG, IgG4 and IgA antibodies, therefore identifying both the immediate and delayed allergic reactions.

One of the key advantages of the ELISA over other laboratory methods is its ability to measure IgG4 antibodies. This subclass of antibody was initially thought to act as a blocking antibody, thereby exerting protective effects against allergy. However, it now appears that IgG4 antibodies are actually involved in producing allergic symptoms.[21] For example, in a study in asthmatics it was demonstrated that asthma in these patients could be produced in response to inhaled antigens that did not bind to IgE antibodies, but did bind to IgG4.[22] These results suggested that IgG4 antibodies play a major role in atopic disease. In short, IgG4 has been shown to act as an allergic antibody, especially to food antigens.[23]

In regard to food allergy testing, it has been shown that the combination of specific IgE and specific IgG4 provides the best answers, especially when compared to skin testing.[24]

Therapeutic Considerations

The simplest and most effective method of treating food allergies is through avoidance of allergenic foods. Elimination of offending antigens from the diet will begin to alleviate associated symptoms after the body has cleared itself of the antigen/antibody complexes and after the intestinal tract has eliminated any remaining food (usually three to five days). Avoidance means not only avoiding the food in its most identifiable state (e.g., eggs in an omelet), but also in its hidden state (e.g., eggs in bread). For severe reactions, closely related foods with similar antigenic components may also need to be eliminated (e.g., rice and millet in patients with severe wheat allergy).

Avoiding allergenic foods may not be simple or practical, for several reasons:

- Common allergenic foods, such as wheat, corn, and soy, are found as components of many processed foods
- When eating away from home, it is often difficult to determine what ingredients are used in purchased foods and prepared meals
- There may have been a dramatic increase in the number of foods to which a given individual is allergic

The latter condition represents a syndrome that may indicate a broad immune-system dysfunction. It may be difficult (psychologically, socially, and nutritionally) to eliminate a large number of common foods from a person's diet.

Rotary Diversified Diet

Many experts believe that the key to dietary control of food allergies is the "Rotary Diversified Diet." The diet was first developed by Dr. Herbert J. Rinkel in 1934.[25] The diet consists of a highly varied selection of foods that are eaten in a definite rotation, in order to prevent the formation of new allergies and to control preexisting ones.

Tolerated foods are eaten at regularly spaced intervals of four to seven days. For example, a person who has wheat on Monday will have to wait until Friday to have anything with wheat in it again. This approach is based on the principle that infrequent consumption of tolerated foods is not likely to induce new allergies or increase any mild allergies, even in highly sensitized and immune-compromised individuals. As tolerance for eliminated foods returns, they may be added back into the rotation schedule without reactivating the allergy (this, of course, applies only to cyclic food allergies; fixed allergenic foods may never be eaten again).

It is not simply a matter of rotating tolerated foods; food families must also be rotated. Foods, whether animal or vegetable, come in families. The reason it is important to rotate food families is that foods in one family can "cross-react" with allergenic foods. In other words, if a person is allergic to wheat they produce antibodies that can react with other grains in the wheat family. Overconsumption or too frequent consumption of foods from the same family can lead to allergies. Food families need not be as strictly rotated as individual foods. It is usually recommended to avoid eating members of the same food family two days in a row in people prone to food allergies.

Table 2 lists family classifications for edible plants and animals, while a simplified four-day rotation diet plan is provided in Table 3.

TABLE 2   Edible Plant and Animal Kingdom Taxonomic List

VEGETABLES

Legumes	Mustard	Parsley	Potato	Grass	Lily
Beans	Broccoli	Anise	Chili	Barley	Asparagus
Cocoa bean	Brussels sprout	Caraway	Eggplant	Corn	Chives
Lentil	Cabbage	Carrot	Peppers	Oat	Garlic
Licorice	Cauliflower	Celery	Potatoes	Rice	Leek
Peanut	Mustard	Coriander	Tomato	Rye	Onions
Peas	Radish	Cumin	Tobacco	Wheat	
Soybean	Turnip	Parsley			
Tamarind	Watercress				

Laurel	Sunflower	Beet	Buckwheat
Avocado	Artichoke	Beet	Buckwheat
Camphor	Lettuce	Chard	Rhubarb
Cinnamon	Sunflower	Spinach	

FRUITS

Gourds	Plums	Citrus	Cashew	Nuts	Beech
Cantaloupe	Almond	Grapefruit	Cashew	Brazil nut	Beechnut
Cucumber	Apricot	Lemon	Mango	Pecan	Chestnut
Honeydew	Cherry	Lime	Pistachio	Walnut	Chinquapin nut
Melons	Peach	Mandarin			
Pumpkin	Plum	Orange			
Squash	Persimmon	Tangerine			
Zucchini					

Banana	Palm	Grape	Pineapple	Rose	Birch
Arrowroot	Coconut	Grape	Pineapple	Blackberry	Filberts
Banana	Date	Raisin		Loganberry	Hazelnuts
Plantain	Date sugar			Raspberry	
				Rosehips	
				Strawberry	

Apple	Blueberry	Pawpaws
Apple	Blueberry	Papaya
Pear	Cranberry	Pawpaw
Quince	Huckleberry	

(continues)

TABLE 2   Edible Plant and Animal Kingdom Taxonomic List, *continued*

ANIMALS

Mammals (Meat/Milk)	Birds (Meat/Egg)	Fish		Crustaceans	Mollusks
Cow	Chicken	Catfish	Salmon	Crab	Abalone
Goat	Duck	Cod	Sardine	Crayfish	Clams
Pig	Goose	Flounder	Snapper	Lobster	Mussels
Rabbit	Hen	Halibut	Trout	Prawn	Oysters
Sheep	Turkey	Mackerel	Tuna	Shrimp	Scallops

TABLE 3   Four-day Rotation Diet

FOOD FAMILY	FOOD
Day 1	
Citrus	Lemon, orange, grapefruit, lime, tangerine, kumquat, citron
Banana	Banana, plantain, arrowroot (musa)
Palm	Coconut, date, date sugar
Parsley	Carrots, parsnips, celery, celery seed, celeriac, anise, dill, fennel, cumin, parsley, coriander, caraway
Spices	Black and white pepper, peppercorn, nutmeg, mace
Subucaya	Brazil nut
Bird	All fowl and game birds, including chicken, turkey, duck, goose, guinea, pigeon, quail, pheasant, eggs
Juices	Juices (preferably fresh) may be made and used from any fruits and vegetables listed above, in any combination desired, without adding sweeteners.
Day 2	
Grape	All varieties of grapes, raisins
Pineapple	Juice-pack, water-pack, or fresh
Rose	Strawberry, raspberry, blackberry, loganberry, rose hips
Gourd	Watermelon, cucumber, cantaloupe, pumpkin, squash, other melons, zucchini, pumpkin or squash seeds
Beet	Beet, spinach, chard
Legume	Pea, black-eyed pea, dry beans, green beans, carob, soybeans, lentils, licorice, peanut, alfalfa
Cashew	Cashew, pistachio, mango
Birch	Filberts, hazelnuts
Flaxseed	Flaxseed
Swine	All pork products
Mollusks	Abalone, snail, squid, clam, mussel, oyster, scallop
Crustaceans	Crab, crayfish, lobster, prawn, shrimp

(continues)

TABLE 3   Four-day Rotation Diet, *continued*

FOOD FAMILY	FOOD
Day 2, continued	
Juices	Juices (preferably fresh) may be made and used without added sweeteners from any fruits, berries, or vegetables listed above, in any combination desired, including fresh alfalfa and some legumes.
Day 3	
Apple	Apple, pear, quince
Gooseberry	Currant, gooseberry
Buckwheat	Buckwheat, rhubarb
Aster	Lettuce, chicory, endive, escarole, globe artichoke, dandelion, sunflower seeds, tarragon
Potato	Potato, tomato, eggplant, peppers (red and green), chili pepper, paprika, cayenne, ground cherries
Lily (onion)	Onion, garlic, asparagus, chives, leeks
Spurge	Tapioca
Herb	Basil, savory, sage, oregano, horehound, catnip, spearmint, peppermint, thyme, marjoram, lemon balm
Walnut	English walnut, black walnut, pecan, hickory nut, butternut
Pedalium	Sesame
Beech	Chestnut
Saltwater fish	Herring, anchovy, cod, sea bass, sea trout, mackerel, tuna, swordfish, flounder, sole
Freshwater fish	Sturgeon, salmon, whitefish, bass, perch
Juices	Juices (preferably fresh) may be made and used without added sweeteners from any fruits and vegetables listed above, in any combination desired.
Day 4	
Plum	Plum, cherry, peach, apricot, nectarine, almond, wild cherry
Blueberry	Blueberry, huckleberry, cranberry, wintergreen
Pawpaws	Pawpaw, papaya, papain
Mustard	Mustard, turnip, radish, horseradish, watercress, cabbage, Chinese cabbage, broccoli, cauliflower, brussels sprouts, kale, kohlrabi, rutabaga
Laurel	Avocado, cinnamon, bay leaf, sassafras, cassia buds or bark
Sweet potato or yam	
Grass	Wheat, corn, rice, oats, barley, rye, wild rice, cane, millet, sorghum, bamboo sprouts
Orchid	Vanilla
Protea	Macadamia nut
Conifer	Pine nut
Fungus	Mushrooms and yeast (brewer's yeast, etc.)
Bovid	Milk products—butter, cheese, yogurt, beef and milk products, oleomargarine, lamb
Juices	Juices (preferably fresh) may be made and used without added sweeteners from any fruits and vegetables listed above, in any combination desired.

TREATMENT SUMMARY

While there is no known simple "cure" for food allergies, there are a number of measures that will help avoid and lessen symptoms and correct the underlying causes. First, all allergenic foods should be identified using one of the methods discussed in this chapter. After identifying allergenic foods, the best approach is clearly avoidance of all major allergens, and rotation of all other foods for at least the first few months. As one improves, the dietary restrictions can be relaxed, although some individuals may require a rotation diet indefinitely. For strongly allergenic foods, all members of the food family should be avoided.

Gallstones

May be without symptoms or may be associated with periods of intense pain in the abdomen that radiates to the upper back

Ultrasound provides definitive diagnosis

In the United States, autopsy studies have shown that gallstones exist in approximately twenty percent of the women and eight percent of the men over age forty. Although gallstones may exist without symptoms, more than 300,000 gallbladders are removed each year in the United States due to the presence of gallstones.[1-4]

Gallstones arise when there is an imbalance among the *bile* components. Bile is composed of: bile salts; bilirubin; cholesterol, phospholipids, and fatty acids; water; electrolytes; and other substances.[5] Bile is an extremely important substance produced by the liver, stored in the gallbladder, and secreted into the small intestine to aid in the absorption of fats, oils, and fat-soluble vitamins. Table 1 shows the characteristics of the major bile components.

Gallstones can be divided into four major categories based on their composition:

1. Pure cholesterol
2. Pure pigment (calcium bilirubinate)
3. Mixed, containing cholesterol and its derivatives along with varying amounts of bile salts, bile pigments, and inorganic salts of calcium
4. Entirely of minerals

Pure stones, either cholesterol or calcium bilirubinate, are extremely rare in the United States, but are found in other parts of the world (e.g., Asia). Recent studies indicate that, in the United States, approximately eighty percent of the stones are of the mixed variety. The remaining twenty percent of the stones are composed entirely of minerals, principally calcium salts, although some stones contain oxides of silicon and aluminum.[1-3]

Causes of Gallstones

The formation of gallstones has been divided into three steps:

1. Bile supersaturation
2. Nucleation and initiation of stone formation
3. Enlargement of the gallstone by accretion

The required step in cholesterol and mixed stone formation is elevations of cholesterol within the gallbladder. The solubility of bile is based on the relative concentrations of cholesterol, bile acids, *phosphatidylcholine* (lecithin) and water. Since free cholesterol is water-insoluble, it must be incorporated into a lecithin-bile salt mixture. Either an increase in cholesterol secretion or a decrease in bile acid or lecithin secretion will result in the bile becoming supersaturated with cholesterol. Once the bile is supersaturated with cholesterol, it sets the stage for any particulate matter to begin attracting the cholesterol and initiate stone formation. Once the stone begins to form, its radius increases at an average rate of 2.6 mm/year, eventually reaching a size of a few millimeters to over a centimeter.

TABLE 1	Characteristics of the Major Bile Components[5]		
COMPONENT	**% OF BILE**	**WATER SOLUBILITY**	**PHYSIOCHEMICAL PROPERTIES**
Cholesterol	5	Very poor	Will precipitate from aqueous solutions
Bile salts	65–90	Soluble; have polar and nonpolar regions	Capable of solubilizing cholesterol and phospholipids in aqueous phase
Phospholipids	2–25	Poor	Fits between bile salt molecules, thus increasing their capacity to solubilize cholesterol

Symptoms occur an average of eight years after formation begins. Gallstones are present in ninety-five percent of patients who have inflammation of the gallbladder (*cholecystitis*).[5]

Risk Factors for Cholesterol and Mixed Stones

The major risk factors for the development of cholesterol and mixed gallstones include diet, sex, race, obesity, high caloric intake, estrogens, gastrointestinal diseases (especially Crohn's disease and cystic fibrosis), drugs, and age.[1–3] The role of a low-fiber, high-fat diet in the development of gallstones, as well as other dietary factors, is discussed under Therapeutic Considerations, while the other factors are briefly discussed here.

Sex The frequency of gallstones is two to four times greater in women than in men. Women are thought to be predisposed to gallstones because of either increased cholesterol synthesis or suppression of bile acids by estrogens. Pregnancy, use of oral contraceptives, or other causes of elevated estrogen levels greatly increase the incidence of gallstones.

Race Gallstone occurrence appears to have some genetic aspects. Gallstones are most common in Native American women over the age of thirty; nearly seventy percent of this group has gallstones. In contrast, only ten percent of black women over thirty have gallstones. The difference in the rates among different ethnic and genetic groups reflects the extent of cholesterol saturation of the bile. However, dietary factors probably outweigh genetic factors.[6]

Obesity Obesity causes an increased secretion of cholesterol in the bile as a result of increased cholesterol synthesis. Therefore, obesity is associated with a significant increased risk for gallstones. However, it is extremely important to recognize that during active weight reduction, the concentration of cholesterol in the bile initially increases.[3] The secretion of all bile components is reduced during weight loss, but the secretion of bile acids decreases more than that of cholesterol. Since one of the functions of bile acids is to keep cholesterol in solution, this scenario greatly increases the risk of gallstone formation or accelerated growth. Once the weight is stabilized, bile acid output returns to normal levels while the cholesterol output remains low. The net effect is a significant improvement in bile solubility with weight loss. We recommend following the guidelines in this chapter for gallstones to anyone on a weight loss program where they are losing more than one pound per week.

Gastrointestinal Tract Diseases Normally, about ninety-eight percent of the bile acids that are secreted during digestion are reabsorbed in the terminal portion of the small intestine (the *ileum*). Impaired reabsorption of bile acids reduces the bile acid pool and the rate of secretion of bile. As a result, the risk for gallstones is greatly increased. Diseases associated with this phenomenon include Crohn's disease and cystic fibrosis.

Drugs In addition to oral contraceptives and other estrogens, some cholesterol-lowering drugs increase the risk of gall-stones. Especially incriminating are the fibric acid derivatives, such as clofibrate and gemfibrozil. These drugs lower blood cholesterol levels but greatly increase the level of cholesterol in the bile.

Age Gallstones have been reported from fetus to extreme old age, but the average patient is forty to fifty years old. The frequency of gallstone occurrence increases with age.

Risk Factors for Pigmented Gallstones

Risk factors for pigmented gallstones are not related to diet as much as they are to geography, sun exposure, and severe diseases. Pigmented gallstones are more common in Asia due to the higher frequency of parasitic infection of the liver and gallbladder by a vari-

QUICK REVIEW

- Gallstones can be prevented through diet and lifestyle measures.
- Fasting or severe calorie restriction can lead to gallstone formation.
- A 1968 study revealed that 100 percent of a group of patients were free from symptoms while they were on a basic elimination diet.
- Coffee can aggravate symptoms of gallstones by causing the gallbladder to contract.
- A low lecithin concentration in the bile may be a causative factor for many individuals with gallstones.
- Vitamin C supplementation (2,000 mg per day) has been shown to produce positive effects on bile composition and reduces cholesterol stone formation.
- Milk thistle extract may help dissolve gallstones via its ability to increase the solubility of the bile.
- A complex of plant terpenes alone or, preferably, in combination with oral bile acids can help dissolve gallstones.

ety of organisms, including the liver fluke (*Clonorchis sinensis*). In the United States, pigmented stones are usually caused by chronic destruction of red blood cells (*hemolysis*) or alcoholic cirrhosis of the liver.

Therapeutic Considerations

Gallstones are easier to prevent than to reverse. Primary treatment, therefore, involves reducing the controllable risk factors discussed above. Once gallstones have formed, therapeutic intervention involves avoiding aggravating foods and employing measures that increase the solubility of cholesterol in bile. If symptoms persist or worsen, surgical removal of the gallbladder should be considered.

A number of dietary factors are important in the prevention and treatment of gallstones. Foremost is the elimination of foods that can produce symptoms. Also important are increasing dietary fiber, eliminating food allergies, and reducing the intake of animal protein.

Other treatment measures involve the use of nutritional lipotropic compounds (described in Lipotropic Factors and Botanical Choleretics, later in this chapter), herbs that promote improved bile flow (*choleretics*), and other natural compounds, in an attempt to increase the solubility of bile.

It must be noted that the level of cholesterol in the bile does not correlate with the total cholesterol levels in the blood.[7] Although some authors have reported that higher levels of HDL cholesterol improve the solubility of the bile, and that a higher LDL cholesterol level reduces the solubility of cholesterol in the bile,[8,9] more detailed research does not appear to support these correlations.[7] There does, however, seem to be an association between increased serum triglyceride levels and less soluble bile.[10]

Silent Gallstones

Elective gallbladder surgery is not warranted in most cases of "silent" (symptom-free) gallstones. While there is a cumulative chance of developing symptoms—ten percent at five years, fifteen percent at ten years, and eighteen percent at fifteen years—if controllable risk factors are eliminated or reduced, a person with a silent gallstone should never experience discomfort.[2]

Diet

Dietary Fiber

Considerable research supports the hypothesis that the main cause of gallstones is the consumption of fiber-depleted refined foods.[3,4] In population studies, gallstones are definitely associated with the "Western diet." Such a diet, high in refined carbohydrates and fat and low in fiber, leads to a reduction in the synthesis of bile acids by the liver and a lower bile acid concentration in the gallbladder.

Another way in which fiber may prevent gallstone formation is by reducing the absorption of *deoxycholic acid*.[3,4] This compound is produced from bile acids by bacteria in the intestine. Deoxycholic acid greatly lessens the solubility of cholesterol in bile.

Dietary fiber has been shown to both decrease the formation of deoxycholic acid and bind to deoxycholic acid and promote its excretion in the feces. This greatly increases the solubility of cholesterol in the bile. A diet high in fiber is extremely important in the prevention as well as the reversal of most gallstones. Especially important are those fibers capable of binding to deoxycholic acid, predominantly the water-soluble fibers found in vegetables, fruits, pectin, oat bran, and guar gum.[4]

Interestingly, diets rich in legumes (beans) with high concentrations of water-soluble fibers are associated with an increased risk for gallstones.[6] Chileans, Pima Indians, and other North American Indians have the highest prevalence rates for cholesterol gallstones. All consume a diet rich in legumes. Evidently, legume intake increases biliary cholesterol saturation as a result of their high content of compounds known as *saponins*.[6] It is therefore recommended that legume intake be restricted in individuals with gallstones.

Vegetarian Diet

A vegetarian diet has been shown to be protective against gallstone formation.[4,11] A recent study in England compared a large group of healthy nonvegetarian women to a group of vegetarian women. Ultrasound diagnosis showed that gallstones occurred significantly less frequently in the vegetarian group.

While this may simply be a result of the increased fiber content of the vegetarian diet, other factors may be equally important. Animal proteins, such as casein from dairy products, have been shown to increase the formation of gallstones in animals while vegetable proteins, such as soy, were shown to be preventive against gallstone formation.[3,4,12]

Food Allergies

Since 1948, Dr. J.C. Breneman, author of *Basics of Food Allergy*, has used a successful therapeutic regime to prevent gallbladder attacks: allergy elimination diets. There is some support in the scientific literature for the theory that food allergies cause gallbladder pain.[13–16] A 1968 study revealed that 100 percent of a group of patients were free from symptoms while they were on a basic elimination diet (consisting of beef, rye, soybean, rice, cherry, peach, apricot, beet, and spinach).[13]

Foods that induced symptoms of gallstones, in decreasing order of their occurrence, were egg, pork, onion, fowl, milk, coffee, citrus, corn, beans, and nuts. Adding eggs to the diet caused gallbladder attacks in ninety-three percent of the patients!

Several mechanisms have been proposed to explain the association of food allergies with gallbladder attacks. Dr. Breneman believes that the ingestion of allergenic substances causes swelling of the bile ducts, resulting in impairment of bile flow from the gallbladder.

Sugar

A high intake of refined sugar may be a risk factor for gallstones as well as biliary tract cancer, based on the relationship between sugars, blood lipids, and gallstone formation.[17] A twenty-five-year follow-up study of 860 men, fifty-four of whom developed symptomatic gallstones, found a positive association between sugar consumption and gallstones.[18]

Caloric Restriction

People with gallstones tend to consume more calories, primarily as a result of an increased intake of refined carbohydrates (sugar) in women and fat in men.[19] Obviously, reducing the intake of these dietary factors is important.

However, as mentioned earlier, rapid weight loss[20] and fasting[21] increase the risk of gallstones. For example, in 179 obese patients, nine percent of whom had preexisting gallstones, a very low-calorie diet (605 calories per day) resulted in eleven percent of the patients developing gallstones either during or within six months of completing the diet.[20] Another study, of a 925-calorie-per-day diet, found that 12.8 percent of the forty-seven women patients displayed gallstones at week seventeen, as determined by ultrasound. Those who developed gallstones had significantly higher initial triglyceride and total cholesterol levels compared to those who didn't. They also had a significantly greater rate of weight loss.[22] The key point is that if a person is going to follow a very low calorie diet and lose more than one pound per week for an extended period of time (e.g., more than two months), and if they have elevated cholesterol and/or triglycerides, they had better follow the recommendations given here for increasing the solubility of the bile to help prevent gallstone formation.

Coffee

Coffee induces gallbladder contractions, so if you have gallstones, you would do best to avoid coffee until the stones are resolved. It doesn't matter if the coffee is decaffeinated, either. Both regular and decaffeinated coffee caused significant gallbladder contractions in six healthy regular coffee drinkers.[23]

Nutritional Factors

Lecithin (phosphatidylcholine) A low lecithin concentration in the bile may be a causative factor for many individuals with gallstones. For example, it takes fifty molecules of a pure bile salt *micelle* (fat droplet) to enclose a single molecule of cholesterol, while only seven mixed bile salt/phospholipid micelles are required.[5]

Studies have shown that taking as little as 100 mg of lecithin three times per day will increase the concentration of lecithin in the bile, while larger doses (up to 10 grams of lecithin) produce even greater increases.[24,25] This is significant, as an increased lecithin content of bile usually increases the solubility of cholesterol. However, no significant effects on dissolving gallstones have been obtained using lecithin supplementation alone.

Nutrient Deficiencies

Deficiencies of either vitamins E or C have been shown to cause gallstones in experimental studies in animals.[26,27] Vitamin C supplementation (2,000 mg per day) has been shown to produce positive effects on bile composition and to reduce cholesterol stone formation.[27]

Olive Oil

A popular lay remedy for gallstones is the so-called olive oil "liver flush." There are several variations. A typical one involves drinking 1 cup of unrefined olive oil with the juice of two lemons in the morning for several days. Many people tell tales of passing huge stones while on the liver flush. However, what they think are gallstones are simply a soft saponified complex of minerals, olive oil, and lemon juice produced within the gastrointestinal tract.

The olive oil liver flush is probably undesirable for patients with gallstones for several reasons. First, consuming a large quantity of any oil will result in contraction of the gallbladder, which may increase the likelihood of a stone blocking the bile duct. This may result in cholecystitis, requiring immediate surgery to prevent death. Second, *oleic acid,* the main component of olive oil, has been shown to increase the development of gallstones in rabbits and rats by increasing the content of cholesterol in the gallbladder.[28,29] Although this effect has not yet been observed in humans, the animal research suggests that it is unwise to use an olive oil liver flush as a treatment for gallbladder disease.[30] This does not mean that the liver flush is invalid as a method of liver detoxification. However, it is not recommended for individuals with gallstones.

Fish Oils

Although human studies appear to be unavailable at this time, some provocative animal studies exist showing that fish-oil supplementation may be of benefit. For example, one study compared a diet high in lard to a diet high in fish oils in twenty-one male African green monkeys. One group was fed 0.8 mg of cholesterol/kcal and forty-two percent of their calories as fat, with half of the fat calories derived from lard. The other group was fed a similar diet, with fish oil substituted for the lard. After two to three years, biopsies were performed and it was found that sixty-seven percent of the animals fed the lard diet had cholesterol gallstones, compared to twenty-two percent of the animals fed the fish oil. There was significantly more lecithin in the bile in the fish-oil-fed animals compared to the lard-fed animals.[31]

A more recent study found similar effects in prairie dogs using a diet more similar to the human diet. Twelve animals consumed a standard control diet while sixteen consumed a 1.2-percent cholesterol diet. One-half of the animals in each group were supplemented with 200 mg/kg per day of fish oils. After fourteen days, those fed the diet with added fish oil showed an inhibition of gallstone formation, accompanied by significant decrease in the calcium and total protein concentration of the bile. This protective effect against gallstones may be due to an enhancement in the stability of biliary phospholipid-cholesterol vesicles.[32]

Lipotropic Factors and Botanical Choleretics

The naturopathic approach to the treatment of gallstones has typically involved the use of *lipotropic* and *choleretic* formulas (see also DETOXIFICATION). Lipotropic factors are, by definition, substances that hasten the removal or decrease the deposit of fat in the liver.

Compounds commonly employed as lipotropic agents include choline, methionine, betaine, folic acid, and vitamin B12.

These nutritional factors are often used with herbal *cholagogues* and *choleretics*. Cholagogues stimulate gallbladder contraction to promote bile flow, while choleretics increase bile secretion by the liver.

Many of the herbal choleretics have a favorable effect on the solubility of bile. Choleretics that are appropriate to use in the treatment of gallstones include extracts of milk thistle (*Silybum marianum*), dandelion (*Taraxacum officinale*), artichoke (*Cynara scolymus*), turmeric (*Curcuma longa*), and boldo (*Peumus boldo*). Of these herbal choleretics, milk thistle extract may offer the greatest benefit.

According to the results of a recent study, milk thistle extract may dissolve gallstones via its ability to increase the solubility of the bile. In the study, the composition of the bile was assayed in nineteen patients with a history of gallstones (four participants) or removal of the gallbladder due to gallstones (fifteen participants) before and after taking milk thistle extract (420 mg of an extract standardized to contain seventy percent silymarin) or a placebo. Patients treated with milk thistle extract experienced significant reductions in the bile cholesterol concentration.

Chemical Dissolution of Gallstones

Several successful nonsurgical alternatives for the treatment of gallstones now exist. These entail using a complex of plant terpenes alone or, preferably, in combination with oral bile acids. As the formation of the stone is dependent on either increased accumulation of cholesterol or reduced levels of bile acids or lecithin, decreasing gallbladder cholesterol levels and/or increasing bile acid or lecithin levels should result in dissolution of the stone. Chemical dissolution of gallstones is especially indicated in the treatment of gallstones in the elderly, who cannot withstand the stress of surgery, and in other cases in which surgery is contraindicated.

Bile Acids

The two primary bile acids used in the treatment of gallstones are chenodeoxycholic acid and ursodeoxycholic acid. Both have shown excellent results. Promoting increased cholesterol solubility through oral *chenodeoxycholic acid* therapy alone (750 mg/d) has resulted in complete dissolution of gallstones in 13.5 percent of patients, and partial dissolution in 27 percent.[33] However, this therapy often takes several years and is associated with mild diarrhea and possible liver damage. *Ursodeoxycholic acid,* alone or in combination with chenodeoxycholic acid, appears to be somewhat more effective and has fewer side effects.[34,35]

Terpenes

Gallstone dissolution by a natural terpene combination (menthol, menthone, pinene, borneol, cineole, and camphene) has been demonstrated in several studies.[36–39] This approach to gallstone removal offers an effective alternative to surgery and has been demonstrated to be safe even when the combination has been consumed for up to four years. The natural terpene combination (Rowachol) is not available in the United States at this time. However, menthol is the major component of this formula; enteric-coated peppermint oil (which is available in the U.S. marketplace) may offer similar benefits.

Combined Therapy

Although terpenes are effective alone, the best results appear to be achieved when plant terpene complexes are used in combination with bile acid therapy.[39–42] This combined approach offers better results than either bile acids or plant terpenes used alone.[40–42] Furthermore, since a lower dose of bile acid can be used, there is a significant reduction in the risk of complications or side effects, as well as in the cost of bile acid therapy.

Lifestyle

Sunbathing

Because almost all cholesterol gallstones contain a central, pigmented nucleus with pigmented bands alternating with layers of crystalline cholesterol, one researcher speculated that the activation of the pigmentary system by sunlight might lead to gallstones. In a study of 206 white-skinned individuals, people who liked to sunbathe had twice the risk of getting gallstones as those who did not like to sunbathe. Furthermore, the association was almost entirely restricted to those who always burn after long sunbathing. In this group, the risk was a remarkable 25.6 times greater compared to people who do not like to lie in the sun.[43]

TREATMENT SUMMARY

As is typical of most diseases, gallstones are much easier to prevent than to reverse. The risk factors and causes of gallstones are well known and, in most cases, a healthy diet rich in dietary fiber will be adequate prevention.

Once gallstones have developed, measures to avoid gallbladder attacks and increase the solubility of the bile are necessary. To limit the incidence of symptoms, allergenic foods must be determined (see FOOD ALLERGIES) and, along with fatty foods, avoided. The solubility of the bile can be increased by following the dietary guidelines and utilizing the nutritional and herbal supplements recommended below.

Diet

Increase intake of vegetables, fruits, and dietary fiber, especially the gel-forming or mucilaginous fibers (flaxseed, oat bran, guar gum, pectin, etc.). Reduce consumption of saturated fats, cholesterol, sugar, and animal proteins. Avoid all fried foods.

Water

Drink six to eight glasses of water each day to maintain the water content of bile.

Nutritional Supplements

- Vitamin C: 500 to 1,000 mg three times daily
- Vitamin E: 200–400 IU per day
- Phosphatidylcholine (lecithin): 100 mg three times per day
- Choline: 1,000 mg per day
- L-Methionine: 1,000 mg per day
- Fiber supplement (guar gum, pectin, psyllium, or oat bran): minimum of 5 g per day
- Bile acids (combination of ursodeoxycholic and chenodeoxycholic acid): 1,000–1,500 mg per day

Botanical Medicines

Dosages are three times per day. Choose one. They are listed in order of effectiveness.

- Gallstone-dissolving formula (dosage: one to three times per day, best if used in combination with ursodeoxycholic acid)
  Menthol: 30 mg
  Menthone: 5 mg
  Pinene: 15 mg
  Borneol: 5 mg
  Camphene: 5 mg
  Cineole: 2 mg
  Citral: 5 mg

  Note: Peppermint oil in an enteric-coated capsule can be used instead of the gallstone-dissolving formula, at a dosage of 1–2 capsules (0.2 ml/capsule) three times per day between meals.

- *Silybum marianum*
  The dosage is based upon the level of silymarin: 70–210 mg of silymarin

- *Cynara scolymus*
  Extract (15% cynarin): 500 mg

- *Peumus boldo*
  Dried leaves (or by infusion): 250–500 mg
  Tincture (1:10): 2–4 ml
  Fluid extract (1:1): 0.5–1.0 ml

- *Curcuma longa*
  Curcumin: 100–200 mg three times per day

- Dandelion (*Taraxicum officinale*)
  Dried root: 4 g
  Fluid extract (1:1): 4–8 ml
  Solid extract (4:1): 250–500 mg

Glaucoma

. . . .

ACUTE GLAUCOMA

Increased pressure within the eye (intraocular), usually on one side only

Severe throbbing pain in eye with markedly blurred vision

Pupil moderately dilated and fixed

Nausea and vomiting is common

CHRONIC GLAUCOMA

Persistent elevation of the pressure within the eye (increased intraocular pressure)

Usually no symptoms are apparent in the early stages

Gradual loss of peripheral vision resulting in tunnel vision

laucoma refers to increased pressure within the eye *(intraocular),* which results from greater production than outflow of the fluid of the eye (the aqueous humor). The normal intraocular pressure is about 10 to 21 mm Hg. In chronic glaucoma, the intraocular pressure is usually mildly to moderately elevated (22 to 40 mm Hg). In acute glaucoma, the intraocular pressure is greater than 40 mm Hg.

In the United States, there are approximately two million people with glaucoma, twenty-five percent of which is undetected.[1] Ninety percent is of the chronic type. Nearly two percent of people over the age of forty have glaucoma, and by age seventy over ten percent have glaucoma. Glaucoma is a major cause of blindness in adults.

The cause of glaucoma appears to be an abnormality in the composition of the supportive structures of the eye. Specifically, biopsy samples indicate that there is a strong correlation between the content and composition of *collagen* and that of the glaucomatous eye.[2] Collagen is the most abundant protein in the body, including the eye. In the eye, it provides support and integrity to all eye structures. Inborn errors of collagen metabolism (e.g., osteogenesis imperfecta, Ehlers-Danlos syndrome, Marfan's syndrome) are often associated with eye disorders such as glaucoma and retinal detachment.[3] Structural changes reflecting poor collagen integrity and function are the hallmark features of glaucoma.[2,4–6] These changes lead to blockage in the flow of the aqeous humour and result in elevated intraocular pressure (IOP) readings and can lead to the progression of peripheral vision loss.

Since patients with glaucoma sometimes have no symptoms, it is important that regular eye exams be included in their annual checkup after the age of sixty. Glaucoma is a serious condition that requires strict attention.

Therapeutic Considerations

Treatment and prevention of both acute and chronic glaucoma is dependent upon:

1. Reduction of IOP
2. Improvement of collagen metabolism within the eye

The role of collagen destruction as a cause of glaucoma is apparent in patients who use corticosteroid drugs such as prednisone.[1,2] These drugs are used in severe allergic and inflammatory conditions. The drugs weaken collagen structures throughout the body including the eye. Use of corticosteroid drugs are a major risk for glaucoma. The individual with glaucoma should do everything possible to avoid corticosteroid drugs.

Vitamin C

Optimal tissue concentrations of vitamin C are central to achieving collagen integrity. Furthermore, vitamin C has been demonstrated to lower IOP levels in many clinical studies.[7-11] For example, in one study a daily dose of 0.5 grams of vitamin C per kilogram (2.2 pounds) of body weight, whether in single or divided doses, reduced the IOP in patients with glaucoma by an average of 16 mm Hg.[11] Using vitamin C, significant improvements have been achieved in some patients who were unresponsive to common glaucoma drugs.[11]

The ability of vitamin C to reduce the IOP lasts only as long as supplementation is continued. Although vitamin C therapy is effective orally, intravenous administration results in an even greater reduction in IOP.[7,9-11] Patient monitoring is required to determine the appropriate individual dose, as some patients respond to as little as 2 grams per day, while others will respond only to extremely high doses (35 grams per day).[7-11] Abdominal discomfort is common when using high doses, but usually tapers off after three to four days.[11]

Bioflavonoids

Bioflavonoid supplementation, particularly with *anthocyanosides* (the blue-red pigments found in berries), further aids normal collagen metabolism. These compounds enhance the effects of vitamin C, improve capillary integrity, and stabilize the collagen matrix by preventing free-radical damage, inhibiting enzymatic cleavage of the collagen matrix, and cross-linking with collagen fibers directly to form a more stable collagen matrix.[12,13,14] European bilberry (*Vaccinium myrtillus*) extract is particularly rich in these flavonoid and anthocyanidin compounds. It has been used in Europe with good results in a variety of eye complaints, and may prove useful in

QUICK REVIEW

- Glaucoma is a major cause of blindness in adults.
- Treatment and prevention of both acute and chronic glaucoma is dependent upon: (1) reduction of intraocular pressure, and (2) improvement of collagen metabolism within the eye.
- Magnesium supplementation lowers intraocular pressure.

the treatment of glaucoma.[15] The citrus bioflavonoid *rutin* has also been demonstrated to lower IOP when used as an adjunct in patients who are unresponsive to glaucoma medications alone.[16]

Allergy

Chronic glaucoma has been successfully treated by eliminating allergies.[17] In one study, of the 113 patients exposed to a food or environmental allergen demonstrated an immediate rise in IOP of up to 20 mm, in addition to other typical allergic symptoms. To treat glaucoma by eliminating food allergens, follow the guidelines given in FOOD ALLERGIES.

Magnesium

Magnesium supplementation lowers IOP in a fashion similar to that of "channel blockers," popular drugs used in the treatment of glaucoma that work by blocking the entry of calcium to produce relaxation of the arteries. In fact, magnesium has been referred to as "nature's calcium-channel blocker." In one study, ten glaucoma patients were given magnesium at a dose of 121.5 mg twice daily for one month. After four weeks of treatment, magnesium supplementation had improved the blood supply (apparently due to relaxing constricted blood vessels) and the visual field in the glaucoma patients.[18]

Chromium

A study of four hundred eye patients demonstrated a strong association between glaucoma and a deficiency of chromium and vitamin C. Chromium increases the ability of insulin receptors that help sustain the ability of eye muscles to focus. Deficiencies of either vitamin C or chromium were associated with elevated IOP, which tends to stretch the normal eye, thereby reducing the capacity for focusing power.[19] Diabetics are at greater risk for glaucoma due to the damaging effects that high blood sugar levels have on collagen structures of the eye.

Omega-3 Oils

In an interesting speculative study, feeding rabbits food soaked with cod liver oil resulted in a significant drop in intraocular pressure. Providing normal rabbits with food soaked in cod liver oil produced a drop in IOP from 25 mm Hg to 11 mm Hg. Intramuscular injections of cod liver oil reduced intraocular pressure in proportion to the dosage. When the rabbits were taken off cod liver oil, their intraocular pressure returned to baseline. Control animals given liquid lard or safflower oil experienced no change in intraocular pressure. The omega-3 oils in the cod liver oil may lower IOP via the same mechanisms by which they lower blood pressure (see HIGH BLOOD PRESSURE).

Ginkgo biloba Extract

Like bilberry extracts, the *Ginkgo biloba* extract (GBE), standardized to contain twenty-four percent ginkgo flavonglycosides, also shows promise in the treatment of glaucoma. In one study of forty-six patients with severe glaucoma, *Ginkgo biloba* extract demonstrated some improvements in IOP and visual field at a dosage of 160 mg/day for four weeks, then 120 mg/day thereafter.[21] Although the improvements were mild, given the poor prognosis for these patients with severe glaucoma the results were deemed relevant.

TREATMENT SUMMARY

Acute glaucoma is a medical emergency. If you are showing any signs of glaucoma, consult an ophthalmologist immediately. Typical signs and symptoms include extreme pain, blurring of vision, reddened eyes, and a fixed and dilated pupil.[1] Unless adequately treated within twelve to forty-eight hours, an individual with acute glaucoma will become permanently blind within two to five days.

Diet

A generally healthful diet is recommended, with a focus on foods high in vitamin C and flavonoids, such as fresh fruits and vegetables. In addition, regular consumption of cold-water fish (e.g., salmon, mackerel, herring, and halibut) is also encouraged due to their high content of omega-3 fatty acids.

Nutritional Supplements

- Vitamin C: minimum of 2,000 mg per day in divided doses (effective dosage may be as high as 35 g per day)
- Bioflavonoids (mixed): 1,000 mg per day
- Magnesium: 200 to 600 mg per day
- Chromium: 200 to 400 mcg per day
- Flaxseed oil: One tablespoon daily

Botanical Medicines

- Bilberry (*Vaccinium myrtillus*) extract (25% anthocyanidin content): 80 mg three times per day
- *Gingko biloba* extract (24% ginkgo flavonglycosides): 40 to 80 mg three times daily

Gout

. . . .

Acute onset of intense joint pain, typically involving the first joint of the big toe (about fifty percent of cases)

Elevated serum uric acid level

Periods without symptoms between acute attacks

Identification of urate crystals in joint fluid

Aggregated deposits of urate crystals in and around the joints of the extremities, but also in subcutaneous tissue, bone, cartilage, and other tissues

Uric acid kidney stones

Gout is a common type of arthritis caused by an increased concentration of *uric acid* (the final breakdown product of purine—one of the units of DNA and RNA—metabolism) in biological fluids. In gout, uric acid crystals (*monosodium urate*) are deposited in joints, tendons, kidneys, and other tissues, where they cause considerable inflammation and damage.[1,2] Gout may lead to debilitation from the uric acid deposits around the joints and tendons, and kidney involvement may result in kidney failure.

The first attack of gout is characterized by intense pain, usually involving only one joint. The first joint of the big toe is affected in nearly half of the first attacks, and is at some time involved in over ninety percent of individuals with gout. If the attack progresses, fever and chills will appear. The first attacks usually occur at night and are usually preceded by a specific event, such as dietary excess, alcohol ingestion, trauma, certain drugs (mainly chemotherapy drugs, certain diuretics, and high dosages of niacin), or surgery.

The classic description of gout was written by an English physician, Sydenham, who suf-

fered from it in 1683.[1] Little has changed in the clinical picture of gout in over three hundred years. Sydenham's classic description:

The victim goes to bed and sleeps in good health. About two o'clock in the morning he is awakened by a severe pain in the great toe; more rarely in the heel, ankle, or instep. The pain is like that of a dislocation, and yet parts feel as if cold water were poured over them. Then follows chills and shivers, and a little fever. The pain which at first was moderate, becomes more intense. With its intensity the chills and fever increase. After a time this comes to a height, accommodating itself to the bones and ligaments of the tarsus and metatarsus. Now it is a violent stretching and tearing of the ligaments, now it is a gnawing pain, and now a pressure and tightening. So exquisite and lively meanwhile is the feeling of the part affected, that it cannot bear the weight of bedclothes nor the jar of a person walking in the room. The night is passed in torture, sleeplessness, turning the part affected, and perpetual change of posture; the tossing about of the body being as incessant as the pain of the tortured joint, and being worse as the fit comes on. Hence the vain effort by change of posture, both in the body and the limb affected, to obtain an abatement of pain.

Subsequent attacks are common, with the majority of gout patients having another attack within one year. However, nearly seven percent never have a second attack. Chronic gout is extremely rare these days, due to the advent of dietary therapy and drugs that lower uric acid levels. Some degree of kidney dysfunction occurs in nearly ninety percent of subjects with gout as a result of uric acid deposits, and there is a higher risk of kidney stones.

Causes of Gout

Gout is classified into two major categories: primary and secondary. Primary gout accounts for about ninety percent of all cases, while secondary gout accounts for only ten percent. The cause of primary gout is usually unknown. There are, however, several genetic defects in which the exact cause of the elevated uric acid is known.

The increased serum uric acid level observed in primary gout can be divided into three categories:

1. Increased synthesis of uric acid, found in a majority of gout patients

2. Reduced ability to excrete uric acid, typical of a smaller group (about thirty percent)

3. Overproduction and underexcretion of uric acid, found in a small minority of gout patients

Although the exact metabolic defect is not known in the majority of cases, gout is one of the most controllable metabolic diseases.

Secondary gout refers to those cases in which the elevated uric acid level is secondary to some other disorder, such as excessive breakdown of cells or some form of kidney disease. Diuretic therapy for high blood pressure and low-dose aspirin therapy are also important causes of secondary gout since they cause decreased uric acid excretion.

CAUSES OF GOUT
METABOLIC
Increased production of purines (primary causes)
    Idiopathic (unknown)
    Increased purine intake
    Specific enzyme defects
Increased production of purines (secondary to another factor)
    Increased turnover of purines
        Cancer

QUICK REVIEW

- Gout is caused by uric acid crystals deposited in joints.
- Several dietary factors are known to be causes of gout: consumption of alcohol, high-purine-content foods, fats, and refined carbohydrates.
- Elimination of alcohol consumption reduces uric acid levels and prevents gouty arthritis in many individuals.
- Liberal fluid intake dilutes the urine and promotes the excretion of uric acid.
- Consuming one-half pound of fresh or canned cherries per day has been found effective in lowering uric acid levels and preventing attacks of gout.

Chronic hemolytic anemia
Cytotoxic drugs
Psoriasis
Increased synthesis
Increased breakdown of purines
  Fructose ingestion or infusion
  Exercise
KIDNEY
Decreased kidney clearance of uric acid (primary)
  Intrinsic kidney disease
Decreased kidney clearance of uric acid (secondary)
  Functional impairment of kidney function
    Drug-induced (e.g., thiazides, salicylates, etc.)
    Increased lactic acid (e.g., lactic acidosis, alcoholism,
      toxemia of pregnancy, etc.)
    Increased ketoacid levels (e.g., diabetic ketoacidosis)
    Chronic lead intoxication

TABLE 1	Prevalence of Gouty Arthritis by Maximum Uric Acid Level		
SERUM URIC ACID LEVEL	**MEN**	**WOMEN**
<6 mg/100 ml	0.6%	0.08%
6.0–6.9	1.9	3.3
7.0–7.9	16.7	17.4
8.0–8.9	25.0	0
9+	90.0	0

About 200 to 600 mg of uric acid is excreted daily in the urine of an adult male, and another 100 to 300 mg is excreted in the bile and other gastrointestinal tract secretions. The dietary contribution to the level of uric acid in the blood is usually only ten percent to twenty percent of the total, but purines and uric acid through the diet can increase crystal formation in tissues nonetheless.

Uric acid is a highly insoluble molecule, and at pH 7.4 and body temperature, the *serum* (blood minus the blood cells) is saturated at 6.4 to 7.0 mg/100 ml. Although higher concentrations do not necessarily result in uric acid crystals being deposited in tissues (some unknown factor in serum appears to inhibit crystal precipitation), the chance of an acute attack of gout is greater than ninety percent when the level is above 9 mg/100 ml.

Lower body temperatures decrease the saturation point of uric acid, which may explain why uric acid deposits tend to form in areas such as the top of the ear, where the temperature is lower than the average body temperature. Uric acid is insoluble below pH 6.0 and can lead to kidney stones, as the urine is concentrated in the collecting ducts of the kidneys and passed to the bladder.

Therapeutic Considerations

The current standard medical treatment for acute gout is administration of colchicine, the anti-inflammatory drug originally isolated from the plant *Colchicum autumnale* (autumn crocus, meadow saffron). Colchicine has no effect on uric acid levels; rather, it stops the inflammatory process by inhibiting neutrophil migration into areas of inflammation.

Over seventy-five percent of patients with gout show major improvement in symptoms within the first twelve hours after receiving colchicine. However, as many as eighty percent of patients are unable to tolerate an optimal dose because of gastrointestinal side effects, which may precede or coincide with clinical improvement.

Colchicine may also cause bone marrow depression, hair loss, liver damage, depression, seizures, respiratory depression, and even death. Other anti-inflammatory agents are also used in acute gout, including: indomethacin, phenylbutazone, naproxen, and fenoprofen.

Once the acute episode has resolved, a number of measures are taken to reduce the likelihood of recurrence:

- Drugs to keep uric acid levels within a normal range
- Controlled weight loss in obese individuals
- Avoidance of known triggering factors, such as heavy alcohol consumption or a diet rich in purines
- Low doses of colchicine to prevent further acute attacks

Several dietary factors are known to be causes of gout, including consumption of:

- Alcohol
- High-purine-content foods (organ meats, meat, yeast, poultry, etc.)
- Fats
- Refined carbohydrates
- Excessive calories[2,3]

Individuals with gout are typically obese, prone to hypertension and diabetes, and at a greater risk for cardiovascular disease. Obesity is probably the most important diet-related factor.[2,3]

In concept, the naturopathic approach for treating chronic gout does not differ substantially from the standard medical approach:

- Dietary and herbal measures are employed, instead of drugs, to keep uric acid levels within the normal range
- Obese individuals are put on a careful weight-loss program
- Known precipitating factors, such as heavy alcohol consumption and numerous dietary factors, are controlled
- Nutritional substances are used to prevent further acute attacks

Dietary Considerations

The dietary treatment of gout involves the following guidelines:

- Elimination of alcohol intake
- Low-purine diet
- Achievement of ideal body weight
- Liberal consumption of complex carbohydrates
- Low fat intake
- Low protein intake
- Liberal fluid intake

Alcohol

Alcohol increases uric acid production by accelerating purine breakdown. It also reduces uric acid excretion by increasing lactate production, which impairs kidney function. The net effect is a significant increase in serum uric acid levels. This explains why alcohol consumption is often a trigger in acute attacks of gout. Elimination of alcohol is all that is needed to reduce uric acid levels and prevent gouty arthritis in many individuals.[2–4]

Low-Purine Diet

A low-purine diet has long been the mainstay of dietary therapy for gout. However, with the advent of potent drugs that lower uric acid levels, many physicians choose to simply write out a prescription rather than educate the patient how to control the gout by dietary measures. Foods with high purine levels should be entirely omitted. These include: organ meats, meats, shellfish, yeast (brewer's and baker's), herring, sardines, mackerel, and anchovies. Foods with moderate levels of protein should be curtailed as well. These include: dried legumes, spinach, asparagus, fish, poultry, and mushrooms.[2,3]

Weight Reduction

Excess weight is associated with an increased rate of gout.[5] Weight reduction in obese individuals significantly reduces serum uric acid levels. Weight reduction should involve the use of a high-fiber, low-fat diet, as this type of diet will help manage the elevated cholesterol and triglyceride levels that are also common in obesity.

Carbohydrates, Fats, and Protein

Consumption of refined carbohydrates, fructose, and saturated fats should be kept to a minimum. Simple sugars (refined sugar, honey, maple syrup, corn syrup, fructose, etc.) increase uric acid production, while saturated fats decrease uric acid excretion.[3,4,6,7] The diet should focus on complex carbohydrates such as legumes, whole grains, and vegetables rather than on simple sugars.

Protein intake should not be excessive (i.e., greater than 0.8 g/kg of body weight), as it has been shown that uric acid synthesis may be accelerated in both normal and gouty patients by a high protein intake.[2] Adequate protein is necessary (0.8 g/kg body weight), however, as amino acids decrease resorption of uric acid in the renal tubules, thus increasing uric acid excretion and reducing serum uric acid concentrations.[2]

Fluid Intake

Liberal fluid intake keeps the urine diluted and promotes the excretion of uric acid. Furthermore, dilution of the urine reduces the risk of kidney stones.[2] Drink at least 48 ounces of water each day.

Nutritional Supplements

Eicosapentaenoic Acid

Supplementation with omega-3 oils appears useful in the treatment of gout. The omega-3 oil *eicosapentaenoic acid* (EPA) limits the production of the inflammatory leukotrienes,

the key mediators of much of the inflammation and tissue damage observed in gout.[8,9]

Vitamin E

Vitamin E is appropriate for the treatment of gout since it also (mildly) inhibits the production of leukotrienes and acts as an antioxidant.[10] Selenium functions synergistically with vitamin E.

Folic Acid

Folic acid has been shown to inhibit *xanthine oxidase*, the enzyme responsible for producing uric acid.[11] In fact, research has demonstrated that a derivative of folic acid is an even greater inhibitor of xanthine oxidase than the drug *allopurinol*—the most widely used drug for gout—suggesting that folic acid at high dosages may be an effective treatment in gout.[12] Positive results in the treatment of gout have been reported, but the data are incomplete at this time.[13] The dosage of folic acid required is in the range of 10 to 40 mg per day.

Folic acid has been used at these high dosages with no reported toxicity and is certainly safer than current drugs used in gout. However, there have been reports of high-dose folic acid interfering with some drugs that are used to treat epilepsy. High doses of folic acid may also mask the symptoms of a vitamin B12 deficiency. Because of these concerns, folic acid therapy should only be utilized under the supervision of a physician.

Bromelain

There are no studies on the use of bromelain in the treatment of gout. However, this proteolytic enzyme complex of pineapple has been demonstrated to be an effective anti-inflammatory agent in both clinical human studies and experimental animal models.[14] Bromelain is a suitable alternative to stronger prescription anti-inflammatory agents used in the treatment of gout. For best results, bromelain should be taken between meals (dosage given below in Treatment Summary).

Quercetin

The flavonoid *quercetin* has demonstrated several effects in experimental studies that indicate its possible benefit to individuals with gout. Quercetin inhibits uric acid production in a similar fashion to the drug allopurinol, as well as inhibiting the manufacture and release of inflammatory compounds.[15-17] Quercetin is widely found in fruits and vegetables, but supplementation can provide higher amounts for the treatment of gout. For best results, 200 to 400 mg of quercetin should be taken with bromelain between meals three times daily. Bromelain may help to enhance the absorption of quercetin as well as exerting anti-inflammatory effects of its own.

Alanine, Aspartic Acid, Glutamic Acid, and Glycine

These amino acids have been shown to lower serum uric acid levels, presumably as a result of decreasing uric acid resorption in the renal tubule. This results in an increase in uric acid excretion.[3] Probably the best way in which to take advantage of this research is to take supplemental minerals like magnesium and calcium bound to aspartate (aspartic acid). The dosage would be based on the level of the mineral (e.g., 1,000 mg of the combination of magnesium and calcium daily).

Niacin and Vitamin C

High doses of niacin (greater than 50 mg per day) and vitamin C (greater than 3,000 mg per day) are probably contraindicated in the treatment of gout, as niacin competes with uric acid for excretion and vitamin C may increase uric acid production in a small percentage of people.[18,19]

Botanical Medicines

Cherries

Consuming one-half pound of fresh or canned cherries per day has been shown to be very effective in lowering uric acid levels and preventing attacks of gout.[20] Cherries, hawthorn berries, blueberries, and other dark red-blue berries are rich sources of anthocyanidins and proanthocyanidins. These compounds are flavonoid molecules that give these fruits their deep red-blue color, and are remarkable in their ability to prevent collagen destruction.[21,22] In addition, these flavonoids are good antioxidants and inhibit the formation of leukotrienes.[23,24] In addition to consuming anthocyanidin- and proanthocyanidin-rich berries, extracts of bilberry (*Vaccinium myrtillus*), grape seed (*Vitis vinifera*), or pine bark (*Pinus maritima*) can be used.

Devil's Claw

Devil's claw (*Harpagophytum procumbens*) has been used in folk medicine for the treatment of a variety of diseases, including gout and rheumatoid arthritis. Clinical research in Europe indicates that devil's claw may be of benefit in the treatment of gout. In addition to relieving joint pain, clinical trials found that devil's claw also reduced serum cholesterol and uric acid levels.[25]

Several pharmacological studies on animals have reported that devil's claw possesses an anti-inflammatory and analgesic effect comparable to the potent drug phenylbutazone.[26] However, other studies have indicated that devil's claw has little, if any, anti-inflammatory activity.[27]

The conflicting experimental results may reflect a mechanism of action that is different than current anti-inflammatory drugs or a lack of quality control (standardization) of the preparations used. Further clinical research is needed to clarify these inconsistencies.

Devil's claw may be useful in the short-term management of gout. However, since gout can be successfully prevented and treated by following simple dietary changes in most instances, the use of devil's claw in long-term management of gout is probably unnecessary.

Lead Toxicity

An additional item of concern relates to lead toxicity. A secondary type of gout, sometimes called *saturnine gout*, can result from lead toxicity.[28,29] Lead in the body can cause a decrease in uric acid secretion, contributing to gout.

Historically, saturnine gout was due to the consumption of alcoholic beverages stored in containers containing lead. An unexpected and fairly common source of lead appears to be leaded crystal, as wine takes on lead when stored in a crystal decanter.[30] Lead concentration increases with storage time, reaching toxic levels after several months. Even a few minutes in a crystal glass results in a measurable increase in the level of lead in the wine.

TREATMENT SUMMARY

The basic treatment goals involve: dietary and herbal measures that maintain uric acid levels within the normal range, controlled weight loss in obese individuals, avoidance of known precipitating factors (such as heavy alcohol consumption and a high-purine diet), the use of nutritional substances to prevent further acute attacks,and the use of herbal and nutritional substances to inhibit the inflammatory process.

Diet

Eliminate alcohol intake, maintain a low-purine diet, increase consumption of complex carbohydrates and decrease consumption of simple carbohydrates, maintain a low fat intake, keep protein intake moderate (0.8 g/kg body weight), and consume liberal quantities of fluid. Urinary twenty-four-hour uric acid levels can be used to monitor effectiveness with diet therapy (maintain below 0.8 g/day).

In addition, liberal amounts of cherries, blueberries, and other anthocyanoside-rich (red-blue) berries or extracts should be consumed (0.5 to 1.0 pound per day).

Nutritional Supplements

- Flaxseed oil: one tablespoon per day or EPA: 1.8 g per day
- Vitamin E: 400–800 IU per day
- Folic acid: 10–40 mg per day
- Bromelain: 200–400 mg two to three times per day between meals

- Quercetin: 200–400 mg two to three times per day between meals

Botanical Medicine

- *Harpagophytum procumbens*
  Dried powdered root: 1–2 grams three times per day
  Tincture (1:5): 4–5 ml three times per day
  Dry solid extract (3:1): 400 mg three times per day
- Flavonoid-rich extracts such as those from bilberry, grape seed, or pine bark: 150–300 mg daily

Headache

Gradual onset of a mild, steady, or dull aching in the head

Pain often described as viselike squeezing or heavy pressure around head

Constant headache (does not throb)

Although a headache may be associated with a serious medical condition, most headaches are not serious. Headaches can be caused by a wide variety of factors, but the overwhelming majority that require medical attention are either tension or migraine headaches. A quick way to differentiate between the two is the nature of the pain. Tension headaches usually have a steady, constant, dull pain that starts at the back of the head or in the forehead and spreads over the entire head, giving the sensation of pressure or a feeling that a vise grip has been applied to the skull. In contrast, migraine headaches are vascular headaches characterized by a throbbing or pounding sharp pain.

A tension headache is usually caused by tightening in the muscles of the face, neck, or scalp as a result of stress or poor posture. The tightening of the muscles results in pinching of the nerve or its blood supply, which results in the sensation of pain and pressure. Relaxation of the muscle usually brings about immediate relief.

Diagnostic Considerations

Tension headache is a straightforward diagnosis. Often the headache can be worsened (or improved) by applying hand pressure to *trigger points* on neck muscles. A trigger point is the central area of tension in the muscle. A tension headache only rarely mimics other types of headaches of a more serious nature, such as those associated with a stroke or brain tumor. The important recommendation is to consult a physician immediately if a headache feels different than a tension headache or migraine, or if the headache is unrelenting.

Therapeutic Considerations

Tension headaches will respond to a number of natural therapies. Particularly helpful are physical treatments, such as massage, chiropractic, and other forms of bodywork (discussed later in this chapter). Therefore, the first therapeutic goal for the chronic tension headache sufferer is to address any structural problem that may trigger a tension headache by consulting a practitioner of "physical medicine." Ask around for a referral. Since headaches are so common, one of your friends has undoubtedly been to someone who provided a real solution to a chronic headache.

In particular, chiropractic care can be quite helpful when misalignment of the spine creates muscular tension in the neck. In

1996, the Rand Corporation analyzed all of the scientific evidence from 1966 to 1996 on chiropractic treatment of tension headaches.[1] Their conclusion was that chiropractic care *probably* provides at least short-term benefits for some patients with neck pain and headaches. It is certainly worth a try.

The next goal is to learn how to relax the tight muscles by alternating tension and then relaxation in the muscle. See the exercise for progressive relaxation given in the chapter STRESS MANAGEMENT. Learning how to relax has been shown in clinical studies to provide exceptional benefits without side effects.[2]

One of the more interesting studies compared the effectiveness of a school-based, nurse-administered relaxation training to no treatment for chronic tension headache in children ten to fifteen years old.[3] Results showed that headache activity in the children treated with relaxation training was significantly reduced compared to that of the no-treatment control group after six weeks, as well as at the six-month follow-up. At the six-week evaluation, sixty-nine percent of the relaxation group, and eight percent of the no-treatment group, had achieved a clinically significant headache improvement (at least a fifty-percent improvement). At six months,

seventy-three percent of the pupils treated with relaxation and twenty-seven percent of the no-treatment control group had achieved improvement. Thus, teaching kids how to relax can be quite effective. We think it gives them a better message: rather than getting relief from a pill (drug), they learn how to control the headache themselves.

The next step is to follow the recommendations given in the chapter on MIGRAINE. These recommendations are also appropriate in the treatment of tension headache. Chronic tension headaches share the following features with migraine headaches:

- Both are often the result of chronic use of aspirin and other pain relievers
- Tension and migraine headaches are often triggered by food allergies
- Magnesium supplementation can help both
- 5-hydroxytryptophan (5-HTP) has been shown to help both

And, finally, occasional use of aspirin (or willow bark extracts standardized for *salicin*—the natural form of aspirin) or acetaminophen is safe and effective in the

QUICK REVIEW

- A tension headache is usually caused by tightening in the muscles of the face, neck, or scalp as a result of stress or poor posture.
- The first therapeutic goal in treating the chronic tension headache sufferer

is to address any structural problem that may trigger a tension headache.
- Learning how to relax and defuse tension goes a long way in the treatment and prevention of tension headache.
- Migraine and tension headaches share many features.

treatment of an acute headache. The key is not to rely too heavily on these medications. After all, a headache is not caused by a lack of aspirin or acetaminophen.

Bodywork, Massage, and Physical Therapy

Bodywork is the term often used to describe healing techniques that work with the structure of the body. Most of these therapies involve hands-on work, such as massage. Virtually all bodywork techniques may be helpful in the treatment of both acute and chronic tension headaches. However, rather than simply getting a massage whenever a headache appears, we recommend physical therapies that teach people to become aware of body tension and posture.

If you suffer from chronic tension headaches and have insurance, getting a referral to a conventional physical therapist (PT) can produce significant benefit. For example, in one study twenty patients with a diagnosis of tension headache were treated for pain relief in a physical therapy clinic once a week for six weeks.[4] The previous three-week period of no treatment served as a control period during which patients recorded their headache frequency, duration, and intensity using a numeric pain scale.

Physical activity level and headache frequency, duration, and intensity were recorded at four points during a one-year period. Measurements were recorded before treatment, after treatment, and at a twelve-month follow-up. Treatment included education for posture at home and in the workplace, home exercise, massage, and stretching of the cervical spine muscles. Results indicated that the frequency of headaches and activity scores were significantly improved over the course of treatment. These benefits were maintained after twelve months.

Given the problems associated with chronic use of aspirin and other pain relievers (see OSTEOARTHRITIS), this study provides evidence that addressing the cause rather than suppressing symptoms is clearly the better approach.

. . . .

TREATMENT SUMMARY

The primary therapy should be addressing the factors that trigger tension in the neck muscles. Since the neck is an area of the body that often holds tension produced by psychological stress, it is especially important to learn to relax neck muscles through techniques such as progressive relaxation. In addition, it is important to address any structural factor that may be triggering tension headaches. Bodywork is an important consideration.

Since tension headaches and migraine headaches share several features, the therapeutic recommendations given in MIGRAINE are appropriate here as well.

Nutritional Supplements

- Magnesium: 250–400 mg three times per day
- Vitamin B6: 25 mg three times per day
- 5-HTP: 100 mg three times per day

Heart Disease

. . . .

Shortness of breath, especially with exertion

Fatigue

Chronic, unproductive cough

Signs of reduced blood flow (blue extremities, swelling of the ankles)

Abnormal finding with electrocardiograph and/or echocardiograph evaluation

eart disease is a term that is most often used to describe *atherosclerosis* (hardening of the artery walls due to a buildup of plaque, which contains cholesterol, fatty material, and cellular debris) of the blood vessels that supply the heart—*the coronary arteries.* However, the focus in this chapter will be on heart diseases such as congestive heart failure, arrhythmias, mitral valve prolapse, and cardiomyopathy, all of which will be defined in this chapter. (Please refer to the chapter HEART AND CARDIOVASCULAR HEALTH for information on atherosclerosis.) Although these diseases of the heart differ from each other, they are grouped in this general chapter on heart disease because the treatment goals with natural measures are basically the same. In some cases, the natural approach to these conditions will provide all the support the heart needs to function effectively. However, in many cases drug therapy will also be necessary.

Congestive Heart Failure

Congestive heart failure (CHF) refers to an inability of the heart to effectively pump

enough blood. Chronic CHF is most often due to long-term effects of high blood pressure, previous myocardial infarction, disorder of a heart valve or the heart muscle, or chronic lung diseases such as asthma or emphysema. Weakness, fatigue, and shortness of breath are the most common symptoms of CHF.

Arrhythmias

Arrhythmia refers to a disturbance in the rhythm of the heartbeat. Some arrhythmias are very mild and nothing to worry about (such as atrial fibrillation and premature ventricular contractions); others are potentially life-threatening (ventricular tachycardia, and severe ventricular arrhythmias). An atrial fibrillation is a minor arrhythmia in which the atria (the upper chambers of the heart) beat irregularly and very rapidly (up to 300 to 500 beats a minute). An atrial fibrillation is minor because the atrium's job is simply to fill the ventricle—the lower chamber. Premature ventricular contractures are because it simply reflects an irregular heartbeat, the heartbeat itself is normal. In contrast, in ventricular tachycardia the beat is too fast (120 to 200 per minute). Other ventricular arrhythmias tend to be even more serious, such as ventricular fibrillation—rapid, uncontrolled, and ineffective contractions of the heart.

Mitral Valve Prolapse

Mitral valve prolapse refers to a loss of tone or a slight deformity of the mitral valve of the heart—the valve that blocks off the left upper chamber (the left atria) from the left ventricle. This deformity causes leakage of the valve and produces a heart murmur that can be heard by a stethoscope.

Cardiomyopathy

Cardiomyopathy refers to any disease of the heart muscle that causes a reduction in the force of heart contraction and a resultant decrease in the efficiency of circulation of blood. Cardiomyopathy may be the result of viral, metabolic, nutritional, toxic, autoimmune, degenerative, genetic, or unknown cause.

Diagnostic Considerations

Individuals who are suspected of having any heart disease should have an extensive cardiovascular evaluation, including: a complete physical exam to look for signs of poor blood flow, an electrocardiogram (which involves a machine that assesses the electrical function of the heart), and an echocardiogram (an ul-

trasound procedure to assess how the heart is functioning from a mechanical perspective, as well as determining the heart's shape and size).

These heart diseases are most effectively treated via natural measures in the early stages. Hence, early diagnosis and prevention by addressing causative factors is imperative. The first symptom of heart disease of any type is usually shortness of breath. A chronic cough may also be the first presenting symptom.

Therapeutic Considerations

The therapeutic goals in the treatment of these heart diseases are identical to the goals given in the treatment of angina: improving energy metabolism within the heart and improving the blood supply to the heart. Not surprisingly, the natural measures used to achieve these goals are also identical to those used in the treatment of angina.

Thiamin and Heart Disease

Thiamin deficiency can result in the cardiovascular manifestations of "wet beriberi," sodium retention, peripheral dilation of blood vessels, and heart failure.

Furosemide (Lasix, the most widely prescribed diuretic) has been shown to cause thiamin deficiency. The association between thiamin deficiency and long-term furosemide use appeared in 1980 when it was shown that, after only four weeks of furosemide use, thiamin concentrations and the activity of the thiamin-dependent enzyme *transketolase* were significantly reduced.

In addition, many elderly Americans do not consume the RDA of 1.5 mg of thiamin. In an attempt to gauge the prevalence of thiamin deficiency in the geriatric population, thirty consecutive outpatients visiting an outpatient clinic in Tampa, Florida, were tested for thiamin levels. Depending upon the thiamin measurement technique (plasma vs. red blood cell thiamin), low levels (defined as a level below the lowest level of the normal range for younger aged groups) were found in fifty-seven and thirty-three percent, respectively.[1]

These results highlight the growing body of evidence that a significant percentage of the geriatric population is deficient in one or more of the B-vitamins. Given the essential role of thiamin and other B vitamins in normal human physiology—especially cardiovascular and brain function—routine B-vitamin supplementation appears to be worthwhile in this age group.

The first study to look at thiamin as a potential adjunct in the treatment of CHF showed only modest benefits. However, several subsequent studies have shown that daily doses of 80 to 240 mg of thiamin per day improved the clinical picture, as best noted by an increase in the left ventricular *ejection fraction* (the amount of blood pumped by the heart) of thirteen to twenty-two percent.[2] The significance of this increase is that an increase in ejection fraction is associated with a greater survival rate in patients with CHF.

Given the possible benefit, lack of risk, and low cost of thiamin supplementation, administration of 200 to 240 mg of thiamin per day appears warranted for patients who have CHF or for anyone who is taking furosemide.

Magnesium

Magnesium and CHF

Many patients with CHF have a magnesium deficiency. The level of magnesium in the blood correlates with the ability of the heart muscle to manufacture enough energy to

. . . .

QUICK REVIEW

- Individuals suspected of having any heart disease should have an extensive cardiovascular evaluation.
- The therapeutic goals in the treatment of heart disease are to improve energy metabolism within the heart and to improve the blood supply to the heart.
- The popular diuretic Lasix (furosemide) can cause a thiamin deficiency.
- Thiamin supplementation improves heart function in patients who are taking Lasix.

- The level of magnesium in the blood correlates with the ability of the heart muscle to manufacture enough energy to beat properly.
- Many disorders of heart rhythm are related to an insufficient level of magnesium in the heart muscle.
- CoQ_{10} is an important natural prescription for all types of heart disease.
- Carnitine improves cardiac function in patients with congestive heart failure.
- Hawthorn (*Crataegus sp.*) preparations are very effective in the early stages of congestive heart failure and minor arrhythmias.

beat properly. In one study, CHF patients with normal levels of magnesium had one- and two-year survival rates of seventy-one and sixty-one percent, respectively, compared with rates of forty-five and forty-two percent, respectively, for patients with lower magnesium levels.[3]

In addition to providing benefits of its own in treating CHF, magnesium supplementation prevents the magnesium depletion caused by the conventional drug therapy for CHF—digitalis, diuretics, and vasodilators (beta-blockers, calcium-channel-blockers, etc.). Magnesium supplementation has been shown to produce positive effects in CHF patients who are receiving conventional drug therapy, even if their serum magnesium levels are normal.[4]

Magnesium and Arrhythmias

Many disorders of heart rhythm are related to an insufficient level of magnesium in the heart muscle. Magnesium was first shown to be of value in the treatment of cardiac arrhythmias in 1935. More than sixty years later, there are now many clinical studies that show magnesium to be of benefit in treating many types of arrhythmias, including atrial fibrillation, ventricular premature contractions, ventricular tachycardia, and severe ventricular arrhythmias. The current concept is that magnesium depletion within the heart muscle leads to potassium depletion as well. Given the importance of these two electrolytes for proper nerve and muscle firings, it is little wonder that an arrhythmia will be produced.[5–8]

According to the results of a recent double-blind, placebo-controlled study, magnesium supplementation may offer significant benefit in the treatment of new-onset atrial fibrillation (AF).[9] The drug of choice for new-onset AF is digoxin; unfortunately, it has been shown to offer no better treatment than a placebo for facilitating proper heart rhythm in AF. Because of the benefits noted in several studies of AF patients who were taking magnesium, researchers decided to conduct a study to determine if magnesium and digoxin were better than digoxin alone in controlling the ventricular response in AF.

Eighteen outpatients with AF of less than seven days duration received either digoxin plus a placebo or digoxin plus magnesium (given in the vein). Those who received magnesium were given twenty percent of a magnesium solution (10 grams of magnesium sulfate in 500 ml of five-percent dextrose in water) during the initial fifteen minutes. The remaining solution was infused over the next six hours.

The benefit of magnesium was obvious within the first fifteen minutes, as heart rate decreased immediately from an average of 130 to 120. After twenty-four hours, the group that received the magnesium had an average heart rate of roughly 80, while the group that received only digoxin had an average heart rate of 105. In the magnesium group, six of ten patients (sixty percent) converted to normal rhythm, whereas only three of eight in the digoxin-only group converted. The results of this study indicate that magnesium either greatly improves the efficacy of digoxin or exerts significant effects on its own.

Because of the lack of effectiveness of digoxin when used as the sole agent, research is focusing on newer drug therapies for new-onset AF, such as esmolol and diltiazem. While these drugs are gaining greater use, it should be pointed out that side effects such as very low blood pressure are quite common. Given the high rate of poor heart function in these patients, the fact that both drugs lower systolic blood pressure is of major concern. In one study with esmolol, almost fifty percent of the subjects had to stop treatment.

The fact that magnesium is both safer and more effective is reason enough for physicians to use it, either alone or in combination with digoxin, for new-onset AF. However, we can add one more factor to the equation: cost. Over a twenty-four-hour period, a patient with new-onset AF would require approximately 6 grams of esmolol (costing four hundred dollars) or 300 mg of diltiazem (costing two hundred dollars). These figures are considerably higher than the cost of 10 grams of magnesium sulfate (one dollar) or 2 mg of digoxin (two dollars) or their combination.

Magnesium and Mitral Valve Prolapse

Since research has shown that eighty-five percent of patients with mitral valve prolapse have chronic magnesium deficiency, magnesium supplementation is indicated. This recommendation is further supported by several studies which show that oral magnesium supplementation actually relieves mitral valve prolapse.[10,11]

Magnesium and Cardiomyopathy

Several studies have shown that magnesium supplementation produces improvements in heart function in patients with a variety of cardiomyopathies.[5–8]

Coenzyme Q₁₀

Many people are also deficient in Coenzyme Q$_{10}$ (CoQ$_{10}$). The research on the role of CoQ$_{10}$ in treating heart disease is even more impressive than the research involving magnesium.

Coenzyme Q₁₀ and CHF

Coenzyme Q$_{10}$ plays a role in energy production. Numerous studies have also shown that CoQ$_{10}$ supplementation is extremely effective in the treatment of CHF, presumably by improving energy production within the heart. Most of these studies utilized CoQ$_{10}$ along with conventional drug therapy. In other words, CoQ$_{10}$ was used as an adjunct. In one of the early studies, seventeen patients with mild congestive heart failure received 30 mg of CoQ$_{10}$ per day. All patients improved, and nine (fifty-three percent) became asymptomatic after four weeks.[12]

In another early study, twenty patients with congestive heart failure, due either to atherosclerosis or high blood pressure, were treated with CoQ$_{10}$ at a dosage of 30 mg/day for one to two months.[13] Fifty-five percent of the patients reported subjective improvement, fifty percent showed a decrease in New York Heart Association (NYHA) classification, and thirty percent showed a "remarkable" decrease in chest congestion, as seen on chest X rays. Patients with mild disease tended to improve more often than those with more severe disease. Subjective improvements in these patients were confirmed by various objective tests, including increased cardiac output, stroke volume, cardiac index, and ejection fraction. These results were consistent with the theory that CoQ$_{10}$ produces an increased force of heart muscle contraction (referred to as a positive inotropic effect). The increase in the force of contraction produced by CoQ$_{10}$ is similar to, but less potent than, digitalis.[14,15]

Three more recent studies have also shown that CoQ$_{10}$ significantly improves heart function in patients with CHF. Results from a Scandinavian study of eighty CHF patients were presented in 1992 at the meeting of the American College of Cardiology.[16] In this double-blind study, patients were given either CoQ$_{10}$ (100 mg/day) or a placebo for three months and then crossed over (those taking CoQ$_{10}$ were then given the placebo, and vice versa). The improvements noted with CoQ$_{10}$ were significant; the results were more positive than those obtained from conventional drug therapy alone.

In another double-blind study, 641 CHF patients received either CoQ_{10} (2 mg/kg of body weight) or a placebo for one year.[17] The number of patients who required hospitalization or who experienced serious consequences due to CHF was significantly reduced in the CoQ_{10} group compared to the placebo group.

In the most recent and largest study to date, performed in Italy, a total of 2,664 patients with mild to moderate CHF were enrolled in an open study.[18] The dosage of CoQ_{10} was 50 to 150 mg orally per day for ninety days, with the majority of patients (seventy-eight percent) receiving 100 mg per day. After three months of CoQ_{10} treatment, the percentages of patients with improvement in clinical signs and symptoms were as follows: *cyanosis* (purple hue of skin) 78.1 percent, *edema* (fluid retention) 78.6 percent, pulmonary edema 77.8 percent, enlargement of the liver area 49.3 percent, venous congestion 71.81 percent, shortness of breath 52.7 percent, heart palpitations 75.4 percent, sweating 79.8 percent, subjective arrhythmia 63.4 percent, insomnia 62.8 percent, vertigo 73.1 percent, and nighttime urination 53.6 percent. Improvement of at least three symptoms occurred in fifty-four percent of patients, indicating a significantly improved quality of life with CoQ_{10} supplementation. The results also showed a low incidence of side effects; only thirty-six patients (1.5 percent) reported mild side effects attributed to CoQ_{10}.

CoQ_{10} and Mitral Valve Prolapse

CoQ_{10} has also been shown to be quite helpful in cases of symptomatic mitral valve prolapse. In one study, eight children received CoQ_{10} (2 mg/kg of body weight) each day for eight weeks, and eight received a placebo. Heart function became normal in seven of the CoQ_{10}-treated patients, and in none of the placebo-treated patients. Relapse frequently occurred in patients who stopped taking the medication within twelve to seventeen months, but rarely occurred in those who took CoQ_{10} for eighteen months or more.[19]

CoQ_{10} and Cardiomyopathy

Regardless of the cause, a deficiency of CoQ_{10} has been found in the blood and heart tissue of most patients who have cardiomyopathy.[20] CoQ_{10} supplementation can raise CoQ_{10} levels and produce improvements in heart function as a result of improved energy production by the heart muscle.

Several double-blind studies in patients with various cardiomyopathies have shown significant benefit with CoQ_{10} supplementation. In one double-blind trial, daily administration of 100 mg of CoQ_{10} for twelve weeks increased cardiac ejection fraction significantly, reduced shortness of breath, and increased muscle strength.[21] These improvements lasted as long as the patients were continuously treated (three years, in this study). However, cardiac function deteriorated when CoQ_{10} was discontinued, indicating that individuals with cardiomyopathy may need to be on CoQ_{10} indefinitely. Of the eighty patients treated, eighty-nine percent improved while taking CoQ_{10}.

Carnitine

Carnitine is a vitamin-like compound that stimulates the breakdown of fats by the *mitochondria*—the energy-producing units in cells. Carnitine is essential in the transport of fatty acids into the mitochondria. A deficiency in carnitine results in a decrease in fatty acid concentrations in the mitochondria and reduced energy production.

Several double-blind clinical studies have shown that carnitine improves cardiac function in patients with congestive heart failure.[22–24] In one double-blind study, after one month of treatment (500 mg three times per day), the patients treated with carnitine showed significant improvement in heart function.[23] The longer carnitine was used, the more dramatic the improvement. After six months of use, the carnitine group demonstrated an increase in the maximum exercise time (25.9 percent) and the amount of blood the heart pumped in one stroke (ventricular ejection fraction) increased by 13.6 percent. In another double-blind study of similar patients, at the end of six months of treatment the maximum exercise time on the treadmill increased 16.4 percent, and the ejection fraction increased by 12.1 percent.[24]

Hawthorn

Hawthorn (*Crataegus sp.*) preparations are very effective in the early stages of congestive heart failure and minor arrhythmias. This effectiveness in CHF has been repeatedly demonstrated in double-blind studies.[25–27]

In one of the most recent studies, thirty patients with congestive heart failure were assessed in a randomized double-blind study.[27] Treatment consisted of a hawthorn extract, standardized to contain 15 mg of procyanidin oligomers per 80-mg capsule. Treatment duration was eight weeks, and the substance was administered at a dose of one capsule taken twice a day. The group receiving the hawthorn extract showed a statistically significant advantage over the placebo group in terms of changes in heart function, as determined by standard testing procedures. Systolic and diastolic blood pressures were also mildly reduced. Like all other studies involving hawthorn extracts, no adverse reactions occurred.

TREATMENT SUMMARY

The primary goals of therapy for CHF, arrhythmias, mitral valve prolapse, and cardiomyopathies are to improve the blood supply to the heart and to improve energy production within the heart muscle. Please consult other chapters in this book as appropriate. For example, if CHF is the result of long-term high blood pressure, please see HIGH BLOOD PRESSURE. Also, please follow the general guidelines on diet and lifestyle given in HEART AND CARDIOVASCULAR HEALTH.

Nutritional Supplements

- High-potency multiple-vitamin-and-mineral supplement
- Vitamin C: 500 mg three times per day
- Vitamin E: 800 IU per day
- Flaxseed oil: 1 tbsp per day
- Magnesium: 200–400 mg three times per day
- Coenzyme Q_{10}: 150–300 mg per day
- L-Carnitine: 300 mg three times per day
- If taking Lasix (furosemide) or other diuretic, thiamin: 200–250 mg per day

Botanical Medicines

- Hawthorn (*Crataegus sp.*) extract (1.8% vitexin-4'-rhamnoside or 10% procyanidin content): 100–250 mg three times daily

Hemorrhoids

. . . .

Abnormally large or painful conglomerates of vessels, supporting tissues, and overlying mucous membrane or skin of the anorectal area

Bright red bleeding on the surface of the stool, on the toilet tissue, and/or in the toilet bowl

In the United States and other industrialized countries, hemorrhoids are extremely common. Estimates have indicated that fifty percent of persons over fifty years of age have symptomatic hemorrhoidal disease, and up to one-third of the total U.S. population has hemorrhoids to some degree. Although most individuals may begin to develop hemorrhoids in their twenties, hemorrhoidal symptoms usually do not become evident until the thirties.

Causes

The causes of hemorrhoids are similar to the causes of varicose veins (see VARICOSE VEINS): genetic weakness of the veins and/or excessive pressure on the veins due to straining during defecation; diarrhea; pregnancy; long periods of standing or sitting; and heavy lifting.

Because the venous system that supplies the rectal area contains no valves, factors that increase venous congestion in the region can lead to hemorrhoid formation. These factors include: increased intra-abdominal pressure (as caused by defecation, pregnancy, coughing, sneezing, vomiting, physical exertion, or portal hypertension due to cirrhosis); an increase in straining during defecation due to a low-fiber diet; diarrhea; and standing or sitting for prolonged periods of time.

Classification of Hemorrhoids

Hemorrhoids are typically classified according to location and degree of severity. *External hemorrhoids* occur below the *anorectal line*—the point in the 3-cm-long anal canal where the skin lining changes to mucous membrane (see Figure 1). They may be full of either blood clots *(thrombotic hemorrhoids)* or connective tissue *(cutaneous hemorrhoids)*. A thrombotic hemorrhoid is produced when a hemorrhoidal vessel has ruptured and formed a blood clot *(thrombus)*, while a cutaneous hemorrhoid consists of fibrous connective tissue covered by anal skin. Cutaneous hemorrhoids can be located at any point on the circumference of the anus. Typically, they are caused by the resolution of a thrombotic hemorrhoid, i.e., the thrombus becomes organized and replaced by connective tissue.

Internal hemorrhoids occur above the anorectal line. Occasionally, an internal hemorrhoid enlarges to such a degree that it prolapses and descends below the anal sphincter.

Internal-external, or *mixed*, hemorrhoids are a combination of contiguous external and internal hemorrhoids that appear as baggy swellings. The following types of mixed hemorrhoids can occur:

507

- *Without prolapse:* bleeding may be present, but there is no pain
- *Prolapsed:* characterized by pain and possibly bleeding
- *Strangulated:* the hemorrhoid has prolapsed to such a degree and for so long that its blood supply is occluded by the anal sphincter's constricting action; strangulated hemorrhoids are very painful and usually become filled with blood clots (thrombosed)

Pain does not usually occur unless there is acute inflammation of external hemorrhoids. As there are no sensory nerves ending above the anorectal line, uncomplicated internal hemorrhoids rarely cause pain. Bleeding is almost always associated with internal hemorrhoids and may occur before, during, or after defecation. When bleeding occurs from an external hemorrhoid, it is due to rupture of an acute thrombotic hemorrhoid. Bleeding hemorrhoids can produce severe anemia due to chronic blood loss.

Diagnostic Considerations

The symptoms most often associated with hemorrhoids include itching, burning, pain, inflammation, irritation, swelling, bleeding, and seepage. Itching is rarely caused by hemorrhoids, except when there is mucous discharge from prolapsing internal hemorrhoids. The common causes of anal itching include tissue trauma resulting from excessive use of harsh toilet paper, *Candida albicans*, parasitic infections, and food allergies.

Therapeutic Considerations

In contrast to the United States, hemorrhoids are rarely seen in parts of the world where diets rich in high-fiber, unrefined foods are consumed.[1] A low-fiber diet, high in refined foods, contributes greatly to the development of hemorrhoids.

Individuals who consume a low-fiber diet tend to strain more during bowel movements since their smaller, harder stools are more

· ·

QUICK REVIEW

- The veins in the rectal area contain no valves, so factors that increase congestion of blood flow in the region can lead to hemorrhoid formation.
- The common causes of anal itching include: tissue trauma from excessive use of harsh toilet paper, *Candida albicans*, parasitic infections, and food allergies.

- A high-fiber diet is perhaps the most important component in the prevention of hemorrhoids.
- Flavonoid preparations have been helpful in relieving hemorrhoids by strengthening the veins.
- Studies suggest that aortic glycosaminoglycan preparations should be used as the "drug of first choice" in the treatment of hemorrhoids.

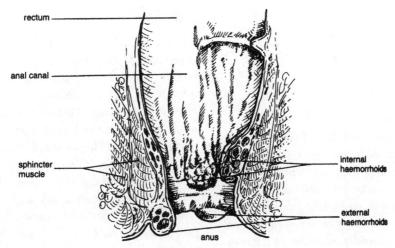

rectum

anal canal

sphincter
muscle

internal
haemorrhoids

external
haemorrhoids

anus

FIGURE 1 Hemorrhoids

difficult to pass. This straining increases the pressure in the abdomen, which obstructs venous blood flow. This intensified pressure increases pelvic congestion and may significantly weaken the veins, causing hemorrhoids to form.

A high-fiber diet is perhaps the most important component in the prevention of hemorrhoids. A diet rich in vegetables, fruits, legumes, and grains promotes peristalsis. Furthermore, many fiber components attract water and form a gelatinous mass that keeps the feces soft, bulky, and easy to pass. The net effect of a high-fiber diet is significantly less straining during defecation. The importance of fiber is discussed in more detail in A HEALTH-PROMOTING DIET.

Bulking Agents

Natural bulking compounds can also be used to reduce fecal straining. These fibrous substances, particularly psyllium seed and guar gum, possess mild laxative action due to their ability to attract water and form a gelatinous mass. They are generally less irritating than wheat bran and other cellulose-fiber prod-

ucts. Several double-blind clinical trials have demonstrated that supplementing the diet with bulk-forming fibers can significantly reduce the symptoms of hemorrhoids (bleeding, pain, itching, and prolapse) and improve bowel habits.[2,3]

Hydrotherapy

A warm sitz bath is an effective noninvasive therapy for uncomplicated hemorrhoids. A *sitz bath* is a partial-immersion bath of the pelvic region. The temperature of the water in the warm sitz bath should be between 100 and 105 degrees Fahrenheit. The warm sitz bath is soothing, but like creams and ointments its relief is short-lived.

Topical Therapy

Topical therapy, in most circumstances, will only provide temporary relief. But even temporary relief is better than no relief at all. Topical treatments include suppositories, ointments, and anorectal pads. Many over-the-counter products for hemorrhoids contain primarily natural ingredients, such as witch hazel (Hamamelis water), shark liver oil, cod liver oil, cocoa butter, Peruvian balsam, zinc oxide, live yeast cell derivative, and allantoin.

Flavonoids

Flavonoid preparations have been shown to relieve hemorrhoids by strengthening the veins. Early studies featured rutin. More recent and much more extensive studies have been performed using hydroxyethylrutosides (HER). Rutin and citrus bioflavonoid preparations can be viewed as providing similar effects to HER, but probably not as potent.

In several double-blind clinical studies, HER has been found helpful in the treatment of varicose veins and hemorrhoids.[4–12] Some of the studies involved pregnant women; HER was shown to be of great benefit in improving venous function and helping relieve hemorrhoidal signs and symptoms during pregnancy. In one study, ninety percent of the women who were given HER (1,000 mg per day for four weeks) experienced relief from symptoms, compared to only twelve percent in the placebo group.[11] Similar results have been reported using HER to treat hemorrhoids not associated with pregnancy.[4,12]

Aortic GAGs

Glycosaminoglycans (GAGs) are structural components essential to maintaining the health of arteries and other blood vessels. A mixture of highly purified bovine-derived glycosaminoglycans (GAGs) that are also naturally present in the human aorta (including dermatan sulfate, heparan sulfate, hyaluronic acid, chondroitin sulfate, and related glycosaminoglycans) has been shown to protect and promote normal artery and vein function. Two double-blind studies have compared aortic GAGs (72 mg per day) to hydroxyethylrutosides (1,000 mg per day) and bilberry extract (320 mg per day) in the treatment of hemorrhoids and varicose veins. The aortic extract produced far better results. In fact, the authors of the hemorrhoids study suggested that aortic GAGs should be used as the "drug of first choice" in the nonsurgical treatment of acute hemorrhoidal pain and disease.[13]

Botanicals

Any of the botanicals described in VARICOSE VEINS, particularly butcher's broom (*Ruscus aculeatus*), are useful for enhancing the integrity of the veins of the rectum.

. . . .

TREATMENT SUMMARY

As with all diseases, the primary treatment for hemorrhoids is prevention. This goal involves reducing the factors that may be responsible for increasing pelvic congestion: straining during defecation, sitting or standing for prolonged periods of time, or underlying liver disease. A high-fiber diet is crucial for the maintenance of proper bowel activity. Fiber supplements, flavonoids, aortic GAGs, and various botanical medicines such as butcher's broom are appropriate supplementary measures.

Warm sitz baths and topical preparations are useful to ameliorate the discomfort, but have only temporary effects.

Diet

A high-complex-carbohydrate diet rich in dietary fiber is recommended. The diet should contain liberal amounts of flavonoid-rich foods, such as blackberries, citrus fruits, cherries, and blueberries to strengthen vein structures.

Nutritional Supplements

- Vitamin C: 500–1,000 mg three times per day
- Flavonoids:
  HER: 1,000–3,000 mg per day

Citrus bioflavonoids, rutin, and/or hesperidin: 3,000–6,000 mg per day
- Aortic GAGs: 100 mg per day

Botanical Medicines

- Butcher's broom (*Ruscus aculeatus*) extract (9–11% ruscogenin content): 100 mg three times per day

Physical Medicine

- Hydrotherapy: warm sitz baths to relieve uncomplicated hemorrhoids

Hepatitis

· ·

During the period before liver involvement a person with viral hepatitis may experience a loss of appetite, nausea, vomiting, fatigue, and flu-like symptoms that can occur two weeks to one month before liver involvement, depending on the incubation period of the virus

Either abrupt or insidious occurrence of symptoms

Tender enlarged liver, fever, jaundice (yellow appearance of the skin)

Dark urine (due to elevated bilirubin levels)

Normal-to-low white blood cell count, markedly elevated liver enzyme level (aminotransaminases) in the blood, elevated bilirubin levels

Hepatitis refers to inflammation of the liver. Hepatitis can be caused by many drugs and toxic chemicals, but in most instances it is caused by a virus. Viral types A, B, and C are the most common. Hepatitis A occurs sporadically or in epidemics, and is transmitted primarily through fecal contamination. Hepatitis B is transmitted through infected blood or blood products, as well as through sexual contact (the virus is shed in saliva, semen, and vaginal secretion).

Hepatitis C (formerly known as hepatitis non-A, non-B) has a primary route of transmission through blood transfusion. In fact, it is responsible for roughly ninety percent of all cases of hepatitis contracted through blood transfusions (about ten percent of people who received blood transfusions developed hepatitis C in the past before the blood supply was checked for the presence of hepatitis C). However, only four percent of cases of hepatitis C are now a result of transfusions. Most cases are due to intravenous drug use, but the source of other cases of hepatitis C infection is unclear. The mortality rate from hepatitis C (one to twelve percent) is much higher than for the other forms. Other viral causes of hepatitis include: hepatitis viruses D, E, and G, as well as Herpes simplex, cytomegalovirus, and Epstein-Barr virus.

Acute viral hepatitis can be an extremely debilitating disease requiring bed rest. It can take anywhere from two to sixteen weeks to recover. Most patients recover completely (usually by nine weeks for type A and sixteen weeks for types B, C, D, and G). However, about one out of one hundred will die, and ten percent of hepatitis B and ten to forty percent of hepatitis C cases now develop into chronic viral hepatitis forms (hepatitis C contracted from a transfusion is associated with a seventy-to-eighty-percent chance of developing into chronic hepatitis). The symptoms of chronic hepatitis vary. The symptoms can be virtually nonexistent, or they can lead to chronic fatigue, serious liver damage, and even death due to cirrhosis of the liver or liver cancer.

Diagnostic Considerations

Diagnosis is made by the appearance of the typical signs and symptoms (see Table 1),

TABLE 1 Incidence of Symptoms in Viral Hepatitis[1]

SYMPTOM	% OF PATIENTS
Dark urine	94
Fatigue	91
Loss of appetite	90
Nausea	87
Fever	76
Vomiting	71
Headache	70
Abdominal discomfort	65
Light stools	52
Muscle pain	52
Drowsiness	49
Irritability	43
Itching	42
Diarrhea	25
Joint pain	21

the body, resulting in the formation of antibodies against them) or the antibodies that bind antigens. The type of virus involved is determined by identifying viral antigens or specific antibodies in the blood.

In cases of chronic hepatitis B or C, it is necessary to perform continued blood evaluation to monitor progression or clearance of the infection. In addition to liver enzymes, hepatitis C is monitored by the presence of the hepatitis C viral-RNA-by-polymerase chain reaction (HCV-RNA[PCR]). The higher the level of HCV-RNA, the more aggressive the chronic infection. Hepatitis B findings and their meaning are listed in Table 2.

along with blood tests showing elevation in liver enzymes (enzymes such as SGPT, GGPT, SGOT, and alkaline phosphatase leak out into the blood when liver cells are damaged) and the presence of viral antigens (compounds recognized as being foreign to

Therapeutic Considerations

Natural therapies can be of great benefit in treating hepatitis. Several nutrients and herbs have been shown to inhibit viral reproduction, improve immune system function, and greatly stimulate regeneration of the damaged liver cells. General therapies to

TABLE 2 Serological Patterns and Their Interpretations in Hepatitis B

HBsAG	ANTI-HBS	ANTI-HBc	HbeAg	ANTI-Hbe	INTERPRETATION
+	−	IgM	+	−	Acute hepatitis B
+	−	IgG	+	−	Chronic active hepatitis B
+	−	IgG	−	+	Chronic nonactive hepatitis B
+	+	IgG	+ or −	+ or −	Chronic hepatitis B
−	−	IgM	+ or −	+ or −	Acute hepatitis B
−	+	IgG	−	+ or −	Recovery from hepatitis B
−	+	−	−	−	Vaccinated against hepatitis B
−	−	IgG	−	−	False positive, or infection in remote past

Table Abbreviations: HBsAG = Hepatitis surface antigen; HBc = Hepatitis B core antigen; HbeAg = Hepatitis B secretory antigen; IgG = Immunoglobulin G; IgM = Immunoglobulin M protect and support the liver are discussed in more detail in the section on DETOXIFICATION. Those recommendations can be used in conjunction with the more specific recommendations given in this chapter.

In regard to chronic hepatitis, it is essential to be aggressive in the treatment of this condition due to the increased risk of liver cancer (hepatocellular carcinoma) and cirrhosis (severe damage to the liver). If cirrhosis is present in chronic hepatitis B, for example, the five-year survival rate is fifty to sixty percent. In other words, forty to fifty percent of people with hepatitis B who show evidence of cirrhosis of the liver die within five years.

Prevention of Hepatitis B

Primary prevention of hepatitis B involves vaccination. Vaccination is a good idea for high-risk occupations, such as members of the medical and dental field who are regularly exposed to blood and other body fluids.

In the case of acute exposure to the hepatitis B virus (HBV), hyperimmune globulin (HBIG)—a concentrated solution of immune globulins specific to HBV—is administered by injection. It is given to individuals who are known to be exposed to HBV (e.g., a medical worker who accidentally comes into contact with a needle used to draw blood from a patient with hepatitis B). It confers immediate, but short-lived immunity against infection. This immunity lasts for three months. Two doses of HBIG are given within two weeks of the exposure, and this is said to confer adequate protective immunity to seventy-five percent of exposed individuals.

HBIG administration is recommended for individuals who are exposed via mucous membranes or through breaks in the skin to material contaminated with HBV surface antigens. Also, newborns with HBsAG-positive mothers should receive the vaccine (0.5ml shortly after birth and at ages three and six months).

Dietary Considerations

During the acute phase, the focus should be on replacing fluids through consumption of

. . . .

QUICK REVIEW

- **Hepatitis is a serious disease, requiring the care of a physician.**
- **Several nutrients and herbs have been shown to inhibit viral reproduction, improve immune system function, and greatly stimulate regeneration of the damaged liver cells.**
- **In the case of acute exposure to the hepatitis B virus (HBV), hyperimmune globulin (HBIG)—a concentrated solution of immune globulins specific to HBV—is administered by injection.**

- The therapeutic goals of natural hepatitis treatment are to protect the liver and to prevent further damage to the liver by supporting the immune system.
- During the acute phase, the focus should be on replacing fluids through consumption of vegetable broths, diluted vegetable juices (diluted fifty percent with water), and herbal teas.
- In chronic cases, the diet should be low in saturated fats, simple carbohydrates (sugar, white flour, fruit juice,

vegetable broths, diluted vegetable juices (diluted by half with water), and herbal teas. Solid foods should be restricted to brown rice, steamed vegetables, and moderate intake of lean protein sources.

In chronic cases, follow the dietary recommendations given in DETOXIFICATION. The diet should be low in saturated fats, simple carbohydrates (sugar, white flour, fruit juice, honey, etc.), oxidized fatty acids (fried oils), and animal products to help aid the liver's detoxification mechanisms. A diet that focuses on plant foods (i.e., a high-fiber diet) has been shown to increase the elimination of bile acids, drugs, and toxic bile substances from the system.

Vitamin C

According to Robert Cathcart, M.D., acute hepatitis is one of the easiest diseases to cure using vitamin C.[2,3] Dr. Cathcart demonstrated that high doses of vitamin C (40 to 100 grams orally or intravenously) were able to greatly diminish acute viral hepatitis in two

to four days. He showed clearing of jaundice within six days.[3] Other studies demonstrated similar benefits.[4-6]

Another controlled study found that two grams or more of vitamin C per day was able to prevent hepatitis B in hospitalized patients—hospitalization is one way to be exposed to hepatitis. While seven percent of the control patients (who received less than 1.5 grams of vitamin C per day) developed hepatitis, none of the treated patients did.[7]

Liver Extracts

The oral administration of liver extracts has been used in the treatment of many chronic liver diseases since 1896. Numerous scientific investigations into the therapeutic effectiveness of liver extracts have demonstrated that these extracts promote hepatic (liver) regeneration and are quite effective in the treatment of chronic liver disease, including chronic active hepatitis.[8-10] For example, in one double-blind study, 556 patients with chronic hepatitis were given either 70 mg

. . . .

honey, etc.), oxidized fatty acids (fried oils), and animal products.

- High doses of vitamin C (40 to 100 grams orally or intravenously) can greatly relieve acute viral hepatitis in two to four days.

- There is good clinical data to support the effectiveness of orally administered bovine (beef) thymus extracts in treating acute and chronic viral hepatitis.

- Licorice exerts many actions that are beneficial in the treatment of acute and chronic hepatitis, including: pro-

tecting the liver; enhancing the immune system; and potentiating interferon.

- Silymarin, the flavonoid complex from milk thistle, is effective in treating both acute and chronic viral hepatitis.

- A growing body of scientific research indicates that silymarin phytosome is better absorbed and produces better clinical results than unbound silymarin.

of liver extracts or a placebo three times per day.[10] At the end of three months of treatment, the group that received the liver extract had far lower liver enzyme levels. Since the level of liver enzymes in the blood reflects damage to the liver, it can be concluded that the liver extract was effective in treating chronic hepatitis, via an ability to improve the function of damaged liver cells and prevent further damage to the liver.

Thymus Extracts

There is good clinical data to support the effectiveness of orally administered bovine (beef) thymus extracts in treating acute and chronic viral hepatitis IMMUNE SUPPORT for information on the thymus gland). The effectiveness of the thymus extract in treating viral hepatitis is reflective of broad-spectrum immune-system enhancement, presumably mediated by improved thymus gland activity. Several double-blind studies of type B viral hepatitis have shown thymus extracts to be effective in both acute and chronic cases. In these studies, therapeutic effect was noted by accelerated decreases of liver enzymes, elimination of the virus, and a higher rate of formation of anti-HBe (signifying clinical remission).[11,12]

Botanicals

Several plant medicines have been investigated for their effects in treating viral hepatitis. The two with the most positive documentation are licorice (*Glycyrrhiza glabra*) and silymarin (the flavonoid complex from milk thistle, *Silybum marianum*). A third, *Phyllanthus amarus*, sparked considerable excitement based on preliminary results, but detailed follow-up studies showed it to provide no benefit.

Licorice (*Glycyrrhiza glabra*)

Licorice exerts many actions that are beneficial in the treatment of acute and chronic hepatitis, including: protecting the liver; enhancing the immune system; potentiating interferon, the body's own antiviral and immune-enhancing agent; and promoting the flow of bile and fat to and from the liver. Clinical studies in Japan using a product that contains glycyrrhizin—the key component of licorice—have shown excellent results in the treatment of acute and chronic hepatitis.[13-17] The product, Stronger Neominophagen C (SNMC), consists of 200 mg of glycyrrhizin, 100 mg of cysteine, and 2,000 mg of glycine in 100 ml of physiological saline solution. It is administered intravenously; oral administration may be just as effective, as discussed below.

SNMC has demonstrated impressive results in treating chronic hepatitis due to either B or C viruses.[13-17] With either form, approximately forty percent of patients will have complete resolution—a statistic that compares favorably to alpha-interferon's forty-to-fifty-percent clearance rate. Like SNMC, alpha-interferon administration has been shown to lead to dramatic reductions in the risk of getting liver cancer.[18] However, alpha-interferon is expensive and associated with side effects (primarily fever, joint pain, nausea, and flu-like symptoms) in 100 percent of patients.

The most recent study involved 453 patients diagnosed with chronic hepatitis C at a hospital in Japan between 1979 and 1984. Eighty-four patients were treated with SNMC at a dosage of 100 ml per day for eight weeks, followed by treatments two to seven times weekly for periods of up to sixteen years.[17] The ten-year cumulative rates of liver cancer and cirrhosis were seven and twelve percent, respectively. The fifteen-year numbers were twelve and twenty-one percent, respectively. The numbers compare quite well to alpha-interferon's success rates in both patients with early stages of the disease (0.6 percent per year progression to liver cancer with alpha-interferon and 0.7 percent for SNMC) and advanced stages (1.5 percent per year progression to liver in alpha-interferon treated patients compared to 1.3 percent for SNMC).[17,18]

Although the studies with SNMC utilized injectable glycyrrhizin, injection may not be necessary, as glycyrrhizin is readily absorbed from licorice. The goal is to achieve a high level of glycyrrhizin in the blood without producing side effects. The dosages given in the Treatment Summary section provide roughly one-half the dosage of glycyrrhizin used in the studies of SNMC. If ingested regularly, licorice root (more than 3 grams per day for more than six weeks) or glycyrrhizin (more than 100 mg/day) may cause sodium and water retention, leading to high blood pressure. Monitoring of blood pressure and increasing dietary potassium intake are suggested.[19,20]

Susceptibility to the blood-pressure-elevating effects of licorice varies greatly among individuals. Adverse effects are rarely observed at levels below 100 mg/day, while they are quite common at levels above 400 mg/day.[19]

Prevention of the side effects associated with licorice may be possible by following a high-potassium, low-sodium diet. Although no formal trial has been performed, patients who normally consume high-potassium foods and restrict sodium intake, even those with high blood pressure and angina, are free from the blood-pressure side effects of licorice. Nonetheless, licorice should probably not be used by patients with a history of hypertension or renal failure, or who are currently using digitalis preparations.

Silymarin

Milk thistle (*Silybum marianum*) contains *silymarin*, a mixture of flavonoids. Silymarin is one of the most potent liver-protecting substances known. Silymarin inhibits hepatic damage by:

- Acting as a direct antioxidant and free-radical scavenger
- Increasing the intracellular levels of glutathione and superoxide dismutase
- Inhibiting the formation of leukotrienes
- Stimulating hepatocyte regeneration

Silymarin is effective in treating both acute and chronic viral hepatitis. In one study of acute viral hepatitis, twenty-nine patients treated with silymarin showed definite improvement in the serum levels of bilirubin (in hepatitis the liver is unable to process this breakdown product of red blood cells; as a result it produces jaundice—a yellowing of the skin—and a dark urine) and liver enzymes compared with a placebo group.[21] The laboratory parameters in the silymarin group improved more than in the placebo group by the fifth day of treatment. The number of patients who attained normal liver values after three weeks' treatment was significantly higher in the silymarin group than in the placebo group.

In a study of chronic viral hepatitis, silymarin was shown to result in dramatic improvement. Used at a high dose (420 mg of silymarin per day) for periods of three to twelve months, silymarin resulted in a reversal of liver cell damage (as noted by biopsy), an increase in protein level in the blood, and a lowering of liver enzymes. Common symptoms of hepatitis (abdominal discomfort, decreased appetite, and fatigue) were all relieved.[22]

Recently, a new form of silymarin has emerged that may provide even greater benefit. The new form binds silymarin to phosphatidylcholine (referred to as silymarin phytosome). A growing body of scientific research indicates that silymarin phytosome is better absorbed and produces better clinical results than unbound silymarin.[23–28] These benefits were demonstrated in one study involving 232 patients with chronic hepatitis (viral, alcohol, or chemical-induced). Subjects were treated with silymarin phytosome at either 120 mg twice daily or 120 mg three times daily for up to 120 days.[28] Liver function tests were compared to a group of controls (49 treated with a commercially available unbound silymarin; 117 untreated or given a placebo). Liver function returned to normal more quickly in the patients given silymarin phytosome than in both the commercially available silymarin and the placebo groups.

Silymarin preparations are widely used in Europe, where a considerable body of evidence points to very low toxicity. When used at high doses for short periods of time, silymarin given by various routes to mice, rats, rabbits, and dogs has shown no toxic effects. Studies in rats receiving silymarin for protracted periods have also demonstrated a complete lack of toxicity.

Because silymarin possesses an ability to increase bile flow (a choleretic effect) and bile can produce a mild laxative effect, silymarin may produce a looser stool. If higher doses are used, it may be appropriate to use bile-sequestering fiber compounds (e.g., guar gum, pectin, psyllium, oat bran, etc.) to prevent mucosal irritation and loose stools. Because of silymarin's lack of toxicity, long-term use is feasible when necessary.

Phyllanthus amarus

Phyllanthus amarus is an Asian herb with a long history of use in treating liver disorders. A preliminary report in 1988 demonstrated that fifty-nine percent of patients with hepatitis B had lost the hepatitis B surface antigen when tested fifteen to twenty days after treatment with a preparation of *Phyllanthus amarus* (200 mg of the dried, powdered, sterilized plant in capsules three times per day).[29] This report was met with a great deal of excitement. In this double-blind study only one in twenty-three (four percent) of the placebo-treated controls tested negative. Unfortunately, these results have not been confirmed by other researchers.[30–32]

For example, in one double-blind study fifty-nine and fifty-seven carriers of hepatitis B virus were given either 400 mg of *P. amarus* or a placebo, respectively, three times per day for thirty days. They were evaluated on days 15, 30, 60, and 180. Hepatitis B surface antigen (HbsAg) was detected during treatment and follow-up in every case but one in each group at day 180.[30] As noted in Table 2, the continued presence of HbsAg indicates chronic infection.

To rule out the possibility that poor-quality herbal material might have caused the poor response, the latest double-blind study utilized a *Phyllanthus amarus* extract in a capsule, standardized to contain 20 mg geraniin per 290 mg of extract.[32] The dosage used was three capsules per day for two months. No effect was noted in the fifty-two patients who received the extract. Specifically, clinical symptoms and hepatitis B surface and core antigen levels did not change.

These results indicate that either the type of extract used is not effective or that phyllanthus itself is not effective. Given the benefits of thymus extracts, licorice, and silymarin in the treatment of chronic hepatitis B as demonstrated in several double-blind studies, it does not seem warranted to use *Phyllanthus amarus* at this time.

TREATMENT SUMMARY

Hepatitis is a serious disease requiring the care of a physician. The therapeutic goals are to prevent further damage to the liver by supporting the immune system and to protect the liver. Bed rest is important during the acute phase of viral hepatitis, with slow resumption of activities as health improves. Strenuous exertion, alcohol, and other liver-toxic drugs and chemicals should be avoided. During the contagious phase (two to three weeks before symptoms appear to three weeks after), careful hygiene and avoiding close contact with others are important. In particular, once diagnosis is made, work in a day care center, restaurant, or similar environs is not recommended.

Diet

During the acute phase, the focus should be on replacing fluids through consumption of vegetable broths, diluted vegetable juices (diluted by half with water), and herbal teas.

In the chronic phase, a natural foods diet, low in saturated fats, simple carbohydrates (sugar, white flour, fruit juice, honey, etc.), oxidized fatty acids (fried oils), and animal fat and high in fiber is recommended.

Nutritional Supplements

Follow the recommendations given in DETOXIFICATION.

- Vitamin C: 1,000 mg three times per day (in acute cases: intravenous vitamin C, 50–100 g per day)
- Liver extracts: 500–1,000 mg crude polypeptides per day
- Thymus extracts: equivalent to 120 mg pure polypeptides with molecular weights less than 10,000, or roughly 750 mg of the crude polypeptide fraction

Botanical Medicines

- *Glycyrrhiza glabra* (licorice):
  Powdered root: 1–2 g three times per day
  Fluid extract (1:1): 2–4 ml three times per day
  Solid (dry powdered) extract (5% glycyrrhetinic acid content): 250–500 mg three times per day

---

NOTE: If licorice is to be used over a long period of time, it is necessary to increase the intake of potassium-rich foods.

- *Silybum marianum* (milk thistle):
  The dose of milk thistle is based on its silymarin content. For this reason, standardized extracts are preferred. The best results are achieved at higher dosages: 140 to 210 mg of silymarin three times per day. The dosage for silymarin phytosome is 120 mg two to three times per day between meals.

Herpes

Recurrent viral infection of the skin or mucous membranes characterized by the appearance of single or multiple clusters of small blisters (*vesicles*) on a reddened base, frequently occurring about the mouth (*herpes gingivostomatitis*), lips (*herpes labialis*), genitals (*herpes genitalis*), and conjunctiva and cornea (*herpes keratoconjunctivitis*)

Incubation period two to twelve days, averaging six to seven

Regional lymph nodes may be tender and swollen

Outbreak recurrences may follow minor infections, trauma, stress (emotional, dietary, and environmental), and sun exposure

More than seventy members compose the *Herpes* family of viruses. Of these, four are important in human disease: *Herpes simplex* (HSV), *Varicella-zoster* (VZV), Epstein-Barr (EBV), and cytomegalovirus (CMV). Serological methods have distinguished two types of HSV, which have been designated HSV-1 and HSV-2. Current estimates indicate that twenty to forty percent of the U.S. population have recurrent HSV infections. Laboratory studies have shown that thirty to one hundred percent of adults have been infected with one or both HSVs, with the greatest frequency among the lower socioeconomic groups. HSV-1 is primarily isolated in "cold sores," while genital infections are primarily caused by HSV-2 (ten to forty percent of genital herpes cases are due to HSV-1). The risk of clinical herpes infection after sexual contact with an individual with herpes lesions is estimated to be seventy-five percent.

After the initial infection, in most people the virus becomes dormant in the nerve cells. In others, however, it can be reactivated. This reactivation causes recurring outbreaks. The reactivation is usually triggered by minor infections, trauma, stress, or sun exposure. HSV-1 genital lesions have a recurrence rate of fourteen percent, while the HSV-2 recurrence rate is sixty percent. Men seem more susceptible to recurrences.

Therapeutic Considerations

Enhancement of the immune status is key to the prevention and control of herpes infection. There is some evidence that a defect of specific cell-mediated immunity is present even in apparently normal subjects with recurrent HSV infection.[1] In addition to general immune support (for a complete discussion see the chapter IMMUNE SUPPORT), one of the key natural measures to strengthen cell-mediated immunity is the use of bovine thymus extracts. Thymus extracts have been shown to be effective in preventing both the number and severity of recurrent infections in immune-suppressed individuals.[2] The thymus extract appears to increase the immune system's response to HSV primarily by potentiating cell-mediated immune responses.

Zinc

Oral supplementation with zinc (50 mg/day) has been shown to be effective in reducing the frequency, duration, and severity of herpes in clinical studies.[3] Although zinc is an effective inhibitor of HSV replication in experiments in test tubes, its clinical effect is probably related to its role in enhancing cell-mediated immunity. The topical application of 0.01–0.025-percent zinc sulfate solutions has also been shown to be effective in both relieving symptoms and inhibiting recurrences of HSV infection.[4]

Vitamin C

Both oral consumption and topical application of vitamin C increase the rate of healing of herpes ulcers. In a randomized, double-blind study, a pharmaceutical formulation that contains ascorbic acid (Ascoxal) was applied to herpes ulcers with a soaked cotton wool pad three times daily for two minutes. Patients subsequently reported fewer days with scabs and fewer cases of worsening of symptoms. In the treatment group, cultures yielded herpes complex viruses significantly less frequently.[5]

In another study, twenty patients with cold sores were treated with a complex of 600 mg of water-soluble bioflavonoids and 600 mg of vitamin C, given in equal increments three times daily. Twenty episodes of cold sores were treated with a complex of 1,000 mg of water-soluble bioflavonoids and 1,000 mg of vitamin C in equal increments five times daily. Ten episodes were treated with a placebo preparation. This approach was maintained for three days after the recognition of symptoms. The water-soluble bioflavonoid-vitamin C complex was shown to reduce blister formation. The therapy was most beneficial when initiated at the beginning of the disease. Those treated with the 1,000-mg regimen had cold-sore lesions for 4.4 days, while those patients treated with a placebo had lesions for ten days.

Lysine and Arginine

A diet high in the amino acid *lysine* and low in *arginine* has become a popular treatment for HSV infections. Foods high in arginine are chocolate, peanuts, seeds, and almonds and other nuts. Foods high in lysine include most vegetables, legumes, fish, turkey, and chicken.

This dietary approach arose from research showing that lysine has antiviral activity in test tube studies due to blocking arginine.[6] HSV replication requires the manufacture of proteins rich in arginine, and arginine itself is suggested to be a stimulator of HSV replication.[6,7] From a theoretical perspective, this approach should be effective, since *in vitro* studies have shown that HSV replication is dependent on adequate levels of arginine and low levels of lysine.

Double-blind studies on the effectiveness of lysine supplementation with uncontrolled avoidance of arginine-rich foods have shown inconsistent results.[7–10] These results may be due to the relatively low levels of lysine used (1,200 mg/day) and the severity of the cases in some of the studies (placebo and treated groups had lesions for forty percent of the time in one negative study).[7,8] In the most recent study, lysine was given at a larger dosage (1 gram three times daily) along with dietary restriction of nuts, chocolate, and gelatin.[10] At six months, lysine was rated as effective or very effective in seventy-four percent of those who received lysine, compared to only twenty-eight percent for those who received the placebo. The mean number of outbreaks was 3.1 in the lysine group, compared to 4.2 in the placebo group.

Topical Preparations

One of the most widely used topical preparations in the treatment and prevention of herpes outbreaks is a concentrated extract (70:1) of *Melissa officinalis* (lemon balm). Rather than any single antiviral chemical, the *Melissa* contains several components that work together to prevent the virus from infecting human cells. When the *Melissa* cream was used on patients at the time of the initial herpes infection, results from comprehensive trials from three German hospitals and a dermatology clinic demonstrated that not a single recurrence occurred.[11] In other words, by using the cream not one patient with a first herpes outbreak developed another cold sore.

Furthermore, it was noted in these studies that the *Melissa* cream produced a rapid interruption of the infection and promoted healing of the herpes blisters much more quickly than normal. The control group receiving other topical creams had a healing period of ten days, while the group receiving the *Melissa* cream was completely healed within five days.

The *Melissa* cream was also studied in patients suffering from recurrent cold sores. Researchers found that, if subjects used the *Melissa* cream regularly, they would either stop having recurrences or they experienced a tremendous reduction in the frequency of recurrences (an average cold-sore-free period of greater than three-and-one-half months).

The *Melissa* cream should be applied to the lips two to four times a day during an active recurrence. It can be applied fairly thickly (1–2 mm). Detailed toxicology studies have demonstrated that it is extremely safe and suitable for long-term use.

Another popular topical treatment for preventing and treating herpes outbreaks is a preparation containing glycyrrhetinic acid. This component of licorice root (*Glycyrrhiza glabra*), inhibits HSV as well as several other viruses.[12] Topical glycyrrhetinic acid has been shown in clinical studies to be quite helpful in reducing the healing time and pain associated with cold sores and genital herpes.[13,14]

. . . .

QUICK REVIEW

- Enhancement of the immune status is key to the prevention and control of herpes infection.
- A diet that avoids arginine-rich foods while promoting lysine-rich foods can be quite effective.
- Oral supplementation with zinc (50 mg/day) has been shown to be effective in reducing the frequency, duration, and severity of herpes in clinical studies.
- Both oral consumption and topical application of vitamin C increase the rate of healing of herpes ulcers.
- One of the most widely used topical preparations in the treatment and prevention of herpes outbreaks is a concentrated extract (70:1) of *Melissa officinalis* (lemon balm).

TREATMENT SUMMARY

The goal of treatment is to shorten the current attack and prevent recurrences. Support of the immune system is of primary importance. Inhibition of HSV replication through manipulation of the lysine/arginine ratio in the diet seems to be appropriate. This combined approach can be very effective at reducing the frequency, duration, and severity of recurrences.

Diet

Follow a diet that avoids arginine-rich foods while promoting lysine-rich foods. Foods high in arginine are chocolate, peanuts, seeds, and almonds and other nuts. Foods high in lysine include most vegetables, legumes, fish, turkey, and chicken.

Nutritional Supplements

- Vitamin C: 2,000 mg per day
- Bioflavonoids: 1,000 mg per day
- Zinc: 30–50 mg per day
- Lysine: 1,000 mg three times per day
- Thymus extract: The equivalent of 120 mg of pure polypeptides with molecular weights less than 10,000, or roughly 500 mg of the crude polypeptide fraction per day

Topical Treatment

- Ice: 10 minutes on, 5 minutes off for up to three cycles every 4 hours during initial symptoms
- Zinc sulfate solution: 0.025% solution three times per day
- Melissa cream: apply twice per day
- Glycyrrhetinic acid: apply twice per day

High Blood Pressure

Borderline high blood pressure: 120–160/90–94

Mild high blood pressure: 140–160/95–104

Moderate high blood pressure: 140–180/105–114

Severe high blood pressure: 160+/115+

Elevated blood pressure is a major risk factor for a heart attack or stroke. In fact, it is generally regarded as the greatest of the risk factors for a stroke. Over sixty million Americans have high blood pressure (also referred to as *hypertension*), including more than half (54.3 percent) of all Americans aged sixty-five to seventy-four years, and almost three fourths (71.8 percent) of all African-Americans in the same age group.

The blood pressure denotes the resistance produced each time the heart beats and sends blood coursing through the arteries. The peak reading of the pressure exerted by this contraction is the *systolic pressure*. Between beats the heart relaxes, and blood pressure drops. The lowest reading is referred to as the *diastolic pressure*. A normal blood pressure reading for an adult is:

120 (systolic) / 80 (diastolic)

High blood pressure is divided into different levels:

- Borderline (120–160/90–94)
- Mild (140–160/95–104)
- Moderate 140–180/105–114)
- Severe (160+/115+)

Although physicians are primarily concerned with diastolic pressure (the second number in the blood pressure reading), systolic pressure is also an important factor. Individuals with a normal diastolic pressure (<82 mm Hg) but elevated systolic pressure (>158 mm Hg) have a twofold increase in their cardiovascular death rates compared to individuals with normal systolic pressures (<130 mm Hg).

Therapeutic Considerations

Since over eighty percent of patients with high blood pressure are in the borderline-to-moderate range, most cases of high blood pressure can be brought under control through changes in diet and lifestyle. In fact, in head-to-head comparisons, many nondrug therapies—such as diet, exercise, and relaxation—have proven superior to drugs in cases of borderline-to-mild hypertension. These nondrug therapies are discussed in detail in this chapter.

Another strike against drugs is the increasing evidence indicating that they may be doing more harm than good. In some people, these drugs may be producing the very thing they are trying to prevent: a heart attack. Several well-designed long-term clinical studies have found that people who take blood-pressure-lowering drugs (typically diuretics and/or beta-blockers) actually suffer from unnecessary side effects (e.g., fatigue,

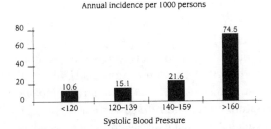

Annual incidence per 1000 persons

FIGURE 1 Blood Pressure and sudden death from heart disease and high blood pressure

headaches, and impotence), including an *increased* risk of heart disease.

Virtually every medical authority (textbook, organization, journal, etc.), including the Joint National Committee on Detection, Evaluation, and Treatment of High Blood Pressure, has recommended that nondrug therapies be used in the treatment of borderline-to-mild hypertension. The drugs carry no benefit, yet they possess significant risks. The two most definitive trials—the Australian and Medical Research Council trials—as well as five other large trials, including the famous Multiple Risk Factor Intervention Trial (MRFIT), have shown that drugs offer no benefit in protecting against heart disease in borderline-to-moderate hypertension.[1-7] Opposed to these seven negative trials, there are two that found treatment was somewhat effective.[8,9] However, upon further examination, both of these studies turn out to be unreliable. The European Working Party on Hypertension in the Elderly Trial was relatively small, and in the Hypertension Detection and Follow-Up Program there was an inadequate control group.

The most startling thing is that these studies compared drug treatment to no treatment (placebo). If the natural alternatives outlined in this chapter were compared to standard drug treatment in borderline-to-moderate hypertension, there is little doubt that the

nondrug approach would yield substantial benefit. A quote from an article in the *American Journal of Cardiology,* examining drug treatment for hypertension, is consistent with current medical opinion: "Few patients with uncomplicated marginal hypertension require drug treatment. . . . There is little evidence these patients (with marginal hypertension) will achieve enough benefit to justify the costs and adverse effects of antihypertensive drug treatment."[10]

Despite this substantial evidence and medical opinion, blood-pressure-lowering drugs are still among the most widely prescribed. Why? According to an article in *JAMA (Journal of the American Medical Association),* "Treatment of hypertension has become the leading reason for visits to physicians as well as for drug prescriptions."[11] In other words, blood-pressure-lowering drugs are big business to the drug companies and to physicians. Yearly sales of blood pressure medications are estimated to be greater than ten billion dollars. Since it is estimated that approximately fifty percent of patients with high blood pressure are in the borderline-to-mild range, if the doctors prescribed the nondrug protocols that have been recommended by the authorities, it could mean a loss of more than five billion dollars to the drug companies each year, as well as a substantial loss to physicians.

Dietary and Lifestyle Factors in High Blood Pressure

High blood pressure is closely related to lifestyle and dietary factors. Some of the important lifestyle factors that may cause high blood pressure include: coffee consumption, alcohol intake, lack of exercise, stress, and smoking. Some of the dietary factors include: obesity; high sodium-to-potassium ratio; low-fiber, high-sugar diet; high saturated-fat and low essential-fatty-acid intake; and a diet low in calcium, magnesium, and vitamin C.

Several of these dietary and lifestyle factors are discussed in HEART AND CARDIOVASCULAR HEALTH, since the health of the artery is critical to maintaining normal blood pressure. When the arteries become hard due to the buildup of plaques that contain cholesterol, blood pressure rises. Therefore, it is important to prevent *atherosclerosis* (hardening of the arteries). The role of potassium and stress in high blood pressure will be discussed in greater detail later in this chapter, followed by a shorter discussion of selected natural blood-pressure-lowering agents.

Some Specific Dietary Recommendations

Next to attaining ideal body weight, perhaps the most important dietary recommendation is to increase the consumption of plant foods in the diet. Vegetarians generally have lower blood pressure, and a lower incidence of high blood pressure and other cardiovascular dis-

eases, than nonvegetarians.[12] While dietary levels of sodium do not differ significantly between these two groups, a vegetarian's diet typically contains more potassium, complex carbohydrates, essential fatty acids, fiber, calcium, magnesium, and vitamin C, and less saturated fat and refined carbohydrate, all of which have a favorable influence on blood pressure.

Special foods for people with high blood pressure include: celery (for its 3-n-butyl phthalide content; see next paragraph); garlic and onions (for their sulfur-containing compounds); nuts and seeds or their oils (for their essential fatty acid content); cold-water fish (salmon, mackerel, etc.); green leafy vegetables (as a rich source of calcium and magnesium); whole grains and legumes (for their fiber); and foods rich in vitamin C, such as broccoli and citrus fruits.

Celery is a particularly interesting recommendation for high blood pressure. Two researchers at the University of Chicago Medical Center have performed studies on a

. . . .

QUICK REVIEW

- Elevated blood pressure is a major risk factor for a heart attack or stroke.
- Since over eighty percent of patients with high blood pressure are in the borderline-to-moderate range, most cases of high blood pressure can be brought under control through changes in diet and lifestyle.
- Virtually every medical authority (textbook, organization, journal, etc.), including the Joint National Committee

on Detection, Evaluation, and Treatment of High Blood Pressure, has recommended that nondrug therapies be used in the treatment of borderline-to-mild hypertension (high blood pressure).

- Vegetarians generally have lower blood pressure levels and a lower incidence of high blood pressure and other cardiovascular diseases than nonvegetarians.
- A high potassium-to-sodium intake is associated with lower blood pressure.

compound found in celery, 3-n-butyl phthalide, and found that it can lower blood pressure. In animals, a very small amount of 3-n-butyl phthalide lowered blood pressure by twelve to fourteen percent, and also lowered cholesterol levels by about seven percent. The equivalent dose in humans can be supplied by about four ribs of celery. The research was prompted by the father of one of the researchers; after eating a quarter-pound of celery every day for one week, he observed that his blood pressure dropped from 158/96 to a normal reading of 118/82. The celery prescription is certainly worth a try.

Garlic and onions are also important foods for lowering blood pressure. Although most recent research has focused on the cholesterol-lowering properties of garlic and onions, both have also been shown to lower blood pressure in cases of hypertension.[13] Both garlic and onion should be used liberally in the diet. Commercial garlic supplements may also be of benefit; follow the dosage recommendations given in CHOLES-

TEROL. The usual response when using garlic is fairly modest: a drop of roughly 8 to 11 mm Hg for the systolic and 5 to 8 mm Hg for the diastolic is common.

Potassium and Blood Pressure

It is a well-established fact that a diet low in potassium and high in sodium is associated with high blood pressure. Potassium, along with sodium and chloride, is an *electrolyte*—a mineral salt that can conduct electricity when dissolved in water. Although sodium and chloride are important, potassium is the most important dietary electrolyte. Potassium functions in the maintenance of:

- water balance and distribution
- blood pressure
- acid-base balance
- muscle and nerve cell function
- heart function
- kidney and adrenal function

Over ninety-five percent of the potassium in the body is found within cells. In contrast,

- -

- Relaxation techniques, such as deep breathing exercises, biofeedback, transcendental meditation, yoga, progressive muscle relaxation, and hypnosis, have all been shown to have some value in lowering blood pressure.

- Population-based and clinical studies have shown that the higher the intake of vitamin C the lower the blood pressure.

- Chronic exposure to lead from environmental sources, including drinking water, is associated with high blood

pressure and increased cardiovascular mortality.

- CoQ$_{10}$ deficiency has been shown to be present in thirty-nine percent of patients with high blood pressure.

- Over sixty double-blind studies have demonstrated that either fish oil supplements or flaxseed oil are very effective in lowering blood pressure.

- Hawthorn extracts exert mild blood-pressure-lowering effects.

most of the sodium in the body is located outside the cells in the blood and other fluids. Cells pump sodium out and potassium in via the *sodium-potassium pump*. This pump is found in the membranes of all cells in the body, and is perhaps the most important aspect of maintaining cellular health. The sodium-potassium pump also functions to maintain the electrical charge within the cell. This is particularly important to muscle and nerve cells.

During nerve transmission and muscle contraction, potassium exits the cell and sodium enters, resulting in a change in electrical charge. This change is what causes a nerve impulse or muscle contraction. It is not surprising that a potassium deficiency affects muscles and nerves first.

In addition to functioning as an electrolyte, potassium is essential for the conversion of blood sugar into *glycogen*— the storage form of blood sugar found in the muscles and liver. A potassium shortage results in lower levels of stored glycogen. Because glycogen is used by exercising muscles for energy, a potassium deficiency will produce great fatigue and muscle weakness. These are typically the first signs of potassium deficiency.

The Sodium-to-Potassium Ratio Just as important as the total potassium content of food, sodium and potassium should be consumed in the proper balance. Too much sodium in the diet can lead to disruption of this balance. Numerous studies have demonstrated that a low-potassium, high-sodium diet plays a major role in the development of cancer and cardiovascular disease (heart disease, high blood pressure, strokes, etc.).[14,15] Conversely, a diet high in potassium and low in sodium is protective against these diseases and, in the case of high blood pressure, it can be therapeutic.[1,16–18]

It is also well-known that excessive consumption of dietary sodium chloride (table salt), coupled with diminished dietary potassium, is a common cause of high blood pressure, especially in "salt-sensitive" individuals. Numerous studies have shown that sodium restriction alone does not improve blood pressure control in most people; it must be accompanied by a high potassium intake.[1,16,17] In our society, only five percent of sodium intake comes from the natural ingredients in food. Prepared foods contribute forty-five percent of our sodium intake, forty-five percent is added in cooking, and another five percent is added as a condiment. All the body requires in most instances is the salt that is supplied in the food.

Most Americans have a potassium-to-sodium (K:Na) ratio of less than 1:2. This 1:2 ratio means that most people ingest twice as much sodium as potassium. Researchers recommend a dietary potassium-to-sodium ratio of greater than 5:1 to maintain health. This is ten times higher than the average intake. However, even this may not be optimal. A natural diet rich in fruits and vegetables can produce a K:Na ratio greater than 100:1, as most fruits and vegetables have a K:Na ratio of at least 50:1. (See Table 4 in A HEALTH PROMOTING DIET.)

Potassium Supplementation in High Blood Pressure Many studies have now shown that increasing dietary potassium intake can lower blood pressure.[1,19] In addition, there are now several studies which show that potassium supplementation alone can produce significant reductions in blood pressure in hypertensive subjects. Typically, these studies have utilized dosages ranging from 2.5 to 5.0 grams of potassium per day. Significant drops in both systolic and diastolic values have been achieved.[19–24]

In one study, thirty-seven adults with mild high blood pressure received either 2.5 grams of potassium per day, 2.5 grams of potassium plus 480 mg of magnesium per day, or a placebo for eight weeks. They were then crossed over to receive one of the other treatments for another eight weeks, and then again for another eight weeks.[23] The results demonstrated that potassium supplementation lowered systolic blood pressure an average of 12 mm Hg and diastolic blood pressure an average of 16 mm Hg. Interestingly, the additional magnesium offered no further reduction in blood pressure. However, magnesium supplementation has been shown to be helpful in other studies (discussed later).

Potassium supplementation may be especially useful in the treatment of high blood pressure in persons over the age of sixty-five. The elderly often do not fully respond to blood-pressure-lowering drugs, making the use of potassium supplementation an exciting possibility. In one double-blind study, eighteen untreated elderly patients (average age seventy-five years), with a systolic blood pressure of greater than 160 mm Hg and/or a diastolic blood pressure of greater than 95 mm Hg, were given either potassium chloride (supplying 2.5 grams of potassium) or a placebo each day for four weeks.[24] After this relatively short treatment period, the group that took potassium was found to experience a drop of 12 mm Hg in the systolic and 7 mm Hg in the diastolic. These results compare favorably to the reduction of blood pressure produced by drug therapy, but without the negative side effects.[25]

Potassium and Magnesium Interactions
Potassium interacts with magnesium in many body systems. Magnesium is second only to potassium in terms of concentration within the individual cells of the body. Low intracel-

lular potassium levels may be the result of low magnesium intake. It is therefore appropriate to supplement magnesium (400 to 1,200 mg per day in divided doses) along with potassium. This suggestion may also lower blood pressure.

For example, in one double-blind clinical study, twenty-one male patients with high blood pressure were given 600 mg of magnesium daily (as magnesium oxide) or a placebo.[26] Mean blood pressure (the average between the systolic and diastolic) decreased from 111 to 102 mm Hg. The patients who responded best were those with reduced red blood cell potassium levels. After therapy with magnesium, the levels of intracellular sodium, potassium, and magnesium normalized, suggesting that one of the ways in which magnesium lowers blood pressure is through activation of the cellular membrane pump that pumps sodium out of and potassium into the cell.

There is considerable evidence from population studies that a high intake of magnesium is associated with lower blood pressure. The principle source of magnesium in early studies was water. Water that is high in minerals like magnesium is often referred to as "hard water." Numerous studies demonstrated that an inverse correlation exists between water hardness and high blood pressure. In other words, where magnesium content of the water was high, there were fewer cases of high blood pressure and heart disease.[27]

These early studies led to more extensive dietary studies looking at the association between magnesium and high blood pressure. These dietary studies found the same results as the hard water studies: when magnesium levels were high, blood pressure was lower. In one of the most extensive studies—the Honolulu Heart Study—systolic blood pressure was 6.4 mm Hg lower, and diastolic blood pressure 3.1 mm Hg lower, in the highest-magnesium-intake group compared to the lowest-magnesium-intake group.[28]

Because of the evidence that magnesium prevents heart disease, researchers began investigating the effect of magnesium supplementation in the treatment of high blood pressure. The results have been mixed. Some of the studies have shown a good blood-pressure-lowering effect; others have not. The distinction as to whether magnesium supplementation will lower blood pressure depends on several factors.

First, if the individual is taking a diuretic, there is a good chance that magnesium supplementation will lower blood pressure by overcoming the magnesium depletion induced by the diuretic. Another scenario in which magnesium supplementation may be of great value is when the high blood pressure is associated with a high level of *renin*— an enzyme released by the kidneys that eventually leads to the formation of angiotensin and the release of aldosterone. These compounds cause the blood vessels to constrict and the blood pressure to increase. And finally, patients with elevated intracellular sodium or decreased intracellular potassium levels (as measured by red blood cell studies) respond better to magnesium supplementation than subjects with normal intracellular potassium and sodium levels.

Rather than performing a blood test to measure renin or intracellular potassium and sodium, we recommend giving magnesium supplementation a four-week trial. We also recommend consuming a high-potassium diet or having your doctor prescribe a potassium supplement.

Dosage Information for Potassium   The estimated safe and adequate daily dietary intake of potassium, as set by the Committee on Recommended Daily Allowances, is 1.9 to 5.6 grams. If body potassium requirements are not being met through diet, supplementation is essential to good health. This statement is particularly true for the elderly, athletes, and people with high blood pressure.

Potassium supplements are available either by prescription or over the counter (OTC). However, the FDA restricts the amount of potassium available in OTC potassium supplements to a mere 99 mg per dose because of problems associated with high-dosage prescription potassium salts. However, so-called salt substitutes, such as the popular brands NoSalt and Nu-Salt, are in fact potassium chloride at a dosage of 530 mg of potassium per one-sixth teaspoon! The prescription and OTC supplements are either potassium salts (chloride and bicarbonate), potassium bound to various mineral chelates (e.g., aspartate, citrate, etc.), or food-based potassium sources.

Potassium chloride preparations are the most popular by prescription and are available in a vast array of formulations (timed-release tablets, liquids, powders, and effervescent tablets) and flavors. Potassium salts are commonly prescribed in the dosage range of 1.5 to 3.0 grams per day. However, potassium salts can cause nausea, vomiting, diarrhea, and ulcers when given in pill form at high dosages. These effects are not seen when potassium levels are increased through the diet only. This difference highlights the advantages of using foods or food-based potassium supplements to meet the human body's high potassium requirements rather than pills.

Dosage Information for Magnesium
Many nutritional experts feel that the ideal intake for magnesium should be based on body weight (6 mg/2.2 pounds of body weight). For a 110-pound person, the recommendation would be 300 mg; for a 154-

pound person, 420 mg, and for a 200-pound person, 540 mg. Rather than relying on dietary intake to achieve this amount of magnesium, for most people we recommend supplementing the diet with additional magnesium corresponding to the recommendation of 6 mg per 2.2 pounds of body weight. In the treatment of the conditions discussed above, we usually recommend twice this amount: 12 mg per 2.2 pounds of body weight.

Magnesium is available in several forms. In general, all forms are equally absorbed. However, we prefer magnesium bound to aspartate or to Krebs-cycle intermediates (malate, succinate, fumarate, and citrate), as opposed to magnesium oxide, gluconate, sulfate, and chloride. Absorption studies indicate that magnesium is easily absorbed orally, especially when it is bound to citrate (and presumably aspartate and other members of the Krebs cycle).[29,30] In addition, magnesium bound to aspartate or Krebs-cycle intermediates may help fight off fatigue. Aspartate feeds into the Krebs cycle—the final common pathway for the conversion of glucose, fatty acids, and amino acids to chemical energy (ATP)—while citrate, fumarate, malate, and succinate are actual components of the Krebs cycle. There is evidence to suggest that minerals chelated to the Krebs-cycle intermediates are better absorbed, utilized, and tolerated than inorganic or relatively insoluble mineral salts (magnesium chloride, oxide, or carbonate). In addition, while inorganic magnesium salts often cause diarrhea at higher dosages, organic forms of magnesium generally do not.

Potassium and Magnesium: Safety Issues

Most people can handle any excess of potassium. The exception is people with kidney disease. These people do not handle potassium in the normal way, and are likely to ex-perience heart disturbances and other consequences of potassium toxicity. Individuals with kidney disorders usually need to restrict their potassium intake and follow the dietary recommendations of their physicians. Also, potassium supplementation is contraindicated when using a number of prescription medications, including digitalis, potassium-sparing diuretics, and the angiotensin-converting-enzyme-inhibitor class of blood-pressure-lowering drugs, unless supervised by a physician. If you are not sure whether you are taking a member of these classes of drugs, check with your physician before taking potassium.

People with kidney disease or severe heart disease (such as high-grade atrioventricular block) should not take magnesium or potassium unless under the direct advice of a physician.

In general, magnesium is well tolerated. Magnesium supplementation can sometimes cause a looser stool, particularly if taken in the forms of magnesium sulfate (Epsom salts), hydroxide, or chloride.

Stress

Stress can cause high blood pressure in many instances. Relaxation techniques, such as deep breathing exercises, biofeedback, autogenics, transcendental meditation, yoga, progressive muscle relaxation, and hypnosis, have all been shown to have some value in lowering blood pressure.[31] Although the effect is only modest, using a stress-reduction technique is a necessary component in a natural blood-pressure-lowering program.

One of the most powerful methods of reducing stress and increasing energy in the body is by breathing with the diaphragm (See STRESS MANAGEMENT for more information). A recent study has shed some light on the effect of breathing on hypertension.[32] Volunteers with normal blood pressure were taught how to breathe very shallowly. Measurement of the amount of sodium and potassium excreted in their urine indicated that shallow breathing led to the retention of sodium in the body. It was suggested that this breathing pattern may play a causative role in some cases of high blood pressure due to the retention of sodium.

Vitamin C and Blood Pressure

Population-based and clinical studies have shown that the higher the intake of vitamin C the lower the blood pressure. Several preliminary studies have shown a modest blood-pressure-lowering effect (a drop of 5 mm Hg) from vitamin C supplementation in people with mild elevations of blood pressure.[33]

One of the ways in which vitamin C may help keep blood pressure in the normal range is by promoting the excretion of lead. Chronic exposure to lead from environmental sources, including drinking water, is associated with high blood pressure and increased cardiovascular mortality.[34] Areas with a soft water supply have higher lead concentrations in drinking water due to the acidity of the water; people who live in these areas may be predisposed to high blood pressure. It should be noted that soft water is also, of course, low in calcium and magnesium—two minerals which also protect against high blood pressure.

Vitamin B6 Supplementation for High Blood Pressure

Vitamin B6 supplementation has been shown to lower blood pressure. In one study, twenty people with high blood pressure were given oral vitamin B6 at a dosage of 5 mg per day per 2.2 pounds of body weight for four weeks. The subjects demonstrated significant reductions in systolic and diastolic blood pressure as well as serum norepinephrine (noradrenaline) levels. These results indicate that vitamin B6 influences the nervous system in a manner

which leads to reduction in blood pressure. The effect on blood pressure may have tremendous clinical significance, as the systolic pressure dropped from 167 to 153 mm Hg and the diastolic pressure dropped from 108 to 98 mm Hg in the study.[35]

Calcium Supplementation for High Blood Pressure

Population-based studies have suggested a link between high blood pressure and a low intake of calcium.[36] However, the association is not as strong as the one for magnesium and potassium. In addition to the epidemiological data, several clinical studies have demonstrated that calcium supplementation can lower blood pressure in cases of hypertension, but the results have been inconsistent.[36]

To clarify the effectiveness of calcium supplementation for patients with hypertension, a recent double-blind placebo-controlled crossover study was performed on forty-six patients with either salt-sensitive or salt-resistant (salt-restriction produces no effect) high blood pressure.[37] During the calcium supplementation phase, patients received 1.5 grams of calcium (as calcium carbonate) per day for eight weeks. The results of the study indicate that calcium supplementation can produce effective reductions in blood pressure in Blacks and in patients who are salt-sensitive, but not in patients who have salt-resistant hypertension. Given the safety and possible benefit of calcium supplementation in the treatment of high blood pressure, it is certainly worth a try. It should be pointed out that better results have been noted for calcium citrate than for calcium carbonate.[38]

Another group that appears to respond to calcium supplementation is elderly hypertensives. One study used twenty-four-hour monitoring of blood pressure to evaluate the effect of calcium supplementation on mild-to-moderate essential hypertension in elderly hospitalized patients. Over a period of twenty-four hours, the mean systolic and diastolic blood pressures declined by 13.6 mm Hg and 5.0 mm Hg, respectively, in patients whose diet was supplemented with 1 gram of elemental calcium.[39]

Coenzyme Q_{10} and High Blood Pressure

Coenzyme Q_{10} (CoQ_{10}), also known as *ubiquinone*, is an essential component of the *mitochondria*—the energy-producing unit of the cells of our body. CoQ_{10} is involved in the manufacture of ATP, the energy currency of all body processes. A good analogy for CoQ_{10}'s role in our body is the role of a spark plug in a car engine. Just as the car cannot function without that initial spark, the human body cannot function without CoQ_{10}.

Although CoQ_{10} can be synthesized within the body, deficiency states have been reported. In fact, CoQ_{10} deficiency has been found in thirty-nine percent of patients with high blood pressure. This finding alone suggests a need for CoQ_{10} supplementation. But CoQ_{10} appears to provide benefits beyond correction of a deficiency.

In several studies, CoQ_{10} has actually been shown to lower blood pressure in patients with hypertension.[40-42] However, the effect of CoQ_{10} on blood pressure is usually not seen until after four to twelve weeks of therapy. Thus, CoQ_{10} is not a typical blood-pressure-lowering drug. Rather, it seems to correct some metabolic abnormality which, in turn, has a favorable influence on blood pressure. In patients with high blood pressure, typical reductions in both systolic and diastolic blood pressure with CoQ_{10} therapy are in the ten-percent range. In other words, in a patient with an initial blood pressure reading of 150/100, CoQ_{10} supplementation would drop the pressure down to 135/90.

While the mechanism of action of CoQ_{10} in angina is well understood (see ANGINA), how CoQ_{10} lowers blood pressure has been a mystery. Blood pressure is similar to water pressure as it passes through a garden hose; if an artery (or a hose) is constricted, pressure will increase. Elevated levels of renin, sodium, or aldosterone are associated with increased resistance to blood flow. When ten patients with high blood pressure were given 100 mg of CoQ_{10} daily for ten weeks, systolic blood pressure in the group dropped from 161.5 to 142 mm Hg and diastolic pressure dropped from 98.5 to 83 mm Hg, but there were no changes in renin, sodium, or aldosterone levels.[40] These three compounds promote constriction of blood vessels and high blood pressure. Cholesterol levels did drop from 227 mg/dl to 204 mg/dl, and a sophisticated test that measures resistance within the arteries of the arms and legs did reveal significant improvements.

These results indicate that CoQ_{10} lowers blood pressure by unusual mechanisms of action: (1) by lowering cholesterol levels and (2) by stabilizing the vascular system via its antioxidant properties. As a result of these actions, resistance to blood flow through the arteries is reduced. An analogy would be that CoQ_{10} acts in a manner similar to opening up the diameter of a sprayer at the end of a garden hose.

Omega-3 Oils and Blood Pressure

Increasing the intake of omega-3 fatty acids can lower blood pressure. Over sixty double-blind studies have demonstrated that either fish oil supplements or flaxseed oil are very effective in lowering blood pressure.[43-46] The fish oils have typically produced a more pronounced effect than flaxseed oil, because the dosage of fish oils used in the studies was quite high (equal to ten fish-oil capsules daily). However, flaxseed oil may be the better choice for lowering blood pressure, especially when cost-effectiveness is considered.

Along with reducing the intake of saturated fat, 1 tablespoon per day of flaxseed oil should lower both the systolic and diastolic readings by up to 9 mm Hg.[45] One study found that for every absolute one-percent increase in body alpha-linolenic acid content, there was a decrease of 5 mm Hg in the systolic, diastolic, and mean blood pressures.[46]

Botanicals

The two most popular herbal recommendations for high blood pressure are garlic (discussed earlier) and hawthorn (*Crataegus monogyna*). Extracts of hawthorn berries and extracts of the flowering tops of hawthorn are widely used by physicians in Europe for their cardiovascular effectiveness. Studies have demonstrated that hawthorn extracts are effective in lowering blood pressure and in improving heart function. However, in general it can be said that the blood-pressure-lowering effect of hawthorn is very mild.[47,48] It usually requires at least two to four weeks before hawthorn begins to exert any effect.

TREATMENT SUMMARY

High blood pressure should not be taken lightly. By keeping your blood pressure in the normal range, you will not only lengthen your life, but you will improve the quality of your life as well. This is especially true if natural measures, rather than drugs, are used to attain proper blood pressure; the drugs carry significant side effects such as fatigue, headaches, and impotence. Here are some concise guidelines for the various classifications of high blood pressure:

For Mild Hypertension (140–160/90–104)

- reduce excess weight
- eliminate salt (sodium chloride) intake
- follow a healthy lifestyle: avoid alcohol, caffeine, and smoking; exercise and use stress-reduction techniques
- follow a high-potassium diet rich in fiber and complex carbohydrates
- increase dietary consumption of celery, garlic, and onions
- reduce or eliminate the intake of animal fats while increasing the intake of vegetable oils
- supplement the diet with the following:
  High-potency multiple-vitamin-and-mineral formula
  Vitamin C: 500–1,000 mg three times per day
  Vitamin E: 400–800 IU per day
  Magnesium: 800–1,200 mg per day
  Garlic: the equivalent of 4,000 mg of fresh garlic per day
  Flaxseed oil: 1 tbsp per day

If, after following the above recommendations for a period of three to six months, blood pressure has not returned to normal, please consult a physician for further nondrug recommendations.

For Moderate Hypertension (140–180/105–114)

- employ all the measures listed for Mild Hypertension
- take Coenzyme Q_{10}: 50 mg two to three times per day
- take hawthorn extract (10% procyanidins or 1.8% vitexin-4'-rhamnoside): 100–250 mg three times per day

Follow these guidelines for one to three months. If your blood pressure has not dropped below 140/105, you will need to work with a physician to select the most appropriate medication. If a prescription drug is necessary, calcium-channel-blockers or ACE-inhibitors appear to be the safest.

For Severe Hypertension (160+/115+)

Consult a physician immediately.

Employ all the measures listed for Mild and Moderate Hypertension. A drug may be necessary to achieve initial control. When satisfactory control over the high blood pressure has been achieved, work with your physician to taper off the medication.

Hives

. . . .

Hives (*urticaria*): raised and swollen welts with blanched centers (*wheals*) that may coalesce to become giant welts. Limited to the superficial portion of the skin.

Angioedema: Similar eruptions to hives, but with larger swollen areas that involve structures beneath the skin.

Chronic versus acute: Recurrent episodes of urticaria and/or angioedema of less than six weeks duration are considered acute, while attacks persisting beyond this period are designated chronic.

Special forms: Special forms have characteristic features (dermographism, cholinergic urticaria, solar urticaria, cold urticaria).

Hives (urticaria) is an allergic reaction in the skin characterized by white or pink welts or large bumps surrounded with redness. These lesions are known as *wheal* and *flare lesions* and are caused primarily by the release of *histamine* (an allergic mediator) in the skin. About fifty percent of patients with hives develop *angioedema*—a deeper, more serious form involving the tissue below the surface of the skin.

Hives and angioedema are relatively common conditions: it is estimated that fifteen to twenty percent of the general population has had hives at some time. Although persons in any age group may experience acute or chronic hives and/or angioedema, young adults (post-adolescence through the third decade of life) are most often affected.[1,2]

The basic cause of hives involves the release of inflammatory mediators from mast cells or basophils—white blood cells that play a key role in allergies. Mast cells are widely distributed throughout the body and are found primarily near small blood vessels, particularly in the skin, while basophils circulate in the blood. The classic allergic reaction oc-

curs as a result of complexes of allergic antibodies (IgE) and antigens (foreign molecules) binding to mast cells and basophils and stimulating the release of histamine and other inflammatory compounds. However, other factors appear to be more important in stimulating the release of histamine in hives.[1,3]

Causes

Fundamental to the treatment of hives is recognition and control of causative factors.

Physical

Hives can be produced as a result of reactions to various physical conditions. The most common forms of physical urticaria are *dermographic, cholinergic,* and *cold urticaria.* These are briefly described below. Less common types of physical urticaria or angioedema are: contact, solar, pressure, heat contact, aquagenic, vibratory, and exercise-induced.[1]

TABLE 1 Clinical Aspects of Physical Urticarias[1]

TYPE	ELICITING FACTOR	TIME OF ONSET	DURATION OF LESION	DIAGNOSTIC TEST	ASSOCIATED SYMPTOMS
Dermographic urticaria (tarda)	Stroking, scratching (rubbing, for red dermographism)	2–5 min (0.5–5 hr)	1–5 hr (48 hr)	Firm stroking of skin	Headache, malaise
Cholinergic urticaria	Physical exercise or overheating mental stress	2–20 min	30–60 min	Bicycling, running, sauna	Headache, nausea, wheezing, salivation, watery eyes, fainting
Cold urticaria	Cold contact	2–5 min	1–2 hr	Ice cube, cold arm bath, cold air	Wheezing, dizziness, fainting
Solar urticaria	Light of varying wavelengths	2–15 min	0.25–3 hr	Phototest	Wheezing, dizziness, fainting
Pressure urticaria creased	Pressure	3–8 min	8–24 hr	Locally applied	Flu-like syndrome, fever, in-weights number of white blood cells, joint pain
Heat-contact urticaria	Contact with heat	2–15 min	30–60 min	Hot arm bath	Gastrointestinal upset, dizziness, fatigue, wheezing, loss of breath
Aquagenic urticaria	Contact with water	2–30 min	30–60 min	Bath, compresses	Faintness, headache
Vibratory angioedema	Vibration	0.5–4 min	1 hr	Vibrating motor	Faintness, headache
Exercise-induced anaphylaxis	Exercise after a heavy meal	2–5 min	10–30 min	Exercise	Flushing, headache, disorientation, glottis edema, dyspnea, collapse
Familial cold urticaria	Cold wind, change from cold to warm air	0.5–3hr	48 hr	Cold wind and subsequent rewarming	Tremor, headache, joint pain, fever

Dermographism

Dermographism, or *dermographic urticaria,* is a readily elicited hive formation that evolves rapidly when moderate amounts of pressure are applied. This pressure may occur as a result of simple contact with another human being, furniture, bracelets, watch bands, towels, or bedding.

The frequency of dermographic urticaria has been estimated at 1.5 to 5 percent in the general population. It is the most common type of physical urticaria and is found twice as frequently in women as in men, with the average age of onset in the third decade. The incidence is much greater among the obese, especially those who wear tight clothing.

Dermographic lesions usually start within one to two minutes of contact as a generalized redness in the area, which is replaced within three to five minutes by a welt and surrounding reflex urticaria. Maximal edema is usually produced within ten to fifteen minutes. While the redness (*erythema*) generally regresses within an hour, the edema can persist for up to three hours.

Dermographism may be associated with other diseases, including parasite infection, insect bites, hormonal changes, thyroid disorders, pregnancy, menopause, diabetes, immunological alterations, other urticarias, drug therapy (during or following), chronic candidiasis, angioedema, and elevated levels of *eosinophils* (another type of white blood cell linked to allergies) in the blood.[1]

Cholinergic Urticaria

Cholinergic, or heat-reflex urticaria, (commonly referred to as "prickly heat rash") is the second most frequent type of physical urticaria. These lesions, which depend upon the stimulation of the sweat gland, consist of pinpoint wheals surrounded by reflex erythema. The wheals arise at or between hair follicles and develop preferentially on the upper trunk and arms.

The three basic types of stimuli that may produce cholinergic urticaria are: (1) passive overheating, (2) physical exercise, and (3) emotional stress. Typical eliciting activities, besides physical exercise, may include taking a warm bath or sauna, eating hot spices, or drinking alcoholic beverages. The lesions usually arise within two to ten minutes after provocation and last for thirty to fifty minutes.

A variety of systemic symptoms may also occur, suggesting a more generalized mast

- -

QUICK REVIEW

- Fundamental to the treatment of hives is recognition and control of causative factors.

- Drug reactions are the leading cause of hives in adults.

- In children, hives are usually due to foods, food additives, or infections.

- Antibiotics, including penicillin and related compounds, are the most common cause of drug-induced hives.

- Although any food can be the causative agent, the most common offenders are: milk, fish, meat, eggs, beans, and nuts.

- Several food additives (e.g., tartrazine, benzoate) and aspirin increase the production of a compound that results in cell release of the mediators than in the skin. Headache, swelling around the eyes, tearing, and burning of the eyes are common symptoms. Less frequent symptoms include nausea, vomiting, abdominal cramps, diarrhea, dizziness, low blood pressure, and asthma attacks.[1]

Cold Urticaria

Cold urticaria is an urticarial reaction of the skin when it comes in contact with cold objects, water, or air. Lesions are usually restricted to the area of exposure, and develop within a few seconds to minutes after the removal of the cold object and rewarming of the skin. The lower the object's or element's temperature, the faster the reaction.

Widespread local exposure and generalized hives can be accompanied by flushing, headaches, chills, dizziness, rapid heartbeat, abdominal pain, nausea, vomiting, muscle pain, shortness of breath, wheezing, or unconsciousness. Cold urticaria has been observed to accompany a variety of clinical conditions, including: viral infections, parasitic infestations, syphilis, multiple insect bites, penicillin injections, dietary changes, and stress.[1]

Drugs

Drugs are the leading cause of hives in adults. In children, hives are usually due to foods, food additives, or infections.[1]

Most drugs are composed of small molecules incapable of inducing antigenic/allergenic activity on their own. Typically, they produce allergic effects by binding to larger molecules and inducing the immune system to develop allergic antibodies to the molecule complex made larger by the drug. Alternatively, drugs can interact directly with mast cells to induce the release of histamine. Many drugs have been shown to produce hives. The two most common drugs that produce hives are penicillin and aspirin.

DRUGS THAT CAN CAUSE URTICARIA

Acetylsalicylic acid
Allopurinol
Antimony
Antipyrines
Barbiturates
Bismuth
Chlorhydrate
Chlorpromazine

• an increase in the number of mast cells throughout the body.
• Elimination of food additives leads to tremendous improvement in chronic hives in children.
• Chronic candidiasis can be an underlying factor in cases of chronic hives.
• Vitamin C prevents the secretion of histamine by white blood cells and increases the breakdown of histamine.
• The flavonoid quercetin inhibits both the manufacture and release of histamine and other allergic/ inflammatory mediators by mast cells and basophils.
• It is important to rule out low thyroid function or the presence of antibodies against the thyroid gland in cases of chronic hives.

Corticotropin (ACTH)
Eucalyptus
Fluorides
Gold
Griseofulvin (cold urticaria)
Insulin
Iodines
Liver extract
Menthol
Meprobamate
Mercury
Morphine, opium
Para-aminosalicylic acid
Penicillin
Phenacetin
Phenobarbital
Pilocarpine
Poliomyelitis vaccine
Potassium sulfocyanate
Procaine
Promethazine
Quinine
Reserpine
Saccharin
Thiamine chloride
Thiouracil

Penicillin

Antibiotics, including penicillin and related compounds, are the most common cause of drug-induced hives. The allergenicity of penicillin in the general population is thought to be at least ten percent. Nearly twenty-five percent of these individuals will display hives, angioedema, or anaphylaxis upon ingestion of penicillin.[1,4]

Penicillin and related contaminants can exist undetected in foods. It is not known to what degree penicillin in the food supply contributes to hives. However, hives and anaphylactic symptoms have been traced to penicillin in milk,[5] soft drinks,[6] and frozen dinners.[7] In one study of 245 patients with chronic hives, twenty-four percent had positive skin tests and twelve percent positive RAST (a blood test for allergies, see FOOD ALLERGIES for further information) tests for penicillin sensitivity.[8] Of the forty-two patients who were sensitive to penicillin, twenty-two improved clinically on a dairy-product-free diet, while only two out of forty patients with negative skin tests improved on the same diet. This study would seem to provide indirect evidence that penicillin in the food supply contributes to hives.

In an attempt to provide direct evidence, penicillin-contaminated pork was given to penicillin-allergic volunteers. No significant reactions were noted, other than transient pruritus in two volunteers.[9] Penicillin in milk appears to be more allergenic than penicillin in meat.[5] Presumably this is due to the fact that penicillin breaks down into more allergenic compounds in the milk.[5]

Aspirin

The frequency of aspirin sensitivity in patients with chronic hives is at least twenty times greater than in normal people without hives.[10–14] Hives is a more common indicator of aspirin sensitivity than is asthma (see ASTHMA). Studies (summarized in Table 2) have demonstrated that two to sixty-seven percent of patients with chronic hives are sensitive to aspirin. In addition to exerting direct effects, aspirin and other nonsteroidal anti-inflammatory drugs (NSAIDs) have been shown to dramatically increase gut permeability and increase the absorption of allergens from the digestive tract.[15,16]

The daily administration of 650 mg of aspirin for three weeks has been shown to desensitize patients with hives who have aspirin sensitivity. While taking the aspirin, patients also became nonresponsive to foods to which

TABLE 2 Provocation Tests with Food Additives in Chronic Hives

					PERCENT POSITIVE TESTS		
AUTHOR & REFERENCE	# PARTICIPANTS	TARTRAZINE	OTHER AZO DYES	ANNATTO	BENZOATES	BHA/BHT	ASPIRIN
August[17]	86	23	—	—	22	—	—
Doeglas[18]	23	30	—	—	23	—	24
Egyedi & Torok[19]	40	37	7	—	17	—	37
Fujita et al.[20]	57	—	—	—	23	—	—
Genton et al.[21]	17	59	—	—	30	—	54
Gibson & Clancy[22]	76	28	—	—	34	—	18
Hannuksela[23]	137	1	—	—	4	—	18
Juhlin[24]	330	—	18	11	11	15	10
Kaaber[25]	65	5	5	8	3	—	—
Kemp & Schembri[26]	23	7	—	—	7	—	36
Kirchoff et al.[27]	100	15	10	—	8	—	—
Lindemayr & Schmidt[28]	90	19	16	—	29	—	—
Merk & Goerz[29]	25	24	—	—	—	—	—
Meynadier et al.[30]	24	24	46	—	25	—	—
Michaelsson & Juhlin[31]	52	36	20	—	44	—	67
Mikkelsen et al.[32]	24	24	46	26	—	—	—
Neuman et al.[33]	30	23	—	—	—	—	—
Ortolani et al.[34]	75	13	—	—	21	10	43
Pigatto et al.[35]	61	10	—	—	—	15	—
Samter & Beers[36]	40	8	—	—	—	—	—
Settipane et al.[37]	38	8	—	—	—	—	—
Simon[38]	25	0	—	—	—	—	—
Supramaniam & Warner[39]	43	26	—	—	15	—	2
Thune & Granhold[40]	100	21	14	—	10	14	33
Warin & Smith[41]	108	12	—	—	16	—	—
Wutrich & Fabro[42]	306	6	—	—	6	—	—
Ziegler & Haustein[43]	100	10	—	—	—	—	—

they usually reacted (pineapple, milk, egg, cheese, fish, chocolate, pork, strawberries, and plums).[44] Others have noted this effect in patients with asthma, but they have also found that the effect disappears within nine days after stopping the treatment, suggesting the loss of effect or a possible placebo response.[45]

Food Allergy

Although any food can be the causative agent, the most common offenders are: milk, fish, meat, eggs, beans, and nuts.[1,4,46–50] Individuals with eczema or asthma are most likely to experience hives as a result of classic allergic (IgE-mediated) mechanisms.

A basic requirement for the development of a food allergy is the absorption of the allergen through the intestinal barrier. Several factors are known to significantly increase gut permeability, including compounds known as *vasoactive amines* ingested in foods or produced by bacterial action on essential amino acids, alcohol, NSAIDs, and possibly many food additives. In addition, several investigators have reported alterations in gastric acidity, *intestinal motility* (contractions of the intestine that propel the food through), and other functions of the digestive tract in up to eighty-five percent of patients with chronic hives.[51–55] These alterations may temporarily or permanently alter the barrier and immune function of the gut wall and predispose an individual to allergic reactions.

In one study of seventy-seven patients with chronic hives, twenty-four (thirty-one percent) were diagnosed as having *achlorhydria* (no gastric acid output), and forty-one (fifty-three percent) were shown to be *hypochlorhydric* (low gastric acid output).[56] Treatment with a hydrochloric acid (HCl) supplement and a vitamin B complex gave impressive clinical results, highlighting the importance of correcting any underlying digestive factor in the treatment of chronic hives. (See DIGESTION AND ELIMINATION for further discussion.)

Food Additives

Food additives are a major factor in many cases of chronic hives in children. Colorants (azo dyes), flavorings (salicylates, aspartame), preservatives (benzoates, nitrites, sorbic acid), antioxidants (hydroxytoluene, sulfite, gallate), and emulsifiers/stabilizers (polysorbates, vegetable gums) have all been shown to produce hives in sensitive individuals.[1,4,57]

The importance controlling food additives is well demonstrated in a recent study of sixty-four patients with common hives. Within two weeks on an additive-free diet, seventy-three percent of the patients had a significant reduction in their symptoms. The diet strictly forbade preservatives, dyes, and antioxidants. No fruits or sweeteners were allowed except honey. Rice, potatoes, and unprocessed cereals were allowed, as well as fresh milk.[58]

Tartrazine

In 1959, the azo dye tartrazine (FD & C Yellow #5) was the first food dye reported to induce hives.[59] Tartrazine is one of the most widely used colorants. It is added to almost every packaged food and to many drugs, including some antihistamines, antibiotics, steroids, and sedatives.[60] Reactions to this food additive are so common that its use has been banned in Sweden.[61]

In the United States, the average daily per capita consumption of certified dyes is 15 mg, of which eighty-five percent is tartrazine. Among children, consumption is usually much higher. Tartrazine sensitivity has been calculated as occurring in 0.1 percent of the population.[60]

Tartrazine sensitivity is extremely common (twenty to fifty percent) in individuals who are sensitive to aspirin.[4,60] Like aspirin, tartrazine is a known inducer of asthma, hives, and other allergic conditions, particularly in children.[60] Both compounds inhibit an enzyme (cyclo-oxygenase) that results in a higher production of allergic compounds known as leukotrienes in some individuals. These compounds are roughly 100 times more potent than histamine in producing an allergic reaction.

In addition, tartrazine, as well as benzoate and aspirin, increases the production of a compound (lymphokine leukocyte inhibitory factor) that results in an increase in the number of mast cells throughout the body.[62] Biopsy examination of patients with hives shows that over ninety-five percent have more mast cells than individuals without hives.[63]

Table 2 summarized the findings of studies that used provocation tests to determine sensitivity to tartrazine and other food additives in patients with hives. Results have shown that from five to ninety percent of participants were sensitive to tartrazine. Diets that eliminate tartrazine, as well as other azo dyes and food additives, have in many cases been shown to be of great benefit to sensitive individuals. These studies are summarized in Table 3.

Food Flavorings

Salicylates   A broad range of salicylic acid esters are used to flavor such foods as cake mixes, puddings, ice cream, chewing gum, and soft drinks. The mechanism of action of these agents is thought to be similar to that of aspirin.[4]

Salicylates (aspirin-like compounds) are also found naturally in many foodstuffs. It is estimated that average salicylate intake from foods is in the range of 10 to 200 mg/day.[68] Dietary salicylate may be a significant factor for aspirin-sensitive individuals. Most fruit,

TABLE 3 Response to a Diet Free of Added Dyes and Benzoates				
			PERCENT	
AUTHOR & REFERENCE NUMBER	**# OF PATIENTS**	**FREE OF HIVES**	**BETTER**	**SAME**
August[17]	22	45	23	32
Doeglas[64]	18	67	67	33
Gibson & Clancy[22]	65	75	15	10
Kaaber[25]	23	44	30	26
Kemp & Schembri[26]	18	39	39	22
Kirchoff et al.[27]	41	44	29	27
Lindemayr & Schmidt[28]	90	20	55	25
Meynadier et al.[30]	98	80	12	8
Michaelsson & Juhlin[31]	16	81	6	13
Ros et al.[65]	75	24	57	19
Thune & Granholt[40]	100	12	50	38
Valverde et al.[66]	258	62	22	16
Verschave et al.[67]	67	73	73	37
Warin & Smith[41]	58	75	75	25
Wuthrich & Fabro[42]	51	31	57	12

especially berries and dried fruits, contains salicylates; raisins and prunes have the highest amounts. Salicylates are also found in appreciable amounts in candies made of licorice and peppermint. Moderate levels of salicylate are found in nuts and seeds. Vegetables, legumes, grains, meat, poultry, fish, eggs, and dairy products typically contain insignificant levels of salicylates. Salicylate levels are especially high in some herbs and condiments, including: curry powder, paprika, thyme, dill, oregano, and turmeric. Although the intake of these herbs and spices is relatively small, they can make a significant contribution to dietary salicylate intake.[68]

Other Flavoring Agents   Other flavoring agents, such as cinnamon, vanilla, menthol, and other volatile compounds, may produce hives in some individuals.[4] The artificial sweetener aspartame (NutraSweet) has also been shown to induce hives.[69]

Food Preservatives

Benzoates   Benzoic acid and benzoates are the most commonly used food preservatives. Although the incidence of adverse reactions to these compounds in the general population is thought to be less than one percent, the frequency of positive challenges in patients with chronic hives varies from four to forty-four percent, as illustrated in Table 2.

Fish and shrimp frequently contain extremely high quantities of added benzoates. This may be one reason why adverse reactions to these foods are so common in patients with hives.

BHT and BHA   Butylated hydroxytoluene (BHT) and butylated hydroxyanisol (BHA) are the primary antioxidants used in prepared and packaged foods. Typically, fifteen percent of patients with chronic hives test positive to oral challenge with BHT.[29,49,54,57] The

use of chewing gum containing BHT was enough to induce hives in one patient.[70]

Sulfites   Like tartrazine, sulfites have been shown to induce asthma, hives, and angioedema in sensitive individuals.[61] The source may be varied, as sulfites are ubiquitous in foods and drugs. They are typically added to processed foods to prevent microbial spoilage and to keep them from browning or changing color. The earliest known use of sulfites was in the treatment of wines with sulfur dioxide by the Romans.

Sulfites are sprayed on fresh foods such as shrimp, fruits, and vegetables. They are also used as antioxidants and preservatives in many pharmaceuticals. Sulfites have caused such a wide range of health problems, including asthma and hives, that their use on fruits and vegetables has been banned in the United States. However, sulfites are still found in many other foods, especially wine and beer. Wine and beer drinkers typically consume up to 10 mg of sulfites per day even with moderate drinking (two to three glasses of wine or beer).

Normally, the enzyme sulfite oxidase metabolizes sulfites to safer sulfates, which are excreted in the urine. Those with a poorly functioning sulfoxidation system, however, have an increased ratio of sulfite to sulfate in their urine. Sulfite oxidase is dependent on the trace mineral molybdenum. Although most nutrition textbooks list molybdenum as an uncommon deficiency, an Austrian study of 1,750 patients found that 41.5 percent were molybdenum deficient.[71] Molybdenum deficiency may produce sulfite sensitivity. If so, supplementation (200 mcg per day) may be beneficial.

Food Emulsifiers and Stabilizers

A variety of compounds are used to emulsify and stabilize many commercial foods to ensure that the solids, oils, and liquids do not separate out. Most of the foods that contain these compounds are heterogeneous as they usually contain antioxidants, preservatives, and dyes as well. Polysorbate in ice cream has been reported to induce hives, and vegetable gums such as acacia, gum arabic, tragacanth, quince, and carrageenan may also induce hives in susceptible individuals.[4]

Infections

Infections are a major cause of hives in children.[1] In adults, immunological tolerance to many microorganisms apparently occurs due to repeated massive antigen exposure. The role of bacteria, viruses, and yeast (*Candida albicans*) in hives is briefly reviewed below. Chronic *Trichomonas* infections have also been found to cause hives.

Bacteria
Bacterial infections contribute to hives in two major settings: in acute streptococcal tonsillitis in children and in chronic dental infections in adults. In the first setting acute hives predominates while in the second, chronic hives predominates.[1]

Viruses
Hepatitis B is the most frequent cause of virally induced hives. One study found that 15.3 percent of patients with chronic hives had antihepatitis B surface antibodies.[72] Hives have also been strongly linked to infectious mononucleosis, and may develop several weeks before clinical manifestation. The incidence of hives during infectious mononucleosis is five percent.[1]

Candida albicans
The association between *Candida albicans* and chronic hives has been suggested in several clinical studies. The number of patients with chronic hives who react positively to an immediate skin test with candida antigens is nineteen to eighty-one percent, compared to ten to fifteen percent of people without hives.[31,73–75] It appears that sensitivity to *Candida albicans* is an important factor in at least twenty-five percent of patients who have chronic hives.[74] Approximately seventy percent of patients who have a positive skin reaction to *Candida* also react to oral provocation tests using foods prepared with yeasts.

Treatment with the drug nystatin has shown that elimination of the *Candida* organism can achieve a cure in a number of *Candida*-sensitive individuals. However, more patients responded to nystatin plus a "yeast-free" diet than to nystatin alone. The yeast-free diet excluded bread, buns, sausage, wine, beer, cider, grapes, raisins, vinegar, tomato, ketchup, pickles, and prepared foods containing yeasts.

In a study of forty-nine patients with positive sensitivity to *Candida*, nine responded to a three-week course of nystatin, while eighteen became symptom-free only after adopting the yeast-free diet in addition.[73] This would seem to support the importance of diet along with elimination of yeast.

Further support for the importance of diet can be found in a study of thirty-six patients with a positive skin-prick test to *Candida*. Only three patients became symptom-free from taking nystatin alone, compared with twenty-three who had diet therapy following the nystatin therapy.[75] Obviously the best approach is to focus on both the elimination of the yeast and avoidance of food allergies.

Stress

In one study involving 236 cases of chronic hives, psychological factors (stress) were reported to be the most frequent primary cause.[76] Stress appears to play an important role by decreasing intestinal secretory IgA levels.

In one study of fifteen patients who had chronic hives, relaxation therapy and hypnosis were shown to provide significant benefit.[77] Patients were given an audiotape and asked to use the relaxation techniques described on the tape at home. At a follow-up examination five to fourteen months after the initial session, six patients were free of hives and an additional seven reported improvement.

Therapeutic Considerations

The treatment goals in hives are straightforward—identify and eliminate the factors that are causing the release of histamine and other allergic compounds. As noted above, allergy to foods, food additives, and drugs, as well as stress are common causes of hives. The best diagnostic test (and therapy) appears to be an elimination diet.

The strictest elimination diets allow only water, lamb, rice, pears, and vegetables. Those foods most commonly associated with inducing hives (milk, eggs, chicken, fruits, nuts, and additives) should definitely be avoided. Foods containing vasoactive amines should be eliminated even if no direct allergy to them is noted. The primary foods to eliminate are cured meat, alcoholic beverages, cheese, chocolate, citrus fruits, and shellfish. Also, the importance of eliminating food additives cannot be overstated. If food additives do, in fact, increase the number of mast cells in the skin, they may also do the same in the small intestine, thereby greatly increasing the risk of developing a "leaky" gut.

In addition to an elimination diet, there are several other factors that can be helpful such as ultraviolet light therapy, vitamin C, vitamin B12, quercetin, and thyroid hormone. These factors are discussed following.

Ultraviolet Light Therapy

Ultraviolet light (e.g., sunlight or tanning beds) has been shown to be of some benefit to patients with chronic hives.[78,79] Both ultraviolet A (UVA), the nonburning type of sunlight, and ultraviolet B (UVB), the one that causes a sunburn, have been used. Patients with cold, cholinergic, and dermographic hives display the greatest therapeutic response.

Vitamin C

High dose vitamin C therapy may also help hives (as well as other allergic conditions) by lowering histamine levels.[80] Vitamin C exerts a number of effects against histamine. Specifically it prevents the secretion of histamine by white blood cells and increases the detoxification of histamine. Dosages of at least 2,000 mg daily appear necessary to produce these effects.

Vitamin B12

Vitamin B12 has been anecdotally reported to be of value in the treatment of acute and chronic hives.[81,82] Although blood levels of B12 are normal in most patients with hives, additional B12 appears to be of value.

Quercetin

The flavonoid *quercetin* inhibits both the manufacture and release of histamine and other allergic/inflammatory mediators by mast cells and basophils.[83,84] These effects suggest that quercetin may be very useful in treating hives. This possibility is strengthened by the observation that the drug sodium cromoglycate, a compound similar to quercetin, offers excellent protection against the development of hives in response to ingested food allergens.[85]

Thyroid

One study reported that thyroid hormone replacement therapy dramatically relieved chronic hives in patients who had normal thyroid function but had evidence of antibodies attacking the thyroid gland (antimicrosomal and antithyroglobulin antibodies).[86] In seven patients with chronic hives, five were started on thyroid hormone and two had their existing dosages increased. Their hives resolved within two to four weeks, at which time the thyroid therapy was discontinued. In five patients, the symptoms returned within four weeks, then resolved within four weeks of resuming the hormone therapy. The message here is that thyroid hormone therapy is essential in an individual with hives who shows any other evidence of low thyroid function (see HYPOTHYROIDISM) or the presence of antithyroid antibodies.

TREATMENT SUMMARY

The first goal of treatment is to identify and control all of the factors that promote the hives. Acute hives is usually a self-limiting disease, especially once the eliciting agent has been removed or reduced. Chronic hives also responds to the removal of the eliciting agent(s).

Diet

An elimination diet is of utmost importance in the treatment of chronic hives (see FOOD ALLERGY). The diet should not only eliminate suspected allergens, but also all food additives.

Nutritional Supplements

- Vitamin C: 1 g three times per day
- Vitamin B12: 1,000 mcg per day orally, or by injection once per week
- Quercetin: 200–400 mg twenty minutes before each meal

Psychological Measures

Perform relaxation techniques daily. Listening to audiotaped relaxation programs may be an appropriate way to induce the desired state.

Physical Medicine

Sunbathe daily for fifteen to twenty minutes or use a UVA solarium, especially in cases of chronic physical urticaria. Obviously sunbathing is contraindicated in solar urticaria.

Hypoglycemia

Blood glucose level below 50 mg/dl

A normal response curve during the first two to three hours of a glucose tolerance test, followed by a decrease of 20 mg or more below the fasting glucose level during the final hours of the test, with symptoms developing during the decrease

ypoglycemia refers to low blood sugar. Normally, the body maintains blood sugar levels within a narrow range through the coordinated effort of several glands and their hormones. If these control mechanisms are disrupted, hypoglycemia (low blood sugar) or diabetes (high blood sugar) may result.

The beta-cells of the pancreas respond to the rise in blood glucose levels after meals by secreting the hormone *insulin,* which lowers blood glucose levels by increasing the rate at which glucose is taken up by cells throughout the body. Declines in blood glucose levels, such as occur during food deprivation or exercise, cause the release of the hormone *glucagon* by the alpha cells of the pancreas. Glucagon stimulates the release of glucose stored in body tissues, especially the liver, as *glycogen.* Rapidly falling blood sugar levels, anger, fright, or stress may stimulate the release of *epinephrine* and *corticosteroids* by the adrenal glands. These hormones provide more rapid breakdown of stored glucose for extra energy during a crisis or an increased need.

Americans over-stress these control mechanisms through improper diet and lifestyle. As a result, diabetes and hypoglycemia are common diseases.

Hypoglycemia is divided into two main categories: *reactive hypoglycemia* and *fasting hypoglycemia.* Reactive hypoglycemia, the most common, is characterized by the development of symptoms of hypoglycemia three to five hours after a meal. Reactive hypoglycemia may also result from taking drugs commonly used in the treatment of diabetes (see DIABETES).

Fasting hypoglycemia is rare, as it usually appears only in severe disease states such as pancreatic tumors, extensive liver damage, prolonged starvation, and various cancers, or as a result of excessive injections of insulin in diabetics.

Because glucose is the primary fuel for the brain, low levels affect the brain first. Symptoms of hypoglycemia can range from mild to severe, including: headache; depression, anxiety, irritability, and other psychological disturbances; blurred vision; excessive sweating; mental confusion; incoherent speech; bizarre behavior; and convulsions.

Diagnostic Considerations

The standard methods of diagnosing hypoglycemia, as well as diabetes, involve the measurement of blood glucose levels. The normal fasting blood glucose level is between 70 and 105 mg/dl. A fasting blood glucose measurement greater than 140 mg/dl on two separate occasions is diagnostic of diabetes.

At levels below 50 mg/dl, the diagnosis is fasting hypoglycemia.[1]

A more functional test of blood sugar control is the oral glucose tolerance test (GTT). The GTT is used in the diagnosis of both reactive hypoglycemia and diabetes, although it is rarely required for the latter. This test is described in DIABETES, along with even more sensitive tests, such as the glucose-insulin tolerance test (G-ITT).[2-5]

Another laboratory parameter that can aid in the diagnosis of hypoglycemia, especially a borderline case, is the *hypoglycemic index*. This value is determined by calculating the fall in blood glucose levels during the ninety-minute period before the lowest point, divided by the value of the lowest point. A hypoglycemic index greater than 0.8 usually indicates reactive hypoglycemia.

When all is considered (especially cost), assessing symptoms remains the most useful way to diagnose hypoglycemia in many cases. In general, when symptoms appear three to four hours after eating and disappear with the ingestion of food, a diagnosis of hypoglycemia should be considered. The questionnaire below is an excellent screening method for hypoglycemia.

HYPOGLYCEMIA QUESTIONNAIRE

	No	Mild	Moderate	Severe
Craving for sweets	0	1	2	3
Irritability if a meal is missed	0	1	2	3
Tired or weak feelings if a meal is missed	0	1	2	3
Dizziness when standing suddenly	0	1	2	3
Frequent headaches	0	1	2	3
Poor memory (forgetfulness) or concentration	0	1	2	3
Tiredness an hour or so after eating	0	1	2	3
Heart palpitations	0	1	2	3
Occasional shakiness	0	1	2	3
Afternoon fatigue	0	1	2	3
Occasional blurry vision	0	1	2	3
Depression or mood swings	0	1	2	3
Overweight	0	1	2	3
Frequent anxiety or nervousness	0	1	2	3

Total: _____

Scoring:
Less than 5 = hypoglycemia is not a likely factor
6–15 = hypoglycemia is a likely factor
Greater than 15 = hypoglycemia is extremely likely

Hypoglycemia: A Historical Perspective

In the 1970s, hypoglycemia was a popular self-diagnosis for a long list of symptoms; every symptom on the hypoglycemia questionnaire above was linked to hypoglycemia. Although all of these symptoms may be due to hypoglycemia, there are obviously other causes in many cases. The tremendous public interest in hypoglycemia and sugar intake was fueled by a number of popular books (such as *Sugar Blues* by William Duffy, *Hope for Hypoglycemia* by Broda Barnes, and *Sweet and Dangerous* by John Yudkin). The popularity of these books and the diagnosis of hypoglycemia was met with much skepticism in the medical community. Editorials in the *Journal of the American Medical Association* and *New England Journal of Medicine* during the 1970s denounced this public interest in hypoglycemia and tried to invalidate the concept of hypoglycemia.[6,7]

Research in the past decade has provided an ever-increasing amount of new information on the role that refined carbohydrates and faulty blood sugar control play in many disease processes. New terminology and descriptions are now used to describe the complex hormonal fluxes that are largely a result of the ingestion of too much refined carbohydrate. For example, the term *syndrome X* has been introduced to describe a cluster of abnormalities that owe their existence largely to a high intake of refined carbohydrates, leading to the development of hypoglycemia, excessive insulin secretion, and glucose intolerance, followed by diminished insulin sensitivity leading to high blood pressure, elevated cholesterol levels, obesity, and, ultimately, Type II diabetes. Syndrome X is discussed in greater detail later in this chapter.

Hypoglycemia is, without question, a valid clinical entity. There exists a substantial amount of information that hypoglycemia is caused by an excessive intake of refined carbohydrates.[8,9] While most medical and health organizations, as well as the U.S. government, have recommended that no more than ten percent of a person's total caloric intake be derived from refined sugars that are added to foods, added sugar accounts for roughly thirty percent of the total calories consumed by most Americans.[10] The average American consumes over 100 pounds of sucrose and 40 pounds of corn syrup each year. This sugar addiction plays a major role in the high prevalence of poor health and chronic disease in the United States.

Consequences of Hypoglycemia

The brain is dependent on glucose as an energy source. When glucose levels are low, as occurs during hypoglycemia, the brain dysfunction results in dizziness, headache, clouding of vision, blunted mental acuity,

QUICK REVIEW

- Hypoglycemia is a complex set of symptoms caused by faulty carbohydrate metabolism induced by a diet too high in refined sugars.
- When all is considered (especially cost), assessing symptoms remains the most useful way to diagnose hypoglycemia in many cases.
- There exists a substantial amount of information that hypoglycemia is caused by an excessive intake of refined carbohydrates.

- *Syndrome X* has been introduced to describe a cluster of abnormalities that owe their existence largely to a high intake of refined carbohydrates, leading to the development of hypoglycemia, excessive insulin secretion, and glucose intolerance, followed by diminished insulin sensitivity leading to high blood pressure, elevated cholesterol levels, obesity, and, ultimately, Type II diabetes.
- When glucose levels are low, as occurs during hypoglycemia, it can result in dizziness, headache, clouding of vision,

emotional instability, confusion, and abnormal behavior. The association between hypoglycemia and impaired mental function is well-known. What is not as well-known is the effect that hypoglycemia plays in various psychological disorders.

For example, despite numerous studies of depressed individuals showing a high percentage of abnormal glucose or insulin tolerance tests, rarely is hypoglycemia considered and rarely are depressed individuals prescribed dietary therapy.[11,12] There is no explanation for this oversight by so many physicians, especially since dietary therapy (usually simply eliminating refined carbohydrate from the diet) is occasionally all that is needed to produce improvement in patients who suffer from depression due to reactive hypoglycemia.

Aggressive and Criminal Behavior

There is a strong, yet controversial, link between hypoglycemia and aggressive or criminal behavior. Several controlled studies of psychiatric patients and habitually violent and impulsive criminals have shown that reactive hypoglycemia (as determined by an oral glucose tolerance test) is a common finding.[13,14] Furthermore, during the GTT, abnormal and sometimes emotionally explosive behavior is often observed in individuals very sensitive to low blood sugar. In one study, reactive hypoglycemia was shown to induce fire-setting behavior in arsonists.[15]

Several large studies, involving over six thousand inmates in ten penal institutions in three states, have now evaluated the effect of dietary intervention—specifically, the elimination of refined sugar—on antisocial or aggressive behavior.[16,17]

In the first study, 174 incarcerated juvenile delinquents were placed on a sugar-restricted diet, while another 102 juvenile offenders were placed on a control diet.[16] During the two-year study, the number of incidents of antisocial behavior was reduced by forty-five percent in the treatment group. The most

- blunted mental acuity, emotional instability, confusion, and abnormal behavior.
- Several controlled studies of psychiatric patients and habitually violent and impulsive criminals have shown that hypoglycemia is a common finding.
- Hypoglycemia has been shown to be a common precipitating factor in migraine headaches since 1933.
- Dietary carbohydrates play a central role in the cause, prevention, and treatment of hypoglycemia.
- Problems with carbohydrates begin when they are refined, which strips them of associated nutrients and increases their rate of absorption.
- Chromium is vital to proper blood sugar control, as it functions in the body as a key constituent of the *glucose tolerance factor.*
- Alcohol consumption severely stresses blood sugar control and is often a contributing factor to hypoglycemia.

significant changes were in the reduction of assaults (eighty-three percent), theft (seventy-seven percent), "horseplay" (sixty-five percent), and refusal to obey an order (fifty-five percent). Antisocial behavior changed the most in those charged with assault, robbery, rape, aggravated assault, auto theft, vandalism, child molestation, arson, and possession of a deadly weapon.

In the largest study, 3,999 incarcerated juveniles were studied over a period of two years.[17] This study limited the dietary revisions to replacing sugary soft drinks with fruit juices, and high-sugar snacks with non-refined carbohydrates snacks (for example, replacing a candy bar with popcorn). When the 1,121 young men on the sugar-restricted diet were compared to the 884 on the control diet, there were significant differences. In the sugar-restricted group, suicide attempts were reduced one hundred percent; the need for restraints to prevent self-injury was reduced seventy-five percent; disruptive behavior was reduced forty-two percent; and assaults and fights were reduced twenty-five percent. Interestingly, the dietary changes did not seem to effect the behavior of female subjects. This lack of effect seems to indicate that men may react to hypoglycemia in a different manner than women. From an anthropological and evolutionary view, this makes sense; low blood sugar levels were undoubtedly an internal signal for men to hunt for food.

The link between hypoglycemia and aggressive behavior also extends to men without a history of criminal activity. In one study, a glucose tolerance test was given to a group of men who did not have a history of aggressive behavior or hypoglycemia.[9] In these subjects, a significant correlation was found between the tendency to become mildly hypoglycemic and scores on questionnaires used to measure aggression. These results in-

dicated that aggressiveness often coincided with hypoglycemia.

Premenstrual Syndrome

Premenstrual syndrome (PMS) is a recurrent condition of women, characterized by troublesome, yet often ill-defined, symptoms that usually appear seven to fourteen days before menstruation. The syndrome affects about one-third of women between thirty and forty years of age, about ten percent of whom may have a significantly debilitating form. Guy Abraham, M.D., an authority on PMS, attempted to clarify the different forms of PMS by subdividing them into four distinct subgroups: A, C, D, and H.[18] Each subgroup is linked to specific symptoms, hormonal patterns, and metabolic abnormalities. PMS-C is associated with hypoglycemia, increased appetite, craving for sweets, headache, fatigue, fainting spells, and heart palpitations.[19] For more information, see PREMENSTRUAL SYNDROME.

Migraine Headaches

Migraine headaches are probably caused by excessive dilation (expansion) of a blood vessel in the head (see MIGRAINE HEADACHE). Hypoglycemia has been shown to be a common precipitating factor in migraine headaches since 1933.[20] Several studies have found that eliminating refined sugar from the diet of migraine sufferers who have confirmed hypoglycemia results in significant improvement. In one study of forty-eight migraine sufferers with reactive hypoglycemia, twenty-seven (fifty-six percent) showed a greater-than-seventy-five-percent improvement in symptoms, seventeen (thirty-five percent) showed a greater-than-fifty-percent improvement, and four (eight percent) showed a greater-than-twenty-five-percent improvement.[21]

Atherosclerosis, Intermittent Claudication, and Angina

There is substantial evidence that reactive hypoglycemia or impaired glucose tolerance is a significant factor in the development of atherosclerosis. Although a high sugar intake leads to elevations in triglyceride and cholesterol levels, the real culprit may be the elevations of insulin.[22] Abnormal glucose tolerance tests and elevations in insulin secretion are common findings in patients with heart disease.[23,24]

In addition to playing a role in atherosclerosis, high sugar consumption and reactive hypoglycemia can be a cause of angina and intermittent claudication (a painful cramp occurring in the calf muscle caused by lack of oxygen).[25,26]

Syndrome X

Syndrome X is a term used to describe a set of cardiovascular risk factors, including glucose or insulin disturbances, high blood cholesterol and triglyceride levels, elevated blood pressure, and android obesity. Other terms to describe this syndrome include "the metabolic cardiovascular risk syndrome" (MCVS), "Reaven's syndrome," "insulin-resistance syndrome," and "atherothrombogenic syndrome." While there is a push to abandon the term "syndrome X," it nevertheless persists.[27,28]

The underlying metabolic denominator in syndrome X is elevated insulin levels. There is little doubt about what contributes to these elevations: an elevated intake of refined carbohydrates. An increased intake of simple sugars leads first to hypoglycemia and later to diabetes. The results from a recent twenty-five-year study add support to the contention that prolonged consumption of refined sugars, and the resulting elevations in insulin, eventually leads to Type II diabetes. In the study, the development of Type II diabetes was shown to be preceded by elevations of serum insulin values and insulin insensitivity.[3] In most cases, these defects presented themselves decades before the development of diabetes.

Hypoglycemia, increased insulin secretion, syndrome X, and Type II diabetes can be viewed as a progression of the same illness—an attempt by the body to adjust to the "Western Diet." The human body was not designed to handle the amount of refined sugar, salt, saturated fats, and other harmful food compounds that many people in the United States and other Western countries feed it. The result is that a metabolic syndrome emerges: elevated insulin levels, obesity, elevated blood cholesterol and triglyceride levels, and high blood pressure.

Therapeutic Considerations

The therapeutic goals in hypoglycemia are straightforward: reestablish proper blood sugar control. This goal is achieved by focusing on dietary factors.

Dietary Factors

Diet control is fundamental to the successful treatment of hypoglycemia. Basically, the dietary guidelines given in DIABETES apply here as well. A diet high in fiber and complex carbohydrates, and low in sugar, has substantial support and validation in the scientific literature as the diet of choice in the treatment of both diabetes and hypoglycemia.[29]

Dietary carbohydrates play a central role in the cause, prevention, and treatment of hypoglycemia. Simple carbohydrates, or sugars, are quickly absorbed by the body, resulting in a rapid elevation in blood sugar level, stimulating a corresponding excessive elevation in serum insulin levels. It is thought by some that the natural, simple sugars found in fruits and vegetables have an advantage over sucrose and other refined sugars, in that they are balanced by a wide range of nutrients which aid in the utilization of the sugars. However, it is more significant that the sugars in whole, unprocessed foods are more slowly absorbed because they are contained within cells and are associated with fiber and other food elements.

Problems with carbohydrates begin when they are refined, which strips them of associated nutrients and increases their rate of absorption. Virtually all of the vitamin and trace-mineral content has been removed from white sugar, white breads and pastries, and many breakfast cereals. When high-sugar foods are eaten alone, blood sugar levels rise quickly, producing a strain on blood sugar control. Eating foods high in simple sugars in any form—sucrose, honey, or maple syrup—is harmful to blood sugar control. Large amounts of fruit juice and even vegetable juice may be a problem for hypoglycemics, as the cell disruption characteristic of juicing increases the absorption rate of the sugars in the juices.

Currently, more than half of the carbohydrates consumed in the United States are in the form of sugars added to processed foods as sweetening agents.[10] Read food labels carefully for clues to sugar content. Beware of the variety of words used to describe refined simple carbohydrates: sucrose, glucose, maltose, lactose, fructose, corn syrup, or white grape juice concentrate may appear on the label.

A Closer Look at Simple Carbohydrates

Glucose is not particularly sweet-tasting compared to fructose and sucrose. It is found in abundant amounts in fruits, honey, sweet corn, and most root vegetables. Glucose is also the primary repeating sugar unit of most complex carbohydrates.

Fructose, or fruit sugar, is the primary carbohydrate in many fruits, maple syrup, and honey. Fructose is very sweet—roughly one-and-one-half times sweeter than sucrose. Although fructose has the same chemical formula as glucose, its structure is quite different. In order to be utilized by the body, fructose must be converted to glucose in the liver.

Many physicians have recommended that individuals with diabetes or hypoglycemia should avoid fruits and fructose. However, recent research challenges this idea. Fructose does not cause a rapid rise in blood sugar levels. Since fructose must be changed to glucose in the liver in order to be utilized by the body, blood glucose levels do not rise as rapidly after fructose consumption, as compared to other simple sugars. For example, the ingestion of sucrose results in an immediate elevation in the blood sugar level. While most diabetics and hypoglycemics cannot tolerate sucrose, most can tolerate moderate amounts of fruits and fructose without loss of blood sugar control. In fact, fructose and fruits are not only much better tolerated than white bread and other refined carbohydrates, they produce less sharp elevations in blood sugar levels compared to most sources of complex carbohydrates (starch).[30] As a bonus, fructose has actually been shown to enhance the sensitivity to insulin.[30,31]

Regular fruit consumption may also help control sugar cravings and promote weight loss in overweight individuals. While studies have shown aspartame (NutraSweet), glucose, and sucrose to increase the appetite, fructose has actually been shown in several double-blind studies to decrease the amount of calories and fat consumed. Typically, study subjects were given food or drink containing equivalent caloric amounts of fructose or another sweetener thirty minutes to two-and-one-half hours before allowing them to consume as much food as they desire at a dinner buffet. Consistently, subjects who received the fructose-sweetened food or drink consumed substantially fewer calories and less fat than the subjects who received aspartame, sucrose, or glucose.[32–34]

The Glycemic Index

The *glycemic index* (not to be confused with the hypoglycemic index discussed earlier in this chapter) was developed in 1981 to express the rise in blood glucose level after eating a particular food.[35] The standard value of 100 is based on the rise seen with the ingestion of glucose. The glycemic index ranges from about 20 for fructose and whole barley to about 98 for a baked potato. The insulin response to carbohydrate-containing foods is similar to the rise in blood sugar level.

The glycemic index is used as a guideline for dietary recommendations for people with either diabetes or hypoglycemia. People who have blood sugar problems are advised to avoid foods with high values, and to choose carbohydrate-containing foods with lower values. However, the glycemic index should not be the only dietary guideline. For example, while high-fat foods such as ice cream and sausage may have a low glycemic index, these foods are not good choices for people with hy-

TABLE 1 Glycemic Index of Same Calorie-content Amounts of Some Common Foods[36]	
FOOD	**GLYCEMIC INDEX**
Sugars	
Glucose	100
Maltose	105
Honey	75
Sucrose	60
Fructose	20
Fruits	
Apples	39
Bananas	62
Oranges	40
Orange juice	46
Raisins	64
Vegetables	
Beets	64
Carrot, raw	31
Carrot, cooked	36
Potato, baked	98
Potato (new), boiled	70
Grains	
Bran cereal	51
Bread, white	69
Bread, whole grain	72
Corn	59
Cornflakes	80
Oatmeal	49
Pasta	45
Rice	70
Rice, puffed	95
Wheat cereal	67
Legumes	
Beans	31
Lentils	29
Peas	39
Other Foods	
Ice cream	36
Milk	34
Nuts	13
Sausages	28

poglycemia or diabetes; a diet high in fat has been shown to impair glucose tolerance.

The Importance of Fiber

Population studies, as well as clinical and experimental data, show that blood sugar disorders are clearly related to inadequate dietary fiber intake.[10,37] These results indicate that, while the intake of refined sugars should be curtailed, the intake of complex carbohydrate sources that are rich in fiber should be increased.

The term *dietary fiber* refers to the components of the plant cell wall as well as the indigestible residues from plant foods. Different types of fiber possess different actions. The water-soluble forms exert the most beneficial effects on blood sugar control. Included in this category are hemicelluloses, mucilages, gums, and pectin substances. These types of fiber are capable of: slowing the digestion and absorption of carbohydrates, thereby preventing rapid rises in blood sugar; increasing cell sensitivity to insulin, thereby preventing the excessive secretion of insulin; and improving uptake of glucose by the liver and other tissues, thereby preventing a sustained elevation of blood sugar.

The majority of fiber in most plant cell walls is water-soluble. Particularly good sources of water-soluble fiber are legumes, oat bran, nuts, seeds, psyllium-seed husks, pears, apples, and most vegetables. In order to obtain adequate levels of dietary fiber, consume a large amount of plant foods. A daily intake of 50 grams of fiber (See A HEALTH-PROMOTING DIET Table 1 for a list of fiber content of food) is a healthful goal.

Chromium

Chromium is vital to proper blood sugar control, as it functions in the body as a key constituent of the *glucose tolerance factor*. Without chromium, insulin's action is blocked and glucose levels are elevated. A chromium deficiency may be an underlying contributing factor in the tremendous number of U.S. cases of hypoglycemia, diabetes, and obesity.[38] There is evidence that marginal chromium deficiency is common in the United States.[39]

In one double-blind crossover study of eight female patients, 200 mcg of chromium (as chromium chloride), given twice daily for three months, alleviated hypoglycemic symptoms and improved the results of glucose tolerance tests.[39]

Alcohol

Alcohol consumption severely stresses blood sugar control and is often a contributing factor to hypoglycemia. Alcohol induces reactive hypoglycemia by interfering with normal glucose utilization and increasing the secretion of insulin. The resultant drop in blood sugar produces a craving for food, particularly foods that quickly elevate blood sugar levels, as well as a craving for more alcohol. The increased sugar consumption aggravates the reactive hypoglycemia, particularly in the presence of more alcohol, again due to alcohol-induced impairment of normal glucose utilization and increased secretion of insulin.

Hypoglycemia is a significant complication of acute and chronic alcohol abuse. Hypoglycemia aggravates the mental and emotional problems of the alcoholic and the withdrawing alcoholic with such symptoms as sweating, tremor, rapid heart beat, anxiety, hunger, dizziness, headache, visual disturbance, decreased mental function, confusion, and depression.[1]

Although acute alcohol ingestion induces hypoglycemia, in the long run it leads to hyperglycemia and diabetes. Eventually, the body becomes insensitive to the augmented insulin release caused by the alcohol. In addition, alcohol itself can cause insulin resistance even in healthy individuals.[40] There is also evidence from large population studies that alcohol intake is strongly correlated with diabetes.[10,41] The higher the alcohol intake, the more likely it is that an individual will have diabetes.

Exercise

An appropriate exercise training program is an important part of a hypoglycemia treatment and prevention plan. Regular exercise has been well-documented to prevent Type II diabetes, and regular exercise improves many aspects of glucose metabolism, including enhancing insulin sensitivity and improving glucose tolerance in existing diabetics. Some of the effects of exercise on blood sugar control may stem from the fact that exercise increases tissue chromium concentrations.[42]

TREATMENT SUMMARY

The primary treatment of hypoglycemia is the use of dietary therapy to stabilize blood sugar levels. Reactive hypoglycemia is not a disease; it is simply a complex set of symptoms caused by faulty carbohydrate metabolism induced by a diet too high in refined carbohydrates.

Diet

All simple, processed, and concentrated carbohydrates must be avoided, while the consumption of complex-carbohydrate, high-fiber foods should be emphasized. Legumes should be consumed regularly. Frequent small meals may be more effective in stabilizing blood sugar levels. Alcohol consumption must be avoided, as it can cause hypoglycemia.

Nutritional Supplements

The recommendations for the daily intake levels of vitamins and minerals given in SUPPLEMENTARY MEASURES are especially important in treating hypoglycemia, as there are many essential nutrients critical to proper carbohydrate metabolism. The recommended levels are most easily attained by taking a multiple-vitamin-and-mineral formula. Chromium (200–400 mcg per day) is critically important.

Exercise

Follow an exercise program that elevates your heart rate to at least sixty percent of maximum for one-half hour three times per week. For a full discussion, see A HEALTHY LIFESTYLE.

Hypothyroidism

. . . .

Depression

Difficulty in losing weight

Dry skin

Headaches

Lethargy or fatigue

Menstrual problems

Recurrent infections

Sensitivity to cold

Hypothyroidism refers to low thyroid gland function. The thyroid gland is situated in the front of the neck, just below the larynx (voice box). Since the hormones of the thyroid gland regulate metabolism in every cell of the body, a deficiency of thyroid hormones can affect virtually all body functions. The severity of symptoms in adults ranges from extremely mild deficiency states that are barely detectable (subclinical hypothyroidism) to severe deficiency states that are life-threatening (myxedema).[1-4]

A deficiency of thyroid hormone may be due to defective hormone synthesis or to lack of stimulation by the pituitary gland. The *pituitary gland* is responsible for secreting a hormone that stimulates the thyroid gland: *thyroid-stimulating hormone* (TSH). When thyroid hormone levels in the blood are low, the pituitary secretes TSH. If a blood test shows that thyroid hormone levels are lowered and TSH levels are elevated in the blood, it usually indicates defective thyroid hormone synthesis. This situation is termed *primary hypothyroidism*. If TSH levels are low and thyroid hormone levels are also

low, this indicates that the pituitary gland is responsible for the low thyroid function. This situation is termed *secondary hypothyroidism.*

Most estimates of the rate of hypothyroidism are based on low levels of thyroid hormone in the blood. As already mentioned, this may mean that a large number of mild cases of hypothyroidism go undetected. Nevertheless, using blood levels of thyroid hormones as the criterion, it is estimated that between one and four percent of the adult population has moderate to severe hypothyroidism, and another ten to twelve percent has mild hypothyroidism.[1-7] The rate of hypothyroidism increases steadily with advancing age.

Some writers of popular books estimate that the rate of hypothyroidism in the general adult population is approximately forty percent, based on medical history, physical examination, basal body temperatures, and blood thyroid levels.[8,9] It is likely that the true rate of hypothyroidism using these criteria is somewhere near twenty-five percent of the population, or about twenty percent of women and five percent of men—an estimate a little more conservative, and probably more realistic.

Causes of Hypothyroidism

About ninety-five percent of all cases of hypothyroidism are primary. In other words, the problem is with the thyroid gland and not the pituitary gland. Most patients with hypothyroidism are not born with it; they develop it as adults. In the past, the most common cause of hypothyroidism was iodine deficiency. Iodine is a trace element required in the manufacture of thyroid hormone. Specifically, the thyroid gland adds iodine to the amino acid tyrosine to create the thyroid hormones.

Iodine deficiency leads to hypothyroidism and/or the development of an enlarged thyroid gland, commonly referred to as a *goiter*. When the level of iodine is low in the diet and blood, it causes the cells of the thyroid gland to become quite large; eventually the entire gland swells at the base of the neck.

Goiters are estimated to affect over two hundred million people worldwide. In all but four percent of these cases, the goiter is caused by an iodine deficiency. Iodine deficiency is now quite rare in the United States and other industrialized countries due to the addition of iodine to table salt. Adding iodine to table salt began in Michigan, where in 1924 the goiter rate was an incredible forty-seven percent.

Few people in the United States are now considered iodine-deficient, yet some people still develop goiters. The goiter in these people is probably a result of the excessive ingestion of certain foods that block iodine utilization. These foods are known as *goitrogens*, and include such foods as turnips,

cabbage, mustard, cassava root, soybeans, peanuts, pine nuts, and millet. Cooking usually inactivates goitrogens.

Currently, the most frequent cause of hypothyroidism in the United States is an autoimmune disease known as Hashimoto's disease. In this disease, antibodies are formed that bind to the thyroid and prevent the manufacture of sufficient levels of thyroid hormone. In addition to binding to thyroid tissue, antibodies may also bind to the adrenal glands, pancreas, and acid-producing cells of the stomach (*parietal cells*).

Manifestations of Adult Hypothyroidism

Since thyroid hormones affect every cell of the body, a deficiency will usually result in a large number of signs and symptoms. The following is a brief review of the common manifestations of hypothyroidism on several body systems.

Metabolic

A lack of thyroid hormones leads to a general decrease in the rate of utilization of fat, protein, and carbohydrate. Moderate weight gain combined with sensitivity to cold weather (demonstrated by cold hands or feet) is a common finding.

Cholesterol and triglyceride levels are increased in even the mildest forms of hypothyroidism.[10] This elevation greatly increases the risk of serious cardiovascular disease. Studies have shown an increased rate of heart disease due to atherosclerosis in individuals with hypothyroidism.[11,12]

Hypothyroidism also leads to increases in capillary permeability and slow lymphatic drainage. This often results in swelling of tissue (*edema*).

Endocrine

A variety of hormonal symptoms can exist in hypothyroidism. Perhaps the most common is a loss of libido (sexual drive) in men and menstrual abnormalities in women.

Women with mild hypothyroidism have prolonged and heavy menstrual bleeding, with a shorter menstrual cycle (the time from the start of one period to the next). Infertility may also be a problem. If the hypothyroid woman does become pregnant, miscarriages, premature deliveries, and stillbirths are common. Rarely does a pregnancy terminate in normal labor and delivery in the hypothyroid woman.

Skin, Hair, and Nails

Dry, rough skin covered with fine, superficial scales is seen in most hypothyroid individuals, while their hair is coarse, dry, and brittle. Hair loss can be quite severe. The nails become thin and brittle and typically show transverse grooves.

Psychological

The brain appears to be quite sensitive to low levels of thyroid hormone. Depression, weakness, and fatigue are usually the first symptoms of hypothyroidism.[13–15] Later, the hypothyroid individual will have difficulty concentrating and become extremely forgetful.

Muscular and Skeletal

Muscle weakness and joint stiffness are a predominant feature of hypothyroidism.[16] Some individuals with hypothyroidism may also experience muscle and joint pain and tenderness.[17]

Cardiovascular

Hypothyroidism is thought to predispose one to hardening of the arteries (atherosclerosis) due to the increase in cholesterol and triglyceride levels.[12–14] Hypothyroidism can also cause hypertension, reduce the function of the heart, and reduce heart rate.

Other Manifestations

Shortness of breath, constipation, and impaired kidney function are some of the other common features of hypothyroidism.

Diagnostic Considerations

There is still controversy over the manner of diagnosing hypothyroidism. Before the use of blood measurements, it was common to diagnose hypothyroidism based on *basal body*

QUICK REVIEW

- Since thyroid hormones affect every cell of the body, a deficiency will usually result in a large number of signs and symptoms.
- Depression, weakness, and fatigue are usually the first symptoms of hypothyroidism.
- The medical treatment of hypothyroidism, in all but its mildest forms, in-

volves the use of desiccated thyroid or synthetic thyroid hormone.
- You can support the thyroid gland by avoiding *goitrogens* (foods that impair the use of iodine) and insuring adequate intake of key nutrients that are required for the manufacture of thyroid hormone.
- In very mild cases, health-food-store thyroid products may provide some benefit.

temperature (the temperature of the body at rest) and Achilles reflex time (reflexes are slowed in hypothyroidism). With the advent of sophisticated laboratory measurement of thyroid hormones in the blood, these "functional" tests of thyroid function fell by the wayside. However, it is now known that the blood tests are not sensitive enough to diagnose milder forms of hypothyroidism in all cases. As mild hypothyroidism is the most common form of hypothyroidism, many people with hypothyroidism are going undiagnosed.

Undiagnosed hypothyroidism is a serious concern, as failure to treat an underlying condition such as hypothyroidism will reduce the effectiveness of nutritional therapies. For example, in most cases, zinc, vitamin A, and essential fatty acids are effective in relieving dry, scaly skin. However, if a person had hypothyroidism, no improvement would occur. It is critical that thyroid function be evaluated, as hypothyroidism is thought to be an underlying factor in a large number of diseases.

Taking Your Basal Body Temperature

The basal body temperature is perhaps the most sensitive functional test of thyroid function.[8,9] Your body temperature reflects your metabolic rate, which is largely determined by hormones secreted by the thyroid gland. The function of the thyroid gland can be determined by simply measuring your basal body temperature. All you need is a thermometer.

Procedure

1. Shake down the thermometer to below 95 degrees Fahrenheit and place it by your bed before going to sleep at night.

2. On waking, place the thermometer in your armpit for a full ten minutes. It is important to move as little as possible; lying and resting with your eyes closed is best. Do not get up until the ten-minute test is completed.

3. After ten minutes, read and record the temperature and date.

4. Record the temperature for at least three mornings (preferably at the same time of day) and give the information to your physician. Menstruating women must perform the test on the second, third, and fourth days of menstruation. Men and postmenopausal women can perform the test at any time.

Interpretation

Your basal body temperature should be between 97.6 and 98.2 degrees Fahrenheit. Low basal body temperatures are quite common and may reflect hypothyroidism. Common signs and symptoms of hypothyroidism are: low basal body temperature, depression, difficulty in losing weight, dry skin, headaches, lethargy or fatigue, menstrual problems, recurrent infections, constipation, and sensitivity to cold.

High basal body temperatures (above 98.6 degrees Fahrenheit) are less common, but may be evidence of hyperthyroidism. Common signs and symptoms of hyperthyroidism include: bulging eyeballs, fast pulse, hyperactivity, inability to gain weight, insomnia, irritability, menstrual problems, and nervousness.

Therapeutic Considerations

The medical treatment of hypothyroidism, in all but its mildest forms, involves the use of desiccated thyroid or synthetic thyroid hormone. Although synthetic hormones have become popular, many physicians (particularly naturopathic physicians) still prefer the use of desiccated natural thyroid, complete with all the thyroid hormones, not just thyroxine—the major thyroid hormone. At this time, it appears that thyroid hormone replacement is necessary in the majority of people who have hypothyroidism. Thyroid hormone replacement therapy consists of using preparations containing active levels of thyroid hormones—either isolated thyroid hormones or natural thyroid extracts.

The thyroid extracts sold in health food stores are required by the Food and Drug Administration (FDA) to be thyroxine-free to prevent the serious consequences (e.g., heart disturbances, insomnia, severe anxiety, etc.) of taking too much of this thyroid hormone. However, it is nearly impossible to remove all the hormone from the gland. In other words, think of health-food-store thyroid preparations as milder forms of desiccated natural thyroid. If you have mild hypothyroidism, these preparations may provide enough support to help you with your thyroid problem.

It is important to nutritionally support the thyroid gland by avoiding goitrogens and insuring adequate intake of key nutrients required in the manufacture of thyroid hormone. For this reason, most health-food-store thyroid products also contain supportive nutrients such as iodine, zinc, and tyrosine.

Iodine and Tyrosine

Thyroid hormones are made from iodine and the amino acid *tyrosine*. The recommended dietary allowance (RDA) for iodine in adults is quite small: 150 micrograms. The average intake of iodine in the United States is estimated to be over 600 micrograms per day.

Too much iodine can actually inhibit thyroid synthesis. For this reason, and because the only function of iodine in the body is for thyroid hormone synthesis, it is recommended that dietary levels or supplementation of iodine not exceed 600 mcg per day for any length of time.

Vitamins and Minerals

Zinc, vitamin E, and vitamin A function together in many body processes, including the manufacture of thyroid hormone. A deficiency of any of these nutrients would result in lower levels of active thyroid hormone being produced. Low zinc levels are common in the elderly, as is hypothyroidism.[18] There may be a correlation.

Vitamin C and the B vitamins riboflavin (B2), niacin (B3), and pyridoxine (B6) are also necessary for normal thyroid hormone manufacture.

Exercise to Improve Thyroid Function

Exercise is particularly important in a treatment program for hypothyroidism. Exercise stimulates thyroid gland secretion and increases tissue sensitivity to thyroid hormone. Many of the health benefits of exercise may be a result of improved thyroid function.

The health benefits of exercise are especially important in overweight hypothyroid individuals who are dieting (restricting food intake). A consistent effect of dieting is a decrease in the metabolic rate as the body strives to conserve fuel. Exercise has been shown to prevent the decline in metabolic rate in response to dieting.[19]

TREATMENT SUMMARY

If you are suffering from symptoms that suggest hypothyroidism, take your basal body temperature and consult a physician for proper evaluation. Support the thyroid gland by insuring adequate intake of key nutrients required in the manufacture of thyroid hormone and by avoiding goitrogens. In very mild cases, health-food-store thyroid products may provide some benefit.

The dosage of health food store preparations really depends on the potency and level of supportive nutrients, especially iodine (no more than 500 mcg daily). A good rule of thumb is to follow the manufacturer's recommendations as provided on the product's label. Use your basal body temperature to determine effectiveness of the product and adjust dosage as necessary.

Impotence

. . . .

Inability to attain or maintain an erection

The term *impotence* has traditionally been used to signify the inability of the male to attain and maintain erection of the penis sufficient to permit satisfactory sexual intercourse. Impotence, in most circumstances, is more precisely referred to as *erectile dysfunction*, as this term differentiates itself from loss of libido, premature ejaculation, or inability to achieve orgasm.[1]

An estimated ten to twenty million American men suffer from erectile dysfunction. This number is expected to increase dramatically as the median age of the population increases. Currently, erectile dysfunction is thought to affect over twenty-five percent of men over the age of fifty.[1,2]

Although the frequency of erectile dysfunction increases with age, it must be stressed that aging itself is not a cause of impotence. Although the amount and force of the ejaculate and the need to ejaculate decrease with age, the capacity for erection is retained. Men are capable of retaining their sexual virility well into their eighties.

The Stages of the Male Sexual Act

The male sexual act is initiated in most instances by an interplay of psychological and physical stimulation. Simply thinking sexual thoughts or dreaming that sexual intercourse is taking place can lead to an erection and even ejaculation. Most men experience nocturnal emissions ("wet dreams") during dreams at some point in their sexual development (usually their teen years).

Although psychological factors obviously contribute to the male sexual response, it is interesting to note that they are not absolutely necessary in the performance of the male sexual act. Appropriate genital stimulation can lead to an erection and ejaculation without psychological stimuli, through an inherent reflex mechanism. For example, some individuals with spinal cord damage that prevents the transmission of nerve impulses from the brain are still capable of achieving an erection and ejaculation.

So either psychological or physical stimulation can initiate the sexual act. Physical stimulation to sensitive tissue—primarily the penis, but also the entire pubic region—sends nerve impulses to the spinal cord, causing a reflex impulse to the penis which leads to dilation of the arteries and engorgement of the erectile tissue. In addition, these same nerve impulses cause the glands in the urethra to secrete mucus which lubricate the urethra and aids in the lubrication of intercourse.

The initial nerve stimulus from the spinal cord during the sexual act is controlled by the parasympathetic nervous system. The parasympathetic controls bodily functions such as digestion, breathing, and heart rate during periods of rest, relaxation, visualization, meditation, and sleep. In contrast, the sympathetic nervous system is designed to protect us against immediate danger and is responsible for the "fight or flight" reaction. While the parasympathetic nervous system is responsible for an erection and lubrication, the sympathetic nervous system controls emission and ejaculation.

Emission and ejaculation are the culmination of the male sexual act. When sexual stimulation becomes extremely intense, the reflex centers of the spinal cord begin to emit sympathetic nerve impulses to initiate *emission*—the forerunner of ejaculation.

Emission begins with contraction of the tubule that transports the sperm from the epididymis to the prostate—the *vas deferens*. This contraction leads to the expulsion of sperm into the ejaculatory duct and urethra. Then, contractions of the prostate and seminal vesicles expel prostatic and seminal fluid into the ejaculatory duct, thus forcing the sperm into the urethra. All of these fluids mix in the internal urethra along with the secretions of the urethral glands to form semen. The process to this point is referred to as emission.

The filling of the urethra then elicits sensory nerve impulses that further excite the rhythmic contractions of the internal organs and also cause the rhythmic contraction of the erectile tissues. Together, these contractions lead to a tremendous increase in pressure, which ejaculates the semen from the urethra. Simultaneously, the pelvic muscles and even muscles of the abdomen cause thrusting movements of the pelvis and penis, which also help propel the semen.

The entire process of emission and ejaculation is known as the male orgasm. After ejaculation, the male sexual excitement disappears almost entirely within one or two minutes, and erection disappears.

Causes of Impotence

Erectile dysfunction may be due to organic or psychogenic factors. In the overwhelming majority of cases the cause is organic, i.e., it is due to some physiological reason. In fact, organic causes are responsible for erectile dysfunction in over ninety percent of men over the age of fifty.[3] In the past, a man with impotence who was able to have nighttime or early morning erections was thought to have psychogenic impotence. However, it is now recognized that this is not a reliable indicator.[2]

CAUSES OF IMPOTENCE

Organic (85%)

Vascular insufficiency
   Atherosclerosis
   Pelvic surgery
   Pelvic trauma
   Venous shunting

Drugs
   Antihistamines
   Antihypertensives
   Anticholinergics
   Antidepressants
   Antipsychotics
   Tranquilizers
   Others

Alcohol and tobacco

Endocrine disorders
   Diabetes
   Hypothyroidism
   Decreased male sex hormones
   Elevated prolactin levels
   High serum estrogen levels

Diseases or trauma to male sexual organs
   Diseases of the penis
   Prostate disorders

Neurological diseases
   Pelvic trauma
   Pelvic surgery
   Multiple sclerosis

Psychological (10%)
Psychiatric illness

Stress
Performance anxiety
Depression
Unknown (5%)

Nighttime penile monitoring
Neurological examination

Since correction of any underlying organic factor is the first step in restoring sexual function, it is critically important that a proper diagnosis be made. A thorough history and physical exam is most often all that is needed. However, there are special noninvasive tests that can be performed to diagnose the cause of erectile dysfunction. These tests are best performed or supervised by a urologist.

PROCEDURES USED TO EVALUATE ERECTILE DYSFUNCTION

Medical history
Physical examination
Laboratory studies
Complete blood count and urinalysis
Biochemical profile
Glucose tolerance test
Serum hormone levels
Psychological evaluation

Vascular Examination

The most common cause of impotence by far is vascular disease. Atherosclerosis of the penile artery is the primary cause of impotence in nearly half the men over the age of fifty who have erectile dysfunction.[1] Atherosclerosis refers to a process of hardening in the artery walls due to a buildup of plaque containing cholesterol, fatty material, and cellular debris. Erectile dysfunction due to atherosclerosis has been shown to be a harbinger of a heart attack or stroke.[3] The process of atherosclerosis occurs systemically throughout the body, not just the arteries supplying the heart or penis. Patients with diseased coronary arteries are much more likely to have erectile dysfunction than individuals without coronary disease. If erectile dysfunction is due to vascular insufficiency, it is imperative to reduce cardiovascular risk factors such as elevated cholesterol and triglyceride levels, high blood pressure, obesity, lack of exercise, and smoking.

QUICK REVIEW

- An estimated ten to twenty million American men suffer from impotence.
- Men are capable of retaining their sexual virility well into their eighties.
- Atherosclerosis of the penile artery is the primary cause of impotence in nearly half the men over the age of fifty who have erectile dysfunction.

- Alcohol and/or tobacco use decrease sexual function.
- Nutrition plays a major role in determining virility.
- If you use yohimbine, use products marketed by reputable companies that clearly state the level of yohimbine per dosage.
- *Ginkgo biloba* extract is quite helpful in cases that result from a lack of blood flow.

The diagnosis of erectile dysfunction due to atherosclerosis can be made with the aid of ultrasound techniques. It is also a good idea to have blood cholesterol and triglyceride levels checked. A total cholesterol level above 200 mg/dl is a strong indicator that atherosclerosis may be responsible for the decreased blood flow.

In many instances, if a vascular cause is suspected, physicians will inject *papaverine* or PGE1 into the penis during the clinical evaluation of erectile dysfunction. These drugs cause the arteries to dilate, thus delivering more blood to erectile tissues. If the erectile dysfunction is due to arterial insufficiency, the penis will become erect and the erection will be sustained. But if the erection cannot be maintained, it is a sign of venous leakage. This form of erectile dysfunction is much more difficult to treat and may require surgery.

Drugs

There is a long list of prescription medications that can interfere with sexual function. If you are on a medication of any sort and have impotence, consult your physician, pharmacist, or *Physician's Desk Reference* to determine if the drug could be responsible. If it is, work with your physician to get off the medication. For most common health conditions, there are natural measures that will produce safer and better clinical results.

Alcohol and Tobacco

Long-term alcohol consumption and/or tobacco use is often a big contributor to impotence. In addition to increasing the risk for atherosclerosis, both of these agents negatively affect sexual function. Alcohol use can produce acute episodes of impotence as well as more permanent impotence due to testicular shrinkage. Smoking just two cigarettes has

been shown to inhibit penile erection produced by injection of low-dose papaverine.[3]

Endocrine Disorders

There are a variety of endocrine and hormonal disorders that can lead to erectile dysfunction. The most common of these disorders is diabetes. Diabetics are at risk for atherosclerosis and nerve damage, both of which can cause impotence. If you are a diabetic, please consult the chapter DIABETES. Other relatively common endocrine disorders associated with impotence include hypothyroidism, excess prolactin, and low levels of testosterone (hypogonadism). Hypothyroidism can often be ruled out by simply taking your basal body temperature (see HYPOTHYROIDISM). Blood measurements are required for the determination of prolactin and testosterone levels. If prolactin levels are high, the herb chasteberry (*Vitex agnus castus*) may be helpful (discussed later). If testosterone levels are low, DHEA may be helpful (follow the recommendations given in LONGEVITY AND LIFE EXTENSION) or try taking *Panax ginseng* (discussed later), although if they are very low it may be necessary to take testosterone as prescribed by a physician.

Diseases or Trauma to Male Sexual Organs

Diseases or trauma to the male sexual organs can cause erectile dysfunction. Diseases of the penis, such as Peyronie's disease, or an enlarged prostate are among the most common findings in this particular category. Since prostate enlargement is discussed fully in the chapter by that name, let's discuss Peyronie's disease

Peyronie's disease is a disorder of the penis in which part of the sheath of fibrous connective tissue within the penis thickens, causing the penis to bend at an angle during an erection. Intercourse is often difficult and quite painful. Although Peyronie's will sometimes improve without any treatment, our recommendation to men with Peyronie's disease is to take the enzyme bromelain along with a concentrated extract of gotu cola *(Centella asiatica)*.

Bromelain is the protein-digesting enzyme of pineapple that prevents the deposition of fibrin. Deposition of fibrin is thought to be responsible for the thickening of the fibrous connective tissue in the penis during Peyronie's disease. For Peyronie's disease, take 750 mg of bromelain three times per day on an empty stomach (twenty minutes before meals is good). As for the gotu cola extract, the dosage is based upon the concentration of active compounds (triterpenic acids). An effective dosage is 60 mg of triterpenic acids twice daily.

Therapeutic Considerations

Although potency is largely dependent on adequate male sex hormones, adequate sensory stimulation, and adequate blood supply to the erectile tissues, all of these factors are dependent on adequate nutrition. Therefore, it can be concluded that nutrition plays a major role in determining virility.

For optimal sexual function, we need optimal nutrition. The diet and nutritional supplementation program in A HEALTH PROMOTING DIET and SUPPLEMENTARY MEASURES, respectively, provides the factors men need to function at their best. A diet rich in whole foods—particularly vegetables, fruits, whole grains, and legumes—is extremely important. Adequate protein is also a must; it is better to

get high-quality protein from fish, chicken, turkey, and lean cuts of beef (preferably hormone-free) than from fat-filled sources such as hamburgers, roasts, and pork.

Special foods often recommended to enhance virility include liver, oysters, nuts, seeds, and legumes. All of these foods are good sources of zinc. Zinc is perhaps the most important nutrient for sexual function. Zinc is concentrated in semen. Frequent ejaculation can greatly diminish body zinc stores. If a zinc deficiency exists, the body appears to respond by reducing sexual drive as a mechanism by which to hold on to this important trace mineral.

Others key nutrients for sexual function include essential fatty acids, vitamin A, vitamin B6, and vitamin E. A high-potency multiple-vitamin-and-mineral formula insures adequate intake of these nutrients as well as others important in health and sexual function.

In addition to nutrition, the natural approach to erectile dysfunction utilizes exercise and herbal medicines.

Reversing Atherosclerosis

Since atherosclerosis is the primary cause of erectile dysfunction, it is especially important to follow the dietary recommendations in the chapter A HEALTH-PROMOTING DIET. For additional help in lowering cholesterol levels, see Cholesterol. These recommendations will prevent or reverse atherosclerosis. The ability of diet to protect against atherosclerosis is well accepted, but evidence is accumulating that diet and lifestyle can also dramatically reverse the blockage of clogged arteries. The dietary guidelines provided in the chapter A HEALTH-PROMOTING DIET are similar to those found to reverse atherosclerosis in the now-famous Lifestyle Heart Trial conducted by Dr. Dean Ornish.[4]

If additional support for lowering cholesterol levels is required, please see the chapter CHOLESTEROL. Niacin is particularly helpful in lowering cholesterol.[5,6] However, an even better recommendation in cases of impotence and high cholesterol levels is the use of inositol hexaniacinate—a safer form of niacin composed of one molecule of inositol (an unofficial B vitamin) and six molecules of niacin. Inositol hexaniacinate has been used in Europe for over thirty years to lower cholesterol levels. It yields slightly better results than standard niacin, but it is much better tolerated—in terms of both flushing and long-term side effects, including effects on blood sugar control.[7-9] Inositol hexaniacinate is available at health food stores. The best dosage for lowering cholesterol levels is 1,000 to 3,000 mg per day.

In the case of erectile dysfunction, inositol hexaniacinate may offer an additional benefit: improving blood flow. In fact, it is used in Europe more for its ability to improve circulation than for its cholesterol-lowering effects.

The nutritional supplement recommendations given in the chapter SUPPLEMENTARY MEASURES are also important, as several of the antioxidant nutrients—vitamins C and E, beta-carotene, and selenium—have been shown to offer significant protection against atherosclerosis and heart disease.

Psychotherapy

Psychological therapies for impotence are useful in some cases, but keep in mind that, in men over the age of fifty, psychological factors are rarely the cause of erectile dysfunction. Nevertheless, impotence itself can lead to psychological disturbances. Even in men with clear-cut organic erectile dysfunction, repeated inability to attain or sustain an erection leads to frustration, anxiety, and anticipation of failure. Learning stress-reduction techniques, such as relaxation exercises, biofeedback, and deep-breathing exercises, may help when anxiety is present. Also, for impotence in men with depression, psychological treatment may be especially beneficial.

Vacuum Constrictive Devices

Vacuum constrictive devices are used to literally pump blood into the erectile tissue. Most of these devices consist of a vacuum chamber, a pump, connector tubing, and penile constrictor bands. The vacuum chamber is large enough to fit over the erect penis. A connector tube runs to the pump from a small opening at the closed end of the container. An elastic constrictor band is placed around the base of the chamber. Water-soluble lubricant is applied to the open end of the cylinder and to the entire penis. The chamber is placed over the flaccid penis, and an airtight seal is obtained.

A vacuum is created by the pump (some are battery-operated) to create negative pressure within the chamber. The suction produced draws blood into the penis to produce an erection-like state. The constrictor band is then guided from the vacuum chamber onto the base of the penis. An erection is maintained because the blood is essentially trapped in the penis.

Although manufacturers and many physicians have stated that vacuum devices have revolutionized the management of erectile dysfunction, patient acceptance does not match this enthusiasm. Vacuum constrictive devices are generally effective and extremely safe, but for some reason they have a significant rate of patient dropout. The reason may be that they are somewhat uncomfortable, cumbersome, and difficult to use: it takes patience and persistence to master the process. Most vacuum devices require both hands or the assistance of the sexual partner. Patients also quit using these devices because they can impair ejaculation and thus lead to some discomfort, and patients and partners complain about the lack of spontaneity. Despite these shortcomings, vacuum constrictive devices have been used successfully by many men with erectile dysfunction.[10]

Exercise

The health benefits of regular exercise cannot be overstated. The immediate effect of exercise is stress on the body. However, with a regular exercise program, the body adapts. The body's response to this regular stress is that it becomes stronger, functions more efficiently, and has greater endurance. Exercise is a vital component of health, especially sexual health.

Regular exercise improves a man's sexual performance. In one study, the effects of nine months of regular exercise on aerobic work capacity (physical fitness), coronary heart disease risk factors, and sexuality were studied in seventy-eight sedentary but healthy men (mean age: forty-eight years).[11] The men exercised in supervised groups for sixty minutes per day, 3.5 days per week on average. Peak sustained exercise intensity was targeted at seventy-five to eighty percent of maximum heart rate (see A HEALTHY LIFESTYLE for description). A control group of seventeen men (mean age: forty-four years) participated in organized walking at a moderate pace for sixty minutes per day, 4.1 days per week on average. Each subject maintained a daily diary of exercise, diet, smoking, and sexuality during the first and last months of the program.

As with many other studies, beneficial effects of regular exercise on fitness and coronary heart disease risk factors were demonstrated. Analysis of diary entries revealed significantly greater sexuality enhancements in the exercise group (frequency of various intimate activities, reliability of adequate functioning during sex, percentage of satisfying orgasms, etc.). Moreover, the degree of sexuality enhancement among exercisers was correlated with the degree of their individual improvement in fitness. In other words, the better physical fitness the men were able to attain, the better their sexuality.

Penile Prosthesis

The "gold standard" for the treatment of erectile dysfunction is the surgical insertion of a penile prosthesis.[1,11] Implantation of these devices is the "treatment of choice in most cases of complete impotence." Three forms are available: semirigid, malleable, and inflatable. The effectiveness, complications, and acceptability vary among the three types. The main problems are mechanical failure, infection, erosions, and irreversible damage to erectile tissue.

Obviously, insertion of a penile prosthesis should be viewed not as a first step in the treatment of erectile dysfunction, but rather as the last step after all other attempts have proved to be futile.

Herbal Medicines

In addition to nutritional measures and exercise, herbal medicines are often used in the natural treatment of erectile dysfunction. Improving sexual desire and function is possible using herbs that (1) improve the activity of the male glandular system, (2) improve the blood supply to erectile tissue, and (3) enhance the transmission or stimulation of the nerve signal.

Yohimbe

The only FDA-approved medicine for treating impotence is *yohimbine*—an alkaloid isolated from the bark of the yohimbe tree (*Pausinystalia johimbe*), native to tropical West Africa. Yohimbine hydrochloride increases libido, but its primary action is to increase blood flow to erectile tissue. Contrary to a popular misconception, yohimbine has no effects on testosterone levels.

When used alone, yohimbine is successful in thirty-four to forty-three percent of cases.[12,13] If combined with strychnine and testosterone, it is much more effective. However, side effects often make yohimbine very difficult to utilize. Yohimbine can induce anxiety, panic attacks, and hallucinations in some individuals. Other side effects include elevations in blood pressure and heart rate, dizziness, headache, and skin flushing. Yohimbine should not be used by women, individuals who have kidney disease, and individuals with psychological disturbances.

Because of the yohimbine content of yohimbe bark, the FDA classifies yohimbe as an unsafe herb.[14] I think there is some validity to this classification. Nevertheless, it is available over the counter without a prescription. It is our opinion that yohimbe and yohimbine are best used under the supervision of a physician. In addition to the problem of side effects with the use of commercial yohimbe preparations, consumers should be very suspicious of the quality of yohimbe products that exist in health food stores. A 1995 analysis showed that, while crude yohimbe bark typically contains six percent yohimbine, most commercial products contained virtually no yohimbine.[14] Compared to authentic yohimbine bark, which contained yohimbine in concentrations of 7,089 parts per million (ppm), concentrations in the commercial products ranged from <0.1 to 489 ppm. Of the twenty-six samples, nine were found to contain absolutely no yohimbine, and seven contained only trace amounts (0.1 to 1ppm). The remaining ten products contained negligible amounts of yohimbine. In other words, there were no legitimate products tested. If you elect to use yohimbine, use products marketed by reputable companies that clearly state the level of yohimbine per dosage. Without knowing the content of yohimbine, it is virtually impossible to prescribe an effective and consistent dosage or to attain any consistent benefit.

Potency Wood (*Muira puama*)

One of the best herbs to use for treating erectile dysfunction or lack of libido is potency wood, which is also known as Muira puama (*Ptychopetalum olacoides*). This shrub is native to Brazil and has long been used as a powerful aphrodisiac and nerve-stimulant in South American folk medicine.[15] A recent clinical study has validated its safety and effectiveness in improving libido and sexual function in some patients.[16]

In 1990, a clinical study was conducted at the Institute of Sexology in Paris, France, under the supervision of one of the world's foremost authorities on sexual function, Dr. Jacques Waynberg. The 262 subjects, who initially complained of lack of sexual desire and the inability to attain or maintain an erection, demonstrated Muira puama extract to be effective in many cases. Within two weeks, at a daily dose of 1 to 1.5 grams of the extract, sixty-two percent of patients with loss of libido claimed that the treatment had a dynamic effect, while fifty-one percent of patients with "erection failures" felt that Muira puama was of benefit.

Presently, the mechanism of action of Muira puama is unknown. From the preliminary information, it appears that it works on enhancing both psychological and physical aspects of sexual function. Future research will undoubtedly shed additional light on this extremely promising herb.

Ginkgo biloba Extract

In addition to its use in increasing blood and oxygen flow to the brain, recent evidence indicates that *Ginkgo biloba* extract may be extremely beneficial in the treatment of erectile dysfunction due to lack of blood flow.[17] In the first study, sixty patients with proven erectile dysfunction who had not reacted to papaverine injections (up to 50 mg) were treated with *Ginkgo biloba* extract at a dose of 60 mg per day for twelve to eighteen months. The penile blood flow was reevaluated by ultrasound techniques every four weeks.

The first signs of improved blood supply were seen after six to eight weeks; after six months' therapy, fifty percent of the patients had regained potency, and in twenty percent a new trial of papaverine injection was then successful; twenty-five percent of the patients showed improved blood flow, but papaverine was still not successful in them. The remaining five percent were unchanged.

According to the results in this preliminary study, *Ginkgo biloba* extract appears to be very effective in the treatment of erectile dysfunction due to lack of blood flow. The improvement of the arterial inflow to erectile tissue is attributed to *Ginkgo biloba* extract's enhancement of blood flow through both arteries and veins without any change in systemic blood pressure.

The second study sought to determine the effectiveness of *Ginkgo biloba* extract when given at a higher dosage (80 mg three times per day).[18] Fifty patients with erectile dysfunction due to arterial insufficiency were divided into two groups. Group 1 (twenty subjects) responded to injection of a drug that improves blood flow to erectile tissue prior to taking the ginkgo. Group 2 (thirty subjects) did not respond to high-dosage injection therapy. After six months of treatment, all twenty patients in the first group responded by regaining the ability to attain and maintain a rigid erection. In Group 2, nineteen patients responded positively to ginkgo in that they were able to attain and maintain an erection with the help of a drug injected into the erectile tissue.

Damiana (Turnera diffusa)

Damiana leaves have been used in the United States since 1874 as an aphrodisiac and "to improve the sexual ability of the enfeebled and aged." Although there are no clinical studies to support this claim, damiana use is very popular. Damiana is thought to slightly irritate the urethra, thereby producing increased sensitivity of the penis.[15] Damiana is seldom used alone; it is typically recommended with other herbs in a commercial preparation. If an individual desires the benefit of damiana on its own, drinking a cup of damiana tea should be sufficient to produce urethral irritation.

Panax ginseng

Although *Panax ginseng* is touted as a "sexual rejuvenator," human studies supporting this belief do not exist. Ginseng has, however, been shown to promote the growth of the testes, increase sperm formation and testosterone levels, and increase sexual activity and mating behavior in studies with animals.[19-21] These results seem to support ginseng's use as a fertility and virility aid.

Chasteberry

Chasteberry (*Vitex agnus castus*) has primarily been used in treating premenstrual syndrome and to lower prolactin levels in women. However, a study exists that shows that chasteberry extract also lowers prolactin levels in men at a dosage of 480 mg per day.[22] Whether this decrease in prolactin levels results in improved sexual performance remains to be seen.

TREATMENT SUMMARY

Restoring potency requires addressing the underlying cause. In the majority of cases, organic factors are the cause. The chief cause is decreased blood flow (vascular insufficiency) due to atherosclerosis.

There are a variety of medical treatments for erectile dysfunction, but each treatment has its drawbacks. The natural approach to erectile dysfunction involves the use of diet, exercise, nutritional supplements, and herbs. This combined approach is designed to restore potency by restoring normal physiology.

Diet

A diet rich in whole foods—particularly vegetables, fruits, whole grains, and legumes—is extremely important. Adequate protein is also a must; it is better to get high-quality protein from fish, chicken, turkey, and lean cuts of beef (preferably hormone-free) than from fat-filled sources such as hamburgers, roasts, and pork.

Special foods often recommended to enhance virility include liver, oysters, nuts, seeds, and legumes. All of these foods are good sources of zinc.

Lifestyle

Avoid health-destroying practices, such as smoking or excessive consumption of al-cohol. Develop a regular exercise program according to the guidelines in the chapter A HEALTHY LIFESTYLE.

Nutritional Supplements

- Multiple-vitamin-and-mineral formula according to the guidelines given in the chapter SUPPLEMENTARY MEASURES
  Vitamin C: 500–1,000 mg three times per day.
  Vitamin E: 400–800 IU per day.
  Flaxseed oil: one tablespoon daily.
- DHEA: please see LONGEVITY AND LIFE EXTENSION for dosage information

Botanical Medicines

For Impotence with Decreased Libido
Choose one of the following or combine them:
- *Panax ginseng*
  The dosage of ginseng is related to the ginsenoside content. The typical dose (taken one to three times daily) should contain a saponin content of at least 5 mg of ginsenosides with a ratio of Rb1 to Rg1 of 2:1. For example, for a high-quality ginseng root powder or extract containing 5% ginsenosides, the dose would be 100 mg. As each individual's response to ginseng is unique, care must be taken to observe possible ginseng toxicity. It is best to begin at lower doses and increase gradually. The Russian approach for long-term administration of either Panax or Siberian ginseng is to use ginseng cycli-

cally for a period of fifteen to twenty days followed by a two-week interval without any ginseng. This recommendation appears prudent.

- Muira puama (*Ptychopetalum olacoides*) extract (6:1): 250 mg three times per day

For Arterial Insufficiency

- *Ginkgo biloba* extract (24% ginkgo flavonglycosides): 80 mg three times per day

For Elevated Prolactin Levels

- Chaste berry (*Vitex agnus castus*) extract (0.5% agnuside content): 350–500 mg daily

For Supportive Therapy

Herbs described in the chapter PROSTATE ENLARGEMENT, especially *Pygeum africanum,* may be helpful. Also, damiana tea may be helpful, as described in this chapter.

Infertility, Male

....

Inability to conceive a child after six months of unprotected sex in the absence of female causes

A total sperm count lower than 5 million/ml

The presence of greater than fifty percent abnormal sperm

Inability of sperm to impregnate egg, as determined by the postcoital or hamster-egg penetration tests

In the United States, it is estimated that as many as fifteen percent of all couples have difficulty conceiving a child. In about one-third of the cases of infertility, it is the man who is responsible; in another one-third, both male and female are responsible; and in another one-third, it is the female who is responsible. Current estimates suggest about six percent of men between the ages of fifteen and fifty are infertile.[1]

Most causes of male infertility reflect an abnormal sperm count or quality. Although it only takes one sperm to fertilize an egg, in an average ejaculate a man will eject nearly two hundred million sperm. However, because of the natural barriers in the female reproductive tract, only about forty sperm will ever reach the vicinity of an egg. There is a strong correlation between fertility and the number of sperm in an ejaculate.

In about ninety percent of the cases of a low sperm count, the reason is deficient sperm production. Unfortunately, in about ninety percent of those cases, the cause for the decreased sperm formation cannot be identified, and the condition is labeled *idio-*

pathic oligospermia or azoospermia.[2] *Oligospermia* means a low sperm count, while *azoospermia* is defined as a complete absence of living sperm in the semen.

CAUSES OF MALE INFERTILITY
Deficient sperm production
Ductal obstruction
    Congenital defects
    Postinfectious obstruction
    Cystic fibrosis
    Vasectomy
Ejaculatory dysfunction
    Premature ejaculation
    Retrograde ejaculation
Disorders of accessory glands
    Infection
    Inflammation
    Antisperm antibodies
Coital disorders
    Defects in technique
    Premature withdrawal
    Erectile dysfunction

Since the overwhelming majority of men who are infertile suffer from deficient sperm production, this will be the major focus of this chapter.

Diagnostic Considerations

Semen analysis is the most widely used test to estimate fertility potential in the male. The semen is analyzed for concentration of sperm and sperm quality. The total sperm count and sperm quality of the general male population has been deteriorating over the last few decades. In 1940, the average sperm count was 113 million/ml; in 1990, that value had dropped to 66 million/ml.[3] Adding to this problem, the amount of semen fell almost twenty percent, from 3.4 ml to 2.75 ml. Altogether, these changes mean that men are now supplying about forty percent of the number of sperm per ejaculate compared to 1940 levels.

The downward trend in sperm count has led to speculation that environmental, dietary, or lifestyle changes in recent decades may be interfering with a man's ability to manufacture sperm. Although controversial, there is substantial evidence that supports this theory. This evidence, as well as methods for improving sperm quality, will be discussed in greater detail in this chapter.

POSSIBLE CAUSES OF FALLING SPERM COUNTS

Increased scrotal temperature
 Tight-fitting clothing and briefs
 Varicoceles (varicose veins that surround the testes) are more common
Environment
 Increased pollution
 Heavy metals (lead, mercury, arsenic, etc.)
 Organic solvents

QUICK REVIEW

- The average sperm count has declined by forty percent since 1940.
- Reducing scrotal temperature in infertile men will often make them fertile.
- Infertile men should wear boxer-type underwear and periodically apply a cold shower or ice to the scrotum.
- If testosterone levels are low or marginal, or if estrogen levels are elevated, a diet rich in legumes (beans), especially soy foods, may be of benefit.
- Free-radical or oxidative damage to sperm is thought to be responsible for many cases of male infertility.
- Antioxidants such as vitamin C, beta-carotene, selenium, and vitamin E, have been shown to be very important in protecting the sperm against damage and improving male fertility.
- Zinc supplementation can be very helpful in achieving fertility, especially in men with low testosterone levels.
- Carnitine supplementation can lead to improvements in sperm counts and sperm motility.

Pesticides (DDT, PCBs, DBCP, etc.)
Diet
    Increased intake of saturated fats
    Reduced intake of fruits, vegetables, and whole grains
    Reduced intake of dietary fiber
    Increased exposure to synthetic estrogens

In diagnosing male infertility on the basis of sperm concentration, it is important to point out that, as sperm counts in the general population have declined, there has been a parallel reduction in the accepted line between infertile and fertile men. The dividing line for sperm count has dropped from 40 million/ml, to 20 million/ml, to 10 million/ml, to 5 million/ml. One of the key reasons these values have dropped so drastically is that researchers are learning that quality is more important than quantity. A high sperm count means nothing if the percentage of healthy sperm is not also high.

Whenever the majority of sperm are abnormally shaped, or are entirely or relatively nonmotile, a man can be infertile despite having a normal sperm concentration. Conversely, a low sperm count does not always mean that a man is infertile. Numerous pregnancies have occurred involving men with very low sperm counts. For example, in studies at fertility clinics, fifty-two percent of couples whose sperm counts were below 10 million/ml achieved pregnancy, and forty per-

cent of those with sperm counts as low as 5 million/ml are able to achieve pregnancy.[1]

Because of these confirmed successes in men with low sperm counts, it is recommended that conventional semen analysis be interpreted with caution regarding the likelihood of conception. More sophisticated functional tests should also be used, especially when screening couples for *in vitro* fertilization.

CAUSES OF TEMPORARY LOW SPERM COUNT
Increased scrotal temperature
Infections, the common cold, the flu, etc.
Increased stress
Lack of sleep
Overuse of alcohol, tobacco, or marijuana
Many prescription drugs
Exposure to radiation
Exposure to solvents, pesticides, and other toxins

Until recently, pregnancy was the only proof of the ability of sperm to achieve fertilization. Now there are several functional tests in use. The postcoital test measures the ability of the sperm to penetrate the cervical mucus after intercourse. *In vitro* variants of this test are also available. One of the most encouraging tests is based on the discovery that human sperm, under appropriate conditions, can penetrate hamster eggs. It was established that fertile males exhibit a range of penetration of ten to one hundred percent, and that penetration less than ten percent is indicative of infertility. The hamster-egg penetration test is considered to predict fertility in sixty-six percent of the cases, compared to about thirty percent for conventional semen analysis.[1]

Another important test in the diagnosis of infertility is the detection of antisperm

TABLE 1 "Normal" Sperm Formation	
CRITERION	**VALUE**
Volume	1.5–5.0 ml
Density	>20 million sperm/ml
Motility	>30% motile
Normal forms	> 60%

antibodies. When produced by the man, these antibodies usually attack the tail of the sperm, thereby impeding the sperm's ability to move and penetrate the cervical mucus. In contrast, the antisperm antibodies produced by women are typically directed against the head of the sperm. The presence of antisperm antibodies in semen analysis is usually a sign of past or current infection in the male reproductive tract.

Therapeutic Considerations

Standard medical treatment of oligospermia can be quite effective when the cause is known, e.g., increased scrotal temperature, chronic infection of male sex glands, prescription medicines, and endocrine disturbances (including hypogonadism and hypothyroidism). However, as stated above, in about ninety percent of the cases of oligospermia, the cause is unknown (idiopathic oligospermia). In regard to azoospermia, if the cause is ductal obstruction, new surgical techniques are showing good results.[1]

In the treatment of idiopathic oligospermia or azoospermia, the rational approach is to focus on enhancing those factors which promote sperm formation. In addition to scrotal temperature, sperm formation is closely linked to nutritional status. Therefore, it is critical that men with low sperm counts have optimal nutritional intake. In addition to consuming a healthful diet, there are several nutritional factors that deserve special mention: vitamin C and other antioxidants, fats and oils, zinc, folate, vitamin B12, arginine, and carnitine. In addition, it appears important for men with low sperm counts to avoid dietary sources of estrogens.

Some herbs, especially *Panax ginseng* and *Eleutherococcus senticosus,* are known to increase sperm counts. And finally, another popular natural treatment of male infertility involves the use of glandular therapy. The concept behind this therapy is discussed in Glandular Therapy, later in this chapter.

Controlling Sperm-Damaging Factors

Scrotal Temperature

The scrotal sac normally keeps the testes at a temperature of between 94 and 96 degrees Fahrenheit.[2] At temperatures above 96 degrees, sperm production is greatly inhibited or stopped completely. Typically, the average scrotal temperature of infertile men is significantly higher than that of fertile men. Reducing scrotal temperature in infertile men will often make them fertile. This temperature reduction is best accomplished by not wearing tight-fitting underwear or tight jeans, and avoiding hot tubs.

Scrotal temperature can be raised by jogging or the use of rowing machines, simulated cross-country ski machines, or treadmills, especially if a man is wearing synthetic fabrics, exceptionally tight shorts, or tight bikini underwear. After exercising, a man should allow his testicles to hang free to allow them to recover from heat buildup.

Infertile men should wear boxer-type underwear and periodically apply a cold shower or ice to the scrotum. They can also choose to use a device called a *testicular hypothermia device* or "testicle cooler" to reduce scrotal temperatures. Still in a primitive stage, the testicle cooler looks like a jock strap from which long, thin tubes have been extended. The tubes are attached to a small fluid reservoir filled with cold water that attaches to a belt around the waist. The fluid reservoir is also a pump that circulates the water. When the water reaches the surface of the scrotum, it evaporates and keeps the scrotum cool. Because of the evaporation, the reservoir must be filled every six hours or so. It is recommended that the testicle cooler be worn daily during waking hours. Most users claim that it is fairly comfortable and easy to conceal.[4]

Increased scrotal temperature can be due to the presence of a *varicocele* (varicose veins that surround the testes). A large varicocele can cause scrotum temperatures high enough to inhibit sperm production and motility. Surgical repair may be necessary, but scrotal cooling should be tried first.

Infections and Infertility

Infections in the male genitourinary tract, including infections of the epididymis, seminal vesicles, prostate, bladder, and urethra, are thought to play a major role in many cases of infertility.[5] The exact extent of their role is largely unknown because of the lack of suitable diagnostic criteria, coupled with the asymptomatic nature of many infections. In the absence of other clinical findings, the presence of antisperm antibodies is considered to a good indicator of a chronic infection.

There is a large number of bacteria, viruses, and other organisms that can infect the male genitourinary system. It is beyond the scope of this chapter to discuss every type of infection, so the discussion will be limited to *Chlamydia trachomatis*. Chlamydia is now recognized as the most common and the most serious of the infections in the male genitourinary tract.[5]

Chlamydia is considered a sexually transmitted disease. In women, chlamydia infection can lead to pelvic inflammatory disease (PID) and scarring of the fallopian tubes. Previous chlamydia infection accounts for a large number of cases of female-factor infertility. In men, chlamydia infection can lead to equally disabling effects. Chlamydia is the major cause of acute nonbacterial prostatitis and urethritis. Typically, the symptoms will be pain or burning sensations upon urination or ejaculation.

More serious is chlamydia infection of the epididymis and vas deferens. The resultant damage to these organs parallels the tubal damage in women; serious scarring and blockage can occur. During an acute chlamydia infection, the use of antibiotics is essential. Chlamydia is sensitive to tetracyclines and erythromycin. Unfortunately, because chlamydia lives within human cells, it may be difficult to totally eradicate the organism with antibiotics alone.

While acute chlamydial infections are usually associated with severe pain, chronic infections of the urethra, seminal vesicles, or prostate can go on with few or no symptoms. It is estimated that twenty-eight to seventy-one percent of infertile men show evidence of a chlamydial infection.[5] Because of the possible link between chlamydia and low sperm counts, there have been several double-blind studies on the effects of antibiotics on sperm counts. These studies have shown only limited improvements in sperm count and sperm quality.[5] However, there have been isolated cases of tremendous increases in sperm counts and sperm quality after antibiotic treatment. If electing this form of treatment, both partners should take the antibiotic. However, it should be used only if there is reason to believe that a chronic infection is present. The presence of antisperm antibodies may indicate a chronic chlamydia infection. In the absence of a positive culture, rectal ultrasonography and the detection of antibodies directed against chlamydia can confirm the diagnosis.

Avoiding Estrogens

According to environmental health experts, we now live in an environment that can be viewed as "a virtual sea of estrogens."[6,7] Increased exposure to estrogens during fetal development, as well as during the reproductive years, is suggested to be a major cause of the tremendous increase in the number of disorders of development and function in the male sexual system.

The relationship between estrogens and male sexual development is best viewed by examining the effects of the synthetic estrogen, diethylstilbestrol (DES). Between 1945 and 1971, several million women were treated with DES during their pregnancy if they had diabetes of pregnancy (gestational diabetes) or were likely to miscarry. By 1970, the side effects of DES became better known. DES given to pregnant mothers carrying a male fetus is now recognized to have led to substantial increases in the number of men suffering from developmental problems of the reproductive tract, as well as decreased semen volume and sperm counts.[5] In addition to being used in humans, DES and other synthetic estrogens were used for twenty to thirty years in the livestock industry to fatten the animals and help them grow faster.

Although many synthetic estrogens like DES are now outlawed, many livestock and poultry are still hormonally manipulated, especially dairy cows. Cow's milk contains substantial amounts of estrogen due to modern farming techniques. The rise in consumption of dairy products since the 1940s inversely parallels the drop in sperm counts. Avoidance of hormone-fed animal products and milk products is important for male sexual vitality, especially in men with low sperm counts or testosterone levels.

There are reports that estrogens have been detected in drinking water.[6,7] Presumably, the estrogens are recycled from excreted synthetic estrogens (birth-control pills) at water treatment plants and eventually find their way into the water supply. These estrogens may be harmful to male sexual vitality. Purified or bottled water may be a suitable option to prevent exposure.

There are other sources of estrogen from the environment (food, water, and air) that can weaken male sexual vitality. For example, many of the chemicals with which we have contaminated our environment in the past fifty years are weakly estrogenic. Most of these chemicals, such as PCBs, dioxin, and DDT, are resistant to biodegradation and are recycled in our environment until they find a safe haven in our bodies. For example, even though DDT has been banned for nearly twenty years, it is still often found in the soil and in root vegetables, such as carrots and potatoes. These toxic chemicals are known to interfere with spermatogenesis, but more important may be their effects during sexual development.

All of the estrogenic factors discussed here are thought to have their greatest impact during fetal development. Based on animal studies, these estrogens inhibit the multiplication of the sperm-producing cells of the testes—the Sertoli cells. The number of Sertoli cells is directly proportional to the amount of sperm that can be produced.

Sertoli cell formation occurs primarily during fetal life and before puberty. It is controlled by follicle-stimulating hormone (FSH). In animal studies, estrogens administered early in life inhibit FSH secretion, resulting in a reduced number of Sertoli cells and, in adult life, reduced sperm counts. Evidence exists to indicate that the same events occur in humans.[6] The best example is the sons of women exposed to DES during pregnancy who, like the animals exposed to estrogens, show reduced sperm counts. Even if a mother didn't take DES, she may have followed the typically low-fiber, high-fat diet of most Americans. Such a diet is associated with higher levels of estrogens because, without the fiber, excreted estrogens are reabsorbed from the intestines.

If testosterone levels are low or marginal, or if estrogen levels are elevated, a diet rich in legumes (beans), especially soy foods, may be of benefit. Soy is a particularly good source of *isoflavonoids*. These compounds are also known as *phytoestrogens*, signifying their mild estrogenic activity. The isoflavonoids in soybeans have about 0.2 percent of the estrogenic activity of *estradiol*, the principal human estrogen. Isoflavononoids (or isoflavones) bind to estrogen receptors. Their weak estrogenic action actually exerts an antiestrogenic effect, as it prevents the binding of the body's own estrogen to the receptor. In addition, phytoestrogens may reduce the effects of estrogens on the body by stimulating the production of SHBG so that the estrogen is bound and subsequently less potent.[8] Soy, as well as other legumes, nuts, and seeds, is also a good source of *phytosterols* (plant compounds similar in structure to human hormones) which may aid in the manufacturer of steroid hormones, including testosterone.

Heavy Metals

Sperm are also particularly susceptible to the damaging effects of heavy metals such as lead, cadmium, arsenic, and mercury. A hair mineral analysis for heavy metals should be performed on all men who have reduced sperm counts to rule out heavy metals as a cause.

Nutritional Considerations

Vitamin C and Other Antioxidants

Free-radical or oxidative damage to sperm is thought to be responsible for many cases of idiopathic oligospermia; high levels of free radicals are found in the semen of forty percent of infertile men.[9–13] Three factors combine to render sperm particularly susceptible to free-radical damage: (1) a high membrane concentration of polyunsaturated fatty acids; (2) active generation of free radicals; and (3) a lack of defensive enzymes. All of these factors make the health of the sperm critically dependent upon antioxidants. Although most free radicals are produced during normal metabolic processes, the environment contributes greatly to the free-radical load. Men exposed to increased levels of sources of free radicals are much more likely to have abnormal sperm and sperm counts.[1,9–12]

Sperm are extremely sensitive to free radicals because they are so dependent upon the integrity and fluidity of their cell membrane for proper function. Without proper membrane fluidity, enzymes are activated, which can lead to impaired motility, abnormal structure, loss of viability, and ultimately death to the sperm.[9] The major determinant of membrane fluidity is the concentration of polyunsaturated fatty acids, particularly omega-3 fatty acids such as docosahexanoic acid, which are very susceptible to free-radical damage. The sperm have a relative lack of the superoxide dismutase and catalase needed to prevent or repair oxidative damage. Adding to this more susceptible state is the fact that sperm generate high quantities of free radicals to help break down barriers to fertilization.

A common source of oxidants is cigarette smoking, which is associated with decreased sperm counts and sperm motility as well as an increased frequency of abnormal sperm.[12] Both cigarette smoking and the increase in environmental pollution are thought to be major contributors to the decrease in sperm counts seen in many industrialized nations during the past few decades.

Antioxidants such as vitamin C, beta-carotene, selenium, and vitamin E, have been shown to be very important in protecting the sperm against damage. Vitamin C plays an especially important role in protecting the sperm's genetic material (DNA) from damage. Ascorbic acid levels are much higher in seminal fluid than in other body fluids, including the blood. When dietary vitamin C was reduced from 250 mg to 5 mg per day in healthy human subjects, the seminal fluid ascorbic acid level decreased by fifty percent and the number of sperm with damage to their DNA increased by ninety-one percent.[14] These results indicate that dietary vitamin C plays a critical role in protecting against sperm damage, and that low dietary vitamin C levels are likely to lead to infertility.

It is now well-documented that cigarette smoking greatly reduces vitamin C levels throughout the body. Even the U.S. Food and Nutrition Board, the organization that calculates the Recommended Dietary Allowances (RDAs), acknowledges that smokers require at least twice as much vitamin C as nonsmokers.[15] In one study, men who smoked one pack of cigarettes per day received either 0, 200, or 1,000 mg of vitamin C. After one month, sperm quality improved proportional to the level of vitamin C supplementation.[16]

Nonsmokers appear to benefit from vitamin C supplementation as much as smokers. In one study, thirty infertile but otherwise healthy men received either 200 mg or 1,000 mg of vitamin C or a placebo daily.[17] There were weekly measurements of sperm count, viability, motility, agglutination, abnormalities, and immaturity. After one week, the 1,000-mg group demonstrated a 140-percent increase in sperm count, the 200 mg group a 112-percent increase, and the placebo group no change. After three weeks, both vitamin C groups continued to improve, with the 200-mg group catching up to the improvement of the 1,000-mg group.

One of the key improvements observed during the study was in the number of *agglutinated* (clumped-together) sperm. Sperm become agglutinated when antibodies produced by the immune system bind to the sperm. Antibodies to sperm are often associated with chronic genitourinary tract or prostatic infection. When more than twenty-five percent of the sperm are agglutinated, fertility is very unlikely. At the beginning of the study, all three groups had over twenty-five percent agglutinated sperm. After three weeks, the agglutinated sperm in the vitamin C groups dropped to eleven percent.

Although this result is significant, the most impressive result of the study was that at the end of sixty days, all of the vitamin C group had impregnated their wives, compared to none for the placebo group. It can be concluded from these results that vitamin C supplementation can be very effective in treating male infertility, particularly if the infertility is due to antibodies against sperm.

Other dietary antioxidants, such as vitamin E, selenium, and beta-carotene are also important and should be supplemented. Vitamin E supplementation appears to be especially warranted, as it is the main antioxidant in various cell membranes, including sperm membranes. Vitamin E has been shown to play an essential role in inhibiting free-radical damage to the unsaturated fatty acids of the sperm membrane.[18] In addition, vitamin E has been shown to enhance the ability of sperm to fertilize an egg in test tubes.

In one study, supplementation with vitamin E decreased the level of lipid peroxide (malondialdehyde levels) concentration in sperm pellet suspensions. Even more important, however, was the fact that eleven of fifty-two treated infertile men impregnated their spouses.[19]

Supplementation appears to be indicated based on its antioxidant effects alone. Vitamin E may prove to exert more beneficial effects on sperm counts or motility when given at higher levels (600 to 800 IU per day).

Fats and Oils

Considering the effects of fats and oils on agglutination and cell membrane function, certain fats are best avoided by infertile men, while intake of others should be increased. Saturated fats, hydrogenated oils, trans-fatty acids, and cottonseed, coconut, and palm oils should be avoided. Coconut and palm oils are primarily saturated fat, while cottonseed may contain toxic residues due to the heavy spraying of cotton and its high levels of *gossypol,* a substance known to inhibit sperm function. In fact, gossypol is being investigated as a "male birth-control pill." Its use as an antifertility agent began after studies demonstrated that men who had used crude cottonseed oil as their cooking oil were shown to have low sperm counts followed by total testicular failure.[20]

Excessive consumption of saturated fats, combined with inadequate intake of essential fatty acids, changes the fatty acid composition of the sperm membranes, thus decreasing fluidity and interfering with sperm motility. Read food labels carefully and avoid all sources of cottonseed oil and other damaging oils.

While the intake of saturated and hydrogenated fats must be eliminated, the intake of essential polyunsaturated oils should be increased. These oils function in all aspects of sexual function, including sperm formation and activity.

Zinc

Zinc is perhaps the most critical trace mineral for male sexual function. It is involved in virtually every aspect of male reproduction, including hormone metabolism, sperm for-

mation, and sperm motility.[21] Among many other problems, zinc deficiency is characterized by decreased testosterone levels and sperm counts. Zinc levels are typically much lower in infertile men with low sperm counts, indicating that a low zinc status may be the contributing factor to the infertility.

Several studies have evaluated the effect of zinc supplementation on sperm counts and motility.[22–24] The results from all of the studies support the use of zinc supplementation in the treatment of oligospermia, especially in the presence of low testosterone levels. The effectiveness of zinc is best illustrated by a study of thirty-seven men who had been infertile for more than five years, and whose sperm counts were less than 25 million/ml.[24] Blood testosterone levels were also measured. The men received a supplement of zinc sulfate (60 mg of elemental zinc daily) for forty-five to fifty days. In the twenty-two patients with initially low testosterone levels, mean sperm count increased significantly, from 8 to 20 million/ml. Testosterone levels also increased, and nine out of the twenty-two wives became pregnant during the study. This result is quite impressive given the long-term nature of the infertility and the rapidity of the results. In contrast, in the fifteen men with normal testosterone levels, although sperm count increased slightly, there was no change in testosterone level and no pregnancies occurred. These results imply that zinc is only effective in increasing male fertility when testosterone levels are low.

Optimal zinc levels must be attained if optimum male sexual vitality is desired. Although severe zinc deficiency is rare in this country, many men consume a diet that does not provide the RDA for zinc (15 mg). Zinc is found in whole grains, legumes, nuts, and seeds. In addition to eating these zinc-containing foods, taking supplementary zinc (45 to 60 mg per day) appears warranted.

Vitamin B12

Vitamin B12 is involved in cellular replication. A deficiency of B12 leads to reduced sperm counts and reduced sperm motility. Even in the absence of a vitamin-B12 deficiency, supplementation appears to be worthwhile in men with sperm counts less than 20 million/ml or a motility rate of less than fifty percent. In one study, twenty-seven percent of men who had sperm counts under 20 million/ml were given 1,000 mcg of vitamin B12 per day. As a result, they were able to achieve a total count in excess of 100 million/ml.[25] In another study, fifty-seven percent of men with low sperm counts who were given 6,000 mcg of vitamin B12 per day demonstrated improvements.[26]

Arginine

The amino acid *arginine* is required for the replication of cells, making it essential in sperm formation. Arginine supplementation is often, but not always, an effective treatment for male infertility. The critical determinant appears to be the level of oligospermia. If sperm counts are less than 20 million/ml, arginine supplementation is less likely to be of benefit. In order to be effective, it appears that the dosage of arginine should be at least 4 grams per day for three months. In perhaps the most favorable study, seventy-four percent of 178 men with low sperm counts had significant improvements in sperm counts and motility with high dose (4 grams per day) arginine therapy.[27] Arginine therapy should be reserved for use after other nutritional measures have been tried.

Carnitine

Carnitine is essential for the transport of fatty acids into the mitochondria. A deficiency of carnitine results in a decrease in fatty acid concentrations in the mitochondria and reduced energy production. Carnitine concentrations are extremely high in the epididymis and sperm, suggesting a role for carnitine in male reproductive function. The epididymis derives the majority of its energy requirements from fatty acids during transport through the epididymis, as do the sperm. After ejaculation, the motility of sperm correlates directly with carnitine content. The higher the carnitine content, the more motile the sperm. Conversely, when carnitine levels are low, sperm development, function, and motility are drastically reduced. One clinical study found that carnitine supplementation (1,000 mg three times daily) led to an increase in sperm count and mobility in thirty-seven of forty-seven men who had abnormal sperm mobility.[28]

Supplementing the diet with L-carnitine may help restore male fertility in some cases. The optimal dosage is 300 to 1,000 mg of L-carnitine three times per day. However, because L-carnitine tends to be relatively expensive, the other nutritional measures should be tried first.

Botanical Medicines

Ginseng

Current scientific investigation suggests that both *Panax ginseng* (Chinese or Korean ginseng) and *Eleutherococcus senticosus* (Siberian ginseng) are probably effective in the treatment of male infertility. Both botanicals have a long history of use as male "tonics." Although human clinical studies are lacking, *Panax ginseng* has been shown to promote the growth of the testes, increase sperm formation and testosterone levels, and increase sexual activity and mating behavior in studies with animals.[29–32] Siberian ginseng may also be of benefit to the male reproductive function, as it has been shown to increase reproductive capacity and sperm counts in bulls.[33] These results seem to support the use of ginseng as a fertility and virility aid.

In general, *Panax ginseng* is regarded as being more potent in effects (particularly stimulant effects) than *Eleutherococcus senticosus*. Although Siberian ginseng contains no ginsenosides and is not a true ginseng, it does possess many of the same effects that *Panax ginseng* exerts, but it is generally regarded as being milder.

Pygeum africanum

Pygeum extracts may be effective in improving fertility in cases where diminished prostatic secretion plays a significant role. Pygeum has been shown to increase prostatic secretions and improve the composition of the seminal fluid.[34–37] Specifically, pygeum administration to men with decreased prostatic secretion has led to increased levels of total seminal fluid as well as increases in alkaline phosphatase (an important enzyme that maintains the proper pH of the seminal fluid) and protein. Pygeum appears to be most effective in cases in which the level of alkaline phosphatase activity is reduced (to less than $400 \ IU/cm^3$) and there is no evidence of inflammation or infection (such as absence of white blood cells or IgA). The lack of IgA in the semen is a good indicator of clinical success. In one study, the patients who had no IgA in their semen demonstrated an alkaline phosphatase increase from 265 to 485 IU/cm^3.[34] In contrast, those subjects with IgA showed only a modest increase from 213 to 281 IU/cm^3.

Pygeum extract has also shown an ability to improve the capacity to achieve an erection in patients with BPH (benign prostate hyperplasia) or prostatitis, as determined by nocturnal penile tumescence in a double-blind clinical trial.[37] BPH and prostatitis are often associated with erectile dysfunction and other sexual disturbances. Presumably, by improving the underlying condition, pygeum can improve sexual function.

Glandular Therapy

For almost as long as historical records have been kept, glandular therapy has been an important form of medicine. The basic concept underlying the medicinal use of glandular substances from animals is that "like heals like." In the case of low testosterone levels or low sperm counts, extracts of bovine (beef) orchic or testicular tissues are often recommended by physicians who practice glandular therapy. It is well established that a number of glandular preparations are effective orally because of active hormones (e.g., thyroid, adrenal, and thymus). Presumably, orchic or testicular products may also be of benefit. Unfortunately, dosage and effectiveness may vary from one manufacturer to another.

. . . .

TREATMENT SUMMARY

Male infertility is most often due to abnormal sperm count or semen quality. As elevated scrotal temperature is a common cause of infertility, scrotal cooling through the use of loose underwear made of cotton, avoidance of activities that elevate testicular temperature (e.g., hot tubs), and application of cold water to the testes should be utilized. Nutritional status should be optimized (especially antioxidants and zinc), environmental pollutants identified and eliminated, and fertility-enhancing botanicals such as one of the ginsengs consumed. We recommend consulting a urologist or fertility specialist for a complete evaluation.

General Measures

- Maintain scrotal temperatures between 94 and 96 degrees Fahrenheit.
- Avoid exposure to free radicals.
- Identify and eliminate environmental pollutants.
- Stop or reduce consumption of all drugs, especially antihypertensives, antineoplastics such as cyclophosphamide, and anti-inflammatory drugs such as sulfasalazine.

Diet

Avoid dietary sources of: free radicals; saturated fats; hydrogenated oils; transfatty acids; and cottonseed oil. Increase consumption of: legumes, especially soy (high in phytoestrogens and phytosterols); good dietary sources of antioxidant vitamins, carotenes, and flavonoids (dark-colored vegetables and fruits); and essential fatty acids and zinc (nuts and seeds).

Consume daily: 8–10 servings of vegetables; 2–4 servings of fresh fruits; and ½ cup of raw nuts or seeds.

Nutritional Supplements

- High-potency multiple-vitamin-and-mineral supplement
- Vitamin C: 500–3,000 mg three times per day
- Vitamin E: 600–800 IU per day
- Beta-carotene: 100,000–200,000 IU per day
- Folic acid: 400 mcg per day
- Vitamin B12: 1,000 mcg per day
- Zinc: 30–60 mg per day

Botanical Medicines

- *Panax ginseng* (three times per day dosages)

  High-quality crude ginseng root: 1.5–2 g three times per day

  Standardized extract (5% ginsenosides): 100–200 mg three times per day

- *Eleutherococcus senticosus* (three times per day dosages)

  Dried root: 2–4 g

  Tincture (1:5): 10–20 ml

  Fluid extract (1:1): 2.0–4.0 ml

  Solid (dry powdered) extract (20:1): 100–200 mg

- *Pygeum africanum*

  The dosage of the fat-soluble extract, standardized to contain fourteen percent triterpenes including beta-sitosterol and 0.5 percent n-docosanol, is 100 to 200 mg per day in divided doses.

Inflammatory Bowel Disease

. . . .

CROHN'S DISEASE

Intermittent bouts of diarrhea, low-grade fever, and pain in the lower right abdomen

Loss of appetite, weight loss, flatulence, and malaise

Abdominal tenderness, especially in the lower right

X rays show abnormality of the terminal portion of the small intestine

ULCERATIVE COLITIS

Bloody diarrhea with cramps in the lower abdomen

Mild abdominal tenderness, weight loss, and fever

Rectal examination may show fissures, hemorrhoids, fistulas, and abscesses

Diagnosis confirmed by X ray and sigmoidoscopy (examination of the colon with a fiber-optic tube)

Inflammatory bowel disease (IBD) is a general term for a group of chronic inflammatory disorders of the intestines. It is divided into two major categories: Crohn's disease and ulcerative colitis. Clinically, IBD is characterized by recurrent inflammation of specific intestinal segments resulting in diverse symptoms.

localized the disease to segments in the *ileum*, the terminal portion of the small intestine. However, the same granulomatous process may involve the mucosa of the mouth, esophagus, stomach, duodenum, jejunum, and colon. Crohn's disease of the small intestine is also known as *regional enteritis*, while involvement of the colon is known as Crohn's disease of the colon or *granulomatous colitis*.

Crohn's Disease

Crohn's disease is characterized by an inflammatory reaction throughout the entire thickness of the bowel wall. In approximately forty percent of cases, however, the inflammatory lesions (*granulomas*) are either poorly developed or totally absent. The original description in 1932 by Crohn and colleagues

Ulcerative Colitis

In ulcerative colitis, there is a nonspecific inflammatory response, limited largely to the lining of the colon. Crohn's disease and ulcerative colitis do share many common features and, where appropriate, will be discussed together. Otherwise they will be discussed as separate entities.

FEATURES SHARED BY CROHN'S DISEASE AND ULCERATIVE COLITIS

1. The colon is frequently involved in Crohn's disease and is invariably involved in ulcerative colitis.

2. Although this is rare, patients with ulcerative colitis who have total colon involvement may develop a so-called backwash ileitis. Thus, both Crohn's disease and ulcerative colitis may cause changes in the small intestine.

3. Patients with Crohn's disease often have close relatives with ulcerative colitis, and vice versa.

4. When there is no granulomatous reaction in Crohn's disease of the colon, the two lesions may resemble each other in both the clinical picture and the biopsy result.

5. The many epidemiological similarities between the two diseases include age, race, sex, and geographic distribution.

6. Both conditions are associated with similar manifestations outside the gastrointestinal tract (extraintestinal).

7. The causative factors appear to be parallel for the two conditions.

8. Both conditions are associated with an increased frequency of colonic carcinoma.

Occurrence

The rates of occurrence of these two diseases differ slightly, with most studies showing ulcerative colitis to be more common than Crohn's disease. It is currently estimated that, in western Europe and the United States, six to eight new cases of ulcerative colitis are diagnosed annually for every 100,000 people. The total estimated number of cases is approximately 70 to 150 per 100,000.

For Crohn's disease, the estimated yearly rate of newly diagnosed cases is approximately two per 100,000, while the total number of cases is estimated at twenty to forty per 100,000. However, the rate of occurrence of Crohn's disease is increasing in Western cultures, possibly due to dietary factors and antibiotic use (discussed below).

Inflammatory bowel disease may occur at any age, but it most often occurs between the ages of fifteen and thirty-five. Females are affected slightly more often than males. Caucasians develop the disease two to five times more often than do people of African or Asian descent, while Jews have a three to six times higher incidence compared with non-Jews.

QUICK REVIEW

- Antibiotic exposure is being linked to Crohn's disease.
- Clinical studies that have utilized an elemental diet, intravenous nutrition, or an exclusion diet have produced great success in the treatment of Crohn's disease and ulcerative colitis.
- Prostaglandin levels are greatly increased in the colonic mucosa, serum, and stools of patients with inflammatory bowel disease (IBD).
- Over 100 disorders, known as extraintestinal lesions (EIL), constitute a diverse group of systemic complications of IBD.

Causes of IBD

Theories about the cause of IBD can be divided into several groups:

1. Genetic predisposition
2. Infectious agent or agents
3. Antibiotic exposure
4. Immune system abnormality
5. Dietary factors

Genetic Predisposition

Although the search for a specific genetic marker for IBD has been futile, several factors suggest a genetic predisposition. As already mentioned, IBD is two to four times more common in Caucasians than non-Caucasians, and four times more common in Jews than non-Jews. In addition, in fifteen to forty percent of the cases, multiple members of a family have Crohn's disease or ulcerative colitis.

Infectious Agents

Many microorganisms have been identified as potential causes of IBD, but the possibility that a microbial agent is responsible for IBD is still a hotly debated subject. Viruses such as rotavirus, Epstein-Barr virus, cytomegalovirus, and mycobacteria continue to be favored candidates. Other candidates include pseudomonas-like organisms, chlamydia, and *Yersinia enterocolitica*.

Antibiootic Exposure

Antibiotic exposure is being linked to Crohn's disease (and possibly ulcerative colitis as well[1]. Prior to the 1950s, Crohn's disease was found in isolated groups and had a strong genetic component. Since then, there has been a rapid climb in the number of cases of Crohn's disease in developed countries, particularly in the United States, and in countries that had previously had virtually no reported cases. In fact, Crohn's disease has spread like an epidemic since 1950. Are antibiotics to blame?

Penicillin and tetracycline have been available in oral form since 1953. The annual increase in prescriptions for antibiotics parallels the annual increase in the incidence of Crohn's disease. Comparative statistics have shown that wherever antibiotics are used early and in large quantities, the incidence of Crohn's disease becomes quite high.

Over the years, researchers have sought to identify Crohn's disease as an infectious process. The problem may arise from an infectious agent that is a component of the

- Many nutritional complications occur during the course of IBD.
- Foremost in nutritional therapy is providing adequate caloric intake.
- Elemental and elimination diets have been shown to be an effective non-toxic primary treatment of acute and chronic IBD.

- Treatment with a high-fiber diet has been shown to have a favorable effect on the course of Crohn's disease.
- The majority of individuals with IBD suffer from nutritional deficiencies.

normal intestinal flora; it might suddenly produce toxins that damage the immune system, or it might become invasive as a direct result of sublethal doses of antibiotics. Administration of antibiotics below the level that kills the target organism has been shown to increase toxin production in intestinal organisms. When microbes are not given a full lethal dose, their usual response is to adapt and become even stronger in virility and numbers.

Immune System Abnormality

An overwhelming amount of evidence points to immune system disturbances in IBD, but whether these disturbances are causal or secondary phenomena remains unclear. Theories linking immune system derangements as causes of IBD have been proposed, but the current evidence seems to indicate that these derangements are probably secondary to the disease process.

Dietary Factors

Despite the fact that a dietary cause of Crohn's disease is hardly considered (if mentioned at all) in most standard medical and gastroenterology texts, several lines of evidence strongly support dietary factors as being the most important causative factor.[2–13]

The incidence of Crohn's disease is increasing in countries where people consume a Western diet (high in saturated fats, refined carbohydrates, and sugar), while it is virtually nonexistent where people consume a more "primitive" diet (one that is high in fiber).[2–6] Because food is the major factor in determining the intestinal environment, the considerable change in dietary habits over the last century could explain the rising rates of Crohn's disease.

Several studies that analyzed the pre-illness diet of patients with Crohn's disease have found that people who develop Crohn's disease habitually eat more refined sugar and less raw fruit and vegetables and dietary fiber than healthy people.[2–6] In one study, the pre-illness intake of refined sugar in Crohn's disease patients was nearly twice that of controls (122 g per day versus 65 g per day).[7] One researcher found that, before the onset of disease, Crohn's disease patients had eaten corn flakes more frequently than controls.[14] Although other researchers could not verify this specific finding, corn flakes are high in refined carbohydrates and are derived from a common allergen (corn).

Much of the controversy over the role of pre-illness diet in the cause of Crohn's disease is due to the fact that the only way to assess diet is from postdiagnostic interviews. Studies in which the interview took place within the first six months of diagnosis tend to be more supportive than studies done more than seven months after diagnosis (it is difficult for people to accurately recall what their diet was like as more time goes by). In contrast, patients with ulcerative colitis do not show an increased consumption of refined carbohydrates when compared with controls.[15]

Another important dietary factor that is entirely overlooked in the standard medical texts is the role of food allergy. However, clinical studies that have utilized an elemental diet, intravenous nutrition, or an exclusion diet have shown great success in the treatment of IBD.[8–13] These restricted diets and the roles of food allergy and dietary fiber are discussed in greater detail later in this chapter (see Correcting Nutritional Deficiencies).

Miscellaneous Factors

Psychosomatic factors, vascular disturbances, and chronic trauma have received consideration in the origin of IBD, but at present are not considered significant mechanisms. While there is little evidence directly relating psychological factors to the initiation of IBD, there is little doubt that emotional factors are important in modifying the course of the disease.

Therapeutic Considerations

Little is known about the natural course of Crohn's disease and ulcerative colitis because virtually all patients with either disease undergo standard medical care (drugs and/or surgery) or alternative therapy. The only exceptions are those patients in clinical trials who are assigned to the placebo group.[16–18] Even these patients do not represent the natural course of the disease, since they are frequently seen by physicians and other members of a health care team and are taking medication, even if it is only in the form of a placebo. However, if proper evaluation of therapies for Crohn's disease is to occur, there must be a greater understanding of its natural history.

It is commonly believed by many alternative health care providers that standard medical care often interferes with the normal efforts of the body to restore itself to health. However, administration of corticosteroids, hospitalization, and even surgical measures do have their place in many instances and should be used when appropriate.

A closer examination of the course of Crohn's disease in experimental studies reveals some interesting information. Researchers in the National Cooperative Crohn's Disease Study (NCCDS) reviewed seventy-seven patients who received placebo therapy in Part 1 of the seventeen-week study.[16,17] They all had active disease, as defined by a Crohn's disease activity index (CDAI; see Crohn's Disease Activity Index

later in this chapter) of above 150. None of the patients who completed the study died; only seven (nine percent) suffered a major worsening of their disease (i.e., they either developed a major fistula [a passageway from the intestines to the skin] or required abdominal surgery); twenty-five (thirty-two percent) suffered a lesser worsening (increase in the CDAI to greater than 450 or presence of a fever of at least 100 degrees Fahrenheit for two weeks); twenty-five (thirty-two percent) were considered failures, because their CDAI remained above 150; and twenty patients (twenty-six percent) achieved clinical remission. On at least one occasion during the seventeen weeks of therapy, forty-nine percent of the patients were found to have a CDAI of below 150.

The patients who responded favorably to the placebo continued to be observed on placebo therapy for up to two years (Part 1, Phase 2). While none of these patients' X rays indicated a worsened condition during Phase 1 or Phase 2, eighteen percent actually showed improvement on their intestinal X rays. Of the patients who responded favorably to the placebo, the majority (seventy percent) remained in remission at one year, and a fair number (forty-five percent) remained in remission at two years. These results indicate that many patients will undergo spontaneous remission—approximately twenty percent at one year and twelve percent at two years.

However, when another factor is considered, the apparent success of the placebo therapy rises dramatically. In patients who had no previous history of steroid therapy, forty-one percent achieved remission after seventeen weeks. In addition, twenty-three percent of this group continued in remission after two years, compared to only four percent of the group with a prior history of steroid use.

The European Cooperative Crohn's Disease Study (ECCDS), although different in some details of method, had similar results to the NCCDS.[16,18] In the ECCDS, 110 patients (sixty-eight patients with prior treatment and forty-two patients with no prior treatment) constituted the placebo group. The results of the study indicated that fifty-five percent of the total placebo group achieved remission by 100 days, thirty-four percent remained in remission at 300 days, and twenty-one percent remained in remission at 700 days. Like the NCCDS, the ECCDS demonstrated that patients with no prior therapy have an increased likelihood of remission.

While one group of researchers did not advocate placebo therapy, they did carefully point out that once remission is achieved, seventy-five percent of the patients will continue in remission at the end of one year, and up to sixty-three percent at the end of two years, regardless of the maintenance therapy used. These results suggest that the key is achieving remission, which, once attained, can be maintained by conservative nondrug therapy rather than the "medicines we are currently using with their limited efficacy and known toxicity."[16]

Prostaglandin Metabolism

Prostaglandins are hormone-like substances manufactured from essential fatty acids that govern many bodily functions, including inflammation. Prostaglandin levels are greatly increased in the colonic mucosa, serum, and stools of patients with IBD. Specifically, these patients show an increase in the synthesis of inflammatory compounds known as *leukotrienes*.[19–22] These compounds are produced by neutrophils and are known to amplify the inflammatory process and cause intestinal cramping and pain.

To reduce the formation of these inflammatory compounds, reduce or eliminate your consumption of meat and dairy products while increasing your consumption of omega-3 fatty acids by increasing your intake of cold-water fish (such as salmon, mackerel, herring, and halibut). These fish are good sources of the longer-chain omega-3 fatty acids, eicosapentaenoic acid (EPA) and docosahexanoic acid (DHA). It is also a good idea to take one tablespoon of flaxseed oil each day. Flaxseed oil contains alpha-linolenic acid, the essential omega-3 fatty acid, which the body can convert to EPA.

Mucin Defects

Mucins are *glycoproteins* (proteins with sugar molecules attached) that are largely responsible for the viscous and elastic characteristics of secreted mucus. Alterations in mucin composition and content in the colonic mucosa have been reported in patients with ulcerative colitis.[23–25] The factors responsible for this appear to be a dramatic decrease in the mucus content of the mucus-producing *(goblet)* cells (proportional to the severity of the disease), as well as a decrease in the major sulfur-containing mucin.

It is significant that, while the mucin content of the goblet cells returns to normal during remission of ulcerative colitis, the sulfur-containing mucin deficiency does not. The specific components of the sulfur-containing mucin and the cause of its lower concentration have not yet been determined. These mucin abnormalities are also thought to be a major factor in the increased risk of colon cancer in these patients.

Many of the herbs used historically in the treatment of ulcerative colitis are *demulcents* (agents that soothe irritated mucous membranes and promote the secretion of mucus). This effect of demulcents appears to be very helpful and supports the use of demulcents such as DGL, marshmallow root, and slippery elm in ulcerative colitis.

These mucin abnormalities are not found in patients with Crohn's disease.

Intestinal Microflora

The fecal flora of patients with Crohn's disease and ulcerative colitis have been found to be greatly disturbed.[26] Indications are that these alterations in fecal flora are not a result of the disease. Alterations in the metabolic activity of the various bacteria are thought to be more important than alterations in the number of bacteria per se. In addition, it is thought that specific bacterial cell components (which vary even within the same species) are responsible for promoting destruction of the intestinal cells.

Carrageenan

Researchers investigating ulcerative colitis often use *carrageenan* (a compound extracted from red seaweeds) to experimentally induce the disease in animals. In the initial experiments reported by Marcus and Watt in 1969, one-percent and five-percent carrageenan solutions were provided as the exclusive source of oral fluids for guinea pigs.[27] Over a period of several days, the animals lost weight, developed anemia, had bloody diarrhea, and developed ulcerative colitis. These results have since been confirmed by numerous investigators and in studies involving other animal species, including primates.[26–30]

In its natural state, this polymer has a molecular weight of 100,000 to 800,000, but in the studies it was degraded by mild acidic hydrolysis to yield products with weights in the vicinity of 30,000. These smaller molecules are thought to be responsible for inducing the ulcerative damage in the animal studies.

Carrageenan compounds are used by the food industry as stabilizing and suspending agents, with different molecular weight polymers being used for a variety of purposes. Typically, carrageenans used in the food industry have a molecular weight greater than 100,000. Carrageenan is widely used in milk and chocolate milk products (ice cream, cottage cheese, milk chocolate, etc.) due to its ability to stabilize milk proteins.

As suggestive as the animal studies are in linking ulcerative colitis with carrageenan, no lesions of IBD were observed in healthy human subjects fed enormous quantities of degraded carrageenan.[31] However, differences in intestinal bacterial flora are probably responsible for this discrepancy, as germ-free animals do not display carrageenan-induced damage either.

The bacteria that has been linked to facilitating the carrageenan-induced damage in animals is a strain of *Bacteroides vulgatus*.[26] This organism is found in much higher concentrations (six times as high) in the fecal cultures of patients with ulcerative colitis. When the data are evaluated, they imply that, while carrageenan can be metabolized into non-damaging components in most human subjects, those individuals with an overgrowth of *Bacteroides vulgatus* may be at risk. Strict avoidance of carrageenan appears warranted at this time for individuals with IBD until further research clarifies its safety for these patients. Read food labels carefully.

Complications of IBD

Over 100 disorders, known as *extraintestinal lesions* (EIL), constitute a diverse group of systemic complications of IBD.[32] The most common EIL in adults is arthritis, which is found in about twenty-five percent of patients. Two types are typically described, the more common being peripheral arthritis affecting the knees, ankles, and wrists. Arthritis is more frequently found in patients with colon involvement. Severity of symptoms is typically proportional to disease activity.

Less frequently, the arthritis affects the spine. Symptoms are low back pain and stiffness with eventual limitation of motion. This EIL occurs predominantly in males and is fairly indistinguishable from typical *ankylosing spondylitis* (rheumatoid arthritis of the spine). In fact, it may precede the bowel symptoms by several years. There is probably a consistent underlying factor in both the progression of ankylosing spondylitis and IBD.

Skin lesions are also common, being seen in approximately fifteen percent of patients. The skin lesions can be quite severe, including gangrene and/or painful, red lumps (e.g., erythema nodosum and pyoderma gangrenosum), but are usually simply annoying, like canker sores. In fact, recurrent canker sores occur in approximately ten percent of patients with IBD.[32]

Serious liver disease (i.e., sclerosing cholangitis, chronic active hepatitis, cirrhosis, etc.) is also a common EIL, affecting three to seven percent of people with IBD. If individuals are demonstrating liver enzyme abnormalities, they should take silymarin, a group of flavonoid compounds derived from milk thistle *(Silybum marianum)*. These compounds exert tremendous effect on protecting the liver from damage as well as enhancing detoxification processes.[33] Silymarin products are available at health food stores. The standard dosage for silymarin is 70 to 210 mg three times daily.

Other common EILs are inflammation of blood vessels, impaired blood flow to the fingers or toes, inflammatory eye manifestations (episcleritis, iritis, and uveitis), kidney stones, gallstones, and, in children, failure to grow, thrive, and mature normally.

IBD's Effects on General Nutrition

Many nutritional complications occur during the course of IBD.[34–36] Because these can have a significant influence on an IBD patient's well-being—and perhaps even mortality—every effort should be made to ensure optimal nutritional status.

CAUSES OF MALNUTRITION IN INFLAMMATORY BOWEL DISEASE

Decreased food intake

Disease-induced (pain, diarrhea, nausea, anorexia)

Doctor-induced (restrictive diets without supplementation)

Malabsorption

Decreased absorptive surface due to disease or surgical resection (removal of diseased segments by surgery)

Bile salt deficiency after surgical resection

Bacterial overgrowth of small intestine (see the DIGESTION section)

Drugs (e.g., corticosteroids, sulfasalazine, cholestyramine)

Increased secretion and nutrient loss

Protein-losing enteropathy (loss of protein due to shedding of intestinal cells)

Electrolyte, mineral, and trace mineral loss in diarrhea

Increased utilization and increased requirements for nutrients

Inflammation, fever, infection

Increased intestinal cell turnover

A decreased food intake is the most significant cause of nutritional deficiency in patients with IBD. It is the most most common nutritional deficit in patients who require hospitalization. Often the IBD patient feels pain, diarrhea, nausea, or other symptoms after a meal, resulting in a subtle decrease in dietary intake. Weight loss is prevalent in sixty-five to seventy-five percent of IBD patients.[34]

Malabsorption—lack of absorption of food and nutrients—can be anticipated in patients with extensive involvement of the small intestine and in patients who have had surgical resection of segments of the small intestine. Particularly common is fat malabsorption, resulting in significant caloric loss as well as loss of fat-soluble vitamins and minerals. Involvement or resection of the ileum of that area typically results in bile acid malabsorption. The laxative effect of bile acids on the colon may result in a chronic watery diarrhea. Patients with a history of chronic diarrhea may develop electrolyte and trace mineral deficiency, while chronic fat malabsorption (*steatorrhea*) may result in calcium and magnesium deficiency.

Increased secretion of tissue components and nutrient loss often occur due to the inflammatory nature of IBD. In particular, there is a significant loss of blood proteins across the damaged and inflamed mucosa. The loss of protein may exceed the ability of the liver to replace blood proteins, even with a high protein intake. The chronic loss of blood often leads to iron depletion and anemia.

The most common drugs used in the allopathic treatment of IBD are corticosteroids (e.g., prednisone) and sulfasalazine, both of which increase nutritional needs. Corticosteroids are known to stimulate protein breakdown (catabolism); depress protein synthesis; decrease the absorption of calcium and phosphorus; increase the urinary excretion of vitamin C, calcium, potassium, and zinc; increase levels of blood glucose, serum triglycerides, and serum cholesterol; increase the requirements for vitamin B6, ascorbic acid, folate, and vitamin D; decrease bone formation; and impair wound healing. Sulfasalazine inhibits the absorption and transport of folate, decreases serum folate and iron, and increases the urinary excretion of ascorbic acid.

A chronic inflammatory and/or infectious disease like IBD also leads to nutritional deficiency because of increased nutritional needs. For example, patients with IBD typically require perhaps as much as, or even more than, twenty-five percent more protein than the usual recommended dietary allowance, especially if a significant amount of protein is being lost (described previously).[34–36]

Correcting Nutritional Deficiencies

The importance of correcting nutritional deficiencies in patients with IBD cannot be overstated. Nutrient deficiencies, both macro and micro, lead to altered gastrointestinal function and structure, which may result in the patient entering a vicious cycle. That is, the secondary effects of malnutrition on the gastrointestinal tract may lead to a further increase in malabsorption, further decreasing nutrient status.

The majority of individuals with IBD suffer from nutritional deficiencies. In addition to the deficiencies listed in Table 1 in the chapter IMMUNE FUNCTION, low levels of vitamin K, copper, niacin, and vitamin E have also been reported.[34]

Providing adequate caloric intake is the most important aspect of nutritional therapy. The next step in dietary treatment involves the use of either an elemental or an elimination diet.

The Elemental Diet

The *elemental diet* is often an effective nontoxic alternative to corticosteroids as the primary treatment of acute IBD.[8–11] An elemental diet is one that contains all essential nutrients, with protein being provided only in the form of predigested or isolated amino acids. However, the improvements seen in patients on an elemental diet are probably not primarily related to nutritional improvement; the elemental diet is probably serving as an allergen-elimination diet. Some

TABLE 1	Frequency of Nutritional Deficiency in Patients with Inflammatory Bowel Disease[34]
DEFICIENCY	**PREVALENCE (%)**
Iron deficiency	40
Low serum vitamin B12	48
Low serum folate	54–64
Low serum magnesium	14–33
Low serum potassium	6–20
Low serum retinol	21
Low serum ascorbate	12
Low serum 25-OH-vitamin D	25–65
Low serum zinc	40–50

improvement may also be the result of alterations in the fecal flora that have been observed in patients consuming an elemental diet.

Hospitalization is often required for satisfactory administration of elemental diets, and relapse is common when patients resume normal eating. An elimination diet may be a more acceptable alternative in the treatment of IBD, particularly chronic cases.

The Elimination Diet

Elimination (oligoantigenic) diets are described in detail in the chapter FOOD ALLERGY. Basically they are diets consisting of foods that have a lower tendency to produce allergic reactions.

Although food allergy has long been considered an important causative factor in the development of IBD, studies have only recently utilized an elimination diet in the treatment of IBD.[11–13] These studies demonstrate that an elimination diet should be the primary therapy in the treatment of chronic IBD. The most common offending foods were found to be wheat and dairy products.

An alternative approach is to determine the actual food allergens by laboratory methods, preferably a method that measures both IgG- and IgE-mediated reactions such as the ELISA test (see FOOD ALLERGY for description). The allergens can then be avoided, or a rotary diversified diet may be appropriate (see FOOD ALLERGY).

The High–Complex Carbohydrate, High-Fiber Diet

Treatment with a high-fiber diet has been shown to have a favorable effect on the course of Crohn's disease and ulcerative colitis.[7] This is in direct contrast to one of the oldest allopathic dietary treatments of IBD: a low-fiber diet. Although some foods, such as wheat bran, may be too "rough" to handle, the dietary treatment of IBD should involve foods rich in fiber and unrefined carbohydrates, combined with a diet that avoids known food allergens or rotary diversified diet. This latter combination is much more effective than a high-fiber diet alone.[12]

Dietary fiber has a profound effect on the intestinal environment and is thought to promote a more optimal intestinal flora composition.[37] However, considering the high degree of intolerance to wheat found in patients with IBD, and the known roughness of wheat bran, supplemental wheat bran is not the fiber of choice for these patients.

A High-Quality Multiple-Vitamin-and-Mineral Formula

It is absolutely essential that patients with IBD take a high-quality multiple-vitamin-and-mineral supplement that provides all of the known vitamins and minerals. Use the recommendations in the chapter SUPPLEMENTARY MEASURES to provide an optimum intake range in selecting a high-quality multiple.

Additional Antioxidants

Along with taking a high-potency multiple-vitamin-and-mineral formula, individuals with IBD will need to take additional antioxidants. The two primary antioxidants in the human body are vitamin C and vitamin E. Vitamin C is an aqueous-phase antioxidant, which means that it is found in body compartments composed of water. In contrast, vitamin E is a lipid-phase antioxidant because it is found in fat-soluble body compartments, such as cell membranes and fatty molecules. For good antioxidant protection, we recommend taking the following dosage each day for patients with IBD (dosages include the amount in the multiple-vitamin-and-mineral formula):

- Vitamin E (d-alpha tocopherol): 400–800 IU
- Vitamin C (ascorbic acid): 1,000–3,000 mg

The Role of Zinc, Folic Acid, and Vitamin B12 in IBD

Three nutrients deserve special mention in the treatment of IBD: zinc, folic acid, and vitamin B12. Zinc deficiency is a well-known complication of Crohn's disease, due to low dietary intake, poor absorption, and excess fecal losses.[38] Evidence of zinc deficiency occurs in approximately forty-five percent of Crohn's disease patients, and in similar numbers for patients with ulcerative colitis. Low zinc concentrations in the blood, low zinc levels in the hair, malabsorption of zinc, altered urinary excretion of zinc, and impaired taste acuity are commonly found in Crohn's disease patients. In addition, many of the complications of the disease may be a direct result of zinc deficiency: poor healing of fissures and fistulas, skin lesions, decreased sexual development (hypogonadism), growth retardation, retinal dysfunction, depressed immunity, and loss of appetite.

Many patients will not respond to oral or even intravenous zinc supplementation; there appears to be a defect in tissue transport. Intravenous supplementation results in a tremendous increase in urinary zinc excretion but has insignificant clinical results. Several clinical trials using oral zinc sulfate have shown the same lack of results.[39] Supplying zinc in the form of *zinc picolinate* may be more advantageous, possibly improving both intestinal absorption and tissue transport. Picolinate is a zinc-binding molecule secreted by the pancreas; it appears to be better absorbed and utilized.

Like zinc deficiency, folic acid deficiency is quite common in IBD, with reports of deficiency occurrence ranging from twenty-five to sixty-four percent of IBD patients.[34,40–42] The reason for this deficiency, in many cases, is the drug sulfasalazine. Correction of folate deficiency is absolutely essential because folate deficiency promotes further malabsorption and diarrhea due to altered structure of the intestinal mucosal cells.[43] These cells have a very rapid turnover (one to four days) and need to have a constant supply of folic acid.

Since vitamin B12 is absorbed at the portion of the intestine most commonly affected with Crohn's disease (the terminal ileum), deficiency of this vitamin is also quite common.[34,44] Overall, abnormal B12 absorption is found in forty-eight percent of patients with Crohn's disease. Often the terminal ileum of a Crohn's disease patient has been surgically removed *(resected)*. If the length of the resection is less than 60 cm, or the extent of the inflammatory lesion is less than 60 cm, adequate absorption may occur. Otherwise, monthly vitamin B12 injections (1,000 mcg, intramuscularly) are recommended.

Take Pancreatic Extracts

Pancreatic extracts can help with digestion as well as reduce some of the inflammation of IBD. See the chapter DIGESTION for a more complete discussion.

An Old Naturopathic Remedy

Although no research has been done to document its efficacy, an old naturopathic remedy—Robert's Formula—has a long history of use by naturopathic physicians for treating IBD. It is composed of several botanical medicines:

- *Althea officinalis* (marshmallow root: a soothing demulcent)
- *Baptisia tinctora* (wild indigo: used for gastrointestinal infections)
- *Echinacea angustifolia* (purple coneflower: antibacterial; used to promote normalization of the immune system)
- *Geranium maculatum* (geranium: used for its astringent action to help heal ulcerations)
- *Hydrastis canadensis* (goldenseal: inhibits the growth of many disease-causing bacteria)
- *Ulmus fulva* (slippery elm: demulcent effect)

Here is a modified version of Robert's Formula that you can mix up yourself using powdered herbs available at health food stores:

8 parts *Althea officinalis*
4 parts *Baptisia tinctora*
8 parts *Echinacea angustifolia*
8 parts *Geranium maculatum*
8 parts *Hydrastis canadensis*
8 parts *Ulmus fulva*
8 parts cabbage powder

You can take 1 to 2 teaspoons of the above three times daily, or you may choose to purchase one of the many commercially available versions marketed as Robert's Formula.

Crohn's Disease Activity Index

The Crohn's Disease Activity Index (CDAI) was developed as a monitoring tool in the National Cooperative Crohn's Disease Study.[45] It met the basic requirements necessary for the study: it provided uniform clinical parameters that could be assessed, and it produced a consistent numerical index for recording the results of the study.

The CDAI is calculated by adding together eight variables. It incorporates both subjective and objective information in determining relative disease activity. Generally speaking, CDAI scores below 150 indicate a better prognosis than higher scores. The CDAI is a useful way to monitor therapeutic progress.

Table 2 outlines the variables and the formula used to calculate the CDAI.

Monitoring the Pediatric IBD Patient

It is often difficult to achieve normal growth and development in a pediatric patient with IBD. Growth failure occurs in seventy-five percent of Crohn's disease pediatric patients, while ulcerative colitis causes growth failure in twenty-five percent.[36] The pediatric patient with IBD should be evaluated at least twice yearly by a physician knowledgeable in all the necessary components of a comprehensive exam for IBD patients, including detailed body and weight measurements and appropriate laboratory testing.

The list below outlines the necessary components of a comprehensive twice-yearly nutritional evaluation of pediatric patients with IBD. An aggressive nutritional program should be instituted, including supplements (it may be necessary to use injectable methods in some patients), that is similar to the approach outlined for the adult patient, with the doses adjusted as appropriate.

Parents of children who have IBD need to know the components necessary to monitor their children. They need not understand the significance of each component, but they do need to make sure that their children are being properly evaluated.

PEDIATRIC IBD MONITORING

- Type and duration of inflammatory bowel disease; frequency of relapses
- Severity and extent of ongoing symptoms
- Medication history
- Three-day diet diary
- Physical examination
- Height, weight, arm circumference, and triceps skin-fold measurements
- Evidence of increased disease activity (e.g., loss of subcutaneous fat, muscle wasting, edema, pallor, skin rash, liver enlargement)
- Laboratory tests:

  CBC and differential, reticulocyte and platelet count, sedimentation rate, urinalysis

  Serum total proteins, albumin, globulin, and retinol binding protein

  Serum electrolytes, calcium, phosphate, ferritin, folate, carotenes, tocopherol, and B12

  Leukocyte ascorbate, magnesium, and zinc

  Creatinine height index, BUN:creatinine ratio

. . . .

TREATMENT SUMMARY

The key recommendation is to identify and control food allergies. Other recommendations are

- Consume a diet that focuses on whole, unprocessed foods (whole grains, legumes, vegetables, fruits, nuts, and seeds).
- Eliminate the intake of alcohol, caffeine, and sugar.
- Get regular exercise.
- Perform a relaxation exercise (deep breathing, meditation, prayer, visualization, etc.) for ten to fifteen minutes each day.
- Drink at least 48 ounces of water daily.

Nutritional Supplements

- High-potency multiple-vitamin-and-mineral formula (see the chapter SUPPLEMENTARY MEASURES)
- Vitamin C: 3,000–8,000 mg per day
- Vitamin E: 200–400 IU per day
- Zinc: 30–45 mg per day
- Flaxseed oil: 1 tablespoon per day
- Pancreatin (8–10X): 350–700 mg three times per day between meals

TABLE 2	Independent Variables and Formula Used to Calculate the CDAI
X1	Number of liquid or very soft stools in one week
X2	Sum of seven daily abdominal pain ratings:
	0 = none, 1 = mild, 2 = moderate, 3 = severe
X3	Sum of seven daily ratings of general well-being:
	0 = well, 1 = slightly below par, 2 = poor, 3 = very poor, 4 = terrible
X4	Symptoms or findings presumed related to Crohn's disease:
	1. Arthritis or arthralgia
	2. Iritis or uveitis
	3. Erythema nodosum, pyoderma gangrenosum, aphthous stomatitis
	4. Anal fissure, fistula, or perirectal abscess
	5. Other bowel-related fistula
	6. Febrile episode > 100 degrees Fahrenheit during past week
	(Add 1 for each category corresponding to patient's symptoms.)
X5	Taking Lomotil or opiates for diarrhea:
	0 = no, 1 = yes
X6	Abdominal mass:
	0 = none, 0.4 = questionable, 1 = present
X7	47 minus hematocrit, males; 42 minus hematocrit, females
X8	100 multi symbol (standard weight according to height and weight charts minus body weight)/standard weight

CDAI = 2 multiplied by X1 + 5 multiplied by X2 + 7 multiplied by X3 + 20 multiplied by X4 + 30 multiplied by X5 + 10 multiplied by X6 + 6 multiplied by X7 + X multiplied by 8.

The CDAI is not as accurate in monitoring IBD in children as it is in adults. To address this shortcoming, Lloyd-Still and Green devised a clinical scoring system for IBD in children.[46] The scoring system has five major divisions (the maximum score is in parentheses):

1. General activity (10)
2. Physical examination and clinical complications (30)
3. Nutrition (20)
4. X rays (15)
5. Laboratory (25)

An elevated score (i.e., scores in the 80s) represents good status, while scores in the 30s and 40s represent severe disease. Table 3 outlines the criteria that are used to determine the clinical score.

Emergency Status of IBD

In some individuals, Crohn's disease and ulcerative colitis are life-threatening diseases, which at times require emergency treatment. A small percentage of patients who have severe disease may require occasional hospitalization. Any serious increase in disease activity requires immediate medical attention. This is particularly true for individuals with IBD who have: a fever of 101 degrees Fahrenheit or higher; profuse, constant, loose, bloody stools; loss of appetite; and a distended abdomen.loose, bloody stools; loss of appetite; and a distended abdomen.

TABLE 3   Clinical Score in Chronic Pediatric IBD

General activity

10: Normal school attendance with less than 3 bowel movements per day
5: Lacks endurance and has 3–5 bowel movements per day
1: Misses more than 4 weeks school/year

Physical examination and complications

Abdomen

10: Normal
5: Mass
1: Distension, tenderness

Proctoscope

10: Normal, no fissures
5: Friable, 1 fissure
1: Ulcers, bleeding, fistulas, multiple fissures

Arthritis

5: None
3: One joint/arthralgia
1: Multiple joints

Skin/mouth/eyes

5: Normal
3: Mild inflammation
4: Erythema nodosum, pyoderma severe canker sores and/or inflammation of the mouth, inflammation of the eyes

Height

10: Growth >2"/year
5: <optimal %
1: No growth

Nutrition

X rays

15: Normal
10: Ileitis, colitis from the rectum to the splenic flexure (the turn of the colon near the spleen)
5: Total colon or ileocecal involvement
1: Toxic megacolon or obstruction

Laboratory

Hematocrit

5: >40
3: 25–35
1: <25

Erythrocyte sedimentation rate

5: Normal
3: 20–40
1: >40

White blood cell count

5: Normal
3: <20,000
1: >20,000

Albumin

10: Normal
5: 3.0 g/dl
1: <2.5 g/dl

Insomnia

Difficulty falling asleep (sleep-onset insomnia)

Frequent or early awakening (sleep-maintenance insomnia)

Within the course of a year, up to thirty percent of the population suffers from insomnia.[1] Many use over-the-counter medications to combat the problem, while others seek stronger sedatives. Each year roughly ten million people in the United States receive prescriptions for sedative hypnotics. Psychological factors, such as depression or anxiety, account for fifty percent of all insomnias evaluated in sleep laboratories.[1] Insomnia is closely associated with depression.[2] The importance of sleep to general health is detailed in A HEALTHY LIFESTYLE.

The Problem with Sleeping Pills

The two primary classes of drugs used in the treatment of insomnia are *antihistamines* and *benzodiazepines*. Antihistamines, like Benadryl and Nytol, are available over the counter, while benzodiazepines, like Valium and Halcion, are available by prescription. While both antihistamines and benzodiazepines are effective in the short term, they cause significant problems in the long term. Benzodiazepines, in particular, are not designed to be used for the long term, as they are addictive, have numerous side effects, and cause abnormal sleep patterns. Antihistamines also interfere with normal sleep patterns. As a result, people who take sleeping pills enter a vicious cycle. They take the drug to induce sleep, but the drug causes further disruption of normal sleep. In the morning,

in an attempt to "get going," they will typically drink large quantities of coffee, which further worsens insomnia.

WARNING: If you have taken a benzodiazepine for more than four weeks, do not stop taking the drug suddenly. It is important to work with your physician to taper off the drug gradually to avoid potentially dangerous withdrawal symptoms. Symptoms of withdrawal can include: anxiety, irritability, panic, insomnia, nausea, headache, impaired concentration, memory loss, depression, extreme sensitivity to the environment, seizures, hallucinations, and paranoia.

Therapeutic Considerations

As with virtually every health condition discussed in this book, the most effective treatment of insomnia is based upon identifying and addressing causative factors. The most common causes of insomnia are psychological: depression, anxiety, and tension. If psychological factors do not seem to be the cause, various foods, drinks, and medications may be responsible. There are numerous compounds in food and drink and in well over three hundred drugs that can interfere with normal sleep.

Insomnia is divided into two primary categories: *sleep-onset insomnia* and *sleep-*

TABLE 1	Causes of Insomnia

SLEEP-ONSET INSOMNIA	SLEEP-MAINTENANCE INSOMNIA
Anxiety or tension	Depression
Environmental change	Environmental change
Emotional arousal	Sleep apnea
Fear of insomnia	Nocturnal myoclonus
Phobia of sleep	Hypoglycemia
Disruptive environment	Parasomnias such as sleep apnea, restless-legs syndrome, etc. (see A HEALTHY LIFESTYLE for more details)
Pain or discomfort	Pain or discomfort
Caffeine	Drugs
Alcohol	Alcohol

maintenance insomnia. In sleep-onset insomnia, individuals have a hard time getting to sleep. In sleep-maintenance insomnia, individuals have a difficult time maintaining sleep. The boundary between these two categories is not entirely distinct in most cases. However, classification is often helpful in identifying causative factors.

Dietary and Lifestyle Factors

There are several dietary and lifestyle factors to consider in relieving insomnia, including: eliminating food and drink compounds that impair sleep processes; avoiding nocturnal hypoglycemia; learning to relax; and getting enough exercise. Each of these factors is discussed in following paragraphs. These possible causes of insomnia should be addressed before resorting to the use of any sedative, even if the sedative is a natural compound.

Eliminating Inhibitors of Sleep
It is essential that the diet be free of natural stimulants such as caffeine and related compounds. Coffee, as well as less obvious caffeine sources such as soft drinks, chocolate,

coffee-flavored ice cream, hot cocoa, and tea, must all be eliminated.

The sensitivity to the stimulant effects of caffeine varies greatly from one person to the next. This is largely a reflection of how quickly the body can eliminate caffeine. In other words, some people are more sensitive to the effects of caffeine than others, due to a slower elimination of these substances from the body. Even small amounts of caffeine such as those found in decaffeinated coffee or chocolate, may be enough to cause insomnia in some people.

Another substance that must be eliminated is alcohol, which produces a number of sleep-impairing effects. In addition to causing the release of adrenaline, alcohol impairs the transport of tryptophan into the brain, and, because the brain is dependent upon tryptophan as the source for serotonin (an important neurotransmitter that initiates sleep), alcohol disrupts serotonin levels.

Avoiding Nocturnal Hypoglycemia
Our experience in clinical practice is that nocturnal hypoglycemia (low nighttime blood glucose level) is an important cause of

TABLE 2	Caffeine Content of Coffee, Tea, and Selected Soft Drinks
BEVERAGE	**CAFFEINE (MG)**
Coffee (7.5-oz cup)	
Drip	115–150
Brewed	80–135
Instant	65–40
Decaffeinated	3–4
Tea (5-oz cup)	
1-minute brew	20
3-minute brew	35
Iced (12 oz)	70
Soft Drinks	
Jolt	100
Mountain Dew	54
Tab	47
Coca-Cola	45
Diet Coke	45
Dr. Pepper	40
Pepsi Cola	38

sleep-maintenance insomnia. When there is a drop in the blood glucose level, it causes the release of hormones that regulate glucose levels, such as adrenaline, glucagon, cortisol, and growth hormone. These compounds stimulate the brain. They are a natural signal that it is time to eat.

Many people in the United States suffer from faulty glucose metabolism, either hypoglycemia or diabetes, because of overeating refined carbohydrates. Good bedtime snacks to keep blood sugar levels steady throughout the night are oatmeal and other whole grain cereals, whole grain breads and muffins, and other complex carbohydrates. These foods will not only help maintain blood sugar levels, they actually can help promote sleep by increasing the level of serotonin within the brain.

Progressive Relaxation

There are numerous techniques that can promote relaxation and prepare the body and mind for sleep. One of the most popular and easy-to-use techniques is progressive relaxation. The technique is based on a simple procedure of comparing tension to relaxation, which teaches the person what it feels like to relax. Many people are not aware of the sensation of relaxation.

To practice progressive relaxation, you will first forcefully contract one muscle group for a period of one to two seconds, then give way to a feeling of relaxation. Since the procedure goes progressively through all the muscles of the body, eventually a deep state of relaxation will result. Begin by contracting the muscles of the face and neck; hold the contraction for

QUICK REVIEW

- Insomnia affects almost one out of every three people in the United States during the course of a year.
- Effective treatment involves identifying and addressing causative factors and eliminating factors that can disrupt sleep.
- In addition to side effects, the major problem with sleeping pills is their interference with normal sleep.
- The most common causes of insomnia are psychological: depression, anxiety, and tension.
- If psychological factors do not seem to be the cause, various foods, drinks, and medications may be responsible.

at least one to two seconds; then relax the muscles. Next, contract and relax the upper arms and chest, followed by the lower arms and hands. Repeat the process progressively down your body, i.e., the abdomen, the buttocks, the thighs, the calves, and the feet. Repeat this whole practice two or three times, or until you fall asleep.

Exercise

Regular physical exercise is known to improve general well-being in addition to promoting improvement in sleep quality.[1] Exercise should be performed in the morning or early evening, not before bedtime, and should be of moderate intensity. Usually twenty minutes of aerobic exercise at a heart rate between sixty and seventy-five percent of maximum (approximately 220 minus age in years) is sufficient. See the chapter A HEALTHY LIFESTYLE for additional information on how to design an exercise program.

Natural Sedatives

The general recommendations just given are often all that is needed to relieve insomnia. When additional support is required, there are several natural sedatives that can produce excellent results without the problems associated with prescription and over-the-counter sedatives. The following topics are discussed as they relate to promoting sleep: serotonin precursor and cofactor therapy, melatonin, restless-legs syndrome, and botanicals with sedative properties.

Serotonin Precursor and Cofactor Therapy

Serotonin is an important initiator of sleep. Serotonin is made from the amino acid *tryptophan* (discussed in more detail in DEPRESSION). Taking tryptophan will raise serotonin levels and promote sleep. Tryptophan is more effective for cases of sleep-onset insomnia, since its greatest effect is to shorten the time required to get to sleep (referred to as sleep latency).[3–5]

More effective than tryptophan is *5-hydroxytryptophan* (5-HTP), a form of tryptophan that is one step closer to serotonin administration. 5-HTP has also been reported, in numerous double-blind clinical studies, to decrease the time required to get to sleep and to decrease the number of awakenings.[6] Because tryptophan is currently available only by prescription, 5-HTP is an obvious substitute. The sedative effects of 5-HTP can be enhanced by taking it near bedtime with a carbohydrate source such as fruit or fruit juice.[3]

• There are numerous compounds in food and drink and well over three hundred drugs that can interfere with normal sleep.

• The two major classifications of insomnia are sleep-onset and sleep-maintenance.

• 5-HTP provides better results than those achieved with L-tryptophan.

• Melatonin is only effective as a sedative when body melatonin levels are low.

• Restless-legs syndrome and myoclonus may respond to folic acid therapy, iron supplementation, and other nutritional therapies.

• Valerian and passionflower can promote improved sleep quality and relief of insomnia.

One of the key benefits of using 5-HTP to treat insomnia is its ability to increase REM sleep (typically by about twenty-five percent) while simultaneously increasing deep-sleep Stages 3 and 4, without increasing total sleep time.[6] The sleep stages that are reduced to compensate for the increases are non-REM Stages 1 and 2, the least important stages of sleep. For more information on normal sleep patterns, see A HEALTHY LIFESTYLE.

It is important to maintain adequate levels of vitamin B_6, niacin, and magnesium when using 5-HTP, as these nutrients serve as essential cofactors in the conversion of 5-HTP to serotonin.

Melatonin

One of the best aids for sleep is *melatonin*—an important hormone secreted by the pineal gland, a small gland in the center of the brain. In several studies, supplementation with melatonin has been found helpful in inducing and maintaining sleep in both children and adults, for both people with normal sleep patterns and those suffering from insomnia. However, it appears that the sleep-promoting effects of melatonin are most apparent only if a person's melatonin levels are low.[7] In other words, taking melatonin is not like taking a sleeping pill or even 5-HTP. It will only produce a sedative effect when melatonin levels are low.

When melatonin is taken by normal subjects just before going to bed, or by insomnia patients who have normal melatonin levels, it produces no sedative effect. That is because, just prior to going to bed, there is normally a rise in melatonin secretion. Melatonin supplementation is only effective as a sedative when the pineal gland's own production of melatonin is very low. Melatonin appears to be most effective in treating insomnia in the elderly, as low melatonin levels are common in this age group.[8]

In one of the most interesting studies, twenty-six elderly insomniacs with lower than normal melatonin levels were given 1 to 2 mg of melatonin two hours prior to their desired bedtime for one week. Both rapid- and slow-release melatonin preparations were used. Both sleep latency and sleep quality were evaluated. While there was no discernible difference in sleep onset and sleep efficiency (percent of time asleep to total time in bed) between the two forms, the timed-release form yielded better results on sleep maintenance.[9]

A dosage of 3 mg at bedtime is more than enough, as dosages as low as 0.1 mg and 0.3 mg have been shown to produce a sedative effect when melatonin levels are low.[10] Although there appear to be no serious side effects at recommended dosages, melatonin supplementation could conceivably disrupt the normal circadian rhythm. In one study, a daily dosage of 8 mg a day for only four days resulted in significant alterations in hormone secretions.[11]

Restless-Legs Syndrome and Nocturnal Myoclonus

The restless-legs syndrome is characterized during waking by an irresistible urge to move the legs. Almost all patients with restless-legs syndrome have nocturnal myoclonus.[1] *Nocturnal myoclonus* is a neuromuscular disorder characterized by repeated contractions of one or more muscle groups, typically of the leg, during sleep. Each jerk usually lasts fewer than ten seconds. The patient is normally unaware of the myoclonus, and only complains of either frequent nocturnal awakenings or excessive daytime sleepiness. However, questioning the sleep partner often reveals the myoclonus. These disorders are significant causes of insomnia.

If there is a family history of restless-legs syndrome (about one-third of all patients with this syndrome have a family history), high-dosage folic acid (35 to 60 mg daily) therapy can be helpful.[12] Dosages in this range will require a prescription, as the FDA limits the amount available per capsule to 800 mcg. In cases of familial restless-legs syndrome, there appears to be a higher need for folic acid.

If there is no family history of restless-legs syndrome, ask your doctor to rule out low iron levels. The best method is to measure the level of the iron-storage protein *ferritin* in the blood; the level of ferritin indicates the level of stored iron. The association between low iron levels and the restless-legs syndrome was documented in clinical studies more than thirty years ago.

The most recent study was conducted in 1994 at the Department of Geriatric Medicine of the Royal Liverpool University in Liverpool, U.K.[13] Levels of ferritin in the blood were found to be lower in the eighteen patients who had restless-legs syndrome than in the eighteen control subjects. Ferritin levels were inversely correlated with the severity of restless-legs syndrome symptoms, meaning that the lower the ferritin level, the more severe the restless legs. Blood levels of iron, vitamin B12, folic acid, and hemoglobin did not differ between the two groups. Fifteen of the patients who had restless-legs syndrome were treated with iron (ferrous sulfate) at a dosage of 200 mg three times daily for two months, with excellent results.

The conclusion of the study: "Iron deficiency, with or without anemia, is an important contributor to the development of RLS [restless legs syndrome] in elderly patients, and iron supplements can produce a significant reduction in symptoms."

If you have nocturnal myoclonus, or muscle cramps that occur at night, try taking magnesium (250 mg at night) and vitamin E (400 to 800 IU per day). If you are over the age of fifty, *Ginkgo biloba* extract (80 mg three times per day) may also be helpful.

Botanicals with Sedative Properties

Numerous plants have sedative action. Plants commonly prescribed as aids in promoting sleep include: passionflower (*Passiflora incarnata*), hops (*Humulus lupulus*), valerian (*Valeriana officinalis*), skullcap (*Scutellaria lateriflora*), and chamomile (*Matricaria chamomilla*).[14–16] Passionflower and valerian, which have research supporting their use, are discussed here.

Passiflora incarnata (Passionflower) Passionflower was widely used by the Aztecs as a sedative and analgesic. Its constituents include *harmine*. Harmine was originally known as telepathine because of its peculiar ability to induce a contemplative state and mild euphoria. It was later used by the Germans in World War II as "truth serum." Harmine and related compounds can inhibit the breakdown of serotonin, therefore their use with 5-HTP would have an additive effect.[14–16]

Valeriana officinalis (Valerian) This plant has also been widely used in folk medicine as a sedative and antihypertensive.[9] An early study involving 128 subjects demonstrated that an aqueous extract of valerian root significantly improved sleep quality.[17] This double-blind study compared the effects of the aqueous extract to a placebo and an over-the-counter preparation of valerian from Switzerland, in both good and poor sleepers. The study measured sleep latency, night awakenings, subjective sleep quality, and sleepiness the next morning. From the results, the following conclusions can be made: the aqueous extract of valerian had its most significant effect among people who considered themselves poor or irregular sleepers (particularly women), smokers, and people with long sleep latencies; the over-the-counter valerian produced little sedative effect compared to the placebo; and the use of the commercially available product produced a significant increase in the degree of sleepiness the next morning compared with the aqueous extract or the placebo.

Several other clinical studies have substantiated valerian's ability to improve sleep quality and relieve insomnia.[18–21] In one study, valerian showed a significant effect compared to the placebo, with forty-four percent reporting perfect sleep and eighty-nine percent reporting improved sleep.[20] In another double-blind study of insomniacs, twenty subjects received either a combination of valerian root extract (160 mg) and *Melissa officinalis* extract (80 mg), benzodiazepine (triazolam 0.125 mg), or a placebo.[21] In the insomniac group, the valerian/melissa preparation showed an effect comparable to that of the benzodiazepines, as well as an ability to increase deep-sleep Stages 3 and 4. The valerian/melissa preparation did not, however, cause daytime sleepiness, and there was no evidence of diminished concentration or impairment of physical performance.

TREATMENT SUMMARY

Effective treatment involves identifying and addressing causative factors. If depression is a possibility, please consult DEPRESSION. Once a normal sleep pattern has been established, the dosages of the recommended supplements and botanicals should be slowly decreased.

Lifestyle

Institute a regular exercise program that elevates heart rate by fifty to seventy-five percent for at least twenty minutes each day. Perform progressive relaxation exercises to help fall asleep.

Nutritional Supplements

Take the following forty-five minutes before bedtime:

- Niacin: 100 mg (decrease dose if uncomfortable flushing interferes with sleep induction)
- Vitamin B6: 50 mg
- Magnesium: 250 mg
- 5-HTP: 100–300 mg
  Or melatonin: 3 mg

Botanical Medicines

Take the following forty-five minutes before bedtime:

- *Valeriana officinalis*
  Dried root (or as tea): 2–3 g
  Tincture (1:5): 4–6 ml (1–1.5 tsp)
  Fluid extract (1:1): 1–2 ml (0.5–1 tsp)
  Dry powdered extract (0.8% valerenic acid): 150–300 mg
- *Passiflora incarnata* (best when used with 5-HTP)
  Dried herb (or as tea): 4–8 g
  Tincture (1:5): 6–8 ml (1.5–2 tsp)
  Fluid extract (1:1): 2–4 ml (0.5–1 tsp)
  Dry powdered extract (2.6% flavonoids): 300–450 mg

Irritable Bowel Syndrome

· ·

Characterized by some combination of
    Abdominal pain or distension
    Altered bowel function, constipation, or diarrhea
    Hypersecretion of colonic mucus
    Dyspeptic symptoms (flatulence, nausea, anorexia)
    Varying degrees of anxiety or depression

Outdated terms include: nervous indigestion, spastic colitis, mucous colitis, and intestinal neurosis.

Irritable bowel syndrome (IBS) is the most common gastrointestinal disorder and represents thirty to fifty percent of all referrals to gastroenterologists.[1,2] Determining the true frequency is virtually impossible, as many sufferers never seek medical attention. It has, however, been estimated that approximately fifteen percent of the population have complaints of IBS, with women predominating two to one (it is likely that an equal number of males have IBS, but that they do not report symptoms as often). IBS has been attributed to physiological, psychological, and dietary factors.

The diagnosis of IBS is often made by exclusion, as a result of ruling out other conditions that can mimic IBS (see box). We recommend that you consult a physician if you have symptoms suggestive of IBS. The physician will decide just how extensive the diagnostic process will be. A detailed medical history and physical examination have been shown to eliminate much of the vagueness involved in diagnosing IBS.[3] Abdominal distension, relief of pain with bowel movements, and the onset of loose or more frequent bowel movements with pain seem to correlate best with the diagnosis of IBS.[1]

CONDITIONS THAT MAY MIMIC IBS

Cancer

Disturbed bacterial microflora as a result of antibiotic or antacid usage

Diverticular disease

Infectious diarrhea, such as amebiasis or giardiasis

Inflammatory bowel disease

Intestinal candidiasis

Lactose intolerance

Laxative abuse

Malabsorption diseases, such as pancreatic insufficiency and celiac disease

Mechanical causes, such as fecal impaction

Metabolic disorders, such as adrenal insufficiency, diabetes, or hyperthyroidism

Response to dietary factors that interfere with digestion, such as excessive consumption of tea, coffee, carbonated beverages, and simple sugars

Therapeutic Considerations

We want to stress the importance of consulting a physician for proper diagnosis of IBS.

Once other conditions have been ruled out, there are four major treatments for IBS, from a natural perspective:

1. Increasing intake of dietary fiber
2. Eliminating allergenic foods
3. Using enteric-coated volatile oils
4. Controlling psychological components

Dietary Fiber

The treatment of irritable bowel syndrome by increasing dietary fiber intake has a long, although irregular, history.[1] Patients with constipation are much more likely to respond to dietary fiber than those with diarrhea. One problem that has not been addressed in studies on the therapeutic use of dietary fiber is the role of food allergy. The type of fiber often used in both research and clinical practice is wheat bran.[4] As wheat and other grains are among the most commonly implicated foods in malabsorptive and allergic conditions, the use of wheat bran is usually not advised since food allergy is a significant causative factor in this condition.

Increasing intake of dietary fiber from fruit and vegetable sources rather than cereal sources may offer more benefit to some individuals. However, in one uncontrolled clinical study there was no significant difference in improvement when a diet composed of 30 grams of fruit and vegetable fiber and 10 grams of cereal fiber was compared to one with the opposite ratio.[5] Although both diets resulted in similar significant improvement in abdominal pain, bowel habits, and state of well-being, the presence of large quantities of potentially allergenic cereal fiber in both diets would probably have obscured any differences. Furthermore, in certain cases fiber may aggravate diarrhea and is therefore not recommended.

Food Allergy or Intolerance

The importance of food allergies as a cause of IBS has been recognized since the early 1900s.[6,7] More recent studies have further documented the association between food allergy and the irritable bowel.[8–11] According to a double-blind challenge, the majority of patients with IBS (approximately two-thirds) have at least one food allergy, and some have multiple allergies.[8] The most common allergens are dairy products (forty to forty-four percent) and grains (forty to sixty percent).[10]

QUICK REVIEW

- Irritable bowel syndrome is a functional disorder of the large intestine with no evidence of accompanying structural defect.
- The four major treatments from a natural perspective are: (1) increasing dietary fiber, (2) eliminating allergenic foods, (3) using enteric-coated volatile oil preparations, and (4) controlling psychological factors through stress reduction and exercise.
- Meals high in refined sugar can contribute to irritable bowel syndrome.
- Enteric-coated peppermint oil is quite beneficial in relieving the symptoms of irritable bowel syndrome.
- The splenic flexure syndrome is a variant of the irritable bowel syndrome in which gas in the bowel leads to pain in the lower chest or the left shoulder

Since, in most cases, the reaction appears to be related to prostaglandin synthesis or IgG- rather than IgE-mediated reactions, skin tests and the IgE-RAST are poor indicators of food intolerance in these patients. The ELISA ACT or ELISA IgE/IgG4 may be better indicators (see FOOD ALLERGY for further discussion), although many sensitivities may still be undetectable by currently available laboratory procedures.[12] Many patients have noted marked clinical improvement when using elimination diets.[8–11]

It is interesting to note that many IBS patients have related symptoms suggestive of vascular instability, such as heart palpitation, hyperventilation, fatigue, excessive sweating, and headaches. This is consistent with food allergy/intolerance reactions.

Sugar

Meals high in refined sugar can contribute to IBS and small intestine bacterial overgrowth by decreasing intestinal motility—the rhythmic contractions of the intestine that propel food through the digestive tract.[13] When blood sugar levels rise too rapidly, the normal rhythmic contractions of the gastrointestinal tract slow down. Since glucose is primarily absorbed in the duodenum and jejunum, the message affects this portion of the gastrointestinal tract the most strongly. The result is that the duodenum and jejunum become paralyzed *(atonic)*. A diet high in refined sugar may be the most important contributing factor to IBS being such a common condition in the United States.

Enteric-Coated Volatile Oils

Peppermint oil, and presumably similar volatile oils, inhibit, gastrointestinal smooth muscle action in both laboratory animal preparations and humans.[14] Clinically, it has been used to reduce colonic spasm during endoscopy (a procedure where a tube with a lens attached is inserted up the rectum to visualize the surface of the colon),[15] and an enteric-coated peppermint oil capsule has been used in treating IBS.[16] Enteric coating is necessary because menthol (the major constituent of peppermint oil) and other volatile compounds in peppermint oil are rapidly absorbed.[17] Menthol, without enteric coating, is rapidly absorbed and results in relaxation of the cardio-esophageal sphincter and common side effects, such as esophageal reflux and heartburn, after administration. A transient hot burning sensation in the rectum during defecation, due to unabsorbed menthol, has been noted in some patients who take the enteric-coated peppermint oil.

Most of the studies have utilized enteric-coated peppermint oil at a dosage of 0.2 ml twice daily between meals.[17] In a more recent double-blind placebo-controlled study, a commercial preparation available in Germany, consisting of 90 mg of peppermint oil and 50 mg of caraway oil in an enteric-coated capsule, provided additional evidence that enteric-coated volatile oil preparations are quite beneficial in relieving the symptoms of irritable bowel syndrome.[18] A total of thirty-nine patients were included in the study. The primary outcomes were the change in the intensity of pain and the degree of improvement as noted during a clinical evaluation by a physician.

After four weeks, significant improvements were noted in both groups, but the group that received the peppermint oil preparation demonstrated the greatest benefit. In regard to pain reduction, at the end of four weeks seventeen out of nineteen (89.5 percent) improved in the treatment group, compared to nine out of twenty (45 percent) in the placebo group. According to the clinical evaluation, eighteen out of nineteen (94.7 percent) had improvements of their pain and other IBS symptoms while on the peppermint preparation compared to eleven out of twenty (55 percent) in the placebo group. These results are quite good for the treatment of the irritable bowel syndrome and appear to be the result of its relaxing and soothing effects on the intestines and antimicrobial effects produced by the volatile oils.

An additional benefit of these volatile oils is their efficacy against *Candida albicans*.[19] This is useful for IBS because an overgrowth of *C. albicans* may be an underlying factor, especially in cases that do not respond to dietary advice and for those who consume large amounts of sugar. In one study, administration of nystatin (600,000 U/day, for ten days) to patients who were unresponsive to an elimination diet produced dramatic clinical improvement.[9]

Psychological Factors

Mental/emotional problems—anxiety, fatigue, hostile feelings, depression, and sleep disturbances—are reported by almost all patients who have IBS.[20] The severity and frequency of symptoms tend to correlate with these psychological factors. Especially significant is sleep quality; poor sleep quality results in an increase in symptom severity.[21]

There are several theories that link psychological factors to the symptoms of IBS. The "learning model" holds that, when exposed to stressful situations, some children learn to develop gastrointestinal symptoms to cope with the stress. Another theory holds that IBS is a manifestation of depression or chronic anxiety, or both. Personality assessments of IBS sufferers have shown them to have higher anxiety levels and a greater feeling of depression than individuals without IBS.[22] However, these studies were based on personality assessments after IBS had developed, and it has since been determined by pre-illness personality assessment that IBS sufferers have normal personality profiles.

Therefore, many of the psychological symptoms may result either from the bowel disturbances (particularly malabsorption of nutrients) or from a common etiological factor (stress, food allergy, candidiasis).

Increased motility of the colon during exposure to stressful situations has been shown to occur in both normal subjects and those suffering from IBS.[23] This apparently accounts for the increased abdominal pain and irregular bowel function seen in patients with IBS and in normal subjects during periods of emotional stress. Some researchers believe that IBS sufferers have difficulty adapting to life events, although this has not been well demonstrated in clinical studies. However, psychotherapy in the form of relaxation therapy,[24] biofeedback,[25] hypnosis,[25] counseling,[26] or stress-management training[27] has been shown to reduce symptom frequency and severity and enhance the results of standard medical treatment of IBS. In contrast, the use of antidepressants, *anxiolytic* (anxiety-reducing) drugs, or a combination of tranquilizers and antispasmodics has not yielded effective results.

Miscellaneous Considerations

Although probably significant, the role of altered microbial flora in IBS has not been investigated. Some of the beneficial effects attributed to increasing dietary fiber may be a result of alterations in colon bacteria concentrations. *Lactobacillus acidophilus* supplementation appears to be indicated in IBS.

An increase in physical exercise also appears helpful. Many people with IBS find that daily leisurely walks markedly reduce symptoms, probably due to the known stress-reduction effects of exercise.

For further related information, please consult the chapter DIGESTION.

TREATMENT SUMMARY

The four primary areas of focus are increasing dietary fiber, elimination of food allergens and sugar, enteric-coated volatile oils, and controlling psychological factors through stress reduction and regular exercise.

Diet

Increase intake of fiber-rich foods and eliminate allergenic foods, refined sugar, and highly processed foods.

Nutritional Supplements

- *Lactobacillus acidophilus:* 1 to 2 billion live organisms per day
- Fiber: 3 to 5 grams per day at bedtime

Botanical Medicines

- Enteric-coated volatile oil preparations (e.g., peppermint oil): 0.2–0.4 ml twice per day between meals

Physical Therapy

Daily, leisurely twenty-minute walks

Counseling

Develop an effective stress-reduction program. Biofeedback may be particularly helpful.

Kidney Stones

Usually without symptoms until stone becomes dislodged

Excruciating intermittent radiating pain originating in the flank or kidney

Nausea, vomiting, and abdominal distension

Chills, fever, and urinary frequency if accompanied by infection

Diagnosed by ultrasound

Stone formation in the urinary tract has been recognized for thousands of years, but during the last few decades the pattern and frequency of the disease have changed. In the past, stone formation was almost exclusively in the bladder, while today most stones form in the kidneys. The frequency of stones has increased dramatically. It is now estimated that ten percent of all American males will experience a kidney stone during their lifetime, with an annual frequency of 0.1 to 6.0 percent of the general population. In the United States, one out of every one thousand hospital admissions is for kidney stones. The frequency has been steadily increasing, paralleling the rise in other diseases associated with the so-called Western diet, e.g., heart disease, high blood pressure, and diabetes.

In the United States, kidney stones are usually composed of calcium salts (seventy-five to eighty-five percent), uric acid (five to eight percent), or struvite (non-calcium-containing crystals, ten to fifteen percent). The frequency varies geographically, reflecting differences in environmental factors, diet, and components of drinking water. Males are affected more than females, and most patients are over thirty years of age.

Components in human urine normally remain in solution due to pH control and the secretion of inhibitors of crystal growth.

However, when there is an increase in stone components or a decrease in protective factors, kidney stones can develop. There are a number of metabolic diseases that lead to kidney stones, including hyperparathyroidism, cystinuria (elevated levels of cystine in the urine), vitamin D excess, milk-alkali syndrome (excessive use of antacids), destructive bone disease, primary oxaluria (increased levels of oxalate being excreted), Cushing's syndrome, and sarcoidosis (a systemic disease characterized by deposits of sarcoid).

Diagnostic Considerations

Diagnosing the type of stone is critical to determining the appropriate therapy. Careful evaluation of a number of criteria (diet; underlying metabolic or disease factors; serum and urinary calcium, uric acid, creatinine, and electrolyte levels; urinalysis; and urine culture) will usually determine the composition of the stone, if one is not available for chemical analysis. Table 1 summarizes the findings in the major types of kidney stones.

Conditions favoring stone formation can be divided into two groups:

1. Factors that increase the concentration of stone crystalloids

TABLE 1	Chemical and Physical Characteristics of Urinary Stones				
COMPOSITION	**CRYSTAL NAME**	**FREQUENCY**	**X RAY APPEARANCE**	**URINE CHARACTERISTICS**	**CRYSTAL CHARACTERISTICS**
Calcium oxalate	Whewellite	30–35%	Opaque	Nonspecific	Small, hempseed or mulberry shaped, brown or black color
Calcium oxalate + calcium phosphate		30–35%	Opaque	pH > 5.5	"
Calcium phosphate	Apatite	6–8%	Opaque	pH > 5.5	Staghorn configuration, light color
Magnesium ammonium phosphate	Struvite Triple phosphate	15–20%	Opaque	pH> 6.2 Infection	Staghorn configuration, light color
Uric acid		6–10%	Translucent	pH < 6.0	Ellipsoid, tan or red-brown
Cystine		2–3%	Opaque	pH < 7.2	Multiple, faceted, Maple sugar color

2. Factors that favor stone formation at normal urinary concentrations

The first group includes reduction in urine volume (dehydration) and an increased rate of excretion of stone constituents. The second group of factors is related to stagnation of urine flow (urinary stasis), pH changes, foreign bodies, and reduction of normal substances that solubilize stone constituents.

Therapeutic Considerations

The high frequency of calcium-containing stones in affluent societies is directly associated with the following dietary patterns: low fiber,[1] highly refined carbohydrates,[2,3] high alcohol consumption,[4] large amounts of animal protein,[4,5] high fat intake,[6] and high intake of high-calcium, low-magnesium, vitamin D–enriched milk products. The classification of most stones as having an "unknown cause" (idiopathic) is reflective of ignorance of dietary factors that lead to stone formation. The cumulative effect of these dietary factors is undoubtedly the reason for the rising incidence of kidney stones.

As a group, vegetarians have a decreased risk of developing stones.[5] Studies have shown that, even among meat eaters, those who ate higher amounts of fresh fruits and vegetables had a lower incidence of stones.[7]

Bran supplementation, as well as the simple change from white to whole wheat bread, has resulted in lowering urinary calcium levels.[1]

Weight Control and Sugar Intake

Weight control and correction of carbohydrate metabolism problems are important, since excess weight and insulin insensitivity (see DIABETES) lead to increased urinary excretion of calcium and are high risk factors for stone formation.[8,9] A meal high in sugar is particularly problematic, since following sugar intake there is a rise in urinary calcium levels. The ingestion of sucrose and other simple sugars causes an exaggerated increase in the urinary calcium oxalate content in approximately seventy percent of people with recurrent kidney stones.[10] Obviously, people with recurrent kidney stones should avoid sugar.

Magnesium and Vitamin B6

A magnesium-deficient diet is one of the quickest ways to cause kidney stones in rats.[11] Magnesium has been shown to increase the solubility of calcium oxalate and inhibit both calcium phosphate and calcium oxalate stone formation.[11–13] A low urinary magnesium-to-calcium ratio is an independent risk factor in stone formation,[14] and supplemental magnesium alone has been shown to be effective in preventing recurrences of kidney stones.[12–14] However, when used in conjunction with vitamin B6, an even greater effect is noted.[15,16]

Many patients with recurrent oxalate stones show laboratory signs of vitamin B6 deficiency. Like magnesium, vitamin B6 deficiency also results in kidney stones. Vitamin B6 is known to reduce the production and urinary excretion of oxalates.[17–19] Supplementing the diet with additional vitamin B6 is important in preventing recurrent kidney stones.

Glutamic Acid

Depressed levels of glutamic acid (due to vitamin B6 deficiency or other reasons) is significant in the formation of kidney stones, since an increased concentration of glutamic acid in the urine causes calcium oxalate to fall out of solution. Glutamic acid supplementation in rats significantly reduces the incidence of

QUICK REVIEW

- Ten percent of all American males will experience a kidney stone during their lifetime.
- Kidney stones have been linked to the following dietary patterns: low intake of fiber; high intake of highly refined carbohydrates, alcohol, animal protein, fat, and high-calcium, low-magnesium, vitamin D–enriched milk products.

- Magnesium and vitamin B6 supplementation can prevent kidney stones.
- Citrate supplementation stops stone formation in nearly ninety percent of cases.
- Cranberry juice has been shown to reduce the amount of ionized calcium in the urine by over fifty percent in patients with recurrent kidney stones.
- It is important to avoid high-purine foods and salt.
- Drink at least 48 ounces of water daily.

kidney stones, and it may do so in humans as well.[20] Supplementation with glutamic acid may, however, be unnecessary if adequate vitamin B6 levels are attained.

Calcium

Most doctors tell their patients to avoid calcium supplements, as calcium restriction actually enhances oxalate absorption. In other words, when calcium intake is restricted, oxalate absorption is increased and calcium oxalate stones still form. A recent study has also shown that calcium supplementation actually reduces oxalate excretion.[21]

The study measured the urinary oxalate excretion after calcium supplementation and the administration of oxalic acid. Calcium was given in the form of calcium carbonate or calcium citrate malate at a dosage of 300 mg of elemental magnesium. Compared to baseline assessment, calcium supplementation significantly reduced oxalate absorption and excretion, indicating that calcium supplementation (300 mg to 1,000 mg) daily may prove to be an effective preventive measure against calcium oxalate kidney stones.

Citrate

Citric acid (citrate) has the ability to reduce urinary saturation of calcium oxalate and calcium phosphate and retard the nucleation and crystal growth of calcium salts. The use of potassium or sodium citrate in the treatment of recurrent calcium oxalate stones has been shown to be quite effective in clinical studies, ceasing stone formation in nearly ninety percent of the subjects.[22,23] For example, in one study, potassium citrate supplementation in recurrent stone-formers resulted in a drop of stone formation from 0.7 to 0.13 per year.[23] However, rather than potassium or sodium

citrate, it appears that magnesium citrate would offer the greatest benefit.

Vitamin K

Vitamin K is necessary in the manufacture of a molecule that is a powerful inhibitor of kidney stone formation.[24] The presence of vitamin K in green leafy vegetables may be one reason vegetarians have a lower incidence of kidney stones.[25]

Uric Acid Metabolism

The level of dietary purine consumption is directly related to the rate of urinary uric acid excretion;[26] this fact is important, since elevation in the purine content of uric acid is a causative factor in recurrent calcium oxalate stones. Foods with high purine levels should be entirely omitted. These include: organ meats, meats, shellfish, yeast (brewer's and baker's), herring, sardines, mackerel, and anchovies. Foods with moderate levels of protein should be curtailed as well. These include: dried legumes, spinach, asparagus, fish, poultry, and mushrooms.

Botanical Medicines

Aloe and Senna
Compounds known as *anthraquinones*, isolated from herbs like senna and *Aloe vera*, bind calcium and significantly reduce the growth rate of urinary crystals when used in oral doses lower than the laxative dose.[27,28] Our recommendation is to use *Aloe vera* or senna at levels just below those which can produce a laxative effect.

Cranberry (Vaccinium macrocarpon)
Cranberry juice or extracts may be useful, as the consumption of cranberry juice has been

shown to reduce the amount of ionized calcium in the urine by over fifty percent in patients with recurrent kidney stones.[29] Since high urinary calcium levels greatly increase the risk of developing a kidney stone, it appears that cranberry juice may offer significant benefit. Because most cranberry juice products on the market are loaded with sugar, many herbal practitioners and physicians recommend taking cranberry juice in pill form. Several manufacturers offer cranberry concentrates. For prevention of kidney stones in those at high risk, take the equivalent of 16 ounces of cranberry juice.

Khella (Ammi visnaga)

In a medical study conducted in the 1930s, Khella was shown to be unusually effective in relaxing the ureter and allowing the stone to pass.[30] This action is due to a relaxing effect on the ureters. Gravel root (Ruta graveolens) contains similar compounds and has also been used in the treatment of kidney stones.

Miscellaneous

Hair mineral analysis may be of value, since many heavy metals (mercury, gold, uranium,

and cadmium) are toxic to the kidneys. Cadmium, in particular, has been shown to greatly increase the incidence of kidney stones. A prospective study of coppersmiths showed a forty-percent incidence of kidney stones, which correlated with elevated serum cadmium levels.[31]

Vitamin C is often cited in the medical literature as a potential factor in the development of calcium oxalate kidney stones. However, numerous studies have now demonstrated that, in persons not on hemodialysis or suffering from recurrent kidney stones, severe kidney disease, or gout, high-dosage vitamin C therapy will not cause kidney stones. Vitamin C administration of up to 10 grams per day has not shown any effect on urinary oxalate levels.[32,33]

Another dietary recommendation is to decrease salt (sodium chloride) consumption. Urinary calcium excretion increases approximately 1 mmol (40 mg) for each 100 mmol (2,300 mg) increase in dietary sodium in normal adults. People who tend to form kidney stones have an even greater increase in urinary calcium with an increase in salt intake.[34]

. . . .

TREATMENT SUMMARY

Prevention of recurrence is the therapeutic goal in the treatment of kidney stones. Since dietary management is effective, inexpensive, and free from side effects, it is the treatment of choice. The specific treatment is determined by the type of stone and may include

- Reducing urinary calcium levels
- Reducing purine intake
- Rvoiding high-oxalate-content foods
- Increasing intake of foods with a high magnesium-to-calcium ratio
- Increasing intake of vitamin-K-rich foods

For all types of stones, increasing urine flow to dilute the urine is vital. Enough fluids should be consumed to produce a daily urinary volume of at least 2,000 ml.

NOTE: In acute cases, surgical removal or breaking up the stone with sound waves *(lithotripsy)* may be necessary.

Calcium Stones

Diet

Increase intake of fiber, complex carbohydrates, and green leafy vegetables, and decrease intake of simple carbohydrates and purines (meat, fish, poultry, yeast). Increase intake of high-magnesium-to-calcium-ratio foods (barley, bran, corn, buckwheat, rye, soy, oats, brown rice, avocado, banana, cashew, coconut, peanuts, sesame seeds, lima beans, potato). If there are oxalate stones, reduce oxalate-containing foods (black tea, cocoa, spinach, beet leaves, rhubarb, parsley, cranberries, nuts). Limit intake of dairy products.

Nutritional Supplements

- Vitamin B6: 25 mg per day
- Vitamin K: 2 mg per day
- Magnesium: 600 mg per day
- Calcium: 300–1,000 mg per day

Botanical Medicines

Use *Aloe vera* or senna at a dosage just below a level that will produce a laxative effect (this will vary from one person to the next).

Miscellaneous

Avoid aluminum-containing antacids.

Uric Acid Stones

Diet

Decrease purine intake (see list under Uric Acid Metabolism in this chapter).

Nutritional Supplements

Folic acid: 5 mg per day

Miscellaneous

Alkalinize urine: citrate, bicarbonate

Magnesium Ammonium Phosphate Stones

Miscellaneous

- Eradicate infection (see BLADDER INFECTIQN)
- Acidify urine: ammonium chloride (100–200 mg three times per day)

Cystine Stones

Diet

Avoid methionine-rich foods (soy, wheat, dairy products [except whole milk], fish, meat, lima beans, garbanzo beans, mushrooms, and all nuts except coconut, hazelnut, and sunflower seeds).

Miscellaneous

Alkalinize urine: optimal pH is 7.5–8.0

Leukoplakia

Adherent white patch or plaque appearing anywhere on the lips or mouth

May be without symptoms until there is ulceration, fissuring, or malignant transformation

Diagnosis confirmed by biopsy

eukoplakia is a clinical term signifying a white plaque-like lesion occurring anywhere on the lips or mouth. It is generally a reaction to irritation, such as cigarette smoking or tobacco or betel nut chewing, and an early sign of impaired immune function in people infected with the human immunodeficiency virus. It appears most frequently in men aged fifty to seventy years.

Leukoplakia is a precancerous lesion.[1] Oral cancer is among the most common malignant cancers, with nearly fifty thousand new cases and twelve thousand deaths reported in the United States each year. Survival rates with chemotherapy, radiation, and surgical procedures are unchanged in the past few decades; it still has a five-year survival rate of fifty percent. In other words, more than half the people who develop oral cancer die within five years of diagnosis. The greatest success in preventing mortality is through prevention of oral cancer. Staying away from tobacco and an increased intake of antioxidant nutrients are the primary preventive measures.

Therapeutic Considerations

Treatment of leukoplakia includes removal of all irritants. Laser surgery, cryosurgery (freezing with liquid nitrogen), and other surgical techniques have not given predictably favorable results.[2]

Vitamin A and Beta-Carotene

Historically, vitamin A supplementation and, more recently, beta-carotene have been found to be clinically effective in the treatment of leukoplakia.[3–8] Population studies and experimental data documenting the protective effect of carotenoids and vitamin A against oral cancers are overwhelming.[9,10]

QUICK REVIEW

- Leukoplakia is a precancerous lesion.
- Staying away from tobacco and increasing one's intake of antioxidant nutrients are the primary preventive measures.
- There have been seven clinical trials showing that beta-carotene produces regression of leukoplakia.

TABLE 1	Beta-Carotene Trials in the Treatment of Leukoplakia	
AUTHOR	**DOSAGE**	**RESPONSE RATE**
Stich[7]	180 mg/week	15%
Stich[8]	180 mg/week	27%
Garewal[13]	30 mg/day	71%
Toma[14]	90 mg/day	44%
Malaker[15]	30 mg/day	50%
Brandt[16]	90 mg/day	60%
Garewal[17]	60 mg/day	56%

Clinical studies that tested vitamin A in the treatment of leukoplakia generally used high dosages (i.e., 150,000 to 900,000 IU/day) but found them extremely effective.[3–6] Since it appears that beta-carotene is as effective as vitamin A and is much safer, it is suggested that beta-carotene be the treatment of choice for this condition.[11,12] Most recent studies have focused on the use of beta-carotene in the treatment of leukoplakia. To date, there have been seven clinical trials showing that beta-carotene produces regression of leukoplakia.[9] The results of these studies are given in Table 1.

Other Antioxidants

In addition to beta-carotene, other antioxidants may be helpful. For example, studies have shown vitamin E (400 mg/day) to produce a sixty-five-percent response rate.[18] However, it makes the most sense to utilize a combination of antioxidant nutrients. Preliminary results using a combination of vitamin C (1,000 mg/day), beta-carotene (30 mg/day), and vitamin E (400 mg/day) are encouraging.[19]

TREATMENT SUMMARY

Since leukoplakia is due to a combination of excessive irritation in the context of marginal or low levels of vitamin A, carotenoids, and/or antioxidants, the approach is simple: eliminate all sources of irritation and establish optimal vitamin A, beta-carotene, and antioxidant levels. Particularly significant irritation results from tobacco smoking and chewing, betel nut chewing, and sunlight exposure.

Nutritional Supplements

- Vitamin A: 5,000 IU per day
- Beta-carotene: 30–90 mg per day
- Vitamin C: 1,000–3,000 mg per day
- Vitamin E: 400 IU per day

Macular Degeneration

. . . .

Progressive visual loss due to degeneration of the macula

Eye exam may reveal spots of pigment near the macula and blurring of the macular borders

The *macula* is the area of the retina where images are focused. It is the portion of the eye responsible for fine vision. Degeneration of the macula is the leading cause of severe visual loss in the United States and Europe in persons aged fifty-five years or older, and is second to cataracts as the leading cause of decreased vision in persons over sixty-five years of age. It is estimated that over 150,000 Americans are legally blind from age-related macular degeneration, with 20,000 new cases occurring each year.[1,2]

The major risk factors for macular degeneration are smoking, aging, *atherosclerosis* (hardening of the arteries), and high blood pressure.[1–3] Apparently, the degeneration is a result of free-radical damage, similar to the type of damage that induces cataracts (see CATARACTS). However, decreased blood and oxygen supply to the retina is the prelude and key factor leading to macular degeneration.

Types of Macular Degeneration

The two most common types of age-related macular degeneration (ARMD) are the *atrophic* ("dry") form, by far the more frequent, and the *neovascular* ("wet") form.[2,3] In either form, patients may experience blurred vision. The patient may note that straight objects appear distorted or bent, that there is a dark spot near or around the center of the visual field, and that, while reading, parts of words are missing.

Dry ARMD

Between eighty and ninety-five percent of people with ARMD have the dry form of the disease. The primary lesions are atrophic changes in the *retinal pigmented epithelium* (RPE), which composes the innermost layer of the retina. Apparently, beginning in early life and continuing throughout life, cells of the RPE gradually accumulate sacs of cellular debris known as *lipofuscin*. The lipofuscin sacs are either remnants of incompletely degraded abnormal molecules from damaged RPE cells or derivatives of damaged membranes of nearby cells. Progressive engorgement of the RPE cells with lipofuscin is associated with the extrusion of other tissue components.[1–3] The hallmark feature of macular degeneration is the appearance of this extrusion beneath the RPE with the aid of an ophthalmoscope—the piece of equipment that physicians use to examine the eye. This extrusion is referred to as *drusen*.

Macular degeneration progresses slowly. Only central vision is lost as peripheral vision remains intact. In other words, people with macular degeneration have good peripheral vision; they just can't see what is directly in front of them. It is rare for anyone to become totally blind from dry ARMD.[1–3] Currently there is no standard medical treatment for this common form of ARMD.

Wet ARMD

The other form of ARMD is the wet, or neovascular, form. This form affects five to twenty percent of those with ARMD. It is characterized by the growth of abnormal blood vessels. Unlike the dry form, wet ARMD can be treated quite effectively with laser photocoagulation therapy. Because the disease can rapidly progress to a point where surgery cannot be utilized, the surgery should be performed as soon as possible.[1–3]

Therapeutic Considerations

The treatment of the wet form of ARMD is straightforward: laser photocoagulation. The treatment of the dry form and prevention of the wet form involve the use of antioxidants and natural substances that correct the underlying disease process, i.e., free-radical damage and poor oxygenation of the macula. This can be accomplished by reducing the risk factors for atherosclerosis (hardening of the arteries), increasing dietary intake of fresh fruits and vegetables, and supplementing with nutritional and botanical antioxidants.

Reducing and Preventing Atherosclerosis

Although atherosclerosis is a well-accepted risk factor for macular degeneration, this association was unconfirmed until 1995.[3] In the confirmation study, 104 subjects with macular degeneration and 1,324 subjects without macular degeneration were evaluated for atherosclerosis by several techniques: ultrasound determination of the thickness of the arterial walls, assessment of the presence of atherosclerotic plaque in the main arteries that supply the head (the carotid arteries), and measuring the ankle-to-arm systolic blood pressure (an indicator of peripheral atherosclerosis). The results indicated that, in subjects younger than eighty-five years, plaques in the carotid arteries were associated with a 4.7 times greater frequency of macular degeneration. Lower-extremity atherosclerosis was associated with a 2.5 times greater risk.

These results indicate that measures designed to reduce the risk of atherosclerosis are of great significance in the prevention

. . . .

QUICK REVIEW

- Degeneration of the macula is the leading cause of severe visual loss in the United States.
- The major risk factors for macular degeneration are smoking, aging, atherosclerosis (hardening of the arteries), and high blood pressure.
- The treatment of the wet form of age-related macular degeneration is immediate laser photocoagulation.
- The treatment goals in the dry form and prevention of the wet form involve

the use of antioxidants and natural substances that protect against free-radical damage and improve blood and oxygen supply to the macula.

- Measures designed to reduce the risk of atherosclerosis are of great significance in the prevention (and treatment) of macular degeneration.
- A diet rich in fruits and vegetables is associated with a lowered risk for macular degeneration.
- Antioxidant formulas have been shown to halt and even reverse macular degeneration.

(and treatment) of macular degeneration. See the chapter HEART AND CARDIOVASCULAR HEALTH for a comprehensive program for prevention and reversal.

Dietary Fruits and Vegetables

A diet rich in fruits and vegetables is associated with a lowered risk for ARMD. Presumably, this protection is the result of increased intake of antioxidant vitamins and minerals.[4-6] However, various "non-essential" food components, such as the nonprovitamin A carotenes (carotenes that are not converted to vitamin A) *lutein, zeaxanthin,* and *lycopene*, along with flavonoids, are proving to be even more significant in protecting against ARMD than traditional nutritional antioxidants such as vitamin C, vitamin E, and selenium. For example, one study compared patients with age-related macular degeneration to healthy controls. Individuals with low levels of lycopene were found to be twice as likely to have age-related macular degeneration.[6]

The macula, especially the central portion (the *fovea*), owes its yellow color to its high concentration of lutein and zeaxanthin. These yellow carotenes function in preventing oxidative damage to the area of the retina responsible for fine vision and obviously play a central role in protecting against the development of macular degeneration.[7]

The best way to protect against ARMD is through diet. In particular, regular consumption of foods rich in the important carotenes for the eye is highly recommended. In addition, lutein and zeaxanthin are also available in pill form.

There are three primary types of carotene supplements on the market:

1. Synthetic all-trans-beta-carotene
2. Beta- and alpha-carotene from the algae *Dunaliella*
3. Mixed carotenes from palm oil

TABLE 1	Food Sources of Important Carotenes for the Eye
CAROTENOID	**FOOD SOURCE**
Lycopene	Tomatoes, carrots, green peppers, apricots, pink grapefruit
Zeaxanthin	Spinach, paprika, corn, fruits
Lutein	Green plants, corn, potatoes, spinach, carrots, tomatoes, fruits

Of these three, palm oil carotenes seem to stand out as the best form. But let's take a look at the antioxidant activities of all three types.

Palm oil carotenes appear to give much better antioxidant protection. The carotene complex of palm oil closely mirrors the pattern in high-carotene foods. In particular, it must be pointed out that, unlike the synthetic version, which only provides one particular form of beta-carotene (the trans configuration), natural carotene sources provide beta-carotene in both naturally occurring forms (trans and cis configurations). Palm oil is composed of

60% beta-carotene (both trans and cis isomers)
34% alpha-carotene
3% gamma-carotene
3% lycopene

Palm oil carotenes have been shown to be about four to ten times better absorbed than synthetic beta-carotene.[8-10] Carotenes from *Dunaliella* have also been shown to be well absorbed.[11]

As a side note, the widespread health concerns about the use of "tropical oils" such as palm and coconut oil do not apply to carotene products extracted from palm oil, as the fat content is minimal. In addition, the real

TABLE 2	Antioxidant Potential of Different Carotene Products			
SOURCE	QUENCHING RATE	% IN SOURCE	MG/ 25,000 IU	ANTIOXIDANT POTENTIAL
Palm oil analysis per 25,000 IU Vitamin A				
Alpha-carotene	1.9	33.00	7.36	2.60
Beta-carotene	1.4	63.00	14.04	3.66
Gamma-carotene	2.5	2.5	0.56	0.26
Lycopene	3.1	0.1	0.02	0.01
Total antioxidant potential				6.53
Algal carotene analysis per 25,000 IU of vitamin A				
Alpha-carotene	1.9	4.0	0.61	0.22
Beta-carotene	1.4	96.0	14.69	3.83
Total antioxidant potential				4.05
Synthetic beta-carotene analysis per 25,000 IU of vitamin A				
Beta-carotene	1.4	100.00	14.97	3.90
Total antioxidant potential				3.90

problem with palm oil occurs when it is processed (partially hydrogenated).

Nutritional Supplements

In addition to recommending a diet high in carotenes and supplemental carotenes, supplementation with nutritional antioxidants such as vitamin C, selenium, and vitamin E is certainly important in the treatment and prevention of macular degeneration. A combination of these nutrients will probably produce better results than any single nutrient, as studies have shown that none of these antioxidants alone accounts for the impaired antioxidant status in ARMD. Instead, the decreased antioxidant status reflects decreases in a combination of nutrients.[4]

Two studies have utilized commercially available broad-based antioxidant formulas, with promising results. For example, a 1½-year study demonstrated that the progression of dry ARMD could be halted (but not reversed) with Ocuguard.[12,13] A study of a nutritional supplement called ICAPS Plus (which contains beta-carotene, vitamins C and E, zinc, copper, manganese, selenium, and riboflavin) compared the thirty-eight who used the preparation regularly to the thirty-seven in the control group, who used only one bottle. Fifteen of the treated patients improved their vision by one line or more, compared to only six of the control group. In addition, three of the thirty-eight in the treatment group lost one line or more of vision, versus thirteen of the control group.[14] In a second clinical trial reported in the same review, vision and contrast sensitivity were evaluated. After six months, visual acuity was the same or better in 36 of 61 controls, versus 168 of 192 treated patients.

Zinc

Zinc plays an essential role in retinal function, and the elderly are at high risk for zinc deficiency. A two-year double-blind, placebo-controlled trial involving 151 subjects with dry ARMD demonstrated that the group taking 200 mg of zinc sulfate (approximately 80 mg of elemental zinc) per day had significantly less vision loss than the placebo group.[15] These results were not confirmed, however, in a more recent double-blind study of 112 patients with wet ARMD.[16]

Although these results are viewed as "inconclusive" until further studies are performed, given the importance of zinc to the human eye, supplementation certainly seems justifiable.

Flavonoid-Rich Extracts

Flavonoid-rich extracts of bilberry (Vaccinium myrtillus), Ginkgo biloba, or grape seed (Vitis vinifera) offer significant benefits in the prevention and treatment of ARMD. In addition to possessing excellent antioxidant activity, all three extracts have been shown to increase blood flow to the retina and improve visual processes. Clinical studies in humans have demonstrated that all three are also capable of halting the progressive vision loss of dry ARMD and possibly even improving visual function.[17–20]

Of the three extracts, bilberry extracts standardized to contain twenty-five percent anthocyanidins appear to be the most useful. The key flavonoids (anthocyanosides) of bilberry have a very strong affinity for the retinal pigmented epithelium (RPE), which composes the optical or functional portion of the retina, reinforcing the supportive structures of the retina and preventing free-radical damage. Since the RPE is the portion of the eye affected in ARMD, it appears that bilberry flavonoids are ideal therapeutic agents in the disorder. However, the Ginkgo biloba extract with a twenty-four-percent ginkgo flavonglycoside content is perhaps a better choice if a person is also demonstrating signs of cerebrovascular insufficiency. Grape seed extract may be the most useful when there is poor night vision or significant sensitivity to bright light (photophobia).

Lifestyle

Because exposure to free radicals is a major factor in macular degeneration, it is not surprising that smoking increases the risk of macular degeneration in both men and women.[21,22] For example, in a twelve-year study of 31,843 registered female nurses, those who currently smoked twenty-five or more cigarettes per day were 2.4 times more likely to get age-related macular degeneration than those who had never smoked. Past smokers of twenty-five cigarettes or more per day still had twice the risk of those who never smoked. Risk did not return to the control level until fifteen years after quitting smoking.[22]

TREATMENT SUMMARY

As with most diseases, prevention and treatment at an early stage are the most effective approaches to ARMD. The treatment of the wet form of ARMD is clearly laser photocoagulation, applied as soon as possible. Since free-radical damage and lack of blood and oxygen supply to the macula appear to be the primary causes of macular degeneration, consumption of antioxidants and promotion of retinal blood flow are the keys to effective treatment.

Anyone with any vision loss should see a physician for complete evaluation, especially if the loss is progressing rapidly.

Diet

Avoid fried and grilled foods and other sources of free radicals. Increase consumption of legumes (high in sulfur-containing amino acids), yellow vegetables (carotenes), flavonoid-rich berries (blueberries, blackberries, cherries, etc.), and foods rich in vitamin E and vitamin C (fresh fruits and vegetables).

Nutritional Supplements

- Vitamin C: 1 g three times per day
- Vitamin E: 600–800 IU per day
- Selenium: 400 mcg per day
- Beta-carotene (mixed carotenoids recommended): 50,000 IU per day
- Lutein: 5 mg per day

Botanical Medicines

Choose one of the following:
- *Ginkgo biloba* extract (24% ginkgo flavonglycosides): 40–80 mg three times per day
- Bilberry *(Vaccinium myrtillus)* extract (25% anthocyanidin content): 40–80 mg three times per day
- Grape seed extract (95% procyanidolic content): 150–300 mg per day

Menopause

. . . .

Defined as: cessation of menstruation in older women for six to twelve months

Average age of onset: fifty-one years

Common complaints of menopause: hot flashes, headaches, atrophic vaginitis, frequent urinary tract infections, cold hands and feet, forgetfulness, and an inability to concentrate

Menopause denotes the cessation of menstruation in women, which usually occurs when a woman reaches the age of fifty but may occur as early as 40 and as late as 55 years of age. Six to twelve months without a menstrual period is the commonly accepted rule for diagnosing menopause. The time period prior to menopause is referred to as *perimenopausal,* while the time period after menopause is referred to as *postmenopausal.* During the perimenopausal period, many women ovulate irregularly due to either inadequate secretion of estrogen or resistance of the remaining follicles to ovulatory stimulus.

The current medical view of menopause is that it is a disease, rather than a normal physiological process. This view is in stark contrast to the perspective of many cultures, where menopause is viewed as a natural part of the life process and a positive event in a woman's life. In fact, in many cultures of the world, most women do not experience the symptoms associated with menopause. This observation raises some interesting questions about menopause being a sociocultural event. However, there are certainly important dietary and environmental factors to consider as well.

Current medical treatment of menopause primarily involves the use of hormone replacement therapy (HRT), utilizing a combination of estrogen and progesterone. The obvious question is: "Is hormone replacement therapy necessary?" The goal of this chapter is to answer that question and provide a natural approach to menopause and the postmenopausal period.

Causes of Menopause

Menopause is thought to occur when there are no longer any eggs left in the ovaries. This "burning out" of the ovaries reflects the natural course of events. At birth, there are about one million eggs *(ova).* This number drops to around 300,000 or 400,000 at puberty, but only about four hundred of these ova will actually mature during reproductive years. By the time a woman reaches the age of fifty, few eggs remain.

With menopause, the absence of active *follicles* (the cellular housing of the egg) results in reduced production of estrogen and progesterone. In response to this drop in estrogen, the pituitary gland increases secretion of *follicle-stimulating hormone* (FSH) and *luteinizing hormone* (LH). After menopause, FSH and LH are secreted in large and continuous quantities.

Although there are no longer any follicles to stimulate in the postmenopausal woman, LH and FSH cause the ovaries and the adrenal glands to secrete increased amounts of androgens, which can be converted to estrogens by the fat cells of the hips and thighs. Converted androgens account for most of the circulating estrogen in the postmenopausal woman, but the total estrogen levels are still far below the levels in women with reproductive function.

Menopause as a Social Construct

While there is undeniably a physiological process involved in menopause, menopause is much more than simply a biological event. Social and cultural factors contribute greatly to how women react to menopause.[1] Modern society has placed great value on the allure of everlasting youth, resulting in a cultural devaluation of older women. This devaluation is deeply entrenched in our mental programming, as it is found in our children's books, fairy tales, television, and movies. Advocates of a social and cultural explanation of menopause often point to this cultural devaluing of older women as the root of the negativity associated with achieving menopause.

In contrast, in many cultures of the world, women look forward to menopause because it brings with it greater respect. Achieving an advanced age is viewed as a sign of divine blessing and great wisdom. Studies of menopausal women in many traditional cultures demonstrate that most will pass through menopause without hot flashes, vaginitis, and other symptoms common to menopausal women in developed countries. Even osteoporosis is extremely rare, despite the fact that the average woman in many traditional societies lives at least thirty years after menopause.

Cross-cultural research clearly demonstrates that the cultural view of menopause is directly related to the symptoms of menopause.[2] If the cultural view of menopause is largely negative, as in the United States, symptoms are quite common. In contrast, if menopause is associated with little negativity or viewed in a positive light, symptoms are far less frequent.

One of the most detailed studies on the effects of culture on menopause involved rural Mayan Indians.[2] Detailed medical histories and examinations, including a physical examination, hormone-level measurement, and bone-density studies, were performed on fifty-two postmenopausal women. According to these results, no woman experienced hot flashes or any other menopausal symptom, and not one single woman showed evidence of osteoporosis, despite the fact that their hormonal patterns (levels of the various female sex hormones) were identical to those of postmenopausal women living in the United States.

The researchers felt that the Mayan women's attitude toward menopause was responsible for their symptomless passage. The Mayan women saw menopause as a positive event that would provide them acceptance as respected elders, as well as relief from childbearing. This attitude is much different from the dominant attitude toward menopause that is common in industrialized societies. If our society adopted a different cultural view of older women, it is likely that the symptoms of menopause would cease to exist.

The Western View of Menopause: Feminine Forever?

In 1966, Robert A. Wilson, M.D., released his landmark book, *Feminine Forever*, which introduced the theory that menopause is an estrogen-deficiency disease that needs to be treated with estrogen to compensate for the normal decline of estrogen levels with aging.[3] According to Wilson, without estrogen replacement therapy women are destined to become sexless "caricatures of their former selves . . . the equivalent of a eunuch."

Wilson's theory of menopause as a disease is now the dominant medical view of menopause. This places women who are entering menopause in a difficult dilemma: should they pass through this period of time naturally, or should they remain "forever feminine"? Before a woman can be counseled, the benefits and risks of estrogen replacement therapy must be considered, as well as the natural alternatives.

Hormone Replacement Therapy

The Evolution of Estrogen Replacement Therapy

During the 1940s and 1950s, estrogen was widely prescribed for ameliorating the symptoms of menopause. By the 1970s, estrogen replacement therapy became firmly entrenched as the medical treatment of choice for women in menopause. Unfortunately, the consequences of long-term estrogen therapy were not well understood.

It is now well established that estrogen replacement therapy is associated with a four- to thirteen-times increased risk of developing endometrial cancer (cancer in the lining of the uterus).[4] To combat this tendency, drug companies and physicians began recommending that estrogen be combined with progesterone. Estrogen replacement therapy thus became hormone replacement therapy. The combination of estrogen and progesterone (or, more accurately, *progestin*, a synthetic version of progesterone) appears to have reduced the risk of endometrial cancer but still carries with it the risk of causing other cancers (discussed in Hormone Replacement Therapy and Cancer, later in this chapter).[5] This stigma looms large in the minds of many women and some physicians.

The Benefits of Hormone Replacement Therapy

Hormone replacement therapy results in undeniable benefits: relief from hot flashes and

QUICK REVIEW

- In many parts of the world, most women do not experience the symptoms associated with menopause in the United States.
- Social and cultural factors contribute greatly to how women react to menopause.
- In the United States, sixty-five to eighty percent of menopausal

women experience hot flashes to some degree.

- Women with atrophic vaginitis (vaginal drying and irritation due to lack of estrogen) should avoid substances that tend to dry the mucous membranes, including antihistamines, alcohol, caffeine, and diuretics.
- Rather than use estrogens to artificially counteract the symptoms of menopause, the natural approach fo-

other menopausal symptoms and a significant reduction in osteoporosis. Furthermore, while early studies showed an increased risk for cardiovascular disease with estrogen use, more recent studies are indicating the estrogen may offer some protection against heart disease and strokes.[6,7]

However, diet, exercise, and lifestyle factors have also been shown to offer identical benefits without the risks. Furthermore, the use of short-term (less than six months) hormone replacement therapy for menopausal symptoms only provides temporary relief. It is not a permanent cure; it only delays the inevitable. Long-term hormone replacement therapy is not justified in most women because the risks outweigh the benefits. The exception is in women who are at high risk of developing osteoporosis.

Since both estrogen and progesterone have been shown to exert beneficial effects against bone loss and, in women with established bone loss, actually increase bone mass, estrogen-progesterone combinations are preferred to estrogen alone.[6,7] However, HRT is not advised for women at high risk for breast cancer or women with a disease aggravated by estrogen, including breast cancer, active liver diseases, and certain cardiovascular diseases. In such cases, the natural approaches described in this chapter are definitely preferable to HRT.

Hormone Replacement Therapy and Cancer

The cancer-causing potential of hormone replacement therapy is a serious concern. Unfortunately, while there have been over fifty studies seeking to determine the cancer risk of hormone replacement therapy, the results have not been clear.[8–11]

Breast cancer is the form of cancer most likely to be exacerbated by hormone replacement therapy. It is also the most common cancer in women. Current estimates are that one in nine women in the United States will develop breast cancer in her lifetime. Since estrogens play a critical role in the development of most breast cancers, it only makes sense that additional estrogens may promote breast cancer.

Several studies of postmenopausal women who take estrogen have shown an increased risk for breast cancer. When all are examined

- -

cuses on improving physiology through diet, exercise, nutritional supplementation, and the use of botanical medicines.

- An especially important dietary recommendation in the relief of hot flashes and atrophic vaginitis, and the prevention of breast cancer, is to increase the consumption of soy foods.

- Several nutrients have been shown to be effective in relieving hot flashes and atrophic vaginitis in clinical studies, including vitamin E, hesperidin (a flavonoid) in combination with vitamin C, and gamma-oryzanol.

- A special extract of black cohosh (*Cimicifuga racemosa*) is the most widely used and thoroughly studied natural alternative to hormone replacement therapy in menopause.

collectively, experts have calculated that estrogen replacement therapy is associated with a one- to thirty-percent increase in the risk of getting breast cancer.[9-11] Most of the studies showing a link between estrogen replacement therapy were conducted in European countries and seem to suggest an association between breast cancer and estrogen replacement therapy that increases with age and length of use. In comparison, only a few studies in the United States have shown that hormone replacement therapy increases the risk of breast cancer. Several hypotheses have been suggested to explain this surprising difference, including American researcher bias and the fact that, since American women are already at such a high risk for breast cancer, the effect is difficult to measure. Defensiveness among the American researchers about the findings of the European studies makes resolution of this issue difficult, as does the years-long U.S. medical establishment's enthusiastic recommendation of estrogen and hormone replacement therapy.

Based on the current evidence, and until the issue of whether hormone replacement therapy increases the risk of breast cancer is cleared up, it can be concluded that women are probably better off avoiding hormone replacement therapy, except in specific cases, such as serious osteoporosis (see Osteoporosis).

Other Side Effects of Hormone Replacement Therapy

The *Physicians' Desk Reference* provides a long list of side effects of HRT, as do the package inserts for estrogen and progesterone products. In addition to the risk of cancer, estrogen and progesterone increase the risk of developing gallstones and blood clots and are absolutely contraindicated during the first four months of pregnancy.

Other side effects of estrogen and progesterone include nausea, breast tenderness, symptoms similar to premenstrual tension syndrome (PMS), depression, liver disorders, enlargement of uterine fibroids, fluid retention, blood sugar disturbances, and headaches. However, these side effects are most often linked to estrogen- and progesterone-containing birth-control pills. Since the doses of estrogen and progesterone used in menopause are much lower than the doses used in oral contraception, these side effects are usually not as common among menopausal women.

A newly recognized side effect was discovered through the evaluation of the more than 23,000 women in the Nurses' Health Study. Women taking postmenopausal hormones were found to be over twice as likely to suffer adult-onset asthma than women who never took hormones.[12] The researchers also found that the effect was dose-related. This finding could help explain why severe adult-onset asthma afflicts more women than men. This finding is not surprising, since the number of asthma cases among women soars at the onset of puberty, when estrogen levels begin to increase.

Types of Hormone Replacement Therapy

If, after weighing all the evidence, a woman elects to utilize hormone replacement therapy for short-term relief, or if she requires long-term therapy because of a high risk for osteoporosis, it is important that she participate in choosing the right combination and dosage pattern for her needs. There is no well-accepted "best program" among many experts. However, based on the current evidence, a strong case could be made for what is known as *combined continuous hormone replacement therapy* as being the best in terms of benefit-to-risk ratio.[6,7]

Combined continuous HRT is best appreciated by gaining an understanding of the other types of HRT. When estrogen is given alone, without a progestin, it is known as *unopposed estrogen therapy*. This regime carries with it the high risk for endometrial cancer and possibly other cancers, including breast cancer. Unopposed estrogen can either be given continuously (every day) or during twenty-five-day cycles, separated by three to six days without estrogen.

In an effort to reduce the risk of endometrial cancer, estrogen is often given in combination with progestin. The hormones can be given either in a cyclical fashion or continuously. The cyclical fashion involves taking estrogen for twenty-five days and progestin for the last ten to twelve days of the cycle. A three- to six-day hormone-free interval follows, during which planned bleeding occurs. In other words, with cyclical administration, menstruation continues in about ninety percent of women.

In order to prevent monthly bleeding, estrogen and progesterone can be taken every day, without a hormone-free interval. This is the regime known as combined continuous hormone replacement therapy. When administered according to recommended guidelines (the lowest dose of estrogen possible along with 2.5 mg of medroxyprogesterone acetate), combined continuous HRT offers several advantages over other regimes.

ADVANTAGES OF COMBINED CONTINUOUS HORMONE REPLACEMENT THERAPY
Avoidance of cyclical bleeding
Avoidance of symptoms of premenstrual syndrome that often accompany estrogen
Continuous protection of the endometrium against the cancer-causing effects of estrogen
Greater convenience and patient compliance
Lower daily and cumulative amounts of progestins required
Prevention of rare conceptions by promoting endometrial atrophy
Prolongation of the synergistic effects of estrogen and progesterone on bone integrity
Regression of uterine fibroids

As for the best type of estrogen to use, natural estrogens are preferred to synthetic versions. Examples of natural estrogens commonly used in hormone replacement therapy include

Conjugated estrogens (Premarin, Genisis)
Esterified estrogen (Evex, Menest)
Micronized 17-beta-estradiol (Estrace)
Transdermal 17-beta-estradiol (Estraderm, Systen)
Triple estrogens (Tri-Est)

The most commonly used forms are the *conjugated estrogens* (mixtures of excreted estrogens obtained from mare's urine) such as Premarin. Conjugated estrogens are metabolized in the body into active forms of estrogen, such as 17-beta-estradiol. Unfortunately, the liver breaks down many of the active estrogens before they have the opportunity to produce their effects. Therefore, relatively large amounts of conjugated estrogens have to be given, especially since the most active estrogen, 17-beta-estradiol, is not well absorbed orally. It is, however, absorbed well through the skin and is the form of estrogen used in the newer estrogen patches and vaginal creams.

Estrogen patches are preferable to conjugated estrogens for several reasons, but primarily because they approximate more accurately the female body's natural estrogen secretions by delivering 17-beta-estradiol into the bloodstream in a slow, sustained manner. Estrogen-containing patches appear to be safer than oral estrogens. The patches are applied to the skin and changed twice per week.

Most naturopathic physicians prefer to use a type of estrogen formulation known as *triple estrogen,* or Tri-Est. This form is a combination of the three major natural forms of estrogen: estriol, estrone, and estradiol.

With regard to the best form of progesterone, natural progesterone is preferred, followed by its natural derivative *medroxyprogesterone acetate,* over the synthetic versions such as megestrol, norethindrone, and norgestrel. Examples of medroxyprogesterone products are Provera, Cycrin, and Amen.

The Major Symptoms of Menopause

The most common complaints of menopause are hot flashes, headaches, atrophic vaginitis, frequent urinary tract infections, cold hands and feet, forgetfulness, and an inability to concentrate.

Hot Flashes

Hot flashes are the most common symptom of menopause. A *hot flash* refers to dilation of the peripheral blood vessels, which leads to a rise in skin temperature and flushing of the skin. In the typical hot flash, the skin, especially of the head and neck, becomes red and warm for a few seconds to two minutes, with cold chills thereafter. Hot flashes can be accompanied by other symptoms, including increased heart rate, headaches, dizziness, weight gain, fatigue, and insomnia.

In the United States, sixty-five to eighty percent of menopausal women experience hot flashes to some degree. Hot flashes are often the first sign that menopause is approaching, as they may begin prior to the cessation of menses. In most cases, hot flashes are at their most uncomfortable in the first and second years after menopause. As the body adapts to decreased estrogen levels, hot flashes typically subside.

Headaches

Headaches often accompany menopause due to increased instability of the blood vessels. Headaches often accompany hot flashes.

Atrophic Vaginitis

After menopause, the vaginal lining may become thin and dry due to the lack of estrogen. As a result, menopausal and postmenopausal women may experience painful intercourse, an increased susceptibility to infection, and symptoms of vaginal itching or burning.

Women with atrophic vaginitis should try to avoid substances that tend to dry the mucous membranes, including antihistamines, alcohol, caffeine, and diuretics. In addition, it is critical that the body stay well hydrated. Drink at least 32 to 48 ounces of water daily.

Clothes made from natural fibers, particularly cotton, are often recommended, as they allow the skin to breathe, thus decreasing the incidence of vaginal infections.

Regular intercourse is also beneficial, as it increases blood flow to vaginal tissues, which helps improve tone and lubrication. However, good lubrication, such as with oil or K-Y Jelly, must be maintained.

Bladder Infections

About fifteen percent of menopausal women experience frequent bladder infections. Apparently, there is a breakdown in the natural defense mechanisms that protect against bacterial growth in the urinary tract. The primary goal in the natural approach to treating bladder infections is to enhance a woman's normal resistance to urinary tract infection. Specifically, this refers to enhancing the flow of urine by achieving and maintaining proper hydration, promoting a pH that will inhibit the growth of the organism, and preventing bacterial adherence to the endothelial cells of the bladder. In addition, there are several botanical medicines that can be employed. See BLADDER INFECTION for further information.

Cold Hands and Feet

Cold hands and feet are common among women in general, not just menopausal women. During the menopausal period they just become even more common. In most instances, there are three major causes of cold hands and feet: hypothyroidism, low iron levels' in the body, and poor circulation. The basal body temperature test (see Taking Your Basal Body Temperature in the chapter HYPOTHYROIDISM) should be performed to evaluate functional thyroid activity. Serum ferritin levels, the best indicator of body iron stores, should also be performed, along with a CBC (complete blood count) and chemistry panel that includes LDL/HDL cholesterol levels. A complete physical exam is also required, paying particular attention to any other signs of decreased blood flow. Once the cause is identified, the treatment is straightforward.

Forgetfulness and Inability to Concentrate

Forgetfulness and an inability to concentrate are common symptoms of menopause. Often these symptoms are simply a result of decreased oxygen and nutrient supply to the brain that occurs not as the result of menopause per se, but rather because of the age of the women and the likelihood they have atherosclerosis (hardening of the arteries) of the blood vessels supplying oxygen and nutrition to the brain.

The brain is highly dependent on a constant supply of oxygen and nutrients. Although it weighs only 3 pounds, the brain utilizes about twenty percent of the oxygen supply of the entire body. In dealing with the forgetfulness of menopause, the goal is to improve the supply of blood, oxygen, and nutrients to the brain.

The Role of the Hypothalamus and Endorphins

Many of the symptoms of menopause, especially hot flashes, appear to be a result of altered function of the *hypothalamus,* a mass of nervous tissue at the center of the brain that serves as the bridge between the nervous system and the hormonal (endocrine) system. The hypothalamus is responsible for the control of many body functions, including body temperature, metabolic rate, sleep patterns, reactions to stress, libido, mood, and the release of pituitary hormones. Critical to proper functioning of the hypothalamus are the *endorphins,* the body's own mood-elevating and pain-relieving compounds. Endorphins are also thought to play a role in hot flashes. Several natural measures are thought to exert some of their beneficial effects against hot flashes by enhancing endorphin output. Some of the most effective measures are exercise and acupuncture.

Therapeutic Considerations

Rather than use estrogens to artificially counteract the symptoms of menopause, the natural approach focuses on improving physiology. This improvement can be accomplished through diet, nutritional supplementation, the use of botanical medicines, and exercise.

Because menopause is such an important time in a woman's life, we recommend consulting a physician to perform the following:

- Detailed personal and family medical history
- Breast exam and instructions on breast self-examination
- Pelvic examination
- The following laboratory tests:
  Complete blood count
  Blood chemistry panel
  Cholesterol evaluation, including HDL, LDL, and VLDL
  Thyroid function panel, including T3, T4, and TSH
  Baseline mammography (if indicated)
  Baseline bone densitometry (see chapter OSTEOPOROSIS)
  Baseline Osteomark-NTX (see chapter OSTEOPOROSIS)

After the initial evaluation, these tests should be repeated every year. The bone-density studies can be used as a gauge of whether hormone replacement therapy is necessary.

Diet

The most important dietary recommendation may be to increase the amount of plant foods, especially those high in phytoestrogens, while reducing the amount of animal foods in the diet. There is also a protective effect that comes from eating fruit and vegetables against chronic degenerative disease like breast cancer, arthritis, heart disease, cataracts, etc.

Phytoestrogen-Containing Foods

Phytoestrogens are plant compounds that are capable of binding to estrogen receptors. Foods high in phytoestrogens include soy, flaxseed and flaxseed oil (highest sources of lignans), nuts, whole grains, apples, fennel, celery, parsley, and alfalfa. A high intake of phytoestrogens is thought to explain why hot flashes and other menopausal symptoms rarely occur in cultures in which people consume a predominantly plant-based diet. Increasing the intake of dietary phytoestrogens helps decrease hot flashes, increase maturation of vaginal cells, and inhibit osteoporosis. In addition, a diet rich in phytoestrogens results in a decreased frequency of breast, colon, and prostate cancer.[13]

Phytoestrogen-containing foods and herbs offer significant advantages over the use of estrogens in the treatment of menopausal symptoms. While both synthetic and natural estrogens may pose significant health risks, including increased risk of cancer, gallbladder disease, and thromboembolic disease (strokes, heart attacks, etc.), phytoestrogens have not been associated with these side effects. In fact, experimental studies with animals have demonstrated that phytoestrogens are extremely effective in inhibiting mammary tumors, not only because they occupy estrogen receptors, but also via other unrelated anticancer mechanisms.[13]

Phytoestrogens in foods and herbs are capable of exerting estrogenic effects, but they are technically referred to as "anti-estrogens" because their activity is only two percent as strong as that of estrogen at the most. They are called anti-estrogens because they can occupy estrogen receptor sites and block estrogen. And, since they are fifty times less potent than estrogen, the net effect is significantly less estrogenic stimulation. However, because of their low estrogen activity, phytoestrogens tend to balance the effects of estrogen. For example, if estrogen levels are low, phytoestrogens will cause an increase in estrogen effect since they have some estrogenic activity. If estrogen levels are high, phytoestrogens will cause a decrease in estrogen effects since they bind to estrogen-receptor sites, thereby competing with estrogen.

Because of the balancing action of phytoestrogens on estrogen effects, it is common to find the same plant or food recommended for conditions of estrogen excess (such as premenstrual syndrome) as well as conditions of estrogen deficiency (such as menopause and menstrual abnormalities). Many of these foods and herbs have been termed *uterine tonics*.

Soy An especially important dietary recommendation for the relief of hot flashes and atrophic vaginitis, and the prevention of breast cancer, is to increase the consumption of soy foods. The isoflavones (such as genistein) and phytosterols of soybeans produce a mild estrogenic effect. One cup of soybeans provides approximately 300 mg of isoflavone. This level would be the equivalent to about 0.45 mg of conjugated estrogens, or one tablet of Premarin.[14] However, while estrogen replacement therapy may increase the risk of getting cancer, the consumption of soy foods is associated with a significant reduction in the risk of getting cancer.[13,14]

In a study of postmenopausal women, the women who consumed enough soy foods to provide about 200 mg of isoflavone demonstrated signs of estrogenic activity in comparison to a control group.[14] Specifically, the women who consumed the soy foods demonstrated an increase in the number of superficial cells that line the vagina. This increase offsets the vaginal drying and irritation that is common in postmenopausal women.

The soybean plant (*Glycine max*) is native to China, where it has been cultivated as food for more than 13,000 years. The ancient Chinese considered the soybean their most important crop and a necessity for life. The soybean, thanks largely to the United States, which accounts for over fifty percent of the world's production, is now the most widely grown and utilized legume; it accounts for well over fifty percent of the world's total legume production.

The increase in soy food consumption is attributed to a number of factors, including economics, health benefits, and environmental concerns.[15] Interestingly, the lower the protein content, the higher the level of isoflavonoids. Products made from whole soybeans are higher in isoflavonoid content than those produced from soy protein concentrates. Therefore, in dealing with the symptoms of menopause, lower-protein-content products made from soy flour and whole soy are superior to high-protein isolates such as those found in many soy-based meal-replacement formulas.

Soy is definitely an important consideration in reducing the risk for breast cancer.[16] In addition, another useful effect of soy is its protection of LDL cholesterol from oxidation, an effect of great significance for the prevention of cardiovascular disease (see HEART AND CARDIOVASCULAR HEALTH).[13]

Nutritional Supplementation

Several nutrients have been shown to be effective in relieving hot flashes and atrophic vaginitis in clinical studies, including vitamin E, hesperidin (a flavonoid) in combination with vitamin C, and gamma-oryzanol.

Vitamin E

In the late 1940s, several clinical studies found vitamin E to be effective in relieving hot flashes and menopausal vaginal complaints when compared to a placebo.[17–19] Unfortunately, there have been no further clinical investigations. In one study, vitamin E supplementation was shown to not only relieve the symptoms, but also improve the blood supply to the vaginal wall when taken for at least four weeks.[17] A follow-up study published in 1949 demonstrated that vitamin E (400 IU per day) was effective in treating about fifty percent of postmenopausal women who had atrophic vaginitis.[18]

Vitamin E oil, creams, ointments, or suppositories can be used topically to provide symptomatic relief of atrophic vaginitis. Vitamin E is usually quite effective in relieving the dryness and irritation of atrophic vaginitis, as well as other forms of vaginitis.[3]

Hesperidin and Vitamin C

Like many other flavonoids, hesperidin is known to improve vascular integrity and relieve capillary permeability. Combined with vitamin C, hesperidin and other citrus flavonoids may be effective in relieving hot flashes.

In one clinical study, ninety-four women who suffered from hot flashes were given a formula containing 900 mg of hesperidin, 300 mg of hesperidin methyl chalcone (another citrus flavonoid), and 1,200 mg of vitamin C daily.[20] At the end of one month, symptoms of hot flashes were relieved in fifty-three percent of the patients and reduced in thirty-four percent. Improvements were also noted in nocturnal leg cramps, nosebleeds, and easy bruising. The only side effect noted was a slightly offensive body odor and a tendency for the perspiration to discolor the clothing.

Gamma-oryzanol

Gamma-oryzanol (ferulic acid) is a growth-promoting substance found in grains and isolated from rice bran oil. In the treatment of hot flashes, its primary action is to enhance pituitary function and promote endorphin release by the hypothalamus. Gamma-oryzanol was first shown to be effective in treating menopausal symptoms, including hot flashes, in the early 1960s.[21] Subsequent studies have further documented its effectiveness.[22]

In one of the earlier studies, eight menopausal women and thirteen women whose ovaries had been surgically removed were given 300 mg of gamma-oryzanol daily. At the end of the thirty-eight-day trial, over sixty-seven percent of the women had a fifty-percent or greater reduction in their menopausal symptoms.[21] In a more recent study, the benefits of a 300-mg-per-day dose of gamma-oryzanol was even more effective; eighty-five percent of the women reported improvement in their symptoms.[22]

Gamma-oryzanol is an extremely safe natural substance. No significant side effects have been produced in experimental and clinical studies. In addition to being helpful in relieving the symptoms of menopause, gamma-oryzanol has been shown to be quite effective in lowering blood cholesterol triglyceride levels.[23]

Botanical Uterine Tonics and Other Medicines

Many plants have been shown to exert a tonic effect on the female glandular system. As a class, these botanicals are often referred to as *uterine tonics*. Much of their effect is thought to be a result of phytoestrogens in the plants and the plants' ability to improve blood flow to the female organs. The botanicals work to nourish and tone the female glandular and organ system rather than exert a drug-like effect. This nonspecific mode of action makes many botanicals useful in a broad range of female conditions.

The four most useful herbs in the treatment of hot flashes are: dong quai *(Angelica sinensis)*, licorice *(Glycyrrhiza glabra)*, chasteberry *(Vitex agnus-castus)*, and black cohosh *(Cimicifuga racemosa)*. These herbs have been used historically to lessen a variety of female complaints, including hot flashes. While these herbs are effective individually, combining them is thought to produce greater benefit.

Ginkgo biloba extract is another useful herbal medicine in menopause because of its effectiveness in dealing with the forgetfulness, as well as cold hands and feet because of its ability to improve blood flow.

Dong Quai (Angelica sinensis)

In Asia, dong quai's reputation is perhaps second only to that of ginseng. Predominantly regarded as a "female" remedy, angelica has been used to treat menopausal symptoms (especially hot flashes), as well as such conditions as dysmenorrhea (painful menstruation), amenorrhea (lack of menstruation), and metrorrhagia (too frequent menstruation), and to assure a healthy pregnancy and easy delivery. Dong quai has demonstrated good uterine tonic activity, causing an initial increase in uterine contraction, followed by relaxation.[24] In addition, administration of dong quai to mice resulted in an increase of uterine weight and increase of glucose utilization by the liver and uterus.[25] These effects reflect estrogenic activities.

Its effectiveness in relieving hot flashes may be a combination of dong quai's mild estrogenic effects coupled with other components that act to stabilize blood vessels.[26]

Licorice (Glycyrrhiza glabra)

The medicinal use of licorice root in both Western and Eastern cultures dates back several thousand years. Licorice is particularly useful in treating premenstrual syndrome (PMS). PMS has been attributed to an increase in the estrogen-to-progesterone ratio. Licorice is believed to lower estrogen levels while simultaneously raising progesterone levels. For menopause, it is thought that the estrogen-like activity of licorice is responsible for many of its beneficial effects, but its effects on progesterone levels may also be important.[27,28]

Chasteberry (Vitex agnus-castus)

The chaste tree is native to the Mediterranean. Its berries have long been used to treat female complaints. As its name suggests, chasteberries were used in suppressing the libido in women of childbearing age. Scientific investigation has shown that chasteberry has profound effects on pituitary function.[29] It is possible that its beneficial effects in menopause are due to altering LH and FSH secretion. It does not appear to reduce libido during menopause.

Black Cohosh (Cimicifuga racemosa)

Black cohosh was widely used by the American Indians and later by American colonists for the relief of menstrual cramps and menopause. Recent scientific investigation has upheld the use of black cohosh in treating both dysmenorrhea and menopause.

A special extract of *Cimicifuga racemosa*, standardized to contain 1 mg of triterpenes calculated as 27-deoxyacteine per tablet (trade name: Remifemin), is the most widely used and thoroughly studied natural alternative to hormone replacement therapy in menopause. In 1997, over ten million monthly units of this extract were sold in Germany, the United States, and Australia. Clinical studies have shown that this cimicifuga extract relieves not only hot flashes, but also depression and vaginal atrophy.[30–33]

In a large open study involving 131 doctors and 629 female patients, cimicifuga extract produced clear improvement in menopausal symptoms in over eighty percent of patients within six to eight weeks.[30] As shown in Table 1, both physical and psychological symptoms were relieved.

Most patients reported noticeable benefits within four weeks after the initiation of

642			
TABLE 1 Cimicifuga in the Treatment of Menopause			
SYMPTOM	% NO LONGER PRESENT	% IMPROVED	TOTAL % IMPROVED
Ringing in the ears	54.8%	38.1%	92.9%
Heart palpitation	54.6%	35.2%	90.4%
Profuse perspiration	49.9%	38.6%	88.5%
Vertigo	51.6%	35.2%	86.8%
Hot flashes	43.3%	43.3%	86.6%
Nervousness/irritability	42.4%	43.2%	85.6%
Headache	45.7%	36.2%	81.9%

cimicifuga therapy. After six to eight weeks, complete resolution of symptoms was achieved in a large percentage of patients. Cimicifuga was well tolerated; there was no discontinuation of therapy, and only seven percent of patients reported mild transitory stomach complaints.

In a double-blind study, sixty patients were given either cimicifuga extract (two tablets twice per day, providing a daily dosage of 4 mg 27-deoxyacteine), conjugated estrogens (0.625 mg daily), or diazepam (a Valium-like drug) (2 mg daily) for twelve weeks.[31] Results from standard indexes of menopausal symptoms indicated a clear advantage of using cimicifuga extract over both drugs. Cimicifuga's effect in relieving the depressive mood and anxiety associated with menopause was far superior to either conjugated estrogens or diazepam.

The Kupperman Menopausal Index is one of the most utilized assessments in clinical studies of menopause. This quantitative assessment of menopausal symptoms is achieved by grading in severity: Severe = 3, Moderate = 2, Mild = 1, Not present = 0. After grading each symptom, the total score is achieved by adding all of the symptom scores together.

Symptoms assessed are

Depressive moods
Feelings of vertigo
Headache
Heart palpitation
Hot flashes
Joint pain
Loss of concentration
Nervousness/irritability
Profuse perspiration
Sleep disturbances

The results on the Kupperman Menopausal Index from the double-blind trial of sixty women clearly demonstrated cimicifuga extract's superiority over conjugated estrogens and diazepam, especially when safety and side effects are taken into consideration.

In another double-blind study, eighty patients were given either cimicifuga extract (two tablets twice daily, providing a daily dosage of 4 mg 27-deoxyacteine), conjugated estrogens (0.625 mg daily), or a placebo for twelve weeks.[32] Cimicifuga produced greater improvement in the vaginal lining and better results on the Kupperman Menopausal Index and the Hamilton Rating Scale for Anxiety (similar to the Hamilton Rating Scale for Depression discussed in DEPRESSION) than estro-

TABLE 2	Effect of Cimicifuga on Kupperman Menopausal Index Compared to Conjugated Estrogens and Diazepam	
TREATMENT GROUP	**BEGINNING**	**AT 12 WEEKS**
Cimicifuga	35	14
Conjugated estrogens	35	16
Diazepam	35	20

gens or placebo. The number of hot flashes experienced each day dropped from an average of 5 to less than 1 in the cimicifuga group. In comparison, the estrogen group only dropped from 5 to 3.5. Even more impressive was the effect of cimicifuga on the vaginal lining. While conjugated estrogens and the placebo produced little effect, a dramatic increase in the number of superficial cells was noted in the cimicifuga group.

The BGA, the German equivalent of the FDA in the United States, lists no contraindications or limitations of use for cimicifuga. Therefore, cimicifuga offers a suitable natural alternative to hormone replacement therapy for menopause, especially where hormone replacement therapy is contraindicated (for women with a history of cancer, unexplained uterine bleeding, liver and gallbladder disease, and pancreatitis, as well as possibly in endometriosis, uterine fibroids, or fibrocystic breast disease).

Since cimicifuga extract shows some estrogenic activity, albeit weak, researchers have sought to determine cimicifuga's effect on established breast tumor cells whose growth *in vitro* depends on the presence of estrogens. The results from these experiments show no stimulatory effects, but rather inhibitory effects.[33] Furthermore, combining Remifemin with tamoxifen (an anti-estrogen drug often used in preventing a recurrence of breast cancer) was shown to potentiate the inhibitory effects of tamoxifen.

Detailed toxicology studies have also been performed on Remifemin. No birth defect–inducing (teratogenic), mutagenic, or carcinogenic effects have been noted. The dosage that showed no effect in a six-month chronic toxicity study in rats was at 1,800 mg/kg body weight—roughly ninety times the therapeutic dose.[34] A six-month toxicological study in rats is comparable to an unlimited treatment time in humans.

What all this toxicology data means is that long-term use, or even indefinite use, of cimicifuga appears to be safe. The German Commission E (the expert panel that sets recommendations on the use of herbal medicines in Germany) has recommended that treatment with cimicifuga be limited to six months (the standard recommendation for hormone replacement therapy as well). However, this recommendation was made prior to the detailed toxicology studies discussed above. Based on currently available data, cimicifuga is appropriate for long-term continued use.

Ginkgo biloba

Ginkgo biloba extract is often appropriate for the menopausal and postmenopausal woman because of its effects on the vascular system. It may be especially useful in relieving both the cold hands and feet and the forgetfulness that often accompany menopause. *Ginkgo biloba* extract has also been shown to improve blood flow to the hands and feet in human clinical trials and has been shown to be effective in the treatment of peripheral vascular disease of the extremities, including Raynaud's syndrome, a disease characterized by extremely cold fingers or toes.[35,36]

Ginkgo biloba extract has repeatedly been used to improve mental health in patients with cerebral vascular insufficiency and may exert similar effects in menopause. *Ginkgo biloba* extract appears to work not only by increasing blood flow to the brain, but also by enhancing energy production within the brain, increasing the uptake of glucose by brain cells and actually improving the transmission of nerve signals.[34]

Improving the transmission rate of nerve signals is critically important to memory. Memory is directly related to the speed at which the nerve impulse can be transmitted. Although the effect of *Ginkgo biloba* extract on menopause-related forgetfulness has not been studied in a controlled fashion, there is ample evidence to suggest that it is worth a clinical trial. Ginkgo has been shown to significantly improve memory in both elderly and college-aged women in double-blind studies.[35,37]

It must be pointed out that, in the treatment of cerebral vascular insufficiency, *Ginkgo biloba* extract should be taken consistently for at least twelve weeks in order to determine effectiveness. Although most people report benefits within a two- to three-week period, some individuals may take longer to respond. It seems that the longer the treatment is continued, the more obvious and lasting the result.

Lifestyle Factors

Exercise

Exercise is very important during menopause for many reasons. In particular, exercise may help reduce the frequency and severity of hot flashes. As a result of the theory that im-paired endorphin activity within the hypothalamus is a major factor in provoking hot flashes, researchers in Sweden designed a study to determine the effect of regular physical exercise on the frequency of hot flashes.[38] In the study, the frequency of moderate and severe hot flashes was investigated in seventy-nine postmenopausal women who took part in physical exercise on a regular basis and was compared to that in a control group of 866 postmenopausal women between fifty-two and fifty-four years old.

The study clearly demonstrated that regular physical exercise decreased the frequency and severity of hot flashes. The women in the exercising group passed through a natural menopause without the use of hormone replacement therapy. The physically active women who had no hot flashes whatsoever spent an average of 3.5 hours per week exercising, while women who exercised less than this amount were more likely to have hot flashes. Similar results, including mood elevation in pre-, peri-, and postmenopausal exercising versus sedentary women, have been reported in other studies.[39] The benefits of exercise were experienced in women both on and off HRT.

Given the many benefits of regular exercise on mood and the health of bone and the cardiovascular system, along with these positive results in reducing the frequency and severity of hot flashes, it is clear that regular physical exercise is a key component of menopause care.

HEALTH BENEFITS OF REGULAR EXERCISE DURING MENOPAUSE

Decreased blood cholesterol levels
Decreased bone loss
Improved ability to deal with stress
Improved circulation
Improved heart function
Improved oxygen and nutrient utilization in all tissues

Increased endurance and energy levels

Increased self-esteem, mood, and frame of mind

Reduced blood pressure

Relief from hot flashes

Cigarette Smoking

Cigarette smoking significantly increases the risk of early menopause, as smokers have approximately double the risk of beginning menopause between the ages of forty-four and fifty-five. Those who were former smokers had a lowered risk, showing that there could be a partial reversal of the effect.[40]

TREATMENT SUMMARY

Many natural measures can help alleviate the most common symptoms of menopause. In most cases, hormone replacement therapy is not necessary. However, in women at high risk for osteoporosis and women who have already experienced significant bone loss, hormone replacement therapy may be appropriate. For the immediate treatment of atrophic vaginitis, topical vitamin E preparations should be considered. If a woman is smoking, she should begin a smoking cessation program.

Diet

Increase the amount of phytoestrogens in the diet by consuming more soy foods, fennel, celery, parsley, high-lignan flaxseed oil, nuts, and seeds.

Nutritional Supplements

- Vitamin E: 800 IU per day until symptoms have improved, then 400 IU per day
- Hesperidin: 900 mg per day
- Vitamin C: 1,200 mg per day
- Gamma-oryzanol: 300 mg per day

Botanical Medicines

All dosages are three times per day.

- Dong quai *(Angelica sinensis)*
  Powdered root or as tea: 1–2 g
  Tincture (1:5): 4 ml (1 tsp)
  Fluid extract: 1 ml (^{1}/4 tsp)
- Licorice *(Glycyrrhiza glabra)*
  Powdered root or as tea: 1–2 g
  Fluid extract (1:1): 4 ml (1 tsp)
  Solid (dry powdered) extract (4:1): 250–500 mg
- Chasteberry *(Vitex agnus-castus)*
  Powdered berries or as tea: 1–2 g
  Fluid extract (1:1): 4 ml (1 tsp)
  Solid (dry powdered) extract (4:1): 250–500 mg
- Black cohosh *(Cimicifuga racemosa)*
  The dosage of cimicifuga is based on its content of 27-deoxyacteine, which serves as an important biochemical marker to indicate therapeutic effect. The dosage of the cimicifuga extract used in the majority of clinical studies has been 2 mg of

27-deoxyacteine twice daily. Here are the approximate dosage recommendations using other forms (nonstandardized) of *Cimicifuga racemosa:*

Powdered rhizome: 1–2 g

Tincture (1:5): 4–6 ml

Fluid extract (1:1): 3–4 ml (1 tsp)

Solid (dry powdered) extract (4:1): 250–500 mg

- *Ginkgo biloba* extract
(24% ginkgo flavonglycoside content):
40 mg

Lifestyle

Exercise regularly—at least thirty minutes three times a week.

Menstrual Blood Loss, Excessive

Excessive menstrual bleeding refers to a blood loss greater than 80 ml, occurring during regular menstrual cycles (cycles are usually of normal length)

Excessive menstrual bleeding, or *menorrhagia*, is a common female complaint that may be entirely prevented in many cases by taking proper nutritional measures. As with any disease, proper determination of the cause is essential for effective treatment. In many cases of "excessive blood loss," it is demonstrated that the amount of blood lost is actually quite normal based upon close questioning of the number of pads/tampons used and how heavy of a flow.[1] If you question whether you have menorrhagia or not, we strongly encourage you to contact your physician for proper evaluation.

The cause of functional menorrhagia (i.e., not caused by the presence of uterine fibroids or endometriosis) involves abnormalities in the biochemical processes of the *endometrium* (the lining of the uterus) that control the supply of the fatty acid *arachidonic acid,* which is needed for prostaglandin synthesis.[2,3] *Prostaglandins* are hormone-like molecules that are manufactured from fatty acids. The endometrium of women who have menorrhagia concentrates arachidonic acid to a much greater extent than normal. The increased arachidonic acid release during menstruation results in increased production of Series 2 prostaglandins, which are thought to be the major factor both in the excessive bleeding and in accompanying menstrual cramps.

Other factors believed to contribute to menorrhagia are iron deficiency, hypothyroidism, vitamin A deficiency, intrauterine devices, and various local factors (e.g., uterine myomas, endometrial polyps, adenomyosis, endometrial hyperplasia, salpingitis, and endometritis).

Therapeutic Considerations

The key consideration is iron. Blood loss above 60 ml during a menstrual period is associated with *negative iron balance*—greater loss of iron than intake.[4] Although menstrual blood loss is well recognized as a major cause of iron deficiency anemia in fertile women, it is not as well known that chronic iron deficiency can be a cause of menorrhagia. This association is based on several observations: (1) response to iron supplementation alone in seventy-four of eighty-three patients in one study; (2) a high rate of uterine fibroids and polyps in the patients who failed to respond to iron supplementation; (3) an associated rise in serum iron levels in forty-four of fifty-seven patients in another study; (4) decreased response to iron therapy when initial serum iron levels were high; (5) correlation of menorrhagia with depleted tissue iron stores

645

(bone marrow) irrespective of serum iron level; and (6) a significant double-blind placebo-controlled study displaying improvement in 75 percent of those on iron supplementation, compared with 32.5 percent for the placebo group.[5]

Iron supplementation, at a daily dose of 100 mg of elemental iron, has been recommended as a preventive therapy by several researchers. This recommendation is based on the observations that chronic iron deficiency appears to promote menorrhagia and that iron-containing enzymes are depleted before changes in the blood (anemia) are observed.[4,5] As a result of the low iron, these iron-dependent enzymes lead to a state of low energy metabolism in the uterine lining and excessive blood loss.

Vitamin A

Vitamin A supplementation may also be valuable. In one study, serum vitamin A levels were found to be significantly lower in seventy-one women with menorrhagia than in healthy controls. After forty of these were given 25,000 IU of vitamin A twice per day for fifteen days, blood loss returned to normal in twenty-three and was reduced in fourteen. All told, 92.5 percent of the women had either complete relief or significant improvement.[6]

Vitamin C and Bioflavonoids

Fragile blood capillaries are believed to play a role in many cases of menorrhagia. Supplementation with vitamin C (200 mg three times per day) and bioflavonoids was shown to reduce menorrhagia in fourteen of sixteen patients.[7] One of the two patients who failed to respond had endometriosis. As vitamin C is known to significantly increase iron absorption, its therapeutic effect could be also due to enhanced iron absorption.

Vitamin E

One group of investigators has suggested that free radicals play a causative role in endometrial bleeding, particularly in the presence of an intrauterine device.[8] Vitamin E supplementation (100 IU every two days) resulted in improvement in all patients by the end of ten weeks.[8] Although vitamin E may have produced its effects via its antioxidant activity, it is equally plausible that it affected prostaglandin metabolism in a manner that would reduce bleeding.

Vitamin K and Chlorophyll

Although women with menorrhagia show no signs of vitamin K deficiency, the use of vitamin K (historically in the form of crude preparations of chlorophyll) has clinical and limited research support.[9] It is certainly worth adding to the program, especially in unresponsive cases.

Thyroid Abnormalities

The association of thyroid problems (hypothyroidism or hyperthyroidism) with menstrual disturbances is well known. However, even minimal thyroid dysfunction—particu-

. . . .

QUICK REVIEW

- Nutritional factors are often responsible for excessive menstrual blood loss.

- Iron therapy is a key consideration in treating menorrhagia.
- Even mild hypothyroidism can lead to excessive menstrual blood loss.

larly minimal, subclinical insufficiency (see HYPOTHYROIDISM)—may be responsible for menorrhagia and other menstrual disturbances.[10] Patients with even mild hypothyroidism and menorrhagia have responded dramatically to thyroid hormone supplementation.[10]

Essential Fatty Acids

Since most of the arachidonic acid in tissues is derived from the diet, it is possible that reducing intake of animal products and/or increasing intake of flaxseed oil could curtail blood loss by decreasing the availability of arachidonic acid.

Botanicals

Numerous botanicals have been used in the treatment of menorrhagia. However, the only plant with any significant clinical research to support its use is shepherd's purse (*Capsella bursa pastoris*). In addition to its long history of use in the management of obstetric and gynecological hemorrhage, a couple of clinical studies have also shown it to be effective in treating menorrhagia.[11,12]

TREATMENT SUMMARY

The first step with menorrhagia is to rule out serious causes. Because excessive menstrual bleeding can reflect a serious condition, it is essential that you consult a physician if you are experiencing excessive menstrual blood loss. When the excessive bleeding has been determined to be functional (not due to a disease state), the following guidelines will usually be of great value.

Diet

The diet should be relatively low in sources of arachidonic acid (animal fats). Green leafy vegetables and other sources of vitamin K should be eaten freely.

Nutritional Supplements

- Vitamin C: 500–1,000 mg three times per day
- Bioflavonoids: 500–1,000 mg per day
- Vitamin A: 25,000 IU twice per day for two weeks, followed by 25,000 IU per day thereafter until the situation normalizes

NOTE: Vitamin A should not be used if there is any chance that a woman is pregnant or at risk of getting pregnant.

- Vitamin E: 200–400 IU per day
- Chlorophyll (fat-soluble): 25 mg per day
- Iron: 100 mg per day

Botanical Medicines

- Shepherd's purse (*Capsella bursa pastoris*), three times per day:
  Dried leaves or by infusion (tea): 1.54 g
  Tincture (1:5): 4–6 ml
  Fluid extract (1:1): 0.5–2.0 ml
  Powdered solid extract (4:1): 250–500 mg

Migraine Headache

. . . .

Headache is typically pounding and on one side

Attacks are often preceded by psychological or visual disturbances; accompanied by anorexia, nausea, and gastrointestinal upset; and followed by drowsiness

Migraine headaches are caused by excessive dilation of blood vessels in the head. Migraines are a surprisingly common disorder; at some time in their lives, fifteen to twenty percent of men and twenty-five to thirty percent of women have migraine headaches.[1] More than half of the patients have a family history of the illness.

Although some migraines come on without warning, many migraine sufferers have warning symptoms ("auras") before the onset of pain. Typical auras last a few minutes and include: blurring or bright spots in the vision, anxiety, fatigue, disturbed thinking, and numbness or tingling on one side of the body.

In vascular headaches, such as migraine headaches, the pain is characterized as a throbbing or pounding sharp pain. In nonvascular headaches, such as tension headaches, the pain is characterized as a steady, constant, dull pain that starts at the back of the head or in the forehead and spreads over the entire head, giving the sensation of pressure, as if a vise grip has been applied to the skull.

The pain of a headache comes from outside the brain, because the brain tissue itself does not have sensory nerves. Pain arises from the lining of the brain (*meninges*) and from the scalp, its blood vessels, and its muscles when these structures are stretched or tensed.

The most common nonvascular headache is the tension headache. This headache is usually caused by tightening in the muscles of the face, neck, or scalp as a result of stress or poor posture. The tightening of the muscles results in pinching of the nerve or its blood supply, which results in the sensation of pain and pressure. Relaxation of the muscle usually brings about immediate relief.

PRIMARY CLASSIFICATIONS OF HEADACHES

Vascular headache
  Migraine headache
    Classic migraine
    Common migraine
    Complicated migraine
    Variant migraine
  Cluster headache
    Episodic cluster
    Chronic cluster
    Chronic paroxysmal hemicrania
  Miscellaneous vascular headaches
    Carotidynia
    Hypertension
    Exertional
    Hangover
    Toxins and drugs
    Occlusive vascular disease
Nonvascular headache
  Tension headache
    Common tension headache
    Temporomandibular joint (TMJ) dysfunction

Increased or decreased intracranial pressure
Brain tumors
Sinus infections
Dental infections
Inner or middle ear infections

Classification

Migraine headache has been subdivided into several types; the three most common (*common, classic,* and *complicated*) comprise the vast majority of patients. Differentiation among these subtypes, while important, does not at this time have any real therapeutic significance.

The *cluster headache* was once considered a migraine-type headache since vasodilation is a key component, but it is now separately classified. Also referred to as a *histamine headache,* it is much less common than migraine.

Another headache to be considered in this chapter is chronic daily headache (CDH). Approximately forty percent of patients seen in headache clinics suffer from CDH. To sim-

plify matters, CDH has now been divided into four major types.

THE FOUR TYPES OF CHRONIC DAILY HEADACHE
1. Transformed migraine
   Drug-induced
   Non-drug-induced
2. Chronic tension headache
3. New daily persistent headache
4. Post-traumatic headache

Causes of Migraine Headache

Considerable evidence supports an association between migraine headache and instability of blood vessels, but the mechanisms are not yet known. Although most clinicians and researchers believe that the sequence of events is excessive constriction of a blood vessel followed by rebound dilation, sophisticated studies of brain blood flow before, during, and after are inconsistent in their support of this hypothesis.[2,3]

TABLE 1 Migraine Classification			
SYMPTOM	**COMMON**	**CLASSIC**	**COMPLICATED**
Incidence	80%	10%	10%
Pain	Frontal, uni/bilateral	Unilateral	Unpredictable, may be absent
Aura	Unusual	Half-hour, striking	Neurological aura, vertigo, syncope, diplopia, hemiparesis
Duration of headache	1–3 days	2–6 hrs	Unpredictable
Physical examination	Unhappiness	Pallor, vomiting	Mild neurological signs, speech disorder, hemiparesis, unsteadiness, cranial nerve III palsy

Vascular Instability

In many cases of migraine headache, the blood vessels of the temple are visibly dilated and local compression of these vessels or the main artery of the neck (the *carotid* artery) temporarily relieves migraine pain.[4] Despite the dilation of blood vessels, the patient with a migraine appears pale during the headache, suggesting dilation of the large blood vessels and constriction of the small vessels. This theory is supported by the observation of lower skin temperature on the same side of the face as the pain.

A majority, but not all, of the studies measuring brain blood flow have confirmed a reduction of blood flow, sometimes to very low and critical levels, during the period prior to a migraine attack. This is followed by a stage of increased blood flow that can persist for more than forty-eight hours. There is significant decrease in regional brain blood flow in classic migraine, but not in common migraine.[5] The abnormal blood flow appears confined to the outer portion of the brain (cerebral cortex), while deeper structures have normal blood supply.

There is some evidence that migraine patients have an inherited abnormality in their control of blood vessel constriction and dilation. Migraine patients suffer more often than normal people from dizziness upon standing suddenly, and they seem to be abnormally sensitive to the effects of physical and chemical factors that cause changes in blood vessels.

Platelet Disorder

Platelets are small blood cells involved in the formation of blood clots. The platelet of migraine sufferers is very different from the normal platelet, both during and between headaches.[8] The differences include a significant increase in spontaneous clumping together (aggregation), highly significant differences in the manner of serotonin release, and significant differences in the structural composition of the platelets.

The biggest factor may be the differences in serotonin metabolism. Serotonin is a compound used in the chemical transfer of information from one cell to another. Serotonin also plays a role in the state of relaxation or constriction of blood vessels. All of the serotonin normally in the blood is stored in the platelets and is released by platelet aggregation. There is no difference in total serotonin content between normal platelets and the

. . . .

QUICK REVIEW

- The first step in treating migraine headache is identifying the precipitating factor.
- Several clinical studies have estimated that approximately seventy percent of patients with chronic daily headaches suffer from drug-induced headaches.

- Many double-blind, placebo-controlled studies have demonstrated that the detection and removal of allergenic foods will eliminate or greatly reduce migraine symptoms in the majority of patients.
- Foods such as chocolate, cheese, beer, and wine precipitate migraine attacks in many people because they contain

platelets of migraine patients. However, the quantity of serotonin released by the platelets of the migraine patient in response to serotonin stimulation (such as a food allergy), while initially normal, becomes progressively higher until a migraine is produced.[6]

The platelet hypothesis is strengthened by the observation that patients with classic migraine have a twofold increase in incidence of mitral valve prolapse.[7] *Mitral valve prolapse* refers to a "leaky" heart valve. This leaky valve can cause damage to blood platelets as they surge through the valve with each beat of the heart. Researchers have found that sixteen percent of migraine patients have definite mitral prolapse, and another fifteen percent have possible prolapse—a rate at least two times higher than normal.[7–9]

Nerve Disorder

A third major hypothesis is that, in migraine, the nervous system plays a role in initiating the vascular events.[1] It has been suggested that the nerve cells in the blood vessels of patients with migraines release a compound known as "substance P."[10] You probably guessed what the "P" stands for: PAIN. In addition to triggering pain, the release of substance P into the arteries is associated with dilating blood vessels and the release of histamine and other allergic compounds by specialized white blood cells known as *mast cells*. Chronic stress is thought to be an important factor in this model.

Migraine as a Serotonin Deficiency Syndrome

The final hypothesis is that migraine headache represents a serotonin deficiency state. The story of serotonin and headaches began in the 1960s, when researchers noted an increase in the serotonin breakdown product 5-hydroxyindoleacetic acid (5-HIAA) in the urine during a migraine.[11] Initially it was thought that serotonin excess was the culprit. However, newer information indicates that the factor responsible for the increase in 5-HIAA is probably increased breakdown of serotonin as a result of increased activity of monoamine oxidase (MAO).[12,13] Because migraine sufferers actually have low levels of serotonin in their tissues, this led researchers to refer to migraine as a "low-serotonin syndrome."[16]

Low serotonin levels are thought to lead to a decrease in the pain threshold in patients with chronic headaches. This contention is

. . . .

histamines and/or other compounds that can trigger migraines in sensitive individuals by causing blood vessels to expand.

- 5-HTP is at least as effective as other pharmacological agents used in the prevention of migraine headaches and is certainly much safer and better tolerated.

- Low magnesium levels may also play a significant role in many cases of headaches.

- Biofeedback and relaxation training have been judged as effective as the drug approach but are without any side effects.

- Feverfew and ginger extracts can help prevent migraine attacks.

strongly supported by over thirty-five years of research, including positive clinical results in double-blind studies with the serotonin precursor 5-hydroxytryptophan (5-HTP).

The link between low serotonin levels and headaches is the basis of many prescription drugs for the treatment and prevention of migraine headaches. For example, the serotonin agonist drug sumatriptan (Imitrex) is now among the most popular migraine prescriptions. In addition to sumatriptan, monoamine oxidase inhibitors (which increase serotonin levels) have also been shown to prevent headaches. The bottom line is there is considerable evidence that increasing serotonin levels leads to relief from chronic migraine headaches.

The effects of 5-HTP, sumatriptan, and other drugs on the serotonin system are extremely complex because of the multiple types of serotonin receptors. Many substances produce their effects on cells by first binding to receptor sites on the cell membrane. Some serotonin receptors are involved in triggering migraines and others prevent them. This situation is quite clear when looking at the different effects that various drugs exert when binding to these different serotonin receptors. Drugs that bind to serotonin receptors designated as 5-HT_{1c} trigger migraines, while drugs such as methysergide that inhibit 5-HT_{1c} are used to prevent migraines.[15] In addition, the serotonin receptor 5-HT_{1d} may prevent migraine headaches, since drugs like sumatriptan that bind to these receptors and mimic the effects of serotonin are quite effective in the acute treatment of migraine.[16]

Because some serotonin receptors appear to undergo desensitization when exposed to higher levels of serotonin, these different receptors come into play with 5-HTP supplementation. It is thought that by increasing serotonin levels, 5-HT_{1c} receptors lose their ability or affinity to bind serotonin, resulting in more serotonin binding to the 5-HT_{1d} receptor. In other words, it is thought that, in the use of 5-HTP for preventive treatment of migraine headache, the higher levels of serotonin produced over time decrease the sensitivity of the 5-HT_{1c} receptors and increase the sensitivity of the 5-HT_{1d} receptors.[17] As a result, there would be a lowered tendency to experience headache. One of the key pieces of evidence to support this concept is the fact that 5-HTP is more effective over time (better results are seen after sixty days of use than at thirty days).

Unified Hypothesis

The mechanism of migraine can be described as a three-stage process: initiation, prodrome (time between initiation and appearance of headache), and headache. Although a particular stressor may be associated with the onset of a specific attack, it appears that initiation is dependent on the accumulation of several stressors over time. These stressors ultimately affect serotonin metabolism. Once a critical point of susceptibility (or threshold) is reached, a "cascade event" is initiated that sets in process a domino-like effect that ultimately produces a headache. This susceptibility is probably a combination of decreased tissue serotonin levels, changes in the platelets, increased sensitivity to compounds such as substance P, and the buildup of histamine and other mediators of inflammation. These events are summarized in Figure 1.

FACTORS THAT TRIGGER MIGRAINE HEADACHES

Low serotonin levels
    Genetics
    Shunting of tryptophan into other pathways
Foods

INITIATION   PRODROME   HEADACHE

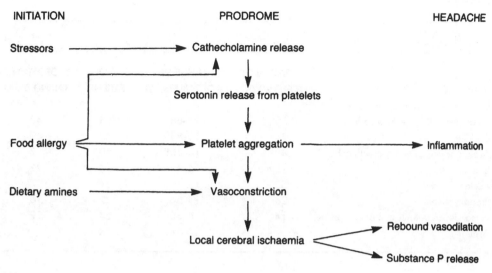

FIGURE 1 Migraine

Food allergies
Histamine-releasing foods
Histamine-containing foods
Alcohol, especially red wine
Chemicals
  Nitrates
  MSG (monosodium glutamate)
  Nitroglycerin
Withdrawal from caffeine or other drugs that constrict
  blood vessels
Stress
Emotional changes, especially let-down after stress, and in-
  tense emotions, such as anger
Hormonal changes, e.g., menstruation, ovulation, birth-
  control pills
Too little or too much sleep
Exhaustion
Poor posture
Muscle tension
Weather changes (barometric pressure changes, exposure
  to sun)
Glare or eyestrain

Therapeutic Considerations

Modern drug treatment of headache, whether migraine or tension, is ultimately doomed because it fails to address the underlying cause. The first step in treating migraine headache is identifying the precipitating factor. Although food intolerance/allergy is the most important, many other factors must be considered as either primary causes or contributors to the migraine process. In particular, it is important to assess the role that headache medications may be playing, especially in chronic headaches.

Drug Reaction

Several clinical studies have estimated that approximately seventy percent of patients with chronic daily headaches suffer from drug-induced headaches.[18] There are two main forms of drug-induced chronic daily headaches: *analgesic-rebound headache* and

TABLE 2 Profile of 200 Patients with Chronic Daily Headache				
MEDICATION	AVERAGE # OF TABLETS/WK	RANGE OF # OF TABLETS/WK	# OF PATIENTS	% OF PATIENTS TAKING DRUG
Butalbital/aspirin, acetaminophen/ caffeine with or without codeine	30	14–86	84	42
Codeine	28	10–84	80	40
Aspirin or acetaminophen with caffeine	42	14–108	50	2
Ergotamine	15 mg	6–42	44	22
Acetaminophen	52	15–105	34	17
Propoxyphene	26	14–56	32	16
Nasal decongestants and antihistamines	14	6–30	24	12
Aspirin		10–64	8	4

ergotamine-rebound headache.[19] Withdrawal of medication results in prompt clinical improvement in most cases. In one study (summarized in Table 2) of two hundred patients suffering from analgesic rebound headache, discontinuation of these headache medications resulted in fifty-two-percent improvement in the total headache index.[21] Improvements in headache frequency and severity, general well-being, and sleep patterns were also noted, as well as a reduction in irritability, depression, and lethargy.

These two hundred patients were typical, in that they sought relief from a variety of drugs. Table 3 lists the types of drugs used for symptomatic relief. Most of these patients took at least three of these preparations at the same time.

Analgesic-Rebound Headache

In the early 1980s, it became apparent in the medical literature that headache medications increase the tendency to get headaches and perpetuate chronic headache. Early reports were labeled "paradoxical," in that heavy analgesic users experienced headaches of much greater frequency and intensity. For example, in one study it was found that sufferers of migraine headaches who took more than thirty analgesic tablets per month had twice as many headache days per month as those who took fewer than thirty tablets.[20] This finding led to the recommendation that analgesic use be restricted in patients with chronic daily headaches.

In another study, seventy patients with daily headaches who were consuming fourteen or more analgesic tablets per week were told to discontinue their use.[21] One month later, sixty-six percent of the patients were improved. At the end of the second month, this percentage had grown to eighty-one percent.

Analgesic-rebound headaches should be suspected in any patient with chronic headaches who is taking large quantities of analgesics and who is experiencing daily predictable headache. The critical dosage that can lead to analgesic-rebound headache is estimated to be 1,000 mg of either acetaminophen or aspirin.

Analgesic medications typically contain substances in addition to the analgesic, such as caffeine or a sedative like butabarbital. These substances further contribute to the problem and may lead to withdrawal headaches and related symptoms, such as nausea, abdominal cramps, diarrhea, restlessness, sleeplessness, and anxiety. Withdrawal symp-

TABLE 3	Drugs Commonly Used to Prevent Migraine Headaches	
DRUG	**ADULT DAILY DOSAGE**	**COMMON SIDE EFFECTS**
Aspirin	650–1950 mg	Gastric irritation, ulcer formation
Propranolol	80–240 mg	Fatigue, lassitude, depression, insomnia, nausea, vomiting, constipation
Amitriptyline and imipramine	10–150 mg	Drowsiness, dry mouth, constipation, weight gain, blurred vision, water retention
Sertraline	50–200 mg	Anxiety, insomnia, sweating, tremor, gastrointestinal disturbances
Fluoxetine	20–60 mg	Similar to those of sertraline
Ergonovine maleate	0.6–2 mg	Nausea, vomiting, abdominal pain, diarrhea
Cyproheptadine	12–20 mg	Sedation, dry mouth, gastrointestinal disturbances
Clonidine	0.2–0.6 mg	Dry mouth, drowsiness, sedation, headache, constipation
Methysergide	4–8 mg	Nausea, vomiting, diarrhea, abdominal pain, cramps, weight gain, insomnia, edema, decreased blood flow to extremities, heart and lung fibrosis
Calcium channel blockers (verapamil, nifedipine, diltiazem, etc.)	80–160 mg	Headache, low blood pressure, flushing, water retention, constipation

toms typically start at twenty-four to forty-eight hours and in most cases subside in five to seven days.

Ergotamine-Rebound Headache

Ergotamine is the most widely used drug in the treatment of severe acute migraine and cluster headaches. Ergotamine works by constricting the blood vessels of the head, thereby preventing or relieving the excessive dilation of the blood vessels that is responsible for the pain of migraine and cluster headaches. Ergotamine is administered intramuscularly, by inhalation, or by suppository since it is poorly absorbed when given orally.

Although usually quite effective, ergotamine (even at prescribed dosages) is also associated with some significant side effects. Symptoms of acute poisoning occur in about ten percent of patients and include: vomiting, diarrhea, dizziness, rise or fall of blood pressure, slow weak pulse, dyspnea (difficulty in breathing), convulsions, and loss of consciousness. Symptoms of chronic poisoning include two types of manifestations. The first type results from blood vessel contraction and reduced circulation and includes: numbness and coldness of the extremities, tingling, pain in the chest, heart valve lesions, hair loss, decreased urination, and gangrene of the fingers and toes. The second type results from nervous system disturbances and includes: vomiting, diarrhea, headache, tremors, contractions of the facial muscles, and convulsions.

Regular use of ergotamine to treat migraine headaches is also associated with a dependency syndrome characterized by severe chronic headache with an increase in headache intensity upon cessation of medication. Because migraine headaches rarely occur more than once or twice a week, the presence of an almost-daily migraine-type headache in individuals who are taking ergotamine is a strong indicator of ergotamine-rebound headache. Dosage of ergotamine can also be a clue. In most cases of ergotamine-rebound headache, individuals take weekly dosages in excess of 10 mg. In some cases, patients may be taking as much as 10 to 15 mg daily.

Quitting ergotamine causes predictable, protracted, and extremely debilitating headache, usually accompanied by nausea and vomiting. These symptoms usually appear within seventy-two hours and may last for another seventy-two hours. However, improvement after going off the medication is very common. Taking ginger (discussed later in this chapter) may lessen ergotamine withdrawal symptoms.

Diet

Food Allergy or Intolerance

There is little doubt that food allergy/intolerance plays a role in many cases of migraine headache. Many double-blind, placebo-controlled studies have demonstrated that the detection and removal of allergenic or untolerated foods will eliminate or greatly reduce migraine symptoms in the majority of patients. What is unclear is the percentage of migraine patients for whom food control is the most important factor. Table 4 summarizes the results of several clinical studies. As can be seen, success rates range from thirty to ninety-three percent, with the majority of studies showing a remarkably high degree of success.[21–26]

These studies found the incidence of food allergy to be similar for the three major types of migraine. The foods most commonly found to induce migraine headaches are listed in Table 5.

Food allergy/intolerance induces a migraine attack largely as a result of platelets releasing serotonin and histamine.[27–32]

There are several methods for detecting food allergies, most of which are described in the FOOD ALLERGIES chapter. Although laboratory procedures are probably the most convenient for the patient, *challenge testing* is thought to be the most reliable. Unfortunately, challenge testing has limitations. Some foods evoke a delayed response, and several days of repeated challenge may be required to elicit recognizable symptoms. Also, ingestion of large amounts of several foods may be necessary to detect those that are

TABLE 4	Food Allergy/Intolerance and Migraine Headache	
STUDY	**% RESPONDING**	**METHOD**
Mansfield et al.[21]	30	Elimination
Carter et al.[22]	93	Oligoantigenic diet
Hughes et al.[23]	80	Fasting, rotation, elimination
Egger et al.[24]	93	Elimination
Monro et al.[25]	70	RAST, elimination, sodium cromoglycate
Grant[26]	85	Elimination

FOOD	EGGER ET AL.	HUGHES ET AL.	MONRO ET AL.
Cow's milk	67%	57%	65%
Wheat	52	43	57
Chocolate	55	57	26
Egg	60	24	22
Orange	52	—	13
Benzoic acid	35	—	—
Cheese	32	—	—
Tomato	32	14	—
Tartrazine	30	—	—
Rye	30	—	—
Rice	—	—	30
Fish	22	29 (shell)	17
Grapes	12	33	—
Onion	—	24	—
Soy	17	24	—
Pork	22	—	17
Peanut	12	29	—
Alcohol	—	29	9
MSG	—	19	—
Walnut	—	19	—
Beef	20	14	—
Tea	17	—	17
Coffee	15	19	17
Nuts	12	19 (cashew)	17
Goat's milk	15	14	—
Corn	20	9	—
Oats	15	—	—
Cane sugar	7	19	—
Yeast	12	14	—
Apple	12	—	—
Peach	12	—	—
Potato	12	—	—
Chicken	7	14	—
Banana	7	—	—
Strawberry	7	—	—
Melon	7	—	—
Carrot	7	—	—

TABLE 5 Foods That Most Commonly Induce Migraine Headaches

marginally allergenic. The recommended procedure for the diagnosis and management of food allergy/intolerance is described later in this chapter under Treatment Summary.

Dietary Amines Foods such as chocolate, cheese, beer, and wine precipitate migraine attacks in many people. This is because they contain histamine and/or other compounds that can trigger migraines in sensitive individuals by causing blood vessels to expand.[30–32]

Red wine is much more likely than white wine to cause a headache because it contains twenty to two hundred times as much histamine and because it stimulates the release of vasoactive compounds by platelets.[8,29,33] Red wine is also much higher in flavonoids—the antioxidant components shown to help prevent heart disease. These compounds can also inhibit the enzyme *(phenolsulphotransferase)* that normally breaks down serotonin and other vasoactive amines in platelets. Many migraine sufferers have been found to have significantly lower levels of this enzyme.[34] Since red wine contains substances that are potent inhibitors of this enzyme, it often triggers migraines in these individuals, especially if it is consumed along with high-vasoactive-amine foods such as cheese and chocolate. The standard treatment for histamine-induced headache is the histamine-free diet along with vitamin B6 supplementation.[31,32]

FACTORS INVOLVED IN HISTAMINE-INDUCED HEADACHES

Histamine levels are increased by
  Histamine in alcoholic beverages (particularly red wine)
  Histamine in food
  Histamine-releasing foods
  Food allergy
  Vitamin B6 deficiency
Histamine breakdown is inhibited by
  Vitamin B6 antagonists
    Alcohol
    Drugs
    Food additives (e.g., yellow dye #5, monosodium glutamate)
  Vitamin C deficiency
Histamine release is prevented by
  Disodium cromoglycate
  Quercetin
  Antioxidants (e.g., vitamin C, vitamin E, selenium, etc.)
Histamine breakdown is promoted by
  Vitamin B6
  Vitamin C

The activity of the enzyme *diamine oxidase,* which breaks down histamine in the lining of the small intestine before it is absorbed into the circulation, appears to play a major role in determining whether a person is going to react to dietary histamine. Individuals sensitive to dietary histamine have about half as much diamine oxidase in their tissues as control subjects.[31]

Diamine oxidase is a vitamin B6–dependent enzyme. Not surprisingly, compounds that inhibit vitamin B6 also inhibit diamine oxidase.[31] These inhibiting factors include food coloring agents (specifically the hydrazine dyes, such as FD&C yellow #5), some drugs (isoniazid, hydralazine, dopamine, and penicillamine), birth-control pills, alcohol, and excessive protein intake. The intake of yellow dye #5 (tartrazine) alone is often greater (per capita intake of 15 grams per day) the RDA for vitamin B6 of 2.0 mg for males and 1.6 mg for females. Since tartrazine blocks vitamin B6, what this means is that many people probably consume more of a B6 blocker than B6 itself.

Vitamin B6 supplementation (usually 1 mg per 2.2 pounds of body weight) has been shown to relieve histamine headaches, presumably by increasing diamine oxidase activtiy.[31,34] Women have lower levels of diamine oxidase, which may explain their higher incidence of histamine-induced headaches. Women are also much more frequently unable to tolerate red wine.[31] Interestingly, the level of diamine oxidase in a woman increases by over five hundred times during pregnancy.[35,36] It is very common for women with histamine-induced headaches to experience complete remission of their headaches during pregnancy.

Nutritional Supplementation

5-HTP

The role of 5-HTP in preventing migraine headaches by increasing serotonin levels was discussed earlier in this chapter. In addition to this mechanism of action, 5-HTP also increases endorphin levels.[37–39] *Endorphins* are the body's own pain-relieving and mood-elevating substances. Typically, endorphin levels are low in migraine sufferers.

The use of 5-HTP in the prevention of migraine headache offers considerable advantages over drug therapy. Although a number of drugs have been shown to be useful in the prevention of migraine headaches, all of the currently used drugs carry significant side effects. 5-HTP is at least as effective as other pharmacological agents used to prevent migraine headaches, and it is certainly much safer and better tolerated. While some studies have used a dosage of 600 mg daily, equally impressive results have been achieved at a dosage as low as 200 mg daily.

The problem with drug therapy in the prevention of migraine headaches is perhaps best exemplified by one of the most commonly used drugs, methysergide (Sansert). Methysergide therapy for the prevention of migraine attacks is effective in about sixty to eighty percent of cases. However, this effectiveness is not without a high price, as side effects are common and can be quite severe.

Several studies have compared 5-HTP to methysergide in the prevention of migraine headaches. In one of the largest double-blind studies, 124 patients received either 5-HTP (600 mg daily) or methysergide (3 mg daily) in identical-looking pills for six months.[40] Treatment was determined to be successful if there was a reduction higher than fifty percent in the frequency of attacks or in the number of severe attacks. Seventy-five percent of the patients (thirty of the remaining forty patients) who were taking methysergide demonstrated significant improvement, compared to seventy-one percent (thirty-two of the forty-five patients) of the patients who were taking 5-HTP. However, this difference was not viewed as being statistically significant. The advantage of 5-HTP over methysergide was demonstrated when researchers looked at side effects. Side effects were more frequent in the group receiving methysergide than in the 5-HTP group. In fact, five patients in the methysergide group had to withdraw during the trial because of side effects.

Two other studies that compared 5-HTP to drugs used in the prevention of migraine headaches (pizotifen and propranolol) demonstrated that 5-HTP performed quite favorably in terms of effectiveness.[41,42] While

TABLE 6 5-HTP vs. Methysergide: Clinical Effects of Treatment in 124 Patients		
	METHYSERGIDE	5-HTP
No attacks (100% reduction)	35%	25%
Improvement (>50% reduction)	40%	46%
No improvement	12.5%	29%
Withdrawal due to side effects	12.5%	0

these drugs have significant side effects, 5-HTP is extremely well tolerated, even at dosages as high as 600 mg daily. One of the other key differences noted in these studies was 5-HTP's ability to improve mood and relieve feelings of depression.

One of the best uses of 5-HTP is in treating chronic headaches in children. These headaches are a big problem because of the tremendous risk of side effects when using the drugs currently used to treat and prevent headaches in children. Fortunately, there have been several studies of 5-HTP in the treatment of chronic headaches in children and adolescents that have shown excellent results.[43–45] Given the risks of current drugs used in chronic childhood headaches, a trial of 5-HTP for two months certainly seems reasonable. If the headaches are also accompanied by sleep disorders, 5-HTP appears to be especially appropriate.

EFAs and Arachidonic Acid

The role of essential fatty acids in the development of a migraine may be quite important, but it does not appear to have received much research attention. Considering the significance of platelet aggregation and arachidonic acid metabolites in the mediation of the events leading to the *prodromal* reduced blood flow to the brain (*cerebral ischemia*) of migraine, manipulation of dietary EFAs may be very useful. It has been well demonstrated that reducing the consumption of animal fats and increasing the consumption of fish will significantly change platelet and membrane EFA ratios and decrease platelet aggregation.[46–48]

Riboflavin

Another hypothesis is that migraine headaches are caused by a reduction of energy production within the blood vessels of the brain. If this is true, riboflavin, which has the potential of increasing cellular energy production, might have preventive effects against migraine. To test this hypothesis, forty-nine patients suffering from migraine were treated with a very large dose (400 mg daily) of riboflavin for at least three months.[49] Overall improvement after therapy was 68.2 percent in the riboflavin group, as determined by the migraine severity score used in the study. No side effects were reported. The results from this preliminary study suggest that high-dose riboflavin could be an effective, low-cost preventive treatment of migraine.

Magnesium

Low magnesium levels may also play a significant role in many cases of headaches, as several researchers have demonstrated substantial links between low magnesium levels and both migraine and tension headaches.[50–53] A magnesium deficiency is known to set the stage for the events that can cause a migraine attack or a tension headache. Low brain and tissue magnesium concentrations have been found in patients with migraines, indicating a need for supplementation since one of magnesium's key functions is to maintain the tone of the blood vessels and prevent overexcitability of nerve cells.

Unfortunately, two recent double-blind studies of people prone to recurrent migraine headaches have produced conflicting results about the use of magnesium in the prevention of migraines. In the first study, 250 mg of magnesium or placebo was given twice daily to sixty-nine patients (thirty-five received magnesium, thirty-four the placebo) for twelve weeks.[54] Ten patients in each group experienced relief (28.6 percent of those taking magnesium, and 29.4 percent of those taking the placebo). There was no benefit from taking magnesium compared to the placebo in the number of migraine days or migraine attacks.

In the other double-blind study, eighty-one patients suffering from recurrent migraines were given either 600 mg of oral magnesium daily for twelve weeks or a placebo.[46] By the ninth week, the attack frequency was reduced by 41.6 percent in the magnesium group, compared to only 15.8 percent in the placebo group.[55] The number of days with migraine and the drug consumption for symptomatic treatment per patient also decreased significantly in the magnesium group. Side effects with magnesium supplementation included diarrhea (18.6 percent) and gastric irritation (4.7 percent).

It appears that magnesium supplementation may only be effective in individuals who have low tissue or low ionized levels of magnesium in the serum (the blood minus all blood cells). Low tissue levels of magnesium are common in patients with migraine, but most cases go unnoticed because most physicians rely on serum magnesium levels to indicate magnesium levels. Serum magnesium is a very unreliable indicator, as most of the body's store of magnesium lies within cells, not in the serum. A low magnesium level in the serum reflects end-stage deficiency. More sensitive tests of magnesium status are the level of magnesium within the red blood cell (erythrocyte magnesium level) and the level of ionized magnesium (the most biologically active form) in serum.

Another possible benefit of magnesium supplementation in migraine sufferers may be its ability to improve mitral valve prolapse. Mitral valve prolapse is linked to migraines because it leads to damage to blood platelets, causing them to release vasoactive substances such as histamine, platelet-activating factor, and serotonin.[9-11] Since research has shown that eighty-five percent of patients with mitral valve prolapse have chronic magnesium deficiency, magnesium supplementation is indicated.[56] This recommendation is further supported by several studies that show that oral magnesium supplementation improves mitral valve prolapse.

Magnesium bound to citrate, malate, or aspartate is better absorbed and better tolerated than inorganic forms such as magnesium sulfate, hydroxide, or oxide, which tend to produce a laxative effect.[57] If magnesium supplementation produces a loose stool or diarrhea, cut back to a level that is tolerable. Also, it is a good idea to take at least 50 mg of vitamin B6 daily, as this B-vitamin has been shown to increase the intracellular accumulation of magnesium.[58]

Intravenous Magnesium for Acute Migraine Headaches Intravenous magnesium has been shown to be an extremely effective treatment in some cases of acute migraine, tension, and cluster headaches in three studies. In several studies, a dosage of 1 to 3 grams of intravenous magnesium (over a ten-minute period) typically resulted in a nearly ninety-percent success rate in patients with low ionized magnesium levels.[59-61]

Physical Medicine

Many forms of physical medicine have been used in the treatment of migraine headache. Although most have been shown effective in shortening the duration and decreasing the intensity of an attack, they appear relatively ineffective in actually curing this disorder. Although very effective for headaches that have a significant muscular contraction component, these methods appear to have more limited success in reducing the frequency of attacks of true migraine.

Chiropractic Manipulation
In a six-month trial in Australia, eighty-five patients were studied to determine the efficacy of manipulation of the cervical spine by

a chiropractor in the treatment of migraine headache. The study was controlled by comparing chiropractic manipulation to manipulation by a medical practitioner or physiotherapist and to simple cervical mobilization. Although the study found no difference in frequency of recurrence, duration, or disability, the chiropractic patients reported greater reduction in the pain associated with the attacks.[62]

Temporomandibular Joint Dysfunction Syndrome

Some researchers and clinicians have claimed that a substantial portion of headaches diagnosed as classic or common migraine are in reality the symptoms of dysfunction of the temporomandibular joint (TMJ)—the jaw joint. However, a careful investigation found that the incidence of migraine in patients with TMJ is similar to that in the general population, while the incidence of headache due to muscle tension is much higher.[63] These results suggest that, while correction of TMJ dysfunction may be of use in the treatment of migraine headaches, it is far more important in muscle tension headaches.

Transcutaneous Electrical Nerve Stimulation

Transcutaneous electrical nerve stimulation (TENS) involves the stimulation of muscles with very low levels of electricity to cause them to contract and then relax. TENS has been shown to be effective in the treatment of patients with migraine and muscle tension headaches (fifty-five percent responded to treatment, versus an eighteen-percent placebo response).[64] Home TENS units are available through doctors.

Acupuncture

The use of acupuncture in the treatment of migraine headache has received considerable research attention. However, assessing its efficacy is difficult since the studies have not been blind, migraine patients were seldom studied separately, and most of the research has been reported in foreign languages, with only summaries available in English.

Despite these limitations, sufficient evidence exists to support use of acupuncture to relieve migraine pain.[65–67] It is interesting to note that the mechanism of relief is apparently not related to raising endorphin levels—a commonly suggested mechanism for the benefits of acupuncture.[68,69] The mechanism of action may instead be through normalization of serotonin levels. One study found that acupuncture was effective in relieving pain when it normalized serotonin levels but was ineffective in relieving pain and in raising serotonin levels in those patients with very low levels of serotonin.[70]

Acupuncture appears to have some success in reducing the frequency of migraine attacks, although, as mentioned previously, limitations in experimental design make interpretation difficult. One study found that forty percent of the subjects experienced a fifty-to-one-hundred-percent reduction in severity and frequency.[68] Although the authors used a double-blind, crossover design, the patients were only followed for two months. Another (uncontrolled) study found that five treatments over a period of one month decreased recurrence in forty-five percent of the patients over a period of six months.[71]

Biofeedback and Relaxation Therapy

The most widely used non-drug therapy for migraine headaches is thermal biofeedback and relaxation training. Thermal biofeedback utilizes a feedback gauge to monitor the temperature of the hands. The patient is then taught how to raise (or lower) the temperature of the hand, with the device providing feedback as to what is affecting the temperature.

Relaxation training involves teaching patients techniques designed to produce the "relaxation response"—a term used to describe the physiological state that is the opposite of the stress response. The effectiveness of biofeedback and relaxation training in reducing the frequency and severity of recurrent migraine headaches has been the subject of over thirty-five clinical studies.[72] When the results from these studies were compared with those of studies using the beta-blocking drug Inderal (propranolol), it was apparent that the non-drug approach was as effective as the drug approach but was without side effects.

Botanicals

Botanical medicines have a long history of use as folk cures for migraine headache. Although many botanicals have been used, few have received careful evaluation. Discussed here are feverfew (*Tanacetum parthenium*) and ginger (*Zingiber officinalis*), as they have the most scientific documentation.

Feverfew (Tanacetum parthenium)

Perhaps the most popular preventive treatment of migraine headaches is the herb feverfew. Scientific interest in feverfew began when a 1983 survey found that seventy percent of 270 migraine sufferers who had eaten feverfew daily for prolonged periods claimed that the herb decreased the frequency and/or intensity of their attacks.[73] Many of these patients had been unresponsive to orthodox medicines. This survey prompted several clinical investigations of the therapeutic and preventive effects of feverfew in the treatment of migraine.[74–77]

The first double-blind study was done at the London Migraine Clinic, using patients who reported being helped by feverfew.[73] Those patients who received the placebo (and as a result stopped using feverfew) had a significant increase in the frequency and severity of headache, nausea, and vomiting during the six months of the study, while patients taking feverfew showed no change in the frequency or severity of their symptoms. Two patients in the placebo group, who had been in complete remission during self-treatment with feverfew leaves, developed recurrence of incapacitating migraine and had to withdraw from the study. The resumption of self-treatment led to renewed remission of symptoms in both patients. The second double-blind study, performed at the University of Nottingham, demonstrated that feverfew was effective in reducing the number and severity of migraine attacks.[74]

Follow-up studies to the clinical results have shown that feverfew works in the treatment and prevention of migraine headaches by inhibiting the release of blood vessel dilating substances from platelets, inhibiting the production of inflammatory substances, and reestablishing proper blood vessel

TABLE 7	Biofeedback/Relaxation Compared to Propranolol: Average Percent Improvement per Patient		
BIOFEEDBACK/RELAXATION	**PROPRANOLOL**	**PLACEBO**	**UNTREATED**
56.4%	55.2%	14.3%	3.2%

tone.[75] The effectiveness of feverfew is dependent upon adequate levels of parthenolide, the active principle.[76]

Ginger (Zingiber officinalis)

The common ginger root has been shown to exert significant effects against inflammation and platelet aggregation.[77,78] Unfortunately, in relation to migraine headache, there is much anecdotal information but little clinical evidence. For example, a 1990 article described a forty-two-year-old woman with a long history of recurrent migraines who discontinued all medications for a three-month period prior to a trial of ginger.[79] For the trial, she took 500 to 600 mg of dried ginger mixed with water at the onset of the migraine and repeated that dosage every four hours for four days. Improvement was evident within thirty minutes, and there were no side effects. The woman subsequently began to use uncooked fresh ginger in her daily diet. Migraines became less frequent, and, when they did occur, they were at a "much lower intensity" than previously.

There remain many questions concerning the best form of ginger and the proper dosage. The most active anti-inflammatory components of ginger are found in fresh preparations and the oil.

TREATMENT SUMMARY

Identification of the precipitating factors, and their avoidance, is important in reducing the frequency of headaches. Due to the high frequency (eighty to ninety percent) of food allergy/intolerance in patients with migraine headache, we recommend beginning treatment by identifying and eliminating food allergies. This can be accomplished through blood analysis or by either a pure water fast or the use of an elemental diet (see FOOD ALLERGY).

Diet

All food allergens must be eliminated and a four-day rotation diet utilized. Foods that contain vasoactive amines should initially be eliminated; after symptoms have been controlled, such foods can be carefully reintroduced. The primary foods to eliminate are alcoholic beverages, cheese, chocolate, citrus fruits, and shellfish. The diet should be low in sources of arachidonic acid (land-animal fats) and high in foods that inhibit platelet aggregation (vegetable oils, fish oils, garlic, and onion).

Nutritional Supplements

- Magnesium: 250–400 mg three times per day
- Vitamin B6: 25 mg three times per day
- 5-HTP: 100–200 mg three times per day

Botanical Medicines

- Feverfew (Tanacetum parthenium): 0.25–0.5 mg parthenolide
- Ginger (Zingiber officinalis): Fresh ginger: approximately 10 g per day (1/4-inch slice)

Dried ginger: 500 mg four times
per day

Extract: standardized to contain 20%
of gingerol and shogaol, 100–200 mg
three times per day for prevention
and 200 mg every two hours (up to
six times per day) in the treatment of
an acute migraine

Physical Medicine

- TENS to control secondary muscle
spasm

- Acupuncture to balance meridians
- Biofeedback:
The Association for Applied Psy-
chophysiology and Biofeedback
10200 West 44th Avenue, Suite 304
Wheat Ridge, CO 80033
303-422-8436
- Guided imagery:
The Academy for Guided Imagery
P.O. Box 2070
Mill Valley, CA 94942
800-726-2070

Multiple Sclerosis

. . . .

Sudden transient motor and sensory disturbances, including blurred vision, dizziness, muscle weakness, and tingling sensations

Evidence of demyelination on MRI

Multiple sclerosis is a syndrome of progressive nerve disturbances that usually occurs early in adult life. It is caused by gradual loss of the myelin sheath that surrounds the nerve cell. This process is called *demyelination*. One of the key functions of this myelin sheath is to facilitate the transmission of the nerve impulse. Without the myelin sheath, nerve function is lost. Symptoms correspond to the nerves that have lost their myelin sheath.

In about two-thirds of the cases, onset is between ages twenty and forty (rarely is the onset after age fifty), and women have a slight edge over men (sixty percent female to forty percent male). The frequency of MS appears to be increasing.

It appears that the initial event in the development of MS may occur in early life. This statement is based on the observation that people who move from a low-risk area to a high-risk area before age fifteen have a higher risk of developing MS, whereas those who make the same move after age fifteen retain their low risk.[2]

One of the more interesting features of MS is the geographic distribution of the disease. Areas with the highest frequency rates are all located in the higher latitudes, in both the northern and southern hemispheres (50 to 100 cases per 100,000 in the higher latitudes versus 5 to 10 per 100,000 in the tropics). These high-risk areas include the northern United States, Canada, Great Britain, Scandinavia, northern Europe, New Zealand, and Tasmania. There are interesting exceptions to this geographic distribution, as the disease is uncommon in Japan.[1,2]

There are many possible reasons for the geographic distribution of MS, such as solar exposure, genetics, diet, and other environmental factors. These factors are discussed more fully later in this chapter.

Causes

The cause of MS remains to be identified conclusively. Many causative factors have been proposed, but the data supporting these candidates are not complete. The following factors represent only a fraction of the possible explanations for the cause of MS.

Viral Infection

There is much information to suggest that MS is the result of a viral infection. Viruses cause several demyelinating diseases in humans and animals that are quite similar to MS.[1-3] The studies, when considered collectively, have clearly demonstrated that demyelination can occur as a result of viral infection. The demyelination may be direct viral damage to the myelin-producing cells, or viral infection leading to formation of antibodies which then attack the myelin.

A number of viruses have been isolated from cultures of material in patients with multiple sclerosis, including rabies virus, herpes simplex virus, scrapie virus, parainfluenza virus, subacute myelo-opticoneuropathy virus, measles virus, and coronavirus.[1–3] However, all of these viruses may simply be bystanders, rather than the cause of MS.

The most suspicious virus is the measles virus. As early as 1962, researchers reported that the blood of patients with multiple sclerosis had elevated levels of antibodies to measles. Subsequent studies confirmed this association, and at one time it was believed that MS was due to an ongoing measles infection. This view has been modified by more recent studies indicating that a high percentage of patients with MS have elevated antibody levels to other viruses. More importantly, studies have shown that the measles-specific antibody in MS patients accounts for only a small percentage of the total antibody level.[1–3]

The *cerebrospinal fluid* (the fluid that surrounds the brain and spinal cord) of most MS patients contains an elevated level of antibodies (protein molecules made by white blood cells that bind to foreign molecules such as bacteria, viruses, and cancer cells) in a pattern that is characteristic of an infectious process. One theory states that this pattern is, in fact, due to an unrecognized infectious agent that causes MS. This theory has been termed the "sense antibody" theory. An alternative theory states that MS is not an infectious disease and that all the IgG in the cerebral spinal fluid is nonspecific, or "nonsense antibody." At present, the available data do not appear to support a common virus as the cause for the increased IgG antibody levels. It is more likely the result of an autoimmune reaction.[1–3]

Autoimmune Reaction

The lesions in the nerve cells of MS patients are quite similar to those seen in *experimental allergic encephalomyelitis* (EAE), an autoimmune disease produced in animals after injecting them with myelin. However, in EAE the autoimmune reaction is the result of sensitivity to a single antigen (myelin basic protein), while in MS sensitivity to myelin basic protein cannot be demonstrated. In other words, even though MS can be produced in animals by injecting them with myelin basic protein, in humans with MS there is no evidence of an increase in antibody levels to myelin basic protein. This indicates that, if MS is an autoimmune disease in humans, it is due to some other antigen. Attempts to find an antigen to which only MS patients react have failed.[1,2] Nevertheless, based on a great deal of circumstantial evidence, MS appears to be an autoimmune disease.

Diet

Many researchers have attempted to correlate various dietary patterns with the geographic distribution of MS. For example, diets high in gluten[4] and milk[5,6] are much more common in areas where there is a high prevalence of MS. As intriguing as these associations are, the majority of research concerning nutrition and MS has focused on the role of dietary fat.[7–10]

Some of the first investigations into diet and MS centered around trying to explain why inland farming communities in Norway had a higher incidence of MS than areas near the coastline.[10] It was discovered that the diets of the farmers were much higher in animal and dairy products than the diets of the coastal dwellers, and the latter group's diet had much higher levels of cold-water fish. Since animal and dairy products are much higher in saturated fatty acids and lower in polyunsaturated fatty acids than fish, researchers explored this association in greater detail. Subsequent studies have upheld a strong association between a diet rich in animal and dairy products and the incidence of MS.[7]

Between 1983 and 1989, population-based studies were performed in thirty-six countries on the relationship between diet and mortality rates from multiple sclerosis. A high intake of saturated fatty acids and animal fat, as well as the degree of latitude, are linked to MS. In addition, the ratio of polyunsaturated fatty acids to saturated fatty acids (P:S ratio) was shown to be particularly suspicious.[8]

To illustrate some of the main findings of population-based studies, let's take a look at the low frequency of MS in Japan. The traditional Japanese diet is high in seafood, seeds, and soyfoods. These foods contain abundant polyunsaturated fatty acids, including the omega-3 oils (alpha-linolenic, eicosapentaenoic, and docosahexaenoic acids). Deficiencies of the omega-3 oils are thought to interfere with elongation of fats that compose the nerve cell membrane and to permanently impair formation of normal myelin.[11] Individuals with MS are thought to have a defect in essential fatty absorption and/or transport, which results in a functional deficiency state. In addition, consumption of saturated fats increases the requirements for the essential fatty acids, creating a relative deficiency state in some individuals. This factor is probably significant in patients with MS. The role of diet in MS is discussed further under Therapeutic Considerations.

Excessive Lipid Peroxidation

Many studies have demonstrated a reduced capacity to detoxify free radicals in patients with MS. The key factor appears to be a reduced activity of the antioxidant enzyme glutathione peroxidase (GSH-Px).[12-15] Since GSH-Px is intricately involved in the protection of cells from free-radical damage, decreased activity level would leave the myelin sheath particularly sensitive to damage. In re-

QUICK REVIEW

- Multiple sclerosis (MS) appears to be an autoimmune disease, based on a great deal of circumstantial evidence.
- A high intake of saturated fatty acids and animal fat is linked to MS.
- Many studies have demonstrated a reduced capacity to detoxify free radicals in patients with MS.
- Dr. Roy Swank, Professor of Neurology at the University of Oregon Medical School, has provided convincing evidence that a diet low in saturated fats, maintained over a long period of time, tends to retard the disease process and reduce the number of attacks.
- Supplementation with sources of the omega-6 essential fatty acid linoleic acid for the treatment of MS has been investigated in at least three double-blind trials.
- Natural alpha-interferon therapy is showing promising results.

sponse to free-radical exposure, lipid peroxides are formed.

GSH-Px is found in two forms: a selenium-dependent enzyme and a non-selenium-dependent enzyme. Since low-selenium areas often overlap with high-frequency-rate areas for MS, it is natural to speculate that there might be a link between selenium levels, GSH-Px activity, and MS. Initial studies seemed to support this link.[12,16] However, subsequent studies indicated that the reduced GSH-Px activity found in MS patients is independent of the selenium concentration and is probably due more to genetic factors.[13–15] There appears to be an increased occurrence of MS among individuals who inherently possess low GSH-Px activity (GSH-PxL), compared with individuals who possess high GSH-Px activity (GSH-PxH).[13]

Diagnostic Considerations

Multiple sclerosis is a difficult disease to diagnose early. The initial symptoms may occur alone or in combination, and they occur in varying frequencies (see Table 1). Typically, they develop over a few days, remain stable for a few weeks, and then recede. Recurrences are common, although the course of the disease is extremely variable.

Although multiple sclerosis is diagnosed primarily by clinical signs and symptoms, some laboratory procedures provide support for the diagnosis. These include measurement of components of the patient's cerebral spinal fluid and nerve function (evoked-potential studies). The concentration of IgG antibodies in the cerebral spinal fluid is elevated in eighty to ninety percent of patients with MS. Unfortunately, these abnormalities are not specific for MS. In other words, there are other neurological conditions that can produce exactly the same symptoms of MS. Nerve function assessment shows abnormalities in ninety-four percent of patients with established MS, and sixty-seven percent of patients with suspected MS. During the past decade, magnetic resonance imaging (MRI) has also become a useful tool for assessing the level of demyelination in the nervous system.

TABLE 1	Early Symptoms of Multiple Sclerosis	
TYPE	**FREQUENCY**	**SYMPTOMS**
Motor	42%	Feeling of heaviness, weakness, leg dragging, stiffness, tendency to drop things, clumsiness
Visual	34%	Blurring, fogginess, haziness, eyeball pain, blindness, double vision
Sensory	18%	Tingling, "pins and needles" sensation, numbness, dead feeling, band-like tightness, electrical sensations
Vestibular	7%	Light-headedness, feeling of spinning, sensation of drunkenness, nausea, vomiting
Genitourinary	4%	Incontinence, loss of bladder sensation, loss of sexual function

Therapeutic Considerations

From a natural therapeutic standpoint, there appear to be three major approaches: dietary therapy, nutritional supplements, and physical therapy. Obviously, including all three provides the most comprehensive treatment plan.

Diet

The Swank Diet

Dr. Roy Swank, Professor of Neurology at the University of Oregon Medical School, has provided convincing evidence that a diet low in saturated fats, maintained over a long period of time, tends to retard the disease process of MS and reduce the number of attacks.[9,17] Swank began successfully treating patients with his lowfat diet in 1948. Dr. Swank recommends:

- A saturated fat intake of no more than 10 grams per day
- A daily intake of 40 to 50 grams of polyunsaturated oils per day (margarine, shortening, and hydrogenated oils are not allowed)
- At least 1 tsp of cod liver oil per day
- A normal allowance of protein
- Consumption of fish three or more times per week[9,17]

A diet low in saturated fats significantly restricts many animal sources of protein. The patient has to derive protein from other sources (legumes, grains, and vegetables). While meat consumption is advised, fish appears to be particularly encouraged due to its excellent protein content and, perhaps more importantly, its oil content. Cold-water fish, such as mackerel, salmon, and herring, are rich in the beneficial oils eicosapentaenoic and docosohexanoic acid (omega-3 oils). These oils are important in maintaining nor-

mal neural function and myelin production.[11] They are incorporated into the myelin sheath, where they may increase fluidity and improve neural transmission.

Swank's diet was originally thought to help patients with MS by overcoming an essential-fatty-acid deficiency. Currently, it is thought that the beneficial effects are probably a result of (1) decreasing platelet aggregation, (2) decreasing an autoimmune response, and (3) normalizing the decreased essential-fatty-acid levels found in the serum, erythrocytes, and, perhaps most importantly, the cerebrospinal fluid in patients with MS.[18,19]

Swank's diet significantly reduces the platelet adhesiveness (stickiness) and aggregation (clumping together) that is observed in atherosclerosis (see HEART AND CARDIOVASCULAR HEALTH) as well as in multiple sclerosis. Excessive platelet aggregation and very small clumps of platelets (micro-emboli) are thought to result in the following abnormalities observed in MS: damage to the blood-brain barrier, alterations in the microcirculation of the central nervous system, and reduced blood flow to the brain.[20,21]

MS patients have been shown to have an abnormal blood-brain barrier, presumably as a result of excessive platelet adhesiveness and aggregation.[21,22] Damage to the blood-brain barrier may allow the passage of blood components that are toxic to myelin into the cerebral spinal fluid; these components include bacteria, viruses, antibodies, toxic chemicals, and other compounds. Reduced blood flow may also be a contributing factor in demyelination, by promoting both cellular death and the release of self-destructing enzymes.[23]

The effect of diet on platelets is important in MS, but probably more important is the effect that fatty acids have on the activity of the immune system. Immune-suppressing compounds, such as adrenal steroids, cyclophosphamide, and methotrexate, have yielded good short-term benefits, but are of limited value in the long run due to their high risk and lack of demonstrable efficacy.[1,3] The idea behind using drugs which suppress the immune system in MS is based upon the theory that MS is an autoimmune condition where the immune system is attacking and destroying the myelin sheath. Currently, new immune-suppressing drugs are being tested for use in treating MS. However, considering the lack of toxicity, Swank's dietary approach and supplementation with linoleic acid (discussed in the Supplementation section) appear to be more appropriate and safer ways of modulating the immune response.

Food Allergy

There is a popular theory that food allergies play a role in the progression and treatment of MS.[24] As mentioned earlier, the consumption of two common allergens—gluten and milk—has been implicated in MS. Small-intestinal biopsy in a small group of MS patients indicated an increased frequency of significant damage to the intestinal lining. The damage was similar to that which occurs in celiac disease and food allergies.[25] Clinical evidence for the efficacy of a gluten-free diet is, however, minimal. A clinical trial of a gluten-free diet in forty patients with MS indicated that the relapse rate was no better than average.[26] Another study demonstrated the absence of gluten antibodies in thirty-five out of thirty-six MS patients.[27] While there is no convincing evidence that gluten-free or allergy-elimination diets are universally beneficial in the management of MS, it certainly is generally healthful to eliminate food allergens (as long as other dietary measures are also included, i.e., the Swank diet); there is anecdotal evidence that specific individuals have been helped.

Supplementation

Linoleic Acid

Supplementation with sources of linoleic acid (an omega-6 essential fatty acid) for the treatment of MS has been investigated in at least three double-blind trials.[28–30] Although the results of the studies were mixed (two showed an effect and one did not), combined analysis indicated that patients who supplemented with linoleic acid had a smaller increase in disability, and reduced severity and duration of relapses, compared with controls.[31,32] These studies used a sunflower seed oil emulsion at a sufficient dosage to provide a daily supplementation of 17.2 grams of linoleic acid. Other vegetable oils that primarily contain linoleic acid include safflower and soy.

Better results would probably have been attained in the double-blind studies if dietary saturated fatty acids had been restricted, larger amounts of linoleic acid had been used (at least 20 g/day),[29] and the studies had been of longer duration; one study found that normalization of red blood cell fatty acid levels required at least two years of supplementation.[33] Better yet would be the use of flaxseed oil for its omega-3 fatty acid content (discussed in the next section).

The effectiveness of linoleic acid supplementation in MS is attributed to suppression of the immune system. As mentioned earlier, MS bears a strong resemblance to experimental allergic encephalomyelitis (EAE), an autoimmune disease induced in animals by immunization with myelin.[34,35] Linoleic acid has been shown to greatly inhibit the severity of EAE in animals with less severe forms of the disease, paralleling the effect of linoleic acid supplementation in humans with MS. In other words, individuals with minimal disability respond better than those with severe disability. Polyunsaturated free fatty acids are known to significantly influence the immune system. At higher dosages they can be used to reduce the autoimmune response.[36,37]

Evidence exists that the beneficial effects of essential fatty acid supplementation are mediated by *prostaglandins* (hormone-like substances made from essential fatty acids) and a factor (tuftsin) secreted by the spleen (one of our important immune system organs). Inhibitors of prostaglandin synthesis (such as aspirin and similar nonsteroidal anti-inflammatory drugs) and surgical removal of the spleen have been shown to prevent the protective effect of linoleic acid in EAE.[38,39] The spleen is considered to be the major site for the production and release of prostaglandins that act upon the immune system. Nonsteroidal anti-inflammatory drugs such as aspirin, ibuprofen, and indomethacin should be avoided by patients with MS.

If the effect of essential fatty acid supplementation is related to correcting the composition of the myelin and nerve cell membranes, several years of supplementation may be required before complete therapeutic benefits are observed. Analysis of red blood cells from subjects with MS indicates that treatment with unsaturated fatty acids must continue for at least two years before they regain normal reactivity.[33] Presumably, since myelin-producing cells have a much longer half-life than red blood cells, it could take several years before the total benefit of supplementation would be observed.

Flaxseed, Evening Primrose, and Fish Oils

Better results in the clinical trials would probably have been obtained if flaxseed oil had been used. Flaxseed oil contains both linoleic and alpha-linolenic acid (an omega-3 oil). Flaxseed oil and other omega-3 oils have a greater effect on platelets[40] than linolenic acid and are required for normal myelin composition.[11,41-43]

Flaxseed oil is also a much better choice for patients with MS than evening primrose, borage, or black currant oil. These oils are good sources of gamma-linolenic acid (GLA) as well as linoleic acid. Supplementation with these oils has been suggested to produce better results than supplementing with omega-6 oils that do not have any significant levels of GLA, such as corn, safflower, sunflower, and soy.[44] However, one study demonstrated that daily supplementation with only 340 mg of gamma-linoleic and 2.92 grams of linoleic acid (the ratio found in evening primrose oil) had no effect on the clinical course of MS.[29] In the same study, those who received 23 grams of linoleic acid demonstrated reduced frequency and severity of acute attacks, even though the study was only twenty-four months in length.

There appears to be a strong rationale for supplementation with flaxseed oil as well as consuming more fish rich in eicosapentaenoic acid (EPA) and docosahexanoic acid (DHA). This recommendation is consistent with Swank's protocol, which included the liberal consumption of fish and supplementation with cod liver oil, a rich source of EPA and DHA.[9,17] Rather than use fish oil supplements or cod liver oil, we recommend flaxseed oil.

Selenium and Vitamin ʟ

The role of selenium as the mineral portion of glutathione peroxidase was discussed earlier in regard to the increased lipid peroxidation observed in people with MS. While selenium supplementation will not increase the activity of glutathione peroxidase (GSH-Px) in the majority of patients with MS, it is a relatively inexpensive supplement that may benefit some.

Vitamin E supplementation is definitely recommended, due to the increased lipid peroxidation previously mentioned and the increased consumption of polyunsaturated fats, which increases vitamin E requirements.

And finally, one study reported that supplementation of eighteen MS patients with high dosages of selenium, vitamin C, and vitamin E for five weeks increased GSH-Px levels fivefold.[44]

Vitamin B12

Acquired deficiency of vitamin B12, as well as inborn errors of metabolism involving this vitamin, are well-known causes of demyelination of nerve fibers in the central nervous system (CNS). There are several reports in the medical literature that vitamin B12 levels in the serum, red blood cells, and CNS are low in multiple sclerosis. The coexistence of a vitamin B12 deficiency in MS may aggravate the disease or promote another cause of progressive demyelination.[45–47]

Recently, researchers in Japan sought to (1) clarify the state of vitamin B12 metabolism in twenty-four Japanese patients with MS and (2) determine if vitamin B12 in massive doses provided any therapeutic benefit in chronic progressive MS.[48] The researchers found that the level of vitamin B12 in the serum was normal, but that there was a significant decrease in the unsaturated vitamin B12 binding capacities in the patients with MS, indicating a defect in the transport of vitamin B12 into cells. In six patients with severe chronic progressive MS, the oral administration of 60 mg of vitamin B12 (methylcobalamin) per day improved both visual and brain-stem auditory evoked potentials by nearly thirty percent. Motor function did not improve, indicating that afferent (to the brain) pathways benefit from vitamin B12 while efferent (from the brain) pathways do not.

The results produced are on a par with those produced by treatment with the combination of high-dose intravenous cyclophosphamide (a very potent immune-suppressing drug) plus steroids. However, while this drug combination is associated with profound immune suppression and toxicity, no side effects have been attributed to high doses of vitamin B12.

The form of vitamin B12 used in this study was methylcobalamin—the most active form of B12—rather than the standard cyanocobalamin. Hydroxocobalamin was tried in an earlier MS study with no apparent benefit.[49] Methylcobalamin is the main form in the body and is directly related to the function of vitamin B12 in methylation reactions.

Evaluation of vitamin B12 in cerebral spinal fluid (the fluid that bathes the brain and spinal cord) and blood levels of sixteen MS patients twenty to sixty-three years of age (twelve females) found that the MS patients were significantly lower in B12 than the healthy subjects.[50] However, another study of thirty-eight patients with MS found no differences in blood levels of B12.[51]

Pancreatic Enzymes

Like other autoimmune diseases, MS is associated with an increased level of circulating immune complexes (antigens bound by antibodies). Experimental and clinical studies have shown that protein-digesting enzyme preparations (e.g., pancreatic extracts, bromelain, and papain) are effective in reducing circulating immune-complex levels in several of these diseases. Furthermore, clinical improvements correspond with decreases in immune-complex levels. In the treatment of multiple sclerosis, pancreatic enzyme preparations have been shown to produce good effects in reducing the severity and frequency of symptom flare-ups.[52] Especially good results were noted in cases of visual disturbance, sensory disturbances, and urinary, bladder, and intestinal malfunction. However, it should be pointed out that little effect on spasticity, dizziness, or tremor was reported.

Other Considerations

Malabsorption

A significant number of people with MS may have some degree of malabsorption.[25,53] In one study, forty-two percent of MS patients were shown to have fat malabsorption, forty-two percent were shown to have high levels of undigested meat fibers in their feces, twenty-seven percent had abnormal sugar absorption, and twelve percent had malabsorption of vitamin B12.[53] Malabsorption appears to be an important factor to consider, since multiple subclinical nutrient deficiencies may result.

Pancreatic enzyme preparations may be helpful to improve absorption as well as reduce the level of circulating immune complexes (antibodies bound to antigens). The presence of immune complexes are thought to contribute greatly to the disease process in MS. Experimental and clinical studies have shown that pancreatic enzyme preparations are extremely effective in reducing circulating immune complex levels in several of these diseases. Furthermore, clinical improvements correspond with decreases in immune complex levels. For example, in the treatment of MS, pancreatic enzyme preparations have been shown to produce good effects in reducing the severity and frequency of symptom flare-ups.[54] Especially good results were noted in cases of visual disturbance, urinary bladder and intestinal malfunction, and sensory disturbances. However, it should be pointed out that there was little effect on spasticity, dizziness, or tremor noted.

Natural Alpha-Interferon

Synthetically produced beta-interferon is emerging as a popular medical treatment for multiple sclerosis. However, naturally derived alpha-interferon from white blood cells may prove to be as advantageous or more so. In three preliminary studies conducted between 1987 and 1991, natural alpha-interferon was evaluated in forty-nine MS patients.[55] In the study, patients received 5 to 30 million IU of alpha-interferon per week for three to twelve months, and were observed for two years after their first injection. Although no major toxicity was observed, thirteen of the forty-nine patients initially reported fatigue, flu-like symptoms, or myalgias. These symptoms tended to abate after one month of treatment.

In the first year, eighty percent of the patients improved or stabilized, and in year two seventy-six percent remained improved or stabilized. Better results were seen with higher dosages for longer periods of time. The eighty-three-percent remission rate in relapsing-remitting patients reported in this study is better than the thirty-percent rate reported for beta-interferon. Further studies with larger patient populations using a double-blind format are needed.

Ginkgo biloba Extract

The increased levels of lipid peroxides and other indicators of free-radical damage in the central nervous system in patients with MS suggests the need for antioxidant support.[56] Ginkgo biloba extract (GBE) demonstrates impressive results as an antioxidant, exerts positive effects on platelet function, improves blood flow to the nervous system, and has been shown to enhance nerve cell functions. This has now been assessed in a clinical study.[57] Unfortunately, the study only lasted seven days—hardly enough time for a suitable evaluation. While the study seemed to demonstrate that ginkgo is not of value for acute flare-ups of symptoms, it is of far too short a duration to assess the value of ginkgo for treating MS in the long term.

Hyperbaric Oxygen

Hyperbaric oxygen therapy involves having a person lie in an oxygen tank that has higher pressure than normal air. Early reports described promising results from the use of hyperbaric oxygen (HBO) in the treatment of MS.[57-59] However, these reports were largely anecdotal or from uncontrolled clinical trials. In 1970, one study reported a small, temporary improvement in sixteen of twenty-six patients treated with HBO.[58] In 1978, another small study reported an improvement in eleven patients treated with HBO.[59] One year later, a large study found minimal to dramatic improvement in ninety-one percent of 250 patients treated with HBO.[60] Several other researchers published similarly encouraging results.

The first double-blind, placebo-controlled trial of HBO indicated an apparent beneficial effect in the treatment of MS.[61] Objective improvement was noted in twelve of seventeen in the study group, compared to only one of twenty in the placebo group. Although the improvements were mild and transient in most of the patients, it appeared that patients with milder forms of MS and a shorter duration of disease derived a more pronounced and longer-lasting benefit. This was an encouraging preliminary study, yet it was criticized for its small sample and short follow-up period.

Subsequently, the Multiple Sclerosis Society commissioned further trials to be performed on a larger number of subjects, with longer periods of follow-up.[62,63] The results showed no significant improvement, apart from a subjective improvement in bowel and bladder functions in one of the studies. The results from these larger well-designed studies cast substantial doubt on the efficacy of HBO treatment of MS.

Recently, a study was published that evaluated the results of fourteen controlled trials of hyperbaric oxygen treatment. Of the eight trials considered of reasonably high quality, only one showed favorable results. The patients in the trials had chronic progressive or chronic stable multiple sclerosis. In most of the trials, hyperbaric oxygen was supplied at pressures of 1.75 to 2 ATA (a unit of atmostpheric pressure) during twenty sessions of ninety minutes each over a period of four weeks. Side effects were generally minor, but included ear and visual problems.[64] In conclusion, we do not feel that HBO therapy is very helpful.

Oral Antigen Therapy

Perhaps the most exciting new therapy for MS is oral antigen therapy. Because of the striking similarity between the clinical and histopathological features of MS and experimental autoimmune encephalomyelitis (EAE), researchers began studying oral administration of myelin basic protein (MBP) in humans. Oral administration of MBP has been shown to exert a profoundly suppressive effect on EAE induced in the rats.[65] This MBP-induced oral tolerance is characterized by an inhibition of EAE clinical neurological signs, reduced demyelination, and a significant decrease in the level of antibodies for MBP.

Preliminary results in humans look equally impressive.[66] However, at this time oral antigen therapy of MS is still in the investigative phase. Hopefully, these preliminary results will be confirmed in subsequent studies.

Physical Therapy and Exercise

We encourage MS patients to try to lead as normal and active a life as possible. Exercise is physically and psychologically beneficial. However, avoid overwork and fatigue. Exercise has been shown to significantly improve fitness and to have a positive impact on quality-of-life factors of multiple sclerosis patients. In an interesting study,[67] MS patients were assigned to either an exercise group or a nonexercise group for fifteen weeks. Aerobic training consisted of three forty-minute sessions per week on a stationary bike that also had arm handles as well. The exercise group improved in all measures of physical function, social interaction, emotional behavior, home management, total sickness impact profile score, and recreation.

For spastic or severely weakened limbs, we recommend assisted movement and massage, both for comfort and circulation.

TREATMENT SUMMARY

Treatment of MS with diet, lifestyle modification, and supplementation should begin as soon as possible, as the earlier in the disease process this therapy is initiated the better the results will be. Several nonspecific measures are important, including avoidance of excessive fatigue, emotional stress, and marked temperature changes.

While not proven highly effective, the natural therapy for MS will help, and it poses no threat to a patient's health. In fact, it is quite healthful since the recommendations decrease the risk of atherosclerosis and other degenerative diseases. However, once MS has progressed to significant disability, it is unlikely to be affected to any great degree by these measures.

Diet

Swank's dietary protocol is recommended:

- Saturated fat intake should be no more than 10 grams per day
- Daily intake of polyunsaturated oils should be 40–50 grams (margarine, shortening, and hydrogenated oils are not allowed)
- Normal amounts of protein are recommended
- Fish should be eaten three or more times a week

Fresh whole foods should be emphasized and consumption of animal foods (with the exception of cold-water fish) should be reduced, if not completely eliminated.

Nutritional Supplements

- High-potency multiple-vitamin-and-mineral formula
- Vitamin E: 800 IU per day
- Selenium: 200–400 mcg per day (including the amount in the multiple)
- Vitamin B12 (methylcobalamin): 2 mg per day in the case of vitamin B12 deficiency; dosages up to 60 mg daily when using it as a therapy
- Flaxseed oil: 1 tbsp per day
- Pancreatin (10X): 350–700 mg three times per day between meals (on an empty stomach)

Botanical Medicines

- *Ginkgo biloba* extract (24% ginkgo flavonglycosides): 40–80 mg three times per day

Nausea and Vomiting of Pregnancy

. . . .

Morning or evening nausea and vomiting, occurring during the first trimester of pregnancy

Many physical and psychological reasons have been suggested to explain the high incidence of nausea and vomiting during pregnancy (morning sickness). It has been estimated that fifty percent of women complain of these symptoms at some time during pregnancy. Considering the many hormonal and metabolic changes that occur during pregnancy, the existence of these symptoms is not surprising. However, emotional factors also play a role in the perception and severity of the nausea and vomiting.

Therapeutic Considerations

The most popular treatment for nausea and vomiting during pregnancy is vitamin B6. This vitamin is extremely important in breaking down and eliminating the increased level of pregnancy-related hormones. In the medical literature prior to the 1990s, support for the use of vitamin B6 in treating the nausea and vomiting of pregnancy consisted primarily of several poorly designed studies in the 1940s.[1,2] In fact, in 1979 the American Medical Association Council on Drugs went so far as to say that "there was no solid evidence that vitamin B6 is effective against nausea." However, two very well-designed double-blind studies in the 1990s appear to provide the necessary support for this popular (and seemingly effective) recommendation to

pregnant women. In the first study, fifty-nine women were randomly assigned to receive either 25 mg of vitamin B6 every eight hours or a placebo. After seventy-two hours, only eight of thirty-one B6-treated patients had nausea, compared to fifteen of twenty-eight in the placebo group.[3]

In the more recent double-blind study, 342 pregnant women (less than seventeen weeks pregnant) were randomized to receive either 30 mg of vitamin B6 or a placebo.[4] Patients graded the severity of their nausea and recorded the number of vomiting episodes over the previous twenty-four hours before treatment, and again during five consecutive days of treatment. Compared to the placebo group, there was a statistically significant reduction in nausea scores and vomiting episodes. Based on the results of this study, vitamin B6 was recommended as a first-line treatment for nausea and vomiting of pregnancy. However, although a positive effect was reported in the trial, the results were not all that impressive. More than one-third of the patients still experienced vomiting and significant nausea with B6 supplementation. Perhaps a larger dosage would have been more effective. Or perhaps ginger (discussed later in this chapter) is a better recommendation, alone or in combination with vitamin B6.

Vitamins K and C

Vitamins K and C, when used together, have shown considerable clinical efficacy;

ninety-one percent of patients in one study showed complete remission within seventy-two hours.[5] The mechanism for this effect is unknown, and both vitamins administered alone showed little effect.

Ginger

Ginger (*Zingiber officinale*) has a long tradition of being very useful in alleviating symptoms of gastrointestinal distress, including the nausea and vomiting typical of pregnancy. Although the mechanism of action has yet to be elucidated, current thought is that this is due more to ginger's effects on the gastrointestinal tract than to any effects on the brain.[6]

Ginger's antivomiting action has been studied in the most severe form of pregnancy-related nausea and vomiting, known as *hyperemesis gravidum*. This condition usually requires hospitalization. In a double-blind trial, ginger root powder at a dose of 250 mg four times per day brought about a significant reduction in both the severity of the nausea and the number of attacks of vomiting in nineteen of twenty-seven women in early pregnancy (less than twenty weeks).[7] These clinical results, along with the safety of ginger, the relatively small dose of ginger required, and the problems associated with antivomiting drugs in pregnancy (e.g., severe birth defects) support the use of ginger to treat nausea and vomiting in pregnancy. This recommendation is becoming accepted even in orthodox obstetrical practices; ginger (as well as vitamin B6) is now often recommended as an effective treatment of early nausea and vomiting of pregnancy in many medical publications.

Psychological Aspects

There appears to be general agreement among experts that mild symptoms of nausea and vomiting during the first trimester have a strong physiological basis (linked to hormone changes during pregnancy) and are predictive of positive pregnancy adjustment and outcome. In other words, many experts consider mild symtoms of nausea and vomiting of pregnancy as a good sign of a healthy pregnancy. More serious or longer-lasting symptoms are thought more likely to have a psychological component.[8]

A study of eighty-six pregnant women showed a significant increase in both nausea and vomiting during the first trimester among women who reported more unplanned, undesired pregnancies and negative

. . . .

QUICK REVIEW

- Vitamin B6 is very important in breaking down and eliminating the inceased level of hormones during pregnancy.
- Vitamin B6 is very effective in most cases of nausea and vomiting of pregnancy.
- Ginger has a long tradition of being very useful in alleviating symptoms of gastrointestinal distress, including the nausea and vomiting typical of pregnancy.
- Clinical studies have shown ginger to be effective even in the most severe form of nausea and vomiting of pregnancy.
- Many experts consider mild symptoms of nausea and vomiting of pregnancy as a good sign of a healthy pregnancy.

relationships with their own mothers. Those whose problems continued into the third trimester were also significantly more negative in their assessments of their relationships with their mothers.[9]

We encourage pregnant women who have severe nausea and vomiting, or whose symptoms extend beyond the first trimester, to explore possible psychological factors. That is not to say that it is "all in the head," but rather to treat the whole person (body and mind).

Acupressure

Acupressure refers to applying pressure to acupuncture points. It may help relieve the nausea and vomiting of pregnancy. In one study, sixteen pregnant women with morning sickness were divided into two groups. Group 1 used acupressure wristbands for five days, followed by five days without therapy. Women in Group 2 had no therapy for five days, followed by five days' use of wristbands. The extent of nausea was assessed at baseline, day five, and day ten. Use of acupressure wristbands (elastic wristbands with hardened plastic balls applied to acupuncture sites on the wrist) relieved morning sickness for twelve of sixteen subjects. Acupressure therapy also resulted in statistically significant reductions in anxiety, depression, behavioral dysfunction, and nausea.[10] These acupuncture wristbands are available at most drug stores.

. . . .

TREATMENT SUMMARY

Diet

Eat dry toast immediately after rising, and small, frequent meals throughout the day.

Nutritional Supplements

- Vitamin B6: 25 mg two to three times per day
- Vitamin C: 250 mg two to three times per day
- Vitamin K: 5 mg per day

Botanical Medicines

There remain many questions concerning the best form of ginger and the proper dosage. Most research studies have utilized 1 gram of dry powdered ginger root—a relatively small dose. For example, ginger is commonly consumed in India at a daily dose of 8 to 10 grams. Furthermore, although most studies have used powdered ginger root, fresh (or possibly freeze-dried) ginger root or extracts concentrated for gingerol at an equivalent dosage may yield even better results.

In the treatment of nausea and vomiting of pregnancy, a dosage of 1 to 2 grams of dry powdered ginger, possibly taken as a tea, may be effective. For ginger extracts standardized to contain 20% gingerol and shogaol, an equivalent dosage would be 100–200 mg.

Counseling

Women who are having an unplanned or undesired pregnancy, or who have a poor relationship with their own mother, should consult a qualified counselor for assistance in resolving these conflicts.

Obesity

Obesity is defined as a state of being more than twenty percent above "normal" weight, or having a body-fat percentage greater than thirty percent for women and twenty-five percent for men

According to the results of The National Health and Nutrition Examination Survey III, one in three adults in the United States is now obese (defined as being more than twenty percent above the ideal weight for height).[1] Even more alarming is the number of obese children; the number doubled between 1960 and 1991, roughly one out of every five children in the United States is overweight.[2] This situation is serious, as the odds are four to one against children ever achieving normal weight as adults if they enter their teenage years obese; the odds are twenty-eight to one if they end their teenage years obese.

Why are so many Americans overweight? Of course there are many factors to consider, but the bottom line is that most Americans have a diet that is high in fat and sugar, and they get little, if any, exercise. If the cause of obesity is dietary and lifestyle practices, then the solution is to make major changes in these areas. In regard to the growing number of obese kids, increases in television viewing and decreased physical activity are the major factors.[2]

Obesity Defined

The simplest definition of *obesity* is an excessive amount of body fat. It must be distinguished from overweight, which refers to an excess of body weight relative to height. A muscular athlete may be overweight, yet have a very low body-fat percentage. With this in mind, it is obvious that using body weight alone as an index of obesity is not entirely accurate. Nevertheless, obesity is classically identified as weighing more than twenty percent over the average desirable weight for men and women of a given height (see the Metropolitan Life Tables in A HEALTH-PROMOTING DIET).

A more accurate measure of whether a person is obese is based on their percentage of body fat. There are several techniques for accomplishing this analysis. The most convenient way for people to measure their body-fat percentage is to weigh themselves on scales that use bioelectrical impedence. The scales look like regular digital bathroom scales. These scales cost $150 to $200. They are expensive, but they do provide valuable information. Physicians often use calculations based on skin-fold thickness to determine body fat percentage, but more and more physicians are opting for the body-fat scales.

In terms of body-fat percentage, obesity is defined as a body-fat percentage greater than thirty percent for women and twenty-five percent for men.[1]

Types of Obesity

Obesity is divided into several categories based on the size and number of fat cells as well as on how the fat is distributed in the body (e.g., in the abdomen versus the hips).

In *hyperplastic obesity* there is an increased number of fat cells throughout the body (*hyper-* means increased, *-plastic* refers to cells). The number of fat cells a person has depends primarily on the diet of the mother while the person was still in the womb, as well as on early infant nutrition. An excess of calories during these early stages of development can lead to the formation of an increased number of fat cells for the rest of the baby's life. Because it is harder to develop new fat cells in adulthood, hyperplastic obesity usually begins in childhood. Fortunately, hyperplastic obesity tends to be associated with fewer serious health effects compared to other types of obesity.

Hypertrophic obesity is characterized by an increase in the size of each individual fat cell and is linked to diabetes, heart disease, high blood pressure, and other serious disturbances of metabolism.[3] In *hyperplastic-hypertrophic obesity* there is both an increase in the number and size of fat cells.

In cases of hypertrophic obesity, the fat distribution is usually around the waist. This distribution is referred to as *male-patterned* or *android,* since it is typically seen in the obese male. If the waist is bigger around than the hips (apple-shaped), a person is said to have *android obesity.* If the hips are larger (pear-shaped), then a person has *female-patterned* or *gynecoid obesity.*

Causes of Obesity

There are basically two areas of focus in trying to understand what causes obesity: psychological factors and physiological factors.

Psychological Factors

Many years ago, it was thought that psychological factors were largely responsible for obesity. A popular theory was that overweight individuals were insensitive to internal signals for hunger and satiety, while being extremely sensitive to external stimuli (sight, smell, and taste) that can increase the appetite. One source of external stimuli that has been shown to be associated with obesity is television watching.

Television watching has been demonstrated to be linked to the onset of obesity, and there is a dose-related effect (i.e., the more TV one watches, the greater the degree of obesity). In addition to leading to childhood obesity,[4] television viewing contributes to excess weight in adults. One study of 4,771 adult women examined the relationship between time spent watching television per week and obesity. The researchers found that twice as many women who reported watching three or more hours of TV per day were obese, compared to the reference group of women who watched less than one hour of television per day.[5]

Although television watching fits nicely with the psychological theory (increased sensitivity to external cues), there are also several physiological effects of watching TV that promote obesity. These include reduced physical activity and the actual lowering of resting (basal) metabolic rate to a level similar to that experienced during trance-like states. In addition to television lowering basal metabolic rate, exercise levels tend to be lower in people who watch a lot of TV. These factors clearly support the physiological view.

Physiological Factors

While the psychological theories primarily propose that obese individuals have a decreased sensitivity to internal cues of hunger and satisfaction, an emerging theory of obesity states almost the opposite: obese individuals appear to be extremely sensitive to specific internal clues.[6] The physiological theories of obesity are tied to brain serotonin levels, diet-induced thermogenesis, the activity of the sympathetic nervous system, the metabolism of the fat cells, and sensitivity to the hormone insulin. All of these models (discussed in the following sections) support the notion that obesity is not just a matter of overeating. They explain why some people can eat large quantities of food and not increase their weight substantially, while for others just the reverse is true.

The Low-Serotonin Theory

A considerable body of scientific evidence demonstrates that brain serotonin levels have a major influence on eating behavior. Much of the initial research was conducted at the Massachusetts Institute of Technology by Judith Wurtman, Ph.D., and her husband, Richard Wurtman, Ph.D. These pioneers in brain chemistry have made many valuable contributions that further our understanding of how amino acids (including melatonin) affect mood and behavior.

What the Wurtmans and other researchers have shown is that, when animals and humans are fed diets that are specially prepared to be deficient in tryptophan, appetite is significantly increased, resulting in binge eating of carbohydrates.[7,8] The diet low in tryptophan leads to low brain serotonin levels; as a result the brain senses that it is starving, so it stimulates the appetite control centers in a powerful way. This stimulation results in a preference for carbohydrates. Researchers discovered that when animals or humans are fed a carbohydrate meal it leads to more tryptophan being delivered to the brain, resulting in the manufacture of more serotonin. This scenario has led to the idea that low

QUICK REVIEW

- A successful program for weight loss must be consistent with the four cornerstones of good health: proper diet, adequate exercise, a positive mental attitude, and the right support for the body through natural measures.

- Most Americans are overweight because they eat too much fat and sugar, and are not physically active enough.

- Television watching has been linked to the onset of obesity, and there is a dose-related effect (i.e., the more TV that is watched, the greater the degree of obesity).

- The physiological theories of obesity are tied to brain serotonin levels, diet-induced thermogenesis, the activity of the sympathetic nervous system, the metabolism of the fat cells, and sensitivity to the hormone insulin.

- 5-hydroxytryptophan reduces the number of calories consumed and promotes weight loss.

- When properly combined, plant stimulants such as ephedrine and caffeine can activate the sympathetic nervous serotonin levels produce "carbohydrate craving" and play a major role in the development of obesity.

Furthermore, it has been demonstrated that concentrations of tryptophan in the bloodstream, and subsequent brain serotonin levels, plummet when a person is dieting.[9] In response to severe drops in serotonin levels, the brain simply puts out such a strong message to eat that no one can ignore it. This explains why most diets do not work.

Cravings for carbohydrate (as well as fat) due to low serotonin levels can be very mild or quite severe. They may range in severity from the desire to nibble on piece of bread to uncontrollable bingeing. At the upper end of the spectrum of carbohydrate addiction is *bulimia,* a potentially serious eating disorder characterized by binge eating followed by purging of the food through forced vomiting or the use of laxatives. The medical consequences of bulimia can be quite severe: rupture of the stomach, erosion of the dental enamel, or heart disturbances due to loss of potassium.

The Set-Point Theory

The *set point* is the weight that a body tries to maintain by regulating the amount of food and calories consumed. Research with animals and humans has indicated that each person has a programmed "set point" weight.[6] It has been postulated that individual fat cells control this set point; when the fat cell becomes smaller, it sends a powerful message to the brain to eat. Since the obese individual often has both more and larger fat cells, the result can be an overpowering urge to eat.

The existence of this set point may also explain why most diets don't work. While the obese individual can fight off the impulse to eat for a time, eventually the signal becomes too strong to ignore. The result is rebound overeating, with individuals often exceeding their previous weight. In addition, their set point is now set at a higher level, making it

· ·

system, thereby increasing the metabolic rate and diet-induced thermogenesis.

- Fiber supplements have been shown to enhance blood sugar control and insulin effects, as well as actually reducing the number of calories absorbed by the body.

- One of the key goals in enhancing weight loss is to increase the sensitivity of cells throughout the body to the hormone insulin.

- Chromium supplementation has been demonstrated to lower body weight yet increase lean body mass, presumably as a result of increased insulin sensitivity.

- Medium-chain triglycerides (MCTs) may promote weight loss by increasing thermogenesis.

- Hydroxycitrate has been shown to be a powerful inhibitor of fat formation in animals.

- Clinical studies have indicated that CoQ_{10} may help promote weight loss.

even more difficult to lose weight. This effect has been termed the "ratchet effect" and "yo-yo dieting."

The set point seems to be related to fat-cell insulin sensitivity. Obesity leads to insulin insensitivity and vice versa. *Insulin* is a hormone produced by the beta-cells of the pancreas; it increases the rate at which blood sugar (*glucose*) is taken up by cells throughout the body. When there is a lack of insulin, or if the cells of the body have become insensitive to insulin, it results in *diabetes*—a chronic disorder of carbohydrate, fat, and protein metabolism characterized by fasting elevations of blood sugar levels and a greatly increased risk of heart disease, stroke, kidney disease, and loss of nerve function. When cells become insensitive to insulin, not only is there impaired transport of blood sugar into the cells, but there is also impaired burning of fat stores for energy. Both obesity and diabetes are strongly linked to the Western diet, presumably due to the negative effects that saturated fats and refined carbohydrates have on internal mechanisms that control blood sugar levels (see DIABETES).

The key to overcoming the fat cell's set point appears to be increasing the sensitivity of the fat cells to insulin. This sensitivity apparently can be improved, and the set point lowered, by exercise, a specially designed diet, and several nutritional supplements which we will discuss below. The set-point theory suggests that a diet that does not improve insulin sensitivity will probably fail to produce long-term results.

Increasing the body's sensitivity to insulin results in less insulin being secreted. This effect is very important for several reasons. When the body's fat cells are pumped up with high levels of fat, insulin triggers the body to manufacture more fat cells. Once a fat cell is formed, it sends signals to the brain to make

the person eat so that it can be filled with fat, thereby producing a long-term stimulus to weight gain. When an overweight individual loses fat, the loss is from each individual fat cell. The fat cell will shrink, but never go away. While the body is able to add new fat cells, it is impossible to reduce the number of existing fat cells via natural means.

It should be clear that the set point of the fat cells not only predisposes an individual to be overweight, it also leads to an increased susceptibility to gain weight following weight loss. This physiology is largely responsible for the "ratchet effect" and "yo-yo dieting," but the loss of muscle mass (the prime burner of fat in the body) caused by dieting is also a factor.

Diet-Induced Thermogenesis

A certain amount of the food we consume is converted immediately to heat. This is known as diet-induced *thermogenesis* (heat production). Diet-induced thermogenesis is the method by which the body "wastes" calories. There is evidence that the level of diet-induced thermogenesis is what determines whether an individual is likely to be overweight. In lean individuals, a meal may stimulate up to a forty-percent increase in heat production. In contrast, overweight individuals often display only a ten-percent or less increase in heat production. The food energy is stored instead of being converted to heat.[10]

A major factor contributing to decreased thermogenesis in overweight people is, again, insulin insensitivity.[11] Therefore, enhancing insulin sensitivity may go a long way toward reestablishing "normal" thermogenesis and resetting the set point in overweight individuals.

Another of the other main reasons for decreased thermogenesis in overweight individuals is impaired sympathetic nervous system activity.[12] The sympathetic nervous system controls many body functions, including metabolism. In other words, the reason why many overweight individuals have a "slow metabolism" is because of a lack of stimulation by the sympathetic nervous system. Several natural plant stimulants will be described in this chapter which can activate the sympathetic nervous system, thereby increasing the metabolic rate and thermogenesis. This increase results in weight loss by addressing one of the underlying defects in the metabolism of overweight individuals.

Researchers have also shown that, even after weight loss has been achieved, individuals predisposed to obesity will still have decreased diet-induced thermogenesis compared to lean individuals.[13] It is therefore important to continue to support insulin sensitivity and proper metabolism indefinitely if weight loss is to be maintained.

In addition to insulin insensitivity and reduced sympathetic nervous system activity, there is another factor that determines diet-induced thermogenesis: the amount of brown fat an individual has. Most fat in the body is *white fat,* consisting of an energy reserve of fats *(triglycerides)* housed in one large droplet. Tissue composed of white fat will look white or pale yellow. *Brown fat* cells are special fat cells that contain multiple compartments instead of the one big compartment of white fat. The triglycerides in brown fat cells are localized in smaller droplets which surround numerous energy-producing compartments known as *mitochondria.* An extensive blood vessel network, along with the density of the mitochondria, gives the tissue its brown appearance and its impressive capacity to burn fat. The mitochondria are to the cell what the furnace is to a steam locomotive; instead of burning wood or coal for energy, the mitochondria burn fat.[14]

Brown fat does not produce energy very efficiently. In other tissues of the body, including white fat, the loss of chemical energy as heat is minimized. In contrast, brown fat wastes energy by burning higher amounts of fat and giving off more heat. Brown fat plays a major role in diet-induced thermogenesis.

Some theories suggest that lean people have a higher percentage of brown fat to white fat than overweight people. There is evidence to support this theory. The amount of brown fat in modern humans is extremely small (estimates are 0.5 to 5 percent of total body weight). However, because of its profound effect on diet-induced thermogenesis as little as 1 ounce of brown fat (0.1 percent of body weight) could make the difference between maintaining body weight and putting on an extra ten pounds per year.[14]

Lean individuals also tend to respond differently to excess caloric intake than overweight individuals. In one experiment, lean individuals were fattened up. In order for these subjects to maintain the excess weight, they had to increase their caloric intake by fifty percent over their previous intake.[15] The opposite appears to be the case for overweight and formerly overweight individuals. In addition to requiring fewer calories to maintain their weight, studies have shown that, in order to maintain a reduced weight, formerly obese persons must restrict their food intake to approximately twenty-five percent less than a lean person of similar weight and body size.[16]

People who are predisposed to obesity because of decreased diet-induced thermogenesis tend to be extremely sensitive to marked weight gain when consuming a high-fat diet compared to lean individuals.[17] These obesity-prone individuals are not only more sensitive to the weight-gain-promoting effects of a high-fat diet, but they tend to consume much more dietary fat compared to lean individuals and they tend to exercise less.

Therapeutic Considerations

Weight loss is one of the most challenging health goals to achieve. Few people want to be overweight, yet only five percent of markedly obese individuals are able to attain and maintain "normal" body weight, while sixty-six percent of people who are just a few pounds overweight are able to do the same.

The successful program for obesity is consistent with the four cornerstones of good health detailed in Part I: a positive mental attitude, a healthy lifestyle (especially important is regular exercise), a health-promoting diet, and supplementary measures. All of these components are interrelated, and no single component is more important than the other. Improvement in one facet (cornerstone) may be enough to result in some positive changes, but impacting all four components yields the greatest results.

There are literally hundreds of diets and diet programs that claim to be the answer to the problem of obesity. Dieters are constantly bombarded with new reports of a "wonder" diet to follow. However, the basic equation for losing weight never changes. In order for an individual to lose weight, energy intake must be less than energy expenditure. This goal can be achieved by decreasing caloric intake (dieting) or by increasing the rate at which calories are burned (exercising).

To lose 1 pound, a person must take in 3,500 fewer calories than he or she expends. To lose 1 pound each week, there must be a negative caloric balance of 500 calories per day. This can be achieved either by decreasing the amount of calories ingested or by exercise. To reduce one's caloric intake by 500 calories is often extremely difficult, as is burning off an additional 500 calories per day by exercise. A person would need to jog for forty-five minutes, play tennis for an hour, or take a brisk walk for one hour and fifteen minutes to burn off that 500 calories. The most sensible approach to weight loss is to simultaneously decrease caloric intake and increase energy expenditure through exercise.

Most individuals will begin to lose weight if they decrease their caloric intake below 1,500 calories per day and do aerobic exercise for fifteen to twenty minutes three to four times per week. Starvation and crash diets usually result in rapid weight loss (largely muscle and water), but cause rebound weight gain. The most successful approach to weight loss is gradual weight reduction (0.5 to 1 pound per week) through adopting long-term dietary and lifestyle modifications.

There are several natural weight loss aids that can help either reduce appetite or enhance metabolism. In order of effect, we would rate these items as follows:

5-Hydroxytryptophan
Thermogenic formulas
Fiber supplements
Chromium
Medium-chain triglycerides
Hydroxycitrate
Coenzyme Q_{10}

5-Hydroxytryptophan

As far back as 1975, researchers demonstrated that administering 5-hydroxytryptophan (5-HTP) to rats that were bred to overeat and be obese resulted in significant reduction in food intake.[4] It turns out that these rats have decreased activity of the enzyme that converts tryptophan to 5-HTP and subsequently to serotonin. In other words, these rats are fat as a result of a genetically determined low level of activity of the enzyme that starts the manufacture of serotonin from tryptophan. As a result, these rats never get the message to stop eating until they have consumed far greater amounts of food than normal rats.

There is much circumstantial evidence that many humans are genetically predisposed to obesity. This predisposition may involve the same mechanism as that observed in rats genetically predisposed to obesity. In other words, many people may be predisposed to being overweight because they have a decreased conversion of tryptophan to 5-HTP and, as a result, decreased serotonin levels. By providing preformed 5-HTP, this genetic defect is bypassed and more serotonin is manufactured. 5-HTP literally turns off hunger.

The early animal studies that used 5-HTP as a weight loss aid have been followed by a series of three human clinical studies of overweight women, conducted at the University of Rome.[18–20] The first study showed that 5-HTP was able to reduce caloric intake and promote weight loss despite the fact that the women made no conscious effort to lose weight.[18] The average amount of weight loss during the five-week period of 5-HTP supplementation was a little more than 3 pounds.

The second study sought to determine whether 5-HTP helped overweight individuals adhere to dietary recommendations.[19] The twelve-week study was divided into two six-week periods. For the first six weeks, there were no dietary recommendations; for the second six weeks the women were placed on a 1,200-calorie diet. As shown in Table 1, the women who took the placebo lost 2.28 pounds, while the women who took the 5-HTP lost 10.34 pounds.

As in the previous study, 5-HTP appeared to promote weight loss by promoting *satiety*—the feeling of satisfaction—leading to fewer calories being consumed at meals. Every woman who took the 5-HTP reported early satiety.

In the third study involving 5-HTP, for the first six weeks there were no dietary restrictions, and for the second six weeks the women were placed on a 1,200-calorie-per-day diet.[20] The results from this study were even more impressive than the previous studies for several reasons. The group that received the 5-HTP had lost an average of 4.39 pounds at six weeks and an average of 11.63 pounds at 12 weeks. In comparison, the placebo group had lost an average of only 0.62 pounds at six weeks and 1.87 pounds at twelve weeks. The lack of weight loss during the second six-week period in the placebo

TABLE 1 Impact of 5-HTP on Weight Loss		
	PLACEBO	5-HTP
Weight (pounds)		
Baseline	207.68	229.46
After 6 weeks	206.58	225.94
After 12 weeks	205.4	219.12
Total weight loss (pounds)		
After 6 weeks	1.1	3.52
After 12 weeks	2.28	10.34

group obviously reflects the fact that the women had difficulty adhering to the diet.

Early satiety was reported by 100 percent of the subjects during the first six-week period. During the second six-week period, even with severe caloric restriction, ninety percent of the women taking 5-HTP reported early satiety. Many of the women who received the 5-HTP (300 mg three times per day) reported mild nausea during the first six weeks of therapy. However, the symptom was never severe enough for any of the women to drop out of the study. No other side effects were reported.

Thermogenic Formulas

When properly combined, plant stimulants such as ephedrine and caffeine can activate the sympathetic nervous system, thereby increasing the metabolic rate and diet-induced thermogenesis. This results in weight loss by addressing the underlying defect in metabolism.

Ephedrine and caffeine combinations are not for everyone, but they do appear to be quite useful in weight-loss programs. However, they should be used in a rational manner and not abused.

Although ephedrine has demonstrated an appetite-suppressing effect, its main mechanism for promoting weight loss appears to be increasing the metabolic rate of adipose tissue.[21,22]

The thermogenic effects of ephedrine can be enhanced by taking *methylxanthines* (caffeine and related compounds). Herbs rich in these active ingredients can be used in a similar fashion to the isolated principles. Good methylxanthine sources include coffee (*Coffea arabica*), tea (*Camellia sinensis*), cola nut (*Cola nitida*), and guarana (*Paullinea cupana*). The optimum dosage of the crude plant preparation or extract depends on the content of active ingredient. Standardized preparations may produce more dependable results.

Although more recent studies have used a daily dosage of 60 mg of ephedrine and 600 mg of caffeine, these high dosages may not be necessary.[21-26] In one study, a daily dosage of 22 mg of ephedrine, 30 mg of caffeine, and 50 mg of theophylline was shown to greatly increase the basal metabolic rate and diet-induced thermogenesis.[27]

One of the key benefits of thermogenic formulas appears to be their ability to promote fat breakdown, and not loss of lean muscle mass. For example, in one study sixteen obese women on a weight-reducing diet were given either a combination of ephedrine (20 mg) and caffeine (200 mg) twice daily or a placebo. No significant differences in overall weight loss were demonstrated.[28] However, upon closer examination it was determined that the ephedrine-caffeine group lost 9.9 pounds more body fat and 6.16 pounds less lean body mass than the placebo group. These results indicate that ephedrine-and-caffeine combinations promote fat loss and preserve lean body mass during weight-reduction diets. As a bonus, subjects in the study who took the ephedrine-caffeine combination had higher energy levels and burned more calories than the placebo group.

A Close Look at the Side Effects

Thermogenic formulas containing ephedrine and caffeine combinations can produce increased blood pressure, increased heart rate, insomnia, and anxiety.

The FDA advisory review panel on nonprescription drugs recommended that ephedrine not be taken by patients who have heart disease, high blood pressure, thyroid disease, diabetes, or difficulty in urination due to enlargement of the prostate. In addition, ephedrine should not be used to treat patients who are taking antihypertensives or anti-depressants.

There is tremendous variation in the response to ephedrine and caffeine. Some people can tolerate high levels quite easily, while others are extremely sensitive to the central-nervous-system-stimulating effects.

It is interesting to examine the side effects reported in the studies that used a daily dosage of 60 mg of ephedrine and 600 mg of caffeine. Surprisingly, side effects were relatively mild. At week four, sixty percent of the subjects who took the ephedrine-caffeine combination typically reported side effects such as dizziness, headache, insomnia, heart palpitations, and headache. However, by week eight the rate of side effects was substantially reduced. In fact, as many people in the placebo group reported symptoms as in the ephedrine-caffeine group.

There were other interesting findings in these studies. Systolic and diastolic blood pressure decreased, indicating that the effect of weight loss more than compensated for any increase in blood pressure caused by the ephedrine and caffeine. Blood glucose, triglyceride, and cholesterol levels also decreased with weight loss and were not affected by ephedrine and caffeine.

Fiber Supplements

Increasing the amount of dietary fiber promotes weight loss. In addition to consuming a high-fiber diet, we recommend supplementing with additional fiber for weight loss. The best fiber sources for weight loss are psyllium, chitin, guar gum, glucomannan, gum karaya, and pectin because they are rich in water-soluble fibers. When taken with water before meals, these fiber sources bind to the water in the stomach to form a gelatinous mass that makes a person feel full. As a result, people will be less likely to overeat.

The benefits of fiber go well beyond this mechanical effect, however. Fiber supplements have been shown to enhance blood sugar control and insulin effects and to actually reduce the number of calories absorbed by the body.[29] In some of the clinical studies on weight loss, fiber supplements were shown to reduce the number of calories absorbed by 30 to 180 calories per day. This reduction in calories may not seem like much, but over the course of a year it would add up to three to eighteen pounds.

There are many water-soluble fiber supplements to choose from. Here are two important recommendations:

1. Avoid products that contain a lot of sugar or other sweeteners added to camouflage the taste
2. Be sure to drink adequate amounts of water when taking any fiber supplement, especially if it is in a pill form

The most impressive results in weight loss studies have been achieved using guar gum, a water-soluble fiber obtained from the Indian cluster bean (*Cyamopsis tetragonoloba*). In one study, nine women who weighed between 160 and 242 pounds were given 10 grams of guar gum immediately before lunch and dinner. They were told not to consciously alter their eating habits. After two months, the women reported an average weight loss of 9.4 pounds—over 1 pound per week. Reductions were also noted in cholesterol and triglyceride levels.[30]

Studies that used soluble fiber to treat elevated cholesterol levels have shown a dose-dependent effect—the higher the dosage, the greater the cholesterol-lowering effect.[29] Dietary fiber supplements appear to exert a dose-dependent effect in weight loss studies as well. Therefore, to achieve the greatest benefit, the dosage should be as high as possible.

TABLE 2   Clinical Studies of Dietary Fiber Supplements

FIBER REFERENCE	# OF SUBJECTS	LENGTH OF STUDY	DOSAGE	CALORIE RESTRICTION	AVG. LOSS W/FIBER	AVG. LOSS W/ PLACEBO
Guar[30]	9	2 months	20 g/day	None	9.4 lbs	No placebo group
Guar[31]	7	1 year	20 g/day	None	61.9 lbs	No placebo group
Guar[32]	21	2 1/2 months	20 g/day	None	15.6 lbs	No placebo group
Guar[33]	33	2.5 months	15 g/day	None	5.5 lbs	0.9 lbs
Glucomannan[34]	20	2 months	3 g/day	None	5.5 lbs	Weight gain of 1.5 lbs
Glucomannan[35]	20	2 months	3 g/day	None	8.14 lbs	0.44 lbs
Citrus Pectin[36]	14	4 weeks	5.56 g/day	Yes	12.8 lbs	No placebo group
Mixture A[37]	60	12 weeks	5 g/day	Yes	18.7 lbs	14.7 lbs
Mixture A[38]	89	11 weeks	10 g/day	Yes	13.9 lbs	9.2 lbs
Mixture B[39]	45	3 months	7 g/day	Yes	13.6 lbs	9 lbs
Mixture B[40]	97	3 months	7 g/day	Yes	10.8 lbs	7.3 lbs
Mixture B[41]	52	6 months	7 g/day	Yes	12.1 lbs	6.1 lbs

Mixture A = 80% fiber from grains, 20% fiber from citrus
Mixture B = 90% insoluble and 10% soluble fiber from beet, barley, and citrus fibers

A word of caution: start out with a small dosage and increase gradually. Water-soluble fibers are fermented by intestinal bacteria. As a result, a great deal of gas can be produced. If a person is not accustomed to a high-fiber diet, an increase in dietary fiber can lead to increased flatulence and abdominal discomfort. Start out with a dosage between 1 and 2 grams before meals and at bedtime, and gradually increase the dosage to 5 grams.

Chromium

One of the key goals for enhancing weight loss is to increase the sensitivity of cells throughout the body to the hormone insulin. Insulin plays a critical role in maintaining proper blood sugar levels and stimulating thermogenesis. Chromium plays a key role in increasing the body's sensitivity to insulin. Without chromium, insulin's action is blocked, blood sugar levels are elevated, and thermogenesis is inhibited.

Chromium has gained a great deal of attention lately as a weight-loss aid. The importance of this trace mineral in human nutrition was not discovered until 1957, when it was shown that it was essential to proper blood sugar control. Although there is no Recommended Dietary Allowance (RDA) for chromium, it appears that we need at least 200 mcg per day in our diet. Chromium levels can be depleted by consumption of refined sugars and white flour products, and by lack of exercise.[42]

In some clinical studies of diabetics, supplementing the diet with chromium has been shown to decrease fasting glucose levels, improve glucose tolerance, lower insulin levels, and decrease total cholesterol and triglyceride levels, while increasing HDL-cholesterol levels.[43] Obviously, chromium is a critical nutrient for treating diabetes, but it is also very important in treating hypoglycemia. In one study, eight female patients with hypoglycemia were given 200 mcg of chromium per day; at the end of three months, their hypoglycemia symptoms were alleviated.[44] In addition, glucose tolerance test results were improved and the number of insulin receptors on red blood cells were increased.

Since increasing insulin sensitivity is a critical goal in promoting weight loss, these studies imply that chromium supplementation would be quite beneficial in people trying to lose weight. In fact, chromium supplementation has been demonstrated to lower body weight yet increase lean body mass, presumably as a result of increased insulin sensitivity.[45] In one study, patients were given chromium bound to picolinic acid (chromium picolinate) in one of the following three doses daily for two and one-half months: 0 mcg (placebo), 200 mcg, or 400 mcg.[46] The patients who took chromium picolinate lost an average of 4.2 pounds of fat. The group that took the placebo lost only 0.4 pounds. Even more impressive was the fact that the chromium groups gained more muscle (1.4 vs. 0.2 pounds) than those taking the placebo. The results were most striking in elderly subjects and in men. The men who took chromium picolinate lost more than seven times as much body fat as those who took the placebo (7.7 vs. 1 pound). The 400-mcg dose was found to be more effective than the 200-mcg dose (by about twenty-five percent).

The results of these preliminary studies using chromium are very encouraging. Particularly interesting is the fact that, in these initial studies, chromium picolinate promoted an increase in lean body weight percentage by producing fat loss and muscle gain.[47] Greater muscle mass means greater fat-burning potential.

All of the effects of chromium appear to result from increased insulin sensitivity. There is evidence that marginal chromium deficiency is common in the United States. Chromium supplementation will often not only improve blood sugar control, but also lower cholesterol and triglyceride levels.[48]

There are several forms of chromium available on the market. Chromium picolinate, chromium polynicotinate, chromium chloride, and chromium-enriched yeast are each touted by their respective suppliers as providing the greatest benefit. Which is the best form? There really is no firm evidence to indicate that one is a significantly better choice than another.

There was one small study, however, of six women and six men who were given 400 mcg of either chromium picolinate or chromium polynicotinate. The test subjects were enrolled in an aerobics class for three months. Those who took the chromium picolinate increased their muscle mass three times as much as those who took chromium polynicotinate (women: 4 lbs vs. 1.3 lbs; men: 4.6 lbs vs. 1.5 lbs).[22]

Medium-Chain Triglycerides

Medium chain triglycerides (MCTs) are special types of saturated fats separated out from

TABLE 3	Effects of Chromium Picolinate on Weight Loss		
DOSAGE	FAT LOSS	MUSCLE GAIN	TOTAL WEIGHT LOSS
200 mcg	–3.3 lbs	+1.5 lbs	–1.8 lbs
400 mcg	–4.6 lbs	+1.1 lbs	–3.5 lbs

coconut oil that range in length from six to twelve carbon chains. MCTs are used by the body differently than the long-chain triglycerides (LCTs) that are the most abundant fats found in nature. LCTs are the storage fat for both humans and plants; they range in length from eighteen to twenty-four carbons. This difference in length makes all the difference in how MCTs and LCTs are utilized. Unlike regular fats, MCTs do not appear to cause weight gain; they actually promote weight loss.

MCTs may promote weight loss by increasing thermogenesis. In contrast, the LCTs are usually stored in the fat deposits and, since their energy is conserved, a high-fat diet actually decreases the metabolic rate. The reason for the difference in how the body handles MCTs and LCTs is due to their size. The larger LCTs are difficult for the body to metabolize, so the body tends to want to store these fats. MCTs, on the other hand, are rapidly burned as energy and actually promote the burning of LCTs.[49]

In one study, the thermogenic effect of a high-calorie diet containing forty-percent fat as MCTs was compared to that of one containing forty-percent fat as LCTs.[50] The thermogenic effect (calories wasted six hours after a meal) of the MCTs was almost twice as great as that of the LCTs: 120 calories vs. 66 calories. The researchers concluded that the excess energy provided by fats in the form of MCTs would not be efficiently stored as fat, but rather would be burned. A follow-up study demonstrated that MCT oil given over a six-day period can increase diet-induced thermogenesis by fifty percent.[50]

In another study, researchers compared single meals of 400 calories composed entirely of MCTs or LTCs.[51] The thermic effect of MCTs over six hours was three times greater than that of LCTs. In addition, while the LCTs elevated blood fat levels by sixty-eight percent, MCTs had no effect on the blood fat level. Researchers concluded that substituting MCTs for LCTs would produce weight loss as long as the calorie level remained the same.

In order to gain the benefit from MCTs, a diet must remain low in LCTs. MCTs can be used as an oil for salad dressing, as a bread spread, or simply taken as a supplement. A good dosage recommendation for MCTs is 1 to 2 tablespoons per day. Products containing MCTs are available in health food stores.

WARNING: Diabetics and individuals with liver disease should be monitored very closely when using MCTs, as they may develop ketoacidosis.

Hydroxycitrate

Hydroxycitrate is a natural substance isolated from the fruit of the Malabar tamarind (*Garcinia cambogia*). It is a powerful lipogenic inhibitor (*lipo* means fat, *-genic* means production; *lipogenic* means fat production). Therefore, a *lipogenic inhibitor* is a substance which helps prevent the production of fat.

The Malabar tamarind is a yellowish fruit that is about the size of an orange, with a thin skin and deep furrows similar to an acorn squash. It is native to southern India, where it is dried and used extensively in curries. The dried fruit contains about thirty percent hydroxycitric acid.

Hydroxycitrate has been shown to be a powerful inhibitor of fat formation in animals.[52,53] Whether it demonstrates this effect in humans has not been proven. The weight-loss-promoting effects in animals are perhaps best exemplified by a study that showed that hydroxycitrate produced a "significant reduction in food intake, and body weight gain" in rats.[54] Hydroxycitrate may be not only a powerful inhibitor of fat production, it may also suppress appetite.

It is critical when using a hydroxycitrate formula that a low-fat diet be maintained. Hydroxycitrate only inhibits the conversion of carbohydrates into fat. Therefore, it will have no effect if a high-fat diet is consumed.

On its own, hydroxycitrate may offer a safe, natural aid for weight loss when taken at a dosage of 500 mg three times per day. However, by combining it with chromium and a thermogenic formula an even greater effect may be noted, because in addition to inhibiting the production of fat, there is likely to be an increase in the burning of fat.

Coenzyme Q10

Coenzyme Q_{10} is an essential compound required in the proper transport and breakdown of fat into energy. Clinical studies have shown that CoQ_{10} may help promote weight loss. For example, in one study coenzyme Q_{10} levels were found to be low in fifty-two percent (fourteen of twenty-seven) of overweight subjects tested.[55] Nine subjects (five with low CoQ_{10} levels, four with normal levels) were given 100 mg of CoQ_{10} per day, along with a low-calorie diet. After nine weeks, mean weight loss in the CoQ_{10}-deficient group was 29.7 pounds, compared with 12.76 in those with initially normal levels of CoQ_{10}. This study suggests that about fifty percent of overweight individuals may be deficient in CoQ_{10}, and that treatment with 100 mg of CoQ_{10} may accelerate weight loss resulting from a low-calorie diet.

TREATMENT SUMMARY

A successful program for weight loss must be consistent with the four cornerstones of good health: proper diet, adequate exercise, a positive mental attitude, and the right support for the body through natural measures. All of these components are critical and interrelated. A successful program must incorporate these four measures, as improvement in one facet may be enough to result in some positive changes, but impacting all four will produce the greatest results.

Diet

Follow the recommendations given in the chapter A HEALTH-PROMOTING Diet.

Psychological Support

It is extremely important to follow the recommendations given in the chapter A POSITIVE MENTAL ATTITUDE. Overweight individuals tend to suffer a great deal of assaults on their self-esteem and self-image.

Lifestyle

Exercise is absolutely critical to an effective weight-loss program. Follow the recommendations given in the chapter A HEALTHY LIFESTYLE.

Nutritional Supplements

Follow the recommendations given in the chapter SUPPLEMENTARY MEASURES.

- 5-HTP: 50–100 mg 20 minutes before meals for the first two weeks; then double the dosage if weight loss is less than 1 pound per week (higher dosages of 5-HTP [e.g., 300 mg)] are associated with nausea, but this symptom disappears after six weeks of use)
- Chromium: 200–400 mcg per day
- Medium-chain triglycerides: 1–2 tbsp per day in the diet
- Hydroxycitrate: 500 mg three times per day
- Coenzyme Q10: 100–300 mg per day

Botanical Medicines

Combinations of an ephedrine source, such as *Ephedra sinica*, with a methylxanthine source, such as coffee *(Coffea arabica)*, tea *(Camellia sinensis)*, cola nut *(Cola nitida)*, and/or guarana *(Paullinea cupana)*, can be used at a dosage that provides 20–30 mg of ephedrine and 80–100 mg of methylxanthines per day.

Osteoarthritis

. . . .

Mild early-morning stiffness, stiffness following periods of rest, pain that worsens on joint use, and loss of joint function

Local tenderness, soft tissue swelling, joint crepitus, bony swelling, restricted mobility, Heberden's nodes, and other signs of degenerative loss of articular cartilage

X ray findings (narrowed joint spaces, cartilage erosion, bone spurs, etc.)

rthritis refers to inflammation of the joint. The most common form of arthritis is *osteoarthritis*, which is also known as *degenerative joint disease* because it is characterized by joint degeneration and loss of *cartilage*—the shock-absorbing gel-like material between joints.

The percentage of people who have osteoarthritis increases dramatically with age. Surveys have indicated that over forty million Americans have osteoarthritis, including eighty percent of those over the age of fifty. Under the age of forty-five, osteoarthritis is much more common in men; after age forty-five it is a little more common in women.[1]

The hands and the weight-bearing joints—the knees, hips, and spine—are the areas most often affected by the degenerative changes of osteoarthritis. These joints are under greater stress because of weight and use.

Osteoarthritis is divided into two categories: primary and secondary. In *primary osteoarthritis,* the degenerative "wear-and-tear" process occurs after the fifth and sixth decades of life, with no apparent predisposing abnormalities. The cumulative effects of decades of use leads to the degenerative changes by stressing the *collagen matrix,* the support structure of the cartilage. Damage to the cartilage results in the release of enzymes that destroy cartilage components. With aging, the ability to restore and synthesize normal cartilage structures decreases.[1-3]

Secondary osteoarthritis is associated with some predisposing factor that is responsible for the degenerative changes. Predisposing factors for secondary osteoarthritis include: inherited abnormalities in joint structure or function; trauma (fractures along joint surfaces, surgery, etc.); presence of abnormal cartilage; and previous inflammatory disease of joints (rheumatoid arthritis, gout, septic arthritis, etc.).

MULTIFACTORIAL CAUSES OF OSTEOARTHRITIS

Age-related changes in collagen-matrix repair mechanisms
Altered biochemistry
Fractures and mechanical damage
Genetic predisposition
Hormonal and sex factors
Hypermobility/joint instability
Inflammation
Inflammatory joint disease
Others

The onset of osteoarthritis can be subtle. Morning joint stiffness is often the first symptom. As the disease progresses, there is pain on motion of the involved joint that is made worse by prolonged activity and

695

relieved by rest. There are usually no signs of inflammation.[1]

The specific symptom picture varies with the joint involved. Disease of the hands leads to pain and limitation of use. Knee involvement produces pain, swelling, and instability. Osteoarthritis of the hip causes local pain and a limp. Spinal osteoarthritis (which is very common) may result in compression of nerves and blood vessels, causing pain and vascular insufficiency.[1]

One of the most interesting clinical features of osteoarthritis is the lack of correlation between severity of osteoarthritis (as determined by degenerative changes apparent on X ray) and the degree of pain. In some cases the joint will appear normal, with little if any joint-space narrowing, yet the pain can be excruciating. On the other hand, there are cases in which there is tremendous deformity, yet very little if any pain. In fact, about forty percent of individuals with the worst X-ray classification for osteoarthritis are pain-free.[3] The exact cause of the pain in osteoarthritis is still not well-defined, but there are numerous potential causes. Depression and anxiety appear to increase the experience of the pain of osteoarthritis.

Therapeutic Considerations

If we examine data collected from the earliest lesions to the most advanced stages of clinical osteoarthritis, the process contributing to osteoarthritis appears to be able to be stopped and, in many cases, reversed.[2] The major therapeutic goal appears to be enhancing repair of the collagen matrix and regeneration by the connective-tissue cells.

Several studies have attempted to determine the "natural course" of osteoarthritis.[2,4] In other words, researchers have sought to determine what happens when people with

QUICK REVIEW

- Osteoarthritis can be halted and even reversed.
- Aspirin and similar drugs may actually contribute to osteoarthritis by inhibiting cartilage repair.
- Nightshade family vegetables, such as tomatoes, potatoes, and eggplants, may trigger osteoarthritis in some cases.
- Antioxidants protect against osteoarthritis.
- Glucosamine sulfate is the most thoroughly researched and most effective natural approach to osteoarthritis.
- Head-to-head studies using arthritis drugs have shown that glucosamine sulfate produces better results without side effects.
- Chondroitin sulfate and cartilage preparations are poorly absorbed.
- Physical therapy and exercise can help relieve osteoarthritis.
- Topically applied menthol or capsaicin preparations can help reduce the pain of osteoarthritis.

osteoarthritis are given no treatment. One group of researchers studied the natural course of osteoarthritis of the hip over a ten-year period. At the beginning of the study, all subjects had X-ray changes suggestive of advanced osteoarthritis, yet the researchers reported marked clinical improvement over time. X rays confirmed these improvements, including complete recovery in fourteen of thirty-one hips.[4] These results, as well as others, raise the serious concern that medical intervention may actually promote disease progression.

Some of the side effects of aspirin and nonsteroidal anti-inflammatory drugs (NSAIDs)—such as ibuprofen (Motrin, Nuprin, Advil), piroxicam (Feldene), diclofenac (Voltaren), fenoprofen (Nalfon), indomethacin (Indocin), naproxen (Naprosyn), tolmetin (Tolectin), and sulindac (Clinoril)—are well-known: gastrointestinal upset, ulcer formation, headaches, dizziness, etc. A less well-known side effect is further degeneration of the joint cartilage. Experimental studies have shown that aspirin and other NSAIDs inhibit cartilage synthesis and accelerate cartilage destruction.[5] Clinical studies have also shown that NSAID use is associated with acceleration of osteoarthritis and increased joint destruction.[6–9]

Simply stated, NSAIDs appear to suppress the symptoms but accelerate the progression of osteoarthritis.

Hormonal Considerations

There is a considerable amount of evidence that hormonal forces may initiate or accelerate the development of osteoarthritis. Specifically, the higher prevalence of osteoarthritis among women suggests that estrogens may play a role. Estradiol worsens experimental osteoarthritis, and tamoxifen (an anti-estrogen drug) relieves it by decreasing erosion of

the cartilage. This suggests a therapeutic role for estrogen blockade. Several botanicals (e.g., *Glycyrrhiza glabra* and *Medicago sativa*) commonly used in the treatment of osteoarthritis contain compounds with phytoestrogen activity capable of binding to estrogen receptors and acting as estrogen antagonists. However, although phytoestrogen-containing herbs may be of value in treating osteoarthritis, perhaps the best way to increase the intake of phytoestrogens is to increase the intake of food sources of phytoestrogens. Good food sources of phytoestrogens include soy, fennel, celery, parsley, nuts, whole grains, and apples.

Growth hormone is becoming an increasing popular "anti-aging" hormone. However, excessive levels of growth hormone can have detrimental effects on bone and joint structures.[10]

And, finally, patients with hypothyroidism have been shown to have an increased risk of osteoarthritis compared with age- and sex-matched population samples.[2] Clearly, correction of underlying endocrine imbalance or liver dysfunction is of critical importance in normalizing cartilage manufacture.

Dietary Considerations

Dietary therapy primarily involves the achievement of normal body weight, as excess weight causes increased stress on the weight-bearing joints affected by osteoarthritis.[11,12] A basic healthy diet, rich in complex carbohydrates and dietary fiber, is recommended. (For further discussion, see OBESITY.)

Nightshade Vegetables

Norman Childers, a horticulturist, popularized a diet that treated osteoarthritis by eliminating foods from the genus *Solanaceae* (nightshade family). He arrived at this method after finding that this simple dietary elimination cured his own osteoarthritis.[13] Childers developed a theory that genetically susceptible individuals might develop arthritis, and other complaints, from long-term, low-level consumption of the alkaloids found in tomatoes, potatoes, eggplant, peppers, and tobacco. Presumably, these alkaloids inhibit normal collagen repair in the joints or promote inflammatory degeneration of the joint. Although as yet unproven, this diet has been of benefit to some individuals and is certainly worth a try. We have seen several patients' osteoarthritis respond well to such a diet.

Antioxidant Nutrients

Results from a very large study (the Framingham Osteoarthritis Cohort Study) indicate that a high intake of antioxidant nutrients, especially vitamin C, may reduce the risk of cartilage loss and inhibit progression of the disease in people who have osteoarthritis.[14] A threefold decrease in the risk of osteoarthritis was found in the groups with higher-than-average vitamin C intake. These results highlight the importance of a diet rich in plant-based antioxidant nutrients, which protects against chronic degenerative diseases, including osteoarthritis.

Glucosamine Sulfate

Glucosamine is a simple molecule composed of glucose and an amine. The main physiological effect of glucosamine on joints is to stimulate the manufacture of glycosaminoglycans.[15,16] Glucosamine also promotes the incorporation of sulfur into cartilage. It appears that, as some people age, they lose the ability to manufacture sufficient levels of glucosamine. The result is that cartilage loses its gel-like nature and its ability to act as a shock absorber. The inability to manufacture glucosamine may be the major factor leading to osteoarthritis.

The clinical benefits of glucosamine sulfate in the treatment of osteoarthritis are impressive. In one of the more recent studies comparing glucosamine sulfate to a placebo, 252 patients with osteoarthritis of the knee were given either a placebo or 500 mg of glucosamine sulfate three times per day for four weeks.[17] Glucosamine sulfate was significantly more effective than the placebo in improving pain and movement after only four weeks of use. Previous studies have shown that the longer glucosamine sulfate is used, the more obvious the therapeutic benefit. The rate and severity of side effects from taking glucosamine did not differ from the placebo. These results are consistent with other double-blind studies that involved a placebo.[18–22]

Head-to-head double-blind studies have shown that glucosamine sulfate produces better long-term results than NSAIDs in relieving the pain and inflammation of osteoarthritis, despite the fact that glucosamine sulfate exhibits very little direct anti-inflammatory effect and no direct analgesic or pain-relieving effects.[23-25] While NSAIDs offer purely symptomatic relief and may actually promote the disease process, glucosamine sulfate appears to address the cause of osteoarthritis. By treating the root of the problem through the promotion of cartilage synthesis, glucosamine sulfate not only relieves the symptoms, including pain, it also helps the body repair damaged joints. The clinical effect is impressive, especially when glucosamine's safety and lack of side effects are considered.

In one of the earlier comparative studies, glucosamine sulfate (1,500 mg/day) was compared to the common anti-inflammatory drug ibuprofen (1,200 mg/day). While pain scores decreased faster in the first two weeks in the ibuprofen group, by week four the group receiving the glucosamine sulfate had improved more than the ibuprofen group.[23]

Physicians rated the overall response as good in forty-four percent of the glucosamine-sulfate-treated patients, as compared to only fifteen percent of the ibuprofen group.

Two more recent studies designed to further evaluate the comparative effectiveness of glucosamine sulfate versus nonsteroidal anti-inflammatory drugs (NSAIDs) provide even better evidence. The first study consisted of two hundred subjects with osteoarthritis of the knee, given either glucosamine sulfate (500 mg three times per day) or ibuprofen (400 mg three times per day) for four weeks.[24] Consistent with previous studies, the ibuprofen group experienced faster pain relief. However, by the end of the second week the group taking glucosamine sulfate experienced results as good as those of the ibuprofen group, with one major exception: while the side effects from taking glucosamine were mild and only affected six percent of the group, ibuprofen produced more significant side effects much more frequently, with thirty-five percent of the group experiencing side effects.

In the second study, 329 patients were given one of the following for ninety days: 1,500 mg of glucosamine sulfate; 20 mg of piroxicam; both compounds; or a placebo.[25]

The results of the study were strikingly in favor of glucosamine sulfate alone. The effectiveness was based on a clinical index known as the Lequesne Index. This index allots numerical values to all the major signs and symptoms of osteoarthritis.

These impressive results from treatment with glucosamine sulfate were achieved without side effects. In fact, patients who took glucosamine sulfate had fewer side effects than the placebo group and no dropouts. Here are the side-effect and dropout values among the four groups:

	PLACEBO	GS	PIROXICAM	GS + PIR
Incidence of side effects	24.4%	14.8%	40.9%	35.9%
Drop outs	3	0	20	3

In addition to showing benefits in double-blind studies, oral glucosamine sulfate was shown to offer significant benefit in an open trial involving 252 doctors and 1,506 patients in Portugal.[26] The patients received 500 mg of glucosamine sulfate three times per day over a mean period of fifty days. Symptoms of pain at rest, on standing, and with exercise and limited active and passive movements

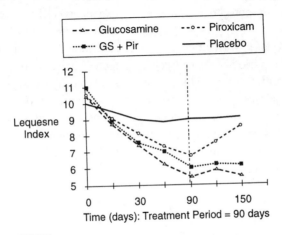

FIGURE 1

improved steadily throughout the treatment period. Objective therapeutic efficacy was rated by doctors as "good" in fifty-nine percent of patients, and "sufficient" in an additional thirty-six percent. Therefore, a total of ninety-five percent of patients achieved benefit from glucosamine sulfate. The results of using glucosamine sulfate were rated by both doctors and patients as being significantly better than those obtained with previous treatment, including NSAIDs, vitamin therapy, and cartilage extracts. Glucosamine sulfate produced good benefit in a significant portion of patients who had not responded to any other medical treatment.

In the study, obesity was associated with a significant shift from "good" to "fair." In other words, being obese reduced the effectiveness of glucosamine sulfate. This finding may indicate that higher dosages may be required for obese individuals or that oral glucosamine is not enough to counteract the stress of obesity on the joints. Patients with peptic ulcers and individuals taking diuretics were also associated with a shift from "good" to "sufficient" in both efficacy and tolerance. Individuals who have current peptic ulcers should try to take glucosamine sulfate with foods. Individuals who are taking diuretics may need to increase the dosage of glucosamine sulfate to compensate for the reduced effectiveness.

The improvement noted with glucosamine treatment lasted for a period of six to twelve weeks after the end of treatment. This result indicates that glucosamine may have to be taken for long periods of time or in repeated short-term courses. Given the safety and excellent tolerability of glucosamine, it is suitable for long-term use, even if continuous.

Chondroitin Sulfate

Chondroitin sulfate—as well as shark cartilage, bovine cartilage extracts, and sea cucumber—contains a mixture of intact or partially hydrolyzed GAGs (glycosaminoglycans), of molecular weights ranging from 14,000 to over 30,000. Chondroitin sulfate is composed of repeating units of derivatives of glucosamine sulfate with attached sugar molecules. Although all of these GAG preparations are popular, they are less effective than glucosamine sulfate. Better results are seen with glucosamine sulfate primarily due to better absorption.

While the absorption rate of glucosamine sulfate is ninety to ninety-eight percent, the absorption of intact chondroitin sulfate is estimated to be anywhere from zero to thirteen percent.[27–29] The difference in absorption is largely due to the difference in size. Chondroitin sulfate molecules are at least fifty to three hundred times larger than glucosamine sulfate molecules and are too large to pass through the normal intact intestinal barrier. If chondroitin sulfate molecules were absorbed intact or partially digested, they would still be unlikely to produce any significant benefit, as the chondroitin sulfate molecules are too large to be delivered to cartilage cells.

One of the key reasons why glucosamine sulfate is so effective is that its small molecular size allows it to penetrate the joint cartilage and be delivered to the chondrocyte (cartilage cell) and stimulate GAG synthesis. It would be nearly impossible for large chondroitin sulfate molecules to produce this effect. Furthermore, chondroitin sulfate levels are typically *elevated* in the joint fluid of patients with osteoarthritis.[30] These absorption problems suggest that any direct effect of these compounds in treating osteoarthritis is highly unlikely.

Any clinical benefit derived from taking chondroitin sulfate is probably due to the absorption of sulfur or smaller GAG molecules broken down by the digestive tract.[23] But even this theory is controversial, because in one human study 1 gram of chondroitin sulfate failed to increase serum GAG concentration at all, based on a highly sensitive measure of intact or depolymerized GAG absorption. These results prompted the researchers to conclude: "We suggest that chondroprotection by orally administered chondroitin sulfate is a biologically and pharmacologically unfounded theory."[28] In a further analysis, these experts on chondroitin sulfate further concluded: "Pooled literature on chondroitin sulfate biochemistry offers enough information to assert that neither intact, nor polymerized chondroitin sulfate is absorbed by the mammalian gastrointestinal tract. Therefore, any *direct* action of orally administered chondroitin sulfate on cartilage and chondrocytes is not possible."[31]

The few clinical studies that have been done using orally administered chondroitin sulfate demonstrate that it is less effective than glucosamine sulfate.[32-35] Far more impressive results have been achieved using glucosamine sulfate; glucosamine sulfate is faster-acting and provides much greater overall benefit.

Niacinamide

In the 1940s and 1950s, Dr. William Kaufman, and later Dr. Abram Hoffer, reported very good clinical results in the treatment of hundreds of patients with rheumatoid arthritis and osteoarthritis using high-dose niacinamide (900 to 4,000 mg per day in divided doses).[36,37] Dr. Kaufman documented improvements in joint function, range of motion, muscle strength, and endurance, and reduction in the sedimentation rate. Most patients achieved noticeable benefits within one to three months of use, with peak benefits noted between one and three years of continuous use.

These clinical results were recently evaluated in a well-designed double-blind, placebo-controlled trial.[38] Seventy-two patients with osteoarthritis were treated with niacinamide (3,000 mg daily in six divided doses) or a placebo for twelve weeks. Outcome measures included evaluation of pain, range of joint motion, and flexibility. The researchers found that niacinamide produced a twenty-nine-percent improvement in all symptoms and signs, compared to a ten-percent worsening in the placebo group. Pain levels did not change, but subjects who took niacinamide reduced their NSAID use. Niacinamide supplementation increased joint mobility by 4.5 degrees over controls (8 degrees vs. 3.5 degrees). Side effects, primarily mild gastrointestinal complaints, were more common in the niacinamide group, but those could be effectively managed by taking the pills with food or fluids. Niacinamide at this high dose can result in significant side effects (e.g., glucose intolerance and liver damage), and therefore requires strict supervision (blood measurement for liver enzymes every three months).

Methionine

A special form of methionine, S-adenosylmethionine (SAM), is an important physiological agent formed in the body by combining the essential amino acid methionine with adenosyl-triphosphate (ATP). A deficiency of SAM in the joint tissue, just like a deficiency of glucosamine, leads to loss of the gel-like nature and shock-absorbing qualities of cartilage. SAM appears to be useful in the treatment of osteoarthritis.

SAM has been shown to be very important in the manufacture of cartilage components.[39] In one double-blind study, supplemental SAM increased cartilage formation, as determined by magnetic resonance imaging (MRI), in fourteen patients with osteoarthritis of the hands.[40] In addition to this effect, SAM has also demonstrated some mild pain-relieving and anti-inflammatory effects in animal studies.

A total of 21,524 patients with osteoarthritis have been treated with SAM in published clinical trials. In double-blind trials, SAM (400 mg three times per day) has demonstrated reductions in pain scores and clinical symptoms similar to NSAIDs such as ibuprofen, indomethacin, naproxen, and piroxicam.[41–49] Unfortunately, as of this writing (November, 1997), SAM is not available commercially in the United States. It is available in Germany, Italy, and several other countries.

Superoxide Dismutase

Injecting the antioxidant enzyme *superoxide dismutase* (SOD) into the joints has demonstrated significant therapeutic effects in the treatment of osteoarthritis.[50,51] Whether oral SOD preparations are absorbed has yet to be determined. Preliminary indications are that they are probably not.[52]

Vitamin E

A clinical trial using 600 IU of vitamin E to treat patients with osteoarthritis demonstrated significant benefit.[53] The benefit was thought to be due to vitamin E's antioxidant and membrane-stabilizing actions. Vitamin E has an ability to inhibit the breakdown of cartilage and to stimulate the formation of new cartilage components.[54]

Vitamin C

Deficient intake of vitamin C is common among the elderly, resulting in altered cartilage synthesis and compromised cartilage repair.[54] Several studies have demonstrated that vitamin C, like vitamin E, protects and enhances cartilage formation.[55,56] Research has confirmed the importance, indeed necessity, of an excess of vitamin C in the cartilage cell.[57] One study of experimental osteoarthri-

tis in guinea pigs found that cartilage erosion was much less in animals kept on high doses of vitamin C.[54] Vitamins C and E appear to possess synergistic effects.[54] The researchers concluded:

Thus, both vitamins E and C appear to enhance the stability of sulfated proteoglycans in the complex structure comprising articular cartilage. Judicious use of these vitamins in the treatment of osteoarthritis, either alone or in combination with other therapeutic means, may thus be of great benefit to the patient population by retarding the erosion of cartilage.

Pantothenic Acid

Acute deficiency of pantothenic acid (vitamin B5) in rats causes a pronounced failure of cartilage growth and eventually produces lesions similar to those of osteoarthritis. In human studies, clinical relief from osteoarthritis symptoms has been reported with the administration of as little as 12.5 mg of pantothenic acid .[58,59] Results in studies often did not manifest until seven to fourteen days. However, a larger double-blind study of patients with primarily rheumatoid arthritis displayed no significant benefit from administration of 500 mg of pantothenic acid.[60]

Vitamins A and B6, Zinc, Copper, and Boron

Vitamins A and B6, zinc, copper, and boron (along with the other nutrients previously described) are required for the manufacture and maintenance of normal cartilage structures. A deficiency of any one of these would allow accelerated joint degeneration. In addition, supplementation at appropriate levels may promote cartilage repair and synthesis. For example, boron supplementation has been used in the treatment of osteoarthritis in Germany since the mid-1970s. This use was recently evaluated in a small double-blind clinical study and an open trial. In the double-blind study, of the patients who were given 6 mg of boron (as sodium tetraborate decahydrate), seventy-one percent improved, compared to only ten percent in the placebo group.[61] In the open trial, boron supplementation (6 to 9 mg per day) produced effective relief in ninety percent of arthritis patients, including patients with osteoarthritis, juvenile arthritis, and rheumatoid arthritis.[62] The preliminary indication is that boron supplements are of value in treating arthritis; many people with osteoarthritis experience complete resolution.

Physical Therapy

Various physical therapy treatments (exercise, heat, cold, diathermy, ultrasound, etc.) are often beneficial in improving joint mobility and reducing the pain of osteoarthritis, especially when administered regularly. Much of the benefit of physical therapy is thought to result from achieving proper hydration within the joint capsule. Clinical and experimental studies seem to indicate that *shortwave diathermy* (a method of administering deep heat) may be of the greatest benefit.[63-65] Combining shortwave diathermy therapy with periodic ice massage, rest, and appropriate exercises appears to be the most effective approach. Ultrasound and laser therapy have also been shown to be helpful.[66,67]

The best exercises are isometrics and swimming. These types of exercise increase circulation to the joint and strengthen surrounding muscles without placing excessive strain on joints. Increasing muscle strength around the joints affected with osteoarthritis has been shown to improve the clinical features and reduce pain.[68] Walking programs help improve functional status and relieve pain in patients with osteoarthritis of the knee.[69]

NONPHARMACOLOGICAL APPROACHES TO PAIN IN OSTEOARTHRITIS

Acupuncture
Exercise
Physical therapy
    Diathermy
    Laser therapy
    Massage
    Thermal baths
    Transcutaneous nerve stimulation
    Ultrasound
Psychological aids
Weight loss

Botanicals

Many herbs have historically been used in the treatment of osteoarthritis. When inflammation is present, the botanicals and nutritional factors that possess anti-inflammatory activity are recommended. Examples include bromelain, curcumin, and ginger. See RHEUMATOID ARTHRITIS for more information.

Yucca

A double-blind clinical trial found that a saponin extract of yucca demonstrated a positive therapeutic effect.[70] Results were of gradual onset, and no direct joint effects of the yucca saponin were noted. The researchers suggested that the clinical improvement was due to indirect effects on the gastrointestinal flora. This is an interesting suggestion, since bacterial endotoxins have been shown to depress the manufacture of cartilage.[71] It is entirely possible that yucca decreases bacterial endotoxin absorption and thus reduces this inhibition of cartilage synthesis. If this is the mechanism of action, then other saponin-containing herbs, and other ways of reducing endotoxin load such as a high-fiber diet, may be useful.

Devil's Claw
(Harpagophytum procumbens)

Several studies utilizing experimental animal models of inflammation have reported that devil's claw possesses anti-inflammatory and pain-relieving effects comparable to those of the potent drug phenylbutazone.[72] However, other studies have indicated that devil's claw has little, if any, anti-inflammatory activity in experimental inflammation.[73,74]

The conflicting research results may reflect a mechanism of action that is inconsistent with current anti-inflammatory models or a lack of quality control (standardization) of the preparations used. Since the main components of devil's claw are saponins, its therapeutic effect on osteoarthritis may be similar to that observed for yucca.

Boswellia serrata

Another herb historically used in the treatment of osteoarthritis is *Boswellia serrata*, a large branching tree native to India. Boswellia yields an exudative gum resin known as salai guggul. Although salai guggul has been used for centuries, newer preparations concentrated for the active components (boswellic acids) are giving better results.

Boswellic acid extracts have demonstrated anti-arthritic effects in a variety of animal models. There are several mechanisms of action, including inhibition of inflammatory mediators, prevention of decreased cartilage synthesis, and improved blood supply to joint tissues.[75,76] Clinical studies using herbal formulas with Boswellia have yielded good results in osteoarthritis as well as rheumatoid arthritis.[77] The standard dosage for boswellic acids in treating arthritis is 400 mg three times per day. No side effects due to taking boswellic acids have been reported.

Topical Treatment

Topical application of menthol-based preparations (e.g., Tiger Balm, White Flower Essence, Ben-Gay, Mineral Ice, etc.) may prove helpful. An alternative to these preparations is products that contain capsaicin—the pungent and irritating compound from cayenne pepper (*Capsicum frutescens*). When applied to the skin, capsaicin is known to stimulate and then block small-diameter nerve fibers that transmit the chemical message of pain by depleting them of the neurotransmitter named *substance P*. Substance P is thought to be the principal chemical responsible for the transmission of pain impulses. In addition, substance P has been shown to activate inflammatory mediators in joint tissues in cases of osteoarthritis and rheumatoid arthritis. Topically applied capsaicin may be effective in relieving the pain of osteoarthritis.[78]

. . . .

TREATMENT SUMMARY

Although glucosamine sulfate has proven remarkably effective on its own, the comprehensive treatment recommended here is based on reducing joint stress and trauma, promoting cartilage repair mechanisms, and eliminating foods and other factors that may inhibit normal cartilage repair.

Non-steroidal anti-inflammatory drugs, such as aspirin, should be avoided as much as possible. If NSAIDs must be used, deglycyrrhizinated licorice (DGL) should be used to help protect the gastrointestinal tract from their damaging effects, and their use should be discontinued as soon as possible. (For information on DGL, see ULCERS).

Diet

All simple, processed, and concentrated carbohydrates must be avoided. Complex-carbohydrate, high-fiber foods should be emphasized, and fats should be kept to a minimum. Plants of the nightshade family should be eliminated (tomatoes, potatoes, eggplant, peppers, and tobacco). Flavonoid-rich berries or extracts should be liberally consumed.

Nutritional Supplements

- Glucosamine sulfate: 1,500 mg per day
- Niacinamide (optional): 500 mg six times per day (under strict supervision; liver enzyme must be regularly checked)
- Vitamin E: 400–800 IU per day
- Vitamin A: 5,000 IU per day
- Vitamin C: 1,000–3,000 mg per day
- Vitamin B6: 50 mg per day
- Pantothenic acid: 12.5 mg per day
- Zinc: 30–45 mg per day
- Copper: 1–2 mg per day
- Boron: 6 mg per day

Botanical Medicines

- Alfalfa (*Medicago sativa*) (optional): equivalent to 5–10 g per day

- Yucca leaves (optional): 2–4 grams three times per day
- Devil's claw (*Harpagophytum procumbens*) (optional):
  Dried powdered root: 1–2 grams three times per day
  Tincture (1:5): 4–5 ml three times per day
  Dry solid extract (3:1): 400 mg three times per day

Topical Treatments

Menthol-based creams or creams containing 0.025 percent or 0.075 percent capsaicin can be applied to affected areas up to four times per day.

Physical Therapy and Exercise

Physical activity that overly strains the joint must be avoided. Chiropractic and other techniques that aid in the normalization of posture, as well as orthopedic correction of structural abnormalities, should be utilized to limit joint strain. Daily nontraumatic exercise (walking, isometrics, or swimming) is important but should be carefully monitored. Short-wave diathermy, hydrotherapy, and other physical therapy modalities that improve joint perfusion are recommended.

Osteoporosis

. . . .

Usually without symptoms until severe backache or hip fracture occurs

Most common in postmenopausal white women

Spontaneous fractures of the hip and vertebra

Decrease in height

Demineralization of spine and pelvis, as confirmed by X-ray techniques

O*steoporosis* literally means "porous bone." Osteoporosis affects more than twenty million people in the United States. Normally there is a decline in bone mass after the age of forty in both sexes (about two percent loss per year), but women are at a much greater risk for osteoporosis because of lower bone density prior to age forty. Many factors can result in excessive bone loss, and different variants of osteoporosis exist, but postmenopausal osteoporosis is the most common form of osteoporosis. Approximately one in four postmenopausal women has osteoporosis.[1] Osteoporosis is very uncommon in men and is most often due to some underlying factor such as long-term corticosteroid use, increased parathyroid hormone levels, or other disease state.

Although the entire skeleton may be involved in postmenopausal osteoporosis, bone loss is usually greatest in the spine, hips, and ribs. Since these bones bear a great deal of weight, they are then susceptible to pain, deformity, or fracture. At least 1.5 million fractures occur each year as a direct result of osteoporosis, including 250,000 hip fractures, the most catastrophic of fractures. Hip fracture leads to death (both directly and indirectly as a result of long-term hospital stays) in twelve to twenty percent of cases and precipitates long-term nursing home care for half of those who survive. Nearly one-third of all women and one-sixth of all men will fracture their hips in their lifetime.[2]

MAJOR RISK FACTORS FOR OSTEOPOROSIS IN WOMEN

Family history of osteoporosis
Gastric or small-bowel resection
Heavy alcohol use
Hyperparathyroidism
Hyperthyroidism
Inactivity
Leanness
Long-term glucocorticosteroid therapy
Long-term use of anticonvulsants
Low calcium intake
Nulliparity (never having been pregnant)
Postmenopause
Premature menopause
Short stature and small bones
Smoking
White or Asian race

Causes

Osteoporosis involves both the mineral (inorganic) and nonmineral (organic matrix, composed primarily of protein) components of bone. This is the first clue that there is more to osteoporosis than a lack of dietary calcium. In fact, lack of dietary calcium in the adult results in a separate condition known as *osteomalacia,* or "softening of the bone." The two conditions, osteomalacia and osteoporosis, are different in that in osteomalacia there is only a deficiency of calcium in the bone. In contrast, in osteoporosis there is a lack of both calcium and other minerals, as well as a decrease in the nonmineral framework (organic matrix) of the bone. Little attention has been given to the important role that this organic matrix plays in maintaining bone structure.

Calcium Metabolism and Hormonal Factors in Osteoporosis

Bone is dynamic living tissue that is constantly being broken down and rebuilt, even in adults. Normal bone metabolism is dependent on an intricate interplay of many nutritional and hormonal factors, with the liver and kidney having a regulatory effect as well. Although over two dozen nutrients are necessary for optimal bone health, it is generally thought that calcium and vitamin D are the most important factors. However, hormones are also critical, as the incorporation of calcium into the bone is dependent upon the hormone estrogen.

In order to understand current theories on how osteoporosis develops, it is necessary to briefly review normal calcium metabolism (absorption, storage, and excretion).

The Importance of Stomach Acid
The absorption of calcium is dependent on its becoming ionized in the intestines. The need to ionize the calcium has been the major problem in using calcium carbonate, the most widely utilized form of calcium for nutritional supplementation. In order for cal-cium carbonate to be absorbed, it must first be solubilized and ionized by stomach acid.

In studies of postmenopausal women, it has been shown that about forty percent are severely deficient in stomach acid.[3] Patients with insufficient stomach acid output have been found to absorb only about four percent of an oral dose of calcium carbonate, while a person with normal stomach acid can typically absorb about twenty-two percent.[3] Patients with low stomach acid secretion need a form of calcium that is already in a soluble and ionized state, such as calcium citrate, calcium lactate, or calcium gluconate. About forty-five percent of the calcium is absorbed from calcium citrate in patients with reduced stomach acid, compared to four percent absorption for calcium carbonate.[4]

This difference in absorption clearly demonstrates that ionized soluble calcium is much more beneficial than insoluble calcium salts like calcium carbonate in patients with reduced stomach acid secretion. It has also been demonstrated that calcium is more bioavailable from calcium citrate in normal subjects than from calcium carbonate.[5] In any event, calcium citrate and other soluble forms (lactate, aspartate, orotate, etc.) appear to be the best to supplement with at this time for optimal absorption (further discussed later in this chapter).

Vitamin D
It is well known that vitamin D stimulates the absorption of calcium. Since vitamin D can be produced in our bodies by the action of sunlight on 7-dehydrocholesterol (a compound the body can manufacture from cholesterol) in the skin, many experts consider it more of a hormone than a vitamin. Strictly defined a vitamin is an essential compound the human body cannot manufacture while a hormone is a compound that the human body manufactures that serves to control a particular function. In the case of vitamin D, it

serves in the role of controlling calcium absorption.

The active form of vitamin D is manufactured in the human. This process begins when sunlight changes the 7-dehydrocholesterol into vitamin D3 (cholecalciferol) in the skin. The vitamin D3 is then transported to the liver and converted by an enzyme into 25-hydroxycholcalciferol (25-OHD3), which is five times more potent than cholecalciferol (D3). The 25-hydroxycholecalciferol is then converted by an enzyme in the kidneys to 1,25-dihydroxycholecalciferol (1,25-$(OH)_2$D3), which is ten times more potent than cholecalciferol and the most potent form of vitamin D3 (see Table 1).

Disorders of the liver or kidneys result in impaired conversion of cholecalciferol to more potent vitamin D compounds. In many patients who have osteoporosis, there are

TABLE 1	Relative Activities of Vitamin D Forms
VITAMIN D FORM	**RELATIVE ACTIVITY LEVEL**
Vitamin D3	1
Vitamin D2	1
25-OH-D3	2 to 5
25-OH-D2	2 to 5
1,25-$(OH)_2$D3	10
1,25-$(OH)_2$D2	10

high levels of 25-OHD3, while the level of 1,25-$(OH)_2$D3 is quite low. This signifies an impairment of the conversion of 25-OHD3 to 1,25-$(OH)_2$D3 within the kidneys of people who have osteoporosis.[6,7] Many theories have been proposed to account for this decreased conversion, including connections to estrogen and magnesium deficiency. Recently, the trace mineral boron has been theorized to

QUICK REVIEW

- Osteoporosis involves both the mineral (inorganic) and nonmineral (organic matrix, composed primarily of protein) components of bone.

- Bone is dynamic living tissue that is constantly being broken down and rebuilt.

- Patients with low stomach acid secretion need a form of calcium that is already in a soluble and ionized state, such as calcium citrate, calcium lactate, or calcium gluconate.

- The concentration of calcium in the blood is strictly maintained within very narrow limits.

- Osteoporosis is best diagnosed by a procedure known as *bone densitometry*.

- The Osteomark-NTX can be used to monitor the rate of bone loss and the success (or failure) of therapy.

- The primary goals in the treatment and prevention of osteoporosis are to:
  - preserve adequate mineral mass
  - prevent loss of the protein matrix and other structural components of bone
  - assure optimal repair mechanisms to remodel damaged areas of bone

- Coffee, alcohol, and smoking cause a *negative calcium balance* (more calcium being lost than taken in) and are associated with an increase risk of developing osteoporosis.

- Although nutritional factors are

play a role in this conversion. All of these theories will be discussed in this chapter.

Hormonal Factors

The concentration of calcium in the blood is strictly maintained within very narrow limits. If levels start to decrease, there is an increase in the secretion of parathyroid hormone by the parathyroid glands (two paired glands located within the thyroid gland in the neck) and a decrease in the secretion of the hormone *calcitonin* by the thyroid and parathyroid glands. If calcium levels in the blood start to increase, there is a decrease in the secretion of parathyroid hormone and an increase in the secretion of calcitonin. An understanding of how these hormones increase (parathyroid hormone) and decrease (calcitonin) serum calcium levels is necessary to understanding osteoporosis.

Parathyroid hormone increases serum calcium levels, primarily by increasing the activity of the cells that break down the bone (*osteoclasts*), although it also decreases the excretion of calcium by the kidneys and increases the absorption of calcium in the intestines. In the kidneys, parathyroid hormone increases the conversion of 25-OHD3 to 1,25-$(OH)_2$D3.

One of the theories that relates bone loss to estrogen deficiency is as follows: an estrogen deficiency makes the osteoclasts more sensitive to parathyroid hormone, resulting in increased bone breakdown, thereby raising blood calcium levels. This elevation in blood calcium level leads to a decreased parathyroid hormone level, which results in diminished levels of active vitamin D and increased calcium excretion. This theory is the most solid explanation of the

important, the best thing a person can do to strengthen their bones is to get physical activity.

- Many general dietary factors have been suggested as a cause of osteoporosis, including: low calcium-high phosphorus intake, high-protein diet, high-acid-ash diet, high salt intake, and trace mineral deficiencies.

- It appears that increased soft-drink consumption is a major factor that contributes to osteoporosis.

- A deficiency of vitamin K leads to impaired mineralization of bone.

- Boron deficiency may contribute greatly to osteoporosis as well as to menopausal symptoms.

- Although calcium supplementation on its own does not completely halt

the process of osteoporosis, it does slow the rate by at least thirty to fifty percent and offers significant protection against hip fracture.

- Avoid natural oyster-shell calcium, dolomite, and bone meal products because of the possibility of high lead content.

- Calcium bound to citrate or other members of the Krebs cycle appears to be the best form for absorption.

- Magnesium supplementation may turn out to be as important as calcium supplementation in the prevention and treatment of osteoporosis.

- A semisynthetic isoflavonoid, similar in structure to soy isoflavonoids, has shown impressive results in a number of clinical studies of osteoporosis.

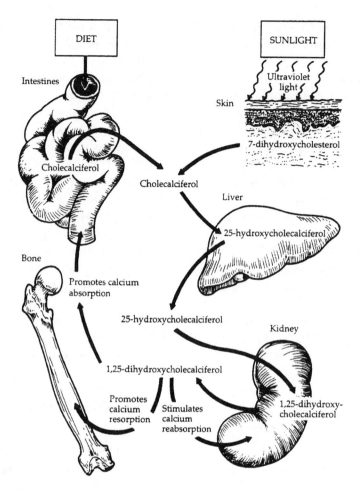

FIGURE 1 Vitamin D Metabolism

ultimate hormonal effects that lead to osteoporosis.

Diagnostic Considerations

Osteoporosis is best diagnosed by a procedure known as *bone densitometry*. There are several bone densitometry techniques, but the one with the greatest support and popularity is *dual energy X-ray absorptiometry* (DEXA).[8] DEXA is currently considered the "gold standard," but there are other promising methods that not only indicate bone density but also bone quality and structure, such as some of the computerized tomography (CT) scans. In addition to providing the most reliable measurement of bone density, the DEXA test also exposes a person to considerably less radiation than other X-ray procedures for measuring bone density. In the DEXA exam, the measurements will usually be of both the hip and the lumbar spine. We recommend that women of high risk get a baseline bone-density measurement and then monitor the rate of bone loss using a urine test known as the Osteomark-NTX.[9] In other words, the DEXA test can be used to measure bone density, while the Osteomark-NTX can be used to measure the rate of bone loss.

The Osteomark-NTX measures the urine levels of a compound linked to bone breakdown (cross-linked N-telopeptide of type I collagen). The Osteomark-NTX can be used to monitor the rate of bone loss and the success (or failure) of therapy. The Osteomark-NTX provides faster feedback than DEXA, which can take up to two years to detect a therapeutic response.[9]

Therapeutic Considerations

Recently there has been an incredible push for increasing dietary calcium intake to prevent osteoporosis. While this appears to be sound medical advice for many, osteoporosis represents much more than a lack of dietary calcium. It is a complex condition involving hormonal, lifestyle, and nutritional factors. A comprehensive plan that addresses these factors offers the greatest protection against developing osteoporosis.

The primary goals in the treatment and prevention of osteoporosis are to:

- Preserve adequate mineral mass
- Prevent loss of the protein matrix and other structural components of bone
- Assure optimal repair mechanisms to remodel damaged areas of bone

Hormone Replacement Therapy

One of the most publicized effects of hormone replacement therapy (a combination of estrogen and progesterone) in menopause is its role in maintaining bone health and preventing osteoporosis. In short, the benefits of hormonal therapy significantly outweigh their risks for women who are susceptible to osteoporosis and women who have already experienced significant bone loss. To determine your risk for osteoporosis and the appropriateness of hormone replacement therapy, please take the following self-test.

Before even taking the self-test, however, it is important to reduce the risk factors over which you have control: start an exercise program; quit smoking; do not drink alcohol, coffee, or soft drinks; take a good calcium supplement; and consume a diet low in protein and high in vegetables. These changes could take as many as 150 points off your total score.

After reducing all these risk factors, if your score is greater than 50, you are at significant risk for osteoporosis. Hormone replacement therapy may be suitable for you, especially if you experienced an early menopause, had your ovaries surgically removed, or never had children.

Since both estrogen and progesterone exert beneficial effects against bone loss and, in women with established bone loss, actually increase bone mass, estrogen-progesterone combinations are preferred to estrogen alone. The exception is for women at high risk for breast cancer or women with a disease aggravated by estrogen, including breast cancer, active liver diseases, and certain cardiovascular diseases, in which case progesterone alone should be used.

Lifestyle Factors

Certain lifestyle factors are extremely important to bone health. For example, coffee, alcohol, and smoking cause a *negative calcium balance* (more calcium being lost than taken in) and are associated with an increased risk

SELF-TEST: Determining Your Risk of Osteoporosis

Choose the item in each category that best describes you, and fill in the point value for that item in the space to the right. You may choose more than one item in categories marked with an asterisk.

	POINTS	SCORE
Frame Size		
Small-boned or petite	10	_____
Medium frame, very lean	5	_____
Medium frame, average or heavy build	0	_____
Large frame, very lean	5	_____
Large frame, heavy build	0	_____
Ethnic Background		
Caucasian	10	_____
Asian	10	_____
Other	0	_____
Activity Level		
How often do you walk briskly, jog, engage in aerobics/sports, or perform hard physical labor, of a duration of at least 30 continuous minutes?		
Seldom	30	_____
1–2 times per week	20	_____
3–4 times per week	5	_____
5 or more times per week	0	_____
Smoking		
Smoke 10 or more cigarettes a day	20	_____
Smoke fewer than 10 cigarettes a day	10	_____
Quit smoking	5	_____
Never smoked	0	_____
*Personal Health Factors**		
Family history of osteoporosis	20	_____
Long-term corticosteroid use	20	_____
Long-term anticonvulsant use	20	_____
Drink more than 3 glasses of alcohol each week	20	_____
Drink more than 1 cup of coffee per day	10	_____
Seldom get outside in the sunlight	10	_____
For women only:		
Had ovaries removed	10	_____
Premature menopause	10	_____
Had no children	10	_____

*If applicable, choose more than one item in this category

(continues)

	POINTS	SCORE
SELF-TEST: Determining Your Risk of Osteoporosis, *continued*		
*Dietary Factors**		
Consume more than 4 oz. of meat on a daily basis	20	_____
Drink soft drinks regularly	20	_____
Consume the equivalent of 3–5 servings of vegetables each day	–10	_____
Consume at least 1 cup of leafy vegetables each day	–10	_____
Take a calcium supplement	–10	_____
Consume a vegetarian diet	–10	_____
Total score		_____

*If applicable, choose more than one item in this category

of developing osteoporosis, while regular exercise reduces that risk.[10,11] In fact, as important as hormonal and dietary factors are, they are not the most critical factors for maintaining healthy bones; exercise is the most critical.

Numerous studies have clearly demonstrated that physical fitness is the major determinant of bone density. Physical exercise, consisting of one hour of moderate activity three times a week, has been shown to prevent bone loss and actually increase bone mass in postmenopausal women.[11–16] In contrast to exercise, immobilization doubles the rate of urinary and fecal calcium excretion, resulting in a significant negative calcium balance.[17] Although nutritional factors are important, the best thing people can do to strengthen their bones is to get physical activity.

General Dietary Factors

Many general dietary factors have been suggested as a cause of osteoporosis: low-calcium-high-phosphorus intake, high-protein diet, high-acid-ash diet, high salt intake, and trace-mineral deficiencies, to name a few.[18,19] A vegetarian diet is associated with a lower risk of having osteoporosis.[20,21] Although bone mass in vegetarians does not differ significantly from that of omnivores in the third, fourth, and fifth decades of life, there are significant differences in the later decades. These findings indicate that the decreased incidence of osteoporosis among vegetarians is not due to increased initial bone mass, but rather to decreased bone loss.

Several factors are probably responsible for this decrease in bone loss observed in vegetarians. Most important is probably a lowered intake of protein. A high-protein diet, or a diet high in phosphates, is associated with increasing the excretion of calcium in the urine. Raising daily protein intake from 47 to 142 grams doubles the excretion of calcium in the urine.[22] A diet this high in protein is common in the United States and may be a significant factor in the increased number of people suffering from osteoporosis in this country.[23]

Another dietary factor that increases the loss of calcium from the body is refined sugar. Following sugar intake, there is an increase in the urinary excretion of calcium.[24] Considering that the average American consumes 150 grams of sucrose in one day, along with other refined simple sugars, carbonated beverages loaded with phosphates, and large quantities of protein, it is little wonder that there are so many people suffering from osteoporosis in this country. When lifestyle factors are also taken into consideration, it is apparent why osteoporosis has become a major medical problem.

Soft Drinks and Osteoporosis

Soft drinks have long been suspected of leading to lower calcium levels and higher phosphate levels in the blood. When phosphate levels are high and calcium levels are low, calcium is pulled out of the bones. The phosphate content of soft drinks like Coca-Cola and Pepsi is very high, and they contain virtually no calcium. The high phosphate level is required for dissolving the sugar and contributing to the taste.

It appears that increased soft-drink consumption is a major factor that contributes to osteoporosis. The United States ranks first among countries in soft-drink consumption. The per-capita consumption of soft drinks is in excess of 150 quarts per year, or about 3 quarts per week.

The link between soft-drink consumption and bone loss is going to become even more significant as children who were practically weaned on soft drinks reach adulthood. Soft-drink consumption in children poses a significant risk factor for impaired calcification of growing bones. Since there is such a strong correlation between maximum bone-mineral density and the risk of osteoporosis, the rate of osteoporosis may reach even greater epidemic proportions.

The severe negative impact that soft drinks exert on bone formation in children was clearly demonstrated in a study that compared fifty-seven children with low blood calcium levels, aged eighteen months to fourteen years, to 171 matched controls (children with normal calcium levels).[25] The goal of the study was to assess whether the intake of at least 1.5 quarts per week of phosphate-containing soft drinks is a risk factor for the development of low blood calcium levels. Not surprisingly, a strong association was found. Of the fifty-seven children who had low blood calcium levels, thirty-eight (66.7 percent) drank more than four bottles (12 to 16 ounces per bottle) of soft drinks per week, but only forty-eight (28 percent) of the 171 children with normal serum calcium levels consumed as much soft drink. For all 228 children, a significant correlation between serum calcium level and the number of bottles of soft drink consumed each week was found. The more soft drinks consumed, the lower the calcium level.

These results more than support the contention that soft-drink consumption leads to lower calcium levels in children. This situation that ultimately leads to poor bone mineralization, which explains the greater risk of broken bones in children who consume soft drinks.[26]

Green Leafy Vegetables

Green leafy vegetables (kale, collard greens, parsley, lettuce, etc.) offer significant protection against osteoporosis. These foods are a rich source of a broad range of vitamins and minerals that are important to maintaining healthy bones, including calcium, vitamin K1, and boron.

Vitamin K1 is the form of vitamin K that is found in plants. A function of vitamin K1 that is often overlooked is its role in converting inactive osteocalcin to its active form. *Osteocalcin* is the major noncollagen protein in bone.

Osteocalcin's role is to anchor calcium molecules and hold them in place within the bone.[27]

A deficiency of vitamin K leads to impaired mineralization of bone due to inadequate osteocalcin levels. In one study, very low blood levels of vitamin K1 were found in patients who had fractures due to osteoporosis.[28] The severity of fracture strongly correlated with the level of circulating vitamin K: the lower the level of vitamin K, the greater the severity of the fracture. Other studies have shown that the lower the level of circulating vitamin K, the lower the bone density.[29] This evidence clearly indicates the importance of vitamin K. And, since vitamin K is found in green leafy vegetables, it may be one of the key protective factors against osteoporosis of a vegetarian diet.

The richest sources of vitamin K1 are dark green leafy vegetables: broccoli, lettuce, cabbage, spinach, and green tea. Other good sources are asparagus, oats, whole wheat, and fresh green peas.

In addition to vitamin K1, the high levels of many minerals in green leafy vegetables, such as calcium and boron, may also be responsible for this protective effect. Boron is a trace mineral that has gained recent attention as a protective factor against osteoporosis.[30] In one study, supplementing the diet of postmenopausal women with 3 mg of boron per day reduced urinary calcium excretion by forty-four percent and dramatically increased the levels of 17-beta-estradiol, the most biologically active estrogen. It appears that boron is required to activate certain hormones, including estrogen and vitamin D. It was mentioned previously that vitamin D is converted to its most active form (1,25-$(OH)_2D3$) within the kidney, and that this conversion was impaired in postmenopausal osteoporosis. Boron is apparently required

for this reaction to occur. A boron deficiency may contribute greatly to osteoporosis and to menopausal symptoms.

Because fruits and vegetables are the main dietary sources of boron, diets low in these foods may be deficient in boron. The standard American diet is severely deficient in these foods. According to several large surveys, including the U.S. Second National Health and Nutrition Examination, fewer than ten percent of Americans meet the minimum recommendation of two fruit servings and three vegetable servings per day, and only fifty-one percent eat one serving of vegetables per day.[31]

In order to guarantee adequate boron levels, supplementing the diet with a daily dose of 3 to 5 mg of boron is recommended. Boron has been shown to mimic some of the effects of estrogen therapy in postmenopausal women.[32]

Nutritional Supplementation to Maintain Bone Health

As stated several times previously, and again here to drive a point home, osteoporosis involves much more than calcium. Bone is dependent on a constant supply of many nutrients. A deficiency of any one of these nutrients will adversely affect bone health. In addition to vitamin K and boron, here is a brief discussion of key nutrients critical to maintaining bone health.

Calcium Supplementation of calcium has been shown to be effective in reducing bone loss in postmenopausal women.[33–39] Although calcium supplementation, on its own, does not completely halt the process, it does slow the rate by at least thirty to fifty percent, and it offers significant protection against hip fractures. Combined with exercise and the dietary recommendations given in this chapter, calcium is clearly part of an effective treatment for most women. While menopausal and postmenopausal women are often told that, without hormone replacement therapy, they will most definitely get osteoporosis, several studies provide strong evidence of the inaccuracy of this commonly held view.

In one study, 118 healthy white women who had experienced the onset of menopause three to six years previously were randomly allocated to receive either 1,700 mg of calcium as calcium carbonate; a placebo; or Premarin and 1,700 mg of calcium.[38] The nearly three-year-long study indicated that calcium supplementation alone prevented bone loss. Using a more absorbable form of calcium, such as calcium citrate or calcium bound to other Krebs-cycle intermediates, may have provided even greater benefit than calcium carbonate due to enhanced absorption. Although calcium alone was less effective than the Premarin-calcium combination, because calcium supplementation carries no significant health risks this study reinforces the opinion that hormone replacement therapy should be reserved for women who are at significant risk for osteoporosis because of the results that were produced with calcium alone.

In another study, eighty-six postmenopausal women received either 1 gram of elemental calcium (from an effervescent form that contains 5.24 grams of calcium-lactate-gluconate and 0.8 grams of calcium carbonate) or a placebo (of an identical effervescent tablet that contained no calcium) for four years.[39] Clinical status, calcium intake, physical activity, and bone mineral density was assessed at baseline and every six months. The results of the study indicated that continued calcium supplementation produces a sustained reduction in the rate of loss of total bone mineral density in healthy postmenopausal women. As a result, the incidence of bone fractures was far lower in the group taking calcium (two out of thirty-eight) compared to the placebo (nine out of forty).

And, finally, in another four-year study, the long-term effect of calcium supplementation on bone density was determined in eighty-four elderly women (fifty-four to seventy-four years of age) for more than ten years past the menopause.[35] A placebo group who did not take calcium supplements at all during the four-year study served as a comparison. Current calcium intake, physical activity, and changes in bone density at the lumbar spine, hip, and ankle sites were monitored. Over the four years, the calcium-supplement group (average calcium intake of nearly 2,000 mg/day) did not lose bone at the hip and ankle sites. The control group (average calcium intake of 950 mg/day) lost significantly more bone than the calcium-supplement group at the hip and ankle sites. No overall bone loss was seen at the spine in either group over the four years of this study. The bottom line was that calcium supplementation produced a sustained reduction in the rate of loss of bone density at the ankle and hip sites of elderly postmenopausal women.

In conclusion, these reviewed studies and others demonstrate that calcium supplementation produces beneficial effects on bone density and significantly reduces the risk of having hip fractures. However, it must be stressed again that calcium is just one piece of the puzzle for healthy bones.

Calcium Supplementation as a Preventive Measure There is a strong correlation between pre-menopausal bone density and the risk of developing osteoporosis. In other words, how dense the bones are prior to menopause is a significant factor in determining whether or not a woman develops osteoporosis. That being the case, building strong bones should be a lifelong goal beginning in childhood. However, the reality is that most women probably are not concerned about osteoporosis until a couple of years before menopause (the perimenopause). Can calcium supplementation improve bone density in perimenopausal women? Yes.

In a two-year study, 214 perimenopausal women received either 1,000 or 2,000 mg of calcium, provided in an effervescent mixture as described previously.[40] While the control group lost 3.2 percent of the bone density of their spine, the calcium-treated groups increased their spinal bone density by 1.6 percent (there was no difference between the two calcium groups). These results highlight the importance of calcium supplementation prior to menopause in the effort to avoid osteoporosis.

What Is the Best Form of Calcium? The best form of calcium is certainly neither oyster shell nor bone meal. Studies have indicated that these calcium supplements may contain substantial amounts of lead.[41] Lead is a toxic metal that primarily affects the brain, kidney, and manufacture of red blood cells. Lead toxicity is a significant problem in industrialized countries, including the United States. The level of lead in the body has been shown to be directly linked to IQ and criminal behavior (see ATTENTION DEFICIT DISORDER). The higher the lead level, the lower the IQ and the greater the risk of delinquent or criminal behavior. Lead is a major problem in children. In 1988, the U.S. Agency for Toxic Substances and Disease Registry estimated that more than three million children younger than twelve years of age (seventeen percent of all children in this age group) had unacceptably high blood lead levels.

In 1981, the FDA cautioned the public to limit their intake of calcium supplements derived from either dolomite or bone meal because of the potentially high lead levels in these calcium supplements. More recent studies have shown that other calcium sources, such as carbonate (from oyster shells) and various chelates, may also contain high amounts of lead.[41]

To determine the extent of the lead problem in calcium supplements, researchers measured the lead level in seventy brands of calcium supplements.[41] The results indicated that lead content is still a major concern in some forms of calcium supplements. The seventy brands were divided into five categories: refined calcium carbonate produced in a laboratory (seventeen brands); unrefined calcium carbonate derived from limestone or oyster shells (twenty-five brands); calcium bound to various organic chelates such as citrate, gluconate, lactate, etc. (thirteen brands); dolomite (nine brands); and bone meal (six brands). Here were the results (lead content in micrograms per 800 mg of calcium):

Refined calcium carbonate	0.92
Calcium chelate	1.64
Dolomite	4.17
Unrefined calcium carbonate	6.05
Bone meal	11.3

None of the products tested in the dolomite and bone-meal groups, and only two out of twenty-five in the unrefined calcium-carbonate group, had lead levels below the recommended level of 1 mcg per 800 mg of calcium. The group that displayed the greatest range of lead content was the unrefined calcium carbonate group (the source was oyster shells); while two products contained very little lead, most contained higher levels, and one product contained a whopping 25 mcg of lead per 800 mg of calcium.

As the total tolerable daily intake of lead for children aged six years and under is less than 6 mcg per day, young children should take refined calcium carbonate or chelated calcium products as calcium supplementation. Since chelated calcium, especially calcium citrate, is better absorbed than calcium carbonate, the best recommendation for calcium supplementation is to take products that feature calcium bound to citrate, gluconate, or some other organic molecule. This recommendation is appropriate for older children and adults as well.

In summary, it appears wise to avoid natural oyster-shell calcium, dolomite, and bone-meal products unless the manufacturer can provide reasonable assurance that lead levels are below acceptable levels (i.e., certificate of analysis for lead content). Refined calcium carbonate has the lowest lead content, but calcium chelates are better absorbed, especially by women with low gastric acid output.

We recommend calcium bound to citrate and other Krebs-cycle intermediates, such as fumarate, malate, succinate, and aspartate. The Krebs cycle is an important energy-producing process in cells that utilizes these intermediate compounds to produce chemical energy. Generally, over ninety-five percent of ingested Krebs-cycle intermediates are used to produce energy, with the remainder being excreted in the urine where they act to prevent kidney stone formation. The Krebs-cycle intermediates fulfill every requirement for an optimum calcium-chelating agent: they are easily ionized, they are almost completely degraded, they have virtually no toxicity, and they have been shown to increase the absorption of not only calcium, but other minerals as well.

On a final note regarding calcium, one popular calcium supplement is calcium hydroxyapatite—basically a purified bone meal. It is interesting to note that, among calcium supplements tested for absorption, this form tested at twenty percent absorption, compared to thirty percent for either calcium carbonate or calcium citrate.[42] Clearly calcium

hydroxyapatite is a poor choice as a calcium supplement, especially in light of the fact that it is derived from bone meal (a high lead source of calcium).

Vitamin D   In addition to studies that utilized calcium supplementation alone, there have been several studies that used calcium in combination with vitamin D (usually vitamin D3) as well as vitamin D alone. In one study that used vitamin D3 alone, it was shown that supplementation with 700 IU daily can reduce the annual rate of hip fracture from 1.3 percent to 0.5 percent—nearly a sixty-percent reduction.[43] In another study, 348 women, ages seventy and older, received either 400 IU of vitamin D3 or a placebo for two years.[44] Bone density at the hip (femoral neck) increased by 1.9 percent in the left hip and 2.6 percent in the right hip in the vitamin-D-treated group. In comparison, the placebo group demonstrated decreases of 0.3 percent in the left hip and 1.4 percent in the right hip.

Studies that combined vitamin D with calcium produced slightly better results. For example, one study monitored 3,270 elderly women living in nursing homes; in those who received 1,200 mg of calcium and 800 IU of vitamin D3, the hip fracture rate was reduced by forty-three percent compared to the placebo group.[45]

In a study published in the *New England Journal of Medicine,* the effects of three years of dietary supplementation with calcium and vitamin D3 on bone mineral density, and the incidence of hip fractures in 176 men and 213 women sixty-five years of age or older who were living at home, was studied.[46] The participants received either 500 mg of calcium plus 700 IU of vitamin D3 (cholecalciferol) per day or a placebo. Bone mineral density was measured by DEXA, and cases of hip fracture were ascertained by means of interviews and verified by hospital records. The average change in bone mineral density in the calcium-vitamin-D group was +0.5 percent for the hip, +2.12 percent for the spine, and +0.06 percent for the whole body. In contrast, the values for the placebo group were -0.70 percent, +1.22 percent, and –1.09 percent, respectively. Of thirty-seven subjects who had hip fractures, twenty-six were in the placebo group and eleven were in the calcium-vitamin-D group.

These studies imply that vitamin D can be helpful. It may be especially helpful for elderly people who don't get sufficient exposure to sunlight (which stimulates the body's manufacture of vitamin D)—those who live in nursing homes or farther away from the equator, or those who do not regularly get outside. We recommend a dosage of 400 IU of vitamin D3 per day rather than higher dosages, as the level of active vitamin D does not differ substantially between 400 and 800 IU. Taking higher dosages offers no significant benefit, and may adversely effect magnesium levels.

Magnesium Magnesium supplementation may turn out to be as important as calcium supplementation in the prevention and treatment of osteoporosis. Women with osteoporosis have lower bone magnesium content and other indicators of magnesium deficiency than people without osteoporosis.[47,48] In human magnesium deficiency, there is a decrease in serum concentration of the most active form of vitamin D $(1,25\text{-}(OH)_2D3)$ which has been observed in osteoporosis.[49] This finding could either be due to the enzyme responsible for the conversion of 25-OHD3 to $1,25\text{-}(OH)_2D3$ being dependent on adequate magnesium levels, or to magnesium's ability to mediate parathyroid hormone and calcitonin secretion.

The benefits of magnesium supplementation were investigated in a small two-year trial involving thirty-one postmenopausal women.[50] The women received an initial dose of either 250 mg of magnesium (as magnesium hydroxide) or a placebo. Dosages were increased to a maximum of 750 mg for the first six months, followed by a maintenance dosage of 250 mg for the remaining eighteen months of the trial. After one year, the women in the magnesium-treated group showed a slight improvement in bone density. In contrast, the placebo group showed a slight decrease in bone density. We hope that there will be follow-up studies to this preliminary study to better assess the benefits of magnesium supplementation in treating osteoporosis.

Vitamin B6, Folic Acid, and Vitamin B12
Low levels of vitamin B6, folic acid, and vitamin B12 are quite common in the elderly population and may contribute to osteoporosis. These vitamins are important in the conversion of the amino acid methionine to cysteine. If a person is deficient in these vitamins, or if a defect exists in the enzymes responsible for this conversion, there will be an increase in homocysteine level. Homocysteine has been implicated in a variety of conditions, including atherosclerosis and osteoporosis.

Increased homocysteine concentrations in the blood have been demonstrated in postmenopausal women, and are thought to play a role in osteoporosis by interfering with collagen cross-linking, leading to a defective bone matrix. Since osteoporosis is known to be a loss of both the organic and inorganic components of bone, the homocysteine theory has much validity as it is one of the few theories that addresses both factors.

Folic acid supplementation has been shown to reduce homocysteine levels in postmenopausal women, even though none of the women were deficient in folic acid by standard laboratory criteria.[51] Vitamins B6 and B12 are also necessary in the metabolism of homocysteine. Combinations of these vitamins will produce better results than any one of them.[52]

Silicon   Silicon is responsible for cross-linking collagen strands, thereby contributing greatly to the strength and integrity of the connective tissue matrix of bone.[53] Since silicon concentrations are increased at calcification sites in growing bone, recalcification in bone remodeling may be dependent on adequate levels of silicon. It is not known whether the typical American diet provides adequate amounts of silicon. In patients who have osteoporosis, or where accelerated bone regeneration is desired, silicon requirements may be increased and therefore supplementation may be appropriate.

Fluoride   Fluoride supplementation is a popular therapy in many parts of the world, but its value is still in question. Early studies showed that fluoride was largely ineffective.[54] Fluoride's predominant effects are stimulation of osteoblastic activity and inducing positive calcium balance. Fluoride is incorporated into the crystalline structure of bone as fluoroapatite, but the resulting bone matrix is poorly formed and weak, and long-term excessive exposure typically results in weak and brittle bones (osteosclerosis).

The therapeutic index (the level between a therapeutic effect and a toxic effect) for fluoride is quite narrow, and at the recommended daily dose of 60 to 75 mg, sodium fluoride causes side effects in one-third to one-half of patients. Joint pain is the most common side effect, but stomach aches, nausea, and vomiting also occur; these are less troublesome if the fluoride is taken with meals.

Newer sodium fluoride preparations (enteric-coated and timed-release to prevent digestion in the stomach) are showing fewer side effects and better clinical results.[55] However, at this time we do not recommend fluoride supplementation in the treatment of osteoporosis.

Phytoestrogens   Plant estrogenic substances, or *phytoestrogens,* are components of many medicinal herbs that have historically been used to treat conditions that are now treated with synthetic estrogens. They may be suitable alternatives to estrogens in the prevention of osteoporosis in menopausal women. See MENOPAUSE for a further description.

A semisynthetic isoflavonoid called *ipriflavone,* similar in structure to soy isoflavonoids, is approved in Japan, Hungary, and Italy as a drug for the treatment and prevention of osteopororis.[56] Ipriflavone has shown impressive results in a number of clinical studies. For example, in one study ipriflavone (200 mg three times per day) increased bone density measurements by 2 percent and 5.8 percent after six and twelve months, respectively, in 100 women with osteoporosis.[57] In another one-year study of women with osteoporosis, ipriflavone (600 mg per day) produced a six-percent increase in bone mineral density after twelve months, while the placebo group lost 0.3 percent in bone density.[58] Longer-term studies are showing equally promising results given the safety and apparent efficacy of ipriflavone.[59,60]

The effectiveness of ipriflavone raises the question of whether naturally occurring isoflavonoids, such as genistein and diadzein from soy, may exert similar benefits. Given the benefits of soy isoflavonoids in combating breast cancer, we encourage the regular consumption of soyfoods.

The mechanism of action appears to be via enhancement of calcitonin effects on calcium metabolism (as previously discussed), because ipriflavone exerts no estrogen-like effects.[61]

TREATMENT SUMMARY

Osteoporosis is a preventable illness if appropriate dietary and lifestyle measures are followed. Women of all ages, from the very young to the very old, should make building healthy and strong bones a lifelong priority. This involves avoiding dietary and lifestyle practices that leach calcium from the bones, and choosing dietary and lifestyle factors that promote bone health.

Although calcium intake is highlighted by most physicians, strong bones require much more than this important mineral. Bone is dynamic, living tissue that requires a constant supply of high-quality nutrients and regular stimulation (exercise).

The primary goal in the treatment of osteoporosis is prevention. In severe cases of osteoporosis, the recommendations given in this chapter should be used in conjunction with appropriate medical care, which may include the use of a variety of prescription drugs; follow the advice of your physician. Although drugs such as Fosamax and natural hormonal therapies such as calcitonin have side effects, the benefits (prevention of hip fracture) usually outweigh the risks in people who already have severe osteoporosis.[62,63]

Diet

Follow the guidelines given in A HEALTH-PROMOTING DIET. Be especially careful to limit dietary factors that promote calcium excretion, such as salt, sugar, protein, and soft drinks.

Nutritional Supplements

- High-potency multiple-vitamin-and-mineral formula, according to the guidelines in the chapter SUPPLEMENTARY MEASURES
- Calcium: 800–1,200 mg per day
- Vitamin D: 400 IU per day
- Magnesium: 400–800 mg per day
- Boron (as sodium tetrahydroborate): 3–5 mg per day

Periodontal Disease

. . . . :

Gingivitis: inflammation of the gums characterized by redness, contour changes, and bleeding

Periodontitis: localized pain, loose teeth, demonstration of dental pockets, redness, swelling, and/or signs of infection

X ray may reveal alveolar bone destruction

Periodontal disease is an inclusive term used to describe an inflammatory condition of the gums *(gingivitis)* and/or support structures *(periodontitis)*. The periodontal disease process typically progresses from gingivitis to periodontitis.[1,2] Periodontal disease may be a manifestation of a more systemic condition, such as diabetes mellitus, collagen diseases, anemia, vitamin deficiency states, or leukemia or other disorders of leukocyte function.[1] An association with hardening of the arteries (atherosclerosis) has also been reported.

Since there can be significant loss of the bone that supports the teeth *(alveolar bone)* without much inflammation, the definition of periodontal disease used in this chapter excludes the processes that cause only tooth loss (the majority of which is due to osteoporosis or endocrine imbalances).[1] These conditions reflect systemic disease, with local factors playing only a minor role. Therefore, the focus in such cases should be on treating the underlying condition rather than the "periodontal disease." In this context, noninflammatory alveolar bone loss should be viewed as a separate entity, as it involves a different cause (see OSTEOPOROSIS).

The focus of this chapter is on the use of nutrition and lifestyle improvement as an adjunctive therapy to aid in control and prevention of the causes of inflammatory periodontal disease. This disease is a good example of a condition that is probably best treated with combined expertise: a dentist or periodontist and a nutritionally minded physician. Although oral hygiene is of great importance in treating and preventing periodontal disease, it is not sufficient in many cases. The patient's immune system and other defense mechanisms must be normalized if development and progression of the disease are to be controlled.[1,3] To a large extent, the nutritional status of the individual determines the status of the host's defense mechanisms.

The frequency of periodontal disease increases directly with age. The rate of periodontal disease is approximately fifteen percent at age ten, thirty-eight percent at age twenty, forty-six percent at age thirty-five, and fifty-four percent at age fifty. As a group, men have a higher prevalence and severity of periodontal disease than women. The occurrence of periodontal disease is inversely related to increasing levels of education and income; rural dwellers have a higher level of severity and prevalence than their urban counterparts.[1]

Disease Process

Understanding the underlying process of any disease leads to a more effective treatment plan. In periodontal disease, this means understanding the normal protective factors in the gums and supporting structures (*periodontium*). It has been concluded by many experts in periodontal disease that: "Clearly bacteria are essential agents, but their presence is in itself insufficient; host factors must be involved if the disease is to develop and progress."[3]

Factors involved in a patient's immune status and other defense mechanisms include:

- The environment of the gingival sulcus
- Bacterial factors
- Neutrophil function
- Complement activation
- IgE and mast cell function
- Amalgam restoration
- Miscellaneous local factors
- The structure and integrity of the collagen matrix of the periodontium and gums

Gingival Sulcus

The *gingival sulcus* is the V-shaped crevice that surrounds each tooth, being bounded by the surface of the tooth on one side and the lining of cells (epithelium) of the free margin of the gingiva (gums) on the other. The anatomy of the gingival sulcus is ideal for growth of bacteria, as it is resistant to the washing and cleaning action of saliva. Furthermore, the gingival fluid (*sulcular fluid*) provides a rich nutrient source for microorganisms. The clinical determination of the depth of the gingival sulcus is an important diagnostic parameter. Individuals who have periodontal disease should see their dentist no less than once every six months for proper evaluation and cleaning.

Bacterial Factors

Bacterial plaque has long been considered the causative agent in most forms of peri-odontal disease.[1] However, an appreciation of immune system factors has now developed.[1,3] Bacteria are known to produce and secrete numerous compounds that are detrimental to the status of a person's defense mechanisms. These compounds include: endotoxins and exotoxins; free radicals and collagen-destroying enzymes; leukotoxins; and bacterial antigens, waste products, and toxic compounds.[1]

Neutrophils

White blood cells known as *neutrophils* constitute a first line of defense against microbial overgrowth. Defects in neutrophil function are catastrophic to the periodontium.[1,3] Neutrophil functions are depressed in the geriatric population as a whole, and in patients with diabetes, Crohn's disease, Chediak Higashi syndrome, Down's syndrome, and juvenile periodontitis.[1,3] These patients are at extremely high risk for developing rapidly progressing periodontal disease, as are people with transient low levels of neutrophils. Temporary defects in neutrophil function may be responsible for the periods of ebb and flow noted in periodontal disease. In addition to serving a vital role in protection against periodontal disease, neutrophils play a major role in tissue destruction. Neutrophils release numerous free radicals, which break down collagen, inflammatory compounds, and a compound that stimulates alveolar bone destruction.[1,3]

Complement Activation

The complement system is composed of at least twenty-two proteins that circulate in the blood. Upon activation, complement components act in a cascade fashion. The complement system plays a critical role in the resistance to infection, but it also plays a big role in the tissue injury of periodontal disease. The products of complement activation regulate a number of events. The net effect is an increase in gingival permeability, resulting in increased penetration of bacteria and bacterial byproducts and, in essence, the initiation of a positive feedback cycle.[1,3,4] In periodontal disease, activation of complement within the periodontal pocket is possibly the major factor in tissue destruction.

Mast Cells and IgE

Mast cells are white blood cells that reside in tissues. They contain histamine and other inflammatory compounds in packets known as *granules*. The release of the content of these packets is a major factor in periodontal disease.[1] Mast-cell degranulation can be initiated by IgE complexes, complement components, mechanical trauma, endotoxins, and/or free radicals. The finding of increased allergy antibody (IgE) concentrations in the gingiva of patients with periodontal disease suggests that allergic reactions may be a factor in the progression of the disease in some patients.[5]

Amalgam Restorations

Faulty dental work is a common cause of gingival inflammation and periodontal destruction.[1] Overhanging margins from a poorly done filling or crown provides an ideal location for the accumulation of plaque and the multiplication of bacteria. If the restoration is a silver amalgam filling, there may be even more involvement due to decreased activities of antioxidant enzymes. Mercury accumulation results in depletion of the free-radical-scavenging enzymes glutathione peroxidase, superoxide dismutase, and catalase.[6] The support structures of the teeth are particularly sensitive to free-radical damage.[7]

Miscellaneous Local Factors

Numerous local factors favor the progression of periodontal disease. These include: food impaction, unreplaced missing teeth, malocclusion, tongue thrusting, bruxism (tooth-grinding), toothbrush trauma, mouth breathing, and tobacco smoking.

. . . .

QUICK REVIEW

- Periodontal disease is best treated with combined expertise: a dentist or periodontist and a nutritionally minded physician.
- Although oral hygiene is of great importance in treating and preventing periodontal disease, it is not sufficient in many cases.
- The patient's immune system and other defense mechanisms must be normalized if development and progression of the disease are to be controlled.
- Faulty dental work is a common cause of gingival inflammation and periodontal destruction.
- Tobacco smoking is associated with increased susceptibility to severe periodontal disease and tooth loss.
- Vitamin C plays a major role in preventing periodontal disease.

Tobacco

Tobacco smoking is associated with increased susceptibility to severe periodontal disease and tooth loss.[1,8,9] (Tobacco smoking is associated with increased susceptibility to virtually every major chronic disease.) Many of the harmful effects of tobacco smoking are a result of free-radical damage, particularly to epithelial cells. Furthermore, smoking greatly reduces ascorbic acid levels, thereby enhancing its damaging effects.[10] Carotenes and flavonoids have been shown to greatly reduce some of the toxic effects of smoking.[11,12]

Structure and Integrity of Collagen Matrix

The collagen matrix of the periodontal membrane serves as the anchor (*periosteum*) to the alveolar bone and allows the dissipation of the tremendous amount of pressure exerted during chewing.[13] The status of the collagen matrix of the periodontium (gums and supportive structures) determines the rate of diffusion and the permeability of inflammatory mediators, bacteria and their byproducts, and destructive enzymes from the oral cavity.[14–16] Due to the high rate of protein turnover in periodontal collagen, the collagen matrix in this area is extremely vulnerable to atrophy when the necessary cofactors for collagen synthesis (protein, zinc, copper, vitamins C, B6, and A, etc.) are absent or deficient.[13]

Therapeutic Considerations

Therapeutic goals in treating periodontal disease from a nutritional perspective are:

- Decrease wound healing time (the time span for wound healing is longer in patients who are more susceptible to periodontal disease)[17]
- Improve membrane and collagen integrity
- Decrease inflammation and free-radical damage (inflammation can induce a vicious cycle and promote periodontal disease)

- Sugar is known to significantly increase plaque accumulation while decreasing white blood cell function.
- Vitamin E has been demonstrated to be of considerable value in treating patients with severe periodontal disease.
- A review of seven studies using Coenzyme Q_{10} found that seventy percent of the 332 patients involved responded favorably to supplementation.

- Flavonoids are extremely effective in reducing inflammation and stabilizing collagen structures of the gums.
- Folic acid, either as a mouthwash or a pill, has produced significant reductions of gingival inflammation in double-blind studies.
- Sanguinarine, an alkaloid derived from bloodroot, demonstrates useful properties in preventing dental plaque formation.

- Enhance immune status (defects in the immune system, particularly white blood cells—especially neutrophils—are catastrophic to the periodontium)

Individual nutrients will be discussed in the following sections in the context of their role in achieving these therapeutic goals.

Vitamin C

Vitamin C (ascorbic acid) plays a major role in preventing periodontal disease, as evident from many experimental studies.[1,18–22] The classical symptom of gingivitis seen in scurvy (severe vitamin C deficiency) illustrates the vital function vitamin C plays in maintaining the integrity and immunocompetence of the periodontal membrane and collagen matrix. Deficiency of vitamin C is associated with defective formation and maintenance of collagen, ground substance, and intercellular cement substances.[1] The effects of deficiency on the bone include osteoporosis and retardation or cessation of bone formation. Subclinical vitamin C deficiency plays a significant role in periodontal disease via these effects and via its role in delaying wound healing.[1,18-22]

Decreased vitamin C levels are also associated with increased permeability of the oral tissues' endotoxin and bacterial byproducts, as well as impaired white blood cell function (particularly neutrophils). The role vitamin C plays in increasing neutrophil function is best exemplified by its effect on Chediak-Higashi syndrome. This inherited disorder is associated with compromised white blood cell function that is responsive to vitamin C supplementation.[23] This syndrome is also associated with an extremely rapidly progressing periodontitis.[1,3] In addition to enhancing the immune system, vitamin C also possesses significant antioxidant and anti-inflammatory properties, and it decreases wound healing time.

Sucrose

Sugar is known to significantly increase plaque accumulation while decreasing white blood cell function.[1,25] The inhibition of neutrophil function is due to competition with vitamin C. Vitamin C and glucose are known to compete for intracellular transport sites, with this intracellular transport being largely insulin-dependent (see IMMUNE SUPPORT for further information on nutrient factors and immune function).

Considering the fact that the average American consumes an excess of 5 ounces of sucrose and other refined carbohydrates per day, it is safe to say that most Americans have a chronically depressed immune status, which puts them at increased risk for periodontal disease.[26]

Vitamin A

Vitamin A deficiency predisposes a person to periodontal disease. Deficiency of vitamin A is associated with abnormal cell structures in the periodontium, inflammatory infiltration and degeneration, periodontal pocket formation, plaque formation, increased susceptibility to infection, and abnormal alveolar bone formation.[1] Vitamin A is necessary for collagen synthesis, wound healing, and enhancing numerous immune functions.[27] Beta-carotene may be a more advantageous supplement due to its potent antioxidant activity.[12]

Zinc

Zinc's importance in treating periodontal disease cannot be overstated. Zinc functions synergistically with vitamin A in many body processes.[28] The severity of periodontal disease is positively associated with decreased zinc levels.[29] In the United States, marginal zinc deficiency is widespread, particularly among the elderly.[29,30] This may be a factor in the increasing prevalence of periodontal disease with age, although the geriatric population as a whole is at higher risk for developing numerous nutrient deficiencies.

The functions of zinc in the gingiva and periodontium include: stabilization of membranes, antioxidant activity, collagen synthesis, inhibition of plaque growth, inhibition of mast-cell degranulation, and numerous immune-enhancing activities.[27,28,30–32] Zinc is also known to significantly reduce wound healing time.[27,28]

Plaque growth can be inhibited by regular, twice-daily use of a mouthwash that contains a five-percent zinc solution.[31] However, lower concentrations or less frequent mouth washing are not particularly successful.

Vitamin E and Selenium

These two nutrients function synergistically in antioxidant mechanisms and seem to potentiate each other's effect. Vitamin E alone has been demonstrated to be of considerable value in treating patients with severe periodontal disease.[1,33] This can largely be attributed to the decreased wound-healing time associated with vitamin E.[34] The antioxidant effects of vitamin E are particularly needed if silver fillings are present. Mercury depletes the tissues of the antioxidant enzymes superoxide dismutase, glutathione peroxidase, and catalase. In animal studies, this toxic effect of mercury is prevented by supplementation with vitamin E.[6] The antioxidant activities of selenium and vitamin E also deter periodontal disease because the effects of free radicals are extremely damaging to gums.[7]

Coenzyme Q$_{10}$

Coenzyme Q$_{10}$ is involved in energy production, and is also an effective antioxidant.[35,36] Coenzyme Q$_{10}$ is widely used in Japan to treat many conditions, including periodontal disease. A review of seven studies that used Coenzyme Q$_{10}$ found that seventy percent of the 332 patients involved responded favorably to supplementation.[37] A double-blind study comprising fifty-six subjects found that the supplemented group responded significantly, while the placebo group displayed very little change in periodontal pocket depth and tooth mobility.

Flavonoids

As a group, these compounds are perhaps the most important components of an antiperiodontal disease program. Flavonoids are extremely effective in reducing inflammation and stabilizing collagen structures. Flavonoids affect collagen structure by: decreasing membrane permeability, thereby decreasing the load of inflammatory mediators and bacterial products; preventing free-radical damage with their potent antioxidant properties; inhibiting destruction to collagen; inhibiting mast-cell degranulation; and cross-linking with collagen fibers directly.[38–43] The more biologically active flavonoids (quercetin, catechin, anthocyanidins, and proanthocyanidins) should be supplemented, as rutin has very little collagen-stabilizing effect compared to these other flavonoids. These are found in flavonoid-rich extracts of bilberry (*Vaccinium myrtillus*), hawthorn (*Crataegus sp.*), grape seed (*Vitis vinifera*), or green tea (*Camellia sinensis*)

Remarkable effects have been displayed by using 3-0-methyl-(+)-catechin in the treatment of hamsters with experimentally induced periodontitis. Large doses of this flavonoid derivative significantly retarded plaque growth and alveolar bone resorption.[44] This flavonoid is not commercially available; the reference is made simply to demonstrate how effective flavonoid therapy may be.

Folic Acid

The use of folic acid in double-blind studies, either as a mouthwash or a pill, has produced significant reductions of gingival inflammation as determined by reduction in color changes, bleeding tendency, and plaque scores.[45–49] Folic acid mouthwash (0.1 percent folic acid) is significantly more effective than the oral supplementation of either 2 or 5 mg of folic acid per day, suggesting a local mechanism of action.[47,48] Folic acid has been demonstrated to bind plaque-derived toxins.[47–49] The use of folic acid mouthwash is particularly indicated for pregnant women, birth-control-pill users, and other conditions associated with exaggerated gingival inflammatory response, or for people taking drugs that interfere with folic acid (e.g., chemotherapy agents, epilepsy drugs, and drugs used in Crohn's disease and ulcerative colitis).

The cells of the oral cavity (as well as the cells that line the cervix) appear to suffer from an "end-organ" deficiency of folic acid under the hormonal influences of pregnancy and oral contraceptive use.[47,48] The blood and white blood cells of pregnant women and oral contraceptive users contain a macromolecule that binds folate, which appears to be the major factor for the "end-organ" folate deficiency, more than malabsorption or decreased intake.[50] (It should be noted, however, that folic acid deficiency is the most common deficiency in the world.[27])

Double-blind studies have shown that the beneficial effects of folic acid are not limited to women.[45,46,49] The positive effects are also not limited to gingivitis, since periodontitis diminishes with folic acid treatment as well.[49]

Botanicals

A number of botanical compounds have shown an ability to inhibit plaque formation, including green tea polyphenols and glycyrrhetinic acid from licorice, but the most extensively studied compound is an alcoholic extract of *Sanguinaria canadensis*.

Bloodroot (Sanguinaria canadensis)

Bloodroot contains a mixture of alkaloids, but chiefly *sanguinarine,* which is available in commercial toothpastes and mouth rinses. Sanguinarine demonstrates properties that are useful in preventing dental plaque formation. It has broad antimicrobial activity and anti-inflammatory properties. *In vitro* studies indicate that the antiplaque action of sanguinaria is due to its ability to inhibit bacterial adherence. Electron-microscope studies demonstrate that bacteria exposed to sanguinarine aggregate and become morphologically irregular.[51]

Sanguinarine appears to be less effective than chlorhexidine mouthwash, but it is effective in many cases and does have the advantage of being a natural compound as opposed to a synthetic.[51,52]

Gotu kola (Centella asiatica)

An extract containing the triterpenoids of gotu kola has demonstrated impressive wound-healing properties. These properties can be put to good use in treating severe periodontal disease or if there is a requirement for surgery. One study demonstrated that centella extract was quite helpful in speeding recovery after laser surgery for severe periodontal disease.[53]

TREATMENT SUMMARY

As discussed above, many factors are involved in the initiation and promotion of periodontal disease. Effective therapy requires that all relevant factors be controlled. Since there are as yet no clear guidelines for determining which factors are most important for a given patient, a general approach is recommended here. If you are a smoker, we strongly encourage you to stop, as continued smoking greatly decreases the success of any therapy for periodontal disease.

Hygiene

Visit a dentist periodically to eliminate plaque and calculus accumulation as needed. Brushing after meals and daily flossing are necessary.

Diet

A diet high in dietary fiber may have a protective effect via increased salivary secretion.[18] Avoidance of sucrose and all refined carbohydrates is extremely important.

Nutritional Supplements

- Vitamin C: 3–5 grams per day in divided doses
- Vitamin E: 400–800 IU per day
- Beta-carotenes: 250,000 IU per day (higher doses if indicated) for up to six months (although not clinically tested in this condition, beta-carotenes are recommended instead of vitamin A due to their similar effects and greater safety)
- Selenium: 400 mcg per day
- Zinc: 30 mg of zinc picolinate per day (60 mg per day if another form); or wash mouth with 1/2 ounce of a 5% zinc solution twice per day
- Folic acid: 2 mg per day; or wash mouth with 1/2 ounce of a 0.1% solution of folic acid twice per day
- Quercetin: 500 mg three times per day

Botanical Medicines

High-flavonoid-content extracts, such as those from bilberry (*Vaccinium myrtillus*), hawthorn (*Crataegus sp.*), grape seed (*Vitis vinifera*), or green tea (*Camellia sinensis*) can be used at a dosage of 150 to 300 mg per day. Of these extracts, green tea extract, or the liberal consumption of green tea as a beverage, may be the most cost-effective. For a green tea extract with a fifty-percent polyphenol content, the dosage would be 200 to 300 mg twice per day.

- *Sanguinaria canadensis:* use toothpaste containing extract
- *Centella asiatica triterpenoids:* 30 mg twice per day of pure triterpenoids

Premenstrual Syndrome

Recurrent signs and symptoms that develop during the seven to fourteen days prior to menstruation

Typical symptoms include: decreased energy level, tension, irritability, depression, headache, altered sex drive, breast pain, backache, abdominal bloating, and edema of the fingers and ankles

remenstrual syndrome (PMS) is a recurrent condition of women, characterized by troublesome symptoms seven to fourteen days before menstruation.[1] Typical symptoms include: decreased energy level, tension, irritability, depression, headache, altered sex drive, breast pain, backache, abdominal bloating, and edema of the fingers and ankles. PMS is estimated to affect between thirty and forty percent of menstruating women, with peak occurrences among women in their thirties and forties. In most cases, symptoms are relatively mild. However, in about ten percent of all women, symptoms can be quite severe. Severe PMS, with depression, irritability, and extreme mood swings, is referred to as *premenstrual dysphoric disorder*.[2]

Although PMS has been a well-defined clinical entity for over sixty years, many physicians still argue that it really does not exist.[3] As a result, many women who suffer from PMS do not receive proper treatment. Instead, they are told that it is "all in your head." This view is gaining momentum, as large pharmaceutical companies have recognized the huge market potential. These companies have sponsored clinical trials using drugs to treat PMS symptoms (e.g., antidepressant drugs such as Prozac and Zoloft, anti-anxiety drugs related to Valium, and go-nadotropin-releasing hormone), despite the fact that risks due to side effects appear to far outweigh the benefits.[4]

A more rational approach to the problem of PMS is identification of the causative factors and appropriate treatment using dietary therapy, nutritional supplementation, and exercise.

SIGNS AND SYMPTOMS OF PREMENSTRUAL SYNDROME

Behavioral
  Nervousness, anxiety, and irritability
  Mood swings and mild-to-severe personality change
  Fatigue, lethargy, and depression
Gastrointestinal
  Abdominal bloating
  Diarrhea and/or constipation
  Change in appetite (usually craving of sugar)
Female
  Tender and enlarged breasts
  Uterine cramping
  Altered libido
General
  Headache
  Backache
  Acne
  Edema of fingers and ankles

The Normal Menstrual Cycle

In order to appreciate the hormonal abnormalities that have been found in some women with PMS, it is important to briefly review the normal menstrual cycle. The menstrual cycle reflects the monthly rhythmic changes in the secretion rates of the female hormones and corresponding changes in the lining of the uterus and other female organs.

The menstrual cycle is controlled by the complex interactions of the hypothalamus, pituitary, and ovaries. Each month during the reproductive years, the secretion of various hormones is designed to accomplish two primary goals: (1) ensure that only a single egg is released by the ovaries each month, and (2) prepare the lining of the uterus (the *endometrium*) for implantation of the fertilized egg. To accomplish these goals, the concentrations of the primary female sexual hormones, estrogen and progesterone, fluctuate during the menstrual cycle.

The control center for the female hormonal system is the *hypothalamus*, a region of the brain roughly the size of a cherry, situated above the *pituitary gland* and below another area of the brain called the *thalamus*. The hypothalamus and pituitary gland are housed in the middle of the head just behind the eyes. The hypothalamus controls the female hormonal system by releasing hormones, such as gonadotropin-releasing hormone (GnRH) and follicle-stimulating-hormone-releasing hormone (FSH-RH), which stimulate the release of pituitary hormones.

In response to the hypothalamus, the pituitary gland releases follicle-stimulating hormone (FSH) and luteinizing hormone (LH). FSH is the hormone primarily responsible for the maturation of the egg *(ovum)* during the first phase of the menstrual cycle. It is called "follicle-stimulating hormone" because each egg within the ovary is housed inside an individual follicle. LH is responsible for initiating ovulation—the release of the fully developed egg.

The release of LH is triggered by increasing estrogen levels as a result of the growing follicle. After ovulation, the eggless follicle is transformed into the *corpus luteum,* which functions primarily to secrete progesterone and estrogen to help a fertilized egg become well-established in the uterine lining. If fertilization does not occur, the corpus luteum recedes, hormone production decreases, menstruation occurs approximately two weeks later, and the entire menstruation process begins anew.

The usual menstrual cycle is completed in about a month. It is divided into three phases, in order of occurrence: follicular, ovulatory, and luteal. The follicular phase lasts for ten to fourteen days, the ovulatory phase lasts for about thirty-six hours and involves the release of the egg, and the luteal phase lasts for fourteen days.

Other Hormones

Because of the complex interrelationships among the components of the endocrine system, disorder of any of the individual members of the system (pituitary, ovaries, adrenals, thyroid, parathyroids, and pancreas) can lead to menstrual abnormalities and/or PMS. For example, low thyroid function *(hypothyroidism)* and elevated *cortisol* (an adrenal hormone) levels are common in women with PMS.

Prolactin, another hormone produced by the pituitary, also plays an important role in PMS and female infertility. Prolactin's chief function is to regulate the development of the mammary gland and milk secretion during and after pregnancy. Increased production of prolactin in lactating women can inhibit the maturation of the follicles in the ovaries. In nonlactating women, elevated levels of prolactin are often linked to cases of PMS, menstrual abnormalities, absence of ovulation, ovarian cysts, and breast tenderness.

Hormonal Patterns in Women with PMS

Although there is a wide spectrum of symptoms, there are common hormonal patterns among PMS patients compared to women who have no symptoms of PMS. The primary finding is that estrogen levels are elevated and plasma progesterone levels are reduced five to ten days before the menses, or the ratio of estrogen to progesterone is increased. In addition to this hormonal abnormality, hypothyroidism and/or elevated prolactin levels are common, FSH levels are typically ele-

vated six to nine days prior to the onset of menses, and *aldosterone* (a hormone produced by the adrenal glands that leads to sodium and water retention) levels are marginally elevated two to eight days prior to the onset of menses.[1,5,6]

Corpus Luteum Insufficiency and PMS

PMS symptoms occur during the luteal phase of the menstrual cycle. This phase signifies the important role that the corpus luteum plays in the production primarily of progesterone, but also of estrogen. Many researchers theorize that PMS reflects *corpus luteum insufficiency*. Corpus luteum insufficiency is usually diagnosed by measuring the level of progesterone in the blood three weeks after onset of menstruation. If the level is below 10 to 12 ng/ml, corpus luteal insufficiency is a strong possibility.

In addition to PMS, corpus luteal insufficiency has been linked to abnormal menstruation (excessive blood loss; absent, persistent, or more frequent menstruation), elevations in prolactin level, and low thyroid function.[7]

· ·

QUICK REVIEW

- Premenstrual Syndrome (PMS) is estimated to affect between thirty and forty percent of menstruating women.
- The primary hormonal disturbance in PMS is that estrogen levels are elevated and progesterone levels are reduced.
- An increased estrogen-to-progesterone ratio leads to impaired liver function,

reduced levels of serotonin (an important mood-elevating neurotransmitter) in the brain, lower endorphin levels, impaired vitamin B6 activity, and alterations in other hormone levels.

- The primary nutritional recommendations for PMS are: increase consumption of plant foods (vegetables, fruits, legumes, whole grains, nuts, and seeds); consume small-to-moderate quantities of meat and dairy products;

Diagnosis and Classification

Diagnosis of PMS is usually made by observation of the symptoms attributed to PMS and their occurrence during the luteal phase of the menstrual cycle. To aid in the diagnosis, symptom questionnaires are often used. Since recalled information loses its accuracy, it is a good idea for a woman with PMS to begin keeping a menstrual symptom diary in addition to answering a symptom questionnaire. The diary will help document improvement and further clarify the symptom pattern. Both a questionnaire and diary are provided in this chapter.

PMS Classifications

In an attempt to bring some order to the clinically and metabolically confusing picture of PMS, several experts have created classification systems that sort PMS sufferers into subgroups.[8] The system with which we have the most experience was developed by Dr. Guy Abraham; it divides PMS into four distinct subgroups.[9] Each subgroup is linked to specific symptoms, hormonal patterns, and metabolic abnormalities. Following is a sample menstrual symptom questionnaire based on Dr. Abraham's classifications, followed by a brief discussion of the individual subgroups. Please note that women rarely experience a particular subgroup in a pure form; usually a woman with PMS experiences aspects of two or more subgroups.

PMS-A

PMS-A (A = anxiety) is the most common symptom category and is found to be strongly associated with excessive estrogen and deficient progesterone levels during the premenstrual phase. Common symptoms of patients in this category are anxiety, irritability, and emotional instability.

PMS-C

PMS-C (C = carbohydrate craving) is associated with increased appetite, craving for sweets, headache, fatigue, fainting spells, and heart palpitations. Glucose tolerance tests (GTT) performed on PMS-C patients during the five to ten days before their menses show a flattening of the early part of the curve

- -

reduce fat and sugar intake; increase consumption of soy foods; eliminate caffeine intake; and keep salt intake low.

- Low thyroid function (hypothyroidism) has been shown to affect a large percentage of women who have PMS.
- Most women who have PMS tend to employ "negative" coping styles.
- Vitamin B6 and magnesium are the two most important nutritional supplements for treating PMS.
- The four most useful herbs in the treatment of PMS are angelica or dong quai, licorice root, black cohosh, and chasteberry.
- The use of progesterone creams should be reserved as the last choice after other natural measures have failed.

Menstrual Syndrome Questionnaire

Date: _____

Grading of Symptoms

1 none
2 mild—present but does not interfere with activities
3 moderate—present and interferes with activities but not disabling
4 severe—disabling (unable to function)

Grade Your Symptoms for Last Menstrual Cycle Only

	SYMPTOMS	WEEK AFTER PERIOD	WEEK BEFORE PERIOD
PMS-A	Nervous tension	_____	_____
	Mood swings	_____	_____
	Irritability	_____	_____
	Anxiety	_____	_____
	TOTAL:	_____	_____
PMS-H	Weight gain	_____	_____
	Swelling of extremities	_____	_____
	Breast tenderness	_____	_____
	Abdominal bloating	_____	_____
	TOTAL:	_____	_____
PMS-C	Headache	_____	_____
	Craving for sweets	_____	_____
	Increased appetite	_____	_____
	Heart pounding	_____	_____
	Fatigue	_____	_____
	Dizziness or fainting	_____	_____
	TOTAL:	_____	_____
PMS-D	Depression	_____	_____
	Forgetfulness	_____	_____
	Crying	_____	_____
	Confusion	_____	_____
	Insomnia	_____	_____
	TOTAL:	_____	_____
Total MSQ score		_____	_____

Other symptoms

	Oily skin	_____	_____
	Acne	_____	_____

During first two days of periods

	Menstrual cramps	_____	_____
	Menstrual backache	_____	_____

(which usually implies excessive secretion of insulin in response to sugar consumption), whereas during other parts of the menstrual cycle their GTT is normal.[2] Currently, there is no clear explanation for this phenomenon, although an increased cellular capacity to bind insulin has been postulated. This increased binding capacity for insulin appears to be hormonally regulated, but other factors may also be involved, such as a high salt intake or decreased magnesium or prostaglandin levels.

PMS-D

PMS-D (D = depression) is the least common type and is relatively rare in its pure form. Its key symptom is depression, which is usually associated with low levels of neurotransmitters in the central nervous system. In PMS-D patients, this is probably due to increased breakdown of the neurotransmitters as a result of decreased levels of estrogen (in contrast to PMS-A, which shows the opposite results). The decreased ovarian estrogen output has been attributed to a stress-induced increase in adrenal androgen and/or progesterone secretion.

PMS-H

PMS-H (H = hyperhydration) is characterized by weight gain (greater than three pounds), abdominal bloating and discomfort, breast tenderness and congestion, and occasional swelling of the face, hands, and ankles. These symptoms are due to an increased fluid volume, secondary to an excess of the hormone aldosterone which causes increased fluid retention. Aldosterone excess during the premenstrual phase of PMS-H patients may arise due to stress, estrogen excess, magnesium deficiency, or excess salt intake.

An Alternative Classification System

Abraham's system is useful for quickly identifying possible causes of a given case of PMS.

However, we prefer to classify patients according to the causative factor. Of course, in order to do so, we must first uncover what the causative factor(s) is/are. The most common causative factors are:

- Excess estrogen
- Progesterone deficiency
- Elevated prolactin levels
- Hypothyroidism
- Stress, endogenous opioid deficiency, and adrenal dysfunction
- Depression
- Nutritional factors
    macronutrient disturbances/excesses
    micronutrient deficiency

The detection of these causative factors involves a diagnostic hierarchy based on the clinical picture and history. Taking the following steps should lead to proper identification of the causative factor, if necessary. This will allow a more effective treatment plan to be tailored to a woman's specific needs, and as a result better relief can be achieved.

1. Determine your basal body temperature (discussed in HYPOTHYROIDISM). If your basal body temperature is below 97.8 degrees Fahrenheit, or if you are suffering from other symptoms associated with PMS, consult your physician for complete thyroid-function testing.

2. Determine whether depression may be a factor by taking the self-test in the DEPRESSION chapter. If it is, follow the recommendations given in that chapter.

3. If you have followed the first two steps and have not improved after two months, consult your physician and ask to have a complete blood count and chemistry panel performed on day twenty-one of your cycle (the first day of menstruation constitutes day one). The tests should include:

- Complete blood count (CBC)
- White blood cell (WBC) count

- Red blood cell (RBC) count
- RBC morphology
- Hemoglobin
- Mean corpuscular volume (MCV)
- Mean corpuscular hemoglobin (MCH)
- Mean corpuscular hemoglobin concentration (MCHC)
- Platelet count
- Differential (Neutrophils, Lymphocytes, Monocytes, and Eosinophils)
- Albumin/Globulin ratio, Lactate dehydrogenase (LDH), Aspartate transaminase (AST or SGOT) Alanine transaminase (ALT or SSGPT, Gamma-glutamyl transpeptidase [GGTP]), Bilirubin (Total and Direct), Alkaline phosphatase, Calcium, Phosphorus, Uric acid, Blood urea nitrogen (BUN)/Creatinine, Glucose, Cholesterol, Triglycerides, Thyroid panel (T3 uptake, Thyroxine, and Free thyroxine index), Ferritin, Progesterone, Estrogen, Prolactin (especially if menstrual cycle is irregular)

4. If there are no apparent abnormalities in the CBC and chemistry panel, additional tests we recommend include:

- Liver detoxification profile (see DETOXIFICATION)
- Adrenal stress index (see STRESS, STRESS MANAGEMENT, and ADRENAL SUPPORT)
- Food allergy panel (see FOOD ALLERGY)

Therapeutic Considerations

PMS represents a multifactorial condition; there is no single cause that explains PMS in every case. Many factors appear to play a role, and some factors are more important in one case than another. However, there is tremendous overlap. The following factors will be discussed in this section:

- Excess estrogen
- Progesterone deficiency
- Elevated prolactin levels
- Hypothyroidism
- Stress, endorphin deficiency, and adrenal dysfunction
- Depression
- Nutritional factors
    macronutrient disturbances/excesses
    micronutrient deficiency

Estrogen and Progesterone in PMS

One of the most common findings in women with PMS is an elevated estrogen-to-progesterone ratio.[1,10–14] Typically this derangement is caused by a combined mild estrogen excess and mild progesterone deficiency. An increased estrogen-to-progesterone ratio contributes to PMS by leading to:

- Impaired liver function
- Reduced manufacture of serotonin
- Decreased action of vitamin B6
- Increased aldosterone secretion
- Increased prolactin secretion

Estrogen Excess and Liver Function

In the early 1940s, Dr. Morton Biskind observed an apparent relationship between B vitamin deficiency and PMS.[15,16] He postulated that PMS, as well as excessive menstruation and fibrocystic breast disease, was due to an excess in estrogen levels caused by decreased detoxification and elimination in the liver due to B vitamin deficiency. The liver utilizes various B vitamins to detoxify estrogen and excrete it in the bile.

There appears to be support for Dr. Biskind's theory. Estrogen excess is known to produce what is known medically as *cholestasis*. This term signifies diminished bile flow or stasis of bile. Naturopathic physicians often refer to this condition as a "sluggish liver." It reflects minimal impairment of liver function, because normal indicators of liver function (such as liver enzymes: alkaline phosphatase, SGOT, SGPT, and GGTP) are not elevated. However, because of the liver's important role in numerous metabolic processes, even minor impairment of liver function can have profound effects.

Cholestasis can be caused by a great number of factors besides estrogen excess (see DETOXIFICATION). Presence of cholestasis may be a predisposing factor to PMS, as with cholestasis there is reduced estrogen detoxification and clearance. Hence, a positive feedback scenario is produced. It is obvious that many American women suffer from cholestasis. All one has to do is look at the tremendous frequency of gallstones.

CAUSES OF CHOLESTASIS
Alcohol
Anabolic steroids
Endotoxins
Estrogen excess or birth-control pills
Hereditary disorders, such as Gilbert's syndrome
Pregnancy
Presence of gallstones
Various chemicals or drugs

Effects of Estrogen on Neurotransmitters
Another possible result of the increase in the estrogen-to-progesterone ratio is impairment of neurotransmitter synthesis and endorphin activity. *Neurotransmitters* are compounds that transmit the nerve impulse. A group of neurotransmitters known as *monoamines* are made from dietary *amino acids*—the building-block molecules of proteins. For example, the amino acid *tryptophan* serves as the precursor to *serotonin* and *melatonin,* while *phenylalanine* and *tyrosine* are precursors to *dopamine, epinephrine,* and *norepinephrine.*

According to the dominant medical view, depression is characterized by imbalances of monoamines. In addition to estrogen-induced alterations, environmental, nutritional, psychological, and genetic factors can all lead to an imbalance in the monoamines, which might result in depression. Different antidepressant drugs act by increasing levels of different monoamines in the brain via blocking either the reuptake or the breakdown, or enhancing the effect of, a specific monoamine.

Antidepressant drug therapy for PMS is gaining popularity among many M.D.s. However, there are other ways to address the alterations in neurotransmitters; chief among them is normalizing estrogen-to-progesterone ratios. It is interesting to note that the majority of the over twelve million patients who take Prozac are women between the ages of twenty-five and fifty—the same population that has a high frequency of PMS. Alternatives to Prozac and other antidepressant drugs are given in the chapter on DEPRESSION.

Estrogen Excess and Endorphin Levels
Estrogen excess during the luteal phase also negatively affects endorphin levels. *Endorphins* are the body's own mood-elevating and pain-relieving substances. One study found a direct correlation between an increased estrogen-to-progesterone ratio and endorphin activity in the brain.[11] In essence, when the estrogen-to-progesterone ratio was increased, there was a decline in endorphin levels. This reduction is significant, considering the known ability of endorphins to normalize or improve mood. Other studies have shown that low endorphin levels during the luteal phase are common among women with PMS.[17] Endorphin levels are lowered by stress and raised by exercise. The role of endorphins is further discussed in Stress, Endorphins, and Exercise in PMS, later in this chapter.

Estrogen Impairs Vitamin B6 Function

The negative impact of estrogen excess on neurotransmitter and endorphin levels during the luteal phase may be secondary to impairment of vitamin B6 action. Vitamin B6 (pyridoxine) is an extremely important B vitamin involved in the formation of body proteins and structural compounds, chemical transmitters in the nervous system, red blood cells, and hormone-like compounds known as *prostaglandins*. Vitamin B6 is critical to maintaining hormonal balance.

It is well known that estrogens negatively affect vitamin B6 function. Vitamin B6 levels are typically quite low in depressed patients, especially women taking estrogens (birth-control pills or Premarin).[18,19] Vitamin B6 supplementation has been shown to exert positive effects on all PMS symptoms (particularly depression) in many women. The improvement is achieved via a combined reduction in mid-luteal estrogen levels and increase in mid-luteal progesterone levels.

Estrogen's Effects on Aldosterone

As stated previously, aldosterone is a hormone produced by the adrenal glands that leads to retention of sodium and water. In many cases of PMS, aldosterone levels are marginally elevated two to eight days prior to the onset of menses. This elevation may be a result of estrogen excess increasing the secretion of aldosterone.

Estrogen and Prolactin Secretion

Excessive levels of prolactin are implicated in many cases of PMS, especially in women experiencing breast pain or fibrocystic breast disease (discussed in FIBROCYSTIC BREAST DISEASE).[20,21] Estrogens, both internally produced and ingested as birth-control pills or Premarin, are known to increase prolactin secretion by the pituitary gland. Following the recommendations (given in the following section, entitled Reducing Estrogen-to-Progesterone Ratio) for lowering the luteal-phase estrogen-to-progesterone ratio may be all that is necessary to lower prolactin levels. In particular, the herb *Vitex agnus-castus* (chasteberry) may prove to be useful in cases of high prolactin levels due to corpus luteum insufficiency (discussed later in Herbal Recommendations for PMS). Vitamin B6 and zinc supplementation also lower prolactin levels and are discussed in subsequent sections of this chapter. Prolactin levels also tend to be elevated in cases of low thyroid function.

Estrogen Excess and Uterine Fibroids

Fibroid tumors are benign (nonmalignant) tumors that consist of uterine muscle cells. Fibroids are one of the most common type of tumor and are thought to be the result of estrogen excess. Most often, fibroids grow silently and cause no problems, especially if they are small. If a fibroid is large (the largest fibroid ever reported weighed an incredible 303 pounds!), it can lead to excessive menstruation (*menorrhagia*), pain, or inability to maintain a pregnancy. The treatment and prevention of uterine fibroids involves the same approach outlined in the next section for reducing the estrogen-to-progesterone ratio.

Reducing Estrogen-to-Progesterone Ratio

Central to effective treatment in most cases of PMS is lowering the luteal-phase estrogen-to-progesterone ratio. An elevation of this ratio may be the underlying factor in the hormonal, neurotransmitter, endorphin, and other physiological disturbances in most cases of PMS. Effective treatment usually involves the following steps:

Step 1: Follow These Dietary Recommendations A number of dietary factors are known to reduce circulating estrogen levels or block the attachment of estrogen to receptor sites. The primary dietary recommendations are:

- Increase consumption of plant foods (vegetables, fruits, legumes, whole grains, nuts, and seeds)
- Consume small-to-moderate quantities of meat and dairy products
- Reduce fat and sugar intake
- Increase consumption of soy foods

In addition, it is important to reduce the load of environmental estrogens by avoiding foods sprayed with pesticides and herbicides.

Step 2: Establish Proper Gastrointestinal Flora One of the key ways in which the liver detoxifies cancer-causing chemicals, as well as the body's hormones such as estrogen, is by attaching *glucuronic acid* to the toxin and excreting it in the bile. *Beta-glucuronidase* is a bacterial enzyme that uncouples (breaks) the bond between excreted toxins and glucuronic acid. Not surprisingly, excess beta-glucuronidase activity is associated with an increased risk of getting cancer, particularly estrogen-dependent breast cancer, and presumably PMS.

The activity of this enzyme can be reduced by establishing proper bacterial flora.[22] The dietary guidelines given in Step 1 go a long way toward this goal. In addition, initial supplementation with probiotics is recommended. *Probiotics* (literally translated, "for life") is a term used to signify the health-promoting effects of "friendly bacteria." The most important friendly bacteria are *Lactobacillus acidophilus* and *Bifidobacterium bifidum*.

The dosage of a commercial probiotic supplement is based on the number of live organisms it contains. One to ten billion viable *L. acidophilus* or *B. bifidum* cells daily is a sufficient dosage for most people. Amounts exceeding this may induce mild gastrointestinal disturbances, while smaller amounts may not be able to colonize the gastrointestinal tract. Probiotics are extremely safe and are not associated with any side effects.

Step 3: Take the Recommended Nutritional Supplements Estrogen excess is known to increase nutritional needs for B vitamins, magnesium, and possibly other nutrients. B vitamins and magnesium are also necessary for the proper detoxification of estrogens. Recommended levels of supplementation are given in Micronutrients and PMS, later in this chapter.

Step 4: Enhance Liver Detoxification Supporting liver function focuses on protecting the liver by following the dietary guidelines listed in Step 1 and the nutritional supplement recommendations mentioned in Step 3. In addition, most naturopathic physicians use formulas that contain *lipotropic factors*. Lipotropic factors are substances that hasten the removal or decrease the deposition of fat and bile in the liver through their interaction with fat metabolism. In essence, they produce a "decongesting" effect on the liver and promote improved liver function and fat metabolism. Compounds commonly employed as lipotropic agents include choline, methionine, betaine, folic acid, and vitamin B12, along with herbal cholagogues and choleretics. Most major manufacturers of nutritional supplements offer lipotropic formulas. The important thing, when taking a lipotropic formula, is to take enough of the formula to provide a daily dose of 1,000 mg of choline and 500 mg of methionine and/or cysteine.

Step 5: Use Chasteberry or Phytoestrogen-Containing Formulas Chasteberry

(*Vitex agnus-castus*) and phytoestrogen-containing herbs, such as dong quai, black cohosh, and licorice, are popular herbal recommendations for treating PMS. Their appropriate use is described later in this chapter, in Herbal Recommendations for PMS.

Step 6: Consider Progesterone Therapy

You may be asking, "If one of the primary features of PMS for most women is an elevated estrogen-to-progesterone ratio, why not simply take progesterone?" Although progesterone administration is a popular recommendation by many physicians (M.D.s and N.D.s alike), we have some reservations. First of all, although progesterone administration has been the most common prescription for PMS by the medical community, controlled clinical trials have failed to consistently demonstrate the superiority of progesterone therapy over a placebo (there is a significant placebo response in PMS, by the way).[23–28]

The studies that demonstrate a beneficial effect of progesterone therapy have used dosages that far exceed the normal levels for progesterone and for the estrogen-to-progesterone ratio (200 to 400 mg twice daily as a vaginal or rectal suppository, from fourteen days before the expected onset of menstruation until the onset of vaginal bleeding).[27,28] Side effects, although generally mild, are common. In one of the more recent double-blind studies that did show a positive effect of progesterone therapy (400 mg twice a day by vaginal or rectal administration), adverse events were reported by fifty-one percent of patients in the progesterone treatment group, compared to forty-three percent in the placebo group.[28] Irregularity of menstruation, vaginal itching, and headache were reported more frequently by the women who took the progesterone.

Secondly, philosophically we would rather help the body naturally improve the estrogen-to-progesterone ratio by addressing the underlying causative factors, such as reduced detoxification or clearance of estrogen, along with reduced corpus luteum function, rather than artificially and drastically tipping the ratio in favor of progesterone.

We do not recommend unsupervised use of progesterone creams as the first step in treating PMS, but rather as a possible last choice after other natural measures have failed. Here are some guidelines if you elect to give a progesterone-containing cream a try:

1. First, make sure that the level (in milligrams) of progesterone per dosage unit is provided so that you can calculate how much of the cream is required to achieve the high dosage required (200 to 400 mg applied twice daily into the vagina). A distinction must be made between prescription progesterone preparations and some of the over-the-counter progesterone-containing creams, including those misrepresented as "yam-concentrates." Mexican yam is a source of a compound known as *diosgenin* that can be converted in a laboratory environment to progesterone and to the hormone DHEA. There is no evidence that such a conversion occurs in the human body. Some companies label a progesterone-containing cream as a yam concentrate, as a marketing ploy, while other companies market a true yam concentrate without any significant levels of progesterone, yet promote it as providing the same benefit as a progesterone-containing cream. In both cases, these representations are wrong.

2. Apply the cream intravaginally; this is more effective than simply applying the cream to the skin. In fact, applying progesterone to the skin (nonmucous membranes) results in poor absorption.

3. Monitor your progesterone levels by ordering a saliva test for progesterone from Aeron Life Cycles Laboratories (800-631-

7900) after one month of use, and adjust your dosage accordingly.

Low Thyroid Function and PMS

Low thyroid function (*hypothyroidism*) has been shown to affect a large percentage of women who have PMS.[29,30] For example, in one study published in the prestigious *New England Journal of Medicine*, fifty-one out of fifty-four PMS subjects demonstrated low thyroid status compared to zero out of twelve in the control group.[29] In another study, it was seven out of ten in the PMS group and zero out of nine in the control group.[30] Other studies have also shown hypothyroidism to be only slightly more common in women with PMS than in controls.[31,32] Many women who have both PMS and confirmed hypothyroidism and who are given thyroid hormone experience complete relief of symptoms.[29] For more information, see HYPOTHYROIDISM.

Stress, Endorphins, and Exercise in PMS

Like many common conditions associated with "modern" living, stress plays a role in PMS. When stress is extreme, unusual, or long-lasting, it triggers biological changes in the brain, largely as a result of altered adrenal gland function and endorphin secretion or action. These changes produce a domino effect that leads to alterations in normal physiology. Effective treatment of PMS must include stress management (see STRESS, STRESS MANAGEMENT, and ADRENAL SUPPORT).

Exercise and PMS

Several studies have shown that women who are engaged in a regular exercise program do not suffer from PMS nearly as often as sedentary women.[33-35] In one of the more thorough studies, mood and physical symptoms during the menstrual cycle were assessed in ninety-seven women who exercised regularly, and in a second group of 159 female nonexercisers.[33] Mood scores and physical symptoms assessed throughout the menstrual cycle revealed that exercise had significant effects on negative mood states and physical symptoms. The regular exercisers obtained significantly lower scores on impaired concentration, negative mood, behavior change, and pain.

In another study, 143 women were monitored for five days in each of the three phases of the cycle (mid-cycle, premenstrual, and menstrual).[34] The women were thirty-five competitive athletes, two groups of exercisers (thirty-three high exercisers and thirty-six low exercisers), and thirty-nine sedentary women. The high exercisers experienced the greatest positive-mood scores, and the sedentary women the least. The high exercisers also reported the least depression and anxiety. The differences were most apparent during the premenstrual and menstrual phases. These results are consistent with the belief that women who frequently exercise (but not competitive athletes) are protected from PMS symptoms. In particular, regular exercise protects against the deterioration of mood before and during menstruation.

These studies provide evidence that women who have PMS need to exercise. One of the ways in which exercise may be positively impacting PMS is through elevations in endorphin levels and lowering of cortisol levels.

Coping Style and PMS

Whether you are currently aware of it or not, you have a pattern for coping with stress. Unfortunately, most women with PMS tend to employ "negative" coping styles.[36] We term them negative because they ultimately do not support good health. If you are to be truly successful in coping with stress, negative coping patterns must be identified and replaced with positive ways of coping. Try to identify from the following list any negative or destructive coping patterns you may have developed:

- Feelings of helplessness
- Overeating
- Watching too much television
- Emotional outbursts
- Overspending
- Excessive behavior
- Dependence on chemicals
    drugs, legal or illicit
    alcohol
    smoking

For some tips on ways to improve coping strategies, see A POSITIVE MENTAL ATTITUDE.

Psychotherapy

Various psychotherapy methods have been used successfully to improve the psychological aspects of PMS. In particular, psychotherapy in the form of biofeedback or short-term individual counseling (especially cognitive therapy, which is further discussed in the chapter DEPRESSION) have documented clinical efficacy.[37,38] One of the advantages of cognitive therapy in the treatment of PMS over antidepressant drug therapy is that learning techniques such as cognitive-behavioral coping skills can produce excellent results that will be maintained over time.

Depression, Low Serotonin Levels, and PMS

There are some important relationships between PMS and depression. Depression is a common feature in many cases of PMS, and PMS symptoms are typically more severe in depressed women.[1] The cause appears to be a decrease in the brain level of various neurotransmitters, with serotonin and gamma-amino-butyric acid (GABA) being the most significant.[39-41] Use of antidepressant drugs such as Prozac is quickly becoming the dominant medical treatment for PMS.[1] As stated

previously, eighty percent of the twelve million Americans taking Prozac are women between the ages of twenty-five and fifty—the age range with the highest frequency of PMS.

Diet and PMS

Women who suffer from PMS typically have a diet that is even worse than the standard American diet. Guy Abraham, M.D., reports that, compared to symptom-free women, PMS patients consume: 62 percent more refined carbohydrates, 275 percent more refined sugar, 79 percent more dairy products, 78 percent more sodium, 53 percent less iron, 77 percent less manganese, and 52 percent less zinc.[9]

In addition to providing benefits in treating PMS symptoms, the following dietary recommendations provide significant protection against the development of breast cancer, other cancers, heart disease, strokes, osteoporosis, diabetes, and virtually every other chronic degenerative disease.

The seven most important dietary recommendations for relieving PMS are:

1. Follow a vegetarian or predominantly vegetarian diet
2. Reduce your intake of fat
3. Eliminate sugar intake
4. Reduce dietary exposure to environmental estrogens
5. Increase your intake of soy foods
6. Eliminate caffeine consumption
7. Keep your salt intake low

Vegetarian Diet and Estrogen Metabolism

Vegetarian women have been shown to excrete two to three times more estrogen in their feces and have fifty-percent-lower levels of free estrogen in their blood than omnivores.[42,43] These differences are thought to be a result of the lower fat and higher fiber intake of the vegetarian women. These dietary differences also may explain the lower incidence of breast cancer, heart disease, and menopausal symptoms in vegetarian women.

At the very least, eat less saturated fat and cholesterol by reducing or eliminating the amounts of animal products in your diet, and increase consumption of fiber-rich plant foods (fruits, vegetables, grains, and legumes). Limit intake of animal protein sources to 4 to 6 ounces per day, and choose fish, skinless poultry, and lean cuts rather than fat-laden meats.

It appears that many of the effects of a vegetarian diet on lowering circulating estrogen levels are related to a higher intake of dietary fiber. The fiber promotes the excretion of estrogens directly and indirectly by promoting a more favorable bacterial flora with lower levels of beta-glucuronidase activity.

Fat Intake and Estrogen Metabolism

Decreasing the percentage of calories consumed as fat, in particular saturated fat, has dramatic effects on reducing circulating estrogen levels.[44,45] In one study, when seventeen women switched from the standard American Diet (SAD), composed of forty percent of calories as fat and only 12 grams of fiber, to a lowfat, high-fiber diet consisting of twenty-five percent of the calories as fat and 40 grams of fiber daily, there was a thirty-six-percent reduction in blood estrogen levels. Sixteen of the seventeen women demonstrated significant reductions in only eight to ten weeks.[46] A lowfat diet has also been shown to relieve PMS symptoms.[46]

Besides possibly relieving PMS symptoms, another reason to reduce intake of fat is that there is a great deal of research linking a diet high in saturated fat and cholesterol to numerous cancers, heart disease, and strokes. Both the American Cancer Society and the American Heart Association have recommended a diet containing less than thirty percent of calories as fat.

The easiest way for most people to achieve this goal is to eat fewer animal products and more plant foods. With the exception of nuts and seeds, most plant foods are very low in fat. In regard to nuts and seeds, while they do contain high levels of fat calories, the calories are derived largely from polyunsaturated essential fatty acids. It is also important to eliminate the intake of margarine and foods that contain trans-fatty acids and partially hydrogenated oils.

Sugar Intake and PMS

Sugar has several detrimental actions in PMS. First of all, when high-sugar foods are eaten alone, blood sugar levels rise quickly, producing a strain on blood sugar control. Eating foods high in simple sugars can be harmful to blood sugar control—especially if you are hypoglycemic or diabetic. Sugar, particularly when combined with caffeine; also has a detrimental effect on PMS and mood (discussed later in Caffeine). The most significant symptom-producing food in PMS appears to be chocolate.[47]

Another detrimental effect of a high intake of sugar is impaired estrogen metabolism. The evidence is based on the higher frequency of PMS symptoms among women who consume a high-sugar diet, and the fact that a high sugar intake is also associated with higher estrogen levels.[48]

Read food labels carefully for clues on sugar content. If the words sucrose, glucose, maltose, lactose, fructose, corn syrup, or white grape juice concentrate appear on the label, extra sugar has been added.

Environmental Estrogens in Food

Widespread environmental contamination by a group of compounds known as *halogenated hydrocarbons* has occurred. Included in this group are the toxic pesticides DDT, DDE, PCB, PCP, dieldrin, and chlordane. These molecules are hard to break down and are stored in fat cells. These chemicals are known to mimic estrogen in the body and are thought to be a major factor in the growing epidemics of estrogen-related health problems, such as PMS, breast cancer, and low sperm counts.[49,50] Follow the guidelines for lowering the level of pesticides given in A HEALTH-PROMOTING DIET.

The presence of pesticides in fruits and vegetables should not deter you from eating a diet high in these foods. The concentrations in fruits and vegetables is much lower than the levels found in animal fats, meat, cheese, whole milk, and eggs. Furthermore, the various antioxidant components of fruits and vegetables help the body deal with the pesticides.

Soy Foods

Soy and soy foods contain compounds referred to as *phytoestrogens* ("plant estrogens") because they are capable of binding to estrogen receptors. Phytoestrogens are also often called *anti-estrogens* because their estrogenic effect is only two percent as strong as estrogen at the most. However, because of this low activity, phytoestrogens have a balancing action on estrogen effects. If estrogen levels are low (as in menopause), since phytoestrogens have some estrogenic activity, they will cause an increase in estrogen effect. If estrogen levels are high (as in PMS), since phytoestrogens bind to estrogen-receptor sites, thereby competing with estrogen, there will be a decrease in estrogen effects.

Caffeine

Caffeine must be avoided by women who have PMS, especially if anxiety or depression or breast tenderness and fibrocystic breast disease are major symptoms.[51] There is con-

siderable evidence that caffeine consumption is strongly related to the presence and severity of PMS. The effect of caffeine is particularly significant in the psychological symptoms associated with PMS, such as anxiety, irritability, insomnia, and depression. The effect of caffeine on fibrocystic breast disease is discussed in FIBROCYSTIC BREAST DISEASE.

Salt Intake

Excessive salt (sodium chloride) consumption, coupled with diminished dietary potassium, greatly stresses the kidneys' ability to maintain proper fluid volume. As a result some people are "salt-sensitive," in that high salt intake causes high blood pressure or, in other cases, water retention. In general, it is a good idea to avoid salt if you have PMS. If you tend to notice more water retention during the midluteal phase, reducing your salt intake is an absolute must. However, it is not simply a matter of reducing salt intake; you must simultaneously increase your intake of potassium. This is easily done by increasing the intake of high-potassium foods (fresh fruits and vegetables, whole grains, and beans) and avoiding high-sodium foods (most processed foods). Read labels carefully, and keep your total daily sodium intake below 1,800 mg.

Micronutrients and PMS

Although all essential nutrients are critical to good health and for dealing with PMS symptomatology, our discussion in this chapter will focus on the following six key nutrients, followed by some practical recommendations:

- Vitamin B6
- Magnesium
- Calcium
- Zinc
- Vitamin E
- Essential fatty acids

Vitamin B6

The first use of vitamin B6 in the management of women's cyclical conditions was in the successful treatment of depression caused by birth control pills, as noted in several studies in the early 1970s. These results led researchers to try to determine the effectiveness of vitamin B6 in relieving PMS symptoms. Since 1975, there have been at least a dozen double-blind clinical trials.[52,53] The majority of these studies have demonstrated a positive effect. For example, in one double-blind cross-over trial, eighty-four percent of the subjects had a lower symptomatology score during the vitamin B6 treatment period.[54] Although PMS has multiple causes, vitamin B6 supplementation alone appears to benefit most patients.

It is important to note, however, that not all double-blind studies of vitamin B6 have been positive.[52,53] These negative results may have been caused by many factors, such as the inability of some women to convert B6 to its active form due to a deficiency in another nutrient (e.g., vitamin B2 or magnesium) that was not supplemented. These results suggest that supplementing pyridoxine by itself may not result in adequate clinical results for all women suffering this disorder, and that some women may have difficulty converting vitamin B6 into its active form, pyridoxal-5-phosphate. To overcome this conversion difficulty, it may be necessary to use a broader-spectrum nutritional supplement or to use injectable pyridoxal-5-phosphate.

Vitamin B6 Dosage Ranges In most situations, the therapeutic dosage of vitamin B6 is 50 to 100 mg per day. This dosage level is generally regarded as safe, even for long-term use. When using a dosage greater than 50 mg per day, it may be important to divide it into 50-mg doses throughout the day. In one study, a single dosage of 100 mg of pyridoxine did not lead to a significant increase in pyridoxal-5-phosphate levels in the blood, indicating that a 50-mg oral dose of pyridoxine is about all the liver can handle at once.[55]

Safety of Vitamin B6 Vitamin B6 is one of the few water-soluble vitamins that is associated with some toxicity when taken in large or moderate dosages for long periods of time. One-time doses greater than 2,000 mg per day can produce symptoms of nerve toxicity in some individuals (tingling sensations in the feet, loss of muscle coordination, and degeneration of nerve tissue). Chronic intake of more than 500 mg of vitamin B6 per day can be toxic over many months or years.[56]

There are also a few rare reports of toxicity occurring at chronic long-term dosages as low as 150 mg a day.[56–58] The toxicity is thought to result from supplemental pyridoxine overwhelming the liver's ability to add a phosphate group to form the active form of vitamin B6 (pyridoxal-5-phosphate). It is speculated that, as a result, pyridoxine is either toxic to the nerve cells or it actually acts as an antimetabolite by binding to pyridoxal-5-phosphate receptors, thereby creating a relative deficiency of vitamin B6. Again, it appears to make sense to limit doses to 50 mg at a time. If more than 50 mg per day is desired, the doses should be spread throughout the day.

Vitamin B6 and Magnesium Interactions There are extensive interactions between vitamin B6 and magnesium, as they work together in many enzyme systems. In fact, one of the ways in which vitamin B6 may relieve the symptoms of PMS is by increasing the accumulation of magnesium within the cells of the body.[59] In fact, without vitamin B6, magnesium will not get inside the cell.

Magnesium and PMS

Magnesium deficiency is strongly implicated as a causative factor in premenstrual syndrome.[60] Red blood cell magnesium levels in PMS patients have been shown to be significantly lower than in normal subjects.[9,61] As magnesium plays such an integral part in normal cell function, magnesium deficiency may account for the wide range of symptoms attributed to PMS. Furthermore, magnesium deficiency and PMS share many features, and magnesium supplementation has been shown to be an effective treatment for PMS.[62]

A recent study set out to explore the association by trying to answer two important questions: (1) do magnesium measures change as a function of menstrual cycle phase, and (2) do magnesium measures change across the menstrual cycle differentially in PMS patients than in controls? Determinations of serum, red blood cell (RBC) and mononuclear blood cell (MBC) magnesium levels were made in twenty-six women with confirmed PMS and in a control group of nineteen women, during the follicular, ovulatory, early luteal, and late luteal phases of the menstrual cycle.[63] RBC and MBC magnesium levels are far more sensitive and reflective of magnesium levels compared to serum.

The principle findings of the study were as follows: (1) there were no significant differences in serum magnesium levels in PMS patients compared with controls, nor was there a menstrual cycle effect on serum magnesium level in either group; (2) PMS patients had significantly lower RBC and MBC magnesium concentrations compared to controls; (3) these lower RBC and MBC magnesium concentrations were consistent across the menstrual cycle; and (4) magnesium measures did not correlate with the severity of mood symptoms.

The observation of low RBC magnesium concentrations in PMS patients has now been confirmed by four independent studies. The low MBC magnesium concentrations are also consistent with other studies. The role that magnesium plays in PMS symptomatology is multifactorial due to magnesium-critical roles in cellular metabolism. In general, it is thought that women with PMS have a vulnerability to luteal-phase mood state destabilization and that chronic intracellular magnesium depletion is a major predisposing factor toward destabilization.

In addition to emotional instability, magnesium deficiency in PMS is characterized by excessive nervous sensitivity, with generalized aches and pains and a lower premenstrual pain threshold. One clinical trial of magnesium in PMS showed a reduction of nervousness in eighty-nine percent of the subjects, breast tenderness in ninety-six percent, and weight gain in ninety-five percent.[9] In another double-blind study, high-dose magnesium supplementation (360 mg three times per day) was shown to dramatically relieve PMS-related mood changes.[62]

While magnesium has been shown to be effective on its own, even better results may be achieved by combining it with vitamin B6 and other nutrients. Several studies have shown that when PMS patients are given a multivitamin-and-mineral supplement containing high doses of magnesium and pyridoxine, they experience a tremendous reduction in PMS symptoms.[64,65]

Magnesium Dosage Ranges Many nutritional experts feel that the ideal intake for magnesium should be based on body weight (6 mg/2.2 pounds of body weight). For a 110-pound person, the recommendation would be 300 mg, for a 154-pound person 420 mg, and for a 200-pound person 540 mg. Rather than relying on dietary intake to achieve this amount of magnesium, for most people we recommend supplementing the diet with additional magnesium, corresponding to the recommendation of 6 mg per 2.2 pounds of body weight. In the treatment of PMS, a dosage of twice this amount—12 mg per 2.2 pounds of body weight—is appropriate.

Magnesium bound to aspartate or the Krebs-cycle intermediates (malate, succinate, fumarate, or citrate) is preferred over magnesium oxide, gluconate, sulfate, or chloride due to better absorption and fewer side effects (laxative effects).[66,67]

Calcium

Calcium appears to be a double-edged sword in treating PMS. High calcium intake due to high milk consumption is a possible causative factor of PMS, perhaps via the combination of calcium, vitamin D, and phosphorus in milk reducing the absorption of magnesium.[9] At the same time, there are studies that show positive improvements in PMS symptomatology with calcium supplementation (1,000 mg to 1,336 mg).[68,69]

In one of the more recent studies, calcium and manganese supplementation (1,336 mg and 5.6 mg, respectively) improved mood, concentration, and behavior. In another study, 1,000 mg of calcium per day improved mood and lowered water retention.[68] It is theorized, based primarily on animal research, that calcium improves the altered hormonal patterns, neurotransmitter levels, and smooth muscle responsiveness noted in PMS.

Further support for the importance of calcium supplementation in treating PMS was the finding that women with PMS have reduced bone mineral density (based on dual-photon absorptiometry).[70]

Zinc

Zinc levels have been shown to be lower in women who have PMS.[71] Zinc is required for proper action of many body hormones, including sex hormones, as well as in the con-

trol of the secretion of hormones. In particular, zinc serves as one of the control factors for prolactin secretion.[72] Low zinc levels promote prolactin release; high zinc levels inhibit prolactin release. Hence, in high prolactin states zinc supplementation is an absolute must since high prolactin levels have been correlated with the presence of PMS symptoms.

For general health support, the dosage range for zinc supplementation is 15 to 20 mg. Since the average American consumes about 10 mg of zinc per day, supplementing an additional 15 to 20 mg results in a daily intake of 25 to 30 mg for most people. When zinc supplementation is being used to address specific needs, such as elevated prolactin levels in women, the dosage range is 30 to 45 mg per day.

Vitamin E

Although vitamin E research concerning PMS has focused primarily on breast tenderness, significant reduction of other PMS symptomatology has also been demonstrated in double-blind studies.[9,73] Nervous tension, headache, fatigue, depression, and insomnia were all significantly reduced with vitamin E supplementation. In one double-blind study, patients who received vitamin E (400 IU per day) demonstrated a thirty-three-percent reduction in physical symptoms (such as weight gain and breast tenderness), a thirty-eight-percent reduction in anxiety, and a twenty-seven-percent reduction in depression after three months of use. In contrast, the placebo group only reported a fourteen-percent reduction in physical symptoms. The group that took vitamin E also noted higher energy levels, fewer headaches, and less cravings for sweets.

A good dosage for vitamin E is 400 IU per day. Make sure the vitamin E is a natural form. Natural forms of vitamin E are designated d-, as in-d-alpha-tocopherol, while synthetic forms are dl-, as in dl-alpha-tocopherol.

Essential Fatty Acids and PMS

Women with PMS have been shown to exhibit essential-fatty-acid and prostaglandin abnormalities. The abnormality most often reported is a decrease in gamma-linolenic acid (GLA) level.[74] Gamma-linolenic acid is derived from linoleic acid. This conversion requires adequate vitamin B6, magnesium, and zinc levels, as these nutrients function in the key enzyme responsible for this conversion: delta-6-desaturase. Given the fact that deficiency of one or more of these nutrients is common in PMS, decreased GLA levels could almost be expected.

GLA Supplements for PMS Evening primrose, black currant, and borage oil contain GLA, with typical levels being nine percent, twelve percent, and twenty-two percent, respectively. Although these essential-fatty-acid sources are quite popular, the research on GLA supplements is controversial and not as strong as the research on omega-3 oils. In general, given all of the benefits of omega-3 fatty acids, we prefer to recommend flaxseed oil over GLA sources.

The double-blind studies on GLA supplements, such as evening primrose oil, in PMS are largely negative in that they showed no greater benefit over a placebo. A meta-analysis of the clinical trials of evening primrose oil for the treatment of PMS concluded that evening primrose oil is of little value in the management of PMS.[75] The three most well-controlled studies failed to show any beneficial effects for evening primrose oil.[76–78]

A better approach to the essential-fatty-acid and prostaglandin abnormalities of PMS may be to provide the necessary nutrients required for proper essential-fatty-acid metab-olism, along with providing adequate levels of essential fatty acids.

Practical Recommendations for Supplementation

There are three primary practical recommendations for nutritional supplementation in PMS:

1. Take a high-quality multiple-vitamin-and-mineral supplement that provides adequate levels of vitamin B6 and magnesium.
2. Take additional antioxidants.
3. Take one tablespoon of flaxseed oil daily.

Multiple-Vitamin-and-Mineral Supplements in PMS Taking a high-quality multiple-vitamin-and-mineral supplement that provides all of the known vitamins and minerals serves as a foundation upon which to build. For women who have PMS, there are two very sound reasons for taking a high-potency multiple:

1. Nutritional deficiency is relatively common among women with PMS.
2. High-potency multiple-vitamin-and-mineral formulations have been shown to produce significant benefits in cases of PMS.

When compared to normal women, the frequency of nutritional supplementation and the calculated intake of selected nutrients by PMS patients has been shown to be much lower. Although women with PMS have been shown to consume vitamins in their food at levels that are close to the Recommended Dietary Allowance, compared to women who did not have PMS, their intake levels were only 2.2 percent as much for thiamin, 2.2 percent for riboflavin, 16.7 percent for niacin, 8.7 percent for pantothenic acid, and 2.7 percent for pyridoxine.[9]

Several double-blind studies have shown that PMS patients who are given a multivitamin-and-mineral supplement that contains high doses of magnesium and pyridoxine typically experience at least a seventy-percent reduction in both pre- and post-menstrual symptoms.[64,65]

Herbal Recommendations for PMS

Although a wide variety of herbs have been used in folk medicine for the many disorders of menstruation, and many have been evaluated for their phytoestrogen effects, few have been specifically evaluated for their efficacy in relieving premenstrual symptoms. The herbs that are most likely to be useful are probably those which exhibit a tonic effect on the female glandular system. This tonic effect is thought to be a result of phytoestrogens or other compounds that help improve the hormonal balance of the female system, as well as the plant's ability to improve blood flow to the female organs.

Because of the balancing action of phytoestrogens on estrogen effects (see Soy Foods, earlier in this chapter, for a description), it is common to find the same plant recommended for conditions of estrogen excess (like PMS) as well as conditions of estrogen deficiency (like menopause, menstrual abnormalities). Many of these herbs have been termed "uterine tonics" because they work to nourish and tone the female glandular and organ system rather than exert a drug-like effect. This nonspecific mode of action makes many herbs useful in treating a broad range of female conditions, including PMS.

The four most useful herbs in the treatment of PMS and related symptoms (as well as menopause) are angelica or Dong quai (*Angelica sinensis*), licorice root (*Glycyrrhiza glabra*), black cohosh (*Cimicifuga racemosa*), and chasteberry (*Vitex agnus-castus*). These herbs have been used historically to lessen a variety of female complaints including hot flashes.

Angelica or Dong Quai

In Asia, angelica's reputation is perhaps second only to that of ginseng. Predominantly regarded as a "female" remedy, angelica has been used to treat menopausal symptoms (especially hot flashes), as well as such conditions as *dysmenorrhea* (painful menstruation), *amenorrhea* (absence of menstruation), and *metrorrhagia* (abnormal menstruation), and to assure a healthy pregnancy and easy delivery.

Angelica has demonstrated good uterine tonic activity, causing an initial increase in uterine contraction followed by relaxation.[79] In addition, administration of angelica to mice resulted in an increase of uterine weight and increase of glucose utilization by the liver and uterus.[80] These effects reflect phytoestrogenic activities. Angelica is particularly helpful if, in addition to PMS, a woman experiences painful menstruation (dysmenorrhea).

When using angelica to treat PMS, we generally recommend that it be taken beginning on day fourteen and continued until menstruation begins. However, if the woman typically experiences dysmenorrhea we recommend that angelica be continued until menstruation has stopped. One of the following may be taken three times per day:

- Powdered root or as tea: 1–2 g
- Tincture (1:5): 4 ml (1 tsp)
- Fluid extract: 1 ml (¼ tsp)

Licorice Root

The medicinal use of licorice in both Western and Eastern cultures dates back several thousand years. In addition to being used to treat a variety of female disorders, it was used primarily as an expectorant and antitussive in respiratory tract infections and asthma. Its other traditional uses include treating peptic ulcers, malaria, abdominal pain, insomnia, and infections. Many of these uses have been substantiated by modern research.

Licorice is particularly useful in treating PMS, as it is believed to lower estrogen levels while raising progesterone levels.[81,82] It raises progesterone levels by inhibiting the enzyme responsible for breaking down progesterone. Licorice is also useful in reducing water retention by blocking the hormone aldosterone. Remember, the adrenal hormone aldosterone is responsible for reducing sodium excretion and, as a result, leads to water retention (edema).

Licorice works to block the effects of aldosterone in much the way it impacts estrogen.[83,84] Its chief component, glycyrrhetinic acid, binds to aldosterone receptors but its activity is only about one-fourth as strong as the body's own aldosterone. This lower level of activity means that, in cases of high aldosterone levels (such as occur often in PMS), licorice may actually reduce the aldosterone effect by competing with aldosterone for binding sites. If aldosterone levels are normal, the chronic ingestion of licorice in large doses may cause symptoms of aldosterone excess, namely high blood pressure due to sodium and water retention.

Prevention of the side effects of glycyrrhizin may be possible by following a high-potassium, low-sodium diet. Although no formal trial has been performed, patients who normally consume high-potassium foods and restrict sodium intake—even those who have high blood pressure and angina—have been reported to be free from the aldosterone-like side effects of glycyrrhizin.[85] Licorice should probably not be used by patients who have a history of hypertension, renal failure, or current use of digitalis preparations.

For PMS, start taking licorice on day fourteen of the cycle and continue till menstruation. Here are dosage recommendations for the various forms of licorice, to be taken three times per day:

- Powdered root or as tea: 1–2 g
- Fluid extract (1:1): 4 ml (1 tsp)
- Solid (dry powdered) extract (4:1): 250–500 mg

Black Cohosh

Black cohosh was widely used by the American Indians and later by American colonists for the relief of menstrual cramps and menopause. Remifemin is a special extract of black cohosh standardized to contain 1 mg of triterpenes (calculated as 1 mg 27-deoxyacteine per tablet) that has been used in Germany for over forty years. Recent scientific investigation of Remifemin has shown that it is a safe and effective natural alternative to hormone replacement therapy in the treatment of menopause and that it may offer some benefits in treating PMS as well. In one study of 135 women, Remifemin was judged to have "performed very well" in treating PMS, in that it reduced feelings of depression, anxiety, tension, and mood swings.[86]

The usual dosage for menopause is two tablets twice per day (4 mg 27-deoxyacteine daily). For PMS the dosage is much less: one tablet once or twice per day.

Chasteberries

The chaste tree (*Vitex agnus-castus*) is native to the Mediterranean. Its berries have long been used for treating female complaints. As its name signifies, chasteberries were used in suppressing the libido.

While Remifemin is the more popular herbal approach to treating menopausal symptoms in Germany, chasteberry extract is probably their most popular herbal approach to PMS. In two surveys of gynecological practices in Germany, physicians graded chasteberry extract as good or very good in the treatment of PMS. More than 1,500 women participated in studies of chasteberry.[87,88] One-third of the women experienced complete resolution of their symptoms, while another fifty-seven percent reported significant improvement; ninety percent reported improvement or resolution.

Chasteberry extract appears to be particularly useful in cases of corpus luteum insufficiency or prolactin excess.[89] It appears that its beneficial effects on PMS and these other conditions are related to altering gonadotropin-releasing hormone (GnRH) and follicle-stimulating-hormone-releasing hormone (FSH-RH). In other words, it appears that chasteberry extract has profound effects on the hypothalamus and on pituitary function. As a result, it is able to normalize the secretion of other hormones; for example, it reduces the secretion of prolactin and lowers the estrogen-to-progesterone ratio.

Chasteberry extract may be useful in certain cases of amenorrhea (absence of menstruation) due to prolactin excess—one of the most frequent causes of amenorrhea. Don't expect immediate results; it takes about three months for chasteberry extract to kick in to lower prolactin levels.[89]

The usual dosage of chasteberry extract (often standardized to contain 0.5 percent agnuside) in tablet or capsule form is 175 to 225 mg per day. If you are using the liquid extract, the typical dosage is 2 ml per day.

TREATMENT SUMMARY

Here are the important steps to take to help you prioritize and implement the various measures detailed above:

1. Evaluate your PMS symptoms by completing the questionnaire in this chapter.

2. Rule out hypothyroidism and/or depression. Determine your basal body temperature (discussed in HYPOTHYROIDISM). If your basal body temperature is below 97.8 degrees Fahrenheit, or if you are suffering from other symptoms associated with PMS, consult your physician for complete thyroid-function testing. Determine whether depression may be a factor by taking the self-test in the DEPRESSION chapter. If it is, follow the recommendations given in that chapter.

3. Begin following the dietary recommendations for PMS:

- Follow a vegetarian or predominantly vegetarian diet
- Reduce your intake of fat
- Eliminate sugar intake
- Reduce exposure to environmental estrogens in foods
- Increase your intake of soy foods
- Eliminate caffeine intake
- Keep salt intake low

4. Follow the guidelines for nutritional supplementation given in this chapter.

5. Select the appropriate herbal support:

- If you have PMS-associated breast pain, infrequent periods, or a history of ovarian cysts, take chasteberry extract [Take one of the following forms daily: fluid extract, 2 ml; dry powdered extract (0.5% agnuside content), 175 to 225 mg)]

- If you typically experience menstrual cramps, take angelica (dong quai) [One of the following forms can be taken three times per day: powdered root or as tea, 1–2 g; tincture (1:5), 4 ml (1 tsp); fluid extract, 1 ml ($^1/_4$ tsp)]

- If you are bothered by PMS water retention, take licorice [One of the following forms can be taken three times per day: powdered root or as tea, 1–2 grams; fluid extract (1:1), 4 ml (1 tsp); solid (dry powdered) extract (4:1), 250–500]

- If you suffer from uterine fibroids, take black cohosh extract at a dosage based on the level of 27-deoxyacteine (1 mg twice daily)

6. Follow the techniques for stress reduction given in STRESS MANAGEMENT, and get regular exercise.

7. If, after at least three complete menstrual periods, you are not experiencing a significant improvement or complete resolution of symptoms, further support is indicated. Our best recommendation is to consult a physician who is familiar with nutritional therapies for PMS. The physician should help you in identifying possible causative factors and more effective treatment strategies tailored specifically for your case.

Prostate Enlargement

. . . .

Symptoms of bladder outlet obstruction (progressive urinary frequency, urgency and nocturia, hesitancy and intermittency with reduced force and caliber of urine)

Enlarged, nontender prostate gland

Uremia if prolonged obstruction

The prostate is a single, doughnut-shaped gland about the size of a walnut that lies below the bladder and surrounds the urethra. The prostate secretes a thin, milky, alkaline fluid that increases sperm motility and lubricates the urethra to prevent infection. Prostate secretions are extremely important to successful fertilization of the egg.

Benign (nonmalignant) enlargement of the prostate gland is known medically as *benign prostatic hyperplasia,* or BPH for short. Because an enlarged prostate can pinch off the flow of urine, BPH is characterized by symptoms of bladder obstruction, such as increased urinary frequency, nighttime awakening to empty the bladder, and reduced force and caliber (speed of flow) of urination.

WARNING: Prostate Disorders Can Only Be Diagnosed by a Physician. Do Not Self-Diagnose. If You Are Experiencing Any Symptoms Associated with BPH or Prostate Cancer, See Your Physician Immediately for Proper Diagnosis.

BPH is an extremely common condition. Current estimates are that it affects over fifty percent of men during their lifetime. The actual frequency increases with advancing age, from approximately five to ten percent at age thirty to over ninety percent in men over eighty-five years of age.[1]

Diagnosing BPH

It is often recommended that men over the age of forty have yearly prostate exams. This exam is not high-tech. It simply involves a doctor inserting a gloved finger into the rectum and feeling the lower part of the prostate for any abnormality. However, in the case of BPH, often the prostate has not enlarged to a point that can be recognized by physical exam. And, in the case of cancer, a digital exam is not reliable enough.

The classic enlarged prostate due to BPH will usually feel softer (boggy) than normal and may be two to three times larger than normal. In BPH, the prostate is not tender; this differentiates it from prostatitis. The classic finding in prostatic cancer is that the prostate feels much harder and its border is not as well-defined as that of a healthy prostate.

The definitive diagnosis of BPH can be made with the aid of ultrasound measurements. However, because the symptoms of BPH and prostate cancer can be similar, a simple blood test is used to differentiate BPH from the more serious prostate cancer. The blood test measures the levels of a protein that is produced in the prostate: prostate-specific antigen (PSA). The PSA test is regarded as a highly significant and sensitive marker for prostate cancer. The normal value for PSA is less than 4 nanograms per milliliter. A level above 10 ng/ml is highly indicative of prostate cancer.

There has been concern that the use of PSA as a screening test for prostate cancer is not reliable enough. Although an elevated level of prostate-specific antigen indicates prostate cancer about ninety percent of the time, it must be kept in mind that midrange elevations in PSA can be caused by BPH, and that in some instances there may be prostate cancer yet PSA levels are not elevated. Despite the fact that this test is not perfect, it is a simple, relatively noninvasive test that can provide valuable information. PSA screening has been endorsed by the American Cancer Society, the American Urological Association, and other physicians' groups.

If you are a man over the age of fifty, and if any of your immediate relatives—father, brother, or uncle—has had prostate cancer, an annual prostate exam and PSA test are a very good idea.

Hormonal Factors in BPH

BPH is largely the result of hormonal changes associated with aging. It is clearly dependent on the actions of male hormones (androgens) within the prostate gland. These changes within the prostate reflect the many significant changes in both male (androgen), female (estrogen), and pituitary hormone levels in aging men. Levels of the main male sex hormone testosterone (T) decrease with advancing age, but estrogen, prolactin, LH, and FSH levels are all increased. The ultimate effect of these changes is that there is an increased concentration of testosterone within the prostate gland and an increased conver-

. . . .

QUICK REVIEW

- Over fifty percent of men will develop an enlarged prostate in their lifetime.
- BPH is largely the result of hormonal changes associated with aging.
- The PSA test can help distinguish BPH from prostate cancer.
- Paramount to an effective BPH treatment plan is adequate zinc intake and absorption.

- Cholesterol damaged by free radicals is particularly toxic and carcinogenic to the prostate.
- Increased consumption of soy and soy foods is associated with a decrease in the risk of getting prostate cancer and may help in treating BPH.
- In Europe, plant-based medicines are the most popular prescriptions for BPH.

sion of this testosterone to an even more potent form known as *dihydrotestosterone* (DHT). The increase in levels of testosterone and DHT is largely due to a decreased rate of removal combined with an increase in the activity of the enzyme 5-alpha-reductase, which converts testosterone to DHT.[2] Elevated estrogen levels are thought to be the key factor that inhibits the elimination of DHT from the prostate gland in cases of BPH.

Therapeutic Considerations

If left untreated, BPH will eventually obstruct the bladder outlet, resulting in the retention of urine and eventually kidney damage. As this situation is potentially life-threatening, proper treatment is crucial. In the past, medical treatment involved a procedure known as a TURP (trans-urethral resection of the prostate). Because this surgery is associated with a high death rate and will often make matters worse, it should be avoided unless there are no viable alternatives.

Dietary Factors

Diet appears to play a critical role in the health of the prostate gland. It is particularly important to avoid pesticides, increase intake of zinc and essential fatty acids, and keep cholesterol levels below 200 mg/dl.

High-Protein Diet

A high-protein diet (total calories: forty-four percent protein, thirty-five percent carbohydrate, twenty-one percent fat) inhibits 5-alpha-reductase (the enzyme that converts testosterone to DHT), while a low-protein diet (ten percent protein, seventy percent carbohydrate, and twenty percent fat) stimulates the enzyme.[3] Since a high-protein diet has not actually been used in the treatment of men with BPH, its use is speculative but may be worth a try.

Zinc

Adequate zinc intake and absorption are paramount to an effective BPH treatment plan. In studies conducted in the 1970s, zinc supplementation was shown to reduce the size of the prostate and to diminish symptoms in the majority of patients.[4,5] The clinical effectiveness

- Saw palmetto extract and other herbal approaches to BPH are most effective in mild to moderate cases.
- Roughly ninety percent of men with mild-to-moderate BPH experience some improvement in symptoms during the first four to six weeks after beginning to take saw palmetto extract.
- Severe BPH, resulting in significant acute urinary retention, may require catheterization for relief; a sufficiently advanced case may not respond to therapy rapidly enough and may require the short-term use of an alpha-1 antagonist drug (e.g., Hytrin or Cordura) or surgical intervention.

of zinc is probably due to its critical involvement in many aspects of hormone metabolism. Intestinal uptake of zinc is impaired by estrogens, but enhanced by androgens. Since estrogen levels are increased in men with BPH, zinc uptake may be low.

Zinc has been shown to inhibit the activity of 5-alpha-reductase, the enzyme that irreversibly converts T to DHT.[6–10] Zinc also inhibits specific binding of androgens to the cytosol and nuclear androgen receptors. These effects imply zinc supplementation may be helpful in BPH.

Zinc has also been shown to inhibit prolactin secretion by the pituitary.[11,12] The hormone prolactin has been shown to increase the uptake of testosterone by the prostate, thereby leading to increased levels of DHT.[12] Drugs like bromocriptine that inhibit the release of prolactin have been shown to reduce many of the symptoms of prostatic hyperplasia. However, these drugs have severe side effects and are of limited value.[13] Beer (but not pure alcohol), tryptophan, and stress all increase prolactin secretion and may therefore be aggravating factors.[14,15]

Alcohol

While only beer raises prolactin levels, and other sources of alcohol do not (it is the hops in the beer that raise prolactin levels), higher alcohol intake of any type is definitely associated with BPH. In a seventeen-year study of 6,581 men in Hawaii, it was noted that intake of at least 25 ounces of alcohol per month was directly correlated with the diagnosis of BPH.[16] The association was most significant for beer, wine, and sake, and less so for distilled spirits.

Essential Fatty Acids

The administration of an essential fatty acids (EFAs) complex has resulted in significant improvement for many BPH patients.[17] All nineteen subjects in an uncontrolled study showed diminution of residual urine, with twelve of the nineteen having no residual urine by the end of several weeks of treatment. These effects appear to be due to the correction of an underlying EFA deficiency, since these patients' prostatic and seminal lipid levels and ratios are often abnormal.[18,19]

Amino Acids

The combination of the amino acids glycine, alanine, and glutamic acid (in the form of two 390-mg capsules administered three times daily for two weeks and one capsule three times daily thereafter) has been shown in several studies to relieve many of the symptoms of BPH. In a controlled study of forty-five men, increased nighttime urination (nocturia) was relieved or reduced in ninety-five percent, urgency reduced in eighty-one percent, frequency reduced in seventy-three percent, and delayed urination alleviated in seventy percent.[20] These results have also been reported in other controlled studies.[21] The mechanism of action is unknown, but is probably related to the amino acids acting as inhibitory neurotransmitters and reducing the feelings of a full bladder. In other words, amino acid therapy only helps with the symptoms.

Cholesterol

Cholesterol damaged by free radicals is particularly toxic and carcinogenic to the prostate. Damaged forms of cholesterol are thought to play a role in stimulating prostrate cell formation in BPH. Drugs that lower cholesterol levels have been shown to have a favorable influence on BPH.[22] Every effort should be made to decrease cholesterol levels by utilizing the principles outlined in CHOLESTEROL.

Soy

Soybeans are especially rich in phytosterols (plant compounds that resemble cholesterol in structure), especially beta-sitosterol. The cholesterol-lowering effects of phytosterols are well documented.[23] Phytosterols have also been shown to relieve BPH. The latest double-blind study consisted of two hundred men who received beta-sitosterol (20 mg) or a placebo three times daily.[24] The beta-sitosterol produced an increase in maximum urine flow rate (a good indicator of bladder obstruction) from a baseline of 9.9 ml/second to 15.2 ml/second and a decrease in the amount of urine left in the bladder after urination from 65.8 to 30.4 ml. No changes were observed in the placebo group. A $3^{1}/_{2}$-ounce serving of soybeans, tofu, or other soy food provides approximately 90 mg of beta-sitosterol.

Increased consumption of soy and soy foods is associated with a decrease in the risk of getting prostate cancer.[25] Much of this protection is due to the isoflavonoids genistein and daidzein, the phytoestrogens of soy.[25,26] In addition to acting on estrogen receptors, these compounds inhibit 5-alpha-reductase. Obviously, this action could have beneficial effects in the treatment of BPH.

Drugs and Pesticides

The diet should be as free as possible of pesticides and other contaminants, since many of these compounds (e.g., dioxin, polyhalogenated biphenyls, hexachlorobenzene, and dibenzofurans) increase 5-alpha-reduction of steroids.[3]

Cadmium

Although cadmium is a known antagonist of zinc and increases the activity of 5-alpha-reductase, its concentration in, and effects on, the prostate are unclear. Several studies have produced conflicting results.[27,28] A major source of cadmium is cigarette smoke.

Botanicals

According to a recent review article published in the *British Journal of Urology*, plant-based medicines are much more popular prescriptions in Europe than their synthetic counterparts.[29] Specifically, in Germany and Austria botanical medicines are considered first-line treatments for BPH; they account for more than ninety percent of all drugs used in the medical management of BPH. In Italy, plant extracts account for roughly fifty percent of all medications prescribed for BPH, while alpha-blockers and 5-alpha-reductase-inhibitors account for only 5.1 percent and 4.8 percent, respectively.[29-31]

There are about thirty different plant-based compounds currently available in Europe for the treatment of BPH. At least fifteen of them contain *Serenoa repens* (saw palmetto) extract. Other popular botanical medicines include *Pygeum Africanum*, *Urtica dioca* (stinging nettle), and Cernilton, a special flower pollen extract. Based on careful examination of the published literature, we would rate the relative effectiveness of these agents as follows: serenoa > Cernilton > pygeum > urtica. However, in certain situations one herbal approach may be more effective than another. In other words, even though we rate urtica lowest, in some cases urtica may produce better results than serenoa. Each plant has a slightly different mechanism of action.

The chance of clinical success with any of the botanical treatments of BPH appears to be determined by the degree of obstruction, as indicated by the residual urine content. For levels below 50 ml, the results are usually excellent. For levels between 50 and 100 ml, the results are usually quite good. For residual urine levels between 100 and 150 ml, it will be tougher to produce significant improvements in the customary four- to six-week period. If the residual urine content is greater than 150 ml, saw palmetto extract and other botanical medicines are not likely to produce any significant improvement.

Serenoa repens (Saw palmetto)

The fat-soluble extract of the fruit of the saw palmetto tree (also known as *Sabal serrulata*), native to Florida, has been shown to significantly diminish the signs and symptoms of BPH in numerous clinical studies (see Table 1). The mechanism of action is related to inhibition of DHT binding to cellular receptors, inhibition of 5-alpha-reductase, and interfering with prostate estrogen receptors. As a result of these effects, excellent results have been produced in numerous clinical studies. In summary, roughly ninety percent of men who have mild to moderate BPH experience some improvement in

TABLE 1	Clinical Studies Demonstrating Efficacy of *Serenoa repens* Extract*			
AUTHORS	**TYPE OF STUDY**	**# OF PATIENTS**	**LENGTH OF STUDY**	**SIGNIFICANT DIFFERENCE IN:**
Boccafoschi et al.[32]	DB** vs placebo	22	60 days	volume voided, max. flow, mean flow, dysuria, nocturia
Cirillo et al.[33]	Open	47	4 months	dysuria, nocturia, urine flow
Tripodi et al.[34]	Open	40	30–90 days	dysuria, nocturia, volume of prostate, voiding rate, residual urine
Emili et al.[35]	DB vs placebo	30	30 days	number of voided, strangury, max. and mean urine flow, residual urine
Greca et al.[36]	Open	14	1–2 months	dysuria, perineal heaviness, nocturia, volume of urine per voiding, interval between two diurnal voidings, sensation of incomplete voiding
Duvia et al.[37]	DB vs Pygeum	30	30 days	voiding rate
Tasca et al.[38]	DB vs placebo	30	31–90 days	frequency, urine flow measurement
Cukier et al.[39]	DB vs placebo	168	60–90 days	dysuria, frequency, residual urine
Crimi et al.[40]	Open	32	4 weeks	dysuria, nocturia, volume of prostate, voiding rate
Champault et al.[41]	DB vs placebo	168	60–90 days	objective and subjective parameters
Champault et al.[42]	DB vs placebo	110	28 days	dysuria, nocturia, flow measurement, residual urine
Mattei et al.[43]	DB vs placebo	40	3 months	dysuria, nocturia, residual urine
Braeckman[44]	Open	305	3 months	maximum urine flow, prostate volume, and international prostate score

*Eighty-five to ninety-five percent fatty acids and sterols at a dosage of 320 mg daily
**DB = double-blind

symptoms during the first four to six weeks of therapy. All major symptoms of BPH have been relieved, especially nocturia.[32–45]

Although saw palmetto extract has shown excellent results in numerous clinical trials, results from a recent study are perhaps the most revealing.[44] In this study, 305 men were given a dosage of 160 mg of the saw palmetto extract twice daily, standardized to contain eighty-five to ninety-five percent fatty acids and sterols. After forty-five days, eighty-three percent of the participants estimated that the drug was effective. After ninety days, the percentage increased to eighty-eight percent. Similarly, global evaluations made by physicians after forty-five and ninety days demonstrated eighty-one percent and eighty-eight percent effectiveness, respectively. The objective evaluations demonstrated remarkable improvements in all measurements. Maximum urinary flow (ml/s) increased from 9.8 to 12.2, mean urinary flow rate (ml/s) increased from 5.8 to 7.4, prostate volume (mm^3) decreased from 40,348 to 36,246, and the international prostate symptom score decreased from 19.0 to 12.4. No serious adverse reactions were reported.

While these results are impressive, perhaps the most interesting changes occurred in the quality-of-life scores, as shown in Table 2.

These improvements in quality-of-life scores demonstrate just how powerful an effect improving bothersome symptoms such as nocturia can have on an individual's mental outlook. Many men who suffer from an enlarged prostate suffer from sleep deprivation. Improving sleep by reducing the number of awakenings for nighttime urination is thought to be the major reason for the improvement in quality-of-life scores with saw palmetto extract. Another important finding from this study was that the saw palmetto extract had no demonstrable effect on serum prostate-specific antigen (PSA) levels.

While the drug finasteride (Proscar) typically takes up to a year to produce significant benefits, saw palmetto extract produces better results in a much shorter period of time. Most patients achieve some relief of symptoms within the first thirty days of treatment with the saw palmetto extract (see Table 3).

Cernilton

Cernilton, an extract of flower pollen, has been used in Europe to treat prostatitis and BPH for more than thirty-five years.[46] It has also been shown to be quite effective in the treatment of BPH in several double-blind clinical studies.[31,32] The overall success rate of Cernilton in patients with BPH is about seventy percent.[47] Patients who respond typically have reductions of nocturia and diurnal frequency of around seventy percent, as well as significant reductions in residual urine volume.[48] The extract has been shown to exert some anti-inflammatory action and to produce a contractile effect on the bladder while relaxing the urethra. In addition, Cernilton contains a substance that inhibits the growth of prostate cells.[49]

In the most recent study, the clinical efficacy of Cernilton in the treatment of symptomatic BPH was examined over a one-year period.[46] Seventy-nine males of an average age of sixty-eight years (ages sixty-two to eighty-nine), with a mean baseline prostatic volume of 33.2 cm^3, were given 63 mg of

TABLE 2	Quality-of-Life Scores with Saw Palmetto Treatment	
EVALUATION	**DAY 0**	**DAY 90**
Delighted	0.6%	5.4%
Happy	2.3%	24.0%
Satisfied	9.7%	36.8%
Mitigated	22.7%	20.9%
Unsatisfied	43.8%	9.5%
Unhappy	18.5%	2.4%
Hopeless	2.3%	1.0%

**TABLE 3   Saw Palmetto Extract vs. Finasteride
Effects on Urine Flow Rate (ml/sec): Pooled Data from Double-Blind Studies**

TIME FRAME	SAW PALMETTO EXTRACT	FINASTERIDE
Initial measurement	9.53	9.6
3 months	13.15*	10.4
12 months	**	11.2
% increase	38% in three months	16% in 12 months

*Many studies on saw palmetto extract lasted fewer than ninety days; final measurements were calculated as ninety-day measurements.
**There are few long-term studies on saw palmetto extract, yet the effect at three months (or less) are obviously superior to those of Proscar.

Cernilton pollen extract twice daily for twelve weeks. Tables 4 and 5 summarize the results.

Overall, eighty-five percent of the test subjects experienced benefit: eleven percent reporting "excellent," thirty-nine percent reporting "good," thirty-five percent reporting "satisfactory," and fifteen percent reporting "poor" as a description of their outcome.

Pygeum Africanum
Pygeum is an evergreen tree native to Africa. Its bark has historically been used in the treatment of urinary tract disorders. The major active components of the bark are fat-soluble sterols and fatty acids. Virtually all of the research on pygeum has featured a pygeum extract standardized to contain fourteen-percent triterpenes, including beta-sitosterol and 0.5-percent n-docosanol. This extract has been extensively studied both in experimental animal studies and clinical trials in humans.[50]

Numerous clinical trials in over six hundred patients have demonstrated pygeum extract to be effective in reducing the symptoms and clinical signs of BPH, especially in early cases.[51-74] However, in a double-blind study that compared the pygeum extract with

TABLE 4   Improvements in Urine Flow with Cernilton

MEASURE	AT BASELINE	AT TWELVE WEEKS
Avg. urine max. flow rate	5.1 ml/s	6.0 ml/s
Avg. flow rate	9.3 ml/s	11 ml/s
Residual urine vol.	54.2 ml	< 30 ml

TABLE 5   Clinical Efficacy of Cernilton Based on Symptoms

SYMPTOM	% IMPROVEMENT
Urgency or discomfort	76.9
Incomplete emptying	66.2
Prolonged voiding	64.1
Delayed voiding	62.2
Intermittency	60.6
Nocturia	56.8
Postvoid dribbling	42.7

TABLE 6 Results with *Pygeum-Africanum* in BPH

				PERCENT OF PATIENTS SHOWING REDUCTION				
AUTHOR	MG/DAY	DAYS	# PATIENTS	DYSURIA	NOCTURIA	FREQUENCY	RES. URINE	PROS. VOL.
Open Trials								
Guillemin[51]	100	30	25	80%	80%	80%	80%	NC
Lange[52]	100	30	25	72%	NC	72%	NC	NC
Wemeau[53]	100	45	27	60%	NC	71%	NC	NC
Violler[54]	75	60	20	64%	NC	64%	NC	NC
Lhez[55]	75	90	52	69%	NC	NC	NC	NC
Thomas[56]	75	50	33	60%	57%	57%	NC	—
Huet[57]	50	30	55	85%	85%	85%	NC	20%
Rometti[58]	100	50	25	72%	72%	72%	NC	25%
Gallizia[59]	100	60	19	90%	85%	70%	20%	NC
Durval[60]	100	90	23	72%	72%	72%	72%	NC
Pansadoro[61]	75	90	35	94%	94%	94%	94%	—
Double-Blind Trials								
Maver[62]	100	60	60	77%	70%	57%	23%	—
Bongi[63]	75	60	50	88%	88%	88%	88%	88%
Doremieuz[64]	100	60	77	85%	NC	NC	NC	NC
Del Valio[65]	100	60	30	—	—	48%	—	—
Colpi[66]	150	45	47	—	70%	—	76%	NC
Donkervoort[67]	150	90	20	80%	80%	80%	NC	NC
Dufour[68]	100	45	120	—	78%	45%	65%	NC
Legromandi[69]	100	45	104	89%	89%	89%	NC	NC
Ranna[70]	200	60	39	75%	75%	75%	NC	NC
Frasseto[71]	200	60	20	—	—	—	—	—
Bassi[72]	200	60	40	70%	70%	70%	70%	70%

— = Not Measured
NC = No change

the extract of saw palmetto, the saw palmetto extract produced a greater reduction of symptoms and was better tolerated.[75] In addition, the effects on objective parameters, especially urine flow rate and residual urine content, were better in the clinical studies using saw palmetto.

However, there may be circumstances in which pygeum is more effective than saw palmetto. For example, saw palmetto has not been shown to produce some of the effects on prostate secretion that pygeum has produced. Of course, as the two extracts have somewhat overlapping mechanisms of actions, they can be used in combination.

Stinging nettle (*Urtica dioca*)
Extracts of stinging nettle have also been shown to be effective in the treatment of BPH. Fewer studies have been done with

stinging nettle extract than with the other botanical medicines discussed. Two double-blind studies have shown it to be more effective than a placebo.[74,75] However, like pygeum, the results with urtica are less impressive than those with saw palmetto extract (or Cernilton). Like the extract of *Serenoa repens*, urtica extracts appear to interact with binding of DHT to cytosolic and nuclear receptors.[76]

TREATMENT SUMMARY

Therapeutic goals for BPH are to normalize prostate nutrient levels, inhibit excessive conversion of testosterone to DHT, inhibit DHT receptor binding, and limit prolactin, which promotes prostate cell growth.

Severe BPH, resulting in significant acute urinary retention, may require catheterization for relief; a sufficiently advanced case may not respond rapidly enough to therapy and may require the short-term use of an alpha-1 antagonist drug (e.g., Hytrin or Cordura) or surgical intervention.

Diet

Since there have been no clinical trials on the use of diet in the treatment of BPH, the following recommendations are somewhat speculative. The diet should be high in protein, low in carbohydrates, low in animal fats, and high in essential fatty acids. Focus on whole, unprocessed foods (whole grains, legumes, vegetables, fruits, nuts, and seeds). Eat a quarter-cup of raw sunflower seeds or pumpkin seeds each day. Eliminate intake of alcohol (especially beer), caffeine, and sugar. Consume soy foods regularly.

Nutritional Supplements

- Zinc: 45–60 mg per day
- Flaxseed oil: 1 tbsp per day
- Amino acid mixture:
  Glycine: 200 mg per day
  Glutamic acid: 200 mg per day
  Alanine: 200 mg per day

Botanical Medicines

- Saw palmetto (*Serenoa repens*) extract (standardized to contain 85–95% fatty acids and sterols): 160 mg twice per day (NOTE: A similar dose using crude berries, fluid extracts, and tinctures would require extremely large quantities and is not reliable. Use the standardized extract for maximum benefit).
- Flower pollen extract (e.g., Cernilton): 63–126 mg two to three times per day
- *Pygeum Africanum* extract (standardized to contain 14% triterpenes including beta-sitosterol and 0.5% n-docosanol): 50–100 mg twice per day
- Stinging nettle (*Urtica dioica*) extract: 300–600 mg per day

Psoriasis

Sharply bordered reddened rash or plaques covered with overlapping silvery scales

Characteristic locations: the scalp; the backside of the wrists, elbows, knees, buttocks, and ankles; and sites of repeated trauma

Family history in fifty percent of cases

Nail involvement results in characteristic "oil drop" stippling (thimble-like appearance)

Possible arthritis

Psoriasis is an extremely common skin disorder. In the United States, it occurs in two to four percent of the population. Psoriasis affects mainly Caucasians. It affects few blacks in tropical zones, but is more common among blacks in temperate zones. It appears commonly among Japanese, but is rare in American Indians. Psoriasis affects men and women equally, and the mean onset is 27.8 years of age, although two percent show onset by two years of age.

In addition to affecting the skin, psoriasis can cause an inflammatory form of arthritis and affect the nails. The nails take on a characteristic thimble-like appearance referred to as "oil drop" stippling.

Causes

Psoriasis is caused by a pileup of skin cells that have replicated too rapidly. The rate at which skin cells divide in psoriasis is roughly one thousand times greater than in normal skin. This high rate of replication is simply too fast for the cells to be shed, so they accumulate, resulting in the characteristic silvery scale of psoriasis.

Psoriasis is the result of a basic defect that lies within the skin cells. The frequency of psoriasis is increased in people with certain genetic markers, reflecting a possible genetic error in the control over how skin cells divide. The genetic link is also confirmed by the observation that thirty-six percent of psoriasis patients have one or more family members with psoriasis.

The rate at which cells divide is controlled by a delicate balance between two internal control compounds: cyclic adenosine monophosphate (AMP) and cyclic guanidine monophosphate (GMP). Increased levels of cyclic GMP (cGMP) are associated with increased cell proliferation; conversely, increased levels of cyclic AMP (cAMP) are associated with enhanced cell maturation and decreased cell replication. Both decreased cAMP and increased cGMP have been measured in the skin of individuals with psoriasis.[1,2] The result is excessive cell replication.

Therapeutic Considerations

Although psoriasis may have a significant genetic component, rebalancing the cyclic

763

AMP:GMP ratio is a prime therapeutic goal. A number of factors appear to cause or contribute to psoriasis, including: incomplete protein digestion, bowel toxemia, impaired liver function, alcohol consumption, excessive consumption of animal fats, nutritional factors, and stress. In addition to addressing these causative factors, the use of ultraviolet light and natural topical preparations are discussed below as well.

Incomplete Protein Digestion

Incomplete protein digestion or poor intestinal absorption of protein breakdown products can result in elevated levels of amino acids and polypeptides in the bowel. These are metabolized by bowel bacteria into several toxic compounds. The toxic metabolites of the amino acids arginine and ornithine are known as polyamines (e.g., putrescine, spermidine, and cadaverine); their levels have been shown to be increased in individuals with psoriasis. Polyamines inhibit the formation of cyclic AMP and therefore contribute to the excessive rate of cell proliferation.[3-5] Lowered skin and urinary levels of polyamines are associated with clinical improvement in psoriasis.[3]

There are a number of natural compounds that can inhibit the formation of polyamines and that may be of benefit in the treatment of psoriasis. For example, vitamin A and the alkaloids of goldenseal *(Hydrastis canadensis)*, such as berberine, inhibit bacterial decarboxylase, the enzyme that converts the amino acids into polyamines.[6,7] However, the best way to prevent the excessive formation of polyamines is to improve digestive function (see DIGESTION and ELIMINATION).

Bowel Toxemia

A number of gut-derived toxins are implicated in the development of psoriasis, including endotoxins (cell-wall components of

QUICK REVIEW

- Psoriasis is caused by a pileup of skin cells that have replicated too rapidly.
- The basic defect is an imbalance in the cellular control compounds cyclic AMP and cyclic GMP.
- Incomplete protein digestion, bowel toxemia, and impaired liver function are linked to psoriasis.
- Reducing the intake of arachidonic acid, a fat found exclusively in animal foods, while increasing the intake of omega-3 fatty acids is a primary nutritional recommendation.
- Several orally administered natural medicines have been shown to be effective in treating psoriasis: omega-3 fatty acids, active vitamin D, fumaric acid, silymarin, and sarsaparilla.
- Sunlight (ultraviolet light) is extremely beneficial for individuals with psoriasis.
- Topical treatments with preparations containing glycyrrhetinic acid from licorice, chamomile extracts, and capsaicin from cayenne pepper can be helpful.

bacteria), byproducts of bacteria, *Candida albicans,* yeast compounds, and immune complexes.[8-10] These compounds lead to increases in cyclic GMP levels within skin cells, thereby increasing the rate of proliferation dramatically. *Candida albicans* overgrowth in the intestines may play a major role in many cases (see CANDIDIASIS, CHRONIC for further information).

A diet low in dietary fiber is associated with increased levels of gut-derived toxins.[8] Dietary fiber is of critical importance in maintaining a healthy colon. Many fiber components bind bowel toxins and promote their excretion in the feces. It is therefore essential that the diet of an individual with psoriasis be rich in fruits and vegetables. Natural compounds that bind endotoxins and promote their excretion may also be used. For example, a 1942 study reported in the *New England Journal of Medicine* found an aqueous extract of *Smilax sarsaparilla* to be effective in treating psoriasis, particularly the more chronic, large plaque-forming variety.[11] In the controlled study of ninety-two patients, sarsaparilla greatly relieved the psoriasis in sixty-two percent of the patients and resulted in complete clearance in another eighteen percent (i.e., eighty percent of the subjects experienced significant benefits). This benefit is apparently due to sarsaparilla components binding to and promoting the excretion of bacterial endotoxins.

Clinical severity and therapeutic response have been shown to correlate well with the level of circulating endotoxins, indicating that gut-derived toxins play a central role in the pathophysiology of psoriasis. Therefore, every effort should be made to promote proper binding and elimination of these compounds through supporting the excretion of absorbed endotoxins in the feces as well as their proper handling by the liver. A diet high in fiber along with sarsaparilla (dosage given below) can help bind the endotoxins in the gut, prevent their absorption, and promote their proper elimination.

Liver Function

Correcting abnormal liver function is of great benefit in the treatment of psoriasis.[12] The connection between the liver and psoriasis relates to one of the liver's basic tasks: filtering and detoxifying the blood. As mentioned, psoriasis has been linked to the presence of several microbial byproducts in the blood. If the liver is overwhelmed by excessive levels of these toxins in the bowel, or if there is a decrease in the liver's detoxification ability, the toxin level in the blood will increase and the psoriasis will get much worse.

Alcohol consumption is known to significantly worsen psoriasis.[13] Alcohol has this effect since it increases the absorption of toxins from the gut and impairs liver function. Alcohol intake must be eliminated in individuals who have psoriasis.

Silymarin, the flavonoid component of *Silybum marianum,* has been reported to be of value in the treatment of psoriasis.[12] Presumably this is a result of its ability to improve liver function, inhibit inflammation, and reduce excessive cellular proliferation.[14,15]

Nutritional Factors

Omega-3 Fatty Acids

The manipulation of dietary oils is extremely important in the management of psoriasis since serum free-fatty-acid levels are typically abnormal in these patients.[16] Of particular benefit are the omega-3 fatty acids. Most of the clinical research has utilized fish oils rich in eicosapentaenoic acid (EPA) and docosohexanoic acid (DHA). Several double-blind clinical studies have demonstrated that supplementing the diet with 10 to 12 grams of fish oils (providing 1.8 g EPA and 1.2 g DHA) results in significant improvement.[17–19] This amount of EPA and DHA would be equivalent to the amount of EPA in about 150 grams of salmon, mackerel, or herring. As discussed in several other chapters, it may be best to frequently consume cold-water fish and supplement daily with 1 tablespoon of flaxseed oil. Fish-oil supplementation is less advantageous as most commercially available fish oils contain very high levels of damaged fats (lipid peroxides) which greatly stress antioxidant defense mechanisms. At this time it makes the most sense to rely on cold-water fish and flaxseed oil for the omega-3 oils rather than fish oil capsules. Hopefully, higher quality fish oil preparations will enter the market.

The improvement noted from taking EPA is largely due to the competition of EPA for arachidonic-acid-binding sites, which results in the inhibition of the production of inflammatory compounds. In the skin of individuals who have psoriasis, the production of inflammatory compounds known as *leukotrienes* is many times greater than normal.[20] These toxic compounds are produced from arachidonic acid, a fat found solely in meat and other animal food sources. Leukotrienes are potent inflammatory agents and promoters of increased GMP levels.

In the involved areas of the skin, the cellular content of free arachidonic acid and 12-HETE (a toxic degradation product of arachidonic acid) are 250 and 810 times greater, respectively, than in uninvolved epidermal tissue.[20] These elevations appear to be due to the presence in the plaques of a yet-to-be-defined inhibitor of the enzyme (cyclo-oxygenase) that normally degrades arachidonic acid. As might be expected, cyclo-oxygenase inhibitors (e.g., aspirin and most other nonsteroidal anti-inflammatory agents) usually worsen psoriasis, while lipoxy-genase inhibitors (e.g., benoxaprofen) may cause improvement.[21] Naturally occurring substances, such as *quercetin* (a flavonoid), vitamin E, onion, and garlic, are known to inhibit lipoxygenase and therefore may be of benefit.

Since arachidonic acid is found only in animal tissues, it is necessary to limit intake of animal products, particularly meat, animal fats, and dairy products.

Fasting and Food-Allergy Control

Psoriatic patients improved on a fasting and vegetarian regime at a Swedish hospital where the effect of such diets on chronic inflammatory disease was being studied.[22] The improvement was probably due to decreased levels of gut-derived toxins and polyamines. Patients have also benefited from gluten-free and elimination diets.[23,24] Following the recommendations given in the chapter FOOD ALLERGY is usually very worthwhile in cases of psoriasis.

Individual Nutrients

Decreased levels of vitamin A and zinc are common in patients with psoriasis.[25-27] Given the critical role of vitamin A and zinc in the health of skin, supplementation appears warranted even without this association.

Chromium supplementation may be indicated to increase insulin-receptor sensitivity, as psoriatics typically have increased serum levels of both insulin and glucose.[28]

Levels of the selenium-containing antioxidant enzyme glutathione peroxidase are low in psoriatic patients, possibly due to such factors as alcohol abuse, malnutrition, and the excessive loss of skin cells, robbing the body of key nutrients. The depressed levels of glutathione peroxidase will normalize with oral selenium and vitamin E therapy.[29]

There is a growing body of evidence that active vitamin D (1,25-dihydroxycholecalciferol) has a role in controlling cellular processes involved with cellular replication. This recognition has led to clinical trials of both oral and topical forms of vitamin D in the treatment of psoriasis. One controlled study found that two to five weeks of topical 1,25-dihydroxycholecalciferol resulted in definite to total improvement in all five patients treated.[30] Another study by the same researchers, this one uncontrolled, found that four of seven patients had complete remission (after one to three months) with daily oral doses of 1.0 ug of 1alpha(OH)D3.[31] Patients with severe psoriasis have also been found to have significantly low serum levels of 1,25-dihydroxycholecalciferol, which normalized after treatment with oral 1alpha(OH)D3.[32]

Fumaric Acid   For the past three decades, fumaric acid therapy has become increasingly popular in Western Europe for psoriasis. Therapy consists of the oral intake of dimethylfumaric acid (240 mg daily) or monoethylfumaric acid (720 mg daily) and the topical application of one to three percent of monoethylfumaric acid. Clinical studies have shown that fumaric acid is useful in treating many patients with psoriasis, but side effects such as flushing of the skin, nausea, diarrhea, general malaise, gastric pain, and mild liver and kidney disturbances can occur.[33] We recommend using fumaric acid therapy only after other natural therapies have proven ineffective.

Stress

A large number (thirty-nine percent) of patients who have psoriasis report that a specific stressful event occurred within one month prior to their initial episode. Patients with a psychological trigger of their psoriasis have a better prognosis than patients whose psoriasis seems unaffected by stress.[34] A few case histories have been reported in the medical literature which document the successful treatment of psoriasis with hypnosis and biofeedback alone.[35]

Ultraviolet Light

Sunlight (ultraviolet light) is extremely beneficial for individuals with psoriasis. The standard medical treatment of psoriasis typically involves the use of the drug psoralen and ultraviolet A (PUVA therapy). However, ultraviolet B (UVB) exposure alone leads to inhibition of cell proliferation and has been shown to be as effective as PUVA therapy with fewer side effects.[36–39]

The induction of localized elevation of temperature (108 degrees Fahrenheit) to the affected area by ultrasound and heating pads has been shown to be an effective treatment for psoriasis.[40,41]

Topical Treatments

A number of natural proprietary formulas and over-the-counter preparations can be used to provide symptomatic relief. Three botanical agents are worth discussing as alternatives to hydrocortisone: glycyrrhetinic acid from licorice (*Glycyrrhiza glabra*); chamomile (*Matricaria chamomilla*); and capsaicin from cayenne pepper (*Capsicum frutescens*).

Glycyrrhetinic acid is a component of licorice which exerts an effect similar to that of topical hydrocortisone in the treatment of psoriasis and eczema. In fact, in several studies glycyrrhetinic acid was shown to be superior to topical cortisone, especially in chronic cases. For example, in one study of patients with eczema, ninety-three percent of the patients who applied glycyrrhetinic acid demonstrated improvement, compared to eighty-three percent who used cortisone.[42]

Glycyrrhetinic acid can also be used to potentiate the effects of topically applied hydrocortisone by inhibiting the 11-beta-hydroxysteroid dehydrogenase which catalyses the conversion of hydrocortisone to an inactive form.[43]

Chamomile preparations are widely used in Europe for the treatment of a variety of common skin complaints, including psoriasis, eczema, and dry, flaky, irritated skin. The flavonoid and essential oil components of chamomile possess significant anti-inflammatory and anti-allergy activity.[44]

Capsaicin is the active component of cayenne pepper (*Capsicum frutescens*). When topically applied, capsaicin is known to stimulate and then block small-diameter pain fibers by depleting them of the neurotransmitter substance P. Substance P is thought to be the principal chemomediator of pain impulses from the periphery. In addition, substance P has been shown to activate inflammatory mediators in psoriasis. Several clinical studies have found that the topical application of 0.025 or 0.075 percent capsaicin is effective in relieving psoriasis.[45,46]

For example, in one study ninety-eight patients applied 0.025-capsaicin cream, while ninety-nine patients applied a placebo cream, four times per day for six weeks.[45] Efficacy was evaluated based on a physician's global evaluation and a combined psoriasis severity score including scaling, thickness, erythema, and pruritus. Capsaicin-treated patients demonstrated significantly greater improvement in global evaluation and in pruritus relief, as well as a significantly greater reduction in combined psoriasis severity scores.

TREATMENT SUMMARY

Despite the complexity of this disease, the therapeutic approach is fairly straightforward.

Diet

Limit consumption of sugar, meat, animal fats, and alcohol. Increase intake of fiber and cold-water fish. Eliminate sources of gluten.

Nutritional Supplements

- High-potency multiple-vitamin-and-mineral formula
- Flaxseed oil: 1 tbsp per day
- Vitamin A: 50,000 IU per day (not to be used by pregnant or women at risk for pregnancy)
- Vitamin E: 400 IU per day
- Chromium: 400 mcg per day
- Selenium: 200 mcg per day
- Zinc: 30 mg per day
- Water-soluble fiber (psyllium, pectin, guar gum, etc.): 5 g at bedtime

Botanical Medicines

- Goldenseal (*Hydrastis canadensis*)
  The dosage should be based on berberine content. As there is a wide range of quality in goldenseal preparations, standardized extracts are preferred. Take one of the following three times per day:

Dried root or as infusion (tea): 2–4 g
Fluid extract (1:1): 2–4 ml ($^1/_2$–1 tsp)
Solid (powdered dry) extract
(4:1 or 8–12% alkaloid content):
250–500 mg

- Sarsaparilla species (one of the following three times per day):
Dried root or by decoction: 1–4 g
Liquid extract (1:1): 8–16 ml (2–4 tsp)
Solid extract (4:1): 250–500 mg
- Silymarin (from *Silybum marianum*):
70–210 mg three times per day

Psychological Factors

Evaluate stress levels and utilize stress-reduction techniques as appropriate.

Physical Medicines

- Ultrasound: 42–45°C for twenty minutes, three times per week
- UVB: 295–305 nm, 2 mw/cm^2 for three minutes, three times per week

Topical Treatment

Preparations that contain one or more of the ingredients described above. Apply to affected areas of the skin two to three times per day.

Rheumatoid Arthritis

. . . .

Fatigue, low-grade fever, weakness, weight loss, joint stiffness, and vague joint pain may precede the appearance of painful, swollen joints by several weeks

Severe joint pain with considerable inflammation that usually begins in the small joints and progresses to eventually affect all joints

X-ray findings usually show soft tissue swelling, erosion of cartilage, and joint-space narrowing

"Rheumatoid factor" is present in the blood

*R*heumatoid arthritis (RA) is a chronic inflammatory condition that affects the entire body, but especially the joints. The joints typically involved are the hands, feet, wrists, ankles, and knees. Between one and three percent of the population is affected, and the number of women with RA exceeds the number of males almost 3:1. The usual age of onset is twenty to forty years, although rheumatoid arthritis may begin at any age.[1,2]

The onset of RA is usually gradual, but occasionally is quite abrupt. Fatigue, low-grade fever, weakness, joint stiffness, and vague joint pain may precede the appearance of painful, swollen joints by several weeks. Several joints are usually involved in the onset, typically in a symmetrical fashion, i.e., both hands, wrists, or ankles. In about one-third of persons with RA, initial involvement is confined to one or a few joints.[1,2]

Involved joints will characteristically be quite warm, tender, and swollen. The skin over the joint will take on a ruddy purplish hue. As the disease progresses, deformities develop in the joints of the hands and feet. The common terms used to describe these deformities include: swan neck, boutonniere, and cock-up toes.[1,2]

Causes

There is abundant evidence that RA is an autoimmune reaction, in which antibodies develop against components of joint tissues. Yet what triggers this autoimmune reaction remains largely unknown. Speculation and investigation have centered around genetic factors, abnormal bowel permeability, lifestyle and nutritional factors, food allergies, and microorganisms. RA is a classic example of a multifactorial disease, wherein an assortment of genetic and environmental factors contribute to the disease process.

Other Autoimmune Diseases Affecting Connective Tissue

In addition to RA, there are several other autoimmune diseases which affect connective tissue (collagen structures which support internal organs as well as cartilage, tendons, muscles, and bone). These diseases include systemic lupus erythematosus (lupus or SLE), ankylosing spondylitis, scleroderma, polymalgia rheumatica, and mixed connective tissue disease. There is tremendous overlap among these diseases in terms of underlying causes, symptoms, and treatment. They share many common features with RA, but the autoimmune and inflammatory process is a bit different in each of these other diseases. From a natural medicine perspective the treatment of any of these other autoimmune diseases involves the same treatment recommendations given here in this chapter for RA.

Genetic Factors

About seventy percent of patients with RA have a specific genetic marker (HLA-DRw4), compared to twenty-eight percent in subjects who do not have RA. The high occurrence of this genetic marker strongly implies that susceptibility to RA is influenced by genetic factors. Severe RA is also found at four times greater frequency in offspring of parents who have RA. However, as strong as these genetic associations are, environmental factors are necessary for the development of the disease. In other words, the fact that a person has a strong genetic predisposition for RA does not mean that he or she will develop RA. The evidence to support this last statement comes from studies in identical twins. In these studies, rarely do both twins get RA.[1] If RA was purely a genetic disease, both twins would be affected every time.

Abnormal Bowel Permeability

There is an interesting association between rheumatoid arthritis and abnormal bowel function. This association may provide a unified theory as to the cause of RA. Individuals with RA have increased intestinal permeability (also referred to as *leaky gut*) to dietary and bacterial components (antigens) against which the body forms antibodies.[3-5] Food allergies may contribute greatly to the increased permeability of the gut in RA.

Nonsteroidal anti-inflammatory drugs such as aspirin and ibuprofen have also been implicated. This altered permeability to gut-derived antigens contributes greatly to the increased levels of circulating *endotoxins* (toxic components of the cell walls of bacteria) and the antibody-antigen complexes (also referred to as *immune complexes*) characteristic of RA.

The increased gut permeability could also result in the absorption of antigens that are similar to antigens found in joint tissues. Antibodies formed to microbial antigens are thought to cross-react with the antigens in the joint tissues. In other words, the antibodies the immune system formed to attack the microbes also attack the body. Increasing evidence appears to support this concept. For example, antibodies to several bacteria (e.g., *Campylobacter, Salmonella, and Shigella*) have been shown to cross-react with *collagen* (the main protein in joint tissue), while antibodies to *Klebsiella pneumoniae, Proteus vulgaris,* and *Yersinia enterocolitica* have been shown to cross-react with other components of joint tissues.[6,7]

Small-Intestinal Bacterial Overgrowth

Perhaps more important than specific causative organisms is that fact that many patients with rheumatoid arthritis exhibit altered microbial flora and *small intestine bacterial overgrowth* (SIBO). In fact, the degree of SIBO has been shown to be associated with the severity of symptoms and disease activity.[6] For more information on SIBO, see DIGESTION and ELIMINATION.

Abnormal Antibodies and Immune Complexes

The serum and joint fluid of nearly all individuals who have RA contain the *rheumatoid factor* (RF)—a number of antibodies that actually attack a specific fragment of IgG antibodies (the Fc fragment of IgG). In other words, in RA antibodies are being formed against antibodies. The level of RF in the blood usually correlates well with the severity of arthritis symptoms.

The presence of circulating immune complexes is one of the major factors thought to contribute to the joint destruction that accompanies RA. Specifically, it is the immune system's response to the immune complexes that leads to much of the tissue destruction seen in RA.

Microbial Hypotheses

A variety of microorganisms (e.g., Epstein-Barr virus, measles virus, amoebic organisms, and mycoplasma) have been suggested as causative factors in RA. However, no microbial agent has been consistently isolated in RA patients.[9] This fact has prompted many researchers who are committed to the "germ theory" to suggest that some atypical virus-like agent(s) may be responsible for RA.[9]

Microbial factors, particularly their role in increasing the level of circulating immune complexes, definitely contribute to the disease process in RA. However, at this time it appears highly unlikely that there is a single causative microbe in RA. Nevertheless, researchers continue to search for a causative agent.

One popular microbial hypothesis that was later disproved involved the Epstein-Barr virus (EBV)—the organism that causes infectious mononucleosis.[10] The link between EBV and RA was initially based on three basic observations:

1. EBV activates white blood cells, which induce autoantibody and rheumatoid-factor production, both *in vitro* and *in vivo*.

2. White blood cells from patients who have RA show evidence of impaired regulation of EBV infection in test tube studies.

3. Levels of antibodies to EBV antigens, such as rheumatoid arthritis nuclear antigen (RANA), are elevated in the blood of patients who have RA.

Researchers have subsequently concluded that EBV is an unlikely etiological agent, based on the prevalence of EBV antibodies in healthy controls.[10] If EBV were solely re-

QUICK REVIEW

- Rheumatoid arthritis (RA) is an autoimmune reaction in which antibodies develop against components of joint tissues.
- RA is a classic example of a multifactorial disease, wherein an assortment of genetic and environmental factors contribute to the disease process.
- Standard medical therapy is of limited value in treating most cases of RA, as it

fails to address the complex underlying causes of this disease.
- Diet has been strongly implicated in rheumatoid arthritis for many years, both in regard to cause and cure.
- Elimination of allergenic foods has been shown to offer significant benefit to some individuals with rheumatoid arthritis.
- Altered gastrointestinal tract flora have been linked to RA and other autoimmune diseases.

sponsible for RA, many more people would have RA.

Microbes known as *mycoplasmas* have also received some attention as possible etiologic factors in RA.[11] Mycoplasmas can infect joints and induce arthritis. Mycoplasmal antigens have been detected in the joint fluid of RA patients, implying that mycoplasmas may lead to immune-complex formation. However, these effects are not specific to mycoplasmas alone.

In summary, it appears that the presence of high levels of circulating immune complexes containing microbial antigens in general, as well as the increased load of microbial antigens observed in RA patients, is of greater significance than antibodies to one particular organism or group of organisms.

Decreased DHEA Levels

Defective manufacture of androgens (male hormones such as testosterone and dehydroepiandrosterone [DHEA]) has been proposed as a potential predisposing factor for rheumatoid arthritis (as well as systemic lupus erythematosus). For example, in one large study, levels of dehydroepiandrosterone sulfate (DHEAS), the main form of DHEA in the blood, were measured in 185 postmenopausal women (aged forty-five to sixty-five years) who had rheumatoid arthritis.[12] Compared with 518 postmenopausal women in the control group, DHEAS levels were below normal in the 120 patients with RA who had never taken corticosteroids, and levels were even lower in the thirty-nine patients who were currently taking corticosteroids.

Supplemental DHEA has shown therapeutic benefits in patients with systemic lupus erythematosus (lupus or SLE) in studies conducted at Stanford Medical Center.[13,14] In the double-blind study, twenty-eight female patients with mild-to-moderate SLE were given DHEA (200 mg per day) or a placebo for three months.[14] Outcomes were assessed using the SLE Disease Activity Index (SLEDAI) score, patients' and physicians' overall assessments of disease activity, and concurrent corticosteroid usage. In the patients who received DHEA, the SLEDAI decreased by nearly two points, while the placebo group's average score increased by

. . . .

- A vegetarian diet has been shown to produce significant benefits in treating RA.

- In the dietary treatment of RA, the importance of consuming a diet rich in fresh fruits and vegetables cannot be overstated.

- Several natural anti-inflammatory compounds (e.g., curcumin, bromelain, and ginger) have shown positive effects in treating RA.

- Physical therapy (i.e., exercise, heat, cold, massage, diathermy, lasers, and paraffin baths) has a major role in the management of RA.

almost a full point. Patient and physician assessments also showed improvements in the SLE group and exacerbation in the placebo group. The average dosage of required corticosteroids decreased by thirty percent in the SLE group, and increased by forty percent in the control group. The number of lupus flare-ups was three in the SLE group, compared to eight in the placebo group. Mild acne was a frequent side effect of DHEA treatment.

Given DHEA's positive effects in treating SLE, even in the absence of double-blind clinical studies in rheumatoid arthritis, DHEA supplementation appears warranted. The dosage required will probably be above 50 mg per day. The major side effect at this dosage and above is mild-to-severe acne in women.

Diagnostic Considerations

RA is easily recognized in its most advanced and characteristic form. However, diagnosis of early RA is often much more difficult. The American Rheumatism Association has established criteria for the diagnosis of "classic," "definite," "probable," and "possible" RA.

CRITERIA FOR THE CLASSIFICATION OF RA
Classic RA
The diagnosis of RA requires that seven of the following criteria be observed by a physician. In criteria 1 through 5, the joint signs or symptoms must be continuous for at least six weeks. Any one of the features listed under Exclusions will exclude a patient from this and other categories.

1. Morning stiffness.
2. Pain on motion or tenderness in at least one joint.
3. Swelling (soft tissue thickening or fluid, not bony overgrowth alone) in at least one joint.

4. Swelling of at least one other joint with any interval free of joint symptoms between the joint involvement may not be more than three months.
5. Symmetric joint swelling with simultaneous involvement of the same joint on both sides of the body.
6. Nodules under the skin over bony prominences on joints.
7. X-ray changes typical of RA, which must include bony decalcification localized to or most marked adjacent to the involved joints and not just degenerative changes.
8. Positive demonstration of the "rheumatoid factor" by an acceptable method.
9. Signs of inflammation on examination of joint fluid.
10. Characteristic biopsy results

Definite RA
This diagnosis requires five of the above criteria. In criteria 1 through 5, the joint signs must be continuous for at least six weeks.

Probable RA
This diagnosis requires three of the above criteria. In at least one of criteria 1 through 5 the joint signs or symptoms must be continuous for at least six weeks.

Possible RA
This diagnosis requires two of the following criteria, and total duration of joint symptoms must be at least three months.

1. Morning stiffness.
2. Tenderness or pain on motion, with history of recurrence or persistence of three weeks.
3. History or observation of joint swelling.
4. Elevated sedimentation rate (a blood test that provides a rough estimation of inflammation)
5. Iritis (inflammation of the eye).

Therapeutic Considerations

Standard medical therapy is of limited value in most cases of RA, as it fails to address the complex underlying causes of this disease. Standard medical treatment of RA involves, in addition to drugs, such physical therapy modalities as exercise, heat, cold, massage, diathermy, lasers, and paraffin baths. The first drug generally employed is aspirin. It is often quite effective in relieving both the pain and inflammation, and is also relatively inexpensive. Since the therapeutic dose required is relatively high, toxicity often occurs. Ringing in the ear (tinnitus) and gastric irritation are early manifestations of toxicity.[1,2]

Other nonsteroidal anti-inflammatory drugs (NSAIDs) are often used as well, especially when aspirin is ineffective or is not well tolerated. Typical representatives of this class of drugs includes: ibuprofen (Motrin, Advil, Nuprin), piroxicam (Feldene), diclofenac (Voltaren), fenoprofen (Nalfon), indomethacin (Indocin), naproxen (Naprosyn), tolmetin (Tolectin), and sulindac (Clinoril).

While more expensive, none of these drugs have demonstrated superior efficacy over aspirin. As with osteoarthritis, use of these drugs in the treatment of rheumatoid arthritis is a classic example of suppression of symptoms accompanied by acceleration of factors that promote the disease process. In the case of rheumatoid arthritis, NSAIDs have been shown to greatly increase the already hyperpermeable gastrointestinal tract of rheumatoid arthritis sufferers.[15] The use of NSAIDs to treat rheumatoid arthritis is also a significant cause of serious gastrointestinal tract reactions, including ulcers, hemorrhage, and perforation. Approximately 20,000 hospitalizations and 2,600 hundred deaths occur each year due to the use of NSAIDs in treating individuals with rheumatoid arthritis.[16]

If NSAIDs are not effective, corticosteroids may be used. However, most experts and medical textbooks clearly state that long-term use of corticosteroids to treat rheumatoid arthritis is not advised due to the side effects. Nonetheless, long-term cortico-steroid use is quite common among RA patients.

When NSAID and cortisone therapies do not offer benefit, more aggressive and potentially more toxic treatments are used, along with continued use of NSAIDs and corticosteroids. Hydroxychloroquine, gold therapy, penicillamine, azathioprine, methotrexate, and cyclophosphamide are examples of drugs currently in use. Unfortunately, in most cases, the benefit produced by these drugs is greatly outweighed by the significant toxicity they possess. The use of these drugs often requires the use of additional drugs to deal with side effects. It is not uncommon for individuals who have rheumatoid arthritis to be on twelve or more prescription drugs at one time. And finally, joint surgery and replacement are reserved for the most severe cases.

There is little argument that rheumatoid arthritis is an aggressive disease that calls for aggressive measures. There is also little argument that current medical treatment of rheumatoid arthritis is aggressive. The big questions are: Is aggressive chemotherapy for rheumatoid arthritis actually providing benefit? And at what cost to the patient?

Research is only beginning to determine the effects of treatment on the long-term outcome of rheumatoid arthritis because, in order to fully answer the questions raised in the previous paragraph, patients must be followed for at least twenty years. Many of the disease-modifying drugs have only been used for the last two or three decades.

A revealing study evaluated the long-term outcome of therapy in 112 RA patients who were being treated with conventional drug therapy.[17] After twenty years, despite aggressive therapy with standard drug regimens, only eighteen percent of all patients were able to lead a normal life. Most patients (fifty-four percent) were either dead (thirty-five percent) or severely disabled (nineteen percent). Most deaths were directly related to rheumatoid arthritis. The results of this study clearly indicate that, although current drug therapy may be effective in providing short-term benefit, this approach is not providing long-term benefits to patients who have rheumatoid arthritis.

Rheumatoid arthritis, as a multifactorial condition, requires a comprehensive therapeutic approach that focuses on reducing the factors known to be involved in the disease process (gut permeability, circulating immune complexes, free radicals, immune dysfunction, etc.), while controlling inflammation and promoting joint regeneration. The natural approach involves addressing poor digestion, food allergies, increased gut permeability, increased levels of circulating immune complexes, and excessive inflammatory processes. Foremost in the natural approach is the use of diet to control inflammation.

Dietary Factors

Diet has been strongly implicated in rheumatoid arthritis for many years, in regard to both cause and cure. In population studies RA has not been found in areas where people eat a more "primitive" diet; it is found at a relatively high rate in places where people consume a so-called "Western" diet.[18] Therefore, a diet rich in whole foods, vegetables, and fiber, and low in sugar, meat, refined carbohydrate, and saturated fat, appears to offer some protection against developing rheumatoid arthritis. In addition, dietary therapy is showing tremendous promise in the treatment of rheumatoid arthritis.[19–21] The major focus in dietary therapy is to eliminate food allergies, follow a vegetarian diet, alter the intake of dietary fats and oils, and increase the intake of antioxidant nutrients.

Food Allergy

Elimination of allergenic foods has been shown to offer significant benefit to some individuals who have rheumatoid arthritis.[22–25]

Virtually any food can aggravate rheumatoid arthritis, but the most common offending foods are wheat, corn, milk and other dairy products, beef, and nightshade-family foods (tomato, potato, eggplant, peppers, and tobacco), as well as food additives.

A well-designed study highlights the effectiveness of eliminating food allergens as part of a healthy diet-and-lifestyle program in the treatment of rheumatoid arthritis.[26] In a thirteen-month study, two groups of patients who suffered from rheumatoid arthritis were studied to determine the effect of diet on their condition. One group followed a therapeutic diet, the other group continued to eat as they wished.

The treatment group began their therapeutic diet by fasting for seven to ten days. Dietary intake during the fast consisted of herbal teas, garlic, vegetable broth, a decoction of potatoes and parsley, and juices of carrots, beets, and celery. No fruit juices were allowed.

Patients with RA have historically benefited from fasting. However, strict water fasting should only be done under direct medical supervision. Fasting decreases absorption of allergenic food components and reduces levels of inflammatory mediators. A juice fast or a fast similar to the one used in this study is probably safer than a water fast and may actually yield better results. Short-term fasts of three to five days' duration are recommended during acute worsening of RA.

After the fast, the patients reintroduced a "new" food item every second day. If they noticed an increase in pain, stiffness, or joint swelling within two to forty-eight hours, this item was omitted from the diet for at least seven days before being reintroduced a second time. If the food caused worsening of symptoms after the second time, it was omitted permanently from the diet.

The results of the study further supported the positive results noted in other studies of

RA, which have shown that short-term fasting, followed by a vegetarian diet, results in "a substantial reduction in disease activity" in many patients.[27-29] The results indicated a therapeutic benefit beyond elimination of food allergies alone. The authors suggested that the additional improvements were due to changes in dietary fatty acids (discussed in the following section on Dietary Fats). In addition, other studies have shown that improvements in RA that result from a vegetarian diet are associated with improvements in fecal flora (discussed in the following section).

In a one-year follow-up to this important study, all the patients who responded to the diet still followed the diet.[30] The majority of these patients remained in complete remission or were significantly better. These long-term results support recommending a vegetarian diet for the treatment of RA.

Fecal Flora

Altered gastrointestinal tract flora have been linked to RA and other autoimmune diseases (see previous discussion of food allergies). Two recent randomized, clinical studies demonstrated that significant changes in microbial flora are associated with clinical improvements.[31,32] In the first study, researchers sought to determine the effect of vegetarian-diet-induced improvement of RA on fecal flora in fifty-three patients.[31] Rather than the traditional method of isolating, identifying, and enumerating different bacterial species in fecal samples, the researchers examined bacterial fatty-acid profiles.

Human fecal flora constitute a complex ecosystem including over four hundred species, making it difficult to isolate and identify the species. Because of the lack of reproducibility and the fact that many bacteria do not grow well on selective culture media, while many others prevent the growth of other species, classic bacteriological techniques are generally unsuitable for studying the microecology of the human gut.

Instead of focusing on particular species, the researchers used another approach to detect overall changes in bacterial flora of stool cultures collected at baseline, four weeks, and thereafter every three months for one year. The technique used was computerized comparison of bacterial fatty-acid profiles of stool samples. The fatty acids measured are structural components of bacterial cell membranes. Each bacterial species has its own characteristic composition. In a stool sample, the profile of fatty acids represents all the bacteria present in the sample. This technique has proven to be more sensitive than classical quantitative culture in detecting microecological changes in stool samples.

In the first study, the fifty-three patients were assigned to either a high-improvement index (HI) or low-improvement index (LI) based on repeated clinical assessments. Significant alteration in the intestinal flora was observed when the patients changed from an omnivorous diet to a vegetarian diet. These results further document a direct association between intestinal flora and disease activity in RA.

The second study, involving forty-three patients, provided additional support for the theory that a vegetarian diet produces clinical improvements in RA.[32] Forty-three RA patients were divided into a treatment group and a control group. The treatment group followed a vegetarian diet for one month, and the control group consumed their normal diet. At the end of only thirty days, positive changes in fecal flora correlated with improvements in RA.

These findings are not surprising. Intestinal flora undoubtedly play a major role in health. The total surface area of the gastrointestinal system is approximately 300 to 400 square meters. Only a single layer of cells separates the bloodstream from enormous amounts of dietary and microbial antigens. Fortunately, the lymphoid tissue in the gut, the largest lymphoid organ, helps protect the individual from antigens that pass through this protective layer. Alterations in intestinal flora change the antigenic challenge. In an autoimmune condition such as RA, this change may significantly impact disease activity.

Digestion

Proper digestion is a requirement for optimum health, and incomplete or disordered digestion can be a major contributor to the development of many diseases, including RA. The problem is not only that ingestion of foods and nutritional substances is of little benefit when breakdown and assimilation are inadequate, but also that incompletely digested food molecules can be inappropriately absorbed. Since many individuals who have RA are deficient in digestive factors, including hydrochloric acid and pancreatic enzymes, incomplete digestion may be a major factor in RA.[33,34]

Supplementation with appropriate digestive aids appears warranted. Beyond their physiological role in digestion, pancreatic enzymes may offer additional benefits. Specifically, the protein-digesting enzymes (pancreases) in pancreatin have been shown to reduce circulating levels of immune complexes in autoimmune diseases such as RA, lupus erythematosus, periarteritis nodosa, scleroderma, ulcerative colitis, Crohn's disease, multiple sclerosis, and AIDS.[35,36] Since clinical improvements usually correspond with decreases in immune-complex levels (the erythrocyte sedimentation rate can be used as a rough indicator), pancreatin or bromelain supplementation (discussed later in this chapter) is often warranted.

Dietary Fats

Fatty acids are important mediators of allergy and inflammation through their role as building blocks for inflammatory compounds known as prostaglandins, thromboxanes, and leukotrienes. Altering dietary oil intake can significantly increase or decrease inflammation, depending on the type of balance of fatty acids. The basic goal is two-fold: (1) reduce the level of arachidonic acid (a fatty acid found only in animal foods) and (2) increase the level of EPA (the key component of fish oils and an important omega-3 fatty acid). Vegetarian diets are often beneficial in the treatment of many chronic allergic and inflammatory conditions, including RA, presumably as a result of decreasing the availability of arachidonic acid for conversion to inflammatory prostaglandins and leukotrienes, while supplying linoleic and linolenic acids.

An important nutritional approach to decreasing the inflammatory response is the consumption of cold-water fish such as mackerel, herring, sardines, and salmon. These fish are rich sources of eicosapentaenoic acid (EPA), which competes with arachidonic acid for prostaglandin and leukotriene production. The net effect of consumption of these fish is a significantly reduced inflammatory/allergic response.

To test the theory that omega-3 fatty acids may protect against the development of RA, a population-based study of women living in the Seattle area compared fish consumption in 324 cases of RA with 1,245 women without RA.[37] Consumption of broiled or baked fish (but not fried fish) was associated with a decreased risk of RA. An apparent dose-dependent response was noted; consuming more than two servings of fish per week offered greater protection than one serving per week.

Based on this study and the one described previously on the benefits of a vegetarian diet, it appears that the best diet for the prevention of RA is a vegetarian diet with the addition of cold-water fish. Also, flaxseed oil supplementation (discussed below under

Nutritional Supplementation) may also be useful.

Nutritional Supplementation

Gamma-Linolenic Acid

Evening primrose, black currant, and borage oils contain gamma-linolenic acid (GLA), an omega-6 fatty acid that eventually acts as a precursor to the anti-inflammatory prostaglandins of the 1 series. Although a popular recommendation by nutrition-oriented physicians, the research on GLA supplements for treating RA is controversial and not as strong as the research on omega-3 oils. Studies have actually shown that, over the long term, GLA supplementation increases tissue arachidonic acid levels while decreasing tissue levels of EPA.[38] Obviously, this effect is contrary to the treatment goal of trying to reduce inflammation by reducing tissue levels of arachidonic acid and raising levels of EPA.

Some studies of RA have shown benefit from GLA supplementation, others have not.[39-41] The key factor appears to be whether subjects are allowed to take their anti-inflammatory drugs. These drugs inhibit the formation of inflammatory prostaglandins and would mask the negative effects of the altered tissue-fatty-acid profile produced by GLA supplements. In other words, the negative effects on arachidonic acid (increased) and EPA (decreased) caused by GLA supplementation are not apparent because the drugs masked or covered up this effect blocking the formation of inflammatory prostaglandins.

Although positive results have been reported from GLA supplementation, closer examination is required. For example, in one double-blind study, thirty-seven patients with RA were given either GLA (1.4 grams per day) or a placebo for twenty-four weeks. GLA supplementation reduced the number of tender joints by thirty-six percent, the tender joint score (severity of tenderness) by forty-five percent, swollen joint count by twenty-eight percent, and the swollen joint score by forty-one percent.[41] In contrast, no patients in the placebo group showed significant improvement in any measure. The superficial results of this study indicate that GLA sources may be useful in reducing the inflammatory process of RA. However, in this study the subjects continued to take their anti-inflammatory drugs and probably masked the detrimental effects on tissue arachidonic acid and EPA levels.

The recommended daily dosage for GLA in the treatment of RA is 1.4 grams. Since evening primrose oil is nine percent GLA, this means that approximately thirty-one 500-mg capsules of evening primrose oil would have to be consumed each day. This dosage would typically cost a person nearly $100 per month to attain. Taking less than the recommended dosage is not likely to produce any benefit. For several reasons, including cost, omega-3 oils appear to be a better choice.

Omega-3 Fatty Acids

The studies of fish oil supplementation in the treatment of RA have demonstrated far better and more consistent responses than the studies that used GLA supplementation. The first double-blind, placebo-controlled study of RA patients, which used 1.8 grams of EPA (from fish oil) per day, showed less morning stiffness and tender joints in the EPA group than in the control group.[42] These results led to considerable scientific interest as well as numerous popular press accounts of the possible benefits of fish oil (as a source of EPA) for treating allergic and inflammatory conditions.

Over a dozen follow-up studies have consistently demonstrated positive benefits.[43-50] In addition to relief of symptoms (morning stiffness and joint tenderness), fish oil supplementation has produced favorable changes in suppressing the production of inflammatory compounds secreted by white blood cells. Unfortunately, most commercially available fish oils contain very high levels of damaged fats (lipid peroxides) and greatly stress antioxidant defense mechanisms. At this time, it makes the most sense to rely on cold-water fish and flaxseed oil for the omega-3 oils rather than fish oil capsules.[51–53] Hopefully, higher-quality fish oil preparations will enter the market.

Although several studies have shown that flaxseed oil is not as effective in increasing tissue concentrations of EPA and lowering tissue concentrations of arachidonic acid as fish oils, these studies failed to address an important factor.[54,55] The studies were all performed on subjects who continued to consume a diet rich in omega-6 fatty acids.

A more recent study was undertaken to determine the potential for dietary flaxseed oil to increase tissue EPA concentration in healthy human subjects.[56] Unlike the previous studies, this study incorporated a diet low in omega-6 oils by restricting the use of other vegetable oils while supplementing the diet with 13 grams (approximately 1 tablespoon) of flaxseed oil daily. The results of the study indicated that flaxseed oil supplementation, along with restriction of linoleic acid intake, raises tissue EPA levels comparably to fish oil supplementation. Furthermore, several human and animal studies have demonstrated that flaxseed oil supplementation can inhibit the autoimmune reaction as well as EPA does.[57]

Unfortunately, a small, twenty-two-patient double-blind study over a two-month period did not show any benefit from taking flaxseed oil (30 grams per day) versus the same amount of safflower oil.[58] However, upon examination of the data, a possible explanation exists. In order to provide clinical benefit, flaxseed oil would have to reduce the tissue concentration of arachidonic acid while increasing the tissue concentration of EPA and DHA. Tissue analysis in patients involved in this study who were taking flaxseed oil did not demonstrate significant changes in tissue levels of either arachidonic acid or EPA and DHA. As mentioned, previous studies have shown that it is possible to raise tissue levels of EPA and DHA and lower levels of arachidonic acid with flaxseed oils if the intake of omega-6 oils (corn, safflower, sunflower, and soy) is restricted. The failure to improve tissue EPA concentrations in this study led to the ineffectiveness of flaxseed oil.

The cause of the failure to improve lipid concentrations was either a failure to restrict the use of other vegetable oils while supplementing the diet with flaxseed oil or a failure to correct an underlying zinc deficiency. Evidence of the former is offered by the fact that there was no significant change in the ratio of alpha-linolenic acid to linoleic acid in test subjects. Evidence to support failure to correct an underlying zinc deficiency comes from serum zinc analysis on test subjects.

Zinc acts as a necessary component in delta-6 desaturase, the enzyme involved in the conversion of alpha-linolenic acid to EPA and DHA. Zinc deficiency is common among people who have RA. In fact, several studies have shown that zinc supplementation relieves RA. The fact that tissue levels of alpha-linolenic acid increased while on the flaxseed oil and that EPA and DHA levels did not increase suggests zinc deficiency. This led researchers to measure serum zinc levels in the patients during the study.

The researchers concluded: "Low conversion of alpha-linolenic acid to EPA and DHA [due to a zinc deficiency], together with a low alpha-linolenic acid to linoleic acid ratio, might explain why a short-term alpha-linolenic acid supplementation did not alter the RA disease activity."

At this time, our recommendation is to follow the dietary recommendations of a vegetarian diet with the addition of cold-water fish, restriction of omega-6 fatty acids, and supplementation with one tablespoon of flaxseed oil daily.

Dietary Antioxidants

The importance of a diet rich in fresh fruits and vegetables in the dietary treatment of RA cannot be overstated. These foods are the best sources of dietary antioxidants. While the benefits of vitamin C, beta-carotene, vitamin E, selenium, and zinc as antioxidant nutrients are becoming well-recognized and well-accepted, there are still other plant compounds that promote healthy joints. Flavonoids are of particular benefit in treating RA due to their neutralization of inflammation and support of collagen structures.[59] In short, the antioxidant benefits of fresh fruits and vegetables go well beyond the antioxidant effects of vitamins and minerals.

Several studies have shown that the risk of RA is highest among people with the lowest levels of nutrient antioxidants (e.g., serum concentrations of vitamin E, beta-carotene, and vitamin C). For example, in one study persons with RA and systemic lupus erythematosus (which developed two to fifteen years after donating blood for a serum bank in 1974) were designated as "cases."[60] For each case, four controls were selected from the serum bank donors, matched for race, sex, and age. Stored serum samples from cases and controls were assayed for alpha tocopherol, beta-carotene, and retinol. Cases of both diseases had lower serum concentrations of vitamin E, beta-carotene, and retinol in 1974 than people who did not develop these diseases.

Selenium and Vitamin E Selenium levels are low in patients who have RA.[61,62] Low selenium levels may be a significant nutritional factor, as selenium plays an important role both as an antioxidant and as the mineral cofactor in the free-radical-scavenging enzyme glutathione peroxidase. This enzyme is especially important in reducing the production of inflammatory prostaglandins and leukotrienes. Since free radicals, oxidants, prostaglandins, and leukotrienes cause much of the damage to tissues seen in RA, a deficiency of selenium would result in even more significant damage.

Clinical studies have not yet clearly demonstrated that selenium supplementation alone relieves the signs and symptoms of RA. However, one clinical study indicated that selenium combined with vitamin E had a positive effect.[63]

Zinc Zinc has antioxidant effects and is a cofactor in the antioxidant enzyme superoxide dismutase (copper-zinc SOD). Zinc levels are typically reduced in patients with RA. Several studies have used zinc in the treatment of RA, with some of the studies demonstrating a slight therapeutic effect.[64-66] Most of the studies utilized zinc in the form of sulfate. Better results may be produced by using a form of zinc with a higher absorption rate, such as zinc picolinate, zinc monomethionine, or zinc citrate. Foods rich in zinc include oysters, whole grains, nuts, and seeds.

Manganese and Superoxide Dismutase
Manganese functions in a different form of the antioxidant enzyme superoxide dismutase (manganese SOD). Levels of manganese-containing SOD are deficient in patients who have RA.[67] The injectable form of this enzyme (available in Europe) has been shown to be effective in the treatment of RA.[68] However, it is not clear if any orally administered SOD can escape digestion in the intestinal tract and exert a therapeutic effect.

In one study, oral SOD was shown to not affect tissue SOD levels.[69]

Perhaps a better and more economical method of raising SOD levels is to supplement the diet with additional manganese. Manganese supplementation has been shown to increase SOD activity.[70] Although no clinical studies have been conducted to determine the effectiveness of manganese supplementation in treating RA, it appears to be indicated based on the low levels seen in patients with RA and on its biochemical functions. Good dietary sources of manganese include nuts, whole grains, dried fruits, and green leafy vegetables. Meats, dairy products, poultry, and seafood are considered poor sources of manganese.

Vitamin C   Vitamin C functions as an important antioxidant. The white-blood-cell and plasma concentrations of vitamin C are significantly decreased in RA patients.[71] Supplementation with vitamin C increases SOD activity, decreases histamine levels, and provides some anti-inflammatory action.[72,73] Foods rich in vitamin C include broccoli, brussels sprouts, cabbage, citrus fruits, tomatoes, and berries.

Pantothenic Acid

Whole-blood pantothenic acid levels have been reported to be lower in RA patients than in normal controls.[74] In addition, disease activity was inversely correlated with pantothenic acid levels. Correction of low pantothenic acid levels to normal brought about some alleviation of symptoms.

In one double-blind study, subjective improvement was noted in patients who received 2 grams of calcium pantothenate daily.[75] Patients noted improvements in duration of morning stiffness, degree of disability, and severity of pain. Good dietary sources of pantothenic acid are whole grains and legumes.

Copper

Copper aspirinate (salicylate) is a form of aspirin that yields better results in reducing pain and inflammation than standard aspirin preparations. These copper-containing substances may be appropriate for RA patients who require aspirin.[76,77]

The wearing of copper bracelets has been a long-time folk remedy that appears to have some scientific support, as found in a double-blind study performed in Australia. Presumably, copper is absorbed through the skin and is chelated to another compound that is able to exert anti-inflammatory action.[78]

Copper is a component, along with zinc, of one type of superoxide dismutase (copper-zinc SOD). Deficiency may result in significant susceptibility to free-radical damage as a result of decreased SOD levels. However, excess intake of copper may be detrimental due to its ability to combine with peroxides and damage joint tissues.[77,79]

Sulfur

The sulfur content of fingernails of arthritis sufferers is lower than that of healthy controls.[80] Normalizing the sulfur content of the nails by using injectable sulfur was reported to alleviate pain and swelling, according to clinical data from the 1930s.[81,82] Presumably, increasing the sulfur content of the body through increased consumption of sulfur-rich foods, such as legumes, garlic, onions, brussels sprouts, and cabbage, or through supplementation may be of equal benefit.

Niacinamide

Drs. William Kaufman and Abram Hoffer have reported very good clinical results in the treatment of hundreds of patients with rheumatoid and osteoarthritis using high-dose niacinamide (i.e., 900 to 4,000 mg per day in divided doses).[83,84] While these promising results have been confirmed in osteoarthritis (see OSTEOARTHRITIS), they have never been fully evaluated in detailed clinical studies of RA patients. Niacinamide has, however, been shown to impact the autoimmune process involved in insulin-dependent diabetes mellitus (see DIABETES MELLITUS). We think niacinamide is quite useful in RA, but long-term supplementation (e.g., more than three months) needs to be monitored by a physician due to the possibility of niacinamide harming the liver.

Botanicals

Many botanicals possess significant anti-inflammatory action and are useful in the treatment of RA. The suggestions given here represent some of the more popular and better researched of these botanical medicines. Several herbs are also discussed in relation to their ability to enhance the function or secretion of endogenous corticosteroids and to prevent or reverse some of the negative effects of orally administered cortisone.

Curcumin

Curcumin, the yellow pigment of *Curcuma longa* (turmeric), exerts excellent anti-inflammatory and antioxidant effects.[85–90] Curcumin is as effective as either cortisone or the potent anti-inflammatory drug phenylbutazone in models of acute inflammation. However, while phenylbutazone and cortisone are associated with significant toxicity, curcumin is without side effects.

Curcumin exhibits many direct anti-inflammatory effects, including inhibiting the formation of the major mediators of inflammation (thromboxanes and leukotrienes).

However, curcumin also appears to exert some indirect effects. In models of chronic inflammation, curcumin is much less active in animals that have had their adrenal glands removed. This observation suggests that curcumin works to enhance the body's own anti-inflammatory mechanisms. Possible mechanisms of action include: (1) stimulation of the release of adrenal corticosteroids; (2) "sensitizing" or priming cortisone receptor sites, thereby potentiating cortisone action; and (3) preventing the breakdown of cortisone.

In human studies, curcumin has demonstrated some beneficial effects that are comparable to those of standard drugs. In one double-blind clinical trial that involved patients with RA, curcumin (1,200 mg per day) was compared to phenylbutazone (300 mg per day).[91] The improvements in the duration of morning stiffness, walking time, and joint swelling were comparable in both groups. However, while phenylbutazone is associated with significant adverse effects, curcumin has not been shown to produce any side effects at the recommended dosage level.

In another study, curcumin was again shown to exert comparable anti-inflammatory action to phenylbutazone in patients recovering from surgery.[92] It must be pointed out that, while curcumin has an anti-inflammatory effect similar to phenylbutazone and various NSAIDs, it does not possess direct analgesic (pain-relieving) action.

The results of these studies indicate that turmeric or curcumin may provide benefit in the treatment of acute flare-ups of inflammation in RA. Furthermore, the safety and excellent tolerability of curcumin compared to standard drug treatment is a major advantage. Toxicity reactions to curcumin have not been reported. Animals fed very high levels of curcumin (3g/kg [1kg = 2.2 pounds] of body weight) have not exhibited any significant adverse effects.[93]

The recommended dosage for curcumin as an anti-inflammatory is 400 to 600 mg three times per day. To achieve a similar amount of curcumin using turmeric would require a dosage of 8,000 to 60,000 mg of turmeric per day. Because there is a question about the absorption of orally administered curcumin, curcumin is often formulated in conjunction with bromelain to possibly enhance absorption. Bromelain also has anti-inflammatory effects (see the next section). If a curcumin-bromelain combination is used, it is important to take it on an empty stomach twenty minutes before meals or between meals. Providing curcumin in a lipid base such as lecithin, fish oils, or essential fatty acids may also increase absorption.

Bromelain

Bromelain is a mixture of enzymes found in pineapple. Bromelain was introduced as a medicinal agent in 1957, and since that time over two hundred scientific papers on its therapeutic applications have appeared in research literature.[94] Bromelain has been reported to exert a wide variety of beneficial effects, including reducing inflammation in cases of RA.[95]

Several mechanisms may account for bromelain's anti-inflammatory effects, including the inhibition of pro-inflammatory compounds. Much of bromelain's anti-swelling effect is due to activating compounds that break down fibrin. Fibrin's role in promotion of the inflammatory response is to form a matrix that walls off the area of inflammation, resulting in blockage of blood vessels and inadequate tissue drainage and edema. Bromelain also blocks the production of kinins—compounds produced during in-

flammation—which increase swelling and cause pain.

Ginger

Ginger (*Zingiber officinale*) possesses numerous therapeutic properties. The most relevant to RA are: its antioxidant effects; inhibition of the formation of inflammatory compounds (e.g., prostaglandins, thromboxanes, and leukotrienes); and direct anti-inflammatory effects. Fresh ginger may be more effective in the treatment of RA than dried preparations, as it contains a protease that may have similar action to bromelain on inflammation.[96]

Ginger's ability to inhibit the formation of inflammatory mediators, along with its strong antioxidant activities and protease component, suggest a possible benefit in treating inflammatory conditions.[97] To test this theory, a clinical study was conducted on seven patients with RA. These patients had not been helped by conventional drugs.[98] All patients were treated with ginger. One patient took 50 grams of lightly cooked ginger per day, while the remaining six took either 5 grams of fresh or 0.1 to 1 gram of powdered ginger daily. Despite the difference in dosage, all patients reported substantial improvement, including pain relief, joint mobility, and decrease in swelling and morning stiffness.

In the follow-up to this preliminary study, twenty-eight patients with RA, eighteen with osteoarthritis, and ten with muscular discomfort who had been taking powdered ginger for periods ranging from 3 months to 2.5 years were evaluated.[99] Based on clinical observations by physicians, it was reported that seventy-five percent of the arthritis patients and one hundred percent of the patients with muscular discomfort experienced relief of pain or swelling. The recommended dosage was 500 to 1,000 mg per day, but many patients took three to four times this amount. Patients who took the higher dosages also reported quicker and better relief.

There remain many questions concerning the best form of ginger and the proper dosage. Most studies have utilized 1 gram of dry powdered ginger root. This is a relatively small dose of ginger compared to the average daily dietary consumption of 8 to 10 grams in India.

Although most scientific studies have used powdered ginger root, fresh (or possibly freeze-dried) ginger root at an equivalent dosage may yield better results because it contains higher levels of gingerol as well as the active protease.

We suggest that a daily dosage of 2 to 4 grams of dry powdered ginger may be effective. This amount would be equivalent to approximately 20 grams (or two-thirds of an ounce) of fresh ginger root—roughly a 1/2-inch slice. These amounts of ginger can easily be incorporated into the diet in fresh fruit and vegetable juices. There do not appear to be any side effects from using ginger at these levels.

Chinese Thoroughwax

Chinese thoroughwax (*Bupleuri falcatum*) root is an important component of various Chinese traditional medicine prescriptions, particularly in remedies for inflammatory conditions. Recently these formulas have also been used in combination with corticosteroid drugs such as prednisone.[100] Chinese thoroughwax has been shown to enhance the activity of cortisone.

The active components of Chinese thoroughwax are steroid-like compounds known as saikosaponins. These compounds have diverse pharmacological activity, including significant anti-inflammatory action.[101] The saikosaponins apparently both increase the release of cortisone and other hormones by the adrenal gland and potentiate their effects. Saikosaponins have also been shown to prevent the adrenal-gland atrophy caused by corticosteroids.[63] It has been recommended that patients who are taking corticosteroid drugs should take herbal formulas containing Chinese thoroughwax to help protect the adrenal gland.[102]

Licorice (*Glycyrrhiza glabra*) and *Panax ginseng* appear to enhance the action of Chinese thoroughwax; the three are almost always used together in traditional Chinese herbal formulas. Both licorice root and ginseng have components with anti-inflammatory activity.[103] In addition, these herbs have been shown to improve the activity of the adrenal glands. Perhaps licorice's major effect is its ability to inhibit the breakdown of adrenal hormones by the liver. When used in combination with Chinese thoroughwax, the net effect is to increase circulating corticosteroid levels. This happens because Chinese thoroughwax promotes secretion of corticosteroids by the adrenal glands, while licorice root inhibits their breakdown in the liver.

Preparations that contain Chinese thoroughwax, licorice, and *Panax ginseng* may help restore adrenal function in patients with a history of long-term or high-dosage corticosteroid use.

Physical Medicine

Physical therapy has a major role in treating RA. While not curative, proper physical management can improve patient comfort and preserve joint and muscle function. Heat is typically used to help relieve stiffness and pain, relax muscles, and increase range of motion. Moist heat (e.g., moist packs, hot baths) is more effective than dry heat (e.g., heating pad), and paraffin (wax) baths are used if skin irritation from regular water immersion develops. Cold packs are of value during acute flare-ups.

Strengthening and range-of-motion exercises are important for improving and maintaining joint function, as well as for general health. Patients with well-developed disease and significant inflammation should begin with progressive, passive range-of-motion and isometric exercises. As inflammation is ameliorated, active range-of-motion and isotonic exercises are more appropriate.

Balneotherapy

Balneotherapy, the therapeutic use of mineral baths and mud packs, is a form of physical therapy often recommended in Europe to treat cases of RA. A study conducted in Israel provides some evidence of benefit.[104] The study was conducted at the Ein Gedi Spa, on the western shore of the Dead Sea. This area along the Dead Sea is renowned for its many hot thermomineral springs and a large natural concentration of mud useful for therapeutic purposes. The area is also popular among persons with RA because of its unique climatic conditions: high barometric pressures, low humidity, high temperatures, paucity of rainfall, and absence of air pollution.

Standard spa therapy for RA in this region consists of mud packs, sulfur baths, and bathing in the waters of the Dead Sea. In a previous study, it was shown that sulfur and mud pack therapy, alone or in combination, are effective in reducing inflammation and pain in active RA. A recent study was conducted to determine whether there was any treatment advantage to sulfur baths or bathing in the Dead Sea, alone or in combination, in the treatment of active RA.

Thirty-six patients with active RA were treated at the spa for twelve days. The patients were divided randomly into four study groups. Group 1 was treated with daily baths in the Dead Sea. Group 2 was treated with daily sulfur baths. Group 3 was treated with a combination of daily Dead Sea bathing and sulfur baths. Group 4 served as a control group (no treatment). All patients were assessed by a rheumatologist who did not know what treatments were being used. Clinical parameters assessed included: duration of morning stiffness, 15-meter walk time, grip strength, activities of daily living assessment, patient's assessment of disease activity, number of active joints, and the Ritchie articular index—an index that takes into consideration all of the signs and symptoms of RA.

The study found a statistically significant improvement, lasting up to three months after treatment, in only the three treatment groups. In morning stiffness, 15-meter walk time, grip strength, activities of daily living assessment, and patient's assessment of disease activity, there was an advantage shown for Dead Sea baths, either alone or in combination with sulfur baths. The number of active joints and the Ritchie index declined (improved) to a similar degree in all three treatment groups, with the group getting the sulfur bath showing the greatest degree of improvement. Table 1 summarizes the results on the Ritchie index by treatment group.

Several research studies have attempted to determine why the Dead Sea baths were so effective. The Dead Sea is extremely saline—ten times more so than the Mediterranean Sea. However, this is not the most likely explanation, as a double-blind study of RA indicated. The study compared Dead Sea salts to regular table salt, dissolved in the patient's home bath heated to 35 degrees Centigrade (95 degrees Fahrenheit), for twenty minutes a day for two weeks. There were statistically significant improvements in most of the clinical variables in the group that used the Dead Sea bath salts compared to the group that used table salt.

TABLE 1	Results of Spa Therapy for Rheumatoid Arthritis			
	BASELINE	**END OF TREATMENT**	**1 MONTH**	**3 MONTHS**
Group 1	27.3	13.1	12.6	15.9
Group 2	23.2	10.1	14.8	11.2
Group 3	21.4	7.8	12.7	19.3
Group 4	25.4	28.0	28.5	27.1

Although muscle tone, joint mobility, and pain intensity are somewhat influenced by hydromechanical and thermal stimuli, the improvement noted from Dead Sea bathing is generally superior to that noted with regular hot baths. A possible explanation may be in the trace-mineral content of the Dead Sea. Trace elements such as zinc and copper (key components of the antioxidant enzyme superoxide dismutase), as well as boron, selenium, rubidium, and other minerals, may be absorbed through the skin. Below-normal levels of several trace minerals have been reported in patients with RA.

The results of the latest study are quite impressive, in that most patients had severe active RA, yet no patient in the treatment group experienced any side effects or aggravation of the disease. Compare this result with standard drug therapy for RA. We hope that there will be further studies to increase our understanding of the beneficial effects of Dead Sea baths.

TREATMENT SUMMARY

RA is a disease known to have many contributing factors. Effective treatment using natural therapies requires controlling as many of these factors as possible. Foremost is the use of dietary measures to reduce the causes and ameliorate the symptoms of RA. Symptomatic relief can also be attained through the use of standard physical therapy techniques (i.e., exercise, heat, cold, massage, diathermy, lasers, and paraffin baths), anti-inflammatory botanicals, and nutrients.

Rheumatoid arthritis is often an aggressive disease that needs aggressive treatment. In mild-to-moderate cases of RA, the physical measures listed in the previous paragraph are extremely effective on their own. In severe cases, NSAIDs and other drugs may be necessary—at least in the acute phase. However, we encourage our patients not to abandon the natural measures, as they will actually enhance the effectiveness of the drugs, resulting in lower dosages. When the drugs are necessary, use deglycyrrhizinated licorice (DGL) to protect against developing peptic ulcers.

Diet

The first step is a therapeutic fast or an elimination diet, followed by careful reintroduction of foods to detect allergens. Virtually any food can aggravate RA, but the most common offenders are wheat, corn, milk and other dairy products, beef, and nightshade family (*Solanaceae*) foods (tomato, potato, eggplant, peppers, and tobacco).

After isolating and eliminating all allergens, a generally healthy diet is recommended: rich in whole foods, vegetables, and fiber, and low in sugar, meat, refined carbohydrates, and animal fats. Foods particularly beneficial for the RA patient include: cold-water fish (mackerel, herring, sardines, and salmon) and flavonoid-rich berries (cherries, hawthorn berries, blueberries, blackberries, etc.).

Nutritional Supplements

- DHEA: 50–200 mg per day
- EPA: 1.8 g per day
  or flaxseed oil: 1 tbsp per day
- Niacinamide: 500 mg four times per day (check liver enzyme values in the blood every six months)
- Pantothenic acid: 500 mg four times per day
- Vitamin C: 1–3 g per day in divided doses
- Vitamin E: 400–800 IU per day
- Copper: 1 mg per day
- Manganese: 15 mg per day
- Selenium: 200 mcg per day
- Zinc: 45 mg per day
- Betaine HCl: 10–70 grains with meals (see the chapter DIGESTION and ELIMINATION for instructions)
- Pancreatin (10 × USP): 350 mg–750 mg between meals three times per day or Bromelain: 250–750 mg (1,800–2,000 mcu) between meals three times per day

Botanical Medicines

The following botanicals may be used alone or in combination with others. Severe inflammation and joint destruction require more aggressive therapy.

Individuals with a history of corticosteroid use (e.g., prednisone) and those being weaned of corticosteroids should take adrenal-supportive herbs such as Chinese thoroughwax (*Bupleuri falcatum*), licorice (*Glycyrrhiza glabra*), and *Panax ginseng*. These herbs support the adrenal glands by preventing and/or reversing the adrenal gland atrophy (shrinkage) induced by these drugs.

- Curcumin: 400 mg three times per day or Ginger: incorporate 8–10 grams of fresh ginger into the diet each day, or recommend ginger extracts standardized to contain 20% gingerol and shogaol at a dosage of 100–200 mg three times per day

- Chinese thoroughwax (*Bupleuri falca-tum*) (dosages to be taken three times per day):
  Dried root: 2–4 g
  Tincture (1:5): 5–10 ml
  Fluid extract (1:1): 2–4 ml
  Solid extract (4:1): 200–400 mg
- *Panax ginseng* (dosages to be taken three times per day)
  Crude herb: 4.5–6 g per day
  Standardized extract (5% ginseno-sides): 500 mg 1–3 times per day
- Licorice (*Glycyrrhiza glabra*) (dosages to be taken three times per day)
  Dried root: 2–4 g
  Tincture (1:5): 10–20 ml
  Fluid extract (1:1): 4–6 ml
  Solid extract (4:1): 250–500 mg

Physical Medicine

- Heat (moist packs, hot baths, etc.): 20–30 minutes one to three times per day
- Cold packs for acute flare-ups
- Paraffin baths (if skin irritation is caused by hot water)
- Active (or, in severe cases, passive) range-of-motion exercises: 3–10 repetitions 1–3 times per day
- Progressive isometric (and isotonic as the joints improve) exercise: 3–10 repetitions several times per day, with generous periods of rest
- Massage: once per week

Rosacea

Chronic acne-like eruption on the face of middle-aged and older adults associated with facial flushing

The primary involvement occurs over the flushed areas of the cheeks and nose

More common in women (3:1), but more severe in men

R*osacea* is a chronic skin disorder in which the nose and cheeks are abnormally red and may be covered with pimples similar to those seen in acne (see ACNE). Rosacea is a relatively common skin disorder among adults between the ages of thirty and fifty, with women being affected about three times as often as men.

Causes

Many factors have been suspected of causing rosacea: alcoholism, menopausal flushing, local infection, B vitamin deficiencies, and gastrointestinal disorders. Most cases are associated with moderate to severe *seborrhea* (excess flow of sebum—a mixture of oils and waxes, which lubricate the skin and prevent the loss of water).

Therapeutic Considerations

The primary therapeutic goals in treating rosacea are to enhance gastric and pancreatic secretions, to minimize intake of food and drinks that cause flushing of the face; and to supplement with B vitamins to try to normalize sebum production by following the recommendations given in ACNE.

Hypochlorhydria

Gastric analysis of rosacea patients has led to the postulate that rosacea results from *hypochlorhydria* (reduced gastric acid output).[1] Psychological factors (i.e., worry, depression, stress, etc.) often reduce gastric acidity. This may explain why sometimes the rosacea is worse than at other times. Hydrochloric acid supplementation results in marked improvement in rosacea patients who

QUICK REVIEW

- Low gastric acid output may be a factor in many cases.

- Lack of B-vitamins, especially vitamin B2 (riboflavin), may cause rosacea.

have insufficient hydrochloric acid secretion.[1] See DIGESTION and ELIMINATION for information on determining whether hydrochloric acid output is sufficient.

Rosacea patients have also been shown to have decreased secretion of the pancreatic enzyme lipase and to benefit from supplementation with pancreatin (pancreatic enzyme preparations made from hog pancreas).[2]

B-Vitamins

The administration of large doses of B-vitamins has been shown to be quite effective in the treatment of rosacea, with riboflavin appearing to be the key factor.[3–5] There is a small organism—a skin mite named *Demodex folliculorum*—that has been considered a causative factor in rosacea. It is interesting to note that researchers were able to infect the skin of riboflavin-deficient rats with *Demodex*, but not the skin of normal rats.[5] This mechanism may be a factor in the clinical improvement noted with B vitamin treatment.

TREATMENT SUMMARY

Although the causes of rosacea have not yet been determined, sufficient information is available to adequately treat most patients. Addressing hypochlorhydria, avoiding foods that can cause flushing of the face, and B vitamin supplementation form the basis of therapy.

General Recommendations

See the chapter ACNE.

Diet

- Avoid coffee, alcohol, hot beverages, spicy foods, and any other food or drink that causes a flush.
- Eliminate all refined and/or concentrated sugars from the diet.

- Do not eat foods that contain trans-fatty acids, such as milk, milk products, margarine, shortening, or other synthetically hydrogenated vegetable oils, as well as fried foods.
- Avoid milk and foods high in iodized salt.

Nutritional Supplements

- Multiple-vitamin-and-mineral formula providing B-complex vitamins according to recommendations given in the chapter SUPPLEMENTARY MEASURES.
- Hydrochloric acid: as recommended in the chapter DIGESTION AND ELIMINATION
- Pancreatin (8–10 × USP): 350–500 mg before meals

Seasonal Affective Disorder

. . . .

Regularly occurring winter depression, frequently associated with summer hypomania

Seasonal affective disorder (SAD) is associated with winter depression and feeling "normal" or very happy in the summer. Typically, individuals with SAD feel depressed; they generally slow down, oversleep, overeat, and crave carbohydrates in the winter. In the summer, these same patients feel elated, active, and energetic.

Although many variables may be responsible for SAD, lack of exposure to full-spectrum natural light appears to be the most logical explanation. Many mammals exhibit seasonal variation in activity level, sleep patterns, and appetite, and are extremely sensitive to changes in day length. The key hormonal change may be a reduced secretion of melatonin by the pineal gland and an increased secretion of cortisol by the adrenal glands. Melatonin supplementation may relieve the symptoms of SAD because it increases brain melatonin levels; it also may suppress cortisol secretion.[1]

Therapeutic Considerations

Please consult the chapter on DEPRESSION. The considerations and therapeutic goals discussed in the DEPRESSION chapter are pertinent here as well. The only difference is that, in addition to the recommendations given for treating Depression, we definitely recommend using light therapy.

Light Therapy

Full-spectrum light therapy, designed to replicate natural sunlight, has been used to treat both SAD and clinical depression. The antidepressive effect of such light therapy has been demonstrated in well-monitored, controlled studies.[2–5] This effect is probably due to restoration of proper melatonin synthesis and secretion by the pineal gland, leading to

. . . .

QUICK REVIEW

- Although many variables may be responsible for SAD, lack of exposure to full-spectrum natural light appears to be the most logical explanation.
- Nighttime melatonin use may be helpful.
- The antidepressive effects of full-spectrum light therapy designed to replicate natural sunlight have been demonstrated in well-monitored, controlled studies.
- The St. John's wort extract standardized to contain 0.3 percent hypericin (see DEPRESSION), at a dosage of 300 mg three times per day, has been shown to relieve SAD.

reestablishment of the proper circadian rhythm—the natural 24-hour rhythmic release of hormones.

Light therapy consists of using full-spectrum lighting (Vitalite is a popular brand). The typical protocol used in clinical studies involved placing full-spectrum fluorescent tubes in regular fluorescent fixtures (eight tubes total). Patients were then instructed to sit three feet away from the light from 5:00 A.M. to 8:00 A.M. and again from 5:30 P.M. to 8:30 P.M. They were free to engage in activities as long as they glanced at the light at least once per minute. Obviously, to adopt this treatment protocol would greatly restrict social activities. Something that may work just as well is simply replacing standard light bulbs with full-spectrum light bulbs—although this recommendation remains to be proven.

St. John's Wort (Hypericum perfoliatum)

The St. John's wort extract, standardized to contain 0.3 percent hypericin (see DEPRES-SION) at a dosage of 300 mg three times per day, has been shown to relieve SAD.[6] However, although effective on its own, St. John's wort extract is more effective when used in combination with light therapy. This was demonstrated by a four-week double-blind study in which patients with SAD were randomly assigned to one of two groups. Both groups were treated with 900 mg of St. John's wort extract (0.3-percent hypericin content) per day; one group was treated with bright light (3000 lux—a unit of light intensity) and the other with dim light (<300 lux). There was a significant reduction in the Hamilton Depression Scale for both groups. The group receiving the bright light had a seventy-two percent reduction while the group getting the dim light had a sixty percent reduction. These results demonstrate that the effectiveness of St. John's wort extract in treating SAD is enhanced with light therapy.

TREATMENT SUMMARY

Since the cause of SAD appears to be light-related, the treatment goal is to extend the length of light exposure on winter days. This can be accomplished by using full-spectrum lighting, as described in this chapter. In addition, we recommend nighttime melatonin supplementation (3 mg forty-five minutes before retiring) and daytime St. John's wort extract (0.3% hypericin content, 300 mg three times per day).

Seborrheic Dermatitis

Superficial reddened small bumps and scaly eruptions occurring on the scalp, cheeks, and skin folds (the armpit, groin, and neck)

Usually does not itch

Seasonal, worse in winter

Seborrheic dermatitis is a common skin condition with an appearance similar to eczema. It may be associated with excessive oiliness (seborrhea) and dandruff. The scale may be yellowish and either dry or greasy. The reddened, scaly bumps may coalesce to form large plaques or patches.

Seborrheic dermatitis occurs either in infancy (usually between two and twelve weeks of age) or in adulthood. It has a prognosis of lifelong recurrence, tending to worsen with advancing age.

The cause of seborrheic dermatitis is unknown. Genetic predisposition, emotional stress, diet, hormones, and infection with yeast-like organisms have all been implicated. Seborrheic dermatitis is now recognized as one of the most common manifestations of AIDS, affecting as many as eighty-three percent. This recent observation has given increased credence to the infection theory of seborrheic dermatitis.

Therapeutic Considerations

Food Allergy

Seborrheic dermatitis usually begins in infancy as "cradle cap" and, although not primarily an allergic disease, has been associated with food allergy; sixty-seven percent of children who get cradle cap develop some form of allergy by age ten.[1]

Biotin

The underlying factor in infants appears to be a biotin deficiency.[2] A syndrome clinically similar to seborrheic dermatitis has been produced by feeding rats a diet high in raw egg white (high in avidin, a protein that binds biotin, making it unavailable for absorption). A large portion of the human biotin supply is provided by intestinal bacteria. It has been

QUICK REVIEW

- Seborrhea may be due to a B vitamin deficiency.
- A biotin deficiency is the most frequent cause of "cradle cap."
- Vitamin B6 ointment can help in treating the sicca variant of seborrheic dermatitis.

postulated that, since newborns are born with a sterile gastrointestinal tract, the absence of normal intestinal flora may be responsible for biotin deficiency in infants.[2] A number of studies have demonstrated successful treatment of seborrheic dermatitis with biotin in both the nursing mother and the infant.[2,3]

In adults, treatment with biotin alone is usually of no value. It is used in combination with other B vitamins that are vital for proper skin metabolism (pyridoxine, pantothenic acid, niacin, thiamin, and the lipotropics—nutritional factors which promote the flow of fat to and from the liver, such as choline, methionine, and inositol).

Vitamin B6

Taking a drug that causes vitamin B6 deficiency (desopyridoxine) can cause skin lesions that are indistinguishable from seborrheic dermatitis.[4] Similar lesions have been produced experimentally in rats by placing them on a vitamin-B6-deficient diet.

Vitamin B6 has been shown to be effective in treating a form of seborrheic dermatitis called the *sicca variant*. It involves only the scalp (dandruff), brow, the nose, and bearded area, with varying degrees of greasy adherent scales on a reddened base. In one study, all patients cleared completely within ten days by locally applying a water-soluble ointment that contained 50 mg of vitamin B6 (pyridoxine) per gram of ointment.[5] Other types of

seborrheic dermatitis did not respond to this mode of therapy.

The improvement may have resulted from correcting a vitamin B6 deficiency, or it may have been due to a reduction in sebaceous secretion rate caused by the vitamin B6 ointment.[4-6]

Vitamin B6 cream can be obtained from a compounding pharmacist. To find a compounding pharmacist in your area, call the International Academy of Compounding Pharmacists (1-800-927-4227).

A person who has seborrheic dermatitis should be checked for exposure to drugs or other factors which can block vitamin B6 function. Possible sources of such exposure include the hydrazine dyes (FD&C yellow #5) and drugs (INH and hydralazine), dopamine, penicillamine, oral contraceptives, and excessive protein intake.[7]

Folic Acid and Vitamin B12

Oral treatment with folic acid has been only moderately successful in cases of seborrheic dermatitis. The best results have been obtained with a special form called *tetrahydrofolate*,[5] which should be used in combination vitamin B12.[8] Injections of vitamin B12, both synthetic and liver-extracted, have been shown to be very effective in many cases.[9] This may be due to vitamin B12's role as a cofactor (with choline) in making tetrahydrofolate from folic acid.

. . . .

TREATMENT SUMMARY

Although the optimal approach to treating all seborrheic dermatitis patients is not clear at this time, effective therapy is

available for most patients. In infants, biotin supplementation and control of food allergies are the keys. If the child is nursing, biotin can be given to the mother and the mother should avoid common food allergens (milk, corn, wheat, citrus, peanuts, and eggs). For adults, supplementing with large doses of vitamin-B-complex is the primary therapy.

Diet

Detect and treat food allergens. In nursing infants, the food allergies of the mother should be considered.

Nutritional Supplements

The following recommendations are for adults.

- Biotin: 3 mg twice per day
- B-complex: Follow the dosage recommendations for the various B vitamins given in the chapter SUPPLEMENTARY MEASURES.
- Zinc: 20–30 mg per day
- Flaxseed oil: 1 tbsp per day

Topical Treatment

- Pyridoxine ointment: 50 mg/g (in water soluble base)

Sinusitis (Bacterial)

History of acute viral respiratory infection, dental infection, or nasal allergy

Nasal congestion and thick discharge

Fever, chills, and frontal headache

Pain, tenderness, redness, and swelling over the involved sinus

Chronic infection may produce no symptoms other than mild postnasal discharge, a musty odor, or a nonproductive cough

Any factor that causes swelling of the lining of the sinuses—the mucous membranes—may result in obstruction of drainage and subsequent infection. The liquid produced by the inflammation and blockage feeds bacteria, which can lead to an infection. The most common predisposing factor to acute bacterial sinusitis is viral upper respiratory infection (the common cold). An underlying dental infection is the causative factor in about one-quarter of the time when sinusitis affects primarily the *maxillary sinuses* (the sinuses of the cheek). In chronic cases, low immune function as well as hay fever (allergic rhinitis) and food allergies are often important factors.

Therapeutic Considerations

Although antibiotic therapy is the dominant treatment for acute and chronic bacterial sinusitis, it is of limited value. In fact, there is considerable doubt that most antibiotics provide any benefit at all. A recent detailed analysis to determine the evidence for the effectiveness of antibiotic treatment in acute sinusitis in adults concluded: "The effectiveness of antibiotic treatment in acute maxillary sinusitis in a general practice population is not based sufficiently on evidence."[1] The same can be said about chronic sinusitis.[2] In other words, there is no evidence that antibiotics provide any benefit.

Nevertheless, in severe or unresponsive cases antibiotics may be appropriate. Newer, more potent antibiotics (e.g., lactam antibiotics) appear to be more effective than penicillin, amoxicillin, and other less potent antibiotics.[3]

In children, there is even less evidence that antimicrobial therapy is of significant benefit. Overuse of antibiotics to treat children who have sinusitis or otitis media is a growing concern, as it is leading to antibiotic-resistant strains of bacterial pathogens. According to a 1997 review article, no studies that show antibiotics to be effective have been published.[4]

Clearly, addressing the underlying cause of chronic sinusitis (e.g., low immune function and respiratory or food allergens), along with supportive therapy (e.g., saline nasal sprays, immune-enhancing herbs, and natural decongestants), appears to be the most rational approach.

In cases of acute sinusitis, the therapeutic goals are to reestablish drainage and to clear the acute infection. Various measures can be used: local application of heat, local use of volatile oils and botanicals with antibacterial properties, and immune system support (see the chapter IMMUNE SUPPORT).

Allergy and Respiratory Tract Irritants

Individuals with chronic sinusitis should avoid environmental and food allergens. Studies have shown that between twenty-five and seventy percent of people with allergies have sinusitis.[5] Environmental control requires the use of air-filtering vacuum cleaners and installation of an air cleaner with a HEPA filter. Some particularly sensitive people may need to have all pets removed from the home, along with carpeting and feather bedding.[6]

In addition to allergens, chemicals in the environment that irritate the respiratory tract can often be a problem for patients who have chronic sinusitis.[7] A small portable air purifier as well as live plants may help purify the air.

Helicobacter pylori

An interesting study involved asthma and eczema patients who had symptoms of peptic ulcer and the presence of *Helicobacter pylori*—the bacteria linked to ulcers (see ULCERS). Elimination of *H. pylori* (using antibiotic therapy) resolved allergy symptoms, including chronic sinusitis, in a significant number of these patients.[8] If you have chronic sinusitis, we recommend asking your doctor to screen for *H. pylori*. For more information, see DIGESTION and ELIMINATION.

Bromelain

Bromelain is a group of sulfur-containing enzymes, obtained from the pineapple plant (*Ananas comusus*), that digest protein (proteolytic enzymes or proteases). Patients with acute sinusitis have responded to bromelain therapy. In one study, good-to-excellent results were obtained in eighty-seven percent of bromelain-treated patients, compared with sixty-eight percent of the placebo group.[9] For more information on treating upper-respiratory-tract infections with bromelain, see BRONCHITIS.

QUICK REVIEW

- Any factor that causes swelling of the mucous membranes that line the sinuses may result in obstruction of drainage and subsequent infection.
- Antibiotic therapy is of limited value.
- Addressing the underlying cause of chronic sinusitis, along with supportive therapy, appears to be the most rational approach.
- Patients with acute sinusitis have responded to bromelain therapy.

TREATMENT SUMMARY

In cases of acute sinusitis, the therapeutic goals are to reestablish drainage and to clear the acute infection. Various measures can be used: local application of heat, local use of volatile oils and botanicals with antibacterial properties, and immune system support (see IMMUNE SUPPORT).

Since chronic sinusitis is often associated with allergy, long-term control is dependent on isolation and elimination of the food or air-borne allergens and correction of the underlying problem that allowed the allergy to develop (see FOOD ALLERGY for a more thorough discussion). During the acute phase, elimination of the common food allergens (milk, wheat, eggs, citrus, corn, and peanut butter) is recommended until a more definitive diagnosis can be made.

Local applications of heat have been shown to be very effective in alleviating both short- and long-term symptoms of allergic rhinitis.[10]

We have found that patients with chronic sinusitis often suffer from yeast syndrome (chronic candidiasis). Take the self-test in CANDIDIASIS to determine whether this situation applies.

Nutritional Supplements
(see IMMUNE SUPPORT for more information)

- Vitamin C: 500 mg every two hours
- Bioflavonoids: 1,000 mg per day
- Vitamin A: 5,000 IU per day
- Beta-carotene: 25,000 IU per day
- Zinc: 20–30 mg per day
- Thymus extract: the equivalent of 120 mg pure polypeptides with molecular weights less than 10,000, or roughly 500 mg of the crude polypeptide fraction

Botanical Medicines
(all dosages three times per day)

- *Echinacea sp.*
  Dried root (or as tea): 0.5–1 g
  Freeze-dried plant: 325–650 mg
  Juice of aerial portion of E. purpurea stabilized in 22% ethanol: 2–3 ml
  Tincture (1:5): 2–4 ml
  Fluid extract (1:1): 2–4 ml
  Solid (dry powdered) extract (6.5:1 or 3.5% echinacoside): 150–300 mg
- *Hydrastis canadensis* (goldenseal)
  The dosage should be based on berberine content. As there is a wide range of quality in goldenseal preparations, standardized extracts are recommended. Three times a day dosages follow:
  Dried root or as infusion (tea): 2–4 g

Tincture (1:5): 6–12 ml (1½–3 tsp)

Fluid extract (1:1): 2–4 ml (½–1 tsp)

Solid (powdered dry) extract (4:1 or
8–12% alkaloid content):
250–500 mg

- Bromelain (1,200–1,800 mcu):
250–500 mg between meals

Topical Treatment

- Intranasal douche with saline solution
(available at pharmacies)

- Swab passages with oil of bitter orange
- Menthol or eucalyptus packs over sinuses (take care to avoid irritation)

Physical Therapy

- Local applications of hot packs (discontinue if pain increases without
drainage)

Sore Throat

. . . .

Sore throat with pain on swallowing

Red throat with swollen tonsils

Tender cervical lymph nodes

Over ninety percent of "sore throats" are caused by viruses. However, if you have a sore throat we recommend consulting a physician to rule out *strep throat* (group A beta-hemolytic streptococci pharyngotonsillitis). You simply cannot tell the difference between the two causes just by looking at the throat and tonsils. Fortunately, physicians now have swabs available that can immediately test for the presence of strep.[1]

These rapid strep screens are a major clinical advance. Since prior to these screening techniques the definitive diagnosis with a positive culture for group A strep usually takes two days, antibiotic therapy during this time for presumed group-A strep throat leads to unnecessary exposure to antibiotics and an increased likelihood of developing antibiotic-resistant organisms.

The hope is that the use of these rapid strep screens will eliminate the unnecessary use of antibiotics. Even in some cases of strep, antibiotics may not be necessary.[2] Strep throat is usually a self-limiting disease. Although most standard medical textbooks strongly assert that antibiotics are very important, recent research has shown that clinical recovery is similar in cases given or not given antibiotics.[3,4] The primary concern with not using antibiotics is the development of rheumatic fever or kidney disease. *Rheumatic fever* develops two to three weeks after a strep throat and is associated with inflammation of the heart, arthritis, and fever. Un-

fortunately, antibiotic administration does not significantly reduce the frequency of these complications.[3]

Our recommendation is that the use of antibiotics should be reserved for those who are suffering from severe infection, or who are unresponsive to therapy (i.e., no response after one week of the natural therapy described in this chapter), and those with a prior history of rheumatic fever or strep-induced kidney disease. Even then, antibiotics such as penicillin fail to kill off all of the streptococci in over twenty percent of patients. The primary reason is the presence of beta-lactase-positive organisms (*Staphylococcus aureus* and *Bacteroides species)*, which shield streptococci by deactivating the penicillin.[5]

As a side note, antibiotics are often praised for their role in effectively eliminating rheumatic fever as a serious concern, but the dramatic decrease in the frequency of rheumatic fever began before the invention of effective antibiotics.[6] Improved socioeconomic, hygienic, and nutritional factors were, as with most infectious diseases, more important than the liberal use of penicillin.

Therapeutic Considerations

The primary therapeutic goal is to enhance the immune system. If a person's immune system is functioning well, the illness will be short-lived. Enhancing general immune function, as described in the chapter IMMUNE SUPPORT may shorten the course. In cases of poor immune function, every effort should be made to strengthen the immune system by following the recommendations given in IMMUNE SYSTEM.

The recommendations given in this chapter are of a general nature; they can be used to treat either strep throat or a sore throat due to a virus, but the focus of discussion will primarily be on strep throat. In cases of viral infection, we encourage you to see COMMON COLD.

Vitamin C

During the 1930s, there was considerable interest in the relationship between malnutrition and the development of rheumatic fever. Both experimental animal work and population surveys demonstrated a correlation between vitamin C deficiency and the development of rheumatic fever. The findings were that rheumatic fever was virtually nonexistent when vitamin C intake was high,

and that eighteen percent of children in high-risk groups had subnormal serum vitamin C levels.

In one study, vitamin C supplementation of streptococcal-infected, vitamin-C-deficient, rheumatic-fever-susceptible guinea pigs, totally prevented their development of rheumatic fever.[7,8] Uncontrolled clinical studies demonstrated very positive results when children were given orange juice supplementation. Unfortunately, this promising line of research appears to have been dropped, probably due to the advent of supposedly effective antibiotics.

Herbal Medicines

The most popular herbal medicines historically used to treat strep throat are goldenseal (*Hydrastis canadensis*) and echinacea (*Echinacea sp.*). The berberine alkaloid of goldenseal exerts antibiotic activity against streptococci and, perhaps more important, has been shown to inhibit the attachment of group-A streptococci to the lining of the throat.[9] To promote the spread of colonies of bacteria, streptococci secrete large amounts

QUICK REVIEW

- Over ninety percent of all cases of sore throat are caused by viruses.
- It is important to see a physician to rule out strep throat as the cause.
- Vitamin C is very important in the prevention of rheumatic fever.
- Goldenseal prevents the adherence of strep bacteria to the lining of the throat.

- Changing to a new toothbrush or washing the toothbrush in the dishwasher every seventeen to thirty-one days has been shown to help many people who are prone to a sore throat.
- If antibiotics are used or have been used, it is important to use a probiotic supplement containing *Lactobacillus acidophilus* and *Bifidobacterium bifidus*.

of hyaluronidase. This enzyme is inhibited by echinacea and bioflavonoids. Echinacea also promotes improved immune function.

Another botanical of value is ginger (*Zingiber officinale*). While not a particularly strong antiviral, it does have analgesic properties and is useful for relieving throat irritation.[10]

Other Considerations

While poor immune function is clearly a factor in people suffering from chronic sore throat, other factors should also be considered. For example, some people experience repeated challenges to their pharynx from microbes residing in their toothbrush. Changing to a new toothbrush or washing the toothbrush in the dishwasher every seventeen to thirty-one days has been shown to help many people who are prone to having a sore throat.[11] Another significant cause of chronic sore throat is food allergy. Typical upper-respiratory-tract symptoms of chronic delayed food allergy include chronic sore throat, runny nose, sinusitis, tonsillitis, and laryngitis.[12]

If antibiotics are used or have been used, it is important to use a probiotic supplement containing *Lactobacillus acidophilus* and *Bifidobacterium bifidus*. Probiotic supplementation helps prevent and treat antibiotic-induced diarrhea, candida overgrowth, and urinary tract infections. Although it is commonly believed that acidophilus supplements are not effective if taken during antibiotic therapy, research actually supports the use of *L. acidophilus* during antibiotic administration.[13,14] Reductions in levels of friendly bacteria, and/or a superinfection with antibiotic-resistant flora, may be prevented by administering *L. acidophilus* products during antibiotic therapy. A dose of at least fifteen to twenty billion organisms per day is required during antibiotic usage. We recommend taking the probiotic supplement as far apart in time from the antibiotic as possible. After the antibiotic course is finished, a dosage of one to two billion live organisms per day is sufficient.

TREATMENT SUMMARY

The time-honored advice to drink plenty of fluids, restrict food intake, and get plenty of rest is very important. We also recommend eliminating concentrated sugars and suspected food allergens from the diet. Because fever is a natural defense mechanism, it should be supported. Drugs to lower fever should not be used unless the body temperature approaches 104 degrees F, at which point the body's ability to control its temperature becomes impaired.

Diet

Eliminate all sources of concentrated simple sugars: sugar, honey, fruit juice, dried fruit, etc. Restrict food intake to less than 1,000 calories per day. Increase fluid intake to 8 ounces per hour, using water and the herbal teas listed below.

Nutritional Supplements

- Vitamin A: 50,000 IU per day for up to two days in infants and up to one week in adults, or beta-carotene: 200,000 IU per day

---

NOTE: Do not use vitamin A in women who are pregnant or at risk for pregnancy, due to a link with birth defects at high dosages.

- Vitamin C: 500 mg every two hours
- Bioflavonoids: 1,000 mg per day
- Zinc: take lozenges that supply 15–25 mg of elemental zinc (gluconate form without citrate mannitol or sorbitol); dissolve in the mouth every two waking hours after an initial double dose; continue for up to 3 days
- Thymus extract: the equivalent of 120 mg pure polypeptides with molecular weights less than 10,000, or roughly 500 mg of the crude polypeptide fraction

Botanical Medicines

- *Echinacea sp.*
  Dried root (or as tea): 0.5–1 g three times per day
  Freeze-dried plant: 325–650 mg three times per day
  Juice of aerial portion of E. purpurea stabilized in 22% ethanol: 2–3 ml three times per day
  Tincture (1:5): 2–4 ml three times per day
  Fluid extract (1:1): 2–4 ml three times per day
  Solid (dry powdered) extract (6.5:1 or 3.5% echinacoside): 150–300 mg three times per day
- Goldenseal (*Hydrastis canadensis*)
  The dosage should be based on berberine content. As there is a wide range of quality in goldenseal preparations, standardized extracts are recommended. Three times per day dosages are:
  Dried root or as infusion (tea): 2–4 g
  Tincture (1:5): 6–12 ml (1 1/2–3 tsp)
  Fluid extract (1:1): 2–4 ml (1/2–1 tsp)
  Solid (powdered dry) extract (4:1 or 8–12% alkaloid content): 250–500 mg

Local Treatment

- Gargle with salt water twice per day: 1 tbsp salt in 8 ounces of warm water
- Ginger (*Zingiber officinalis*): strong tea made with fresh root

Sports Injuries, Tendinitis, and Bursitis

Tendinitis
  Acute or chronic pain localized in a tendon
  Limited range of motion

Bursitis
  Severe pain of the affected joint, particularly on movement
  Limited range of motion

This chapter deals with sports injuries (e.g., sprains, strains, and bruises), tendinitis, and bursitis. *Tendinitis* is an inflammatory condition of a *tendon*—the connective tissue that connects muscles to bones. Tendinitis usually results from a strain. Although acute tendinitis usually heals within a few days to two weeks, it may become chronic, in which case calcium salts will typically deposit along the tendon fibers. The tendons most commonly affected are the Achilles (back of ankle), the biceps (front of shoulder), the pollicis brevis and longus (thumb), the upper patella (knee), the posterior tibial (inside of foot), and the rotator cuff (shoulder).

Bursitis is inflammation of the *bursa,* the sac-like membrane that contains fluid which lubricates the joints. Bursitis may result from trauma, strain, infection, or arthritic conditions. The most common locations are shoulder, elbow, hip, and lower knee. Occasionally the bursa can develop calcified deposits and become a chronic problem.

Cause

The most common cause of sports injury is sudden excessive tension on a tendon or bursa, producing a strain or sprain. Repeated muscle contraction, leading to exhaustion of the muscle, can result in similar injury. Sometimes tendinitis develops when the grooves in which the tendons move develop bone spurs or other mechanical abnormalities. Proper stretching and warm-up before exercise are important preventive measures.

Therapeutic Considerations

After an injury or sprain, immediate injury first-aid is very important. The acronym RICE summarizes the approach:

- **R**est the injured part as soon as it is hurt, to avoid further injury
- **I**ce the area of pain to decrease swelling and bleeding
- **C**ompress the area with an elastic bandage, also to limit swelling and bleeding
- **E**levate the injured part above the level of the heart to increase drainage of fluids out of the injured area

Proper application of these procedures is important for optimal results. When icing, first cover the injured area with a towel, then place an ice pack on it. It is important to not wrap the injured part so tightly that circulation is impaired. The ice and compress should be applied for thirty minutes, followed by fifteen minutes without the ice to allow recirculation.

Of course, for any serious injury, a physician should be consulted immediately. Conditions that indicate the need to see a physician include: severe pain, injury to a joint, loss of function, or pain that persists for more than two weeks.[1]

After the acute inflammatory stage (twenty-four to forty-eight hours), gradually increasing range-of-motion and stretching exercises should be used to maintain and improve mobility and prevent adhesions (abnormal scar formation).

General Nutritional Support

Several nutrients are important for the promotion of healing. For example, vitamin C supplementation is important since vitamin C plays a major role in the prevention and repair of injuries. Deficiency of vitamin C is associated with defective formation and maintenance of tendon and bursal tissues. In addition to vitamin C, Vitamin A, zinc, vita-

QUICK REVIEW

- **Proper stretching and warm-up before exercise are important preventive measures.**
- **After an injury or sprain, immediate first-aid to the injured area (rest, ice, compression, and elevation) is very important.**
- **Deficiency of vitamin C is associated with defective formation and maintenance of tendon and bursal tissues.**
- **Vitamin A, zinc, vitamin E, and selenium, as well as vitamin C, are important not only for their wound-healing** properties, but also for their antioxidant effects.
- **Bromelain has been reported in scientific studies to exert a wide variety of beneficial effects, including reducing inflammation in cases of sports injury or trauma.**
- **Curcumin, the yellow pigment of *Curcuma longa* (turmeric), exerts excellent anti-inflammatory and antioxidant effects.**
- **Physical therapy can aid in pain relief and recovery from injury.**

min E, and selenium are important not only for their wound healing properties, but also for their antioxidant effects.

Flavonoids

Flavonoids, a group of plant pigments responsible for the colors of many fruits and flowers, are extremely effective in reducing inflammation and stabilizing collagen structures. Collagen is the major protein in tendons and other connective tissues. Flavonoids help maintain a healthy collagen structure by: (1) decreasing blood vessel permeability, thereby decreasing the influx of inflammatory mediators into areas of damage; (2) preventing free-radical damage via their potent antioxidant properties; (3) inhibiting damage to collagen tissue caused by enzymes that break down collagen; (4) inhibiting the release of inflammatory chemicals; and (5) reinforcing the natural cross-linking of collagen fibers to make them stronger.[1–3]

Double-blind, placebo-controlled studies have shown that supplemental citrus flavonoids cut in half the time needed to recover from sports injuries.[4,5]

Vitamin B12

An uncontrolled study found that intramuscular injections of vitamin B12 (daily for the first week and then less frequently according to response) gave rapid relief from bursitis pain for most patients. Subsequent X rays of patients with bursitis that had formed calcium deposits showed considerable breaking down of the calcium deposits.[6]

Bromelain

Bromelain (the protein-digesting enzyme complex of pineapple) was introduced as a medicinal agent in 1957, and since that time over four hundred scientific papers on its therapeutic applications have appeared in medical literature. In these studies, bromelain has been reported to exert a wide variety of beneficial effects, including reducing inflammation in cases of sports injury or trauma and prevention of swelling after trauma or surgery.[7]

One of the most interesting studies that used bromelain to treat sports-related injuries was a 1960 study that involved 146 boxers.[8] Seventy-four boxers received bromelain; in fifty-eight, all signs of bruising cleared completely within four days. In the remainder, complete clearance took eight to ten days. Among the seventy-two boxers who did not take bromelain, at the end of four days only ten showed bruises completely cleared; the remainder took seven to fourteen days. These results indicate that bromelain goes a long way in reducing bruising, inflammation, and swelling due to trauma.

It is important to recognize that, while bromelain has been shown to effectively reduce pain, this probably is the result of a reduction in tissue inflammation and edema, rather than a direct analgesic effect.

Curcumin

Curcumin—the yellow pigment of *Curcuma longa* (turmeric)—exerts excellent anti-inflammatory and antioxidant effects. Curcumin is as effective as cortisone or the potent anti-inflammatory drug phenylbutazone in animal studies. However, while phenylbutazone and cortisone are associated with significant toxicity, curcumin is without side effects. Curcumin has also demonstrated beneficial effects in human studies comparable to those of standard drugs. See RHEUMATOID ARTHRITIS for more information on curcumin.

Physical Therapy

There are a number of physical therapy techniques that can be quite helpful in speeding recovery and relieving pain. Perhaps the two most popular techniques are *transcutaneous electrical nerve stimulation* (TENS) and ultrasound. TENS involves the use of electricity to stimulate muscular contractions. The use of TENS to control pain has been well documented. Individuals with tendinitis have been found to respond well to TENS.[9] TENS therapy may be applied by a physical therapist or physician. In addition, there are also home units now available.

Ultrasound is a form of high-frequency sound vibration used to heat an area and increase its blood supply and lymphatic drainage. While it is useful during the acute stage (the first twenty-four to forty-eight hours) of an injury, it offers the greatest benefit in the recovery phase. It is particularly useful when the bursitis or tendinitis forms calcium deposits, or when *adhesions* (scar tissue) have formed inappropriately.[10]

TREATMENT SUMMARY

Treatment of the muscle, joint, tendon, or bursal damage caused by acute and chronic injuries involves two phases: inflammation inhibition and protection of the injured tissues, followed by promotion of healing after the acute phase has resolved. For any serious injury, a physician should be consulted immediately. Indications for a physician include: severe pain, injuries to the joints, loss of function, and pain which persists for more than two weeks.

RICE:

- **R**est the injured part
- **I**ce the painful area
- **C**ompress the injured area with an elastic bandage
- **E**levate the injured part above the level of the heart

The ice and compress should be applied for thirty minutes, followed by fifteen minutes without either to allow blood flow to return. After the acute inflammatory stage (twenty-four to forty-eight hours), gradually increasing range-of-motion and stretching exercises should be used to maintain and improve mobility and prevent adhesions (abnormal scar formation).

Nutritional Supplements

- High-potency multiple-vitamin-and-mineral formula, as described in the chapter SUPPLEMENTARY MEASURES
- Vitamin C: 500–1,000 mg three to four times per day
- Flavonoids (choose one):
  Grape seed or pine bark extract: 50–100 mg three times per day
  Citrus bioflavonoids: 500–1,000 mg three times per day

Botanical Medicines

- Curcumin (from turmeric): 200–400 mg three times per day between meals
- Bromelain (1,800–2,000 milk-clotting or gelatin-digesting units, mcu and gdu, respectively): 250–750 mg three times per day between meals

Physical Medicines

- TENS: if needed for pain control
- Ultrasound: three times per week during the recovery phase and if adhesions or contractures develop

Ulcers (Duodenal and Gastric)

. . . .

Abdominal distress forty-five to sixty minutes after meals or during the night; both relieved by food, antacids, or vomiting

Abdominal tenderness

Chronic but periodic symptoms

Ulcer crater or deformity in the stomach or upper small intestine visible on X ray or fiber-optic (endoscopic) exam

Positive test for blood in the stool

eptic ulcers (an ulcer is an erosion of the tissue, producing a crater-like lesion) occur in the stomach *(gastric ulcer)* or the first portion of the small intestine *(duodenal ulcer)*. Duodenal ulcers are more common, occurring in an estimated six to twelve percent of the adult population in the United States. In other words, approximately ten percent of the U.S. population has clinical evidence of duodenal ulcer at some time in their lifetime. Duodenal ulcers are four times more common in men than in women, and four to five times more common than gastric ulcers.

Although symptoms of a peptic ulcer may be absent or quite vague, most peptic ulcers are associated with abdominal discomfort noted forty-five to sixty minutes after meals or during the night. In the typical case, the pain is described as gnawing, burning, cramp-like, or aching, or as "heartburn." Eating or taking antacids usually results in great relief.

Even though duodenal and gastric ulcers occur at different locations, they appear to be the result of similar mechanisms. Specifically, the development of a duodenal or gastric ulcer is a result of damage to the protective factors that line the stomach and duodenum.

In the past, the focus has primarily been on the acidic secretions of the stomach as the primary cause of both gastric and duodenal ulcers. However, more recently the focus has been on the bacterium *Helicobacter pylori* and non-steroidal anti-inflammatory drugs.

Gastric acid is extremely corrosive. The pH of gastric acid (pH 1 to 3) would eat an ulcer right through the skin. To protect against ulcers, the lining of the stomach and small intestine has a layer of *mucin*, a slippery layer of mucus (mucopolysaccharides). In addition, the constant renewing of intestinal cells and the secretion of factors that neutralize the acid when it comes in contact with the stomach and intestinal linings also protect against ulcer formation. Gastric acid is designed to digest the food we eat, not the stomach or small intestine.

Contrary to popular opinion, oversecretion of gastric acid output is rarely a factor in the development of gastric ulcers. In fact, patients who have gastric ulcers tend to secrete normal or even reduced levels of gastric acid. In duodenal ulcer patients, almost half have increased gastric acid output. This increase may be due to an increased number of acid-producing cells, known as *parietal cells*. As a group, patients with duodenal ulcers have twice as many parietal cells in their stomach as people without ulcers.

Even with an increase in gastric acid output, under normal circumstances there are enough protective factors to prevent either gastric or duodenal ulcer formation. However, when the integrity of these protective factors is impaired, an ulcer can form. A loss of integrity can be a result *of H. pylori*, aspirin and other non-steroidal anti-inflammatory drugs (NSAIDs), alcohol, nutrient deficiency, stress, and many other factors. Of these factors, *H. pylori* and NSAIDs are by far the most significant.

Helicobacter pylori

The role of the bacterium *H. pylori* in peptic ulcer disease has been extensively investigated. It has been shown that ninety to one hundred percent of patients with duodenal ulcers, seventy percent with gastric ulcers, and about fifty percent of people over the age of fifty test positive for this bacterium.[1] Physicians can determine the presence of *H. pylori* by measuring the level of antibodies to *H. pylori* in the blood or saliva, or by culturing material collected during an *endoscopy* (the process of examination of the stomach or duodenum with a fiber-optic tube with a lens attached to it).

Predisposing factors for *H. pylori* infection are low gastric acid output and low antioxidant content in the gastrointestinal lining. *H. pylori* infection increases gastric pH, thereby setting up a positive-feedback scenario.[2] In other words, *H. pylori* infection leads to ulcer formation, and ulcer formation leads to *H. pylori* infection. For more information on *H. pylori*, see DIGESTION and ELIMINATION.

Aspirin and Other NSAIDs

Aspirin and other nonsteroidal anti-inflammatory drugs (NSAIDs) are associated with a significant risk of developing a peptic ulcer. Most studies that document the relative frequency of peptic ulcers as a consequence of aspirin and NSAID use have focused on their use in the treatment of arthritis and headaches. But recently the risk of gastrointestinal bleeding due to peptic ulcers was evaluated as a result of taking aspirin at daily dosages of 300 mg, 150 mg, and 75 mg—dosages commonly recommended to prevent heart attacks and strokes.[3]

One study, conducted at five test hospitals in England, found an increased risk of gastrointestinal bleeding due to peptic ulcer at all dosage levels. However, the dosage of 75 mg per day was associated with forty percent less bleeding than 300 mg per day, and thirty percent less than 150 mg per day. The researchers concluded: "No conventionally used prophylactic aspirin regimen seems free of the risk of peptic ulcer complications."

The combination of NSAID use and smoking is particularly harmful to the ulcer patient.[4] The NSAID use causes an ulcer and the smoking stimulates gastric acid output which subsequently worsens the symptoms and the severity of the ulcer.

Therapeutic Considerations

Individuals who experience any symptoms of a peptic ulcer need competent medical care. Peptic ulcer complications such as hemorrhage, perforation, and obstruction represent medical emergencies that require immediate hospitalization. Individuals with peptic ulcer must be monitored by a physician, even if they are following the natural approaches discussed below.

Lifestyle Factors

Stress and Emotions

Stress is universally believed to be an important causative factor in peptic ulcers. However, this link is quite controversial in the medical literature. One of the big problems is that studies attempting to examine this assumption about stress and ulcers have been poorly designed.[5] Several studies have shown that the number of stressful life events is not significantly different in peptic ulcer patients than in carefully selected, ulcer-free controls. These data suggest that it is not simply the amount of stress, but rather the patient's response to it, that is the significant factor. A large study of 4,000 persons who had no history of peptic ulcer disease revealed that those who perceived stress in their lives were at increased risk of developing peptic ulcers.[6] (See STRESS, STRESS MANAGEMENT, AND ADRENAL SUPPORT for a more complete discussion.)

Psychological factors are probably important in some patients with peptic ulcer disease, but not in others. As a group, ulcer patients have been characterized as tending to repress emotions. At the very least, we encourage our patients with ulcers to discover enjoyable outlets of self-expression and emotions.

Smoking

Smoking is a significant factor in the occurrence and severity of peptic ulcers. Increased frequency, decreased response to peptic ulcer therapy, and an increased mortality due to peptic ulcers are all related to smoking. Smoking causes ulcers by at least three mechanisms. First of all, smoking increases the backflow (*reflux*) of bile salts into the stomach. Bile salts are extremely irritating to the stomach and initial portions of the duodenum. Bile salt reflux induced by smoking appears to be the most significant factor responsible for the increased peptic ulcer

---

QUICK REVIEW

- Individuals with peptic ulcer must be monitored by a physician due to potential serious consequences if not effectively treated.
- Ulcers are usually the result of a breakdown in protective factors that line the stomach or small intestine.
- The bacterium *Helicobacter pylori* has been linked to both duodenal and gastric ulcers.

- Aspirin and other nonsteroidal anti-inflammatory drugs (NSAIDs) are associated with a significant risk of developing an ulcer.
- Smoking is a significant factor in the occurrence and severity of peptic ulcers.
- An allergy to milk may be a causative factor in many cases of ulcers.
- A diet rich in fiber is associated with a reduced rate of duodenal ulcers as compared with a low-fiber diet.

rate in smokers. Smoking also decreases the secretion of *bicarbonate* (an important neutralizer of gastric acid) by the pancreas, and accelerates the passage of food from the stomach into the duodenum.[6]

The psychological aspects of smoking are also important, since the chronic anxiety and psychological stress associated with smoking appear to worsen ulcer activity.

Nutritional Considerations

Food Allergy

Clinical and experimental evidence points to food allergy as a primary factor in many cases of peptic ulcer.[7-10] In one study, ninety-eight percent of patients who had X-ray evidence of peptic ulcer had coexisting lower- and upper-respiratory-tract allergic disease.[9] In another study, twenty-five of forty-three allergic children had peptic ulcers as diagnosed by X rays.[10] A diet that eliminates food allergens has been used with great success in treating and preventing recurrent ulcers.[8,9] It is ironic that many people with peptic ulcers

soothe themselves by consuming milk, a highly allergenic food. Milk should be avoided on this basis alone. However, there is additional evidence that milk should be avoided by patients with peptic ulcers; population studies show that the higher the milk consumption, the greater the likelihood of ulcer. Milk significantly increases stomach acid production.[11]

Fiber

A diet rich in fiber is associated with a reduced rate of ulcers, as compared with a low-fiber diet. The therapeutic use of a high-fiber diet by patients with recently healed duodenal ulcers reduces the recurrence rate by half.[12] Although several fibers that are often used to supplement the diet (pectin, guar gum, psyllium, etc.) have been shown to produce beneficial effects, a diet rich in plant foods is the best way to consume fiber.[13,14]

Cabbage

Raw cabbage juice is well documented as having remarkable success in treating peptic

---

- Raw cabbage juice is well documented as having remarkable success in treating peptic ulcers.

- Bismuth is a naturally occurring mineral that can act as an antacid and exert activity against *H. pylori*.

- DGL, a special form of licorice, has been shown to be more effective than Tagamet or Zantac in head-to-head comparison studies.

- Rhubarb or aloe vera preparations can be used to stop the bleeding of an ulcer.

ulcers.[15–17] In one study, 1 liter of the fresh juice per day, taken in divided doses, resulted in total ulcer healing in an average of only ten days. Further research has shown that the high glutamine content of the juice is probably responsible for the efficacy of cabbage in treating these ulcers.

In a double-blind clinical study of fifty-seven patients, twenty-four took 1.6 grams of glutamine per day, and the rest used conventional therapy (antacids, antispasmodics, diet, milk, and bland diet); glutamine proved to be the more effective treatment. Half of the glutamine patients showed complete healing (according to radiographic analysis) within two weeks, and twenty-two of the twenty-four showed complete relief and healing within four weeks.[17] Although the mechanism for these results is not known, the authors attributed them to the role of glutamine in the manufacture of compounds that line and protect the stomach and small intestine.

Bismuth Subcitrate

Bismuth is a naturally occurring mineral that can act as an antacid and exert activity against *H. pylori*. The best-known and most widely used bismuth preparation is bismuth subsalicylate—Pepto-Bismol. However, bismuth subcitrate has produced the best results against *H. pylori* and in the treatment of peptic ulcers.[18,19] In the United States, bismuth subcitrate preparations are primarily available through compounding pharmacies (pharmacies that still make up medications on site). To find a compounding pharmacist in your area, call the International Academy of Compounding Pharmacists (1-800-927-4227).

One of the key advantages of bismuth preparations over standard antibiotic approaches to eradicating *H. pylori* is that, while the bacteria may develop resistance to various antibiotics, they are unlikely to develop resistance to bismuth.

The usual dosage for bismuth subcitrate is 240 mg twice per day before meals. For bismuth subsalycilate, the dosage is 500 mg four times per day. Bismuth preparations are extremely safe when taken at prescribed dosages. Bismuth subcitrate may cause a temporary and harmless darkening of the tongue and/or stool. Bismuth subsalicylate should not be taken by children who are recovering from the flu, chicken pox, or other viral infection, as it may mask the nausea and vomiting associated with Reye's syndrome, a rare but serious illness.

Flavonoids

Flavonoids are known to counteract both the production and secretion of histamine, which is an important factor in ulcer formation since histamine stimulates the release of gastric acid. Experimental studies on guinea pigs and rats have demonstrated that flavonoids (e.g., catechin) exert significant anti-ulcer activity.[20,21]

In a human clinical study, oral administration of catechin at a dosage of 1,000 mg five times per day resulted in reduced histamine levels in the gastric tissue (determined by biopsy) of both normal patients and those with gastric and duodenal ulcers and acute gastritis.[21] In addition, in a recent study, several flavonoids were shown to inhibit *H. pylori* in a clear-cut concentration-dependent manner.[22] In addition, unlike antibiotics, the flavonoids were also shown to augment natural defense factors that prevent ulcer formation. The activity of flavone, the most potent flavonoid in the study, was shown to be similar to that of bismuth subcitrate.

Miscellaneous Nutrients

Vitamins A and E have been shown to inhibit the development of stress ulcers in rats, and are important factors in maintaining the integrity of the mucosal barrier.[23,24]

Zinc increases mucin production and has been shown to have a protective effect against peptic ulcers in animals[25] and a curative effect in humans.[26]

Botanical Medicines

Licorice (Glycyrrhiza glabra)

Licorice has historically been regarded as an excellent medicine for treating peptic ulcer. However, due to the side effects of the licorice compound glycyrrhetinic acid (it causes elevations in blood pressure in some cases), a procedure was developed to remove this compound from licorice and form deglycyrrhizinated licorice (DGL). The result is a very successful anti-ulcer agent without any known side effects. [27-32]

The proposed mechanism of DGL is that it stimulates and/or accelerates the protective factors that protect against ulcer formation.[27] This mechanism of action is much different than that of antacids and drugs such as Tagamet, Zantac, and Pepcid, which work by neutralizing or suppressing gastric acid.

Numerous studies over the years have found DGL to be an effective anti-ulcer compound. In several head-to-head comparison studies, DGL has been shown to be more effective than either Tagamet, Zantac, or antacids in both short-term treatment and maintenance therapy of peptic ulcers.[28,29] However, while these drugs are associated with significant side effects, DGL is extremely safe and costs only a fraction as much. For example, while Tagamet and Zantac typically cost well over $100 for a month's supply, DGL is available in health food stores at $15 for a month's supply.

DGL and Gastric Ulcers In one study, thirty-three gastric ulcer patients were treated with either DGL (760 mg three times per day) or a placebo for one month.[30] There

was a significantly greater reduction in ulcer size in the DGL group (seventy-eight percent), than in the placebo group (thirty-four percent). Complete healing occurred in forty-four percent of those who received DGL, but in only six percent of the placebo group.

Another study compared DGL to Tagamet: one hundred patients received either DGL (760 mg three times per day between meals) or Tagamet (200 mg three times per day and 400 mg at bedtime).[28] The percentage of ulcers healed after six and twelve weeks was similar in both groups. Yet while Tagamet is associated with some toxicity, DGL is extremely safe to use.

Gastric ulcers are often a result of the use of alcohol, aspirin or other nonsteroidal anti-inflammatory drugs, caffeine, or other factors that decrease the integrity of the gastric lining. As DGL has been shown to reduce the gastric bleeding caused by aspirin, DGL is recommended for the prevention of gastric ulcers in patients who require long-term treatment with ulcer-causing drugs, such as aspirin, other NSAIDs, and corticosteroids.[31]

DGL and Duodenal Ulcers DGL is also effective in treating duodenal ulcers. This is perhaps best illustrated by one study of patients with severe duodenal ulcers. In the study, forty patients with chronic duodenal ulcers of four to twelve years duration and more than six relapses during the previous year were treated with DGL.[32] All of the patients had been referred for surgery because of relentless pain, sometimes with frequent vomiting, despite treatment with bed rest, antacids, and powerful drugs. Half of the patients received 3 grams of DGL per day for eight weeks; the other half received 4.5 grams per day for sixteen weeks. All forty patients showed substantial improvement, usually within five to seven days, and none required surgery during the one-year follow-up.

Although both dosages were effective, the higher dose was significantly more effective than the lower dose.

In another more recent study, the therapeutic effect of DGL was compared to that of antacids or cimetidine in 874 patients with confirmed chronic duodenal ulcers.[29] Ninety-one percent of all ulcers healed within twelve weeks; there was no significant difference in healing rate among the groups. However, there were fewer relapses in the DGL group (8.2 percent) than in those who received cimetidine (12.9 percent), or antacids (16.4 percent). These results, coupled with DGL's protective effects, suggest that DGL is a superior treatment for duodenal ulcers.

An obvious question is: "Does DGL have any effect on *Helicobacter pylori?*" The answer appears to be "Yes," as DGL is composed of several flavonoids which have been shown to inhibit *H. pylori.*[22]

Rhubarb and Aloe vera

In cases of active intestinal bleeding, rhubarb (*Rheum species*) and aloe vera preparations can be extremely effective. In one double-blind study, the effectiveness of alcohol-extracted rhubarb tablets in stopping intestinal bleeding was evaluated. Of the 312 cases of bleeding gastric and duodenal ulcers, rhubarb stopped the bleeding in over ninety percent.[33] The time taken for evidence of bleeding (the presence of blood in the stool) to change from positive to negative was under sixty hours.

The beneficial actions of rhubarb are due to the presence of anthraquinones and flavonoids, which stop the bleeding by acting as *astringents* (basically, drying agents). Aloe vera contains similar compounds. In cases of active gastrointestinal bleeding, we recommend that rhubarb or aloe vera preparations be used. The most accessible treatment may be drinking aloe vera juice, about 1 liter per day, during these times.

TREATMENT SUMMARY

The first step is to identify and eliminate or reduce all factors implicated in the etiology of peptic ulcers: food allergy, cigarette smoking, stress, and drugs—especially aspirin and other NSAIDs. Once the causative factors have been controlled, attention should be directed at healing the ulcer, inhibiting factors that aggravate the ulcer (e.g., reducing excess acid secretion if present), and promoting tissue resistance. Finally, the proper diet and lifestyle should be developed to prevent further recurrence.

Antacids can be used as part of the initial treatment for symptomatic relief. All antacids are relatively safe when used on an occasional basis, but avoid antacids that contain aluminum. We recommend following label instructions and avoiding the regular use or overuse of antacids. Taken regularly, antacids can lead to malabsorption of nutrients, bowel irregularities, kidney stones, and other side effects.

We recommend holding off on the bismuth subcitrate until the other recommendations have failed, including a one-month trial of DGL. We have had particularly good results when using DGL to treat both gastric and duodenal ulcers. For the rare patient who simply cannot get past the taste of licorice, we recommend bismuth subcitrate or Robert's formula (see CROHN'S DISEASE AND ULCERATIVE COLITIS).

Psychological

Develop an effective stress-reduction program; eliminate or control stressors, and design a regular relaxation plan.

Diet

Eliminate allergenic foods, especially milk. Eat a diet high in dietary fiber, and consume fresh cabbage juice and other vegetable juices on a regular basis.

Nutritional Supplements

- Vitamin A: 5,000 IU per day
- Vitamin C: 500 mg three times per day
- Vitamin E: 100 IU three times per day
- Flavonoids: 500 mg three times per day
- Zinc: 20–30 mg per day

- Glutamine: 500 mg three times per day
- Bismuth subcitrate: 240 mg twice per day before meals

Botanical Medicines

Deglyrrhizinated Licorice (DGL)
The standard dosage for DGL in acute cases is two to four 380-mg chewable tablets between or twenty minutes before meals. For more mild chronic cases, or for maintenance, the dosage is one to two tablets twenty minutes before meals. Taking DGL after meals is associated with poor results. DGL therapy should be continued for at least eight to sixteen weeks after there is a full therapeutic response.

It appears that, in order to be effective in healing peptic ulcers, DGL must mix with saliva. DGL may promote the release of salivary compounds that stimulate the growth and regeneration of stomach and intestinal cells. DGL in capsule form has not been shown to be effective.

Aloe vera
Drink 1 liter per day when there is active bleeding of an ulcer.

Vaginitis

· ·

Increased volume of vaginal secretions

Abnormal color, consistency, or odor of vaginal secretions

Vaginal and vulval itching, burning, or irritation

Pelvic area may show patchy redness, and the vaginal mucosa may be inflamed

Painful urination or pain with intercourse

Infection of the vaginal tract *(vaginitis)* is one of the most common reasons for women to seek medical attention. Vaginitis accounts for approximately seven percent of all visits to gynecologists.[1] A recent study reported that seventy-two percent of young sexually active females had one or more forms of vulvovaginitis.[2] Another study of 821 women found vaginal infections to be six times more common than urinary tract infections.[3] In fact, women who experience painful urination are much more likely to have vaginitis than a bladder infection (see BLADDER INFECTION). Chronic vaginal infections are often the underlying cause of recurrent urinary tract infections due to their action as a reservoir of the infectious bacteria.[4,5]

In addition to causing physical discomfort and embarrassment, vaginitis is medically important for two primary reasons:

1. It may be a symptom of a more serious underlying problem, such as chronic inflammation of the cervix *(cervicitis)* or a sexually transmitted disease

2. The infection may travel up the vagina to deeper tissues and lead to *pelvic inflammatory disease*—a serious situation that can result in infertility due to scarring of the fallopian tubes

Causes of Vaginitis

Infectious vaginitis may be sexually transmitted or may arise from a disturbance to the delicate ecology of a healthy vagina. In many instances, vaginal "infections" involve common organisms normally found in the vagina of many healthy women.[6] In other words, in normal situations these microbes do not cause any problems, but when there is a disturbance in the vaginal environment a normally present microbe can overgrow and produce an infection.

Factors that influence the vaginal environment include the pH, tissue sugar (glycogen) content, blood sugar (glucose) level, the presence of "friendly" organisms (particularly *Lactobacillus acidophilus),* the natural flushing action of vaginal secretions, the presence of blood (menstruation), and the presence of antibodies and other compounds in the vaginal secretions.

These factors are, in turn, affected by such factors as diabetes, wearing synthetic panty hose (which tend to retain moisture), or low immune function as a result of nutritional deficiencies, medications (e.g., steroids, birth control pills), pregnancy, or serious illness.[7] Vaginal yeast infections are three times more prevalent among women who wear panty hose than among those who wear cotton underwear, because the panty hose prevent drying of the area.[8]

Risk factors for sexually transmitted infections include increased numbers of sexual partners, unusual sexual practices, and the type of birth control (barrier methods reduce risk of infection; birth-control pills increase the risk by suppressing the immune system).

Approximately ninety percent of vulvovaginitis *is* associated with one of three organisms: *Trichomonas vaginalis, Candida albicans,* or *Gardnerella vaginalis*.[9] The relative frequency of each form varies with the population studied, as well as with sexual activity levels. Less frequent causes of vaginitis include *Neisseria gonorrhea, Herpes simplex,* and *Chlamydia trachomatis*. Table 1 summarizes the diagnostic differentiation of the most common causes of infectious vaginitis.

Trichomonas vaginalis

Trichomonas vaginalis is a single-celled organism that is transmitted via sexual intercourse. *Trichomonas* does not invade tissues and rarely causes serious complications. The most frequent symptom is vaginal discharge with itching and burning. The discharge is frequently smelly, greenish yellow and frothy. This organism grows optimally at a pH of 5.5 to 5.8.[9] Thus, a vaginal pH of 4.5 in a woman with vaginitis is suggestive of an agent other than trichomonas. Looking at vaginal fluid under a microscope will confirm the diagnosis in eighty to ninety percent of cases.[10,11]

Candida albicans

The relative frequency and the total incidence of vaginal yeast infections (candidal vaginitis) has increased dramatically in the past forty years. Several factors have contributed to this increased incidence, chief among them being the increased use of antibiotics. The problem of vaginal yeast infections as a result of antibiotic use is well-known by virtually all women.

Most cases of recurrent candidal vaginitis are due either to transmission of candida from the gastrointestinal tract or failure to recognize and treat the presence of one or more predisposing factors.[12] In extremely persistent cases, sexual partners may be a source of reinfection. Allergies have also been reported to cause recurrent candidiasis, which resolves when the allergies are treated.[13]

PREDISPOSING FACTORS TO CANDIDAL VAGINITIS

Allergies
Antibiotics
Diabetes mellitus
Elevated vaginal pH
Gastrointestinal candidiasis
Oral contraceptives
Panty hose
Pregnancy
Steroids

The primary symptom of a vaginal yeast infection is vulval itching, which can be quite severe. Candidal vaginitis is often associated with the presence of a thick, curdy, or "cottage cheese" discharge, which may reveal pinpoint bleeding when removed. The presence of such a discharge is strong evidence of a yeast infection, but its absence does not rule out candida.

Nonspecific Vaginitis

This category is defined as "vaginitis not due to trichomonas, gonorrhea, or candida."

Whereas itching is the predominant symptom of candidal vaginitis, the presence of a discharge and odor are the keynotes to nonspecific vaginitis (NSV). The odor is variously described as fishy, foul, or rotten, and reflects the breakdown of proteins by bacteria. The discharge is nonirritating, gray, and usually of even consistency; occasionally it is frothy or even thick and pasty. The pH will be elevated to 5.0 to 5.5 in most cases, and there appears to be a correlation between elevated pH and the presence of odor: the higher the pH, the stronger the odor.[14]

The organism most frequently cited as responsible for NSV is *Gardnerella vaginalis* (formerly *Haemophilus vaginalis*). However, although this bacteria is found in ninety-five percent of women who have NSV, it is also found in forty percent of women who do not have vaginitis.[1] When purified cultures of *Gardnerella* were placed in the vaginas of thirteen volunteers, only one of the women developed signs of vaginitis.[15]

There is growing evidence that *Gardnerella* prospers under the conditions of NSV. However, the responsible organisms may be the other microorganisms found in cases of NSV, or the combination of *Gardnerella* and these other microorganisms (particularly anaerobic bacteria). This argument is furthered by the fact that *Gardnerella* lacks the enzymes to produce the amines characteristic of NSV, whereas the anaerobes do possess them. Additionally, the antibiotic most effective in treating NSV appears to be more active against anaerobes than *Gardnerella*, lending credence to the newer theories that downplay the causative role of *Gardnerella*.[15–17]

Gonorrhea

Neisseria gonorrhea is an uncommon cause of vaginitis, responsible for less than four percent of cases.[3] Gonorrhea is a sexually transmitted disease. It is more common among young girls because the vaginal epithelium is thinner before puberty. During reproductive years, severe infection of the cervix is the primary symptom (painful, bloody, pus-filled discharge).

Gonorrhea, either alone or in combination with other organisms, is cultured in forty to sixty percent of cases of pelvic inflammatory

. . . .

QUICK REVIEW

- Consult a physician for immediate and accurate diagnosis.
- Infectious vaginitis may be sexually transmitted or may arise from a disturbance to the delicate ecology of the healthy vagina.
- Approximately ninety percent of vulvovaginitis will be associated with one of three organisms: *Trichomonas vaginalis*, *Candida albicans*, or *Gardnerella vaginalis*.
- The goals of therapy are to identify and eliminate or reduce contributing factors, to improve immune function and defense mechanisms, and to reestablish proper bacterial flora using *Lactobacillus acidophilus*.
- Iodine, boric acid, or gentian violet can be used as vaginal antiseptics.

TABLE 1 Diagnostic Differentiation of Common Causes of Infectious Vaginitis

	CANDIDA	*NSV*	*TRICHOMONAS*	*GONORRHEA*	*HERPES*	*CHLAMYDIA*
Key symptoms	Itching	Odor	Odor & itching	No symptoms or painful cervicitis	Vesicles (small blisters) or ulcers	Usually without symptoms
Discharge:						
pH	<4.5	>4.5	>5.0	<4.5	<4.5	<4.5
Odor	None	Fishy/amines	May be fishy	None	None	None
Appearance	Curdy, adher-ent, scant to thick	Gray, even consistency	Greenish-yellow, frothy	Bloody and pus-filled	None	None
Pelvic exam	Adherent white patches with a reddened border	Unremarkable	May show reddened bumps on cervix— a "strawberry" cervix— or vaginal lining	Cervical discharge, may have pelvic tenderness	Small, multiple vesicles or ulcers on cervix or labia	May show signs of pelvic inflammatory disease

disease (PID), a severe infectious condition of the female genital tract that is a major cause of infertility. Because of the potential for serious consequences, sexually active women who experience any symptoms suggestive of gonorrhea must consult a physician immediately.

Herpes simplex

Herpes simplex infection is the most common cause of genital ulcers in the United States. For a more thorough discussion, see HERPES.

Chlamydia trachomatis

Chlamydia trachomatis is a parasite that lives within human cells. It rarely causes vaginitis on its own, but is frequently found in association with other common causes, such as *Candida albicans*. *Chlamydia* is another sexually transmitted disease that is now recognized as a major health problem in the United States.[18]

Chlamydia infects five to ten percent of sexually active women and is usually without symptoms until the development of complications, such as infections of the cervix, fallopian tubes, or urethra. *Chlamydia* is the organism most frequently found in cultures of women who have pelvic inflammatory disease.[19] *Chlamydia* infections are the major cause of infertility due to scarring of the fallopian tubes.

Chlamydial infection during pregnancy increases risk of prematurity and infant death. If a healthy baby is born to an infected woman, there is a fifty-percent chance that it will develop chlamydial infection of the eyes, and a ten-percent chance of pneumonia.[18] Because of the considerable risks from untreated chlamydia, we again recommend consulting a physician immediately if you are suffering from any suspicious symptoms.

Therapeutic Considerations

Although vaginitis is usually due to *Candida albicans* and is almost always self-treated with over-the-counter preparations, given the possibility for a more serious cause of vaginitis, we strongly recommend consulting a physician for a definitive diagnosis. The natural treatments described below are recommended only after consultation with a health care provider. The focus is on the treatment of candidal vaginitis, but the same principles apply to trichomonas and NSV. For chlamydial and gonorrheal vaginitis, we recommend conventional antibiotic therapy given the serious risk of tubal scarring and other complications.

The goals of therapy are to identify and eliminate or reduce contributing factors, to improve immune function and defense mechanisms, and to reestablish proper bacterial flora.

Dietary Considerations

The recommendations given in the chapter CANDIDIASIS are appropriate here, especially when dealing with candidal vaginitis. Do not eat refined or simple sugars. Do not drink milk or consume other dairy products. Do not eat foods with a high content of yeast or mold, including alcoholic beverages, cheeses, dried fruits, melons, and peanuts. Avoid all known or suspected food allergens. In addition, follow the guidelines for taking a high-quality multiple-vitamin-and-mineral supplement and extra antioxidants given in the chapter SUPPLEMENTARY MEASURES.

Lactobacillus acidophilus

One of the primary goals in successfully treating vaginal infections is reestablishing the normal vaginal flora. In particular, it is important to reestablish the adequate presence of *Lactobacillus acidophilus*. This desirable bacterium is an integral component of the normal vaginal flora and helps to prevent the overgrowth of *Candida albicans* and less desirable bacterial species. *L. acidophilus* does this by producing lactic acid and natural antibiotic substances. In addition *L. acidophilus* competes with other bacteria and *Candida albicans* for the utilization of glucose.

Reestablishment of normal vaginal lactobacilli can be accomplished by douching twice a day with an acidophilus-containing solution. The solution is best prepared by using a high-quality acidophilus supplement or active-culture yogurt (careful reading of labels is important, since most commercially available yogurts do not use live lactobacilli). Dissolve enough of either choice in 10 ml of water to provide one billion organisms. Use a syringe to douche the material into the vagina. Since lactobacilli are normal inhabitants of the vaginal flora, the douche can be retained in the vagina as long as desired.

In addition, we recommend taking an oral supplement of *L. acidophilus*. Take enough to provide one to two billion live organisms.

Local Antiseptics

There are a number of natural antiseptic compounds that can be used during the infectious stage to get rid of the offending organisms. The following discussion will focus on iodine, boric acid, and gentian violet, as these appear to be the most effective. In fact, their effectiveness has been shown to be as good as or better than standard antibiotic therapy for treating the common causes of vaginitis (*Trichomonas vaginalis*, *Candida albicans*, or *Gardnerella vaginalis*).

Iodine

Iodine, used topically as a douche, is effective against a wide range of infectious agents linked to vaginal infections, including those due to trichomonas, candida, chlamydia, and nonspecific vaginitis. Povidone iodine (Betadine) has all the advantages of iodine without the disadvantages of stinging and staining; Betadine is available at any pharmacy. A study published in 1969 showed povidone iodine to be effective in treating 100 percent of cases of candidal vaginitis, eighty percent of trichomonas, and ninety-three percent of combination infections. A douching solution diluted to one part iodine in 100 parts water, used twice daily for fourteen days, is effective against most organisms.[20-23] However, excessive use must be avoided since some iodine will be absorbed into the system and can cause suppression of thyroid function.

Boric Acid

Capsules of boric acid inserted into the vagina have been used to treat candidiasis with success rates equal to or better than

TABLE 2 Outcome of Therapy with Conventional Antifungal Agents and Boric Acid		
AGENT	LOSS OF SYMPTOMS (% OF PATIENTS)	ABNORMAL MICROSCOPIC FINDINGS (% OF PATIENTS)
Antifungals	52%	100%
Boric Acid	98%	2%

those of nystatin and creams containing miconazole, clotrimazole, or butoconazole.[24-26] Boric acid treatment offers an inexpensive, easily accessible therapy for vaginal yeast infections. In the most recent study, involving ninety-two women with chronic vaginal yeast infections, boric acid was shown to be significantly more effective.[26] The dosage was 600 mg of boric acid in a vaginal suppository twice daily for two weeks.

In addition to being more effective in relieving symptoms, boric acid demonstrated more significant improvements in microscopic examination of vaginal swabs. In fact, no patient who received antifungal drugs had a normal microscopic exam; all exams of these patients demonstrated continued presence of yeast, damaged cells that lined the vagina, or some other abnormality.

It appears that standard antifungal agents are often ineffective in treating chronic cases of vaginal yeast infection. In these cases, it is recommended that boric acid (600 mg) be used twice a day for four months. After this time, further use may not be necessary, but we do recommend using boric acid during menstruation.

Side effects from using boric acid are quite rare. The most common side effect is burning of the labia due to boric acid leaking out of the vagina. If this occurs, reduce the amount of boric acid or discontinue use.

Gentian Violet

Gentian violet is a purple dye that possesses activity against *Candida albicans*. In fact, it has been stated that swabbing the vagina with gentian violet is "as close to a specific treatment for candida as exists."[26] However, despite this proclamation we prefer to recommend other measures because it is extremely messy; it is nearly impossible to remove gentian violet from fabrics, it is, after all, a dye. If you elect to give it a try, be careful. The best way to apply gentian violet is to soak a tampon in it and then insert the tampon into the vagina.

TREATMENT SUMMARY

Since approximately ninety percent of all cases of vaginitis are due to candida, trichomonas, or gardnerella infections, the following recommendations are primarily directed toward treatment of these organisms. Immune support (through proper diet, nutritional supplementation, and botanical medicines) is an important aspect of the therapy. In recurrent infections, please follow the recommendations given in the chapter IMMUNE SUPPORT.

General Recommendations

1. Consult a physician for accurate diagnosis.

2. Treatment failures may be due to incorrect diagnosis, reinfection, failure to treat predisposing factors, or resistance to the treatment used.

3. In all cases of vaginitis, it is important to use live *Lactobacillus* preparations to reestablish a healthy colony of these desirable organisms in the vagina.

4. Sexual activity should be avoided during treatment to prevent reinfection and to reduce trauma to inflamed tissues. If

this is not possible, at least assure that condoms are used.

5. In recurrent cases, consider having sexual partners treated.

6. Wear cotton underwear.

Diet

For all causes of vaginitis, a nutrient-dense diet is recommended. All refined foods and simple carbohydrates should be eliminated. The focus should be on high-quality whole foods. If food allergies are suspected, allergens should be determined and eliminated.

Nutritional Supplements

- High-potency multiple-vitamin-and-mineral formula according to the guidelines given in the chapter SUP-PLEMENTARY MEASURES
- *Lactobacillus sp.:* one to two billion live organisms per day

Local Treatment

Douches and saturated tampons are effective methods of achieving high concentrations of therapeutic agents in the vagina. The following agents are useful in treatment of the common forms of vaginitis. The list is by no means exhaustive.

Only the agents that have been mentioned in several articles or texts are included. Many other agents are doubtlessly also effective. Choose one or more of the agents below; do not try to use all at once. The variety provides alternatives for use in resistant cases.

- Betadine: various gels, suppositories, and fluids are available; a 1:100 dilution in a retention douche kills most organisms within 30 seconds
- Boric Acid Caps: 600 mg placed in capsules

Repeated use may cause irritation, and use for more than seven days may result in problems from systemic absorption

---

- Gentian Violet: swab or soak tampon as described in

Sensitivity reactions are common, and staining of clothes can occur if a pad is not used

---

- *Lactobacillus sp.:* dissolve enough in 10 ml of water to provide one billion organisms; use a syringe to douche the material into the vagina

Varicose Veins

. . . .

Dilated, tortuous, superficial veins in the legs

May be without symptoms or may be associated with fatigue, aching discomfort, feelings of heaviness, or pain in the legs

Fluid retention (*edema*), discoloration, and ulceration of the skin may develop

Women are affected four times as frequently as men

Veins are fairly frail structures. Defects in the wall of a vein lead to dilation of the vein and damage to the valves that prevent blood from backing up and flowing away from the heart.[1] When the valves become damaged, blood pools and causes the bulging veins known as varicose veins.

Varicose veins affect nearly fifty percent of middle-aged adults. Varicose veins affect the legs, largely due to the gravitational pressure that standing exerts on the veins. When an individual stands for long periods of time, the pressure buildup in the veins can increase up to ten times. Hence, individuals with occupations that require long periods of standing are at greatest risk for developing varicose veins.[2] Women are affected about four times as frequently as men; obese individuals have a much greater risk; and the risk increases with age due to loss of tissue tone, loss of muscle mass, and weakening of the walls of the veins. Pregnancy may also lead to the development of varicose veins, as pregnancy increases venous pressure in the legs.[2]

In general, varicose veins pose little harm if the involved vein is near the surface. These types of varicose veins are, however, cosmetically unappealing. Although significant symptoms are not common with this type, the legs may feel heavy, tight, and tired.

A more serious form of varicose vein involves obstruction and valve defects of the deeper veins of the leg. This type of varicose vein can lead to problems such as thrombophlebitis (severe inflammation of a vein), pulmonary embolism (blood clot in the lungs), heart attack, or stroke. Ultrasound evaluation is the most accurate method of diagnosis of deep-vein involvement.

Causes of Varicose Veins

Several theories exist to explain the cause of varicose veins: genetic weakness of the vein walls or their valves; excessive pressure within the vein due to a low-fiber-induced increase in straining during defecation; long periods of standing and/or heavy lifting; damage to the veins or venous valves resulting from inflammation (e.g., thrombophlebitis); and weakness of the vein walls due to either abnormalities in the structural components (e.g., proteoglycans) or excessive release of enzymes that break down the proteoglycans, resulting in loss of integrity of the vein.

Therapeutic Considerations

The natural treatments discussed below are very effective in improving vein function and relieving the symptoms of varicose veins. However, while small "spider veins" may resolve entirely, well-formed large varicose veins should not be expected to magically go away. In these cases, elastic compression stockings are occasionally beneficial, but they are a nuisance to put on and take off.

Fortunately, the natural program outlined in this chapter produces results as good as or better than compression stockings in most cases, without the hassle. In cases of severe or very large varicose veins, surgical stripping (the surgical removal of the entire vein) of the vein or *sclerotherapy* (injection of an agent that will cause the vein to form a clot and pinch off the vein), performed by a vascular surgeon or *phlebologist* (a doctor who specializes in treating varicose veins), are appropriate treatments.

Dietary Fiber

In contrast to the United States and many other developed countries, varicose veins are rarely seen in parts of the world where high-fiber, unrefined diets are consumed.[3,4] A low-fiber diet, high in refined foods, contributes to the development of varicose veins.

Individuals who consume a low-fiber diet tend to strain more during bowel movements since their smaller and harder stools are more difficult to pass. This straining increases the pressure in the abdomen, which obstructs the flow of blood up the legs. The increased pressure may, over a period of time, significantly weaken the vein wall, leading to the formation of varicose veins or hemorrhoids, or it may weaken the wall of the large intestine and produce diverticuli (small outpouchings) in the large intestine.[5]

A high-fiber diet is the most important component in the treatment and prevention of varicose veins (and hemorrhoids). A diet rich in vegetables, fruits, legumes, and grains promotes peristalsis; many fiber components attract water and form a gelatinous mass that keeps the feces soft, bulky, and easy to pass. The net effect of a high-fiber diet is significantly less straining during defecation.

Bulking Agents

Natural bulking compounds can also be used. These substances, particularly psyllium seed, pectin, and guar gum, possess mild laxative action due to their ability to attract water and form a gelatinous mass. This, as mentioned in regard to dietary fiber, keeps the feces soft and promotes peristalsis, significantly reducing straining during defecation. These types of fibers are generally less irritating than wheat bran and other cellulose fiber products.

Nutritional Supplements

There are a number of key nutrients involved in supporting the health of the vein. Most notable are vitamin C and E, bioflavonoids, and zinc. Supplementation with sufficient levels of these key nutrients is important in insuring optimal nutritional support.

Physical Measures

Exercise and avoidance of standing for long periods of time will reduce the risk of developing varicose veins. Exercise, especially walking, riding a bike, or jogging, is particularly beneficial, as the contraction of leg muscles pushes pooled blood back into circulation.

Botanical Medicines

Several herbal medicines have been shown to be useful in improving vein structure and function. Those with the greatest amount of support in the scientific literature are presented here.

Gotu Kola (Centella asiatica)

An extract of centella containing seventy percent triterpenic acids (asiatic acid, madecassic acid, and asiaticoside) has demonstrated impressive clinical results in the treatment of cellulite, venous insufficiency of the lower limbs, and varicose veins.[6-10] Its effect on venous insufficiency and varicose veins appears to be related to its ability to enhance connective tissue structure, reduce sclerosis, and improve blood flow through the affected limbs.[6-10] A key benefit of centella extracts is its ability to increase the integrity of the perivascular sheath—the connective tissue structure that surrounds the frail vein—giving it at least some support. By increasing the support structure's integrity, the function of the vein is also improved.

Horse chestnut (Aesculus hippocastanum)

Extracts of horse-chestnut seed standardized for escin (a key compound) appear to be as effective as compression stockings without the nuisance. For example, in a well-designed study, the effectiveness of horse-chestnut-seed extract versus leg-compression stockings was examined in 240 patients with varicose veins.[11] Patients received either horse-chestnut-seed extract (50 mg of escin per day), compression stockings, or a placebo. Patients were treated over a period of twelve weeks. Effectiveness was evaluated by a machine that measures the volume of fluid in the leg (a *phlethysmograph*). After the twelve-week trial, lower-leg volume of the more severely affected leg decreased an average of 56.5 ml with compression therapy and 53.6 ml with horse-chestnut-seed extract, while it increased by 9.8 ml with the placebo.

Compression stockings and horse-chestnut-seed extract produced nearly identical reductions in edema. So why take the horse-chestnut-seed extract rather than wear the stockings? These are not regular stockings; they are made of special material, cost about seventy dollars each, and are quite difficult to put on, not to mention uncomfortable to wear.

Horse-chestnut-seed extracts standardized for escin exert anti-edema and anti-inflammatory properties, and decrease capillary permeability by reducing the number and size of the small pores in the capillary walls. The reduction in capillary permeability and edema appears to result from inhibition of the enzymes that break down the support structures of the vein.

Investigators have also demonstrated that escin has venotonic activity.[12] A *venotonic* is a substance that improves venous tone by increasing the contractile potential of the elastic fibers in the vein wall. Relaxation of the venous wall contributes greatly to the devel-

. . . .

QUICK REVIEW

- A diet high in fiber prevents varicose veins.
- Veins can be strengthened with flavonoid-rich extracts.
- Several herbal extracts have been shown to act as *venotonics*—agents that enhance the structure, function, and tone of veins—and produce excellent clinical results.

opment of varicose veins. This venotonic activity may be the key factor in the positive effects of horse-chestnut-seed extracts in the treatment of varicose veins.[11,13,14]

Butcher's Broom (Ruscus aculeatus)

Butcher's broom has a long history of use in treating venous disorders such as hemorrhoids and varicose veins. The active ingredients in butcher's broom are *ruscogenins*. These compounds have demonstrated a wide range of pharmacological actions, including anti-inflammatory and vasoconstrictor effects.[15] In Europe, butcher's broom extracts are used extensively, both internally and externally, to treat varicose veins and hemorrhoids. Most of the clinical research has been on butcher's broom extracts in combination with *hesperidin* (a bioflavonoid) and vitamin C.[16,17]

Flavonoid-Rich Extracts

Since increasing the integrity of the wall of the vein may also reduce the risk of developing varicose veins, it appears that flavonoid-rich berries, such as hawthorn berries, cherries, blueberries, and blackberries, are beneficial in the prevention and treatment of varicose veins. These berries are very rich sources of proanthocyanidins and anthocyanidins.[18-20] These bioflavonoids give the berries their blue-red color. Proanthocyanidins and anthocyanidins also improve the integrity of support structures of the veins and entire vascular system. Extracts of several of these berries are used widely in Europe as medications for various circulatory conditions, including varicose veins. Grape seed extract and pine bark extracts are the most popular and possibly the most effective.[21]

If you are looking for a flavonoid-rich tea that may provide some benefit, look to buckwheat tea (*Fagopyrum esculentum*). In one double-blind study, seventy-seven patients with varicose veins were given placebo tea or buckwheat tea for twelve weeks. The tea was standardized to contain five percent total flavonoids, yielding a daily dosage of 270 mg of *rutin*—the key bioflavonoid in buckwheat. A statistically significant decrease in total leg volume was seen in the treated group, along with statistically insignificant improvements in capillary permeability and symptoms. No adverse effects were noted.[22]

The efficacy of flavonoids and flavonoid-rich extracts in treating varicose veins is related to their ability to: (1) reduce capillary fragility, (2) increase the integrity of the venous wall, (3) inhibit the breakdown of the compounds composing the ground substance, and (4) increase the muscular tone of the vein.[19-21]

Consumption of flavonoid-rich foods (such as berries) or extracts is recommended for individuals with varicose veins, as well as for those who wish to prevent them.

Bromelain and Other Fibrinolytic Compounds

Individuals with varicose veins have a decreased ability to break down fibrin, one of the compounds involved in clot and scar formation.[23] This is extremely important, as fibrin is deposited in the tissue near the varicose veins. The skin then becomes hard and lumpy due to the presence of the fibrin and fat. In addition, decreased fibrinolytic activity increases the risk of thrombus formation, which may result in thrombophlebitis, myocardial infarction, pulmonary embolism, or stroke.

Herbs that increase the fibrinolytic activity of the blood are therefore helpful. Capsicum (cayenne),[24] garlic,[25] onion,[26] and ginger[27] all increase fibrin breakdown. Liberal consumption of these spices in foods is recommended for individuals with varicose veins and other disorders of the cardiovascular system.

Bromelain, the proteolytic enzyme from pineapple, also appears appropriate for the treatment of varicose veins. Vein walls are an important source of *plasminogen activator,* which promotes the breakdown of fibrin. Veins that have become varicosed have decreased levels of plasminogen activator. Bromelain acts in a similar manner to plasminogen activator to cause fibrin break-down.[28] Bromelain may help prevent the development of the hard and lumpy skin (*lipodermatosclerosis*) found around varicosed veins.

TREATMENT SUMMARY

Varicose veins are extremely common in our society, largely due to dietary and lifestyle factors. The supplements and botanicals are recommended to strengthen the walls of the vein and increase fibrinolytic activity. To treat or reduce the risk of developing varicose veins, we recommend that you:

1. Consume a diet high in fiber
2. Exercise regularly
3. Avoid standing in one place for long periods of time (use elastic support stocking if standing is necessary)
4. Avoid being obese
5. Employ measures to increase the integrity of the connective tissue and vein wall
6. Enhance fibrinolytic activity

Diet

Consume a high-complex-carbohydrate diet rich in dietary fiber. The diet should contain liberal amounts of proantho-cyanidin- and anthocyanidin-rich foods, such as blackberries, cherries, blueberries, etc. Garlic, onions, ginger, and cayenne should also be consumed liberally.

Nutritional Supplements

- Vitamin C: 500–3,000 mg per day
- Vitamin E: 200–600 IU per day
- Bioflavonoids: 100–1,000 mg per day
- Zinc: 15–30 mg per day

Botanical Medicines

Choose one or more:
- Horse chestnut (*Aesculus hippocas-tanum*): use extracts that provide a daily dosage of 50 mg escin
- Gotu kola (*Centella asiatica*): use extracts that provide a daily dosage of 30–60 mg triterpenic acids
- Butcher's broom (*Ruscus aculeatus*): use extracts standardized to contain 9–11% ruscogenin at a dosage of 100 mg three times per day
- Bilberry (*Vaccinium myrtillus*): use extracts standardized to contain 25% anthocyanoside; 80–160 mg three times per day
- Grape seed (*Vitis vinifera*) or pine bark (*Pinus maritima*): use extracts standardized to contain 95% or more procyanidolic oligomers (PCOs or OPCs); 150–300 mg per day
- Bromelain (1,200–1,800 mcu): 500–750 mg two to three times per day between meals

GLOSSARY

Abortifacient A substance that induces abortion.

Abscess A localized collection of pus and liquefied tissue in a cavity.

Acetylcholine One of the chemicals that transmits impulses between nerves and between nerves and muscle cells.

Acrid A pungent biting taste that causes irritation.

Acute Having a rapid onset, severe symptoms, and a short course; not *chronic*.

Adaptogen A substance that is safe, increases resistance to stress, and has a balancing effect on body functions.

Adjuvant A substance that enhances the effect of the medicinal agent or increases the antigenicity of a cancer cell.

Adrenaline A hormone secreted by the adrenal gland that produces the "fight or flight" response. Also called *epinephrine*.

Aldosterone A hormone secreted by the adrenal gland that causes the retention of sodium and water.

Alkaloids Naturally occurring *amines*, arising from heterocyclic and often complex structures, that display pharmacological activity. Their common names usually end in *ine*. They are usually classified according to the chemical structure of their main nucleus: phenylalkylamines (ephedrine), pyridine (nicotine), tropine (atropine, cocaine), quinoline (quinine), isoquinolone (papaverine), phenan-threne (morphine), purine (caffeine), imidazole (pilocarpine), and indole (physostigmine, yohimbine).

Allopathy The conventional approach to medicine, which combats disease by using substances and techniques targeted specifically against the disease.

Alterative A substance that produces a balancing effect on a particular body function.

Amebiasis An intestinal infection characterized by severe diarrhea, caused by the parasite *Entamoeba histolytica*.

Amines Nitrogen-containing compounds.

Amino acids A group of nitrogen-containing chemical compounds that form the basic structural units of proteins.

Analgesic A substance that reduces the sensation of pain.

Androgen A hormone that stimulates male characteristics.

Anthelminthic A substance that causes the elimination of intestinal worms.

Anthocyanidin A class of flavonoids that gives plants, fruits, and flowers colors that range from red to blue.

Antibody A protein manufactured by the body which binds to an antigen to neutralize, inhibit, or destroy it.

Antidote A substance that neutralizes or counteracts the effects of a poison.

Antigen   Any substance that, when introduced into the body, causes the formation of antibodies against it.

Antihypertensive   A substance that exerts a blood-pressure-lowering effect.

Antioxidant   A compound that prevents free-radical or oxidative damage.

Aphrodisiac   A substance that increases sexual desire.

Artery   A blood vessel that carries oxygen-rich blood away from the heart.

Astringent   An agent that causes the contraction of tissue.

Atherosclerosis   A process in which fatty substances (cholesterol and triglycerides) are deposited in the walls of medium-to-large arteries, eventually leading to blockage of the artery.

Atopy   A predisposition to various allergic conditions, including eczema and asthma.

Autoimmune   A process in which antibodies develop against the body's own tissues.

Balm   A soothing or healing medicine applied to the skin.

Basal metabolic rate   The rate of metabolism when the body is at rest.

Basophil   A type of white blood cell that is involved in allergic reactions.

Benign   Harmless; mild, not fatal.

Beta-carotene   Provitamin A. A plant carotene that can be converted to two vitamin A molecules.

Beta-cells   The cells in the pancreas that manufacture insulin.

Bilirubin   The breakdown product of the hemoglobin molecule of red blood cells.

Biopsy   A diagnostic test in which tissue or cells are removed from the body for examination under a microscope.

Bleeding time   The time required for the cessation of bleeding from a small skin puncture as a result of platelet disintegration and blood vessel constriction. Ranges from one to four minutes.

Blood-brain barrier   A special barrier that prevents the passage of materials from the blood to the brain.

Blood pressure   The force exerted by blood as it presses against and attempts to stretch blood vessels.

Bromelain   The protein-digesting enzyme found in pineapple.

Bursa   A sac or pouch that contains a special fluid which lubricates joints.

Bursitis   Inflammation of a bursa.

Calorie   A unit of heat. A nutritional calorie is the amount of heat necessary to raise 1 kg of water 1 degree C.

Candida albicans   A yeast common to the intestinal tract.

Candidiasis   A complex medical syndrome produced by a chronic overgrowth of the yeast *Candida albicans*.

Carbohydrates   Sugars and starches.

Carcinogen   Any agent or substance capable of causing cancer.

Carcinogenesis   The development of cancer, caused by the actions of certain chemicals, viruses, and unknown factors on primarily normal cells.

Cardiac output   The volume of blood pumped from the heart in one minute.

Cardiopulmonary   Pertaining to the heart and lungs.

Cardiotonic   A compound that tones and strengthens the heart.

Carminative   A substance that promotes the elimination of intestinal gas.

Carotenes   Fat-soluble plant pigments, some of which can be converted into vitamin A by the body.

Cartilage   A type of connective tissue that acts as a shock absorber at joint interfaces.

Cathartic   A substance that stimulates the movement of the bowels; more powerful than a laxative.

Cholagogue   A compound that stimulates the contraction of the gallbladder.

Cholecystitis   Inflammation of the gallbladder.

Cholelithiasis   Production of gallstones; having gallstones.

Choleretic   A compound that promotes the flow of bile.

Cholestasis   The stagnation of bile within the liver.

Cholinergic   Pertaining to the parasympathetic portion of the autonomic nervous system and the release of acetylcholine as a transmitter substance.

Chronic   Long-term or frequently recurring.

Cirrhosis   A severe disease of the liver characterized by the replacement of liver cells with scar tissue.

Coenzyme   A necessary nonprotein component of an enzyme, usually a vitamin or mineral.

Cold sore   A small skin blister anywhere around the mouth caused by the *Herpes simplex* virus.

Colic   Severe, spasmodic pain that occurs in waves of increasing intensity, reaches a peak, then abates for a short time before returning.

Colitis   Inflammation of the colon; usually associated with diarrhea with blood and mucus.

Collagen   The protein that is the main component of connective tissue.

Compress   A pad of linen applied under pressure to an area of the skin and held in place.

Congestive heart failure   Chronic disease that results when the heart is not capable of supplying the oxygen demands of the body.

Connective tissue   The type of tissue that provides support, structure, and cellular cement to the body.

Contagious   Capable of being transferred from one person to another by social contact, such as by sharing a home or workplace.

Coronary artery disease   A condition in which the heart receives an inadequate supply of blood and oxygen due to atherosclerosis.

Corticosteroid drugs   A group of drugs, similar to the natural corticosteroid hormones, that are used predominantly in the treatment of inflammation and to suppress the immune system.

Corticosteroid hormones   A group of hormones produced by the adrenal glands that control the body's use of nutrients and the excretion of salt and water in the urine.

Cushing's syndrome   A condition caused by a hypersecretion of cortisone, characterized by spindly legs, "moon face," "buffalo hump," abdominal obesity, flushed facial skin, and poor wound healing.

Cyst   An abnormal lump or swelling, filled with fluid or semisolid material, in any body organ or tissue.

Cystitis   Inflammation of the inner lining of the bladder; usually caused by a bacterial infection.

Decoctions   Teas prepared by boiling the botanical with water for a specified period of time, followed by straining or filtering.

Dehydration   Excessive loss of water from the body.

Dementia   Senility; loss of mental function.

Demineralization   Loss of minerals from the bone.

Demulcent   A substance that is soothing to irritated mucous membranes.

Dermatitis   Inflammation of the skin, sometimes due to allergy.

Diastolic pressure   The second number in a blood pressure reading; the measure of the pressure in the arteries during the relaxation phase of the heartbeat.

Disaccharide A sugar composed of two monosaccharide units.

Diuretic A compound that causes increased urination.

Diverticuli Saclike outpouchings of the wall of the colon.

Double-blind study A way of controlling against experimental bias by insuring that neither the researcher nor the subject knows when an active agent or a placebo is being used.

Douche Introduction of water and/or a cleansing agent into the vagina, with the aid of a bag with a tube and nozzle attached.

Dysplasia Any abnormality of growth.

Dysfunction Abnormal function.

Edema Accumulation of fluid in tissues (swelling).

Eicosapentaenoic acid (EPA) A fatty acid found primarily in cold-water fish.

Electroencephalograph A machine that measures and records brain waves.

Elimination diet A diet that eliminates allergenic foods.

Emulsify To disperse large fat globules into smaller, uniformly distributed particles.

Encephalitis Inflammation of the brain, usually due to viral infection.

Endometrium The mucous membrane lining of the uterus.

Enteric-coated A tablet or capsule coated to ensure that it does not dissolve in the stomach so that it can reach the intestinal tract.

Enzyme An organic catalyst that speeds a chemical reaction.

Epidemiology The study of the occurrence and distribution of diseases in human populations.

Epinephrine See adrenaline.

Epithelium The cells that cover the entire surface of the body and that line most of the internal organs.

Epstein-Barr virus The virus that causes infectious mononucleosis and is associated with Burkitt's lymphoma and nasopharyngeal cancer.

Essential fatty acids Fatty acids that the body cannot manufacture; linoleic and linolenic acids.

Essential oils Also known as volatile oils, ethereal oils, or essences. They are usually complex mixtures of a wide variety of organic compounds (e.g., alcohols, ketones, phenols, acids, ethers, esters, aldehydes, oxides, etc.) that evaporate when exposed to air. They generally represent the odoriferous principles of plants.

Estrogens Hormones that exert female characteristics.

Excretion The process of eliminating waste products from a cell, tissue, or the entire body.

Extracts Concentrated forms of natural products obtained by treating crude materials containing these substances with a solvent and then removing the solvent completely or partially from the preparation. The most commonly used extracts are fluid extracts, solid extracts, powdered extracts, tinctures, and native extracts.

Extracellular The space outside the cell, composed of fluid.

Exudate Escaping fluid or semifluid material that oozes from a space that may contain serum, pus, or cellular debris.

Fibrin A white insoluble protein formed by the clotting of blood which serves as the starting point for wound repair and scar formation.

Fibrinolysis The dissolution of fibrin or a blood clot by the action of enzymes which convert insoluble fibrin into soluble particles.

Flavonoid A generic term for a group of flavone-containing compounds that are found widely in nature. They include many of the compounds that account for plant pigments (anthocyanins, anthoxanthins, apigenins, flavones, flavonols, bioflavonols, etc.). These plant pigments exert a wide variety of physiological effects in the human body.

Fluid extracts These extracts are typically hydro-alcoholic solutions with a strength of 1 part solvent to 1 part herb. The alcohol content varies with each product. They are, in essence, concentrated tinctures.

Free radicals Highly reactive molecules, characterized by an unpaired electron, that can bind to and destroy cellular compounds.

Furuncle Another name for a boil that involves a hair follicle.

Gerontology The study of aging.

Giardiasis An infection of the small intestine caused by the protozoan (single-celled organism) *Giardia lamblia*.

Gingivitis Inflammation of the gums.

Glaucoma A condition in which the pressure of the fluid in the eye is so high that it causes damage.

Glucose A monosaccharide found in the blood; one of the body's primary energy sources.

Gluten One of the proteins in wheat and certain other grains that gives dough its tough, elastic character.

Glycosides Sugar-containing compounds composed of a glycone (sugar component) and an aglycone (non-sugar-containing component) that can be cleaved on hydrolysis. The glycone portion may be glucose, rhamnose, xylose, fructose, arabinose, or any other sugar. The aglycone portion can be any kind of compound (e.g., sterols, triterpenes, anthraquinones, hydroquinones, tannins, carotenoids, or anthocyanidins).

Goblet cell A goblet-shaped cell that secretes mucus.

Ground substance The thick, gel-like material in which the cells, fibers, and blood capillaries of cartilage, bone, and connective tissue are embedded.

Helper T cells Lymphocytes that help in the immune response.

Hematocrit An expression of the percentage of blood occupied by blood cells.

Hemorrhoids Distended veins in the lining of the anus.

Hepatic Pertaining to the liver.

Hepatomegaly Enlargement of the liver.

Holistic medicine A form of therapy aimed at treating the whole person, not just the part or parts in which symptoms occur.

Hormone A secretion of an endocrine gland that controls and regulates body functions.

Hyperglycemia High blood sugar.

Hypersecretion Excessive secretion.

Hypertension High blood pressure.

Hypochlorhydria Insufficient gastric acid output.

Hypoglycemia Low blood sugar.

Hypolipidemic Having elevated levels of cholesterol and triglycerides in the blood.

Hypotension Low blood pressure.

Hypoxia An inadequate supply of oxygen.

Iatrogenic Meaning literally "physician produced," the term can be applied to any medical condition, disease, or other adverse occurrence that results from medical treatment.

Idiopathic Of unknown cause.

Immunoglobulins Antibodies.

Incidence The number of new cases of a disease that occurs during a given period (usually years) in a defined population.

Incontinence The inability to control urination or defecation.

Infarction Death to a localized area of tissue due to lack of oxygen supply.

Infusions Teas produced by steeping a botanical in hot water.

Insulin A hormone secreted by the pancreas which lowers blood sugar levels.

Interferon A potent immune-enhancing substance that is produced by the body's cells to fight off viral infection and cancer.

In vitro   Outside a living body and in an artificial environment.

In vivo   In a living body of an animal or plant.

Jaundice   A condition caused by elevation of bilirubin levels in the body and characterized by yellowing of the skin.

Keratin   An insoluble protein found in hair, skin, and nails.

Lactase   An enzyme that breaks down lactose into the monosaccharides glucose and galactose.

Lactose   One of the sugars present in milk; a *disaccharide*.

Laxative   A substance that promotes the evacuation of the bowels.

LD50   The dosage that will kill fifty percent of the animals that take the substance.

Lesion   Any localized, abnormal change in tissue formation.

Leukocyte   A white blood cell.

Lethargy   A feeling of tiredness, drowsiness, or lack of energy.

Leukotrienes   Inflammatory compounds produced when oxygen interacts with polyunsaturated fatty acids.

Lipids   Fats, phospholipids, steroids, and prostaglandins.

Lipotropic   Promoting the flow of lipids to and from the liver.

Lymph   Fluid contained in lymphatic vessels that flows through the lymphatic system to be returned to the blood.

Lymphocyte   A type of white blood cell found primarily in lymph nodes.

Malabsorption   Impaired absorption of nutrients, most often due to diarrhea.

Malaise   A vague feeling of being sick or of physical discomfort.

Malignant   A term used to describe a condition that tends to worsen and eventually causes death.

Manipulation   As a therapy, the skillful use of the hands to move a part of the body or a specific joint or muscle.

Mast cell   A cell found in many tissues of the body that contributes greatly to allergic and inflammatory processes by secreting histamine and other inflammatory particles.

Menorrhagia   Excessive loss of blood during menstrual periods.

Menstruum   Solvent used for extraction (water, alcohol, acetone, etc.).

Metabolism   A collective term for all the chemical processes that take place in the body.

Metabolite   A product of a chemical reaction.

Metalloenzyme   An enzyme that contains a metal at its active site.

Microbe   A popular term for a microorganism.

Microflora   The microbial inhabitants of a particular region (e.g., the colon).

Mites   Small eight-legged animals, less than one-twentieth of an inch (1.2 mm) long; similar to tiny spiders.

Molecule   The smallest complete unit of a substance that can exist independently and still retain the characteristic properties of the substance.

Monoclonal antibodies   Genetically engineered antibodies specific for one particular antibody.

Monosaccharide   A simple, one-unit sugar such as fructose or glucose.

Mortality rate   The number of deaths per 100,000 of the population per year.

Mucosa   Another term for mucous membranes.

Mucous membrane   The soft, pink, tissue that lines most of the cavities and tubes in the body, including the respiratory tract, gastrointestinal tract, genitourinary tract, and eyelids. The mucous membranes secrete *mucus*.

Mucus The slick, slimy fluid secreted by the mucous membranes which acts as a lubricant and mechanical protector of the mucous membranes.

Mycotoxins Toxins from yeast and fungi.

Myelin sheath A white fatty substance that surrounds nerve cells to aid in nerve impulse transmission.

Neoplasia A medical term for a tumor formation, characterized by a progressive, abnormal replication of cells.

Neurofibrillary tangles Clusters of degenerated nerves.

Neurotransmitters Substances that modify or transmit nerve impulses.

Night blindness The inability to see well in dim light or at night.

Nocturia The disturbance of a person's sleep at night by the need to pass urine.

Oleoresins Primarily mixtures of resins and volatile oils. They either occur naturally or are made by extracting the oily and resinous materials from botanicals with organic solvents (e.g., hexane, acetone, ether, alcohol). The solvent is then removed under vacuum, leaving behind a viscous, semisolid extract which is the oleoresin. Examples of prepared oleoresins are paprika, ginger, and capsicum.

Oligoantigenic diet See *Elimination diet*.

Otitis media Acute infection of the middle ear.

Pancreatin A special extract of pork pancreas.

Papain The protein-digesting enzyme of papaya.

Parkinson's disease A slowly progressive, degenerating nervous system disease characterized by resting tremor, pill-rolling of the fingers, a mask-like facial expression, shuffling gait, and muscle rigidity and weakness.

Pathogen Any agent, particularly a microorganism, that causes disease.

Pathogenesis The processes by which a disease originates and develops, particularly the cellular and physiological processes.

Peristalsis Successive muscular contractions of the intestines that move food through the intestinal tract.

Physiology The study of the functioning of the body, including the physical and chemical processes of its cells, tissues, organs, and systems.

Physostigmine A drug that blocks the breakdown of acetylcholine.

Phytoestrogens Plant compounds that exert estrogenic effects.

Placebo An inert or inactive substance used to test the efficacy of another substance.

Polysaccharide A molecule composed of many sugar molecules linked together.

Powdered extract A solid extract that has been dried as a powder.

Prostaglandins Hormone-like compounds manufactured from essential fatty acids.

Psychosomatic Pertaining to the relationship between the mind and body. Commonly used to refer to those physiological disorders thought to be caused entirely or partly by psychological factors.

Putrefaction The process of breaking down protein compounds by rotting.

Recommended Dietary Allowance (RDA) Recommended Dietary Allowance.

Resins Complex oxidative products of terpenes that occur naturally as plant exudates, or that are prepared by alcohol extraction of botanicals that contain resinous principles.

Saccharide A sugar molecule.

Saponins Non-nitrogenous glycosides, typically with sterol or triterpenes as the aglycone, that possess the common property of foaming or making suds when strongly agitated in aqueous solution.

Satiety A feeling of fullness or gratification.

Saturated fat   A fat whose carbon atoms are bonded to the maximum number of hydrogen atoms; found in animal products such as meat, milk, milk products, and eggs.

Sclerosis   The process of hardening or scarring.

Senile dementia   Mental deterioration associated with aging.

Slow-reacting substance of anaphylaxis (SRSA)   A potent allergic mediator produced and released by mast cells.

Solid extracts   Extracts that have had all of their residual solvent or liquid removed.

Submucosa   The tissues just below the mucous membrane.

Suppressor T cells   Lymphocytes controlled by the thymus gland which suppress the immune response.

Syndrome   A group of signs and symptoms that occur together in a pattern characteristic of a particular disease or abnormal condition.

T cell   A lymphocyte that is under the control of the thymus gland.

Tinctures   Alcoholic or hydro-alcoholic solutions usually containing the active principles of botanicals in low concentrations. They are usu-ally prepared by maceration, percolation, or dilution of their corresponding fluid or native extracts. The strengths of tinctures are typically 1:10 or 1:5. Alcohol content will vary.

Tonic   A substance that exerts a gentle strengthening effect on the body.

Trans-fatty acid   The type of fat found in margarine.

Uremia   The retention of urine by the body and the presence of high levels of urine components in the blood.

Urinalysis   The analysis of urine.

Urticaria   Hives.

Vasoconstriction   The constriction of blood vessels.

Vasodilation   The dilation of blood vessels.

Vitamin   An essential compound necessary to act as a catalyst in normal processes of the body.

Western diet   A diet characteristic of Western societies (i.e., a diet high in fat, refined carbohydrates, and processed foods, and low in dietary fiber).

Wheal   The characteristic lesion of hives; a small welt.

REFERENCES

What Is Natural Medicine?

1. G. Cody, "History of Naturopathic Medicine," in *A Textbook of Natural Medicine*, eds. J.E. Pizzorno and M.T. Murray (Seattle, WA: Bastyr College Publications, 1985).

2. B. Lust, *Universal Naturopathic Directory and Buyer's Guide* (New York: American Naturopathic Association, 1918).

3. F. Campion, *AMA and U.S. Health Policy Since 1940* (Chicago, IL: AMA Publications, 1984).

4. World Health Organization, *Fighting Disease, Fostering Development: Report of the Director General* (London: HMSO, 1996).

5. M. Woodhead, "Antibiotic Resistance," *Brit J Hosp Med* 56 (1996): 314–5.

6. M. Cohen, "Epidemiology of Drug Resistance: Implications for a Post-Antibiotic Era," *Science* 257 (1992): 1050–5.

7. J.T. Dingle, "The Effect of NSAIDs on Human Articular Cartilage Glycosaminoglycan Synthesis," *Eur J Rheumatol Inflammation* 16 (1996): 47–52.

8. K.D. Brandt, "Effects of Nonsteroidal Anti-Inflammatory Drugs on Chondrocyte Metabolism In Vitro and In Vivo," *Am J Med* 83, Suppl. 5A (1987): 29–34.

9. M.J. Shield, "Anti-Inflammatory Drugs and Their Effects on Cartilage Synthesis and Renal Function," *Eur J Rheumatol Inflam* 13 (1993): 7–16.

10. P.M. Brooks, S.R. Potter, and W.W. Buchanan, "NSAID and Osteoarthritis—Help or Hindrance?" *J Rheumatol* 9 (1982): 3–5.

11. N.M. Newman and R.S.M. Ling, "Acetabular Bone Destruction Related to Non-Steroidal Anti-Inflammatory Drugs," *Lancet* ii (1985): 11–13.

12. Solomon, "Drug-Induced Arthropathy and Necrosis of the Femoral Head," *J Bone Joint Surg* 55B (1973): 246–51.

13. H. Ronningen and N. Langeland, "Indomethacin Treatment in Osteoarthritis of the Hip Joint," *Acta Orthop Scand* 50 (1979): 169–74.

14. G. Crolle and E. D'este, "Glucosamine Sulfate for the Management of Arthrosis: A Controlled Clinical Investigation," *Curr Med Res Opin* 7 (1980): 104–9.

15. J.M. Pujalte, E.P. Llavore, and F.R. Ylescupidez, "Double-Blind Clinical Evaluation of Oral Glucosamine Sulphate in the Basic Treatment of Osteoarthrosis," *Curr Med Res Opin* 7 (1980): 110–4.

16. A. Drovanti, A.A. Bignamini, and L.A. Rovati, "Therapeutic Activity of Oral Glucosamine Sulfate in Osteoarthrosis: A Placebo-Controlled Double-Blind Investigation," *Clin Ther* 3 (1980): 260–72.

17. Y. Vajaradul, "Double-Blind Clinical Evaluation of Intra-Articular Glucosamine in Outpatients with Gonarthrosis," *Clin Ther* 3 (1981): 336–43.

18. E.D. D'Ambrosia, et al., "Glucosamine Sulphate: A Controlled Clinical Investigation in Arthrosis," *Pharmatherapeutica* 2 (1982): 504–8.

19. W. Noack, et al., "Glucosamine Sulfate in Osteoarthritis of the Knee," *Osteoarthritis Cartilage* 2 (1994): 51–9.

20. A.L. Vaz, "Double-Blind Clinical Evaluation of the Relative Efficacy of Ibuprofen and Glucosamine Sulfate in the Management of Osteoarthrosis of the Knee in Outpatients," *Curr Med Res Opin* 8 (1982): 145–9.

21. H. Muller-Fassbender, et al., "Glucosamine Sulfate Compared to Ibuprofen in Osteoarthritis of the Knee," *Osteoarthritis Cartilage* 2 (1994): 61–9.

22. L.C. Rovati, et al., "A Large, Randomized, Placebo-Controlled, Double-Blind Study of Glucosamine Sulfate vs Piroxicam and vs Their Association, on the Kinetics of the Symptomatic Effect in Knee Osteoarthritis," *Osteoarthritis Cartilage* 2, Suppl. 1 (1994): 56.

23. D. Leslie and M. Gheorghiade, "Is There a Role for Thiamine Supplementation in the Management of Heart Failure?" *Am Heart J* 131 (1996): 1248–50.

24. K.L. Goa and R.N. Brogden, "L-Carnitine—A Preliminary Review of Its Pharmacokinetics, and Its Therapeutic Use in Ischemic Cardiac Disease and Primary and Secondary Carnitine Deficiencies in Relationship to Its Role in Fatty Acid Metabolism," *Drugs* 34 (1987): 1–24.

25. M. Mancini, et al., "Controlled Study on the Therapeutic Efficacy of Propionyl-L-Carnitine in Patients with Congestive Heart Failure," *Arzneim Forsch* 42 (1992): 1101–4.

26. G. Pucciarelli, "The Clinical and Hemodynamic Effects of Propionyl-L-Carnitine in the Treatment of Congestive Heart Failure," *Clin Ter* 141 (1992): 379–84.

839

27. C. Hofman-Bang, N. Rehnquist, and K. Swedberg, "Coenzyme Q10 as an Adjunctive Treatment of Congestive Heart Failure," *J Am Coll Cardiol* 19 (1992): 216A.

28. C. Morisco, B. Trimarco, and M. Condorelli, "Effect of Coenzyme Q10 Therapy in Patients with Congestive Heart Failure: A Long-Term Multicenter Randomized Study," *Clin Investig* 71, Suppl. 8 (1993): S134–6.

29. E. Baggio, et al., "Italian Multicenter Study on the Safety and Efficacy of Coenzyme Q10 as Adjunctive Therapy in Heart Failure," CoQ10 Drug Surveillance Investigators. *Mol Aspects Med* 15, Suppl. (1994): s287–94.

30. K.R. Pelletier, "A Review and Analysis of the Health and Cost-Effective Outcome of Comprehensive Health Promotion and Disease Promotion at the Worksite: 1991–1993 Update," *Am J Health Promotion* 8 (1993): 50–61.

31. J.P. Geyman and G. Hart, "Family Practice and the Health Care System, Primary Care at a Crossroads: Progress, Problems and Future Projections," *JABFP* 7 (1994): 60–70.

32. L.L. Leape, "Unnecessary Surgery," *Health Serv Res* 24 (1989): 351–7.

33. T.B. Graboys, et al., "Results of Second-Opinion Trial Among Patients Recommended for Coronary Angiography," *JAMA* 268 (1992): 2537–40.

34. A.C. Monheit and J.P. Vistnes, "Implicit Pooling of Workers from Large and Small Firms," *Health Affairs* 13 (1994): 30–4.

35. L.M. Verbrugge and D.L. Patrick, "Seven Chronic Conditions: Their Impact on U.S. Adults' Activity Levels and Use of Medical Services," *Am J Pub Health* 85 (1995): 173–82.

36. W.T. Oojendijk, et al., *What Is Better? An Investigation into the Use and Satisfaction with Complementary and Official Medicine in the Netherlands* (Netherlands: Institute of Preventive Medicine and the Technical Industrial Organization, 1980).

A Positive Mental Attitude

1. M.E.P. Seligman, *Learned Optimism* (New York: Knopf, 1981).

2. C. Peterson, M. Seligman and G. Valliant, "Pessimistic Explanatory Style as a Risk Factor for Physical Illness: A Thirty-Five Year Longitudinal Study," *J Person Soc Psych* 55 (1988): 23–7.

3. C. Peterson, "Explanatory Style as a Risk Factor for Illness," *Cognitive Therapy and Research* 12 (1988): 117–30.

A Healthy Lifestyle

1. U.S. Dept. of Health and Human Services, *The Surgeon General's Report on Nutrition and Health* (Rocklin, CA: Prima, 1988).

2. M. Law and J.L. Tang, "An Analysis of the Effectiveness of Interventions Intended to Help People Stop Smoking," *Arch Intern Med* 155 (1995): 1933–41.

3. M.L. Pollack, J.H. Wilmore, and S.M. Fox, *Exercise in Health and Disease* (Philadelphia: W.B. Saunders, 1984).

4. W.H. Dietz and S.L. Gortmaker, "Do We Fatten Our Children at the Television Set?" *Pediatrics* 75 (1985): 807–12.

5. M.E. Farmer, B.Z. Locke, E.K. Mosciki, et al., "Physical Activity and Depressive Symptomatology: The NHANES 1 Epidemiologic Follow-Up Study," *Am J Epidemiol* 1328 (1988): 1340–51.

6. Daniel Carr et al., "Physical Conditioning Facilitates the Exercised-Induced Secretion of Beta-Endorphin and Beta-Lipoprotein in Women," *New Engl J Med* 305 (1981): 560–5.

7. D. Lobstein, B.J. Mosbacher, and A.H. Ismail, "Depression as a Powerful Discriminator between Physically Active and Sedentary Middle-Aged Men," *J Psychosom Res* 27 (1983): 69–76.

8. S.N. Blair et al., "Changes in Physical Fitness and All-Cause on Mortality: A Prospective Study of Healthy and Unhealthy Men," *JAMA* 273 (1995): 1093–8.

9. I.M. Lee, C.C. Hsieh, and R.S. Paffenbarger, "Exercise Intensity and Longevity in Men: The Harvard Alumni Health Study," *JAMA* 273 (1995): 1179–84.

10. P. Koch-Sheras and A. Lemley, *The Dream Sourcebook* (Los Angeles: Lowell House, 1996).

A Health-Promoting Diet

1. S.B. Eaton and M. Konner, "Paleolithic Nutrition: A Consideration of Its Nature and Current Implications," *New Engl J Med* 312 (1985): 283–9.

2. D. Ryde, "What Should Humans Eat?" *Practitioner* 232 (1985): 415–8.

3. National Research Council, *Diet and Health: Implications for Reducing Chronic Disease Risk* (Washington, D.C.: National Academy Press, 1989).

4. H. Trowell and D. Burkitt, *Western Diseases: Their Emergence and Prevention* (Cambridge, MA: Harvard University Press, 1981); H. Trowell, D. Burkitt and K. Heaton, *Dietary Fibre, Fibre-Depleted Foods, and Disease* (New York: Academic Press, 1985).

5. U.S. Department of Health and Human Services, *The Surgeon General's Report on Nutrition and Health* (Rocklin, CA: Prima Publishing, 1988).

6. W.C. Willett et al., "Intake of Trans Fatty Acids and Risk of Coronary Heart Disease Among Women," *Lancet* 341 (1993): 581–5.

7. M.P. Longnecker, "Do Trans Fatty Acids in Margarine and Other Foods Increase the Risk of Coronary Heart Disease?" *Epidemiology* 4 (1993): 492–5.

8. J. Booyens and C.F. Van Der Merwe, "Margarines and Coronary Artery Disease," *Med Hypothesis* 37 (1992): 241–4.

9. R.P. Mensink and M.B. Katan, "Effect of Dietary Trans Fatty Acids on High-Density and Low-Density Lipoprotein Cholesterol Levels in Healthy Subjects" *New Engl J Med* 323 (1990): 439–45.

10. P. Quillin, *Safe Eating* (New York: Evans, 1990).

11. A.M. Fan and R.J. Jackson, "Pesticides and Food Safety," *Regulatory Toxicol Pharmacol* 9 (1989): 158–74.

12. T. Sterling and A.V. Arundel, "Health Effects of Phenoxy Herbicides," *Scand J Work Environ Health* 12 (1986): 161–73.

13. D.T. Wigle, R.M. Semenciw, K. Wilkins, et al., "Mortality Study of Canadian Male Farm Operators: Non-Hodgkin's Lymphoma Mortal-

ity and Agricultural Practices in Saskatchewan." *J Nat Canc Inst* 82 (1990): 575–582.

14. L. Mott and M. Broad, *Pesticides in Food* (San Francisco: National Resources Defense Council, 1984).

15. F. Falck et al., "Pesticides and Polychlorinated Biphenyl Residues in Human Breast Lipids and Their Relation to Breast Cancer," *Archives of Environmental Health* 47 (1992): 143–6.

16. R.M. Sharpe and N.E. Skakkebaek, "Are Oestrogens Involved in Falling Sperm Counts and Disorders of the Male Reproduction Tract?" *Lancet* 341 (1993): 1392–5.

17. P. Newberne and M.W. Conner, "Food Additives and Contaminants: An Update," *Cancer* 58 (1986): 1851–62.

18. T. Furia, ed., *CRC Handbook of Food Additives*, Volumes 1 and 2 (Boca Raton, FL: CRC Press, 1980).

19. L.K. Golightly, et al., "Pharmaceutical Excipients: Adverse Effects Associated with Inactive Ingredients in Drug Products," *Med Toxicol* 3 (1988): 128–65.

20. C. Collins-Williams, "Clinical Spectrum of Adverse Reactions to Tartrazine," *J Asthma* 22 (1985): 139–43.

21. I. Neuman, R. Elian, H. Nahum, et al., "The Danger of 'Yellow Dyes' (Tartrazine) to Allergic Subjects," *Clin Allergy* 8 (1978): 65–8.

22. S.F. Natbony, M.E. Phillips, J.M. Elias, et al., "Histologic Studies of Chronic Idiopathic Urticaria," *J Allergy Clin Immunol* 71 (1983): 177–83.

23. R.J. Warrington, P.J. Sauder, and S. McPhillips, "Cell-Mediated Immune Responses to Artificial Food Additives in Chronic Urticaria," 16 (1986): 527–33.

24. G. Michaelsson and L. Juhlin, "Urticaria Induced by Preservatives and Dye Additives in Food and Drugs," *Br J Derm* 88 (1973): 525–34.

25. P. Thune and A. Granhold, "Provocation Tests with Anti-Phlogistic and Food Additives in Recurrent Urticaria," *Dermatologica* 151 (1975): 360–72.

26. A.M. Ros, L. Juhlin, and G. Michaelsson, "A Follow-Up Study of Patients with Recurrent Urticaria and Hypersensitivity to Aspirin,

Benzoates, and Azo Dyes," *Br J Derm* 95 (1976): 19–24.

27. R.P. Warin and R.J. Smith, "Challenge Test Battery in Chronic Urticaria," *Br J Derm* 94 (1976): 401–10.

28. K. Kaaber, "Colouring and Preservative Agents and Chronic Urticaria: Value of a Provocative Trial and Elimination Diet," *Ugeskr Laeger* 140 (1978): 1473–6.

29. J. Meynadier, J. Guilhou, J. Meynadier, et al., "Chronic Urticaria," *Ann Derm Venereol* 106 (1979): 153–8.

30. H. Lindemayr and J. Schmidt, "Intolerance to Acetylsalicylic Acid and Food Additives in Patients Suffering from Chronic Urticaria," *Wien Klin Wochenschr* 91 (1979): 817–22.

31. A. Gibson and R. Clancy, "Management of Chronic Idiopathic Urticaria by the Identification and Exclusion of Dietary Factors," *Clin Allergy* 10 (1980): 699–704.

32. H.M.G. Doeglas, "Reactions to Aspirin and Food Additives in Patients with Chronic Urticaria, Including the Physical Urticaria," *Br J Derm* 93 (1975): 135–44.

33. G.A. Settipane et al., "Significance of Tartrazine Sensitivity in Chronic Urticaria of Unknown Etiology," *J Allergy Clin Immunol* 57 (1976): 541–9.

34. L. Juhlin, "Recurrent Urticaria: Clinical Investigation of 330 Patients," *Br J Derm* 104 (1981): 369–81.

35. C. Ortolani et al., "Diagnosis of Intolerance to Food Additives," *Ann Allergy* 53 (1984): 587–91.

36. L. Juhlin, "Additives and Chronic Urticaria," *Ann Allergy* 59 (1987): 119–23.

37. G. Supramaniam and J.O. Warner, "Artificial Food Additive Intolerance in Patients with Angio-Oedema and Urticaria," *Lancet* ii (1986): 907–9.

38. J.G. Llaurado, "The Saga of BHT and BHA in Life-Extension Myths," *J Am Coll Nutr* 4 (1985): 481–4.

39. R.A. Simon, "Sulfite Sensitivity," *Annals Allergy* 56 (1986): 281–8.

40. N. Feingold, *Why Your Child Is Hyperactive* (New York: Random House, 1975).

41. American Medical Association, *Drinking Water and Human Health* (Chicago: American Medical Association, 1984).

42. J.L. Stanto and D.R. Keast, "Serum Cholesterol, Fat Intake, and Breakfast Consumption in the United States Adult Population," *J Am Coll Nutr* 8 (1989): 567–72.

43. National Research Council, *Recommended Dietary Allowances,* 10th ed. (Washington, D.C.: National Academy Press, 1989).

Supplementary Measures

1. G. Block et al., "Vitamin Supplement Use, by Demographic Characteristics," *Am J Epidemiol* 127 (1988): 297–309.

2. National Research Council, *Diet and Health: Implications for Reducing Chronic Disease Risk* (Washington, DC: National Academy Press, 1989).

3. National Research Council, *Recommended Dietary Allowances,* 10th ed. (Washington, DC: National Academy Press, 1989).

Heart and Cardiovascular Health

1. National Research Council, *Diet and Health: Implications for Reducing Chronic Disease Risk* (Washington, DC: National Academy Press, 1989).

2. U.S. Dept. of Health and Human Services, *The Surgeon General's Report on Nutrition and Health* (Rocklin, CA: Prima, 1988).

3. H. Imamura et al., "Relationship of Cigarette Smoking to Blood Pressure and Serum Lipids and Lipoproteins in Men," *Clin Exp Pharmacol Physiol* 23 (1996): 397–402.

4. J. Levenson et al., "Cigarette Smoking and Hypertension," *Arteriosclerosis* 7 (1987): 572–7.

5. H. Kritz, P. Schmid, and H. Sinzinger, "Passive Smoking and Cardiovascular Risk," *Arch Intern Med* 155 (1995): 1942–8.

6. M. Law and J.L. Tang, "An Analysis of the Effectiveness of Interventions Intended to Help People Stop Smoking," *Arch Intern Med* 155 (1995): 1933–41.

7. P.W.F. Wilson, "High-Density Lipoprotein, Low-Density Lipoprotein,

and Coronary Artery Disease," *Am J Cardiol* 66 (1990): 7A–10A.

8. A.M. Scanu and G.M. Fless, "Lipoprotein(a): A Genetic Risk Factor for Premature Coronary Heart Disease," *JAMA* 267 (1992): 3326–9.

9. E.J. Schaefer et al., "Lipo-protein(a) Levels and Risk of Coronary Heart Disease in Men: The Lipid Research Clinics Coronary Primary Prevention Trial," *JAMA* 271 (1994): 999–1003.

10. H.M.G. Princen et al., "Supplementation with Low Doses of Vitamin E Protects LDL from Lipid Peroxidation in Men and Women," *Arterioscler Thromb Vasc Biol* 15 (1995): 325–33.

11. M. Abbey, P.J. Nestel, and P. Baghurst, "Antioxidant Vitamins and Low-Density Lipoprotein Oxidation," *Am J Clin Nutr* 58 (1993): 525–32.

12. H.M.G. Princen et al., "Supplementation with Vitamin E, but Not Beta-Carotene, in Vivo Effects Low Density Lipoprotein from Lipid Peroxidation in Vitro: Effect of Cigarette Smoking," *Arterioscler Thromb* 12 (1992): 554–62.

13. K.F. Gey et al., "Inverse Correlation between Plasma Vitamin E and Mortality from Ischemic Heart Disease in Cross-Cultural Epidemiology," *Am J Clin Nutr* 53 (1991): 326S–4S.

14. M.J. Stampfer et al., "Vitamin E Consumption and the Risk of Coronary Heart Disease in Women," *New Engl J Med* 328 (1993): 1444–9.

15. E.B. Rimm et al., "Vitamin E Consumption and the Risk of Coronary Heart Disease in Men," *New Engl J Med* 328 (1993): 1450–6.

16. M.C. Bellizzi et al., "Vitamin E and Coronary Heart Disease: The European Paradox," *Eur J Clin Nutr* 48 (1994): 822–31.

17. M.J. Stampfer et al., "Vitamin E Consumption and the Risk of Coronary Disease in Women," 328 (1993): 1444–8.

18. E.B. Rimm, "Vitamin E Consumption and the Risk of Coronary Heart Disease in Men," *New Engl J Med* 328 (1993): 1450–5.

19. H.N. Hodis et al., "Serial Coronary Angiographic Evidence That Antioxidant Vitamin Intake Reduces Progression of Coronary Artery Atherosclerosis," *JAMA* 273 (1995): 1849–54.

20. B. Frei, L. England, and B.N. Ames, "Ascorbate Is an Outstanding Antioxidant in Human Blood Plasma," *Proc Natl Acad Sci* 86 (1989): 6377–81.

21. S. Whitehead et al., "Effect of Red Wine Ingestion on the Antioxidant Capacity of Serum," *Clin Chem* 41 (1995): 32–5.

22. J.A. Simon, "Vitamin C and Cardiovascular Disease: A Review," *J Am Coll Nutr* 11 (1992): 107–25.

23. J.E. Engstrom, L.E. Kanim, and M.A. Klein, "Vitamin C Intake and Mortality Among a Sample of the United States Population," *Epidemiol* 3 (1992): 194–202.

24. D. Harats et al., "Effect of Vitamin C and E Supplementation on Susceptibility of Plasma Lipoproteins to Peroxidation Induced by Acute Smoking," *Atherosclerosis* 85 (1990): 47–54.

25. P.A. Howard and D.G. Meyers, "Effect of Vitamin C on Plasma Lipids," *Pharmacother* 29 (1995): 1129–36.

26. P.F. Jacques et al., "Ascorbic Acid and Plasma Lipids," *Epidemiol* 5 (1994): 19–26.

27. J. Hallfrisch et al., "High Plasma Vitamin C Associated with High Plasma HDL and HDL2 Cholesterol," *Am J Clin Nutr* 60 (1994): 100–5.

28. B. Schwitters and J. Masquelier, *OPC in Practice: Bioflavanols and Their Application* (Rome: Alfa Omega, 1993).

29. M.G. Hertog et al., "Dietary Antioxidant Flavonoids and Risk of Coronary Heart Disease: The Zutphen Elderly Study," *Lancet* 342 (1993): 1007–11.

30. R.M. Facino et al., "Free Radicals Scavenging Action and Anti-Enzyme Activities of Procyanidines from *Vitis vinifera*: A Mechanism for their Capillary Protective Action," *Arzneim Forsch* 44 (1994): 592–601.

31. W.C. Chang and F.L. Hsu, "Inhibition of Platelet Aggregation and Arachidonate Metabolism in Platelets by Procyanidins," *Prostagland Leukotri Essential Fatty Acids* 38 (1989): 181–8.

32. M.T. Meunier et al., "Inhibition of Angiotensin I Converting Enzyme

by Flavanolic Compounds: In Vitro and in Vivo Studies," *Planta Med* 54 (1987): 12–5.

33. N. Kromann and A. Green, "Epidemiological Studies in the Upernavik District, Greenland," *Acta Med Scand* 208 (1980): 401–6.

34. D. Kromhout, E.B. Bosscheiter, and C. De Lezenne-Coulander, "Inverse Relation between Fish Oil Consumption and 20 Year Mortality from Coronary Heart Disease," *N Engl J Med* 312 (1985): 1205–9.

35. K.N. Seidelin, B. Myrup, and B. Fischer-Hansen, "n-3 Fatty Acids in Adipose Tissue and Coronary Artery Disease Are Inversely Correlated," *Am J Clin Nutr* 55 (1992): 1117–9.

36. G.N. Sandker et al., "Serum Cholesterol Ester Fatty Acids and Their Relation with Serum Lipids in Elderly Men in Crete and the Netherlands," *Eur J Clin Nutr* 47 (1993): 201–8.

37. Y. Kagawa et al., "Eicosapolyenoic Acids of Serum Lipids of Japanese Islanders with Low Incidence of Cardiovascular Diseases," *J Nutr Sci Vitaminol* 28 (1982): 441–53.

38. R.M. McLean, "Magnesium and Its Therapeutic Uses: A Review," *Am J Med* 96 (1994): 63–76.

39. B.M. Altura, "Basic Biochemistry and Physiology of Magnesium: A Brief Review," *Magnes Trace Elem* 10 (1991): 167–71.

40. J.R. Purvis and A. Movahed, "Magnesium Disorders and Cardiovascular Disease," *Clin Cardiol* 15 (1992): 556–68.

41. B.M. Altura, "Ischemic Heart Disease and Magnesium," *Magnesium* 7 (1988): 57–67.

42. E.M. Hampton, D.D. Whang, and R. Whang, "Intravenous Magnesium Therapy in Acute Myocardial Infarction," *Ann Pharmacother* 28 (1994): 212–9.

43. K.K. Teo and S. Yusuf, "Role of Magnesium in Reducing Mortality in Acute Myocardial Infarction: A Review of the Evidence," *Drugs* 46 (1993): 347–59.

44. M. Schecter, E. Kaplinsky, and B. Rabinowitz, "The Rationale of Magnesium Supplementation in Acute Myocardial Infarction: A Review of the Literature," *Arch Intern Med* 152 (1992): 2189–96.

45. S.C.-T. Lam, E.J. Harfenist, M.A. Packham, et al., "Investigation of Possible Mechanisms of Pyridoxal 5'-Phosphate Inhibition of Platelet Reactions," *Thrombosis Res* 20 (1980): 633–45.

46. A. Sermet et al., "Effect of Oral Pyridoxine Hydrochloride Supplementation on in Vitro Platelet Sensitivity to Different Agonists," *Arzneim Forsch* 45 (1995): 19–21.

47. H. Kiesewetter et al., "Effect of Garlic on Thrombocyte Aggregation, Microcirculation, and Other Risk Factors," *Int J Clin Pharmacol Ther Toxicol* 29 (1991): 151–5.

48. E. Ernst, "Fibrinogen: An Important Risk Factor for Atherothrombotic Diseases," *Annals Med* 26 (1994): 15–22.

49. C.J. Glueck et al., "Evidence That Homocysteine Is an Independent Risk Factor for Atherosclerosis in Hyperlipidemic Patients," *Am J Cardiol* 75 (1995): 132–6.

50. R. Clarke et al., "Hyperhomocysteinemia: An Independent Risk Factor for Vascular Disease," *New Engl J Med* 324 (1991): 1149–55.

51. F. Landgren et al., "Plasma Homocysteine in Acute Myocardial Infarction: Homocysteine-Lowering Effect of Folic Acid," *J Int Med* 237 (1995): 381–8.

52. J.B. Ubbink et al., "Vitamin B-12, Vitamin B-6, and Folate Nutritional Status in Men with Hyperhomocysteinemia," *Am J Clin Nutr* 57 (1993): 47–53.

53. J.B. Ubbink, W.J. van der Merwe, and R. Delport, "Hyperhomocysteinemia and the Response to Vitamin Supplementation," *Clin Invest* 71 (1993): 993–8.

54. K.A. Matthews and S.G. Haynes, "Type A Behavior Pattern and Coronary Disease Risk," *Am J Epidemiol* 123 (1986): 923–60.

55. U. Lundberg et al., "Type A Behavior in Healthy Males and Females as Related to Physiologic Reactivity and Blood Lipids," *Psychosomatic Med* 51 (1989): 113–22.

56. M.M. Muller et al., "The Relationship between Habitual Anger Coping Style and Serum Lipid and Lipoprotein Concentrations," *Biol Psychol* 41 (1995): 69–81.

57. L.D. Kubzansky et al., "Is Worrying Bad for Your Heart? A Prospective Study of Worry and Coronary Heart Disease in Normative Aging Study," *Circulation* 95 (1997): 818–24.

58. J.F. Desforges, "The Use of Aspirin in Ischemic Heart Disease," *New Engl J Med* 327 (1992): 175–181.

59. J. Weil et al., "Prophylactic Aspirin and Risk of Peptic Ulcer Bleeding," *BMJ* 310 (1995): 827–30.

60. D. Ornish et al., "Can Lifestyle Changes Reverse Coronary Heart Disease?" *Lancet* 336 (1990): 129–33.

61. D. Kromhout, E.B. Bosscheiter, and C. De Lezenne-Coulander, "Inverse Relation between Fish Oil Consumption and 20 Year Mortality from Coronary Heart Disease." *N Engl J Med* (1985):1205–9.

62. K.N. Seidelin, B. Myrup and B. Fischer-Hansen, "n-3 Fatty Acids in Adipose Tissue and Coronary Artery Disease Are Inversely Correlated *Am J Clin Nutr* 55 (1992): 1117–9..

63. M.L. Burr et al., "Effects of Changes in Fat, Fish, and Fiber Intakes on Death and Myocardial Reinfarction: Diet and Reinfarction Trial (DART)," *Lancet* 334 (1989): 757–61.

64. M. de Lorgeril et al., "Mediterranean Alpha-Linolenic Acid-Rich Diet in Secondary Prevention of Coronary Heart Disease," *Lancet* 343 (1994): 1454–9.

65. G. Abate et al., "Controlled Multicenter Study on the Therapeutic Effectiveness of Mesoglycan in Patients with Cerebrovascular Disease," *Minerva Med* 82(3) (1991): 101–5.

66. D. Mansi et al., "Open Trial of Mesoglycan in the Treatment of Cerebrovascular Ischemic Disease," *Acta Neurologica* 10 (1988): 108–12.

67. G. Laurora et al., "Delayed Arteriosclerosis Progression in High Risk Subjects Treated with Mesoglycan: Evaluation of Intima-Media Thickness," *J Cardiovasc Surg* 34(4) (1993): 313–8.

68. F. Vecchio et al., "Mesoglycan in Treatment of Patients with Cerebral Ischemia: Effects on Hemorrheologic and Hematochemical Parameters," *Acta Neurol* 15(6) (1993): 449–56.

69. G. De Donato and P. Sangiuolo, "Instrumental Evaluation of the Mesoglycan Effects in Phlebopathic Patients: Prospective Randomized Double-Blind Study," *Minerva Medica* 77 (1986): 1927–31.

70. K. Nakazawa and K. Murata, "The Therapeutic Effect of Chondroitin Polysulphate in Elderly Atherosclerotic Patients," *J Int Med Res* 6 (1978): 217–25.

71. F.V. DeFeudis, ed., *Ginkgo Biloba Extract (EGb 761): Pharmacological Activities and Clinical Applications* (Paris: Elsevier, 1991).

72. E.W. Funfgeld, ed., *Rokan (Ginkgo Biloba): Recent Results in Pharmacology and Clinic* (New York: Springer-Verlag, 1988).

73. J. Kleijnen and P. Knipschild, "Ginkgo biloba," *Lancet* 340 (1992): 1136–9.

74. J. Kleijnen and P. Knipschild, "Ginkgo biloba for Cerebral Insufficiency," *Br J Clinical Pharmacol* 34 (1992): 352–8.

75. T.D. Graboys et al., "Results of a Second-Opinion Program for Coronary Artery Bypass Surgery," *JAMA* 268 (1992): 2537–40; T.D. Graboys et al., "Results of a Second-Opinion Program for Coronary Artery Bypass Surgery," *JAMA* 258 (1987): 1611–4.

76. E.L. Alderman et al., "Ten-Year Follow-Up of Survival and Myocardial Infarction in the Randomized Coronary Artery Surgery Study (CASS)," *Circulation* 82 (1990): 1629–46.

77. CASS Principle Investigators and Their Associates, "Myocardial Infarction and Mortality in the Coronary Artery Surgery Study (CASS) Randomized Trial," *New Engl J Med* 310 (1984): 750–8.

78. CASS Principle Investigators and Their Associates, "Coronary Artery Surgery (CASS): A Randomized Trial of Coronary Artery Bypass Surgery," *Circulation* 68 (1983): 939–50.

79. W. Hueb, "Two- to Eight-Year Survival Rates in Patients who Refused Coronary Artery Bypass Grafting," *Am J Cardiol* 63 (1989): 155–9.

80. C.W. White et al., "Does Visual Interpretation of the Coronary Angiogram Predict the Physiologic Importance of a Coronary Stenosis?" *New Eng J Med* 310 (1984): 819–24.

81. C.M. Winslow et al., "The Appropriateness of Performing Coronary Artery Bypass Surgery," *JAMA* 260 (1988): 505.

82. N.E. Clarke et al., "Treatment of Angina Pectoris with Disodium Ethylene Diamine Tetraacetic Acid," *Am J Med Sci* 232 (1956): 654–66.

83. N.E. Clarke, "Atherosclerosis, Occlusive Vascular Disease, and EDTA," *Am J Cardiol* 6 (1960): 233–6.

84. D. Steinberg et al., "Beyond Cholesterol. Modifications of Low-Density Lipoprotein That Increase Its Atherogenicity," *N Engl J Med* 320 (1989): 915–24.

85. E.M. Cranton and J.P. Frackelton, "Current Status of EDTA Chelation Therapy in Occlusive Arterial Disease," *J Adv Med* 2 (1989): 107–19.

86. E. Olszwer and J.P. Carter, "EDTA Chelation Therapy: A Retrospective Study of 2,870 Patients," *J Adv Med* 2 (1989): 197–211.

87. E. Olszewer, F.C. Sabbag, and J.P. Carter, "A Pilot Double-Blind Study of Sodium-Magnesium EDTA in Peripheral Vascular Disease," *J Nat Med Assoc* 82 (1988): 173–7.

88. P.E. Ballmer et al., "Depletion of Plasma Vitamin C but Not Vitamin E in Response to Cardiac Operations," *J Thorac Cardiovasc Surg* 108 (1994): 308–11.

89. M. Chello et al., "Protection of Coenzyme Q10 from Myocardial Reperfusion Injury during Coronary Artery Bypass Grafting," *Ann Thorac Surg* 58 (1994): 1427–32.

90. W.J. Elliott, "Earlobe Crease and Coronary Artery Disease," *Am J Med* 75 (1983): 1024–32.

91. W.J. Elliott and L.H. Powell, "Diagonal Earlobe Creases and Prognosis in Patients with Suspected Coronary Artery Disease," *Am J Med* 100 (1996): 205–11.

Detoxification

1. R.A. Passwater and E.M. Cranton, *Trace Elements, Hair Analysis, and Nutrition* (New Canaan, CT: Keats, 1983).

2. M. Rutter and R. Russell-Jones, eds., *Lead versus Health: Sources and Effects of Low-Level Lead Exposure* (New York: John Wiley, 1983).

3. K.J. Yost, "Cadmium, the Environment and Human Health: An Overview," *Experentia* 40 (1984): 157–64.

4. B.G. Gerstner and J.E. Huff, "Clinical Toxicology of Mercury," *J Toxicol Environ Health* 2 (1977): 471–526.

5. J.R. Nation et al., "Dietary Administration of Nickel: Effects on Behaviour and Metallothionein Levels," *Physiol Behavior* 34 (1985): 349–53.

6. Anonymous, "Toxicologic Consequences of Oral Aluminum," *Nutrition Reviews* 45 (1987): 72–4.

7. M. Marlowe et al., "Hair Mineral Content as a Predictor of Learning Disabilities," *J Learn Disabil* 17 (1977): 418–421.

8. R. Pihl and M. Parkes, "Hair Element Content in Learning Disabled Children," *Science* 198 (1977): 204–6.

9. O. David, J. Clark, and K. Voeller, "Lead and Hyperactivity," *Lancet* ii (1972): 900–3.

10. O. David, S. Hoffman, and J. Sverd, "Lead and Hyperactivity. Behavioral Response to Chelation: A Pilot Study," *Am J Psychiatry* 133 (1976): 1155–1188.

11. V. Benignus et al., "Effects of Age and Body Lead Burden on CNS Function in Young Children: EEG Spectra," *EEG and Clin Neurophys* 52 (1981): 240–8.

12. B. Rimland and G. Larson, "Hair Mineral Analysis and Behavior: An Analysis of 51 Studies," *J Learn Disabil* 16 (1983): 279–285.

13. S.J.S. Flora et al., "Protective Role of Trace Metals in Lead Intoxication," *Toxicology Letters* 13 (1982): 51–6.

14. H.S. Hsu et al., "Interaction of Dietary Calcium with Toxic Levels of Lead and Zinc in Pigs," *J Nutrit* 105 (1975): 112–68.

15. H.G. Petering, "Some Observations on the Interaction of Zinc, Copper and Iron Metabolism in Lead and Cadmium Toxicity," *Environ Health Perspect* 25 (1978): 141–5.

16. R. Papaioannou, A. Sohler, and C.C. Pfeiffer, "Reduction of Blood Lead Levels in Battery Workers by Zinc and Vitamin C," *J Orthomol Psychiatry* 7 (1978): 94–106.

17. S.J.S. Flora, S. Singh, and S.K. Tandon, "Role of Selenium in Protection Against Lead Intoxication," *Acta Pharmacol et Toxicol* 53 (1983): 28–32.

18. S.K. Tandon et al., "Vitamin B Complex in Treatment of Cadmium Intoxication," *Annals Clin Lab Sci* 14 (1984): 487–92.

19. G.R. Bratton et al., "Thiamin (Vitamin B1) Effects on Lead Intoxication and Deposition of Lead in Tissue: Therapeutic Potential," *Toxicol Appl Pharmacol* 59 (1981): 164–72.

20. S.J.S. Flora, S. Singh, and S.K. Tandon, "Prevention of Lead Intoxication by Vitamin B Complex," *Z Ges Hyg* 30 (1984): 409–11.

21. N. Ballatori and T.W. Clarkson, "Dependence of Biliary Excretion of Inorganic Mercury on the Biliary Transport of Glutathione," *Biochem Pharmacol* 33 (1984): 1093–8.

22. M. Murakami and M.A. Webb, "A Morphological and Biochemical Study of the Effects of L-Cysteine on the Renal Uptake and Nephrotoxicity of Cadmium," *Br J Exp Pathol* 62 (1981): 115–30.

23. C.W. Cha, "A Study on the Effect of Garlic to the Heavy Metal Poisoning of Rat," *J Korean Med Sci* 2 (1987): 213–23.

24. B. Hunter, "Some Food Additives as Neuroexcitors and Neurotoxins," *Clinical Ecology* 2 (1984): 83–9.

25. M.R. Cullen, ed., *Workers with Multiple Chemical Sensitivities* (Philadelphia: Hanley & Belfus, 1987).

26. L.T. Stayner, L. Elliott, L. Blade, et al., "A Retrospective Cohort Mortality Study of Workers Exposed to Formaldehyde in the Garment Industry," *Am J Ind Med* 13 (1988): 667–81.

27. K.H. Kilburn, R. Warshaw, C.T. Boylen, et al., "Pulmonary and Neurobehavioral Effects of Formaldehyde Exposure," *Archiv Environ Health* 40 (1985): 254–60.

28. T.D. Sterling and A.V. Arundel, "Health Effects of Phenoxy Herbicides," *Scand J Work Environ Health* 12 (1986): 161–73.

29. L. Dickey, ed., *Clinical Ecology* (Springfield, IL: C.C. Thomas, 1976).

30. K. Lindstrom, H. Riihimaki, and K. Hannininen, "Occupational Solvent Exposure and Neuropsychiatric Disorders," *Scand J Work Environ Health* 10 (1984): 321–3.

31. G. Talska et al., "Genetically Based n-Acetyltransferase Metabolic Poly-

morphism and Low-Level Environmental Exposure to Carcinogens," *Nature* 369 (1994): 154–56.

32. J.E. Gallagher et al., "Comparison of DNA Adduct Levels in Human Placenta from Polychlorinated Biphenyl Exposed Women and Smokers in Which CYP 1A1 Levels Are Similarly Elevated," *Terato Carcino Mutagen* 14 (1994): 183–92.

33. M.E. Campbell et al., "Biotransformation of Caffeine, Paraxanthine, Theophylline, and Theobromine by Polycyclic Aromatic Hydrocarbon-Inducable Cytochrome P-450 in Human Liver Microsomes," *Drug Metab Disp* 15 (1987): 237–49.

34. C.W.W. Beecher, "Cancer Preventive Properties of Varieties of *Brassica oleracea*: A Review." *Am J Clin Nutr* 59(suppl.) (1994): 1166S–70S.

35. P.L. Crowell and M.N. Gould, "Chemoprevention and Therapy of Cancer by d-Limonene," *Critical Rev Oncogenesis* 5 (1994): 1–22.

36. G.C. Yee et al., "Effect of Grapefruit Juice on Blood Cyclosporin Concentration," *Lancet* 345 (1995): 955–56.

37. M. Nagabhushan and S.V. Bhide, "Curcumin as an Inhibitor of Cancer," *J Am Coll Nutr* 11 (1992): 192–98.

38. K. Polasa et al., "Effect of Turmeric on Urinary Mutagens in Smokers," *Mutagenesis* 7 (1992): 107–9.

39. T.M. Hagen et al., "Fate of Dietary Glutathione: Disposition in the Gastrointestinal Tract," *Am J Physiol* 259 (1990): G524–9.

40. B. Ketter et al., "The Human Glutathione S-Transferase Supergene Family: Its Polymorphism, and Its Effects on Susceptibility to Lung Cancer," *Env Health Persp* 98 (1992): 87–94.

41. A.C. White et al., "Glutathi-one Deficiency in Human Disease," *J Nutr Biochem* 5 (1994): 218–26.

42. P. Peristeris et al., "N-Acetylcysteine and Glutathione as Inhibitors of Tumor Necrosis Factor Production," *Cell Immunol* 140 (1992): 390–99.

43. A. Witschi et al., "The Systemic Availability of Oral Glutathione," *Eur J Clin Pharmacol* 43 (1992): 667–9.

44. C.J. Johnston, C.G. Meyer, and J.C. Srilakshmi, "Vitamin C Elevates Red Blood Cell Glutathione in Healthy Adults," *Am J Clin Nutr* 58 (1993): 103–5.

45. A. Jain et al., "Effect of Ascorbate or N-Acetylcysteine Treatment in a Patient with Hereditary Glutathione Synthetase Deficiency," *J Pediatr* 124 (1994): 229–33.

46. H.A. Kleinveld, P.N.M. Demacker, and A.F.H. Stalenhoef, "Failure of N-Acetylcystein to Reduce Low-Density Lipoprotein Oxidizability in Healthy Subjects," *Eur J Clin Pharmacol* 43 (1992): 639–42.

47. A.J. Quick, "Clinical Value of the Test for Hippuric Acid in Cases of Disease of the Liver," *Arch Int Med* 57 (1936): 544–56.

48. M. Frezza et al., "Reversal of Intrahepatic Cholestasis of Pregnancy in Women after High Dose S-Adenosyl-L-Methionine (SAMe) Administration," *Hepatology* 4 (1984): 274–78.

49. S. Gregus et al., "Nutritionally and Chemically Induced Impairment of Sulfate Activation and Sulfation of Xenobiotics *in vivo*," *Chem-Biol Interactions* 92 (1994): 169–77.

50. R. Barzatt and J.D. Beckman, "Inhibition of Phenol Sulfotransferase by Pyridoxal Phosphate," *Biochem Pharmacol* 47 (1994): 2087–95.

51. R.I. Skvortsova et al., "Role of Vitamin Factor in Preventing Phenol Poisoning," *Vopr Pitan* 2 (1981): 32–35.

52. G. Bombardieri et al., "Effects of S-Adenosyl-Methionine (SAMe) in the Treatment of Gilbert's Syndrome," *Curr Ther Res* 37 (1985): 580–5.

53. J.G.D. Birkmayer and W. Beyer, "Biological and Clinical Relevance of Trace Elements," *Arztl Lab* 36 (1990): 284–87.

54. C. Padova et al., "S-Adenosyl-L-Methionine Antagonizes Oral Contraceptive-Induced Bile Cholesterol Supersaturation in Healthy Women: Preliminary Report of a Controlled Randomized Trial," *Am J Gastroenterol* 79 (1984): 941–44.

55. S.J.S. Flora, S. Singh, and S.K. Tandon, "Prevention of Lead Intoxication by Vitamin B Complex," *Z Ges Hyg* 30 (1984): 409–11.

56. R.A. Shakman, "Nutritional Influences on the Toxicity of Environmental Pollutants: A Review," *Arch Env Health* 28 (1974): 105–33.

57. S.J.S. Flora et al., "Protective Role of Trace Metals in Lead Intoxication," *Toxicology Letters* 13 (1982): 51–6.

58. J. Wisniewska-Knypl et al., "Protective Effect of Methionine Against Vinyl Chloride-Mediated Depression of Non-Protein Sulfhydryls and Cytochrome P-450," *Toxicol Lett* 8 (1981): 147–52.

59. A.J. Barak et al., "Dietary Betaine Promotes Generation of Hepatic S-Adenosylmethionine and Protects the Liver from Ethanol-Induced Fatty Infiltration," *Alcohol Clin Exp Res* 17 (1993): 552–5.

60. S.H. Zeisel et al., "Choline, an Essential Nutrient for Humans," *FASEB J* 5 (1991): 2093–8.

61. H. Hikino et al., "Antihepatotoxic Actions of Flavonolignans from *Silybum marianum* Fruits," *Planta Medica* 50 (1984): 248–50.

62. G. Vogel et al., "Studies on Pharmacodynamics, Site and Mechanism of Action of Silymarin, the Antihepatotoxic Principle from *Silybum marianum* (L.) Gaert," *Arzneim.-Forsch* 25 (1975): 179–85.

63. H. Wagner, "Antihepatotoxic Flavonoids," in V. Cody, E. Middleton, and J.B. Harbourne, eds., *Plant Flavonoids in Biology and Medicine: Biochemical, Pharmacological, and Structure-Activity Relationships* (New York: Alan R. Liss, Inc., 1986), 545–558.

64. A. Valenzuela et al., "Selectivity of Silymarin on the Increase of the Glutathione Content in Different Tissues of the Rat," *Planta Med* 55 (1989): 420–2.

65. H. Sarre, "Experience in the Treatment of Chronic Hepatopathies with Silymarin," *Arzneim.-Forsch* 21 (1971): 1209–12.

66. F. Canini, Bartolucci, E. Cristallini, et al., "Use of Silymarin in the Treatment of Alcoholic Hepatic Steatosis," *Clin Ter* 114 (1985): 307–14.

67. H.A. Salmi and S. Sarna, "Effect of Silymarin on Chemical, Functional, and Morphological Alteration of the Liver: A Double-Blind Controlled Study," *Scand J Gastroenterol* 17 (1982): 417–21.

68. C. Boari et al., "Occupational Toxic Liver Diseases: Therapeutic Effects of Silymarin," *Min Med* 72 (1985): 2679–88.

69. P. Ferenci et al., "Randomized Controlled Trial of Silymarin Treatment in Patients with Cirrhosis of the Liver," *J Hepatol* 9 (1989): 105–13.

70. M. Imamura and T. Tung, "A Trial of Fasting Cure for PCB Poisoned Patients in Taiwan," *Am J Ind Med* 5 (1984): 147–53.

Digestion and Elimination

1. D.Y. Graham, J.L. Smith, and D.J. Patterson, "Why Do Apparently Healthy People Use Antacid Tablets? *Am J Gastroenterol* 78 (1983): 257–60.

2. G.W. Bray, "The Hypochlorhydria of Asthma in Childhood," *Br Med J* i (1930): 181–97.

3. I.M. Rabinowitch, "Achlorhydria and Its Clinical Significance in Diabetes Mellitus," *Am J Dig Dis* 18 (1949): 322–33.

4. W.M. Carper, T.J. Butler, J.O. Kilby, and M.J. Gibson, "Gallstones, Gastric Secretion and Flatulent Dyspepsia," *Lancet* i (1967): 413–5.

5. W.B. Rawls and V.C. Ancona, "Chronic Urticaria Associated with Hypochlorhydria or Achlorhydria," *Rev Gastroent* Oct (1950): 267–71.

6. R.A. Gianella, S.A. Broitman, and N. Zamcheck, "Influence of Gastric Acidity on Bacterial and Parasitic Enteric Infections," *Ann Int Med* 78 (1973): 271–6.

7. T.J. De Witte, P.J. Geerdink, and C.B. Lamers, "Hypochlorhydria and Hypergastrinaemia in Rheumatoid Arthritis," *Ann Rheum Dis* 38 (1979): 14–17.

8. J.A. Ryle and H.W. Barber, "Gastric Analysis in Acne Rosacea," *Lancet* ii (1920): 1195–6.

9. S. Ayres, "Gastric Secretion in Psoriasis, Eczema and Dermatitis Herpetiformis," *Arch Derm* Jul (1929): 854–9.

10. G. Dotevall and A. Walan, "Gastric Secretion of Acid and Intrinsic Factor in Patients with Hyper and Hypothyroidism," *Acta Med Scand* 186 (1969): 529–33.

11. J. Howitz and M. Schwartz, "Vitiligo, Achlorhydria, and Pernicious Anemia," *Lancet* i (1971): 1331–4.

12. C.V. Howden and R.H. Hunt, "Relationship Between Gastric Secretion and Infection," *Gut* 28 (1987): 96–107.

13. H.A. Rafsky and M. Weingarten, "A Study of the Gastric Secretory Response in the Aged," *Gastroent* May (1946): 348–52.

14. S.A. Barrie, "Heidelberg pH Capsule Gastric Analysis," in: *A Textbook of Natural Medicine,* J.E. Pizzorno and M.T. Murray, eds. (Seattle, WA: JBC Publications, 1985).

15. D. Davies and T.G. James, "An Investigation into the Gastric Secretion of a Hundred Normal Persons over the Age of Sixty," *Brit J Med* i (1930): 1–14.

16. J.H. Baron, "Studies of Basal and Peak Acid Output with an Augmented Histamine Meal," *Gut* 3 (1963): 136–44.

17 P. Mojaverian et al., "Estimation of Gastric Residence Time of the Heidelberg Capsule in Humans," *Gastroenterology* 89 (1985): 392–7.

18. J. Wright, "A Proposal for Standardized Challenge Testing of Gastric Acid Secretory Capacity Using the Heidelberg Capsule Radiotelemetry System," *J John Bastyr Col Nat Med* 1:2 (1979): 3–11.

19. K. Berstad and A. Berstad, "*Helicobacter pylori* Infection in Peptic Ulcer Disease," *Scand J Gasroenterol* 28 (1993): 561–7.

20. S.A. Sarker and K. Gyr, "Non-Immunological Defense Mechanisms of the Gut," *Gut* 33 (1992): 987–93.

21. R.W. Stockbrueger, et al., "Intragastric Nitrites, Nitrosamines, and Bacterial Overgrowth during Cimetidine Therapy," *Gut* 23 (1982): 1048–54.

22. T. Shibata et al., "High Acid Output May Protect the Gastric Mucosa from Injury Caused by *Helicobacter pylori* in Duodenal Ulcer Patients," *J Gastroenterol Hepatol* 11 (1996): 674–80.

23. T. Rokkas et al., "*Helicobacter pylori* Infection and Gastric Juice Vitamin C Levels," *Digestive Dis Sci* 40 (1995): 615–21.

24. P.S. Phull et al., "Vitamin E Concentrations in the Human Stomach and Duodenum: Correlation with *Helicobacter pylori* Infection," *Gut* 39 (1996): 31–5.

25. S.C. Baik et al., "Increased Oxidative DNA Damage in *Helicobacter pylori*-Infected Human Gastric Mucosa," *Cancer Res* 56 (1996): 1279–82.

26. J. van Marle et al., "Deglycyrrhizinised Liquorice (DGL) and the Renewal of Rat Stomach Epithelium," *Eur J Pharmacol* 72 (1981): 219–25.

27. B. Johnson and R. McIssac, "Effect of Some Anti-Ulcer Agents on Mucosal Blood Flow," *Br J Pharmacol* 1 (1981): 308.

28. W. Beil, J. Birkholz, and K.F. Sewing, "Effects of Flavonoids on Parietal Cell Acid Secretion, Gastric Mucosal Prostaglandin Production, and *Helicobacter pylori* Growth," *Arzneim Forsch* 45 (1995): 697–700.

29. J.Y. Kang et al., "Effect of Colloidal Bismuth Subcitrate on Symptoms of Gastric Histology in Non-Ulcer Dyspepsia: A Double-Blind Placebo Controlled Study," *Gut* 31 (1990): 476–80.

30. B.J. Marshall et al., "Bismuth Subsalicylate Suppression of *Helicobacteria pylori* in Non-Ulcer Dyspepsia: A Double-Blind Placebo-Controlled Trial," *Dig Dis Sci* 38 (1993): 1674–80.

31. A.W. Oelgoetz et al., "The Treatment of Food Allergy and Indigestion of Pancreatic Origin with Pancreatic Enzymes," *Am J Dig Dis Nutr* 2 (1935): 422–6.

32. Y. Sawada et al., "Polyamines in the Intestinal Lumen of Patients with Small Bowel Bacterial Overgrowth," *Biochem Soc Trans* 22 (1994): 392(S).

33. A.E.K. Henriksson et al., "Small Intestinal Bacterial Overgrowth in Patients with Rheumatoid Arthritis," *Annals Rheumatic Dis* 52 (1993): 503–10.

34. S.A. Sarker and R. Gyr, "Non-Immunological Defense Mechanisms of the Gut," *Gut* 33 (1990): 1331–7.

35. J.R. Saltzman et al., "Bacterial Overgrowth without Clinical Malabsorption in Elderly Hypochlorhydric Subjects," *Gastroenterol* 106 (1994): 615–23.

36. E. Rubinstein et al., "Antibacterial Activity of the Pancreatic Fluid," *Gastroenterol* 88 (1985): 927–32.

37. E. Husebye, "Gastrointestinal Motility Disorders and Bacterial Overgrowth," *J Intern Med* 237 (1995): 419–27.

39. A. Russo, R. Fraser, and M. Horowitz, "The Effect of Acute Hy-

perglycemia on Small Intestinal Motility in Normal Subjects," *Diabetologia* 39 (1996): 984–9.

40. A. Watanabe, T. Obata, and H. Nagashima, "Berberine Therapy of Hypertyraminemia in Patients with Liver Cirrhosis," *Acta Med Okayama* 36 (1982): 277–81.

41. E. Rubinstein et al., "Antibacterial Activity of the Pancreatic Fluid," *Gastroenterol* 88 (1985): 927–32.

42. A. Sonnenberg and T.R. Koch, "Epidemiology of Constipation in the United States," *Dis Colon Rectum* 32 (1989): 1–8.

43. D.J. Hentges, ed., "Human Intestinal Microflora," *In: Health and Disease* (New York: Academic Press, , 1983.

44. E. Metchnikoff, *The Prolongation of Life* (New York: Arna Press, 1908; 1977 reprint).

Immune Support

1. L.T. Vollhardt, "Psychoneuroimmunology: A Literature Review," *Am J Orthopsychiatry* 61 (1991): 35–47.

2. R.W. Bartrop, et al., "Depressed Lymphocyte Function After Bereavement," *Lancet* i (1977): 834–6.

3. S.J. Schleifer et al., "Suppression of Lymphocyte Stimulation Following Bereavement," *JAMA* 250 (1983): 374–7.

4. N. Cousins, *Anatomy of an Illness* (New York: Bantam Books, 1979).

5. K.M. Dillon and B. Minchoff, "Positive Emotional States and Enhancement of the Immune System," *Intern J Psychiatry Med* 15 (1986): 13–7.

6. R.A. Martin and J.P. Dobbin, "Sense of Humor, Hassles, and Immunoglobulin A: Evidence for a Stress-Moderating Effect of Humor," *Int J Psychiatry Med* 18 (1988): 93–105.

7. J.K. Kiecolt-Glaser and R. Glaser, "Psychoneuroimmunology: Can Psychological Interventions Modulate Immunity?" *J Consult Clin Psychol* 60 (1992): 569–75.

8. M. Irwin et al., "Reduction of Immune Function in Life Stress and Depression," *Biol Psych* 27 (1990): 22–30.

9. H. Moldofsky et al., "The Relationship of Interleukin-1 and Immune Functions to Sleep in Humans,"

Psychosomatic Medicine 48 (1986): 309–18.

10. Y. Kusaka, H. Kondou, and K. Morimoto, "Healthy Lifestyles Are Associated with Higher Natural Killer Cell Activity," *Prev Med* 21 (1992): 602–15.

11. K. Nekachi and K. Imai, "Environmental and Physiological Influences on Human Natural Killer Cell Activity in Relation to Good Health Practices," *Jap J Cancer Res* 83 (1992): 789–805.

12. K. Tucker, "Micronutrient Status and Aging," *Nutr Rev* 53 (1995): S9–15.

13. J.D. Bogden, "Studies on Micronutrient Supplements and Immunity in Older People," *Nutr Rev* 53 (1995): S59–65.

14. J. Pike and R.K. Chandra, "Effect of Vitamin and Trace Element Supplementation on Immune Indices in Healthy Elderly," *Internat J Vit Nutr Res* 65 (1995): 117–20.

15. R. Chandra and R. Newberne, *Nutrition, Immunity, and Infection* (New York: Pleneum Press, 1977).

16. A. Sanchez, J. Reeser, H. Lau, et al., "Role of Sugars in Human Neutrophilic Phagocytosis," *Am J Clin Nutr* 26 (1973): 1180–4.

17. W. Ringsdorf, E. Cheraskin, and R. Ramsay, "Sucrose, Neutrophil Phagocytosis, and Resistance to Disease," *Dent Surv* 52 (1976): 46–8.

18. J. Bernstein, S. Alpert, K. Nauss, and R. Suskind, "Depression of Lymphocyte Transformation Following Oral Glucose Ingestion," *Am J Clin Nutr* 30 (1977): 613.

19. G. Mann, "Hypothesis: The Role of Vitamin C in Diabetic Angiopathy," *Pers Biol Med* 17 (1974): 210–7.

20. G. Mann and P. Newton, "The Membrane Transport of Ascorbic Acid," *Ann N Y Acad Sci* 258 (1975): 243–51.

21. J. Palmblad, D. Hallberg, and S. Rossner, "Obesity, Plasma Lipids, and Polymorphonuclear (PMN) Granulocyte Functions," *Scand J Hematol* 19 (1977): 293–303.

22. C. Waddell, D. Tauton, and J. Twomey, "Inhibition of Lymphoproliferation by Hyperlipoproteinemic Plasma," *J Clin Invest* 58 (1976): 950–4.

23. L. Gianni, F. Padova, M. Zuin, and M. Podda, "Bile Acid-Induced Inhi-

bition of the Lymphoproliferative Response to Phytohemagglutinin and Pokeweed Mitogen: An In Vitro Study," *Gastroenterol* 78 (1980): 231–5.

24. M. Dianzani, M. Torriella, R. Canuto, et al., "The Influence of Enrichment with Cholesterol on the Phagocytic Activity of Rat Macrophages," *J Path* 118 (1976): 193–9.

25. C. Simone, M. Ferrari, A. Lozzi, et al., "Vitamins and Immunity II: Influence of L-Carnitine on the Immune System," *Acta Vit Enz* 4 (1982): 135–40.

26. D. Simone, M. Ferrari, D. Meli, et al., "Reversibility by L-Carnitine of Immunosuppression Induced by an Emulsion of Soya Bean Oil, Glycerol, and Egg Lecithin," *Arzneim Forsch* 32 (1982): 1488–8.

27. R. Brayton, P. Stokes, M. Schwartz, and D. Louria, "Effect of Alcohol and Various Diseases on Leukocyte Mobilization, Phagocytosis and Intracellular Bacterial Killing," *NEJM* 282 (1970): 123–8.

28. R.D. Semba, "Vitamin A, Immunity, and Infection," *Clin Inf Dis* 19 (1994): 489–99.

29. W.W. Fawzi, et al., "Vitamin A Supplementation and Child Mortality," *JAMA* 269 (1993): 898–903.

30. A.C. Arrieta et al., "Vitamin A Levels in Children with Measles in Long Beach, California," *J Pediatr* 121 (1992): 75–8.

31. G.D. Hussey and M. Klein, "A Randomized, Controlled Trial of Vitamin A in Children with Severe Measles," *N Engl J Med* 323 (1990): 160–4.

32. K.M. Neuzil et al., "Safety and Pharmacokinetics of Vitamin A Therapy for Infants with Respiratory Syncytial Infections," *Antimicrob Agents Chemother* 39 (1995): 1191–3.

33. A. Bendich, "Beta-Carotene and the Immune Response," *Proc Nutr Soc* 50 (1991): 263–74.

34. S.W. Clausen, "Carotenemia and Resistance to Infection," *Trans Am Pediatr Soc* 43 (1931): 27–30.

35. M. Alexander, H. Newmark, and R.G. Miller, "Oral Beta-Carotene Can Increase the Number of OKT4+ Cells in Human Blood," *Immunol Letters* 9 (1985): 221–4.

36. P.B. Brevard, "Beta-Carotene Affects White Blood Cells in Human

Peripheral Blood," *Nutr Rep Internat* 40 (1989): 139–50.

37. E.D. Brown et al., "Plasma Carotenoids in Normal Men After a Single Ingestion of Vegetables or Purified Beta-Carotene," *Am J Clin Nutr* 49 (1989): 1258–65.

38. W. Beisel, R. Edelman, K. Nauss, and R. Suskind, "Single-Nutrient Effects of Immunologic Functions," *JAMA* 245 (1981): 53–8.

39. P. Dowd and R. Heatley, "The Influence of Undernutrition on Immunity," *Clin Sci* 66 (1984): 241–8.

40. K. Tachibana, S. Sone, E. Tsubura, and Y. Kishino, "Stimulation Effect of Vitamin A on Tumoricidal Activity of Rat Alveolar Macrophages," *Br J Cancer* 49 (1984): 343–8.

41. R.D. Semba, "Vitamin A, Immunity, and Infection," *Clin Inf Dis* 19 (1994): 489–99.

42. E. Seifter, G. Rettura, J. Seiter, et al., "Thymotrophic Action of Vitamin A," *Fed Proc* 32 (1973): 947.

43. A. Reinhardt, D. Auperin, and J. Sands, "Mechanism of Viricidal Activity of Retinoids: Protein Removal from Bacteriophage 6 Envelope," *Antimicrob Agents Chemother* 17 (1980): 1034–7.

44. A. Bendich, "Beta-Carotene and the Immune Response," *Proc Nutr Soc* 50 (1991): 263–74.

45. A. Bendich, "Vitamin C and Immune Responses," *Food Technol* 41 (1987): 112–4.

46. J. Scott, "On the Biochemical Similarities of Ascorbic Acid and Interferon," *J Theor Biol* 98 (1982): 235–8.

47. H. Hemila, "Vitamin C and the Common Cold," *Br J Nutr* 67 (1992): 3–16.

48. H. Hemila and W. Herman, "Vitamin C and the Common Cold: A Retrospective Analysis of Chalmers' Review," *J Am Coll Nutr* 14 (1995): 116–23.

49. C. Hunt et al., "The Clinical Effects of Vitamin C Supplementation in Elderly Hospitalized Patients with Acute Respiratory Infections," *Int J Vit Nutr Res* 64 (1994): 212–9.

50. R.F. Cathcart, "The Third Face of Vitamin C," *J Orthomol Med* 7 (1992): 197–200.

51. H. Baur and H. Staub, "Treatment of Hepatitis with Infusions of Ascorbic Acid: Comparison with Other Therapies," *JAMA* 156 (1954): 565.

52. E. Ginter, "Optimum Intake of Vitamin C for the Human Organism," *Nutr Health* 1 (1982): 66–77.

53. B. Havsteen, "Flavonoids: A Class of Natural Products of High Pharmacological Potency," *Biochem Pharmacol* 32 (1983): 1141–8.

54. J. Kelleher, "Vitamin E and the Immune Response," *Proceedings Nutr Soc* 50 (1991): 245–9.

55. S.N. Meydani et al., "Vitamin E Supplementation and In Vivo Immune Response in Healthy Elderly Subjects: A Randomized Controlled Trial," *JAMA* 277 (1997): 1380–6.

56. J. Stockman, "Infections and Iron: Too Much of a Good Thing?" *Am J Dis Child* 135 (1981): 18–20.

57. J.W. Hadden, "The Treatment of Zinc Deficiency Is an Immunotherapy," *Int J Immunopharmac* 17 (1995): 697-701.

58. M. Dardenne, J. Pleau, B. Nabarra, et al., "Contribution of Zinc and Other Metals to the Biological Activity of the Serum Thymic Factor," *Proc Natl Acad Sci* 79 (1982): 5370–3.

59. S. Eaterbrook-Smith, "Activation of the Binding of C1q to Immune Complexes by Zinc," *FEBS Letters* 162 (1983): 117–9.

60. E. Katz and E. Margalith, "Inhibition of Vaccinia Virus Maturation by Zinc Chloride," *Antimicrobial Agents Chemotherapy* 19 (1981): 213–7.

61. M. Gershwin, R. Beach, and L. Hurley, "Trace Metals, Aging, and Immunity," *J Am Ger Soc* 31 (1983): 374–8.

62. G.A. Eby, D.R. Davis, and W.W. Halcomb, "Reduction in Duration of Common Colds by Zinc Gluconate Lozenges in a Double-Blind Study," *Antimicrob Agents Chemother* 25 (1984): 20–4.

63. S.B. Mossad, et al., "Zinc Gluconate Lozenges for Treating the Common Cold: A Randomized, Double-Blind, Placebo-Controlled Study," *Annals Intern Med* 125 (1996): 81–8.

64. L. Kiremidjian-Schumacher and G. Stotsky, "Selenium and Immune Responses," *Environmental Res* 42 (1987): 277–303.

65. L. Kiremidjian-Schumacher et al., "Supplementation with Selenium and Human Immune Cell Functions II: Effect on Cytotoxic Lymphocytes and Natural Killer Cells," *Biol Trace Elem Res* 41 (1994): 115–27.

66. M. Roy, "Supplementation with Selenium and Human Immune Cell Functions I: Effect on Lymphocyte Proliferation and Interleukin 2 Receptor Expression," *Biol Trace Elem Res* 41 (1994): 103–14.

67. H. Hasselbalch et al., "Decreased Thymus Size in Formula-Fed Infants Compared with Breast-Fed Infants," *Acta Periatr* 85 (1996): 1029–32.

68. J.D. Bogden et al., "Zinc and Immunocompetence in the Elderly: Baseline Data on Zinc Nutriture and Immunity in Unsupplemented Subjects," *Am J Clin Nutr* 46 (1987): 101–9.

69. P. Cazzola, P. Mazzanti, and G. Bossi, "In Vivo Modulating Effect of a Calf Thymus Acid Lysate on Human T Lymphocyte Subsets and CD4+/CD8+ Ratio in the Course of Different Diseases," *Curr Ther Res* 42 (1987): 1011–7.

70. N.M. Kouttab, M. Prada, and P. Cazzola, "Thymomodulin: Biological Properties and Clinical Applications," *Medical Oncology Tumor Pharmacotherapy* 6 (1989): 5–9.

71. A. Fiocchi et al., "A Double-Blind Clinical Trial for the Evaluation of the Therapeutic Effectiveness of a Calf Thymus Derivative (Thymomodulin) in Children with Recurrent Respiratory Infections," *Thymus* 8 (1986): 831–9.

72. M. Fridkin and V.A. Najjar, "Tuftsin: Its Chemistry, Biology, and Clinical Potential," *Crit Rev Biochem Mol Biol* 24 (1989): 1–40.

73. W. Diezel et al., "The Effect of Splenopentin (DA SP-5) on In Vitro Myelopoiesis and on AZT-Induced Bone Marrow Toxicity," *Int J Immunopharmac* 15 (1993): 269–73.

74. M.M. Minter, "Agranulocytic Angina: Treatment of a Case with Fetal Calf Spleen," *Texas State J Med* 2 (1933): 338–43.

75. G.A. Gray, "The Treatment of Agranulocytic Angina with Fetal Calf Spleen," *Texas State J Med* 29 (1933): 366–9.

76. A.E. Greer, "Use of Fetal Spleen in Agranulocytosis: Preliminary Report," *Texas State J Med* 28 (1932): 338–43.

77. A. Rastogi et al., "Augmentation of Human Natural Killer Cells by Splenopentin Analogs," *FEBS Lett* 317 (1993): 93–5.

78. H.D. Volk et al., "Immunorestitution by a Bovine Spleen Hydrosylate and Ultrafiltrate," *Arzneim Forsch* 41 (1991): 1281–5.

79. R. Bauer and H. Wagner, "Echinacea Species as Potential Immunostimulatory Drugs," *Econ Med Plant Res* 5 (1991): 253–321.

80. M. Erhard et al., "Effect of Echinacea, Aconitum, Lachesis, and Apis Extracts, and Their Combinations on Phagocytosis of Human Granulocytes," *Phytother Res* 8 (1994): 14–7.

81. A. Wildfeuer and D. Meyerhofer, "Study of the Influence of Phytopreparation on the Cellular Function of Bodily Defense," *Arzneim Forsch* 44 (1994): 361–6.

82. H.M. Chang and P.P.H. But, eds., *Pharmacology and Applications of Chinese Materia Medica* (Singapore: World Scientific, 1987), 1041–6.

83. K.S. Zhao et al., "Enhancement of the Immune Response in Mice by *Astragalus membranaceus*," *Immunopharmacol* 20 (1988): 225–33.

84. D.T. Chu, W.L. Wong, and G.M. Mavlight, "Immunotherapy with Chinese Medicinal Herbs," *J Clin Lab Immunol* 25 (1988): 119–29.

Longevity and Life Extension

1. "Changes in U.S. Life Expectancy," *Statistical Bull* Jul/Sept (1994): 11–17.

2. "Report of Final Mortality Statistics, 1995," *Monthly Vital Statistics Report* 45(11) (1995): S2.

3. A.E. Harper, "Nutrition, Aging, and Longevity," *Am J Clin Nutr* 36 (1982): 737–49.

4. R.B. Mazess and S.H. Forman, "Longevity and Age Exaggeration in Vilcabamba, Ecuador," *J Gerontol* 34 (1979): 94–8.

5. Z.A. Medvedev, "Myths about the Caucasian Mountain Centers of Longevity," *Geriatric Med Today* 5 (1986): 96–112.

6. L.B. Taubman, "Theories of Aging," *Resident and Staff Physician* 32 (1986): 31–7.

7. L. Hayflick, "The Cell Biology of Human Aging," *N Eng J Med* 295 (1976): 302–8.

8. R.G. Cutler, "Peroxide-Producing Potential of Tissues: Inverse Correlation with Longevity of Mammalian Species," *Proc Natl Acad Sci* 82 (1985): 4798–802.

9. M. Fossel, *Reversing Human Aging* (New York, NY: Morrow, 1996).

10. C.B. Harley, A.B. Futcher, and C.W. Greider, "Telomeres Shorten During Aging of Human Fibroblasts," *Nature* 345 (1990): 458–60.

11. D. Harman, "Free-Radical Theory of Aging: The Free-Radical Diseases," *Age* 7 (1984): 111–31.

12. A.T. Diplock, "Antioxidant Nutrients and Disease Prevention: An Overview," *Am J Clini Nutr* 53 (1991): 189S–93S.

13. R.G. Cutler, "Peroxide-Producing Potential of Tissues: Inverse Correlation with Longevity of Mammalian Species," *Proc Natl Acad Sci* 82 (1985): 4798–4802.

14. O. Chappey et al., "Advanced Glycation Endproducts, Oxidant Stress, and Vascular Lesions," *Eur J Clin Invest* 27 (1997): 97–108.

15. B.P. Yu, E.J. Masoro, and C.A. McMahan, "Nutritional Influences on Aging of Fischer 344 Rats, I: Physical, Metabolic, and Longevity Characteristics," *J Gerontol* 40 (1985): 657–70.

16. R.G. Cutler, "Carotenoids and Retinol: Their Possible Importance in Determining Longevity of Primate Species," *Proc Natl Acad Sci* 81 (1984): 7627–31.

17. H. Gerster, "Anticarcinogenic Effect of Common Carotenoids," *Internat J Vit Nutr Res* 63 (1993): 93–121.

18. V. Cody, E. Middleton, and J.B. Harborne, *Plant Flavonoids in Biology and Medicine: Biochemical, Pharmacological, and Structure-Activity Relationships* (New York: Alan R Liss, 1986).

19. J. Kuhnau, "The Flavonoids: A Class of Semi-Essential Food Components: Their Role in Human Nutrition," *Wld Rev Nutr Diet* 24 (1976): 117–91.

20. E. Middleton, "The Flavonoids," *Trends in Pharmaceut Sci* 5 (1984): 335–8.

21. F.V. DeFeudis, ed., *Ginkgo Biloba Extract (EGb 761): Pharmacological Activities and Clinical Applications* (Paris: Elsevier, 1991).

22. E.L. Schneider and J.D. Reed, "Life Extension," *New Eng J Med* 312 (1985): 1159–68.

23. S.S. Yen, A.J. Morales, and O. Khorram, "Replacement of DHEA in Aging Men and Women: Potential Remedial Effects," *Ann NY Acad Sci* 774 (1995): 128–42.

24. R.J. Reiter et al., "A Review of the Evidence Supporting Melatonin's Role as an Antioxidant," *J Pineal Res* 18(1) (1995): 1–11.

25. C. Mallo et al., "Effects of a Four-Day Nocturnal Melatonin Treatment on the 24 h Plasma Melatonin, Cortisol, and Prolactin Profiles in Humans," *Acta Endocrinologia* 119 (1995): 474–80.

Stress Managment

1. H. Selye, *The Stress of Life* (New York: McGraw Hill, 1978).

2. T.H. Holmes and R.H. Rahe, "The Social Readjustment Scale," *J Psychosomatic Res* 11 (1967): 213–8.

3. H. Benson, *The Relaxation Response* (New York: William Morrow, 1975).

4. T. Chou, "Wake Up and Smell the Coffee: Caffeine, Coffee, and the Medical Consequences," *West J Med* 157 (1992): 544–53.

5. M.G. Montiero et al., "Subjective Feelings of Anxiety in Young Men after Ethanol and Diazepam Infusions," *J Clin Psychiatry* 51 (1990): 12–6.

6. A. Winokur et al., "Insulin Resistance after Glucose Tolerance Testing in Patients with Major Depression," *Am J Psychiatry* 145 (1988): 325–30.

7. J.H. Wright et al., "Glucose Metabolism in Unipolar Depression," *Br J Psychiatry* 132 (1978): 386–93.

8. A.H. Rowe and A. Rowe, Jr., *Food Allergy: Its Manifestations and Control and the Elimination Diets: A*

Compendium (Springfield, IL: Charles C. Thomas, 1972).

9. N.R. Farnsworth et al., "Siberian Ginseng (*Eleutherococcus senticosus*): Current Status as an Adaptogen," *Economic Medicinal Plant Research* 1 (1985): 156–215.

10. H. Hikino, "Traditional Remedies and Modern Assessment: The Case of Ginseng," in R.O.B. Wijeskera, ed., *The Medicinal Plant Industry* (Boca Raton, FL: CRC Press, 1991), 149–66.

11. S. Shibata et al., "Chemistry and Pharmacology of Panax," *Econ Med Plant Research* 1 (1985): 217–84.

12. C. Hallstrom, S. Fulder, and M. Carruthers, "Effect of Ginseng on the Performance of Nurses on Night Duty," *Comp Med East & West* 6 (1982): 277–82.

13. S.K. Bhattacharya and S.K. Mitra, "Anxiolytic Activity of Panax Ginseng Roots: An Experimental Study," *J Ethnopharmacol* 34 (1991): 87–92.

Acne

1. P. Pochi, "Acne: Endocrinological Aspects," *Cutis* 30 (1982): 212–22.

2. F. Schiavone, R. Rietschel, D. Squotas, and R. Harris, "Elevated Free Testosterone Levels in Women with Acne," *Arch Dermatol* 119 (1983): 799–802.

3. C. Darley, J. Moore, G. Besser, et al., ìAndrogen Status in Women with Late Onset or Persistent Acne Vulgaris," *Clin Exp Dermatol* 9 (1984): 28–35.

4. S. Takayasu, H. Wakimoto, S. Itami, and S. Sano, "Activity of Testosterone 5-alpha-reductase in Various Tissues of Human Skin," *J Invest Dermatol* 74 (1980): 187–91.

5. G. Sansone and R. Reisner, "Differential Rates of Conversion of Testosterone to Dihydrotestosterone in Acne and Normal Human Skin: A Possible Pathogenic Factor in Acne," *J Invest Dermatol* 56 (1971): 366–72.

6. L. Juhlin and G. Michaelson, "Fibrin Microclot Formation in Patients with Acne," *Acta Derm Venerol* 63 (1983): 538–40.

7. S. Ayres and R. Mihan, "Acne Vulgaris: Therapy Directed at Patho-

physiological Defects," *Cutis* 28 (1981): 41–2.

8. A. Kappas, K. Anderson, A. Conney, et al., "Nutrition-Endocrine Interactions: Induction of Reciprocal Changes in the delta-5-alpha-reduction of Testosterone and the Cytochrome P-450-Dependent Oxidation of Estradiol by Dietary Macronutrients in Man," *Proc Natl Acad Sci USA* 80 (1983): 7646–9.

9. H. Semon and F. Herrmann, "Some Observations on the Sugar Metabolism in Acne Vulgaris, and Its Treatment by Insulin," *Br J Derm* 52 (1940): 123–8.

10. R. Grover and N. Arikan, "The Effect of Intralesional Insulin and Glucagon in Acne Vulgaris," *L Invest Derm* 40 (1963): 259–61.

11. K.M. Abdel, A. El Mofty, A. Ismail, and F. Bassili, "Glucose Tolerance in Blood and Skin of Patients with Acne Vulgaris," *Ind J Derm* 22 (1977): 139–49.

12. J. Cohen and A. Cohen, "Pustular Acne Staphyloderma and Its Treatment with Tolbutamide," *Can Med Assoc J* 80 (1959): 629–32.

13. M. McCarthy, "High Chromium Yeast for Acne?" *Med Hypoth* 14 (1984): 307–10.

14. A. Kugman, O. Mills, J. Leyden, et al., "Oral Vitamin A in Acne Vulgaris," *Int J Dermatol* 20 (1981): 278–85.

15. G. Michaelsson, A. Vahlquist, and L. Juhlin, "Serum Zinc and Retinol-Binding Protein in Acne," *Br J Dermatol* 96 (1977): 283–6.

16. G. Michaelson, L. Juhlin, and K. Ljunghall, "A Double-Blind Study of the Effect of Zinc and Oxytetracycline in Acne Vulgaris," *Br J Dermatol* 97 (1977): 561–5.

17. V. Weimar, S. Puhl, W. Smith, and J. Broeke, "Zinc Sulphate in Acne Vulgaris," *Arch Dermatol* 114 (1978): 1776–8.

18. G. Michaelson, L. Juhlin, and A. Vahlquist, "Effects of Oral Zinc and Vitamin A on Acne," *Arch Dermatol* 113 (1977): 31–6.

19. B. Dreno et al., "Low Doses of Zinc Gluconate for Inflammatory Acne," *Acta Derm Venerol* 69 (1989): 541–3.

20. G. Michaelson and L. Edqvist, "Erythrocyte Glutathione Peroxidase Activity in Acne Vulgaris and the Effect

of Selenium and Vitamin E Treatment," *Acta Derm Venerol* 64 (1984): 9–14.

21. B. Snider and D. Dieteman, "Pyridoxine Therapy for Premenstrual Acne Flare," *Arch Dermatol* 110 (1974): 103–1.

22. E. Symes, D. Bender, J. Bowen, and W. Coulson, "Increased Target Tissue Uptake of, and Sensitivity to, Testosterone in the Vitamin-B6-Deficient Rat," *J Steroid Biochem* 20 (1984): 1089–93.

23. L.H. Leung, "Pantothenic Acid Deficiency as the Pathogenesis of Acne Vulgaris," *Med Hypoth* 44 (1995): 490–2.

24. B. Barnes, "Thyroid Therapy in Dermatology," *Cutis* 8 (1971): 581–3.

25. C.F. Carson and T.V. Riley, "The Antimicrobial Activity of Tea Tree Oil," *Med J Australia* 160 (1994): 236.

26. I.B. Bassett, D.L. Pannowitz, and R.S.C. Barnetson, "A Comparative Study of Tea-Tree Oil versus Benzoyl Peroxide in the Treatment of Acne," *Med J Australia* 153 (1990): 455–8.

27. M. Nazzaro-Porro, "Azelaic Acid," *J Am Acad Dermatol* 17 (1987): 1033–41.

AIDS

1. H. Hollander and M.H. Katz, "HIV Infection," in L.M. Tierney, S.J. McPhee, and M.A. Papdakis, eds. *Current Medical Diagnosis and Treatment*, 36th ed. (Stamford, CT: Appleton & Lange, 1997), 1178–1202.

2. P. Duesberg, "Infectious AIDS—Stretching the Germ Theory Beyond Its Limits," *Int Arch Allergy Immunol* 103 (1994): 118–127.

3. J. Lindenmann, "Duesberg on AIDS—Stretching Our Benevolence Beyond Its Limits,". *Int Arch Allergy Immunol* 103 (1994): 128–30.

4. J.H. Skurnick et al., "Micronutrient Profiles in HIV-1-Infected Heterosexual Adults," *J AIDS Human Retrovirol* 12 (1996): 75–83.

5. K.M. Casey, "Malnutrition Associated with HIV/AIDS, Part One: Definition and Scope, Epidemiology, and Pathophysiology," *J Assoc Nurses AIDS Care* 8 (1997): 24–32.

6. G. Babameto and D.P. Kotler, "Malnutrition in HIV Infection," *Gastroenterol Clin North Am* 26 (1997): 393–415.

7. B. Liang et al., "Vitamins and Immunomodulation in AIDS," *Nutr* 12 (1996): 1–7.

8. G.W. Pace and C.D. Leaf, "The Role of Oxidative Stress in HIV Disease," *Free Radical Biology Med* 19 (1995): 523–8.

9. A. Favier et al., "Antioxidant Status and Lipid Peroxidation in Patients Infected with HIV," *Chem Biol Interact* 91(2–3) (1994): 165–80.

10. F.J. Staal et al., "Glutathione Deficiency and Human Immunodeficiency Virus Infection," *Lancet* 339 (1992): 909–12.

11. A. Witschi et al., "Supplementation of N-Acetylcysteine Fails to Increase Glutathione in Lymphocytes and Plasma of Patients with AIDS," *AIDS Res Hum Retroviruses* 11 (1995): 141–3.

12. Y. Wang and R.R. Watson, "Potential Therapeutics of Vitamin E (Tocopherol) in AIDS and HIV," *Drugs* 48 (1994): 327–38.

13. A.M. Tang et al., "Association between Serum Vitamin A and E Levels and HIV-1 Disease Progression," *AIDS* 11 (1997): 613–20.

14. S. Harakeh and R.J. Jariwalla, "Ascorbate Effect on Cytokine Stimulation of HIV Production," *Nutrition* 11(Suppl.5) (1995): 684–7.

15. E. Eylar et al., "Sustained Levels of Ascorbic Acid Are Toxic and Immunosuppressive for Human T Cells," *P R Health Sci J* 15 (1996): 309–10.

16. C.J. Johnston, C.G. Meyer, and J.C. Srilakshmi, "Vitamin C Elevates Red Blood Cell Glutathione in Healthy Adults," *Am J Clin Nutr* 58 (1993): 103–5.

17. R.D. Semba et al., "Increased Mortality Associated with Vitamin A Deficiency during Human Immunodeficiency Virus Type 1 Infection," *Arch Intern Med* 153 (1993): 2149–54.

18. R. Ullrich et al., "Serum Carotene Deficiency in HIV-Infected Patients," *AIDS* 8 (1994): 661–5.

19. J.A. Omene et al., "Serum Beta-Carotene Deficiency in HIV-Infected Children," *J Natl Med Assoc* 88 (1996): 789–93.

20. G.O. Coodley et al., "Beta-Carotene in HIV Infection," *J Acquir Immune Defic Syndr* 6 (1993): 272–6.

21. A. Bianchi-Santamaria et al., "Short Communication: Possible Activity of Beta-Carotene in Patients with the AIDS Related Complex: A Pilot Study," *Med Oncol Tumor Pharmacother* 9 (1992): 151–3.

22. H.S. Garewal et al., "A Preliminary Trial of Beta-Carotene in Subjects Infected with the Human Immunodeficiency Virus," *J Nutr* 122 (1992): 728–32.

23. D.A. Fryburg et al., "The Effect of Supplemental Beta-Carotene on Immunologic Indices in Patients with AIDS: A Pilot Study," *Yale J Biol Med* 68 (1995): 19–23.

24. G.O. Coodley et al., "Beta-Carotene in HIV Infection: An Extended Evaluation," *AIDS* 10 (1996): 967–73.

25. M.C. Delmas-Beauvieux et al., "The Enzymatic Antioxidant System in Blood and Glutathione Status in Human Immunodeficiency Virus (HIV)-Infected Patients: Effects of Supplementation with Selenium or Beta-Carotene," *Am J Clin Nutr* 64 (1996): 101–7.

26. M. Marmor et al., "Low Serum Thiol Levels Predict Shorter Times-to-Death among HIV-Infected Injecting Drug Users," *AIDS* 11 (1997): 1389–93.

27. C. Allavena et al., "Relationship of Trace Element, Immunological Markers, and HIV-1 Infection Progression," *Biol Trace Elem Res* 47 (1995): 133–8.

28. V.E. Kagan et al., "Dihydrolipoic Acid—A Universal Antioxidant Both in the Membrane and in the Aqueous Phase," *Biochemical Pharmacol* 44 (1992): 1637–49.

29. A. Baur et al., "Alpha-Lipoic Acid Is an Effective Inhibitor of Human Immuno-Deficiency Virus (HIV-1) Replication," *Klin Wochenschr* 69 (1991): 722–4.

30. Y.J. Suzuki, B.B. Aggarwal, and L. Packer, "Alpha-Lipoic Acid Is a Potent Inhibitor of NF-kB Activation in Human T Cells," *Biochem Biophys Res Commun* 189 (1992): 1709–15.

31. J. Fuchs et al., "Studies on Lipoate Effects on Blood Redox State in Human Immunodeficiency Virus Infected Patients," *Arzneim Forsch* 43 (1993): 1359–62.

32. E. Mocchegiani et al., "Benefit of Oral Zinc Supplementation As an Adjunct to Zidovudine (AZT) Therapy against Opportunistic Inffections in AIDS," *Int J Immunopharmacol* 17 (1995): 719–27.

33. M.K. Bum et al., "Association of Vitamin B6 Status with Parameters of Immune Function in Early HIV-1 Infection," *J AIDS* 4 (1991): 122–32.

34. K.R. Robertson et al., "Vitamin B12 Deficiency and Nervous System Disease in HIV Infection," *Arch Neurol* 50 (1993): 807–11.

35. O. Palteil et al., "Clinical Correlates of Subnormal Vitamin B12 Levels in Patients Infected with the Human Immunodeficiency Virus," *Am J Hematol* 49 (1995): 318–22.

36. S.A.J. Rule, "Serum Vitamin B12 and Transcobalamin Levels in Early HIV Disease," *Am J Hematol* 47 (1994): 167–71.

37. A.M. Tang et al., "Low Serum Vitamin B12 Concentrations Are Associated with Faster Human Immunodeficiency Virus Type 1 (HIV-1) Disease Progression," *J Nutr* 127 (1997): 345–51.

38. M.K. Baum et al., "Micronutrients and HIV-1 Disease Progression," *AIDS* 9 (1995): 1051–6.

39. J.B. Weinberg et al., "Inhibition of Productive Human Immunodeficiency Virus-1 Infection by Cobalamins," *Blood* 86 (1995): 1281–7.

40. C. De Simone et al., "Carnitine Depletion in Peripheral Blood Mononuclear Cells from Patients with AIDS: Effect of Oral L-Carnitine," *AIDS* 8 (1994): 655–60.

41. M.C. Semino-Mora et al., "Effect of L-Carnitine on the Zidovidine-Induced Destruction of Human Myotubes," *Lab Invest* 71 (1994): 102–12.

42. C. De Simone et al., "High Dose L-Carnitine Improves Immunologic and Metabolic Parameters in AIDS Patients," *Immunopharmacol Immunotoxicol* 15 (1993): 1–12.

43. G. Valesini et al., "A Calf Thymus Lysate Improves Clinical Symptoms and T-Cell Defects in the Early Stages of HIV Infection: Second Report," *Eur. J Cancer Clin Oncol* 23 (1987): 1915–9.

44. C.J. Li et al., "Three Inhibitors of Human Type 1 Immunodeficiency Virus Long Terminal Repeat

Directed Gene Expression and Virus Replication," *Proc Natl Acad Sci* 90 (1993): 1839–41.

45. A. Mazumder et al., "Inhibition of Human Immunodeficiency Virus Type-1 Integrase by Curcumin," *Biochemical Pharmacol* 49 (1995): 1165–70.

46. M.C. Jiang, J.K. Lin, S.S. Chen, "Inhibition of HIV-1 Tat-Mediated Transactivation by Quinacrine and Chloroquine," *Biochem Biophys Res Commun* 226 (1995): 1–7.

47. M.M. Chan, "Inhibition of Tumor Necrosis Factor by Curcumin, a Phytochemical," *Biochem Pharmacol* 49(11) (26 May 1995): 1551–6.

48. S. Singh, B.B. Aggarwal, "Activation of Transcription Factor NF-Kappa B Is Suppressed by Curcumin (Diferulolymethane)," *J Biol Chem* 270(42) (20 Oct. 1995): 24995–5000.

49. S. Rao and M.N.A. Rao, "Curcuminoids As Potent Inhibitors of Lipid Peroxidation," *J Pharm Pharmacol* 46 (1994): 1013–6.

50. R. Copeland et al., "Curcumin Therapy in HIV-Infected Patients," *Int Conf AIDS* 10 (1994): 216 (abstract no. PB0876).

51. D. Noever, "Naturally Occurring Protease Inhibitors Potent against the Human," *Biochemical Biophys Res Commun* 227 (1996): 125–30

52. N. Ikegami et al., "Prophylactic Effect of Long-Term Oral Administration of Glycyrrhizin on AIDS Development of Asymptomatic Patients," *Int Conf AIDS* 9(1) (1993): 234 (abstract no. PO-A25-0596).

53. N. Ikegami et al., "Clinical Evaluation of Glycyrrhizin on HIV-Infected Asymptomatic Hemophiliac Patients in Japan," *Fifth International Conference on AIDS* (June 1989): Abstract W.B.P. 298; cited in *AIDS Treatment News* 103 (May 18, 1990).

54. T. Hattori et al., "Preliminary Evidence for Inhibitory Effect of Glycyrrhizin on HIV Replication in Patients with AIDS," *Antiviral Res* 11 (1989): 255–61.

55. K. Mori et al., "Effects of Glycyrrhizin (SNMC: Stronger Neo-Minophagen C) in Hemophilia Patients with HIV-1 Infection," *Tohoku J Exp Med* 162 (1990): 183–93.

Alcoholism

1. S.E. Hyman and N.H. Casseman, "Alcoholism," in E. Rubenstein and D. Federman, eds., *Scientific American Textbook of Medicine* (New York: Scientific American Inc, 1997), 13: III:1–14.

2. R. Cruz-Coke, "Genetics and Alcoholism," *Neurobeh Toxicol Teratol* 5 (1983): 179–80.

3. D.B. Goldstein, *Pharmacology of Ethanol* (New York: Oxford University Press, 1983).

4. K.F. Tipton, G.T.M. Heneman, and J.M. McCrodden, "Metabolic and Nutritional Aspects of Alcohol," *Biochem Soc Trans* 11 (1983): 59–61.

5. C.S. Lieber, "Alcohol, Liver, and Nutrition," *J Am Coll Nutr* 10 (1991): 602–32.

6. I. Das, R.E. Burch, and H.K.J. Hahn, "Effects of Zinc Deficiency on Ethanol Metabolism and Alcohol and Aldehyde Dehydrogenase Activities," *J Lab Clin Med* 104 (1984): 610–7.

7. C.T. Wu, J.N. Lee, W.W. Shen, and S.L. Lee, "Serum Zinc, Copper, and Ceruloplasmin Levels in Male Alcoholics," *Biol Psy* 19 (1982): 1333–8.

8. J. Scholmerich, E. Lohle, E. Kottgen, and W. Gerok, "Zinc and Vitamin A Deficiency in Liver Cirrhosis," *Hepato-Gastroenterol* 30 (1983): 119–25.

9. A.A. Yunice and R.D. Lindeman, "Effect of Ascorbic Acid and Zinc Sulphate on Ethanol Toxicity and Metabolism," *Proc Soc Exp Biol Med* 154 (1977): 146–50.

10. F.S. Messiha, "Vitamin A, Gender and Ethanol Interactions," *Neuorbehav Toxicol Teratol* 5 (1983): 233–6.

11. L.P. Morin and N.G. Forger, "Endocrine Control of Ethanol Intake by Rats or Hamsters: Relative Contributions of the Ovaries, Adrenals and Steroids," *Pharmac Biochem Behav* 17 (1982): 529–37.

12. E. Lecomte et al., "Effect of Alcohol Consumption of Blood Antioxidant Nutrients and Oxidative Stress Indicators," *Am J Clin Nutr* 60 (1994): 255–61.

13. T. Suematsu, T. Matsumura, N. Sato et al., "Lipid Peroxidation in Alcoholic Liver Disease in Humans," *Al-*

coholism Clin Exp Res 5 (1981): 427–30.

14. N.R. DiLuzio, "A Mechanism of the Acute Ethanol-Induced Fatty Liver and the Modification of Liver Injury by Antioxidants," *Lab Invest* 15 (1966): 50–61.

15. R.T. Stanko, H. Mendelow, H. Shinozuka, and S.A. Adibi, "Prevention of Alcohol-Induced Fatty Liver by Natural Metabolites and Riboflavin," *J Lab Clin Med* 91 (1978): 228–35.

16. W.S. Hartroft, E.A. Porta, and M. Suzuki, "Effects of Choline Chloride on Hepatic Lipids after Acute Ethanol Intoxication," *Q J Stuc Alcohol* 25 (1964): 427–37.

17. D.S. Sachan, T.H. Rhew, and R.A. Ruark, "Ameliorating Effects of Carnitine and Its Precursors on Alcohol-Induced Fatty Liver," *Am J Clin Nutr* 39 (1984): 738–44.

18. E.A. Hosein and B. Bexton, "Protective Action of Carnitine on Liver Lipid Metabolism after Ethanol Administration to Rats," *Biochem Pharm* 24 (1975): 1859–63.

19. D.A. Sachan and T.H. Rhew, "Lipotropic Effect of Carnitine on Alcohol-Induced Hepatic Stenosis," *Nutr Rep Int* 27 (1983): 1221–6.

20. S.K. Majumdar, G.K. Shaw, and A.D. Thomson, "Changes in Plasma Amino Acid Patterns in Chronic Alcoholic Patients during Ethanol Withdrawal Syndrome: Their Clinical Applications," *Med Hypoth* 12 (1983): 239–51.

21. L. Branchey, M. Branchey, S. Shaw, and C.S. Lieber, "Relationship between Changes in Plasma Amino Acids and Depression in Alcoholic Patients," *Am J Psych* 141 (1984): 1212–5.

22. H.M. Rosen, N. Yoshimura, J.M. Hodgman, and J.E. Fischer, "Plasma Amino Acid Patterns in Hepatic Encephalopathy of Differing Etiology," *Gastro* 72 (1977): 483–7.

23. J.E. Fischer, H.M. Rosen, A.M. Ebeid et al., "The Effect of Normalization of Plasma Amino Acids on Hepatic Encephalopathy," *Surgery* 80 (1976): 77–91.

24. M. Baines, "Detection and Incidence of B and C Vitamin Deficiency in Alcohol-Related Illness," *Ann Clin Biochem* 15 (1978): 307–12.

25. A.A. Yunice, J.M. Hsu, A. Fahmy, and S. Henry, "Ethanol-Ascorbate Interrelationship in Acute and Chronic Alcoholism in the Guinea Pig," *Proc Soc Exp Biol Med* 177 (1984): 262–71.

26. S.M. Zimatkin and Zimatkina, "Thiamine Deficiency As Predisposition to, and Consequence of, Increased Alcohol Consumption," *Alcohol Alcoholism* 31 (1996): 421–7.

27. L. Lumeng, "The Role of Acetaldehyde in Mediating the Deleterious Effect of Ethanol on Pyridoxal 5'-Phosphate Metabolism," *J Clin Invest* 62 (1978): 286–93.

28. K.E. McMartin et al., "Cumulative Excess Urinary Excretion of Folate in Rats after Repeated Ethanol Treatment," *J Nutr* 116 (1986): 1316–25.

29. D.M. Jermain, M.L. Crismon, and R.B. Nisbet "Controversies over the Use of Magnesium Sulfate in Delirium Tremens," *Ann Pharmacother* 26 (1992): 650–2.

30. L. Abbott, J. Nadler, and R.K. Rude, "Magnesium Deficiency in Alcoholism," *Alcoholism Clin Exp Res* 18 (1994): 1076–82.

31. D.F. Horrobin, "A Biochemical Basis for Alcoholism and Alcohol-Induced Damage Including the Fetal Alcohol Syndrome and Cirrhosis: Interference with Essential Fatty Acid and Prostaglandin Metabolism," *Med Hypothesis* 6 (1980): 929–42; 12 (1983): 217–22.

32. L.L. Rogers and R.B. Pelton, "Glutamine in the Treatment of Alcoholism," *J Biol Chem* 214 (1955): 503–6.

33. L.L. Rogers and R.B. Pelton, "Glutamine in the Treatment of Alcoholism," *Q J Studies in Alcoholism* 18 (1957): 581–7.

34. J.M. Ravel, B. Felsing, E. Lansford et al., "Reversal of Alcohol Toxicity by Glutamine," *J Biol Chem* 214 (1955): 497–502.

35. L.L. Rogers, R.B. Pelton, and R.J. Williams, "Voluntary Alcohol Consumption by Rats Following Administration of Glutamine," *J Biol Chem* 214 (1955): 503–7.

36. J.C. Bode, C. Bode, R. Heidelbach, et al., "Jejunal Microflora in Patients with Chronic Alcohol Abuse," *Hepato-Gastro* 31 (1984): 30–4.

37. B.S. Worthington, L. Meserole, and J.A. Syrotuck, "Effect of Daily Ethanol Ingestion on Intestinal Permeability to Macromolecules," *Dig Dis* 23 (1978): 23–32.

38. D. Sinyor, T. Brown, L. Rostant, and P. Seraganian, "The Role of a Physical Fitness Program in the Treatment of Alcoholism," *J Stud Alcohol* 43 (1982): 380–6.

39. P. Ferenci et al., "Randomized Controlled Trial of Silymarin Treatment in Patients with Cirrhosis of the Liver," *J Hepatology* 9 (1989): 105–13.

40. G. Deak et al., "Immunomodulator Effect of Silymarin Therapy in Chronic Alcoholic Liver Diseases," *Orv Hetil* 131 (1990): 1291–2; 1295–6.

Alzheimer's Disease

1. A.R. Dmasio, "Alzheimer's Disease and Related Dementias," in C.J. Bennett and F. Plum, eds., *Cecil Textbook of Medicine*, 20th ed (Philadelphia: W.B. Saunders, 1996), 1992–6.

2. W.R. Markesbery, "Oxidative Stress Hypothesis in Alzheimer's Disease," *Free Radical Biol Med* 23 (1997): 134–47.

3. R.W. Shin, "Interaction of Aluminum with Paired Helical Filament Tau Is Involved in Neurofibrillary Pathology of Alzheimer's Disease," *Gerontol* 43 (Suppl.1) (1997): 16–23.

4. M.D. Zapatero et al., "Serum Aluminum Levels in Alzheimer's Disease and Other Senile Dementias," *Biol Trace Element Res* 47 (1995): 235–40.

5. L. Frolich and P. Riederer, "Free Radical Mechanisms in Dementia of the Alzheimer's Type and the Potential for Antioxidative Treatment," *Drug Res* 45 (1995): 443–46.

6. J. Walton et al., "Uptake of Trace Amounts of Aluminum into the Brain from Drinking Water," *Neurotoxicology* 16 (1995): 187–90.

7. C.A. Garcia, M.J. Reding, and J.P. Blass, "Overdiagnosis of Dementia," *J Am Ger Soc* 29 (1981): 407–10.

8. J.S. Smith and L.G. Kiloh, "The Investigation of Dementia: Results in 200 Consecutive Admissions," *Lancet* 1 (1981): 824–7.

9. H.J. Weinreb, "Fingerprint Patterns in Alzheimer's Disease," *Arch Neurol* 42 (1985): 50–4.

10. B.N. Ames, M.K. Shigenaga, and T.M. Hagen, "Oxidants, Antioxidants, and the Degenerative Diseases of Aging," *Proc Natl Acad Sci* 90 (1993): 7915–22.

11. M.A. Smith et al., "Oxidative Damage in Alzheimer's Disease," *Nature* 382 (1996): 120–1.

12. J.W. Jama et al., "Dietary Antioxidants and Cognitive Function in a Population-Based Sample of Older Persons," *Am J Epidem* 144 (1996): 275–80.

13. D.A. Evans and M.C. Morris, "Is a Randomized Trial of Antioxidants in the Primary Prevention of Alzheimer Disease Warranted?" *Alzheimer Dis Assoc Disorders* 10 (Suppl.1) (1996): 45–9.

14. S. Fahn, "A Pilot Trial of High-Dose Alpha-Tocopherol and Ascorbate in Early Parkinson's Disease," *Annals of Neurology* 32 (1992): S128–32.

15. L.H. Kuller, "Hormone Replacement Therapy and Its Potential Relationship to Dementia," *JAGS* 44 (1996): 878–80.

16. A. Paganini-Hill, "Oestrogen Replacement Therapy and Alzheimer's Disease," *Br J Obstet Gyn* 103 (Suppl.13) (1996): 80–6.

17. H. Honjo et al., "Senile Dementia-Alzheimer's Type and Estrogen," *Horm Metab Res* 27 (1995): 204–7.

18. N.R. Smalheiser and D.R. Swansom, "Linking Estrogen to Alzheimer's Disease: An Informatics Approach," *Neurology* 47 (1996): 809–10.

19. K.A. Matthews et al., "Prior to Use of Estrogen Replacement Therapy, Are Users Healthier than Nonusers?" *Am J Epidemiol* 143 (1996): 971–8.

20. C.R. Nolan et al., "Aluminum and Lead Absorption from Dietary Sources in Women Ingesting Calcium Citrate," *Southern Med J* 87 (1994): 894–98.

21. J.L. Glick, "Dementias: The Role of Magnesium Deficiency and Hypothesis Concerning the Pathogenesis of Alzheimer's Disease," *Med Hypoth* 31 (1990): 211–25.

22. D.M. Tucer et al., "Nutrition Status and Brain Function in Aging," *Am J Clin Nutr* 52 (1990): 93–102.

23. M.F. Chen et al., "Plasma and Erythrocyte Thiamin Concentration in Geriatric Outpatients," *J Am Coll Nutr* 15 (1996): 231–6.

24. K.J. Meador et al., "Evidence for a Central Cholinergic Effect of High-Dose Thiamine," *Ann Neurol* 34 (1993): 724–6.

25. K. Meador, "Preliminary Findings of High-Dose Thiamine in Dementia of Alzheimer's Type," *J Geriatr Psychiatry Neurol* 6 (1993): 222–9.

26. D. Benton, J. Fordy, and J. Haller, "The Impact of Long-Term Vitamin Supplementation on Cognitive Functioning," *Psychopharmacol* 117 (1995): 298–305.

27. H. Van Goor et al., "Review: Cobalamin Deficiency and Mental Impairment in Elderly People," *Age Ageing* 24 (1995): 536–42.

28. M.I. Shevell and D.S. Rosenblatt, "The Neurology of Cobalamin," *Can J Neurol Sci* 19 (1992): 472–86.

29. Y. Yao et al., "Decline of Serum Cobalamin Levels with Increasing Age Among Geriatric Outpatients," *Arch Fam Med* 3 (1994): 918–22.

30. D.G. Savage et al., "Sensitivity of Serum Methylmalonic Acid and Total Homocysteine Determinations for Diagnosing Cobalamin Deficiency," *Am J Med* 96 (1994): 239–46.

31. E.J. Norman and J.A. Morrison, "Screening Elderly Populations for Cobalamin (Vitamin B12) Deficiency Using the Urinary Methylmalonic Acid Assay by Gas Chromatography Mass Spectrophotometry," *Am J Med* 94 (1993): 589–4.

32. K. Nilsson et al., "Plasma Homocysteine in Relationship to Serum Cobalamin and Blood Folate in a Psychogeriatric Population," *Eur J Clin Invest* 24 (1994): 600–6.

33. E.B. Healton et al., "Neurologic Aspects of Cobalamin Deficiency," *Medicine* 70 (1991): 229–45.

34. D.C. Martin et al., "Time Dependency of Cognitive Recovery with Cobalamin Replacement: A Report of a Pilot Study," *J Am Geriatric Soc* 40 (1992): 168–72.

35. A.J. Levitt and H. Karlinsky, "Folate, Vitamin B12, and Cognitive Impairment in Patients with Alzheimer's Disease," *Acta Psychiatr Scand* 86 (1992): 301–5.

36. A.J. Levitt et al., "Folate, Vitamin B12, and Cognitive Impairment in Patients with Alzheimer's Disease," *Acta Psychiatr Scand* 86 (1992): 301–5.

37. M.O. Kristensen et al., "Serum Cobalamin and Methylmalonic Acid in Alzheimer Dementia," *Acta Neurol Scand* 87 (1993): 475–81.

38. J. Constantinidis, "The Hypothesis of Zinc Deficiency in the Pathogenesis of Neurofibrillary Tangles," *Med Hypoth* 35 (1991): 319–23.

39. F.M. Burnet, "A Possible Role of Zinc in the Pathology of Dementia," *Lancet* 1 (1981): 186–8.

40. J. Constantinidis, "Treatment of Alzheimer's Disease by Zinc Compounds," *Drug Develop Res* 27 (1992): 1–14.

41. G. Rosenberg and K.L. Davis, "The Use of Cholinergic Precursors in Neuropsychiatric Diseases," *Am J Clin Nutr* 36 (1982): 709–20.

42. R. Levy, A. Little, P. Chuaqui, and M. Reith, "Early Results from Double-Blind, Placebo-Controlled Trial of High-Dose Phosphatydylcholine in Alzheimer's Disease," *Lancet* 1 (1982): 474–6.

43. N. Sitaram, B. Weingartner, E.D. Gaine, and J.C. Cillin, "Choline: Selective Enhancement of Serial Learning and Encoding of Low Imagery Words in Man," *Life Sci* 22 (1978): 1555–60.

44. T. Cenacchi et al., "Cognitive Decline in the Elderly: A Double-Blind, Placebo-Controlled Multicenter Study on Efficacy of Phosphatidylserine Administration," *Aging* 5 (1993): 123–33.

45. R.R. Engel et al., "Double-Blind Cross-Over Study of Phosphatidylserine vs. Placebo in Patients with Early Dementia of the Alzheimer Type," *Eur Neuropsychopharmacol* 2 (1992): 149–55.

46. T. Crook et al., "Effects of Phosphatidylserine in Alzheimer's Disease," *Psychopharmacol Bull* 28 (1992): 61–6.

47. T.H. Crook et al., "Effects of Phosphatidylserine in Age-Associated Memory Impairment," *Neurology* 41 (1991): 644–9.

48. E.W. Funfgeld et al., "Double-Blind Study with Phosphatidylserine (PS) in Parkinsonian Patients with Senile Dementia of Alzheimer's Type (SDAT)," *Prog Clin Biol Res* 317 (1989): 1235–46.

49. L. Amaducci et al., "Phosphatidylserine in the Treatment of Alzheimer's Disease: Results of a Multicenter Study," *Psychopharmacol Bull* 24 (1988): 1030–4.

50. D. Nerozzi et al., "Phosphatidylserine in Age-Related Disturbance of Memory," *Clin Terapeutica* 120 (1987): 399–404.

51. G. Palmieri et al., "Double-Blind Controlled Trial of Phosphatidylserine in Patients with Senile Mental Deterioration," *Clin Trials J* 24 (1987): 73–83.

52. C. Villardita et al., "Multicentre Clinical Trial of Brain Phosphatidylserine in Elderly Patients with Intellectual Deterioration," *Clin Trials J* 24 (1987): 84–93.

53. P.J. Delwaide et al., "Effect of Phosphatidylserine in Demented Patients," *Acta Neurol Scand* 73 (1986): 136–40.

54. B. Bowman, "Acetyl-Carnitine and Alzheimer's Disease," *Nutrition Reviews* 50 (1992): 142–4.

55. A. Carta et al., "Acetyl-L-Carnitine and Alzheimer's Disease: Pharmacological Considerations beyond the Cholinergic Sphere," *Ann NY Acad Sci* 695 (1993): 324–6.

56. M. Calvani et al., "Action of acetyl-L-carnitine in Neurodegeneration and Alzheimer's Disease," *Ann NY Acad Sci* 663 (1993): 483–6.

57. J.W. Pettegrew et al., "Clinical and Neurochemical Effects of acetyl-L-carnitine in Alzheimer's Disease," *Neurobiol Aging* 16 (1995): 1–4.

58. M. Sano et al., "Double-Blind Parallel Design Pilot Study of Acetyl Levocarnitine in Patients with Alzheimer's Disease," *Arch Neurol* 49 (1992): 1137–41.

59. A. Spagnoli et al., "Long-Term acetyl-L-carnitine Treatment in Alzheimer's Disease," *Neurology* 41 (1991): 1726–32.

60. G.P. Vecchi et al., "Acetyl-L-carnitine Treatment of Mental Impairment in the Elderly: Evidence from a Multicenter Study," *Arch Gerontol Geriatr* 2 (Suppl.) (1991): 159–68.

61. G. Salvioli and M. Neri, "L-acetyl-carnitine Treatment of Mental De-

cline in the Elderly," *Drugs Exp Clin Res* 20 (1994): 169–76.

62. C. Cipolli and G. Chiari, "Effects of L-acetylcarnitine on Mental Deterioration in the Aged: Initial Results," *Clin Ter* 132 (1990): 479–510.

63. M. Kalimi and W. Regelson, *The Biological Role of Dehydroepiandrosterone* (New York: de Gruyter, 1990).

64. S.S. Yen, A.J. Morales, and O. Khorram, "Replacement of DHEA in Aging Men and Women: Potential Remedial Effects," *Ann NY Acad Sci* 774 (1995): 128–42.

65. A.J. Morales et al., "Effects of Replacement Dose of Dehydroepiandrosterone in Men and Women of Advancing Age," *J Clin Endocrinol Metab* 78(6) (1994): 1360–7.

66. F.V. DeFeudis, ed., *Ginkgo biloba Extract (EGb 761): Pharmacological Activities and Clinical Applications* (Paris: Elsevier, 1991).

67. E.W. Funfgeld, ed., *Rokan (Ginkgo biloba): Recent Results in Pharmacology and Clinic* (New York: Springer-Verlag, 1988).

68. J. Kleijnen and P. Knipschild, "Ginkgo biloba," *Lancet* 340 (1992): 1136–9.

69. B. Hofferberth, "The Efficacy of EGb 761 in Patients with Senile Dementia of the Alzheimer Type, A Double-Blind, Placebo-Controlled Study on Different Levels of Investigation," *Human Psychopharmacol* 9 (1994): 215–22.

70. S. Kanowski et al., "Proof of the Efficacy of the Ginkgo biloba Special Extract Egb 761 in Outpatients Suffering from Mild to Moderate Primary Degenerative Dementia of the Alzheimer Type of Multi-Infarct Dementia," *Phytomedicine* 4 (1997): 3–13.

71. P.L. Le Bars, et al., "A Placebo-Controlled, Double-Blind, Randomized Trial of an Extract of Ginkgo biloba for Dementia," *JAMA* 278 (1997): 1327–32.

Anemia

1. V.F. Fairbanks and E. Beutler, "Iron," in M.E. Shils and V.R. Young, eds., *Modern Nutrition in Health and Disease*, 7th ed. (Phila-

delphia, PA: Lea and Febiger, 1988), 193–226.

2. J.E. Morley, "Nutritional Status of the Elderly," *Am J Med* 81 (1986): 679–95.

3. A.M. Jacobs and G.M. Owen, "The Effect of Age on Iron Absorption," *J Gerontol* 24 (1969): 95–6.

4. W. Bezwoda et al., "The Importance of Gastric Hydrochloric Acid in the Absorption of Nonheme Iron," *J Lab Clin Med* 92 (1978): 108–16.

5. J.D. Cook and S.R. Lynch, "The Liabilities of Iron Deficiency," *Blood* 68 (1986): 803–9.

6. F.E. Viteri and B. Torun, "Anaemia and Physical Work Capacity," *Clin Haematol* 3 (1974): 609–26.

7. S.S. Basta et al., "Iron Deficiency Anemia and the Productivity of Adult Males in Indonesia," *Am J Clin Nutr* 32 (1979): 6–25.

8. G.W. Gardner et al., "Physical Work Capacity and Metabolic Stress in Subjects with Iron Deficiency Anemia," *Am J Clin Nutr* 30 (1977): 910–7.

9. M.M. Werler, S. Shapiro, and A.A. Mitchell, "Periconceptional Folic Acid Exposure and Risk of Occurrent Neural Tube Defects," *JAMA* 269 (1993): 1257–61.

10. C.S. Tsao and K. Myashita, "Influence of Cobalamin on the Survival of Mice Bearing Ascites Tumor," *Pathobiology* 61 (1993): 104–8.

11. F.A. Lederly, "Oral Cobalamin for Pernicious Anemia: Medicine's Best Kept Secret," *JAMA* 265 (1991): 94–5.

13. A. Doscherholmen et al., "A Dual Mechanism of Vitamin B12 Plasma Absorption," *J Clin Invest* 36 (1957): 1551–7.

14. E.H. Reisner et al., "Oral Treatment of Pernicious Anemia with Vitamin B12 Without Intrinsic Factor," *N Eng J Med* 253 (1955): 502–6.

15. P.A. McIntyre et al., "Treatment of Pernicious Anemia with Orally Administered Cyanocobalamin (Vitamin B12)," *Arch Intern Med* 106 (1960): 280–92.

16. S.O. Waife et al., "Oral Vitamin B12 without Intrinsic Factor in the Treatment of Pernicious Anemia," *Ann Intern Med* 58 (1963): 810–7.

17. H. Berlin, R. Berlin, and G. Brante, "Oral Treatment of Pernicious Anemia with High Doses of Vitamin B12

without Intrinsic Factor," *Acta Med Scand* 184 (1968): 247–8.

18. R. Berlin et al., "Vitamin B12 Body Stores during Oral and Parenteral Treatment of Pernicious Anemia," *Acta Med Scand* 204 (1978): 81–4.

19. F.H. Bethell et al., "Present Status of Treatment of Pernicious Anemia: Ninth Announcement of USP Anti-Anemia Preparations Advisory Board," *JAMA* 171 (1959): 2092–4.

20. L.B. Bailey, *Folate in Health and Disease* (New York: Marcel Dekker, 1995).

Angina

1. S. Bansal, S.H. Toh, and K.A. LaBresh, "Chest Pain as a Presentation of Reactive Hypoglycemia," *CHEST* 84 (1983): 641–2.

2. T.D. Graboys et al., "Results of a Second-Opinion Program for Coronary Artery Bypass Surgery," *JAMA* 268 (1992): 2537–40; T.D. Graboys et al., "Results of a Second-Opinion Program for Coronary Artery Bypass Surgery," *JAMA* 258 (1987): 1611–4.

3. E.L. Alderman et al., "Ten-Year Follow-Up of Survival and Myocardial Infarction in the Randomized Coronary Artery Surgery Study (CASS)," *Circulation* 82 (1990): 1629–46.

4. CASS Principle Investigators and Their Associates, "Myocardial Infarction and Mortality in the Coronary Artery Surgery Study (CASS) Randomized Trial," *New Engl J Med* 310 (1984): 750–8.

5. CASS Principle Investigators and Their Associates, "Coronary Artery Surgery (CASS): A Randomized Trial of Coronary Artery Bypass Surgery," *Circulation* 68 (1983): 939–50.

6. W. Hueb, "Two- to Eight-Year Survival Rates in Patients Who Refused Coronary Artery Bypass Grafting," *Am J Cardiol* 63 (1989): 155–9.

7. C.W. White et al., "Does Visual Interpretation of the Coronary Angiogram Predict the Physiologic Importance of a Coronary Stenosis?" *New Eng J Med* 310 (1984): 819–24.

8. C.M. Winslow et al., "The Appropriateness of Performing Coronary Artery Bypass Surgery," *JAMA* 260 (1988): 505.

9. P.J. Shaw et al., "Neurological Complications of Coronary Artery Bypass Graft Surgery: Six-Month Follow-Up Study," *Br Med J* 293 (1986): 165–7.

10. European Coronary Surgery Study Group, "Long-Term Results of Prospective Randomized Study of Coronary Artery Bypass Surgery in Stable Angina Pectoris," *Lancet* ii (1982): 1173–80.

11. P.E. Ballmer et al., "Depletion of Plasma Vitamin C but Not Vitamin E in Response to Cardiac Operations," *J Thorac Cardiovasc Surg* 108 (1994): 308–11.

12. M. Chello et al., "Protection of Coenzyme Q_{10} from Myocardial Reperfusion Injury During Coronary Artery Bypass Grafting," *Ann Thorac Surg* 58 (1994): 1427–32.

13. G. Laurora et al., "Delayed Arteriosclerosis Progression in High-Risk Subjects Treated with Mesoglycan: Evaluation of Intima-Media Thickness," *J Cardiovasc Surg* 34 (1993): 313–8.

14. R. Lagioia et al., "Propionyl-L-Carnitine: A New Compound in the Metabolic Approach to the Treatment of Effort Angina," *Int J Cardiol* 34 (1992): 167–72.

15. G.L. Bartels et al., "Effects of L-Propionylcarnitine on Ischemia-Induced Myocardial Dysfunction in Men with Angina Pectoris," *Am J Cardiol* 74 (1994): 125–30.

16. L. Cacciatore et al., "The Therapeutic Effect of L-Carnitine in Patients with Exercise-Induced Stable Angina: A Controlled Study," *Drugs Exptl Clin Res* 17 (1991): 225–335.

17. P. Davini et al., "Controlled Study on L-Carnitine Therapeutic Efficacy in Post-Infarction," *Drugs Exptl Clin Res* 18 (1992): 355–65.

18. T. Kamikawa, Y. Suzuki, A. Kobayashi, et al., "Effects of L-Carnitine on Exercise Tolerance in Patients with Stable Angina Pectoris," *Jap Heart J* 25 (1984): 587–97.

19. A.G. Rebuzzi, G. Schiavoni, C.M. Amico, et al., "Beneficial Effects of L-Carnitine in the Reduction of the Necrotic Area in Acute Myocardial Infarction," *Drugs Exp Clin Res* 10 (1984): 219–23.

20. L. Arsenio, P. Bodria, G. Magnati, et al., "Effectiveness of Long-Term Treatment with Pantethine in Patients with Dyslipidemias," *Clin Ther* 8 (1986): 537–45.

21. R. Miccoli, P. Marchetti, T. Sampietro, et al., "Effects of Pantethine on Lipids and Apolipoproteins in Hypercholesterolemic Diabetic and Non-Diabetic Patients," *Curr Ther Res* 36 (1984): 545–9.

22. A. Gaddi et al., "Controlled Evaluation of Pantethine, a Natural Hypolipidemic Compound, in Patients with Different Forms of Hyperlipoproteinemia," *Atheroscl* 50 (1984): 73–83.

23. H. Hayashi et al., "Effects of Pantethine on Action Potential of Canine Papillary Muscle During Hypoxic Perfusion," *Jap Heart J* 26 (1985): 289–96.

24. K. Folkers and Y. Yamamura, eds., *Biomedical and Clinical Aspects of Coenzyme Q_{10}*, Volumes 1–4 (Amsterdam: Elsevier Science Publishers, Vol 1: 1977, Vol 2: 1980, Vol 3: 1982, Vol 4: 1984).

25. T. Kamikawa et al., "Effects of Coenzyme Q_{10} on Exercise Tolerance in Chronic Stable Angina Pectoris," *Am J Cardiol* 56 (1985): 247.

26. P.D.M.V. Turlapaty and B.M. Altura, "Magnesium Deficiency Produces Spasms of Coronary Arteries: Relationship to Etiology of Sudden Death Ischemic Heart Disease," *Sci* 208 (1980): 199–200.

27. B.M. Altura, "Ischemic Heart Disease and Magnesium," *Magnesium* 7 (1988): 57–67.

28. R.M. McLean, "Magnesium and Its Therapeutic Uses: A Review," *Am J Med* 96 (1994): 63–76.

29. J.R. Purvis and A. Movahed, "Magnesium Disorders and Cardiovascular Disease," *Clin Cardiol* 15 (1992): 556–68.

30. E.M. Hampton, D.D. Whang, and R. Whang, "Intravenous Magnesium Therapy in Acute Myocardial Infarction," *Ann Pharmacother* 28 (1994): 212–9.

31. K.K. Teo and S. Yusuf, "Role of Magnesium in Reducing Mortality in Acute Myocardial Infarction: A Review of the Evidence," *Drugs* 46 (1993): 347–59.

32. M. Schecter, E. Kaplinsky, and B. Rabinowitz, "The Rationale of Magnesium Supplementation in Acute Myocardial Infarction: A Review of the Literature," *Arch Intern Med* 152 (1992): 2189–96.

33. H.P.T. Ammon and M. Handel, "Crataegus, Toxicology and Pharmacology, Part I: Toxicity," *Planta Med* 43 (1981): 105–20; "Part II: Pharmacodynamics," *Planta Med* 43 (1981): 209–39; "Part III: Pharmacodynamics and Pharmacokinetics," *Planta Med* 43 (1981): 313–22.

34. R. Blesken, "Crataegus in Cardiology," *Fortschr Med* 110 (1992): 290–2.

35. Y. Nasa et al., "Protective Effect of Crataegus Extract on the Cardiac Mechanical Dysfunction in Isolated Perfused Working Rat Heart," *Arzneim Forsch* 43 (1993): 945–9.

36. H.L. Osher, K.H. Katz, and D.J. Wagner, "Khellin in the Treatment of Angina Pectoris," *New Eng J Med* 244 (1951): 315–21.

37. G.V. Anrep, M.R. Kenawy, and G.S. Barsoum, "Coronary Vasodilator Action of Khellin," *Am Heart J* 37 (1949): 531–42.

38. J.J. Conn et al., "Treatment of Angina Pectoris with Khellin," *Ann Int Med* 36 (1952): 1173–8.

39. N.E. Clarke et al., "Treatment of Angina Pectoris with Disodium Ethylene Diamine Tetraacetic Acid," *Am J Med Sci* 232 (1956): 654–66.

40. N.E. Clarke, "Atherosclerosis, Occlusive Vascular Disease, and EDTA," *Am J Cardiol* 6 (1960): 233–6.

41. D. Steinberg et al., "Beyond Cholesterol: Modifications of Low-Density Lipoprotein That Increase Its Atherogenicity," *N Engl J Med* 320 (1989): 915–24.

42. E.M. Cranton and J.P. Frackelton, "Current Status of EDTA Chelation Therapy in Occlusive Arterial Disease," *J Adv Med* 2 (1989): 107–19.

43. E. Olszwer and J.P. Carter, "EDTA Chelation Therapy: A Retrospective Study of 2,870 Patients," *J Adv Med* 2 (1989): 197–211.

44. E. Olszewer, F.C. Sabbag, and J.P. Carter, "A Pilot Double-Blind Study of Sodium-Magnesium EDTA in Peripheral Vascular Disease," *J Nat Med Assoc* 82 (1988): 173–7.

45. E. Olszewer and J.P. Carter, "EDTA Chelation Therapy in Chronic Degenerative Disease," *Med Hypothesis* 27 (1988): 41–9.

46. H.R. Casdorph, "EDTA Chelation Therapy: Efficacy in Arteriosclerotic Heart Disease," *J Holistic Med* 3 (1981): 53–9.

Anxiety

1. M. Werbach, *Nutritional Influences on Mental Illness: A Sourcebook of Clinical Research* (Tarzana, CA: Third Line Press, 1991).

2. M. Bruce and M. Lader, "Caffeine Abstention in the Management of Anxiety Disorders," *Psychol Med* 19 (1989): 211–4.

3. D.O. Rudin, "The Major Psychoses and Neuroses as Omega-3 Essential Fatty Acid Deficiency Syndrome: Substrate Pellagra," *Biol Psychiatry* 16 (1981): 837–50.

4. Y. Singh, "Kava: An Overview," *J Ethnopharmacol* 37 (1992): 13–45.

5. W.E. Scholing and H.D. Clausen, "On the Effect of d,l-kavain: Experience with Neuronika," *Med Klin* 72 (1977): 1301–6.

6. D. Lindenberg and H. Pitule-Schodel, "D,L-kavain in Comparison with Oxazepam in Anxiety Disorders: A Double-Blind Study of Clinical Effectiveness," *Forschr Med* 108 (1990): 49–50, 53–4.

7. H.J. Meyer, "Pharmacology of Kava," in B. Holmstedt and N.S. Kline, eds., *Ethnopharmacological Search for Psychoactive Drugs* (New York: Raven Press, 1979), 133–40.

8. J. Keledjian et al., "Uptake into Mouse Brain of Four Compounds Present in the Psychoactive Beverage Kava," *J Pharm Sci* 77 (1988): 1003–6.

9. E. Kinzler, J. Kromer, and E. Lehmann, "Clinical Efficacy of a Kava Extract in Patients with Anxiety Syndrome: Double-Blind Placebo Controlled Study over 4 Weeks," *Arzneim Forsch* 41 (1991): 584–8.

10. G. Warnecke, "Neurovegetative Dystonia in the Female Climacteric: Studies on the Clinical Efficacy and Tolerance of Kava Extract WS 1490," *Fortschr Med* 109 (1991): 120–2.

11. K.W. Herberg, "The Influence of Kava-Special Extract WS 1490 on Safety-Relevant Performance Alone and in Combination with Ethylalcohol," *Blutalkohol* 30 (1993): 96–105.

12. T.F. Munte et al., "Effects of Oxazepam and an Extract of Kava Roots *(Piper methysticum)* on Event-Related Potentials in a Word Recognition Task," *Neuropyschobiol* 27 (1993): 46–53.

13. L. Schelosky et al., "Kava and Dopamine Antagonism [Letter]," *J Neurol Neurosurg Psychiatry* 58 (1995): 639–40.

14. J.C. Almeida and E.W. Grimsley, "Coma from the Health Food Store: Interaction between Kava and Alprazolam," *Annals Int Med* 125 (1996): 940–1.

15. S.A. Norton and P. Ruze, "Kava Dermopathy," *J Am Acad Dermatol* 31 (1994): 89–97.

16. P. Ruze, "Kava-Induced Dermopathy: A Niacin Deficiency," *Lancet* 335 (1990): 1442–5.

17. J.D. Mathews et al., "Effects of the Heavy Usage of Kava on Physical Health: Summary of a Pilot Survey in an Aboriginal Community," *Med J Aust* 148 (1988): 548–55.

Asthma and Hay Fever

1. M.R. Odent, E.E. Culpin, and T. Kimmel, "Pertussis vaccination and asthma: Is there a link?" *JAMA* 272 (1994): 592–3.

2. S.S. Yen and H.G. Morris, "An imbalance of arachidonic acid metabolism in asthma," *Biochem Biophys Res Com* 103 (1981): 774–9.

3. Y. Tan and C. Collins-Williams, "Aspirin-induced asthma in children," *Ann Allergy* 48 (1982): 1–5.

4. J.Y. Vanderhoek, S.L. Ekborg, and J.M. Bailey, "Nonsteroidal anti-inflammatory drugs stimulate 15-lipoxygenase/leukotriene pathway in human polymorphonuclear leukocytes," *J Allergy Clin Immunol* 74 (1984): 412–7.

5. T. Shirakawa and K. Morimoto, "Lifestyle effect on total IgE," *Allergy* 46 (1991): 561–9.

6. S.A. Bock, "Food-related asthma and basic nutrition," *J Asthma* 20 (1983): 377–81.

7. A. Oehling, "Importance of food allergy in childhood asthma," *Allergol Immunopathol Suppl* IX (1981): 71–3.

8. K.A. Ogle and J.D. Bullocks, "Children with allergic rhinitis and/or bronchial asthma treated with elimination diet: A five-year follow-up," *Ann Allergy* 44 (1980): 273–8.

9. L. Businco et al., "Food allergy and asthma," *Pediatr Pulmonol Suppl* 11 (1995): 59–60.

10. A.J. Bircher et al., "IgE to food allergens are highly prevalent in patients allergic to pollens, with and without symptoms of food allergy," *Clin Exp Allergy* 24(4) (1994): 367–74.

11. L. Hodge et al., "Assessment of food chemical intolerance in adult asthmatic subjects," *Thorax* 51 (1996): 805–9.

12. D.W. Hide et al., "Effect of allergen avoidance in infancy on allergic manifestations at age two years," *J Allergy Clin Immunol* 93 (1994): 842–6.

13. G.W. Bray, "The hypochlorhydria of asthma in childhood," *Quart J Med* 24 (1931): 181–97.

14. A. Benard et al., "Increased intestinal permeability in bronchial asthma," *J Allergy Clin Immunol* 97 (1996): 1173–8.

15. K. Akiyama et al., "Atopic asthma caused by *Candida albicans* acid protease: Case reports," *Allergy* 49 (1994): 778–81.

16. O. Lindahl et al., "Vegan diet regimen with reduced medication in the treatment of bronchial asthma," *J Asthma* 22 (1985): 45–55.

17. L. Hodge et al., "Consumption of oily fish and childhood asthma risk," *MJA* 164 (1996): 137–40.

18. J.P. Arm et al., "The effects of dietary supplementation with fish oil lipids on the airway response to inhaled allergen in bronchial asthma," *Am Rev Respiratory Dis* 139 (1989): 1395–1400.

19. J. Dry and D. Vincent "Effect of a fish oil diet on asthma: Results of a 1-year double-blind study," *Int Arch Allergy Apply Immunol* 95 (1991): 156–7.

20. K.S. Broughton et al., "Reduced asthma symptoms with n-3 fatty acid ingestion are related to 5-series leukotriene production," *Am J Clin Nutr* 65 (1997): 1011–7.

21. B.J. Freedman, "A diet free from additives in the management of allergic disease," *Clin Allergy* 7 (1977): 417–21.

22. D.D. Stevenson and R.A. Simon "Sensitivity to ingested metabisulfites in asthmatic subjects," *J Allergy Clin Immunol* 68 (1981): 26–32.

23. R. Papaioannou and C.C. Pfeiffer "Sulfite sensitivity—Unrecognized threat: Is molybdenum deficiency the cause?" *J Orthomol Psych* 13 (1984): 105–10.

24. G. Unge, J. Grubbstrom, P. Olsson et al., "Effect of dietary tryptophan restrictions on clinical symptoms in patients with endogenous asthma," *Allergy* 38 (1983): 211–2.

25. R.D. Reynolds and C.L. Natta, "Depressed plasma pyridoxal phosphate concentrations in adult asthmatics," *Am J Clin Nutr* 41 (1985): 684–8.

26. P.J. Collip, S. Goldzier, N. Weiss, et al., "Pyridoxine treatment of childhood asthma," *Ann Allergy* 35 (1975): 93–7.

27. S. Sur et al., "Double-blind trial of pyridoxine (vitamin B_6) in the treatment of steroid-dependent asthma," *Annals Allergy* 70 (1993): 147–52.

28. T. Shimizu et al., "Theophylline attenuates circulating vitamin B_6 levels in children with asthma," *Pharmacol* 49 (1994): 392–7.

29. P.R. Bartel et al., "Vitamin B_6 supplementation and theophylline-related effects in humans," *Am J Clin Nutr* 60 (1994): 93–9.

30. A. Seaton, D.J. Godden, and K. Brown, "Increase in asthma: A more toxic environment or a more susceptible population," *Thorax* 49 (1994): 171–4.

31. G.E. Hatch, "Asthma, inhaled oxidants, and dietary antioxidants," *Am J Clin Nutr* 61(Suppl.) (1995): 625S–30S.

32. S.O. Olusi, O.O. Ojutiku, W.J.E. Jessop, and M.I. Iboko, "Plasma and white blood cell ascorbic acid concentrations in patients with bronchial asthma," *Clinica Chimica Acta* 92 (1979): 161–6.

33. L. Bielory and R. Gandhi, "Asthma and vitamin C," *Annals Allergy* 73 (1994): 89–96.

34. C.S. Johnston, L.J. Martin, and X. Cai, "Antihistamine effect of supplemental ascorbic acid and neutrophil

35. C.M.S. Fewtrell and B.D. Gomperts, "Effect of flavone inhibitors of transport ATPase on histamine secretion from rat mast cells," *Nature* 265 (1977): 635–6.

36. E. Middleton, G. Drzewiecki, and D. Krishnarao, "Quercetin: An inhibitor of antigen-induced human basophil histamine release," *J Immunol* 127 (1981): 546–50.

37. J.C. Foreman, "Mast cells and the actions of flavonoids," *J Allergy Clin Immunol* 73 (1984): 769–74.

38. W.C. Hope et al., "In vitro inhibition of the biosynthesis of slow reacting substance of anaphylaxis (SRS-A) and lipoxygenase activity by quercetin," *Biochem Pharmacol* 32 (1983): 367–71.

39. W. Grosch and G. Laskawy, "Co-oxidation of carotenes requires one soybean lipoxygenase isoenzyme," *Biochem Biophys Acta* 575 (1979): 439–45.

40. R.V. Panganamala and D.G. Cornwell, "The effects of vitamin E on arachidonic acid metabolism," *Ann NY Acad Sci* 393 (1982): 376–91.

41. N.L.A. Misso et al., "Reduced platelet glutathione peroxidase activity and serum selenium concentration in atopic asthmatic patients," *Clinical Exp Allergy* 26 (1996): 838–47.

42. J. Stone, "Reduced selenium status of patients with asthma," *Clinical Science* 77 (1989): 495–500.

43. J. Kadrabova et al., "Selenium status is decreased in patients with intrinsic asthma," *Biological Trace Element Research* 52 (1996): 241–8.

44. Personal communication with Jonathan Wright, M.D.

45. S.W. Simon, "Vitamin B_{12} therapy in allergy and chronic dermatoses," *J Allergy* 2 (1951): 183–5.

46. R. Garrison and E. Somer, "Vitamin Research: Selected Topics," *The Nutrition Desk Reference* (New Canann, CT: Keats, 1985), 93–4.

47. P. Trendelenburg, "Physiologische und pharmakologische untersuchungen an der isolierten bronchial muskulatur," *Arch Exp Pharmacol Ther* CI: (1912): 79.

48. V.G. Haury, "Blood serum magnesium in bronchial asthma and its

treatment by the administration of magnesium sulfate," *J Lab Clin Med* 26 (1940): 340–4.

49. E.M. Skobeloff et al., "Intravenous magnesium sulfate for the treatment of acute asthma in the emergency department," *JAMA* 262 (1989): 1210–3.

50. H. Okayama et al., "Bronchodilating effect of intravenous magnesium sulfate in bronchial asthma," *JAMA* 257 (1987): 1076–8.

51. M. Noppen et al., "Bronchodilating effect of intravenous magnesium sulfate in acute severe bronchial asthma," *Chest* 97 (1990): 373–6.

52. M.S. Skorodin et al., "Magnesium sulfate in exacerbations of chronic obstructive pulmonary disease," *Arch Intern Med* 155(1995): 496–500.

53. R.M. McLean, "Magnesium and its therapeutic uses: A review," *Am J Med* 96 (1994): 63–76.

54. L. Gullestad et al., "Oral versus intravenous magnesium supplementation in patients with magnesium deficiency," *Magnes Trace Elem* 10 (1991): 6–11.

55. J. Britton et al., "Dietary magnesium, lung function, wheezing, and airway hyper-reactivity in a random adult population sample," *Lancet* 344 (1994): 357–62.

56. O.J. Carrey, C. Locke, and J.B. Cookson, "Effect of alterations of dietary sodium on the severity of asthma in men," *Thorax* 48 (1993): 714–8.

57. P.G.J. Burney, "A diet rich in sodium may potentiate asthma: Epidemiological evidence for a new hypothesis," *Chest* 91 (1987): 143–8.

58. R.E. Weinstein et al., "Decreased adrenal sex steroid levels in the absence of glucocorticoid suppression in postmenopausal asthmatic women," *J Allergy Clin Immunol* 97 (1996): 1–8.

59. A.G. Gilman, A.S. Goodman, and A. Gilman, *The Pharmacologic Basis of Therapeutics* (New York: MacMillan, 1980)

60. American Pharmaceutical Association, *Handbook of Nonprescription Drugs*, 8th ed., (Washington, DC: American Pharmaceutical Association, 1986).

61. E. Okimasu, Y. Moromizato, S. Watanabe et al., "Inhibition of phospholipase A2 and platelet aggregation by glycyrrhizin, an anti-inflammatory drug," *Acta Med Okayama* 37 (1983): 385–91.

62. P. Cambar, S. Shore, and D. Aviado, "Bronchopulmonary and gastrointestinal effects of lobeline," *Arch Int Pharmacodyn* 177 (1969): 1–27.

63. D.F.J. Halmagyi, A. Kovacs, and P. Neumann, "Adrenalcortical pathway of lobeline protection in some forms of experimental lung edema in the rat," *Dis Chest* 33 (1958): 285–96

64. J.M. Lundberg and A. Saria, "Capsaicin-Induced Desensitization of Airway Mucosa to Cigarette Smoke, Mechanical and Chemical Irritants," *Nature* 302 (1983): 251–53.

65. J. Vanderhoek, A. Makheja, and J. Bailey, "Inhibition of fatty acid lipoxygenases by onion and garlic oils: Evidence for the mechanism by which these oils inhibit platelet aggregation," *Bioch Pharmacol* 29 (1980): 3169–73.

66. W. Dorsch and J. Weber, "Prevention of allergen-induced bronchial constriction in sensitized guinea pigs by crude alcohol onion extract," *Agents Actions* 14 (1984): 626–30.

67. W. Dorsch, O. Adam, J. Weber, and T. Ziegeltrum, "Antiasthmatic effects of onion extracts—Detection of benzyl- and other isothiocyanates in mustard oils as antiasthmatic compounds of plant origin," *Euro J Pharmacol* 107 (1985): 17–24.

68. A.L. Udupa, S.L. Udupa, and M.N. Guruswamy, "The possible site of anti-asthmatic action of *Tylophora asthmatica* on pituitary-adrenal axis in albino rats," *Planta Med* 57 (1991): 409–13.

69. C. Gopalakrishnan et al., "Effect of tylophorine, a major alkaloid of *Tylophora indica*, on immunopathological and inflammatory reactions," *Ind J Med Res* 71 (1980): 940–8.

70. S. Gupta et al., "*Tylophora indica* in bronchial asthma—a double blind study," *Ind J Med Res* 69 (1979): 981–9.

71. K.V. Thiruvengadam et al., "*Tylophora indica* in bronchial asthma (a controlled comparison with a standard anti-asthmatic drug," *J Indian Med Assoc* 71 (1978): 172–6.

72. D.N. Shivpuri, S.C. Singhal, and D. Parkash, "Treatment of asthma with an alcoholic extract of *Tylophora indica*: A cross-over, double-blind study," *Ann Allergy* 30 (1972): 407–12.

73. D.N. Shivpuri, M.P. Menon, and D. Prakash, "A crossover double-blind study on *Tylophora indica* in the treatment of asthma and allergic rhinitis," *J Allergy* 43 (1969): 145–50.

74. J.H. Wilkens et al., "Effects of a PAF-antagonist (BN 52063) on bronchoconstriction and platelet activation during exercise induced asthma," *Br J Clin Pharmacol* 29 (1990): 85–91.

75. P. Guinot et al., "Effect of BN 52063, a specific PAF-acether antagonist, on bronchial provocation test to allergens in asthmatic patients: A preliminary study," *Prostaglandins* 34 (1987): 723–31.

76. T. Shida et al., "Effect of aloe extract on peripheral phagocytosis in adult bronchial asthma," *Planta Med* 51 (1985): 273–5.

77. J. Lichey, T. Friedrich, M. Priesnitz et al., "Effect of forskolin on methacholine-induced bronchoconstriction in extrinsic asthmatics," *Lancet* II (1984): 167.

78. K. Bauer et al., "Pharmacodynamic effects of inhaled dry powder formulations of fenoterol and colforsin in asthma," *Clin Pharmacol Ther* 53 (1993): 76–83.

Attention Deficit Disorders

1. B.A. Shaywitz, J.M. Fletcher, and S.E. Shaywitz, "Attention-Deficit/Hyperactivity Disorder," *Adv Pediatr* 44 (1997): 331–67.

2. T.E. Tuormaa, "The Adverse Effects of Food Additives on Health: A Review of the Literature with Special Emphasis on Childhood Hyperactivity." *J Orthomolecular Med* 4 (1994):225–38.

3. N. Feingold, *Why Your Child Is Hyperactive* (New York: Random House, 1975).

4. C. Conners, C. Goyette, D. Southwick, J. Lees, and P. Andrulonis, "Food Additives and Hyperkinesis: A Double-Blind Experiment," *Pediatrics* 58 (1976): 154–166.

5. C. Goyette, C. Conners, T. Petti, and L. Curtis, "Effects of Artificial Colors on Hyperkinetic Children: A Double-Blind Challenge Study," *Psychopharmacol Bull* 14 (1978): 39–40.

6. C. Conners, *Food Additives and Hyperactive Children* (New York: Plenum Press, 1980).

7. J. Harley, R. Ray, L. Tomasi, et al., "Hyperkinesis and Food Additives: Testing the Feingold Hypothesis," *Pediatrics* 61 (1978): 811–7.

8. K. Rowe, I. Hopkins, and B. Lynch, "Artificial Food Colourings and Hyperkinesis," *Aust Paediatr J* 15 (1979): 202.

9. F. Levy, S. Dumbrell, G. Hobbes, et al., "Hyperkinesis and Diet: A Double-Blind Crossover Trial with Tartrazine Challenge," *Med J Aust* 1 (1978): 61–4.

10. K. Rowe, "Food Additives," *Aust Paediatr J* 20 (1984): 171–4.

11. A. Schauss, "Nutrition and Behavior: Complex Interdisciplinary Research," *Nutr Health* 3 (1984): 9–37.

12. V. Rippere, "Food Additives and Hyperactive Children: A Critique of Conners," *Br J Clin Psych* 22 (1983): 19–32.

13. J. Swanson and M. Kinsbourne, "Food Dyes Impair Performance of Children on a Laboratory Learning Task," *Science* 207 (1980): 1485–7.

14. B. Weiss, J. Williams, S. Margen, et al., "Behavioral Responses to Artificial Food Colours," *Science* 207 (1980): 1487–9.

15. B. Weiss, "Food Additives and Environmental Chemicals as Sources of Childhood Behavior Disorders," *J Am Acad Child Psychiatry* 21 (1982): 144–152.

16. B. Rimland, "The Feingold Diet: An Assessment of the Reviews by Mattes, by Kavale and Forness and Others," *J Learn Disabil* 16 (1983): 331–3.

17. M. Lipton and J. Mayo, "Diet and Hyperkinesis: An Update," *J Am Diet Assoc* 83 (1983): 132–4.

18. Anonymous, "Defined Diets and Childhood Hyperactivity. Consensus Conference: Office for Medical Applications of Research, National In-

stitutes of Health," *JAMA* 248 (1982): 290–2.

19. L. Mayron, J. Ott, R. Nations, and E. Mayron, "Light, Radiation, and Academic Behavior," *Academic Therapy* 10 (1974): 33–47.

20. J. Mattes, "The Feingold Diet: A Current Reappraisal," *J Learn Disabil* 16 (1983): 319–323.

21. P. Cook and J. Woodhill, "The Feingold Dietary Treatment of the Hyperkinetic Syndrome," *Med J Aust* 2 (1976): 85–90.

22. J. Noonan and H. Meggos, "Synthetic Food Colors," in T. Furia, ed., *CRC Handbook of Food Additives,* vol 2 (Boca Raton, FL: CRC Press, 1980), 339–83.

23. R. Prinz, W. Roberts, and E. Hantman, "Dietary Correlates of Hyperactive Behavior in Children," *J Counsult Clin Psych* 48 (1980): 760–9.

24. L. Langseth and J. Dowd, "Glucose Tolerance and Hyperkinesis," *Food Cosmet Toxicol* 16 (1978): 129–33.

25. J. Egger, C. Carter, P. Graham, D. Gumley, and J. Soothill, "Controlled Trial of Oligoantigenic Treatment in the Hyperkinetic Syndrome," *Lancet* (1985): 540–5.

26. J. O'Shea and S. Porter, "Double-Blind Study of Children with Hyperkinetic Syndrome Treated with Multi-Allergen Extract Sublingually," *J Learn Disabil* 14 (1981): 189–91.

27. J. Egger et al., "Controlled Trial of Hyposensitization in Children with Food-Induced Hyperkinetic Syndrome," *Lancet* 339 (1992): 1150–3.

28. M. Boris and F.S. Mande, "Food and Additives Are Common Causes of the Attention Deficit Hyperactive Disorder in Children," *Ann All* 72 (1994): 462–468.

29. L. Salzman, "Allergy Testing, Psychological Assessment, and Dietary Treatment of the Hyperactive Child Syndrome," *Med J Aust* 2 (1976): 248–251.

30. K.S. Rowe and K.J. Rowe, "Synthetic Food Coloring and Behavior: A Dose Response Effect in a Double-Blind, Placebo-Controlled, Repeated-Measures Study," *J Pediatr* 125 (1994): 691–8.

31. M. Boris and F.S. Mandel, "Foods and Additives are Common Causes

of Attention Deficit Hyperactive Disorder in Children," *Annals Allergy* 72 (1994): 462–7.

32. C.M. Carter et al. "Effects of a Few-Food Diet in Attention Deficit Disorder," *Archives Dis Child* 69 (1993): 564–8.

33. L. Sanders, F. Hofeldt, M. Kirk, and J. Levin, "Refined Carbohydrate as a Contributing Factor in Reactive Hypoglycemia," *Southern Med J* 75 (1982): 1972–5.

34. J. Reichman and W. Healey, "Learning Disabilities and Conductive Hearing Loss Involving Otitis Media," *J Learn Disabil* 16 (1983): 272–8.

35. P. Silva, C. Kirkland, A. Simpson, I. Stewart, and S. Williams, "Some Developmental and Behavioral Problems with Bilateral Otitis Media with Effusion," *J Learn Disabil* 15 (1982): 417–21.

36. M. Krause and L. Mahan, "Nutritional Care in Disease of the Nervous System and Behavioral Disorders," *Food, Nutrition and Diet Therapy* (Philadelphia: W.B. Saunders, 1984), 654–670.

37. R. Tseng, J. Mellon, and K. Bammer, *The Relationship Between Nutrition and Student Achievement, Behavior, and Health: A Review of the Literature* (Sacramento, CA: California State Department of Education, 1980).

38. E. Pollitt and R. Leibel, "Iron Deficiency and Behavior," *J Pediatrics* 88 (1976): 372–381.

39. T. Webb and F. Oski, "Iron Deficiency Anemia and Scholastic Achievement in Young Adolescents," *J Pediatrics* 82 (1973): 827–830.

40. M. Colgan and L. Colgan, "Do Nutrient Supplements and Dietary Changes Affect Learning and Emotional Reactions of Children with Learning Difficulties? A Controlled Series of 16 Cases," *Nutr Health* 3 (1984): 69–77.

41. J. Kerschner and W. Hawke, "Megavitamins and Learning Disorders: A Controlled Double-Blind Experiment," *J Nutr* 109 (1979): 819–826.

42. S. Perkins, "Malnutrition: A Selected Review of Its Effects on the Learning and Behavior of Children,"

Int J Early Childhood 5 (1977): 173–9.

43. M. Marlowe, A. Coissairt, K. Welch, and J. Errera, "Hair Mineral Content as a Predictor of Learning Disabilities," *J Learn Disabil* 17 (1977): 418–421.

44. R. Pihl and M. Parkes, "Hair Element Content in Learning Disabled Children," *Science* 198 (1977): 204–6.

45. O. David, J. Clark, and K. Voeller, "Lead and Hyperactivity," *Lancet* ii (1972): 900–3.

46. O. David, S. Hoffman, and J. Sverd, "Lead and Hyperactivity. Behavioral Response to Chelation: A Pilot Study," *Am J Psychiatry* 133 (1976): 1155–1188.

47. V. Benignus, D. Otto, K. Muller, and K. Seipple, "Effects of Age and Body Lead Burden on CNS Function in Young Children: EEG Spectra," *EEG and Clin Neurophys* 52 (1981): 240–8.

48. B. Rimland and G. Larson, "Hair Mineral Analysis and Behavior: An Analysis of 51 Studies," *J Learn Disabil* 16 (1983): 279–285.

49. D. Bryce-Smith, "Lead-Induced Disorders of Mentation in Children," *Nutr Health* 1 (1983): 179–184.

50. C.A. Kahn, P.C. Kelly, and W.O. Walker, "Lead Screening in Children with Attention Deficit Hyperactivity Disorder and Developmental Delay," *Clinical Pediatr* Sept (1995): 498–501.

51. R.W. Tuthill, "Hair Lead Levels Related to Children's Classroom Attention-Deficit Behavior," *Arch Environ Health* 51 (1996): 214–20.

52. D. Benton and G. Roberts, "Effect of Vitamin and Mineral Supplementation on Intelligence of a Sample of Schoolchildren," *Lancet* i (1988): 140–3.

Bipolar (Manic) Depression

1. J. Growden, "Neurotransmitter Precursors in the Diets: Their Use in the Treatment of Brain Diseases," in R. Wurtman and J. Wurtman, eds., *Nutrition and the Brain,* vol 3 (New York: Raven Press, 1979), 117–82.

2. G. Chouinard et al., "Tryptophan in the Treatment of Depression and Mania," *Adv Biol Psychiat* 10 (1983): 47–66.

3. I. Sano, "L-5-hydroxytryptophan Therapy," *Folia Psychiatr Neurol Japan* 26 (1972): 7–17.

4. H.M. van Praag, "Central Monoamine Metabolism in Depressions, I: Serotonin and Related Compounds," *Compr Psychiatry* 21 (1980): 30–43.

5. W.R. Millington and R. Wurtman, "Choline Administration Elevates Brain Phosphorylcholine Concentrations," *J Neurochem* 38 (1982): 1748–52.

6. B. Cohen, A. Miller, J. Lipinski, and H. Pope, "Lecithin in Mania: A Preliminary Report," *Am J Psychiat* 137 (1980): 242–3.

7. B. Cohen, J. Lipinski, and R. Altesman, "Lecithin in the Treatment of Mania: Double-Blind, Placebo-Controlled Trials," *Am J Psychiat* 139 (1982): 1162–4.

8. R. Jope et al., "Biochemical RBC Abnormalities in Drug-Free and Lithium-Treated Manic Patients," *Am J Psychiat* 142 (1985): 356–8.

9. D. Jenden, R. Jope, and S. Fraser, "A Mechanism for the Accumulation of Choline in Erythrocytes during Treatment with Lithium," *Commun Psychopharmacol* 4 (1980): 339–44.

10. G. Naylor, A. Smith, D. Bryce-Smith, and N. Ward, "Tissue Vanadium Levels in Manic-Depressive Psychosis," *Psychol Med* 14 (1984): 767–72.

11. G. Naylor, "Vanadium and Manic Depressive Psychosis," *Nutr Health* 3 (1984): 79–85.

12. G. Naylor, "Vanadium and Affective Disorders," *Biol Psychiat* 18 (1983): 103–12.

13. D. Myron, S. Givand, and F. Nielsen, "Vanadium Content of Selected Foods as Determined by Flameless Atomic Absorption Spectroscopy," *J Agr Food Chem* 25 (1977): 297–300.

14. A. Lewy, T. Wehr, F. Goodwin, et al., "Manic-Depressive Patients May Be Supersensitive to Light," *Lancet* i (1981) 383–4.

15. C. Tamminga, R. Smith, S. Chang, et al., "Depression Associated with Oral Choline," *Lancet* ii (1976): 905.

Bladder Infection

1. W.T. Branch, *Office Practice of Medicine* (Philadelphia: W.B. Saunders, 1982), 488–504, 679–85.

2. R.H. Rubin, "Infections of the Urinary Tract," in *Scientific American Medicine,* ed. by D.C. Dale and D.D. Federman (New York: Scientific American, 1997).

3. G. Reid, A.W. Bruce, and R.L. Cook, "Effect on Urogenital Flora of Antibiotic Therapy of Urinary Tract Infection," *Scand J Infect Dis* 22 (1990): 43–7.

4. K.J. Lidefelt, I. Bollgren, and C.E. Nord, "Changes in Periurethral Microflora after Antimicrobial Drugs," *Arch Dis Child* 66 (1991): 683–5.

5. F.F. Marshall and A.W. Middleton, "Eosinophilic Cystitis," *J Urol* 112 (1974): 225–8.

6. M. Goldstein, "Eosinophilic Cystitis," *J Urol* 106 (1972): 854–7.

7. A.S. Palacios et al., "Eosinophilic Food-Induced Cystitis," *Allergol Et Immunopathol* 12 (1984): 463–9.

8. A. Aziz-Fam, "Use of Titrated Extract of *Centella asiatica* (TECA) in Bilharzial Bladder Lesions," *Int Surg* 58 (1973): 451–2.

9. A. Etrebi, A. Ibrahim, and K. Zaki, "Treatment of Bladder Ulcer with Asiaticoside," *J Egypt Med Assoc* 58 (1975): 324–7.

10. P.N. Prodromos, C.A. Brusch, and G.C. Ceresia, "Cranberry Juice in the Treatment of Urinary Tract Infections," *Southwest Med* 47 (1968): 17.

11. P. Sternlieb, "Cranberry Juice in Renal Disease," *New Engl J Med* 268 (1963): 57.

12. D.V. Moen, "Observations on the Effectiveness of Cranberry Juice in Urinary Infections," *Wisconsin Med J* 61 (1962): 282.

13. D.H. Kahn et al., "Effect of Cranberry Juice on Urine," *J Am Diet Assoc* 51 (1967): 251.

14. P.T. Bodel, R. Cotran, and E.H. Kass, "Cranberry Juice and the Antibacterial Action of Hippuric Acid," *J Lab Clin Med* 54 (1959): 881.

15. A.E. Sobota, "Inhibition of Bacterial Adherence by Cranberry Juice: Potential Use for the Treatment of Urinary Tract Infections," *J Urology* 131 (1984): 1013–6.

16. I. Ofek et al., "Anti-Escherichia Activity of Cranberry and Blueberry Juices," *New Eng J Med* 324 (1991): 1599.

17. A. Sanchez et al., "Role of Sugars in Human Neutrophilic Phagocytosis," *Am J Clin Nutr* 26 (1973): 1180–4.

18. W. Ringsdorf, E. Cheraskin, and R. Ramsay, "Sucrose, Neutrophil Phagocytosis, and Resistance to Disease, "*Dent Surv* 52 (1976): 46–8.

19. J. Bernstein et al., "Depression of Lymphocyte Transformation Following Oral Glucose Ingestion," *Am J Clin Nutr* 30 (1977): 613.

20. P.E. Munday and S. Savage, "Cymalon in the Management of Urinary Tract Symptoms," *Genitourin Med* 66 (1990): 461.

21. J.B. Spooner, "Alkalinization in the Management of Cystitis," *J Int Med Res* 12 (1984): 30–4.

22. The *Merck Index,* 10th ed. (Rahway, NJ: Merck & Co, 1983) 112–3, 699.

23. V. Frohne, "Untersuchungen Zur Frage der Harndesifizierenden Wirkungen von Barentraubenblatt-Extracten," *Planta Medica* 18 (1970): 1–25.

24. B. Larsson, A. Jonasson, and S. Fianu, "Prophylactic Effect of UVA-E in Women with Recurrent Cystitis: A Preliminary Report," *Curr Ther Res* 53 (1993): 441–3.

25. L. Avorn, M. Monane, et al., "Reduction of Bacteriuria and Pyuria after Ingestion of Cranberry Juice," *JAMA* 271 (1994): 751–4.

26. A.H. Amin, T.V. Subbaiah, and K.M. Abbasi, "Berberine Sulfate: Antimicrobial Activity, Bioassay, and Mode of Action," *Can J Microbiol* 15 (1969): 1067–76.

27. C.C. Johnson, G. Johnson, and C.F. Poe, "Toxicity of Alkaloids to Certain Bacteria," *Acta Pharmacol Toxicol* 8 (1952): 71–8.

Boils

1. L.M. Tierney, S.J. McPhee, and M.A. Papadakis, eds., *Current Medical Diagnosis and Treatment* (Los Altos, CA: Lange Medical Publications, 1997), 161–2.

2. P.M. Altman, "Australian Tea Tree Oil," *Australian J Pharmacy* 69 (1988): 276–8.

3. H.M. Feinblatt, "Cajeput-Type Oil for the Treatment of Furunculosis," *J Nat Med Assoc* 52 (1960): 32–4.

4. F.E. Hahn and J. Ciak, "Berberine," *Antibiotics* 3 (1976): 577–88.

5. C.C. Johnson, G. Johnson, and C.F. Poe, "Toxicity of Alkaloids to Certain Bacteria," *Acta Pharmacol Toxicol* 8 (1952): 71–8.

6. Y. Kumazawa, A. Itagaki, M. Fukumoto, et al., "Activation of Peritoneal Macrophages by Berberine Alkaloids in Terms of Induction of Cytostatic Activity," *Int J Immunopharmacol* 6 (1984): 587–92.

7. M. Sabir, M.H. Akhter, and N.K. Bhide, "Further Studies on Pharmacology of Berberine," *Ind J Physiol Pharmacol* 22 (1978): 9–23.

Bronchitis and Pneumonia

1. P.H. Orr et al., "Randomized Placebo-Controlled Trials of Antibiotics for Acute Bronchitis: A Critical Review of the Literature," *J Fam Practice* 36 (1993): 507–12.

2. R. Gonzales and M. Sande, "What Will It Take to Stop Physicians from Prescribing Antibiotics in Acute Bronchitis?" *Lancet* 345 (1995): 665.

3. F. Bicknell and F. Prescott, *The Vitamins in Medicine* (Minneapolis: Lee Foundation, 1953), 420, 473.

4. C. Hunt et al., "The Clinical Effects of Vitamin C Supplementation in Elderly Hospitalized Patients with Acute Respiratory Infections," *Internat J Vit Nutr Res* 64 (1994): 212–9.

5. R. Rimoldi, F. Ginesu, and R. Giura, "The Use of Bromelain in Pneumological Therapy," *Drugs Exp Clin Res* 4 (1978): 55–66.

6. R. Ryan, "A Double-Blind Clinical Evaluation of Bromelains in the Treatment of Acute Sinusitis," *Headache* 7 (1967): 13–7.

Candidiasis, Chronic

1. O. Truss, *The Missing Diagnosis* (Birmingham, AL: P.O. Box 26508, 1983).

2. W.G. Crook, *The Yeast Connection,* 2nd ed. (Jackson, TN: Professional Books, 1984).

3. G.F. Kroker, "Chronic Candidiasis and Allergy," in J. Brostoff and S.J. Challacombe, eds., *Food Allergy and Intolerance* (Philadelphia: W.B. Saunders, 1987), 850–72.

4. W.G. Crook, *The Yeast Connection and the Woman* (Jackson, TN: Professional Books, 1995).

5. D.S. Bauman and H.E. Hagglund, "Correlation Between Certain Polysystem Chronic Complaints and an Enzyme Immunoassay with Antigens of Candida albicans," *J Advancement Med* 4 (1991): 5–19.

6. M. Woodhead, "Antibiotic Resistance," *Brit J Hosp Med* 56 (1996): 314–5.

7. M. Cohen, "Epidemiology of Drug Resistance: Implications for a Post-Antibiotic Era," *Science* 257 (1992): 1050–5.

8. World Health Organization, *Fighting Disease, Fostering Development: Report of the Director General* (London: HMSO, 1996).

9. L. Demling, "Is Crohn's Disease Caused by Antibiotics?" *Hepato-Gastroenterol* 41 (1994): 549–51.

10. M. Boero et al., "Candida Overgrowth in Gastric Juice of Peptic Ulcer Subjects on Short- and Long-Term Treatment with H_2-Receptor Antagonists," *Digestion* 28 (1983): 158–63.

11. E. Rubinstein et al., "Antibacterial Activity of the Pancreatic Fluid," *Gastroenterol* 88 (1985): 927–32.

12. S.A. Sarker and R. Gyr, "Nonimmunological Defense Mechanisms of the Gut," *Gut* 33 (1990): 1331–7.

13. K. Iwata, "Toxins Produced by Candida albicans," *Contr Microbiol Immunol* 4 (1977): 77–85.

14. N.H. Axelson, "Analysis of Human Candida Precipitins by Quantitative Immunoelectrophoresis," *Scand J Immunol* 5 (1976): 177–90.

15. P. Cazzola, P. Mazzanti, and G. Bossi, "In Vivo Modulating Effect of a Calf Thymus Acid Lysate on Human T Lymphocyte Subsets and CD4+/CD8+ Ratio in the Course of Different Diseases," *Curr Ther Res* 42 (1987): 1011–7.

16. N.M. Kouttab, M. Prada, and P. Cazzola, "Thymomodulin: Biological Properties and Clinical Applications," *Medical Oncology and Tumor Pharmacotherapy* 6 (1989): 5–9.

17. A. Klein et al., "The Effect of Nonviral Liver Damage on the T-Lymphocyte Helper/Suppressor Ratio," *Clin Immunol Immunopathol* 46 (1988): 214–20.

18. F. Abe, S. Nagata, and M. Hotchi, "Experimental Candidiasis in Liver Injury," *Mycopathologica* 100 (1987): 37–42.

19. A.J. Barak et al., "Dietary Betaine Promotes Generation of Hepatic S-adenosylmethionine and Protects the Liver from Ethanol-Induced Fatty Infiltration," *Alcohol Clin Exp Res* 17 (1993): 552–5.

20. S.H. Zeisel et al., "Choline, an Essential Nutrient for Humans," *FASEB J* 5 (1991): 2093–8.

21. H.A. Salmi and S. Sarna, "Effect of Silymarin on Chemical, Functional, and Morphological Alteration of the Liver: A Double-Blind Controlled Study," *Scand J Gastroenterol* 17 (1982): 417–21.

22. C. Boari et al., "Occupational Toxic Liver Diseases: Therapeutic Effects of Silymarin," *Min Med* 72 (1985): 2679–88.

23. P. Ferenci et al., "Randomized Controlled Trial of Silymarin Treatment in Patients with Cirrhosis of the Liver," *J Hepatol* 9 (1989): 105–13.

24. D.J. Hentges, ed., "Human Intestinal Microflora," in *Health and Disease* (New York: Academic Press, 1983).

25. K.M. Shahani and B.A. Friend, "Nutritional and Therapeutic Aspects of Lactobacilli," *J Appl Nutr* 36 (1984): 125–52.

26. E.L. Keeney, "Sodium Caprylate: A New and Effective Treatment of Moniliasis of the Skin and Mucous Membrane," *Bull Johns Hopkins Hosp* 78 (1946): 333–9.

27. I. Neuhauser and E.L. Gustus, "Successful Treatment of Intestinal Moniliasis with Fatty Acid Resin Complex," *Arch Intern Med* 93 (1954): 53–60.

28. A.D. Scwhabe, L.R. Bennett, and L.P. Bowman, "Octanoic Acid Absorption and Oxidation in Humans," *J Applied Physiol* 19 (1964): 335–7.

29. F.E. Hahn and J. Ciak, "Berberine," *Antibiotics* 3 (1976): 577–88.

30. A.H. Amin, T.V. Subbaiah, and K.M. Abbasi, "Berberine Sulfate: Antimicrobial Activity, Bioassay, and Mode of Action," *Can J Microbiol* 15 (1969): 1067–76.

31. C.C. Johnson, G. Johnson, and C.F. Poe, "Toxicity of Alkaloids to Certain Bacteria," *Acta Pharmacol Toxicol* 8 (1952): 71–8.

32. Y. Kaneda et al., "In Vitro Effects of Berberine Sulfate on the Growth of *Entamoeba histolytica, Giardia lamblia,* and *Trichomonas vaginalis*," *Annals Trop Med Parasitol* 85 (1991): 417–25.

33. T.V. Subbaiah and A.H. Amin, "Effect of Berberine Sulfate on *Entamoeba histolytica*," *Nature* 215 (1967): 527–8.

34. A.K. Ghosh, "Effect of Berberine Chloride on *Leishmania donovani*," *Ind J Med Res* 78 (1983): 407–16.

35. V.M. Majahan, A. Sharma, and A. Rattan, "Antimycotic Activity of Berberine Sulphate: An Alkaloid from an Indian Medicinal Herb," *Sabouraudia* 20 (1982): 79–81.

36. S. Gupta, "Use of Berberine in the Treatment of Giardiasis," *Am J Dis Child* 129 (1975): 866.

37. M.P. Bhakat et al., "Therapeutic Trial of Berberine Sulphate in Non-Specific Gastroenteritis," *Ind Med J* 68 (1974): 19–23.

38. S.A. Kamat, "Clinical Trial with Berberine Hydrochloride for the Control of Diarrhoea in Acute Gastroenteritis," *J Assoc Physicians India* 15 (1967): 525–9.

39. A.B. Desai, K.M. Shah, and D.M. Shah, "Berberine in the Treatment of Diarrhoea," *Ind Pediatr* 8 (1971): 462–5.

40. R. Sharma, C.K. Joshi, and R.K. Goyal, "Berberine Tannate in Acute Diarrhea," *Ind Pediatr* 7 (1970): 496–501.

41. V.P. Choudry, M. Sabir, and V.N. Bhide, "Berberine in Giardiasis," *Ind Pediatr* 9 (1972): 143–6.

42. S.A. Kamat, "Clinical Trial with Berberine Hydrochloride for the Control of Diarrhoea in Acute Gastroenteritis," *J Assoc Physicians India* 15 (1967): 525–9.

43. S. Gupta, "Use of Berberine in Treatment of Giardiasis," *Am J Dis Child* 129 (1975): 866.

44. G.H. Rabbani et al., "Randomized Controlled Trial of Berberine Sulfate Therapy for Diarrhea due to Enterotoxigenic *Escherichia coli* and *Vibrio cholerae*," *J Infect Dis* 155 (1987): 979–84.

45. B. Hladon, "Toxicity of Berberine Sulfate," *Acta Pol Pharm* 32 (1975): 113–20.

46. G.S. Moore and R.D. Atkins, "The Fungicidal and Fungistatic Effects of an Aqueous Garlic Extract on Medically Important Yeast-Like Fungi," *Mycologia* 69 (1977): 341–8.

47. D.K. Sandhu, M.K. Warraich, and S. Singh, "Sensitivity of Yeasts Isolated from Cases of Vaginitis to Aqueous Extracts of Garlic," *Mykosen* 23 (1980): 691–8.

48. G. Prasad and V.D. Sharma, "Efficacy of Garlic (*Allium sativum*) Treatment Against Experimental Candidiasis in Chicks," *Br Vet J* 136 (1980): 448–51.

49. J.C. Stiles et al., "The Inhibition of *Candida albicans* by Oregano," *J Applied Nutr* 47 (1995): 96–102.

Canker Sores

1. C.W.M. Wilson, "Food Sensitivities, Taste Changes, Aphthous Ulcers, and Atopic Symptoms in Allergic Disease," *Ann Allergy* 44 (1980): 302–7.

2. R.A. Rays, F. Hamerlinck, and R.H. Cormane, "Immunoglobulin-Bearing Lymphocytes and Polymorphonuclear Leukocytes in Recurrent Aphthous Ulcers in Man," *Arch Oral Biol* 22 (1977): 147–53.

3. J.W. Little, "Food Allergens and Basophil Histamine Release in Recurrent Aphthous Stomatitis," *Oral Surgery* 54 (1982): 388–95.

4. K.D. Hay and P.C. Reade, "The Use of an Elimination Diet in the Treatment of Recurrent Aphthous Ulceration of the Oral Cavity," *Oral Surg* 57 (1984): 504–7.

5. A. Nolan et al., "Recurrent Aphthous Ulceration and Food Sensitivity," *J Oral Pathol Med* 20 (1991): 473–5.

6. R. Ferguson et al., "Jejunal Mucosal Abnormalities in Patients with Recurrent Aphthous Ulceration," *Br Med J* 1 (1975): 11–3.

7. M.M. Ferguson, D. Wray, H.A. Carmichael, et al., "Coeliac Disease Associated with Recurrent Aphthae," *Gut* 21 (1980): 223–6.

8. D. Wray, "Gluten-Sensitive Recurrent Aphthous Stomatitis," *Dig Dis Sci* 26 (1981): 737–40.

9. D.M. Walker et al., "Gluten Hypersensitivity in Recurrent Aphthous Ulceration," *J Dent Res* 58, Special Issue C (1979): 1271.

10. C. O'Farrelly et al., "Gliadin Antibodies Identify Gluten-Sensitive Oral Ulceration in the Absences of Villous Atrophy," *J Oral Pathol Med* 20 (1991): 476–8.

11. I.I. Ship, A.D. Merritt, and H.R. Stanley, "Recurrent Aphthous Ulcers," *Am J Med* 32 (1962): 32–43.

12. M. Haisraeli et al., "Recurrent Aphthous Stomatitis and Thiamine Deficiency," *Oral Surg Oral Med Oral Pathol Oral Radiol Endod* 82 (1996): 634–6.

13. D.W. Wray et al., "Nutritional Deficiencies in Recurrent Aphthae," *J Oral Path* 7 (1978): 418–23.

14. A. Nolan et al., "Recurrent Aphthous Ulceration: Vitamin B1, B2, and B6 Status and Response to Replacement Therapy," *J Oral Pathol Med* 20 (1991): 389–91.

15. D. Wray et al., "Recurrent Aphthae: Treatment with Vitamin B12, Folic Acid, and Iron," *Br Med J* 2 (1975): 490–3.

16. F.L. Pearce, A.D. Befus, and J. Bienenstock, "Mucosal Mast Cells III: Effect of Quercetin and Other Flavonoids on Antigen-Induced Histamine Secretion from Rat Intestinal Mast Cells," *J Allergy Clin Immunol* 73 (1984): 819–23.

17. M.J. Kowolik, K.F. Muir, and I.T. MacPhee, "Disodium Cromoglycate in the Treatment of Recurrent Aphthous Ulceration," *Br Dent J* 144 (1978): 384–9.

18. S.K. Das, A.K. Gulati, and V.P. Singh, "Deglycyrrhizinated Liquorice in Aphthous Ulcers," *J Assoc Physicians India* 37 (1989): 647.

Carpal Tunnel Syndrome

1. J.M. Ellis, K. Folkers, S. Shizukuishi, et al., "Response of Vitamin B6 Deficiency and the Carpal

Tunnel Syndrome to Pyridoxine," *Proc Natl Acad Sci USA* 79 (1982): 7494–8.

2. J.E. Fuhr, A. Farrow, and H.S. Nelson, Jr., "Vitamin B6 Levels in Patients with Carpal Tunnel Syndrome," *Arch Surg* 124 (1989): 1329–30.

3. G. Stransky, E. Wenger, L. Dimitrov, and S. Weis, "Collagen Dysplasia in Idiopathic Carpal Tunnel Syndrome," *Path Res Pract* 185 (1989): 795–98.

4. M.C.T.F.M. de Krom, A.D.M. Kester, P.G. Knipschild, and F. Spaans, "Risk Factors for Carpal Tunnel Syndrome," *AM J Epidemiol* 132 (1990): 1102–10.

6. J.N. Katz and C.R. Stirrat, "A Self-Administered Hand Diagram for the Diagnosis of Carpal Tunnel Syndrome," *J Hand Surg* 15A (1990): 360–3.

7. K. Folkers and J. Ellis, "Successful Therapy with Vitamin B6 and Vitamin B2 of the Carpal Tunnel Syndrome and Need for Determination of the RDAs for Vitamin B6 and B2 Disease States," *Annals NY Acad Sci* 585 (1990): 295–301.

8. J.M. Ellis and K. Folkers, "Clinical Aspects of Treatment of Carpal Tunnel Syndrome with B_6," *Annals NY Acad Sci* 585 (1990): 302–20.

9. K.A. Folkers, A. Wolaniuk, and S. Vadhanavikit, "Enzymology of the Response of Carpal Tunnel Syndrome to Riboflavin and to Combined Riboflavin and Pyridoxine," *Proc Nat Acad Sci* 81 (1984): 7076–78.

10. G.S. Phalen, "The Birth of a Syndrome, or Carpal Tunnel Syndrome Revisited," *J Hand Surg* 6 (1981): 109–10.

11. A. Franzblau et al., "The Relationship of Vitamin B6 Status to Median Nerve Function and Carpal Tunnel Syndrome Among Active Industrial Workers," *JOEM* 38 (1996): 485–91.

12. G.S. Chen, "The Effect of Acupuncture Treatment on Carpal Tunnel Syndrome," *Am J Acupunct* 18 (1990): 5–9.

13. H. Seradge, "Splints Aren't Enough; Hand Exercises Improve Carpal Tunnel Treatment," *Modern Med* 64 (1996):14–15.

14. G. Tassman, J. Zafran, and G. Zayon, "Evaluation of a Plant Proteolytic

Enzyme for the Control of Inflammation and Pain," *J Dent Med* 19 (1964): 73–7.

15. G. Tassman, J. Zafran, and G. Zayon, "A Double-Blind Crossover Study of a Plant Proteolytic Enzyme in Oral Surgery," *J Dent Med* 20 (1965): 51–4.

16. R. Howat and G. Lewis, "The Effect of Bromelain Therapy on Episiotomy Wounds: A Double-Blind Controlled Clinical Trial," *J Ob Gyn Br Commonwealth* 79 (1972): 951–3.

17. G. Zatuchni and D. Colombi, "Bromelaine Therapy for the Prevention of Episiotomy Pain," *Ob Gyn* 29 (1967): 275–8.

Cataracts

1. A. Taylor, "Cataract: Relationships Between Nutrition and Oxidation," *J Am Coll Nutr* 12 (1993): 138–46.

2. S. Bouton, "Vitamin C and the Aging Eye, "*Arch Int Med* 63 (1939): 930–45.

3. D. Atkinson, "Malnutrition as an Etiological Factor in Senile Cataract," *Eye, Ear, Nose and Throat Monthly* 31 (1952): 79–83.

4. A. Ringvold, H. Johnsen, and S. Blika, "Senile Cataract and Ascorbic Acid Loading," *Acta Ophthalmol* 63 (1985): 277–80.

5. W. Rathbun and S. Hanson, "Glutathione Metabolic Pathway as a Scavenging System in the Lens," *Ophthal Res* 11 (1979): 172–6.

6. A. Swanson and A. Truesdale, "Elemental Analysis in Normal and Cataractous Human Lens Tissue," *Biochem Biophys Res Comm* 45 (1971): 1488–96.

7. S. Karakucuk et al., "Selenium Concentrations in Serum, Lens, and Aqueous Humor of Patients with Senile Cataract," *Arch Opthalmol Scand* 73 (1995): 329–32.

8. P. Whanger and P. Weswig, "Effects of Selenium, Chromium, and Antioxidants on Growth, Eye Cataracts, Plasma Choles-terol, and Blood Glucose in Selenium-Deficient, Vitamin-E-Supplemented Rats," *Nutr Rep Int* 12 (1975): 345–58.

9. A. Swanson and A. Truesdale, "Elemental Analysis in Normal and

Cataractous Human Lens Tissue," *Biochem Biophys Res Comm* 45 (1971): 1488–96.

10. G.N. Rao and R.C. Cotlier, "The Enzymatic Activities of GTP Cyclohydrolase, Sepiapterin Reductase, Dihydropteridine Reductase, and Dihydrofolate Reductase; and Tetrahydrobiopterin Content in Mammalian Ocular Tissues and in Human Senile Cataracts," *Comp Biochem Physiol* 80B (1985): 61–6.

11. H. Skalka and J. Prchal, "Cataracts and Riboflavin Deficiency," *Am J Clin Nutr* 34 (1981): 861–3.

12. J. Prchal, M. Conrad, and H. Skalka, "Association of Pre-Senile Cataracts with Heterozygousity for Galactosemic States and Riboflavin Deficiency," *Lancet* 1 (1978): 12–3.

13. O. Hockwin, *Drug Treatment of Senile Lens Opacities: Analysis of Possible Ways and Means From the Aging Lens* (Paris: Elsevier/ North-Holland Biomedical Press, 1980), 281.

14. G. Burton and K. Ingold, "Beta-Carotene: An Unusual Type of Lipid Antioxidant," *Science* 224 (1984): 569–73.

15. R.J. Reiter et al., "Oxygen Radical Detoxification Processes During Aging: The Functional Importance of Melatonin," *Aging Clinical Exp Res* 7 (1995): 340–351.

16. A. Tavani et al., "Food and Nutrient Intake and Risk of Cataract," *Ann Epidem* 6 (1996): 41–46.

17. H. Hess, J.J. Knapka, D.A. Newsome, et al., "Dietary Prevention of Cataracts in the Pink-Eyed RCS Rat," *Lag Anim Sci* 35 (1985): 47–53.

18. E.L. Pautler, J.A. Maga, and C. Tengerdy, "A Pharmacologically Potent Natural Product in the Bovine Retina," *Exp Eye Res* 42 (1986): 285–8.

19. G. Bravetti, "Preventive Medical Treatment of Senile Cataract with Vitamin E and Anthocyanosides: Clinical Evaluation," *Ann Ottalmol Clin Ocul* 115 (1989): 109.

20. K. Fujihira, "Treatment of Cataract of Ba-wei-wan," *J Soc Oriental Med Jap* 24 (1974): 465–79.

21. H. Yoshida, "The Effects of Bawei-wan (Hachimijiogan) on Plasma Levels of High-Density Lipoprotein-Cholesterol and Lipoperoxide

in Aged Individuals," *Am J Chin Med* 13 (1985): 71–6.

Celiac Disease

1. S. Auricchio, "Gluten-Sensitive Enteropathy and Infant Nutrition," *J Ped Gastroenterol Nutr* 2(Suppl 1) (1983): S304–9.
2. S. Auricchio, D. Follo, G. deRitis et al., "Does Breast-Feeding Protect Against the Development of Clinical Symptoms of Celiac Disease in Children?" *J Ped Gastroenterol Nutr* 2 (1983): 428–33.
3. S.G. Cole and M.F. Kagnoff, "Celiac Disease," *Ann Rev Nutr* 5 (1985): 241–66.
4. S.P. Fallstrom, J. Winberg, and H.J. Anderson, "Cow's Milk Malabsorption as a Precursor of Gluten Intolerance," *Acta Paediatrica Scand* 54 (1965): 101–15.
5. B. McNicholl, B. Egan-Mitchell, F.M. Stevens, et al., "History, Genetics, and Natural History of Celiac Disease: Gluten Enteropathy," in *Food, Nutrition, and Evolution*, D.N. Walker and N. Kretchmer, eds. (New York: Masson Publishers, 1981), 169–78.
6. F.J. Simoons, "Celiac Disease as a Geographic Problem," in *Food, Nutrition, and Evolution*, D.N. Walker and N. Kretchmer, eds. (New York: Masson Publishers, 1981), 179–200.
7. D.D. Kasarda, "Toxic Proteins and Peptides in Celiac Disease: Relations to Cereal Genetics," in *Food, Nutrition, and Evolution*, D.N. Walker and N. Kretchmer, eds. (New York: Masson Publishers, 1981), 201–16.
8. J.E. Morley, A. Levine, T. Yamada, et al., "Effect of Exorphins on Gastrointestinal Function, Hormonal Release, and Appetite," *Gastroenterol* 84 (1983): 1517–23.
9. J.E. Morley, "Food Peptides: A New Class of Hormones," *JAMA* 247 (1982): 2379–80.
10. M.M. Singh and S.R. Kay, "Wheat Gluten as a Pathogenic Factor in Schizophrenia," *Science* 191 (1976): 401–2.
11. F.C. Dohan and J.C. Gasberger, "Relapsed Schizophrenics: Earlier Discharge from the Hospital After

Cereal-Free, Milk-Free Diet," *Am J Psychiatry* 130 (1973): 685–8.
12. F.C. Dohan, E.H. Harper, M.H. Clark, et al., "Is Schizophrenia Rare If Grain Is Rare?" *Biol Psychiatry* 19 (1984): 385–99.
13. S.L. Robbins, R.S. Cotran, and V. Kumar, *Pathologic Basis of Disease* (Philadelphia: W.B. Saunders, 1984), 847–8.
14. A. Ferguson, K. Ziegler, and S. Strobel, "Gluten Intolerance (Coeliac Disease)," *Annals Allergy* 53 (1984): 637–42.
15. C.M. Swinson, G. Slavin, E.C. Coles, and C.C. Booth, "Coeliac Disease and Malignancy," *Lancet* i (1983): 111–5.
16. B.T. Cooper, K.Y. Holmes, R. Ferguson, et al., "Celiac Disease and Malignancy," *Medicine* 59 (1980): 249–61.
17. C. O'Farrelly, C.A. Whelan, C.F. Feighery, D.G. Weir, "Suppressor-Cell Activity in Coeliac Disease Induced by Alpha-Gliadin, a Dietary Antigen," *Lancet* ii (1984): 1305–6.
18. L. Stenhammar, A.F. Kilander, L.A. Nilsson, et al., "Serum Gliadin Antibodies for Detection and Control of Childhood Coeliac Disease," *Acta Paediatr Scand* 73 (1984): 657–63.
19. A. Burgin-Wolff, R.M. Bertele, R. Berger, et al., "A Reliable Screening Test for Childhood Celiac Disease: Fluorescent Immunosorbent Test for Gliadin Antibodies," *J Pediatr* 102 (1983): 655–60.
20. G. Ferfoglia et al., "Do Dietary Antibodies Still Play a Role in the Diagnosis and Follow-Up of Coeliac Disease? A Comparison among Different Serological Tests," *Panminerva Med* 37 (1995): 55–9.
21. E.K. Janatuinen et al., "A Comparison of Diets with and without Oats in Adults with Celiac Disease," *New Eng J Med* 333 (1995): 1033–8.
22. M.V. Krause and K.L. Mahan, *Food, Nutrition, and Diet Therapy*, 7th ed. (Philadelphia: W.B. Saunders, 1984), 452–7.
23. A.H.G. Love, A. Elmes, M. Golden, et al., "Zinc Deficiency and Celiac Disease," in B. McNicholl, C.F. McCarthy, and P.F. Fotrell, eds., *Perspectives in Celiac Disease* (Baltimore, MD: University Press, 1978), 335–42.
24. A. Carroccio et al., "Pancreatic Enzyme Therapy in Childhood Celiac

Disease: A Double-Blind Prospective Randomized Study," *Dig Dis Sci* 40 (1995): 2555–2560.
25. A.H. Corwin, "The Rotating Diet and Taxonomy," in L.D. Dickey, *Clinical Ecology* (Springfield, IL: C.C. Thomas, 1976), 122–48.

Cellulite

1. C. Scherwitz and O. Braun-Falco, "So-Called Cellulite," *J Dermatol Surg Oncol* 4 (1978): 230–4.
2. F. Nurnberger and G. Muller, "So-Called Cellulite: An Invented Disease," *J Dermatol Surg Oncol* 4 (1978): 221–9.
3. F. Nurnberger, H. Mende, and P. Roedel,"Behandlungsergebnisse bei der Sog. 'Cellulitis' mit Verteilerenzymen im Einfachen Blindversuch," *Arch Dermatol Forsch* 29 (1972): 173–81.
4. F. Nurnberger and B. Schroter, "Behandlungsergebnisse bei der Sog. Zellulitis mit Verteilerenzymen im Doppelblindversuch," *Z Hautkr* 48 (1973): 1009–17.
5. D. Bourguignon, "Study of the Action of Titrated Extract of *Centella asiatica*," *Gaz Med Fr* 82 (1975): 4579–83.
6. A. Tenailleau, "On 80 Cases of Cellulitis Treated with the Standard Extract of *Centella asiatica*," *Quest Med* 31 (1978): 919–24.
7. G.F. Bonnett, "Treatment of Localized Cellulitis with Asiaticoside Madecassol," *Progr Med* 102 (1974): 109–10.
8. C. Allegra, "Comparative Capillaroscopic Study of Certain Bioflavonoids and Total Triterpenic Fractions of *Centella asiatica* in Venous Insufficiency," *Clin Terap* 110 (1984): 555–9.
9. J.P. Pointel, H. Boccalon, M. Cloarec, et al., "Titrated Extract of *Centella asiatica* (TECA) in the Treatment of Venous Insufficiency of the Lower Limbs," *Angiology* 38 (1987): 46–50.
10. *Monograph: Escin* (Milan, Italy: Indena S.p.A., 1987).
11. F. Aichinger, G. Giss, and G. Vogel, "Neue Befunde zur Pharmakodynamik von Bioflavoiden und des Rosskastanien Saponins Aescin als

Grundlage Ihrer Anwendung in der Therapie," *Arzneim Forsch* 14 (1964): 892.

12. P. Manca and E. Passarelli, "Aspetti Farmacologici Dell'Escina, Principio Attivo Dell'*Aesculus hyppocastanum*," *Clin Terap* (1965): 297–328.

13. *Monograph: Bladderwrack* (Milan, Italy: Indena S.p.A., 1987).

Cerebral Vascular Insufficiency

1. H.J.M. Barnett, R.W. Barnes, and J.T. Robertson, "The Uncertainties Surrounding Carotic Endarterectomy," *JAMA* 268 (1992): 3120–1.

2. N.C. Fode et al., "Multicenter Retrospective Review of Results and Complications of Carotid Endarterectomy," *Stroke* 17 (1986): 370–6.

3. C.M. Winslow et al., "The Appropriateness of Carotid Endarterectomy," *N Engl J Med* 318 (1988): 721–7.

4. NASCET Collaborators, "Beneficial Effect of Carotid Endarterectomy in Symptomatic Patients with High-Grade Carotid Stenosis," *N Eng J Med* 325 (1991): 445–53.

5. European Carotid Surgery Trialists Collaborative Group, "MRC European Surgery Trial: Interim Results for Symptomatic Patients with Severe (70-99%) or with Mild (0-29%) Carotid Stenosis," *Lancet* 337 (1991): 1235–43.

6. J.D. Easton and J.L. Wilterdink, "Carotid Endarterectomy: Trials and Tribulations," *Ann Neurol* 35 (1994): 5–17.

7. G. Abate et al., "Controlled Multicenter Study on the Therapeutic Effectiveness of Mesoglycan in Patients with Cerebrovascular Disease," *Minerva Med* 82(3) (1991): 101–5.

8. D. Mansi et al., "Open Trial of Mesoglycan in the Treatment of Cerebrovascular Ischemic Disease," *Acta Neurologica* 10 (1988): 108–12.

9. F. Vecchio et al., "Mesoglycan in Treatment of Patients with Cerebral Ischemia: Effects on Hemorrheologic and Hematochemical Parameters," *Acta Neurol* 15(6) (1993): 449–56.

10. J. Kleijnen and P. Knipschild, "*Ginkgo biloba* for Cerebral Insufficiency," *Br J Clinical Pharmacol* 34 (1992): 352–8.

11. U. Schmidt, K. Rabinovici, and S. Lande, "Einfluss eines *Ginkgo biloba* specialextraktes auf doe befomdlickeit bei zerebraler onsuffiizienz," *Munch Med Wockenschr* 133(suppl.1) (1991): S15–8.

12. E. Bruchert, S.E. Heinrich, and P. Ruf-Kohler, "Wirksamkeit von LI 1370 bei alteren Patienten mit Himleistungsschwache. Multizentrische Doppelblindstudie des fachverbandes deutscher Allgmeinaezte," *Munch Med Wockenschr* 133 (suppl.1) (1991) S9–S14.

13. B. Meyer, "Etude multicentrique randomisee a double insu face au placebo due traitment des acouphenes par l'extrait de *Gingko biloba*," *Presse Med* 15 (1986): 1562–4.

14. J. Taillandier et al., "Traitment des troubles du vidillissement cerebral pal l'extrait *Ginkgo biloba*," *Presse Med* 15 (1986): 1583–7.

15. J.P. Haguenauer et al., "Traitment des troubles de l'equilibre par l'extrai *Ginkgo biloba*," *Presse Med* 15 (1986): 1569–72.

16. G. Vorberg, U. Schmidt, and N. Schenk, "Wirksamkeit eines neuen *Ginkgo biloba* extraktes bei 100 patienten mit zerebraler insuffizienz," *Herg + Gefasse* 9 (1989): 936–41.

17. F. Eckmann, "Himleistungsstorungen—Behandlung mit *Ginkgo biloba* extrakt," *Fortsch Med* 108 (1990): 557–60.

18. K. Wesnes et al., "A Double-Blind Placebo-Controlled Trial of Tanakan in the Treatment of Idiopathic Cognitive Impairment in the Elderly," *Hum Psychopharmacol* 2 (1987): 159–69.

19. I. Anadere, H. Chmiel, and S. Witte, "Hemorrheological Findings in Patients with Completed Stroke and the Influence of *Ginkgo biloba* Extract," *Clin Hemorrheo* 4 (1985): 411–20.

Cervical Dysplasia

1. S. Robbins and R. Cotran, *Pathologic Basis of Disease*, 3rd ed.

(Philadelphia: W.B. Saunders, 1984), 1123–8.

2. P. Rubin, *Clinical Oncology*, 6th ed. (Philadelphia: American Cancer Society, 1983), 458–67.

3. E. Clarke, R. Morgan, and A. Newman, "Smoking as a Risk Factor in Cancer of the Cervix: Additional Evidence from a Case-Control Study," *Am J Epid* 115 (1982): 59–66.

4. J. Lyon, J. Gardner, D. West, et al., "Smoking and Carcinoma *in situ* of the Uterine Cervix," *Am J Public Health* 73 (1983): 558–562.

5. J. Marshall, S. Graham, T. Byers, M. Swanson, and J. Brasure, "Diet and Smoking in the Epidemiology of Cancer of the Cervix," *J Natl Cancer Instit* 70 (1983): 847–851.

6. E. Clarke, J. Hatcher, G. McKeown-Eyssen, and G. Liekrish, "Cervical Dysplasia: Association with Sexual Behavior, Smoking, and Oral Contraceptive Use," *Am J Ob Gyn* 151 (1985): 612–6.

7. O. Pelleter, "Vitamin C and Tobacco," *Int J Vit Nutr Res* 16 (1977): 147–169.

8. R. Hoover, C. Bain, P. Cole, and B. Macmahon, "Oral Contraceptive Use: Association with Frequency of Hospitalization and Chronic Disease Risk Indicators," *Am J Public Health* 68 (1978): 335–341.

9. "World Health Organization Collaborative Study of Neoplasia and Steroid Contraceptives: Invasive Cervical Cancer and Combined Oral Contraceptives," *Br Med J* 290 (1983): 961–3.

10. M. Vessey, M. Lawless, K. McPherson, and D. Yeates, "Neoplasia of the Cervix Uteri and Contraception: A Possible Adverse Effect of the Pill," *Lancet* ii (1983): 930–4.

11. M. Krause and L. Mahan, *Food, Nutrition, and Diet Therapy*, 7th ed. (Philadelphia: W.B. Saunders, 1984).

12. J. Orr, K. Wilson, C. Bodiford, et al., "Nutritional Status of Patients with Untreated Cervical Cancer, I: Biochemical and Immunologic Assessment," *Am J Ob Gyn* 151 (1985): 625–631.

13. J. Orr, K. Wilson, C. Bodiford, et al., "Nutritional Status of Patients with Untreated Cervical Cancer, II: Vitamin Assessment," *Am J Ob Gyn* 151 (1985): 632–5.

14. C. La Vecchia, S. Franceshi, A. De-carlli, et al., "Dietary Vitamin A and the Risk of Invasive Cervical Cancer," *Int J Cancer* 34 (1984): 319–22.

15. S. Romney, P. Palan, C. Duttagupta, et al., "Retinoids and the Prevention of Cervical Dysplasia," *Am J Ob Gyn* 141 (1981): 890–4.

16. J. Wylie-Rosett, S. Romney, S. Slagel, et al., "Influence of Vitamin A on Cervical Dysplasia and Carcinoma *in situ*," *Nutr Cancer* 6 (1984): 49–57.

17. S. Wassertheil-Smoller, S. Romney, J. Wylie-Rosett, et al., "Dietary Vitamin C and Uterine Cervical Dysplasia," *Am J Epid* 114 (1981): 714–24.

18. S. Romney, C. Duttagupta, J. Basu, et al., "Plasma Vitamin C and Uterine Cervical Dysplasia," *Am J Ob Gyn* 151 (1985): 978–80.

19. W. Van Niekerk, "Cervical Cytological Abnormalities Caused by Folic Acid Deficiency," *Acta Cytol* 10 (1966): 67–73.

20. D. Kitay and B. Wentz, "Cervical Cytology in Folic Acid Deficiency of Pregnancy," *Am J Ob Gyn* 104 (1969): 931–8.

21. R. Streiff, "Folate Deficiency and Oral Contraceptives," *JAMA* 214 (1970): 105–8.

22. N. Whitehead, F. Reyner, and J. Lindenbaum, "Megaloblastic Changes in the Cervical Epithelium Association with Oral Contraceptive Therapy and Reversal with Folic Acid," *JAMA* 226 (1973): 1421–4.

23. C.E. Butterworth et al., "Folate Deficiency and Cervical Dysplasia," *JAMA* 267 (1992): 528–33.

24. J.M. Harper et al., "Erythrocyte Folate Levels, Oral Contraceptive Use, and Abnormal Cervical Cytology," *Acta Cytol* 38 (1994): 324–30.

25. C.E. Butterworth et al., "Oral Folic Acid Supplementation for Cervical Dysplasia: A Clinical Intervention Trial," *Am J Obstet Gynecol* 166 (1992): 803–9.

26. C. Butterworth et al., "Improvement in Cervical Dysplasia Associated with Folic Acid Therapy in Users of Oral Contraceptives," *Am J Clin Nutr* 35 (1982): 73–82.

27. P. Ramaswamy and R. Natarajan, "Vitamin B6 Status in Patients with Cancer of the Uterine Cervix," *Nutr Cancer* 6 (1984): 176–180.

28. K. Prasad, ed., *Vitamins, Nutrition, and Cancer* (New York: Karger, 1984).

29. E. Dawson, J. Nosovitch, and E. Hannigan, "Serum Vitamin and Selenium Changes in Cervical Dysplasia," *Fed Proc* 43 (1984): 612.

Cholesterol

1. National Research Council, *Diet and Health: Implications for Reducing Chronic Disease Risk* (Washington, DC: National Academy Press, 1989).

2. P.W.F. Wilson, "High-Density Lipoprotein, Low-Density Lipoprotein, and Coronary Artery Disease," *Am J Cardiol* 66 (1990): 7A–10A.

3. A.M. Scanu and G.M. Fless, "Lipoprotein(a): A Genetic Risk Factor for Premature Coronary Heart Disease," *JAMA* 267 (1992): 3326–9.

4. E.J. Schaefer et al., "Lipoprotein(a) Levels and Risk of Coronary Heart Disease in Men: The Lipid Research Clinics Coronary Primary Prevention Trial," *JAMA* 271 (1994): 999–1003.

5. A.W.C. Kung, R.W.C. Pang, and E.D. Janus, "Elevated Serum Lipoprotein(a) in Subclinical Hypothyroidism," *Clin Endocrinol* 43 (1995): 445–9.

6. T.B. Neman and S.B. Hulley, "Carcinogenicity of Lipid-Lowering Drugs," *JAMA* 275 (1996): 55–60.

7. P.L. Canner et al., "Fifteen-Year Mortality in Coronary Drug Project Patients: Long-Term Benefit with Niacin," *J Am Coll Cardiol* 8 (1986): 1245–55.

8. J.R. DiPalma and W.S. Thayer, "Use of Niacin as a Drug," *Ann Rev Nutr* 11 (1991): 169–87.

9. Committee of Principal Investigators, "World Health Organization Clofibrate Trial: A Co-Operative Trial in the Primary Prevention of Ischemic Heart Disease Using Clofibrate," *Br Heart J* 40 (1978): 1069–1118.

10. Lovastatin Study Groups I through IV, "Lovastatin 5-Year Safety and Efficacy Study," *Arch Intern Med* 153 (1993): 1079–87.

11. D.R. Illingworth et al., "Comparative Effects of Lovastatin and Niacin in Primary Hypercholesterolemia," *Arch Intern Med* 154 (1994): 1586–95.

12. L.A. Carlson, A. Hamsten, and A. Asplund, "Pronounced Lowering of Serum Levels of Lipoprotein Lp(a) in Hyperlipidaemic Subjects Treated with Nicotinic Acid," *J Intern Med* 226 (1989): 271–6.

13. G.L. Vega and S.M. Grundy, "Lipoprotein Responses to Treatment with Lovastatin, Gemfibrozil, and Nicotinic Acid in Normolipidemic Patients with Hypoalphalipoproteinemia," *Arch Intern Med* 154 (1994): 73–82.

14. J.M. McKenney et al., "A Comparison of the Efficacy and Toxic Effects of Sustained- vs Immediate-Release Niacin in Hypercholesterolemic Patients," *JAMA* 271 (1994): 672–7.

15. A.L. Welsh and M. Ede, "Inositol Hexanicotinate for Improved Nicotinic Acid Therapy," *Int Record Med* 174 (1961): 9–15.

16. A.M.A. El-Enein et al., "The Role of Nicotinic Acid and Inositol Hexaniacinate as Anticholesterolemic and Antilipemic Agents," *Nutr Rep Intl* 28 (1983): 899–911.

17. G.T. Sunderland, J.J.F. Belch, R.D. Sturrock, et al., "A Double-Blind Randomised Placebo Controlled Trial of Hexopal in Primary Raynaud's Disease," *Clin Rheumatol* 7 (1988): 9.

18. L. Arsenio, P. Bodria, G. Magnati, et al., "Effectiveness of Long-Term Treatment with Pantethine in Patients with Dyslipidemias," *Clin Ther* 8 (1986): 537–45.

19. A. Gaddi, et al., "Controlled Evaluation of Pantethine, a Natural Hypolipidemic Compound, in Patients with Different Forms of Hyperlipoproteinemia," *Atheroscl* 50 (1984): 73–83.

20. F. Coronel et al., "Treatment of Hyperlipidemia in Diabetic Patients on Dialysis with a Physiological Substance," *Am J Nephrol* 11(1) (1991): 32–6.

21. C. Donati, R.S. Bertieri, and G. Barbi, "Pantethine, Diabetes Mellitus, and Atherosclerosis: Clinical Study of 1045 Patients," *Clin Ter* 128(6) (1989): 411–22.

22. K. Hiramatsu, H. Nozaki, and S. Arimori, "Influence of Pantethine on

Platelet Volume, Microviscosity, Lipid Composition, and Functions in Diabetes Mellitus with Hyperlipidemia," *Tokai J Exp Clin Med* 6(1) (1981): 49–57.

23. J.A. Simon, "Vitamin C and Cardiovascular Disease: A Review," *J Am Coll Nutr* 11 (1992): 107–25.

24. P.A. Howard and D.G. Meyers, "Effect of Vitamin C on Plasma Lipids," *Pharmacother* 29 (1995): 1129–36.

25. P.F. Jacques et al., "Ascorbic Acid and Plasma Lipids," *Epidemiol* 5 (1994): 19–26.

26. J. Hallfrisch et al., "High Plasma Vitamin C Associated with High Plasma HDL- and HDL2 Cholesterol," *Am J Clin Nutr* 60 (1994): 100–5.

27. H. Kock and L. Lawson, eds., *Garlic: The Science and Therapeutic Application of Allium Sativum L and Related Species,* 2nd ed. (Baltimore, MD: Williams & Wilkins, 1996).

28. M. Steiner et al., "A Double-Blind Crossover Study in Moderately Hypercholesterolemic Men That Compared the Effect of Aged Garlic Extract and Placebo Administration on Blood Lipids," *Am J Clin Nutr* 64 (1996): 866–70.

29. J. Kleijnen et al., "Garlic, Onions, and Cardiovascular Risk Factors: A Review of the Evidence from Human Experiments with Emphasis on Commercially Available Preparations," *Br J Clin Pharmacol* 28 (1989): 535–44.

30. S. Warshafsky, R.S. Kamer, and S.L. Sivak, "Effect of Garlic on Total Serum Cholesterol," *Ann Intern Med* 119 (1993): 599–605.

31. A.K. Jain et al., "Can Garlic Reduce Levels of Serum Lipids? A Controlled Clinical Study," *Am J Med* 94 (1993): 632–5.

32. W. Rotzch et al., "Postprandial Lipaemia under Treatment with *Allium sativum:* Controlled Double-Blind Study in Healthy Volunteers with Reduced HDL$_2$- Cholesterol Levels," *Arzneim Forsch* 42 (1992): 1223–7.

33. F.H. Mader, "Treatment of Hyperlipidemia with Garlic-Powder Tablets," *Arzneim Forsch* 40 (1990): 1111–6.

34. C.A. Silagy and H.A. Neil, "A Meta-Analysis of the Effect of Garlic on Blood Pressure," *J Hypertens* 12 (1994): 463–8.

35. H.D. Reuter, "*Allium sativum* and *Allium ursinum,* Part 2: Pharmacology and Medicinal Application," *Phytomed* 2 (1995): 73–91.

36. B.S. Kendler, "Garlic *(Allium sativum)* and Onion *(Allium cepa):* A Review of Their Relationship to Cardiovascular Disease," *Prev Med* 16 (1987): 670–85.

37. E. Ernst, "Cardiovascular Effects of Garlic *(Allium sativum):* A Review," *Pharmatherapeutica* 5 (1987): 83–9.

38. G.S. Sainani et al., "Effect of Dietary Garlic and Onion on Serum Lipid Profile in the Jain Community," *Ind J Med Res* 69 (1979): 776–80.

39. G.V. Satyavati, "Gugulipid: A Promising Hypolipidaemic Agent from Gum Guggul *(Commiphora wightii),*" *Econ Med Plant Res* 5 (1991): 47–82.

40. S. Nityanand, J.S. Srivastava, and O.P. Asthana, "Clinical Trials with Gugulipid, a New Hypolipidaemic Agent," *J Assoc Phys India* 37 (1989): 321–8.

Chronic Fatigue Syndrome

1. G.P. Holmes et al., "Chronic Fatigue Syndrome: A Working Case Definition," *Ann Intern Med* 108 (1988): 387–9.

2. D.W. Bates et al., "Prevalence of Fatigue and Chronic Fatigue Syndrome in a Primary Care Practice," *Arch Int Med* 153 (1993): 2759–65.

3. S.D. Shafran, "The Chronic Fatigue Syndrome," *Am J Med* 90 (1991): 731–9.

4. D.V. Kyle and R.D. Deshazo, "Chronic Fatigue Syndrome: A Conundrum," *Am J Med Sci* 303 (1992): 28–34.

5. A.L. Komaroff, "Chronic Fatigue Syndromes: Relationship to Chronic Viral Infections," *J Virol Meth* 21 (1988): 3–10.

6. J.F. Jones et al., "Evidence for Active Epstein-Barr Virus Infection in Patients with Persistent Unexplained Illness: Elevated Anti-Early Antigen Antibodies," *Ann Intern Med* 102 (1985): 1–7.

7. S.E. Straus et al., "Persisting Illness and Fatigue in Adults with Evidence of Epstein-Barr Virus Infection," *Ann Intern Med* 102 (1985): 7–16.

8. G.P. Holmes et al., "A Cluster of Patients with a Chronic Mononucleosis-Like Syndrome: Is Epstein-Barr Virus the Cause?" *JAMA* 257 (1987): 2297–302.

9. M. Caligiuri et al., "Phenotypic and Functional Deficiency of Natural Killer Cells in Patients with Chronic Fatigue Syndrome," *J Immunol* 139 (1987): 3306–13.

10. S. Gupta and B. Vayuvegula, "A Comprehensive Immunological Analysis in Chronic Fatigue Syndrome," *Scand J Immunol* 33 (1991): 319–27.

11. A. Komaroff and D. Goldenberg, "The Chronic Fatigue Syndrome: Definition, Current Studies, and Lessons for Fibromyalgia Research," *J Rheumatol* 16 (Suppl.19) (1989): 23–7.

12. D.S. Bell, "Chronic Fatigue Syndrome Update," *Postgrad Med* 96 (1994): 73–81.

13. D. Buchwald, D.L. Garrity, "Comparison of Patients with Chronic Fatigue Syndrome, Fibromyalgia, and Multiple Chemical Sensitivities," *Arch Int Med* 154 (1994): 2049–53.

14. J.S. Bland, E. Barrager, R.G. Reedy, and K. Bland, "A Medical Food-Supplemented Detoxification Program in the Management of Chronic Health Problems," *Alt Ther* 1 (1995): 62–71.

15. A.H. Rowe and A. Rowe, Jr., *Food Allergy: Its Manifestations and Control and the Elimination Diets: A Compendium* (Springfield, IL: Charles C. Thomas, 1972).

16. J.C. Breneman, *Basics of Food Allergy* (Springfield, IL: Charles C. Thomas, 1977).

17. B.O. Barnes and L. Galton, *Hypothyroidism: The Unsuspected Illness* (New York: Thomas Crowell, 1976).

18. S.E. Langer and J.F. Scheer, *Solved: The Riddle of Illness* (New Canaan, CT: Keats, 1984).

19. M. Gold, A. Pottash, and I. Extein, "Hypothyroidism and Depression, Evidence from Complete Thyroid Function Evaluation," *JAMA* 245 (1981): 1919–22.

20. A. Winokur et al., "Insulin Resistance after Glucose Tolerance Testing in Patients with Major Depression," *Am J Psychiatry* 145 (1988): 325–30.

21. J.H. Wright et al., "Glucose Metabolism in Unipolar Depression," *Br J Psychiatry* 132 (1978): 386–93.

22. J.W. Tinera, "The Hypoadrenocortical State and Its Management," *NY State Med J* 55 (1955): 1869–76.

23. M.A. Demitrack, "Chronic Fatigue Syndrome: A Disease of the Hypothalamic-Pituitary-Adrenal Axis?" *Ann Med* 26 (1994): 1–3.

24. C.J. Estler, H.P. Ammon, and C. Herzog, "Swimming Capacity of Mice After Prolonged Treatment with Psychostimulants, I: Effects of Caffeine on Swimming Performance and Cold Stress," *Psychopharmacol* 58 (1978): 161–6.

25. J.R. Hughes et al., "Caffeine Self-Administration, Withdrawal, and Adverse Effects among Coffee Drinkers," *Arch Gen Psych* 48 (1991): 611–7.

26. I.M. Cox, M.J. Campbell, and D. Dowson, "Red Blood Cell Magnesium and Chronic Fatigue Syndrome," *Lancet* 337 (1991): 757–60.

27. H. Ahlborg, L.G. Ekelund, and C.G. Nilsson, "Effect of Potassium-Magnesium Aspartate on the Capacity for Prolonged Exercise in Man," *Acta Physiologica Scandinavia* 74 (1968): 238–45.

28. J.T. Hicks, "Treatment of Fatigue in General Practice: A Double Blind Study," *Clin Med* Jan (1964): 85–90.

29. H.S. Friedlander, "Fatigue as a Presenting Symptom: Management in General Practice," *Curr Ther Res* 4 (1962): 441–9.

30. D.L. Shaw, "Management of Fatigue: A Physiologic Approach," *Am J Med Sci* 243 (1962): 758–69.

31. L. Gullestad et al., "Oral Versus Intravenous Magnesium Supplementation in Patients with Magnesium Deficiency," *Magnes Trace Elem* 10 (1991): 11–6.

32. J.S. Lindberg et al., "Magnesium Bioavailability from Magnesium Citrate and Magnesium Oxide," *J Am Coll Nutr* 9 (1990): 48–55.

33. M.E. Farmer et al., "Physical Activity and Depressive Symptomatology: The NHANES 1 Epidemiologic Follow-Up Study," *Am J Epidemiol* 1328 (1988): 1340–51.

34. M.A. Fiatarone et al., "The Effect of Exercise on Natural Killer Cells Activity in Young and Old Subjects," *J Gerontol* 44 (1989): M37–45.

35. L.T. Makinnon, "Exercise and Natural Killer Cells: What Is Their Relationship?" *Sports Med* 7 (1989): 141–9.

36. S. Xusheng, X. Yugi, and X. Yunjian, "Determination of E-Rosette-Forming Lymphocytes in Aged Subjects with Tai Chi Quan Exercise," *Int J Sport Med* 10 (1989): 217–9.

37. L. Fitzgerald, "Exercise and the Immune System," *Immunol Today* 9 (1988): 337–9.

38. B. Bohn, C.T. Nebe, and C. Birr, "Flow-Cytometric Studies with *Eleutherococcus senticosus* Extract as an Immunomodulatory Agent," *Arzneim Forsch* 37 (1987): 1193–6.

39. R. Baschetti, "Chronic Fatigue Syndrome and Liquorice (Letter)," *New Zealand Med J* 108 (1995): 156–7.

40. F.C. Stormer, R. Reistad, and J. Alexander, "Glycyrrhizic Acid in Liqourice: Evaluation of Health Hazard," *Fd Chem Toxicol* 31 (1993): 303–12.

41. J. Baron et al., "Metabolic Studies, Aldosterone Secretion Rate and Plasma Renin after Carbonoxolone Sodium as Biogastrone," *Br Med J* 2 (1969):

Common Cold

1. A. Sanchez et al., "Role of Sugars in Human Neutrophilic Phagocytosis," *Am J Clin Nutr* 26 (1973): 1180–4.

2. W. Ringsdorf, E. Cheraskin, and R. Ramsay, "Sucrose, Neutrophil Phagocytosis, and Resistance to Disease," *Dent Surv* 52 (1976): 46–8.

3. J. Bernstein et al., "Depression of Lymphocyte Transformation Following Oral Glucose Ingestion," *Am J Clin Nutr* 30 (1977): 613.

4. L. Pauling, *Vitamin C and the Common Cold* (San Francisco: Freeman, 1970).

5. H. Hemila, "Vitamin C and the Common Cold," *Br J Nutr* 67 (1992): 3–16.

6. H. Hemila and W. Herman, "Vitamin C and the Common Cold: A Retrospective Analysis of Chalmers' Review," *J Am Coll Nutr* 14 (1995): 116–23.

7. E. Katz and E. Margalith, "Inhibition of Vaccinia Virus Maturation by Zinc Chloride," *Antimicrobial Agents Chemotherapy* 19 (1981): 213–7.

8. G.A. Eby, D.R. Davis, and W.W. Halcomb, "Reduction in Duration of Common Colds by Zinc Gluconate Lozenges in a Double-Blind Study," *Antimicrob Agents Chemother* 25 (1984): 20–4.

9. S.B. Mossad et al., "Zinc Gluconate Lozenges for Treating the Common Cold: A Randomized, Double-Blind, Placebo-Controlled Study," *Ann Int Med* 125 (1996): 142–4.

10. J.E. Zarembo et al., "Zinc (II) in Saliva: Determination of Concentrations Produced by Different Formulations of Zinc Gluconate Lozenges Containing Common Excipients," *J Pharm Sci* 81 (1992): 128–30.

11. D. Melchart et al., "Immunomodulation with Echinacea: A Systemic Review of Controlled Clinical Trials," *Phytomed* 1 (1994): 245–54.

12. B. Braunig et al., "*Echinacea purpurea radix* for Strengthening the Immune Response in Flu-Like Infections," *Z Phytother* 13 (1992): 7–13.

13. D. Schoneberger, "The Influence of Immune-Stimulating Effects of Pressed Juice from Echinacea purpurea on the Course and Severity of Colds: Results of a Double-Blind Study," *Forum Immunologie* 8 (1992): 2–12.

Depression

1. M. Seligman, *Learned Optimism* (New York: Knopf, 1991).

2. C. Peterson, M. Seligman, and G. Valliant, "Pessimistic Explanatory Style as a Risk Factor for Physical Illness: A Thirty-Five Year Longitudinal Study," *J Person Soc Psych* 55 (1988): 23–7.

3. C. Peterson, "Explanatory Style as a Risk Factor for Illness," *Cognitive Therapy and Research* 12 (1988): 117–30.

4. R.B. Jarrett and A.J. Rush, "Short-Term Psychotherapy of Depressive Disorders: Current Status and Future Directions," *Psychiatry* 57 (1994): 115–32.

5. C.J. Robins and A.M. Hayes, "An Appraisal of Cognitive Therapy," *J Consult Clin Psychol* 61 (1993): 205–14.

6. M. Evans et al., "Differential Relapse Following Cognitive Therapy and Pharmacotherapy for Depression," *Arch Gen Psychiatry* 49 (1992): 802–8.

7. M. Gold, A. Pottash, and I. Extein, "Hypothyroidism and Depression, Evidence from Complete Thyroid Function Evaluation," *JAMA* 245 (1981): 1919–22.

8. R. Joffe, P. Roy-Byrne, and T. Udhe, "Thyroid Function and Affective Illness: A Reappraisal," *Biol Psychiatry* 19 (1984): 1685–91.

9. B.J. Carroll, G.C. Curtis, and J. Mendels, "Cerebrospinal Fluid and Plasma Free Cortisol Concentrations in Depression," *Psychol Med* 6 (1976): 235–44.

10. R. Baldessarini and G. Arana, "Does the Dexamethasone Suppression Test Have Clinical Utility in Psychiatry?" *J Clin Psychiatry* 46 (1985): 25–9.

11. C. Banki, M. Arato and Z. Papp, "Thyroid Stimulation Test in Healthy Subjects and Psychiatric Patients," *Acta Psychiatr Scand* 70 (1984): 295–303.

12. C. Altar et al., "Glucocorticoid Induction of Tryptophan Oxygenase," *Biochem Pharmacol* 32 (1983): 979–84.

13. R.S. Schottenfeld and M.R. Cullen, "Organic Affective Illness Associated with Lead Intoxication," *Am J Psychiat* 141 (1984): 1423–6.

14. M. Rutter and R. Russell-Jones, eds., *Lead versus Health: Sources and Effects of Low Level Lead Exposure* (New York: John Wiley, 1983).

15. A. Seaton, E.H. Jeelinek, and P. Kennedy, "Major Neurological Disease and Occupational Exposure to Organic Solvents," *Quart J Med* 305 (1992): 707–12.

16. R. Kinsman and J. Hood, "Some Behavioral Effects of Ascorbic Acid Deficiency," *Am J Clin Nutr* 24 (1971): 455–64.

17. T. Chou, "Wake Up and Smell the Coffee: Caffeine, Coffee, and the Medical Consequences," *West J Med* 157 (1992): 544–53.

18. K. Gilliand and W. Bullick, "Caffeine: A Potential Drug of Abuse," *Adv Alcohol Subst Abuse* 3 (1984): 53–73.

19. J. Greden et al., "Anxiety and Depression Associated with Caffeinism among Psychiatric Patients," *Am J Psychiatry* 131 (1979): 1089–94.

20. J.F. Neil et al., "Caffeinism Complicating Hypersomnic Depressive Disorders," *Compr Psychiatry* 19 (1978): 377–85.

21. D. Charney, G. Henninger, and P. Jatlow, "Increased Anxiogenic Effects of Caffeine in Panic Disorders," *Arch Gen Psychiatry* 42 (1984): 233–43.

22. S. Bolton and G. Null, "Caffeine, Psychological Effects, Use, and Abuse," *J Orthomol Psychiatry* 10 (1981): 202–11.

23. K. Kreitsch et al., "Prevalence, Presenting Symptoms, and Psychological Characteristics of Individuals Experiencing a Diet-Related Mood Disturbance," *Behav Ther* 19 (1985): 593–4.

24. L. Christensen, "Psychological Distress and Diet: Effects of Sucrose and Caffeine," *J Apl Nutr* 40 (1988): 44–50.

25. J.E. Martin and P.M. Dubbert, "Exercise Applications and Promotion in Behavioral Medicine," *J Consult Clin Psychol* 50 (1982): 1004–17.

26. S. Weyerer and B. Kupfer, "Physical Exercise and Psychological Health," *Sports Med* 17 (1994): 108–16.

27. Daniel Carr et al., "Physical Conditioning Facilitates the Exercised-Induced Secretion of Beta-Endorphin and Beta-Lipoprotein in Women," *New Engl J Med* 305 (1981): 560–5.

28. D. Lobstein, B.J. Mosbacher, and A.H. Ismail, "Depression as a Powerful Discriminator between Physically Active and Sedentary Middle-Aged Men," *J Psychosom Res* 27 (1983): 69–76.

29. C.H. Folkins and W.E. Sime, "Physical Fitness Training and Mental Health," *Am Psychologist* 36 (1981): 375–88.

30. E.W. Martinsen, "The Role of Aerobic Exercise in the Treatment of Depression," *Stress Med* 3 (1987): 93–100.

31. S. Weyerer and B. Kupfer, "Physical Exercise and Psychological Health," *Sports Med* 17 (1994): 108–16.

32. A. Byrne and D.G. Byrne, "The Effect of Exercise on Depression, Anxiety, and Other Mood States: A Review," *J Psychosom Res* 37 (1993): 565–74.

33. R.C. Casper, "Exercise and Mood," *World Rev Nutr Diet* 71 (1993): 115–43.

34. A. Winokur et al., "Insulin Resistance after Glucose Tolerance Testing in Patients with Major Depression," *Am J Psychiatry* 145 (1988): 325–30.

35. J.H. Wright, J.J. Jacisin, N.S. Radin, et al., "Glucose Metabolism in Unipolar Depression," *Br J Psychiatry* 132 (1978): 386–93.

36. A. Hadji-Georgopoulus et al., "Elevated Hypoglycemic Index and Late Hyperinsulinism in Symptomatic Postprandial Hypoglycemia," *J Clin Endocrinol Metabol* 50 (1980): 371–6.

37. M. Fabrykant, "The Problem of Functional Hyperinsulinism on Functional Hypoglycemia Attributed to Nervous Causes, 1: Laboratory and Clinical Correlations," *Metabolism* 4 (1955): 469–79.

38. M. Werbach, *Nutritional Influences on Mental Illness: A Sourcebook of Clinical Research* (Tarzana, CA: Third Line Press, 1991).

39. R. Crellin, T. Bottiglieri, and E.H. Reynolds, "Folates and Psychiatric Disorders: Clinical Potential," *Drugs* 45 (1993): 623–36.

40. M.W.P. Carney et al., "Red Cell Folate Concentrations in Psychiatric Patients," *J Affective Disorders* 19 (1990): 207–13.

41. P.S.A. Godfrey et al., "Enhancement of Recovery from Psychiatric Illness by Methyl Folate," *Lancet* 336 (1990): 392–5.

42. E. Reynolds et al., "Folate Deficiency in Depressive Illness," *Br J Psychiat* 117 (1970): 287–92.

43. W.E. Thornton and B.P. Thornton, "Geriatric Mental Function and Folic Acid: A Review and Survey," *Southern Med J* 70 (1977): 919–22.

44. F. Abalan et al., "Frequency of Deficiencies of Vitamin B12 and Folic Acid in Patients Admitted to a Geriatric-Psychiatry Unit," *Encephale* 10 (1984): 9–12.

45. D. Zucker et al., "B12 Deficiency and Psychiatric Disorders: A Case Report and Literature Review," *Biol Psychiatry* 16 (1981): 197–205.

46. S.L. Kivela, K. Pahkala, and A. Eronen, "Depression in the Aged: Relation to Folate and Vitamins C and B12," *Biol Psychiatry* 26 (1989): 209–13.

47. H. Curtius, H. Muldner, and A. Niederwieser, "Tetrahydrobiopterin: Efficacy in Endogenous Depression and Parkinson's Disease," *J Neural Trans* 55 (1982): 301–8.

48. H. Curtius et al., "Successful Treatment of Depression with Tetrahydrobiopterin," *Lancet* (1983): 657–8.

49. R. Leeming et al., "Tetrahydrofolate and Hydroxycobalamin in the Management of Dihydropteridine Reductase Deficiency," *J Ment Def Res* 26 (1982): 21–5.

50. M. Botez et al., "Effect of Folic Acid and Vitamin B12 Deficiencies on 5-hydroxyindoleacetic Acid in Human Cerebrospinal Fluid," *Ann Neurol* 12 (1982): 479–84.

51. E. Reynolds and G. Stramentinoli, "Folic Acid, S-Adenosylmethionine and Affective Disorder," *Psychol Med* 13 (1983): 705–10.

52. E. Reynolds, M. Carney, and B. Toone, "Methylation and Mood," *Lancet* ii (1983): 196–9.

53. R. Crellin, T. Bottiglieri, and E.H. Reynolds, "Folates and Psychiatric Disorders: Clinical Potential," *Drugs* 45 (1993): 623–36.

54. C. Russ, T. Hendricks, B. Chrisley, N. Kalin, and J. Driskell, "Vitamin B6 Status of Depressed and Obsessive-Compulsive Patients," *Nutr Rep Intl* 27 (1983): 867–73.

55. M. Carney, D. Williams, and B. Sheffield, "Thiamin and Pyridoxine Lack in Newly-Admitted Psychiatric Patients," *Br J Psychiatr* 135 (1979): 249–54.

56. B. Nobbs, "Pyridoxal Phosphate Status in Clinical Depression," *Lancet* i (1974): 405.

57. W.M.W.P. Carney, D.G. Williams, and B.F. Sheffield, "Thiamin and Pyridoxine Lack in Newly-Admitted Psychiatric Patients," *Br J Psychiat* 135 (1979): 249–54.

58. J.W. Stewart, W. Harrison, F. Quitkin, and H. Baker, "Low-Level B6 Levels in Depressed Outpatients," *Biolog Psychiat* 19 (1984): 613–6.

59. J.R. Hibbeln and N. Salem, "Dietary Polyunsaturated Fatty Acids and Depression: When Cholesterol Does Not Satisfy," *Am J Clin Nutr* 62 (1995): 1–9.

60. A.H. Rowe and A. Rowe, Jr., *Food Allergy: Its Manifestations and Control and the Elimination Diets: A Compendium* (Springfield, IL: Charles C. Thomas, 1972).

61. J. Brostoff and S.J. Challacombe, eds., *Food Allergy and Intolerance* (Philadelphia, PA: W.B. Saunders, 1987).

62. P.A. Hertzman et al., "Association of the Eosinophilia-Myalgia Syndrome with the Ingestion of Tryptophan," *N Engl J Med* 322 (1990): 869–73.

63. E.M. Kilbourne, "Eosinophilia-Myalgia Syndrome: Coming to Grips with a New Illness," *Epidemiologic Rev* 14 (1992): 16–36.

64. E.M. Kilbourne et al., "Tryptophan Produced by Showa Denko and Epidemic Eosinophilia-Myalgia Syndrome," *J Rheumatol Suppl* 46 (1996): 81–8.

65. G.A. Filippini, C.V.L. Costa, and A. Bertazzo, eds., "Recent Advances in Tryptophan Research: Tryptophan and Serotonin Pathways," *Exp Biol Med* 398 (1996): 1–762.

66. "Proceedings: Eosinophilic-Myalgia Syndrome: Review and Reappraisal of Clinical, Epidemiologic and Animal Studies Symposium. Washington, D.C., December 7–8, 1994," *J Rheumatol Suppl* 46 (1996): 1–110.

67. E.A. Belongia et al., "An Investigation of the Cause of the Eosinophilia-Myalgia Syndrome Associated with Tryptophan Use," *N Engl J Med* 323 (1990): 357–65.

68. R.M. Silver et al., "Tryptophan Metabolism via the Kynurenine Pathway in Patients with the Eosinophilia-Myalgia Syndrome," *Arthritis Rheum* 35 (1992): 1097–1105.

69. P.A. Hertzman, "The Eosinophilia-Myalgia Syndrome and the Toxic Oil Syndrome: Pursuing Parallels," *Exp Biol Med* 398 (1996): 339–42.

70. D.L. Hatch and L.R. Goldman, "Reduced Severity of Eosinophilia-Myalgia Syndrome Associated with the Consumption of Vitamin-Containing Supplements before Illness," *Arch Intern Med* 153 (1993): 2368–73.

71. B. Boman, "L-tryptophan: A Rational Antidepressant and a Natural Hypnotic?" *Aust NZ J Psychiatry* 22 (1988): 83–97.

72. S. Moller et al., "Tryptophan Availability in Endogenous Depression: Relation to Efficacy of l-tryptophan Treatment," *Adv Biol Psychiat* 10 (1983): 30–46.

73. G. D'Elia, L. Hanson, and H. Raotma, "L-tryptophan and 5-hydroxytryptophan in the Treatment of Depression: A Review," *Acta Psychiatr Scand* 57 (1978): 239–52.

74. B.J. Carroll, "Monoamine Precursors in the Treatment of Depression," *Clin Pharmacol Ther* 12 (1971): 743–61.

75. H.M. van Praag, "Studies on the Mechanism of Action with Serotonin Precursors in Depression," *Psychopharmacol Bull* 20 (1984): 599–602.

76. H.M. van Praag, "Central Monoamine Metabolism in Depressions, I: Serotonin and Related Compounds," *Compr Psychiatry* 21 (1980): 30–43.

77. J.J. van Hiele, "L-5-hydroxytryptophan in Depression: The First Substitution Therapy in Psychiatry?" *Neuropsychobiology* 6 (1980): 230–40.

78. W.F. Byerley et al., "5-hydroxytryptophan: A Review of Its Antidepressant Efficacy and Adverse Effects," *J Clin Psychopharmacol* 7 (1987): 127–37.

79. H.M. van Praag, "Management of Depression with Serotonin Precursors," *Biol Psychiatry* 16 (1981): 291–310.

80. W. Poldinger, B. Calanchini, and W. Schwarz, "A Functional-Dimensional Approach to Depression: Serotonin Deficiency as a Target Syndrome in a Comparison of 5-hydroxytryptophan and Fluvoxamine," *Psychopathology* 24 (1991): 53–81.

81. H.M. van Praag and C. Lemus, "Monoamine Precursors in the Treatment of Psychiatric Disorders," in R.J. Wurtman and J.J. Wurtman, eds., *Nutrition and the Brain*, vol. 7 (New York: Raven Press, 1986), 89–139.

82. C. Gibson and A. Gelenberg, "Tyrosine for Depression," *Adv Biol Psychiat* 10 (1983): 148–59.

83. H. Beckman, "Phenylalanine in Affective Disorders," *Adv Biol Psychiat* 10 (1983): 137–47.

84. H.M. van Praag et al., "In Search of the Mode of Action of Antidepressants: 5-HTP/Tyrosine Mixtures in Depression," *Adv*

Biochem Psychopharmacol 39 (1984): 301–14.

85. R.J. Baldessarini, "Neuropharmacology of S-Adenosyl-L-Methionine," *Am J Med* 83 (Suppl.5A) (1987): 95–103.

86. E. Reynolds, M. Carney, and B. Toone, "Methylation and Mood," *Lancet* ii (1983): 196–9.

87. T. Bottiglieri, M. Laundry, R. Martin et al., "S-Adenosylmeth-ionine Influences Monoamine Metabolism," *Lancet* ii (1984): 224.

88. P.G. Janicak et al., "Parenteral S-Adenosylmethionine in Depression: A Literature Review and Preliminary Report," *Psychopharmacology Bulletin* 25 (1989): 238–41.

89. H.A. Friedel, K.L. Goa, and P. Benfield, "S-Adenosylmethionine," *Drugs* 38 (1989): 3889–417.

90. M.W.P. Carney, B.K. Toone, and E.H. Reynolds, "S-adenosylmethionine and Affective Disorder," *Am J Med* 83 (Suppl A) (1987): 104–6.

91. S.A. Vahora and P. Malek-Ahmadi, "S-adenosylmethionine in Depression," *Neurosci Biobehav Rev* 12 (1988): 139–41.

92. B.L. Kagan et al., "Oral S-adenosylmethionine in Depression: A Randomized, Double-Blind Placebo-Controlled Trial," *Am J Psychiatry* 147 (1990): 591–5.

93. J.F. Rosenbaum et al., "An Open-Label Pilot Study of Oral S-adenosylmethionine in Major Depression," *Psychopharmacol Bull* 24 (1988): 189–94.

94. M. De Vanna and R. Rigamonti, "Oral S-adenosyl-L-methionine in Depression," *Curr Ther Res* 52 (1992): 478–85.

95. P. Salmaggi et al., "Double-Blind, Placebo-Controlled Study of S-adenosyl-L-methionine in Depressed Postmenopausal Women," *Psychother Psychosom* 59 (1993): 34–40.

96. K.M. Bell et al., "S-adenosylmethionine Blood Levels in Major Depression: Changes with Drug Treatment," *Acta Neurol Scand* 154 (Suppl.) (1994): 15–8.

97. P. Morazzoni and E. Bombardelli, "Hypericum perforatum," *Fitoterapia* 66 (1995): 43–68.

98. G. Harrer and V. Schulz, "Clinical Investigation of the Antidepressant Effectiveness of *Hypericum*," *J Geriatr Psychiatry Neurol* 7(Suppl 1) (1994): S6–8.

99. P.A.G. De Smet and W. Nolen, "St. Johnswort as an Antidepressant," *BMJ* 313 (1996): 241–2.

100. P. Halama, "Efficacy of the *Hypericum* Extract LI 160 in the Treatment of 50 Patients of a Psychiatrist," *Nervenheilkunde* 10 (1991): 305–7.

101. D. Hansgren, J. Vesper, and M. Ploch, "Multicenter Double-Blind Study Examining the Antidepressant Effectiveness of the Hypericum Extract LI 160," *J Geriatr Psychiatry Neurol* 7(Suppl 1) (1994): S15–8.

102. G. Harrer and H. Sommer, "Treatment of Mild/Moderate Depressions with Hypericum," *Phytomed* 1 (1994): 3–8.

103. W.D. Hubner, S. Lande, and H. Podzuweit, "Hypericum Treatment of Mild Depressions with Somatic Symptoms," *J Geriatry Psychiatry Neurol* 7(Suppl 1) (1994): S12–4.

104. J. Quandt, U. Schmidt and N. Schenk, "Ambulante Behandlung Leichter und Mittelschwerer Depressiver Verstimmungen," *Der Allgemeinarzt* 2 (1993): 97–102.

105. C. Reh, P. Laux, and N. Schenk, "Hypericum-Extrakt Bei Depressionen: Eine Wirksame Alternative," *Therapiewoche* 42 (1992): 1576–81.

106. U. Schmidt and H. Sommer, "St. Johnswort Extract in the Ambulatory Therapy of Depression: Attention and Reaction Ability Are Preserved," *Fortschr Med* 111 (1993): 339–42.

107. U. Schmidt et al., "The Therapy of Depressive Moods," *Psycho* 15 (1989): 665–71.

108. H. Sommer and G. Harrer, "Placebo-Controlled Double-Blind Study Examining the Effectiveness of an Hypericum Preparation in 105 Mildly Depressed Patients," *J Geriatr Psychiatry Neurol* 7(Suppl 1) (1994): S9–11.

109. R. Bergman, J. Nubner, and J. Demling, "Behandlung Leichter gis Mittelschwerer Depressionen," *Therapiewoch Neurologie/Psychiatrie* 7 (1993): 235–40.

110. G. Harrer, W.D. Hubner, and H. Podzuweit, "Effectiveness and Tolerance of the Hypericum Extract LI 160 Compared to Maprotiline: A Multicenter Double-Blind Study," *J Geriatr Psychiatry Neurol* 7(Suppl 1) (1994): S24–8.

111. E.U. Vorbach, W.D. Hubner, and K.H. Arnoldt, "Effectiveness and Tolerance of the Hypericum Extract LI 160 in Comparison with Imipramine: Randomized Double-Blind Study with 135 Outpatients," *J Geriatr Psychiatry Neurol* 7(Suppl 1) (1994): S19–23.

112. Y. Singh, "Kava: An Overview," *J Ethnopharmacol* 37 (1992): 13–45.

113. D. Lindenberg and H. Pitule-Schodel, "D,L-kavain in Comparison with Oxazepam in Anxiety Disorders: A Double-Blind Study of Clinical Effectiveness," *Forschr Med* 108 (1990): 49–50, 53–4.

114. E. Kinzler, J. Kromer, and E. Lehmann, "Clinical Efficacy of a Kava Extract in Patients with Anxiety Syndrome: Double-Blind Placebo Controlled Study over 4 Weeks," *Arzneim Forsch* 41 (1991): 584–8.

115. F.V. DeFeudis, ed., *Ginkgo biloba Extract (EGb 761): Pharmacological Activities and Clinical Applications* (Paris: Elsevier, 1991).

116. E.W. Funfgeld, ed., *Rokan (Ginkgo biloba). Recent Results in Pharmacology and Clinic* (New York: Springer-Verlag, 1988).

117. J. Kleijnen and P. Knipschild, "Ginkgo biloba," *Lancet* 340 (1992): 1136–9.

118. J. Kleijnen and P. Knipschild, "Ginkgo biloba for Cerebral Insufficiency," *Br J Clinical Pharmacol* 34 (1992): 352–8.

119. H. Schubert and P. Halama, "Depressive Episode Primarily Unresponsive to Therapy in Elderly Patients: Efficacy of Ginkgo biloba (Egb 761) in Combination with Antidepressants," *Geriatr Forsch* 3 (1993): 45–53.

120. F. Huguet et al., "Decreased Cerebral 5-HT1a Receptors During Aging: Reversal by Ginkgo biloba Extract (Egb 761)," *J Pharm Pharmacol* 46 (1994): 316–8.

Diabetes

1. J.B. Wyngaarden, L.H. Smith, and J.C. Bennett, eds., *Cecil Textbook of*

Medicine (Philadelphia: W.B. Saunders, 1992).

2. R.J. Rubin et al., "Health Care Expenditures for People with Diabetes Mellitus, 1992," *J Clin Endocrinol Metab* 78 (1994): 809A–809F.

3. D. Burkitt and H. Trowell, *Western Diseases: Their Emergence and Prevention* (Cambridge, MA: Harvard University Press, 1981).

4. G. Vahouny and D. Kritchevsky, *Dietary Fiber in Health and Disease* (New York: Plenum Press, 1982).

5. T. Hughs, J. Gwynne, B. Switzer, et al., "Effects of Caloric Restriction and Weight Loss on Glycemic Control, Insulin Release and Resistance and Atherosclerotic Risk in Obese Patients with Type II Diabetes Mellitus," *Am J Med* 77 (1984): 7–17.

6. R.D.G. Leslie and R.B. Elliott, "Early Environmental Events as a Cause of IDDM," *Diabetes* 43 (1994): 843–50.

7. T. Helgason and M.R. Johasson, "Evidence for a Food Additive as a Cause of Ketosis-Prone Diabetes," *Lancet* 2 (1981): 716–20.

8. M.A. Krupp, L.M. Tierney, and S.J. McPhee, *Current Medical Diagnosis and Treatment* (Los Altos, CA: Lange Medical Publications, 1997).

9. H.C. Gerstein, "Cow's Milk Exposure and Type I Diabetes Mellitus: A Critical Review of the Clinical Literature," *Diabetes Care* 17 (1994): 13–19.

10. P.J. Campbell and M.G. Carlson, "Impact of Obesity on Insulin Action in NIDDM," *Diabetes* 42 (1993): 405–10.

11. U. Smith, "Insulin Resistance in Obesity, Type II Diabetes and Stress," *Acta Endocrin* suppl. 262 (1984): 67–69.

12. M. Krotkiewski et al., "Impact of Obesity on Metabolism in Men and Women," *J Clin Invest* 72 (1983): 1150–62.

13. J.A. Marshall, R.F. Hamman, and J. Baxter, "High-Fat, Low-Carbohydrate Diet and the Etiology of Non-Insulin-Dependent Diabetes Mellitus: The San Luis Valley Diabetes Study," *Am J Epidemiol* 134 (1991): 590–603.

14. J.A. Marshall et al., "Dietary Fat Predicts Conversion from Impaired Glucose Tolerance to NIDDM," *Diabetes Care* 17 (1994): 50–6.

15. R. Anderson et al., "Beneficial Effect of Chromium for People with Type II Diabetes," *Diabetes* 45 Suppl. 2 (1996): 124A/454.

16. E. Offenbacher and F. Stunyer, "Beneficial Effect of Chromium-Rich Yeast on Glucose Tolerance and Blood Lipids in Elderly Patients," *Diabetes* 29 (1980): 919–25.

17. M. Mertz, "Chromium Occurrence and Function in Biological Systems," *Physiol Rev* 49 (1969): 163–237.

18. R. Levine, D. Streeten, and R. Doisy, "Effect of Oral Chromium Supplementation on the Glucose Tolerance of Elderly Human Subjects," *Metabolism* 17 (1968): 114–25.

19. A.D. Mooradian et al., "Selected Vitamin and Mineral in Diabetes," *Diabetes Care* 17 (1994): 464–79.

20. B. Baker, "Chromium Supplements Tied to Glucose Control," *Family Practice News* (July 15, 1996): 5.

21. G. Drner, A. Mohnike, and H. Thoelke, "Further Evidence for the Dependence of Diabetes Prevalence on Nutrition in Perinatal Life," *Exp Clin Endocrinol* 84 (1984): 129–33.

22. G. Drner, E. Steindel, H. Thoelke, and V. Schliack, "Evidence for Decreasing Prevalence of Diabetes Mellitus in Childhood Apparently Produced by Prevention of Hyperinsulinism in the Foetus and Newborn," *Exp Clin Endocrinol* 84 (1984): 134–42.

23. S.A. Amiel, "Intensified Insulin Therapy," *Diabetes Metab Rev* 9 (1993): 3–24.

24. University Group Diabetes Program, "A Story of the Effectiveness of Hypoglycemic Agents on Vascular Complications in Patients with Adult-Onset Diabetes, II: Mortality Results," *Diabetes* 19 (1970): 789–830.

25. M. Brownlee, H. Vlassara, and A. Cerami, "Nonenzymatic Glycosylation and the Pathogenesis of Diabetic Complications," *Ann Int Med* 101 (1984): 527–37.

26. D.G. Cogan, J.H. Kinoshita, P.F. Kador, et al., "Aldose Reductase and Complications of Diabetes," *Ann Int Med* 101 (1984): 82–91.

27. D.K. Yue, M.A. Hanwell, P.M. Satshell, et al., The Effects of Aldose Reductase Inhibition on Nerve Sor-

bitol and Myoinositol Concentrations in Diabetic and Galactosemic Rats," *Metabolism* 33 (1984): 1119–22.

28. G. Gegersen, H. Harb, A. Helles, and J. Christensen, "Oral Supplementation of Myoinositol: Effects on Peripheral Nerve Function in Human Diabetics and on the Concentration in Plasma, Erythrocytes, Urine, and Muscle Tissue in Human Diabetics and Normals," *Acta Neurol Scand* 67 (1983): 164–71.

29. P.W.F. Wilson, W.P. Castelli, and W.B. Kannel, "Coronary Risk Predictors in Adults," *Am J Cardiol* 59 (1987): 91G–94G.

30. National Research Council, *Diet and Health: Implications for Reducing Chronic Disease Risk* (Washington, DC: National Academy Press, 1989).

31. J. Anderson, "Nutrition Management of Diabetes Mellitus," in R. Goodhart and V.R. Young, eds., *Modern Nutrition in Health and Disease* (Philadelphia: Lea and Febiger, 1988), 1201–29.

32. J.W. Anderson and K. Ward, "High-Carbohydrate, High-Fiber Diets for Insulin-Treated Men with Diabetes Mellitus," *Am J Clin Nutr* 32 (1979): 2312–21.

33. J.W. Anderson, "High Polysaccharide Diet Studies in Patients with Diabetes and Vascular Disease," *Cereal Foods World* 22 (1977): 12–22.

34. R. Kay, W. Grobin, and N. Trace, "Diets Rich in Natural Fiber Improve Carbohydrate Tolerance in Maturity Onset, Noninsulin Dependent Diabetics," *Diabetologia* 20 (1981): 12–23.

35. H.C.R. Simpson, R.W. Simpson, S. Lousley, et al., "A High Carbohydrate Leguminous Fiber Diet Improves All Aspects of Diabetic Control," *Lancet* 1 (1981): 1–5.

36. D.J.A. Jenkins, T.M.S. Wolever, S. Bacon, et al., "Diabetic Diets: High Carbohydrate Combined with High Fiber," *Am J Clin Nutr* 33 (1980): 1729–33.

37. C.B. Hollenbeck, J.E. Lecklem, M.C. Riddle, and W.E. Conner, "The Composition and Nutritional Adequacy of Subject-Selected High Carbohydrate, Low Fat Diets in Insulin-Dependent Diabetes

Mellitus," *Am J Clin Nutr* 38 (1983): 41–51.

38. J. Anderson, *Diabetes: A Practical Approach to Daily Living* (New York: Arco Press, 1981).

39. N. Pritikin and P. McGrandy, *The Pritikin Program for Diet and Exercise* (New York: Grosset and Dunlap, 1979).

40. D.J.A. Jenkins, T.M.S. Wolever, R.H. Taylor, et al., "Glycemic Index of Foods: A Physiological Basis for Carbohydrate Exchange," *Am J Clin Nutr* 24 (1981): 362–66.

41. V.A. Koivisto and H. Yki-Jarvinen, "Fructose and Insulin Sensitivity in Patients with Type II Diabetes," *Journal of Internal Medicine* 233 (1993): 145–53.

42. J. Cunningham, "Reduced Mononuclear Leukocyte Ascorbic Acid Content in Adults with Insulin-Dependent Diabetes Mellitus Consuming Adequate Dietary Vitamin C," *Metabolism* 40 (1991): 146–49.

43. S.J. Davie, B.J. Gould, and J.S. Yudkin, "Effect of Vitamin C on Glycosylation of Proteins," *Diabetes* 41 (1992): 167–73.

44. J.A. Vinson, et al., "In Vitro and in Vivo Reduction of Erythrocyte Sorbitol by Ascorbic Acid," *Diabetes* 38 (1989): 1036–41.

45. J.J. Cunningham, P.L. Mearkle, and R.G. Brown, "Vitamin C: An Aldose Reductase Inhibitor that Normalizes Erythrocyte Sorbitol in Insulin-Dependent Diabetes Mellitus," *J Am Coll Nutr* 4 (1994): 344–50.

46. M. Urberg and M.B. Zemel, "Evidence for Synergism Between Chromium and Nicotinic Acid in the Control of Glucose Tolerance in Elderly Humans," *Metabolism* 36 (1987): 896–99.

47. F. Pocoit, J.I. Reimers, and H.U. Andersen, "Nicotinamide: Biological Actions and Therapeutic Potential in Diabetes Prevention," *Diabetologia* 36 (1993): 574–76.

48. J.P. Cleary, "Vitamin B_3 in the Treatment of Diabetes Mellitus: Case Reports and Review of the Literature," *J Nutr Med* 1 (1990): 217–25.

49. P. Pozzilli and D. Andreani, "The Potential Role of Nicotinamide in the Secondary Prevention of IDDM," *Diabetes Metabol Rev* 9 (1993): 219–30.

50. T. Mandrup Paulsen et al., "Nicotinamide in the Prevention of Insulin Dependent Diabetes Mellitus," *Diabetes Metabol Rev* 9 (1993): 295–309.

51. H.U. Andersen et al., "Nicotinamide Prevents Interleukin-1 Effects on Accumulated Insulin Release and Nitric Oxide Production in Rat Islets of Langerhans," *Diabetes* 43 (1994): 770–77.

52. The Expert Panel, "Report of the National Cholesterol Education Program Expert Panel on Detection, Evaluation, and Treatment of High Cholesterol in Adults," *Arch Intern Med* 148 (1988): 136–69.

53. The Coronary Drug Project Group, "Clofibrate and Niacin in Coronary Heart Disease," *JAMA* 231 (1975): 360–81.

54. P.L. Canner and the Coronary Drug Project Group, "Mortality in Coronary Drug Project Patients During a Nine-Year Post-Treatment Period," *J Am Coll Cardiol* 8 (1986): 1245–55.

55. Y. Henkin, K.C. Johnson, and J.P. Segrest, "Rechallenge with Crystalline Niacin after Drug-Induced Hepatitis from Sustained-Release Niacin," *JAMA* 264 (1990): 241–43.

56. A.L. Welsh and M. Ede, "Inositol Hexanicotinate for Improved Nicotinic Acid Therapy," *Int Record Med* 174 (1961): 9–15.

57. A.M.A. El-Enein, Y.S. Hafez, H. Salem, and M. Abdel, "The Role of Nicotinic Acid and Inositol Hexaniacinate as Anticholesterolemic and Antilipemic Agents," *Nutr Rep Intl* 28 (1983): 899–911.

58. G.T. Sunderland, J.J.F. Belch, R.D. Sturrock, et al., "A Double-Blind Randomized Placebo-Controlled Trial of Hexopal in Primary Raynaud's Disease," *Clin Rheumatol* 7 (1988): 46–49.

59. A. Reddi, B. DeAngelis, O. Frank, et al., "Biotin Supplementation Improves Glucose and Insulin Tolerances in Genetically Diabetic KK Mice," *Life Sci* 42 (1988): 1323–30.

60. M. Maebashi, Y. Makino, Y. Furukawa, et al., "Therapeutic Evaluation of the Effect of Biotin on Hyperglycemia in Patients with Non-Insulin Dependent Diabetes Mellitus," *J Clin Biochem Nutr* 14 (1993): 211–8.

61. C.L. Jones and V. Gonzalez, "Pyridoxine Deficiency: A New Factor in Diabetic Neuropathy," *J Am Pod Assoc* 68 (1978): 646–53.

62. L.R. Solomon and K. Cohen, "Erythrocyte O_2 Transport and Metabolism and Effects of Vitamin B_6 Therapy in Type II Diabetes Mellitus," *Diabetes* 38 (1989): 881–86.

63. H.J.T. Coelingh-Bennink and W.H.P. Schreurs, "Improvement of Oral Glucose Tolerance in Gestational Diabetes," *Br Med J* 3 (1975): 13–15.

64. S. Davidson, "The Use of Vitamin B_{12} in the Treatment of Diabetic Neuropathy," *J Flor Med Assoc* 15 (1954): 717–20.

65. S.M. Sancetta, P.R. Ayres, and R.W. Scott, "The Use of Vitamin B_{12} in the Management of the Neurological Manifestations of Diabetes Mellitus, with Notes on the Administration of Massive Doses," *Ann Int Med* 35 (1951): 1028–48.

66. H.R. Bhatt, J.C. Linnell, and D.M. Matt, "Can Faulty Vitamin B_{12} (Cobalamin) Metabolism Produce Diabetic Retinopathy?" *Lancet* 2 (1983): 572.

67. G. Paolisso et al., "Chronic Intake of Pharmacological Doses of Vitamin E Might be Useful in the Therapy of Elderly Patients with Coronary Heart Disease," *Am J Clin Nutr* 61 (1995): 848–52.

68. J.T. Salonen et al., "Increased Risk of Non-Insulin Diabetes Mellitus at Low Plasma Vitamin E Concentrations: A Four-Year Follow-up Study in Men," *Br Med J* 311 (1995): 1124–27.

69. J.R. White and R.K. Campbell, "Magnesium and Diabetes: A Review," *Ann Pharmacother* 27 (1993): 775–80.

70. G. Norbiato, M. Bevilacqua, R. Merino, et al., "Effects of Potassium Supplementation on Insulin Binding and Insulin Action in Human Obesity: Protein-Modified Fast and Refeeding," *Europ J Clin Invest* 44 (1984): 414–19.

71. K.T. Khaw and J.T. Barrett-Connor, "Dietary Potassium and Blood Pressure in a Population," *Am J Clin Nutr* 39 (1984): 963–68.

72. J.M. Wimhurst and K.L. Manchester, "Comparison of Ability of Mg and Mn to Activate the Key En-

zymes of Glycolysis," *FEBS Letters* 27 (1972): 321–26.

73. Anonymous, "Manganese and Glucose Tolerance," *Nutr Rev* 26 (1968): 207–10.

74. A.D. Mooradian and J.E. Morley, "Micronutrient Status in Diabetes Mellitus," *Am J Clin Nutr* 45 (1987): 877–95.

75. S.M. Hegazi et al., "Effect of Zinc Supplementation on Serum Glucose, Insulin, Glucagon, Glucose-6-Phosphatase, and Mineral Levels in Diabetics," *J Clin Biochem Nutr* 12 (1992): 209–15.

76. E.D. Engel, N.E. Erlich, and R.H. Davis, "Diabetes Mellitus: Impaired Wound Healing from Zinc Deficiency," *J Am Pod Assoc* 71 (1981): 536–44.

77. V. Cody, E. Middleton, and J.B. Harborne, *Plant Flavonoids in Biology and Medicine: Biochemical, Pharmacological, and Structure-Activity Relationships* (New York: Alan R .Liss, 1986).

78. V. Cody, E. Middleton, J.B. Harborne, and A. Beretz, *Plant Flavonoids in Biology and Medicine II: Biochemical, Pharmacological, and Structure-Activity Relationships* (New York: Alan R. Liss, 1988).

79. J. Kuhnau, "The Flavonoids: A Class Of Semi-Essential Food Components: Their Role in Human Nutrition," *Wld Rev Nutr Diet* 24 (1976): 117–91.

80. G.A. Jamal, "The Use of Gamma Linolenic Acid in the Prevention and Treatment of Diabetic Neuropathy," *Diabetic Med* 11 (1994): 145–49.

81. H. Keen et al., "Treatment of Diabetic Neuropathy with Gamma-Linolenic Acid," *Diabetes Care* 16 (1993): 8–13.

82. E.B. Schmidt and J. Dyerberg, "Omega-3 Fatty Acids: Current Status in Cardiovascular Medicine," *Drugs* 47 (1994): 405–24.

83. E.B Schmidt, "Omega-3 Polyunsaturated Fatty Acids and Ischaemic Heart Disease," *Curr Opin Lipidol* 4 (1993): 27–33.

84. L. Axelrod, "Effects of a Small Quantity of Omega-3 Fatty Acids on Cardiovascular Risk Factors in NIDDM," *Diabetes Care* 17 (1994): 37–45.

85. H.T. Westervel et al., "Effects of Low-Dose EPA-E on Glycemic Control, Lipid Profile, Lipoprotein (a), Platelet Aggregation, Viscos ty, and Platelet and Vessel Wall Interaction in NIDDM," *Diabetes Care* 16 (1993): 683–88.

86. L. Cobias, P.S. Clifton, M. Abbey, et al., "Lipid, Lipoprotein, and Hemostatic Effects of Fish vs Fish Oil w-3 Fatty Acids in Mildly Hyperlipidemic Males," *Am J Clin Nutr* 53 (1991): 1210–16.

87. E.J.M. Feskens, C.H. Bowles, and D. Kromhout, "Inverse Association between Fish Intake and Risk of Glucose Intolerance in Normoglycemic Elderly Men and Women," *Diabetes Care* 14 (1991): 935–41.

88. K.S. Bjerve et al., "Clinical Studies with Alpha-Linolenic Acid and Long Chain n-3 Fatty Acids," *Nutrition* 8 (1992): 130–32.

89. E. Mantzioris et al., "Dietary Substitution with Alpha-Linolenic Acid-Rich Vegetable Oil Increases Eicosapentaenoic Acid Concentrations in Tissues," *Am J Clin Nutr* 59 (1994): 1304–9.

90. M.T. Abdel-Aziz, M.S. Abdou, K. Soliman, et al., "Effect of Carnitine on Blood Lipid Patterns in Diabetic Patients," *Nutr Rep Int* 29 (1984): 1071–79.

91. C.G. Sheela and K.T. Augusti, "Antidiabetic Effects of S-allyl Cysteine Sulphoxide Isolated from Garlic (*Allium sativum*, Linn.)," *Indian J Exp Biol* 30 (1992): 523–26.

92. K.K. Sharma, R.K. Gupta, S. Gupta, and K.C. Samuel, "Antihyperglycemic Effect of Onion: Effect on Fasting Blood Sugar and Induced Hyperglycemia in Man," *Ind J Med Res* 65 (1977): 422–29.

93. J. Welihinda, E.H. Karunanaya, M.H.R. Sheriff, and K.S.A. Jayasinghe, "Effect of *Momardica charantia* on the Glucose Tolerance in Maturity Onset Diabetes," *J Ethnopharmacol* 17 (1986): 277–82.

94. Y. Srivastava, H. Venkatakrishna-Bhatt, Y. Verma, et al., "Antidiabetic and Adaptogenic Properties of *Momordica_charantia* Extract: An Experimental and Clinical Evaluation," *Phytotherapy Res* 7 (1993): 285–89.

95. J. Welihinda, G. Arvidson, E. Gylfe, et al., "The Insulin-Releasing Activity of the Tropical Plant *Momordica*

charantia," *Acta Biol Med Germ* 41 (1982): 1229–40.

96. E.R.B. Shanmugasundaram, G. Rajeswari, K. Baskaran, et al., "Use of *Gymnema sylvestre* Leaf Extract in the Control of Blood Glucose in Insulin-Dependent Diabetes Mellitus," *J Ethnopharmacol* 30 (1990): 281–94.

97. K. Baskaran, B.K. Ahamath, K.R. Shanmugasundaram, and E.R.B. Shanmugasundaram, "Antidiabetic Effect of a Leaf Extract from *Gymnema_sylvestre* in Non-Insulin Dependent Diabetes Mellitus Patients," *J Ethnopharmacol* 30 (1990): 295–305.

98. G. Ribes, Y. Sauvaire, J.C. Baccou, et al., "Effects of Fenugreek Seeds on Endocrine Pancreatic Secretions in Dogs," *Ann Nutr Metab* 28 (1984): 37–43.

99. R.D. Sharma, T.C. Raghuram, and N.S. Rao, "Effect of Fenugreek Seeds on Blood Glucose and Serum Lipids in Type I Diabetes," *Eur J Clin Nutr* 44 (1990): 301–6.

100. Z. Mada, R. Abel, S. Samish, and J. Arad, "Glucose-Lowering Effect of Fenugreek in Non-Insulin Dependent Diabetics," *Eur J Clin Nutr* 42 (1988): 51–54.

101. E. Stern, "Successful Use of *Atriplex Halimus* in the Treatment of Type II Diabetic Patients: A Preliminary Study." Unpublished study conducted at the Zamenhoff Medical Center, Tel Aviv, Israel.

102. G. Earon, E. Stern, and H. Lavosky, "Successful Use of *Atriplex Halimus* in the Treatment of Type II Diabetic Patients: Controlled Clinical Research Report on the Subject of *Atriplex*." Unpublished study conducted at the Hebrew University of Jerusalem, Israel.

103. B.K. Chakravarthy, S. Gupta, S.S. Gambhir, and K.D. Gode, "Pancreatic Beta-Cell Regeneration in Rats by (-)-Epicatechin," *Lancet* 2 (1981): 759–60.

104. B.K. Chakravarthy, S. Gupta, and K.D. Gode, "Functional Beta-Cell Regeneration in the Islets of Pancreas in Alloxan Induced Diabetic Rats by (-)-Epicatechin," *Life Sci* 31 (1982): 2693–97.

105. S.S. Subramanian, "(-)-Epicatechin as an Anti-Diabetic Drug," *Ind Drugs* 18 (1981): 259.

106. T. Okuda, Y. Kimura, T. Yoshida, et al., "Studies of the Activities of Tannins and Related Compounds from Medicinal Plants and Products, I: Inhibitory Effects on Lipid Peroxidation in Mitochondria and Microsomes of Liver," *Chem Pharm Bull* 31 (1983): 1625–31.

107. F.M. Allen, "Blueberry Leaf Extract: Physiologic and Clinical Properties in Relation to Carbohydrate Metabolism," *JAMA* 89 (1927): 1577–81.

108. B. Bever and G. Zahnd, "Plants with Oral Hypoglycemic Action," *Quart J Crude Drug Res* 17 (1979): 139–96.

109. L. Caselli, "Clinical and Electroretinographic Study on Activity of Anthocyanosides," *Arch Med Int* 37 (1985): 29–35.

110. N. Passariello, V. Bisesti, and S. Sgambato, "Influence of Anthocyanosides on the Microcirculation and Lipid Picture in Diabetic and Dyslipidic Subjects," *Gazz Med Ital* 138 (1979): 563–66.

111. J.M. Coget and J.F. Merlen, "Anthocyanosides and Microcirculation," *J Mal Vasc* 5 (1980): 43–46.

112. A. Scharrer and M. Ober, "Anthocyanosides in the Treatment of Retinopathies," *Klin Monatsbl Augenheilkd* 178 (1981): 386–89.

113. J. Kleijnen and P. Knipschild, "Ginkgo biloba for Cerebral Insufficiency," *Br J Clin Pharm* 34 (1992): 352–58.

114. E.W. Funfgeld, ed., *Rokan (Ginkgo Biloba): Recent Results in Pharmacology and Clinic* (New York: Springer-Verlag, 1988), 32–36.

115. U. Bauer, "6-Month Double-Blind Randomized Clinical Trial of *Ginkgo Biloba* Extract versus Placebo in Two Parallel Groups in Patients Suffering from Peripheral Arterial Insufficiency," *Arzneim-Forsch* 34 (1984): 716–21.

116. V.G. Rudofsky, "The Effect of *Ginkgo Biloba* Extract in Cases of Arterial Occlusive Disease: A Randomized Placebo Controlled Double-Blind Cross-Over Study," *Fortschr Med* 105 (1987): 397–400.

117. M. Doly, M.T. Droy-Lefaix, B. Bonhomme, and P. Braquet, "Effect of *Ginkgo Biloba* Extract on the Electrophysiology of the Isolated Diabetic Rat Retina," in E.W. Funfgeld, ed., *Rokan* (Ginkgo Biloba): *Recent Results in Pharmacology and Clinic* (New York: Springer-Verlag, 1988), 83–90.

118. E. Sotaniemi et al., "Ginseng Therapy in Non-Insulin-Dependent Diabetic Patients," *Diabetes Care* 18 (1995): 1373–75.

119. V.A. Koivisto and R.A. DeFronzo, "Exercise in the Treatment of Type II Diabetes," *Acta Endocrin* suppl 262 (1984): 107–111.

120. J.V. Selby, B. Newman, M.C. King, et al., "Environmental and Behavioral Determinants of Fasting Plasma Glucose in Women: A Matched Co-Twin Analysis," *Am J Epidem* 125 (1987): 979–88.

121. M.L. Pollack, J.H. Wilmore, and S.M. Fox, *Exercise in Health and Disease* (Philadelphia: W.B. Saunders, 1984).

122. A.L. Vallerand, J.P. Cuerrier, D. Shapcott, et al., "Influence of Exercise Training on Tissue Chromium Concentrations in the Rat," *Am J Clin Nutr* 39 (1984): 402–9.

123. O. Pedersen, H. Beck-Nielsen, and L. Heding, "Increased Insulin Receptors after Exercise in Patients with Insulin-Dependent Diabetes Mellitus," *N Engl J Med* 302 (1980): 886–92.

Diarrhea

1. H. Loeb et al., "Tannin-Rich Carob Pod for the Treatment of Acute-Onset Diarrhea," *J Ped Gastroenterol Nutr* 8 (1989): 480–5.

2. S. Gupta, "Use of Berberine in the Treatment of Giardiasis," *Am J Dis Child* 129 (1975): 866.

3. M.P. Bhakat et al., "Therapeutic Trial of Berberine Sulphate in Non-Specific Gastroenteritis," *Ind Med J* 68 (1974): 19–23.

4. S.A. Kamat, "Clinical Trial with Berberine Hydrochloride for the Control of Diarrhoea in Acute Gastroenteritis," *J Assoc Physicians India* 15 (1967): 525–9.

5. A.B. Desai, K.M. Shah, and D.M. Shah, "Berberine in the Treatment of Diarrhoea," *Ind Pediatr* 8 (1971): 462–5.

6. R. Sharma, C.K. Joshi, and R.K. Goyal, "Berberine Tannate in Acute Diarrhea," *Ind Pediatr* 7 (1970): 496–501.

7. V.P. Choudry, M. Sabir, and V.N. Bhide, "Berberine in Giardiasis," *Ind Pediatr* 9 (1972): 143–6.

8. S.A. Kamat, "Clinical Trial with Berberine Hydrochloride for the Control of Diarrhoea in Acute Gastroenteritis," *J Assoc Physicians India* 15 (1967): 525–9.

9. S. Gupte, "Use of Berberine in Treatment of Giardiasis," *Am J Dis Child* 129 (1975): 866.

10. R.B. Sack and J.L. Froehlich, "Berberine Inhibits Intestinal Secretory Response of Vibrio Cholerae Toxins and Escherichia Coli Enterotoxins," *Infect Immun* 35 (1982): 471–5.

11. U. Khin-Maung et al., "Clinical Trial of Berberine in Acute Watery Diarrhoea," *Br Med J* 291 (1985): 1601–5.

12. G.H. Rabbani et al., "Randomized Controlled Trial of Berberine Sulfate Therapy for Diarrhea Due to Enterotoxigenic Escherichia Coli and Vibrio Cholerae," *J Infect Dis* 155 (1987): 979–84.

13. M.H. Akhter, M. Sabir, and N.K. Bhide, "Possible Mechanism of Antidiarrhoeal Effect of Berberine," *Ind J Med Res* 70 (1979): 233–41.

14. Y.H. Tai, J.F. Feser, W.G. Mernane, and J.F. Desjeux, "Antisecretory Effects of Berberine in Rat Ileum," *Am J Physiol* 241 (1981): G253–8.

15. M.L. Clements, M.M. Levine, and P.A. Ristaino, "Exogenous Lactobacilli Fed to Man: Their Fate and Ability to Prevent Diarrheal Disease," *Prog Food Nutr Sci* 7 (1983): 29–37.

16. G. Zoppi, A. Deganello, G. Benoni, and F. Saccomani, "Oral Bacteriotherapy in Clinical Practice I: The Use of Different Preparations in Infants Treated with Antibiotics," *Eur J Ped* 139 (1982): 18–21.

17. V.P. Gotz, J.A. Romankiewics, J. Moss, and H.W. Murray, "Prophylaxis against Ampicillin-Induced Diarrhea with a Lactobacillus Preparation," *Am J Hosp Pharm* 36 (1979): 754–7.

18. G. Zoppi, V. Balsamo, A. Deganello et al., "Oral Bacteriotherapy in Clinical Practice: I. The Use of Different Preparations in the Treatment of Acute Diarrhea," *Eur J Ped* 139 (1982): 22–4.

Ear Infection

1. K.A. Daly, "Epidemiology of Otitis Media," *Otolaryngol Clin North Am* 24 (1991): 775–86.
2. L.C. Kleinman et al., "The Medical Appropriateness of Tympanostomy Tubes Proposed for Children Younger than 16 Years in the United States," *JAMA* 271 (1994): 1250–5.
3. C.D. Bluestone, "Otitis Media in Children: To Treat or Not to Treat," *NEJM* 306 (1982): 1399–404.
4. F.L. Van Buchen, J.H. Dunk, and M.A. van Hof, "Therapy of Acute Otitis Media: Myringotomy, Antibiotics, or Neither?" *Lancet* 2 (1981): 883–7.
5. R.L. Williams et al., "Use of Antibiotics in Preventing Recurrent Acute Otitis Media and in Treating Otitis Media with Effusion," *JAMA* 270 (1993): 1344–51.
6. R.M. Rosenfeld et al., "Clinical Efficacy of Antimicrobial Drugs for Acute Otitis Media: Meta-analysis of 5400 Children from Thirty-Three Randomized Trials," *J Pediatr* 124 (1994): 355–67.
7. J. Froom et al., "Antimicrobials for Acute Otitis Media? A Review from the International Primary Care Network," *BMJ* 315 (1997): 98–102.
8. M. Woodhead, "Antibiotic Resistance," *Brit J Hosp Med* 56 (1996): 314–5.
9. U.M. Saarinen, "Prolonged Breast Feeding As Prophylaxis for Recurrent Otitis Media," *Acta Ped Scand* 71 (1982): 567–71.
10. Editor: "Breast Feeding Prevents Otitis Media," *Nutr Rev* 41 (1983): 241–2.
11. H. Hasselbalch et al., "Decreased Thymus Size in Formula-Fed Infants Compared with Breastfed Infants," *Acta Periatr* 85 (1996): 1029–32.
12. J.T. McMahan, E. Calenoff, D.J. Croft et al., "Chronic Otitis Media with Effusion and Allergy: Modified RAST Analysis of 119 Cases," *Otol Head Neck Surg* 89 (1981): 427–31.
13. G.J. Viscomi, "Allergic Secretory Otitis Media: An Approach to Management," *Laryngoscope* 85 (1975): 751–8.
14. P.B. Van Cauwenberge, "The Role of Allergy in Otitis Media with Effusion," *Ther Umschau* 39 (1982): 1011–6.
15. P. Bellionin, A. Cantani, and F. Salvinelli, "Allergy: A Leading Role in Otitis Media with Effusion," *Allergol Immunol* 15 (1987): 205–8.
16. D.S. Hurst, "Association of Otitis Media with Effusion and Allergy As Demonstrated by Intradermal Skin Testing and Eostinophil Cationin Protein Levels in Both Middle Ear Effusions and Mucosal Biopsies," *Laryngoscope* 106 (1996): 1128–37.
17. T.M. Nsouli et al., "Role of Food Allergy in Serous Otitis Media," *Annals Allergy* 73 (1994): 215–9.
18. A. Fiocchi, E. Borella, E. Riva et al., "A Double-Blind Clinical Trial for the Evaluation of the Therapeutic Effectiveness of a Calf Thymus Derivative (Thymomodulin) in Children with Recurrent Respiratory Infections," *Thymus* 8 (1986): 831–9.
19. R. Genova and A. Guerra, "Thymomodulin in Management of Food Allergy in Children," *Int J Tissue Reac* 8 (1986): 239–42.
20. P. Cazzola, P. Mazzanti, and G. Bossi, "In Vivo Modulating Effect of a Calf Thymus Acid Lysate on Human T Lymphocyte Subsets and CD4+/CD8+ Ratio in the Course of Different Diseases," *Curr Ther Res* 42 (1987): 1011–7.
21. H.M. Lovejoy et al., "Effects of Low Humidity on the Rat Middle Ear," *Laryngoscope* 104 (1994): 1055–8.

Eczema

1. N. Soter and H. Baden, *Pathophysiology of Dermatologic Disease* (New York: McGraw-Hill, 1984).
2. A. Siccardi, A. Fortunato, M. Marconi, et al., "Defective Bactericidal Reaction by the Alternative Pathway of Complement in Atopic Patients," *Infect Immun* 33 (1981): 710–3.
3. P.D. Cooper and M. Carter, "Anti-Complementary Action of Polymorphic 'Solubility Forms' of Particulate Inulin," *Molecular Immunol* 23 (1986): 895–901.
4. U.M. Saarinen and M. Kajosaari, "Breastfeeding as Prophylaxis Against Atopic Disease: Prospective Follow-Up Study until 17 Years Old," *Lancet* 346 (1995): 1065–9.
5. A.J. Cant et al., "Effect of Maternal Dietary Exclusion on Breast-Fed Infants with Eczema: Two Controlled Studies," *Br Med J* 293 (1986): 231–3.
6. A.W. Burks et al., "Peanut Protein as a Major Cause of Adverse Food Reaction in Patients with Atopic Dermatitis," *Allergy Proceed* 10 (1989): 265–9.
7. F. de Maat-Bleeker and C. Bruijnzeel-Koomen, "Food Allergy in Adults with Atopic Dermatitis," *Highlights Food Allergy* 32 (1996): 157–163.
8. H.P. Van Bever, M. Docx, and W.J. Stevens, "Food and Food Additives in Severe Atopic Dermatitis," *Allergy* 44 (1989): 588–94.
9. A. Gondo, N. Saeki, and Y. Tokuda, "IgG4 Antibodies in Patients with Atopic Dermatitis," *Br J Dermatol* 117 (1987): 301–10.
10. H. Majamaa and E. Isolauri, "Evaluation of the Gut Mucosal Barrier: Evidence for Increased Antigen Transfer in Children with Atopic Eczema," *J Allergy Clin Immunol* 97 (1996): 985–90.
11. H. Agata et al., "Effect of Elimination on Food-Specific IgE Antibodies and Lymphocyte Proliferative Responses to Food Antigens in Atopic Dermatitis Patients Exhibiting Sensitivity to Food Allergens," *J Allergy Clin Immunol* 91 (1993): 668–79.
12. H.A. Sampson and S.M. Scanlon, "Natural History of Food Hypersensitivity in Children with Atopic Dermatitis," *J Pediatr* 115 (1989): 23–7.
13. J. Savolainen et al., "*Candida albicans* and Atopic Dermatitis," *Clin Exp Allergy* 23 (1993): 332–9.
14. M. Manku, D. Horrobin, N. Morse, et al., "Reduced Levels of Prostaglandin Precursors in the Blood of Atopic Patients: Defective delta-6-desaturase Function as a Biochemical Basis for Atopy," *Prostaglandins Leukotrienes and Medicine* 9 (1982): 615–28.
15. R. Lindskov and G. Holmer, "Polyunsaturated Fatty Acids in Plasma, Red Blood Cells, and Mononuclear Cell Phospho-lipids of Patients with

Atopic Dermatitis," *Allergy* 47 (1992): 517–22.

16. J.C.M. Stewart et al., "Treatment of Severe and Moderately Severe Atopic Dermatitis with Evening Primrose Oil (Epogam): A Multi-Center Study," *J Nutr Med* 2 (1991): 9–15.

17. C.A. Hederos and A. Berg, "Epogam Evening Primrose Oil Treatment in Atopic Dermatitis and Asthma," *Arch Dis Child* 75(6) (1996): 494–7.

18. A. Fiocchi et al., "The Efficacy and Safety of Gamma-Linolenic Acid in the Treatment of Infantile Atopic Dermatitis," *J Int Med Res* 22(1) (1994): 24–32.

19. J. Berth-Jones and R.A.C. Graham-Brown, "Placebo-Controlled Trial of Essential Fatty Acid Supplementation in Atopic Dermatitis," *Lancet* 341 (1993): 1557–60.

20. A. Bjorneboe et al., "Effect of Dietary Supplementation of Eicosapentaenoic Acid in the Treatment of Atopic Dermatitis," *Br J Dermatol* 117 (1987): 463–9.

21. K. Sakai et al., "Fatty Acid Compositions of Plasma Lipids in Atopic Dermatitis/Asthma Patients," *Arerugi* 43(1) (1994): 37–43.

22. E. Soyland et al., "Dietary Supplementation with Very Long-Chain n-3 Fatty Acids in Patients with Atopic Dermatitis: A Double-Blind, Multicentre Study," *Brit J Dermatol* 130 (1994): 757–64.

23. K. Seamon, W. Padgett, and J. Daly, "Forskolin: Unique Diterpine Activator of Adenylate Cyclase in Membranes and Intact Cells," *Proc Natl Acad Sci USA* 78 (1981): 3363–7.

24. T. Nikaido, T. Ohmoto, H. Noguchi, et al., "Inhibitors of Cyclic AMP Phosphodiesterase in Medicinal Plants," *J Med Plant Res* 43 (1981): 18–23.

25. E. Petkov, N. Nikolov, and J. Uzunov, "Inhibitory Effects of Some Flavonoids and Flavonoid Mixtures on Cyclic AMP Phosphodiesterase Activity of Rat Heart," *J Med Plant Res* 43 (1981): 183–6.

26. A. Beretz et al., "Role of Cyclic AMP in the Inhibition of Human Platelet Aggregation by Quercetin, a Flavonoid That Potentiates the Effect of Prostacyclin," *Biochem Pharm* 31 (1981): 3597–3600.

27. M. Amellal et al., "Inhibition of Mast Cell Histamine Release by Flavonoids and Bioflavonoids," *Planta Med* 51 (1985): 16–20.

28. M. Koltai et al., "Platelet Activating Factor (PAF): A Review of Its Effects, Antagonists, and Possible Future Clinical Implications (Part I)," *Drugs* 42(1) (1991): 9–29.

29. M. Koltai et al., "PAF: A Review of Its Effects, Antagonists, and Possible Future Clinical Implications (Part II)," *Drugs* 42(2) (1991): 174–204.

30. T.J. David, "Serum Levels of Trace Metals in Children with Atopic Eczema," *Br J Dermatol* 122 (1990): 485–9.

31. D.J. Atherton et al., "Treatment of Atopic Eczema with Traditional Chinese Medicinal Plants," *Pediatr Dermatol* 9(4) (1992): 373–5.

32. M.P. Sheehan et al., "Efficacy of Traditional Chinese Herbal Therapy in Adult Atopic Dermatitis," *Lancet* 340 (1992): 13–7.

33. M.P. Sheehan and D.J. Atherton, "A Controlled Trial of Traditional Chinese Medicinal Plants in Widespread Non-Exudative Atopic Eczema," *Br J Dermatol* 126(2) (1992): 179–84.

34. F.Q. Evans, "The Rational Use of Glycyrrhetinic Acid in Dermatology," *Br J Clin Pract* 12 (1958): 269–79.

35. B. Barnes, "Thyroid Therapy in Dermatology," *Cutis* 8 (1971): 581–3.

36. J. Jordan and F. Whitlock, "Emotions and the Skin: The Conditioning of Scratch Responses in Cases of Atopic Dermatitis," *Br J Dermatol* 86 (1972): 574–84.

37. C. Mann and E.J. Staba, "The Chemistry, Pharmacology, and Commercial Formulations of Chamomile," *Herbs, Spices, and Medicinal Plants* 1 (1984): 235–80.

38. R. Pfister, "Problems in the Treatment and After Care of Chronic Dermatoses: A Clinical Study on Hametum Ointment," *Fortschr Med* 99 (1981): 1264–8.

Fibrocystic Breast Disease

1. E.N. Cole, R.A. Sellwood, P.G. England, and K. Griffiths, "Serum Prolactin Concentrations in Benign Breast Disease Throughout the Menstrual Cycle," *J Cancer* 13 (1977): 597–603.

2. F. Peters, W. Schuth, B. Scheurich, and M. Breckwoldt, "Serum Prolactin Levels in Patients with Fibrocystic Breast Disease," *Obstet Gynecol* 64 (1984): 381–5.

3. C.A. Boyle, G.S. Berkowitz, V.A. LiVolsi, et al., "Caffeine Consumption and Fibrocystic Breast Disease: A Case-Control Epidemiologic Study," *JNCI* 72 (1984): 1015–9.

4. J.P. Minton, H. Abou-Issa, N. Reiches, J.M. Roseman, "Clinical and Biochemical Studies on Methylxanthine-Related Fibrocystic Breast Disease," *Surgery* 90 (1981): 299–304.

5. J.P. Minton, M.K. Foecking, D.J.T. Webster, and R.H. Matthews, "Caffeine, Cyclic Nucleotides, and Breast Disease," *Surgery* 86 (1979): 105–9.

6. V.L. Ernster, L. Mason, W.H. Goodson, et al., "Effects of Caffeine-Free Diet on Benign Breast Disease: A Random Trial," *Surgery* 91 (1982): 263–7.

7. C. Welsh, K. Scieska, E. Senn, and J. Dehoog, "Caffeine (1,3,7-tri-methylxanthine): A Temperate Promoter of DMBA-Induced Rat Mammary Gland Carcinogenesis," *Int J Ca* 32 (1983): 479–83.

8. R.S. London, G.S. Sundaram, M. Schultz, et al., "Endocrine Parameters and Alpha-Tocopherol Therapy of Patients with Mammary Dysplasia," *Cancer Res* 41 (1981): 3811–3.

9. R.S. London, G. Sundaram, S. Manimekalai, et al., "The Effect of Alpha-Tocopherol on Premenstrual Symptomatology: A Double-Blind Study. II: Endocrine Correlates," *J Am Col Nutr* 3 (1984): 351–6.

10. G.S. Sundaram, R. London, S. Margolis, et al, "Serum Hormones and Lipoproteins in Benign Breast Disease," *Cancer Res* 41 (1981): 3814–6.

11. P.R. Band, M. Deschamps, M. Falardeau, et al., "Treatment of Benign Breast Disease with Vitamin A," *Prev Med* 13 (1984): 549–54.

12. B.A. Eskin, D.G. Bartushka, M.R. Dunn, et al., "Mammary Gland Dysplasia in Iodine Deficiency," *JAMA* 200 (1967): 691–5.

13. N.C. Estes, "Mastodynia Due to Fibrocystic Disease of the Breast Controlled with Thyroid Hormone," *A J Surg* 142 (1981): 764–6.

14. W.R. Ghent et al., "Iodine Replacement in Fibrocystic Disease of the Breast," *Can J Surg* 36 (1993): 453–60.

15. Z.E. Mielens, J. Rozitis, Jr., and V.J. Sansone, Jr., "The Effect of Oral Iodides on Inflammation," *Texas Rep Biol Med* 26 (1968): 117–21.

16. N.L. Petrakis and E.B. King, "Cytological Abnormalities in Nipple Aspirates of Breast Fluid from Women with Severe Constipation," *Lancet* 2 (1981): 1203–5.

17. D.J. Hentges, "Does Diet Influence Human Fecal Microflora Composition?" *Nutr Rev* 38 (1980): 329–6.

18. B. Goldin, H. Aldercreutz, J. Dwyer, et al., "Effect of Diet on Excretion of Estrogens in Pre- and Postmenopausal Women," *Cancer Res* 41 (1981): 3771–3.

19. B. Goldin and S. Gorback, "The Effect of Milk and Lactobacillus Feeding on Human Intestinal Bacterial Activity," *Am J Clin Nutr* 39 (1984): 256–61.

20. P.A. Baghurst and T.E. Rohan, "Dietary Fiber and Risk of Benign Proliferative Epithelial Disorders of the Breast," *Int J Cancer* 63 (1995): 481–485.

Fibromyalgia

1. D. Buchwald and D. Garrity, "Comparison of Patients with Chronic Fatigue Syndrome, Fibromyalgia, and Multiple Chemical Sensitivities," *Arch Intern Med* 154 (1994): 2049–53.

2. K.P. White and M. Harth, "An Analytical Review of 24 Controlled Clinical Trials for Fibromyalgia Syndrome (FMS)," *Pain* 64 (1996): 211–9.

3. G. Affleck et al., "Sequential Daily Relations of Sleep, Pain Intensity, and Attention to Pain among Women with Fibromyalgia," *Pain* 68 (1996): 363–8.

4. F. Sicuteri, "The Ingestion of Serotonin Precursors (L-5-hydroxytryptophan and L-tryptophan) Improves Migraine," *Headache* 13 (1973): 19–22.

5. M. Nicolodi and F. Sicuteri, "Fibromyalgia and Migraine, Two Faces of the Same Mechanism: Serotonin As the Common Clue for Pathogenesis and Therapy," *Adv Exp Med Biol* 398 (1996): 373–9.

6. M. Nicolodi and F. Sicuteri, "Eosinophilia Myalgia Syndrome [Food and Drink]: The Role of Contaminants, the Role of Serotonergic Set Up," *Exp Biol Med* 398 (1996): 351–7.

7. I. Caruso et al., "Double-Blind Study of 5-Hydroxytryptophan versus Placebo in the Treatment of Primary Fibromyalgia Syndrome," *J Int Med Res* 18 (1990): 201–9.

8. P.S. Puttini and I. Caruso, "Primary Fibromyalgia Syndrome and 5-Hydroxy-L-Tryptophan: A 90-Day Open Study," *J Int Med Res* 20 (1992): 182–9.

9. D. Goldenberg et al., "A Randomized, Double-Blind Crossover Trial of Fluoxetine and Amitriptyline in the Treatment of Fibromyalgia," *Arthritis Rheum* 39 (1996): 1852–9.

10. T.J. Romano and J.W. Stiller, "Magnesium Deficiency in Fibromyalgia Syndrome," *J Nutr Med* 4 (1994): 165–7.

11. I.M. Cox, M.J. Campbell, and D. Dowson, "Red Blood Cell Magnesium and Chronic Fatigue Syndrome," *Lancet* 337 (1991): 757–60.

12. G. Abraham, "Management of Fibromyalgia: Rationale for the Use of Magnesium and Malic Acid," *J Nutr Med* 3 (1992): 49–59.

13. J.T. Hicks, "Treatment of Fatigue in General Practice: A Double Blind Study," *Clin Med* (January 1964): 85–90.

Food Allergies

1. F. Adams, *The Genuine Works of Hippocrates* (Baltimore, MD: Williams & Williams, 1939).

2. H.A. Sampson, "Eczema and Food Hypersensitivity," in D.D. Metcalfe, H.A. Sampson, and R.A. Simon, eds., *Food Allergy: Adverse Reactions to Foods and Food Additives* (Boston: Blackwell Scientific Publications, 1991), 113–128.

3. H.A. Sampson, "Food Hypersensitivity and Dietary Management in Atopic Dermatitis," *Pediatric Dermatology* 9 (1992): 376–379.

4. N.I. Kjellman, "Natural History and Prevention of Food Sensitivity," in D.D. Metcalfe, H.A. Sampson, and R.A. Simon, eds., *Food Allergy: Adverse Reactions to Foods and Food Additives* (Boston: Blackwell Scientific Publications, 1991), 319–331.

5. F. Andre, C. Andre, L. Colin, F. Cacaraci, S. Cavagna, "Role of New Allergens and of Allergens Consumption in the Increased Incidence of Food Sensitizations in France," *Toxicology* 93 (1994): 77–83.

6. J.W. Gerrard, C.G. Ko, and P. Vickers, "The Familial Incidence of Allergic Disease," *Ann All* 36 (1976): 10.

7. J.J. McGovern, "Correlation of Clinical Food Allergy Symptoms with Serial Pharmacological and Immunological Changes in the Patient's Plasma," *Ann Allergy* 44 (1980): 57.

8. R.J. Trevino, "Immunologic Mechanisms in the Production of Food Sensitivities," *Laryngoscope* 91 (1981): 1913.

9. W.A. Commings and E.W. Williams, "Transport of Large Breakdown Products of Dietary Protein through the Gut Wall," *Gut* 19 (1978): 715.

10. W.A. Walker, "Uptake and Transport of Macromolecules by the Intestine—Possible Role in Clinical Disorders," *Gastroenter* 67 (1974): 531.

11. S.E. Keller, J.M. Weiss, S.J. Schleifer et al., "Suppression of Immunity by Stress: Effect of Graded Series of Stressors on Lymphocyte Stimulation in the Rat," *Science* 213 (1981): 1397.

12. R. Ader, Ed., *Psychoimmunology* (New York: Academic Press, 1981).

13. J.D. Minor, S.G. Tolber, and O.L. Frick, "Leukocyte Inhibition Factor in Delayed-Onset Food Sensitivity," *J Allergy Clin Immunol* 6 (1980): 314.

14. J. Brostoff and S.J. Challacombe, eds., *Food Allergy and Intolerance* (Philadelphia: WB Saunders, 1987).

15. J.J. McGovern, "Correlation of Clinical Food Allergy Symptoms with Serial Pharmacological and Immunological Changes in the Patient's Plasma," *Ann Allergy* 44 (1980): 57.

16. R.J. Dockhorn and T.C. Smith, "Use of a Chemically Defined Hypoaller-

genic Diet in the Management of Patients with Suspected Food Allergy," *Ann Allergy* 47 (1981): 264–66.

17. A.H. Rowe and A. Rowe, *Food Allergy: Its Manifestations and Control and the Elimination Diets* (IL: CC Thomas, 1972).

18. D. Metcalfe, "Food Hypersensitivity," *J All Clin Imm* 73 (1984): 749–61.

19. A.F. Coca, "Art of Investigating Pulse Diet Record in Familial Nonreagenic Food Allergy," *Ann Allergy* 2 (1944): 1.

20. H.J. Rinkel, T. Randolph, and M. Zeller, *Food Allergy* (IL: CC Thomas, 1951).

21. AAAI Board of Directors, "Measurement of Specific and Nonspecific IgG4 Levels As Diagnostic and Prognostic Tests for Clinical Allergy," *J Allergy Clin Immunol* 95 (1995): 652–4.

22. C.M. Gwynn et al., "Bronchial Provocation Tests in Atopic Patients with Allergen Specific IgG4 Antibodies," *Lancet* 1 (1982): 254–6.

23. F. Shakib et al., "Study of IgG Sub-Class Antibodies in Patients with Milk Intolerance," *Clin Allergy* 16 (1986): 451–8.

24. A.E. Rafei et al., "Diagnostic Value of IgG4 Measurements in Patients with Food Allergy," *Annals Allergy* 62 (1989): 94–99.

25. R.J. Rinkel, "Food Allergy IV: The Function and Clinical Application of the Rotary Diversified Diet," *J Pediat* 32 (1948): 266.

Gallstones

1. S.L. Robbins, R.S. Cotran, and V. Kumar, *Pathologic Basis of Disease* (Philadelphia: W.B. Saunders, 1984), 942–50.

2. R. Petersdorf et al., eds., *Harrison's Principles of Internal Medicine* (New York: McGraw-Hill, 1983), 1821–321.

3. H.F. Weisberg, "Pathogenesis of Gallstones," *Ann Clin Lab Sci* 14 (1984): 243–51.

4. H. Trowell, D. Burkitt, and K. Heaton, *Dietary Fibre, Fibre-Depleted Foods, and Disease* (New York: Academic Press, 1985), 289–304.

5. E. Rubenstein and D.D. Federman, *Scientific American Medicine* (New York: Scientific American, 1986), 4:VI–1–10.

6. F. Nervi, C. Covarubias, P. Bravo, et al., "Influence of Legume Intake on Biliary Lipids and Cholesterol Saturation in Young Chilean Men," *Gastroenterol* 96 (1989): 825–30.

7. J.W. Marks, P.A. Cleary, and J.J. Albers, "Lack of Correlation between Serum Lipoproteins and Biliary Cholesterol Saturation in Patients with Gallstones," *Dig Dis Sci* 29 (1984): 1118–22.

8. D.B. Petitti, G.D. Friedman, and A.L. Klatsky, "Association of a History of Gallbladder Disease with a Reduced Concentration of High-Density Lipoprotein Cholesterol," *NEJM* 304 (1981): 1396–8.

9. J.R. Thornton, K.W. Heaton, and D.G. MacFarland, "A Relation between High-Density-Lipoprotein Cholesterol and Bile Cholesterol Saturation," *Lancet* i (1981): 1352–4.

10. W. Van der Linder and F. Bergman, "An Analysis of Data on Human Hepatic Bile: Relationship between Main Bile Components, Serum Cholesterol, and Serum Triglycerides," *Scand J Clin Lab Invest* 37 (1977): 741–7.

11. F. Pixley, D. Wilson, K. McPherson, et al., "Effect of Vegetarianism on Development of Gallstones in Women," *Br Med J* 291 (1985): 11–22.

12. D. Kritchevsky and D.M. Klurfeld, "Gallstone Formation in Hamsters: Effect of Varying Animal and Vegetable Protein Levels," *Am J Clin Nutr* 37 (1983): 802–4.

13. J.C. Breneman, "Allergy Elimination Diet as the Most Effective Gallbladder Diet," *Ann All* 26 (1968): 83–7.

14. H. Necheles, B.Z. Rappaport, R. Green, et al., "Allergy of the Gallbladder," *Am J Dig Dis* 7 (1949): 238–41.

15. M. Walzer, I. Gray, M. Harten, et al, "The Allergic Reaction in the Gallbladder: Experimental Studies in Rhesus Monkeys," *Gastroenterol* 1 (1943): 565–72.

16. P. De Muro and A. Ficari, "Experimental Studies on Allergic Cholecystitis," *Gastroenterol* 6 (1946): 302–14.

17. C.J. Moerman, et al., "Dietary Sugar Intake in the Etiology of Biliary Tract Cancer," *Int J Epidem* 22 (1993): 207–13.

18. C.J. Moerman, et al., "Dietary Risk Factors for Clinically Diagnosed Gallstones in Middle-Aged Men: A 25-Year Follow-Up Study (The Zutphen Study)," *Ann Epidem* 4 (1994): 248–54.

19. R.K. Tandon et al., "Dietary Habits of Gallstone Patients in Northern India: A Case Control Study," *J Clin Gastroenterol* 22 (1996): 23–7.

20. R.O. Kamrath et al., "Cholelithiasis in Patients Treated With a Very Low Calorie Diet," *Am J Clin Nutr* 56 (1992): 255S–7S.

21. Anonymous: "Fasting May Cause Stones," *Med Trib* (July 25, 1991): 13.

22. B.A. Spirt et al., "Gallstone Formation in Obese Women Treated by a Low-Calorie Diet," *Int J Obesity* 19 (1995): 593–5.

23. B.R. Douglas et al, "Coffee Stimulation of Cholecystokinin Release and Gallbladder Contraction in Humans," *Am J Clin Nutr* 52 (1990): 553–6.

24. S.A. Tuzhilin, D.A. Drieling, R.V. Narodetskaja, and L.K. Lukash, "The Treatment of Patients with Gallstones by Lecithin," *Am J Gastroenterol* 65 (1976): 231.

25. I. Hanin and G.B. Ansell, *Lecithin: Technological, Biological, and Therapeutic Aspects* (New York: Plenum Press, 1987).

26. S.A. Jenkins, "Vitamin C and Gallstone Formation: A Preliminary Report," *Experentia* 33 (1977): 1616–7.

27. U. Gustafsson et al., "The Effect of Vitamin C in High Doses on Plasma and Biliary Lipid Composition in Patients with Cholesterol Gallstones: Prolongation of the Nucleation Time," *Eur J Clin Invest* 27 (1997): 387–91.

28. S.P. Lee, C. Tassman-Jones, and V. Carlisle, "Oleic Acid-Induced Cholelithiasis in Rabbits," *Am J Pathol* 124 (1986): 18–24.

29. A.C. Beynen, "Dietary Monounsaturated Fatty Acids and Liver Cholesterol," *Artery* 15 (1988): 170–5.

30. G. Baggio, A. Pagnan, M. Muraca, et al., "Olive-Oil-Enriched Diet: Effect on Serum Lipoprotein Levels and Biliary Cholesterol Saturation," *Am J Clin Nutr* 47 (1988): 960–4.

31. M. Scobey et al., "Dietary Fish Oil Effects on Biliary Lipid Secretion and Cholesterol Gallstone Formation in the African Green Monkey," *Hepatology* 14 (4/ Pt.1) (1991): 679–84.

32. T.H. Magnuson et al., "Dietary Fish Oil Inhibits Cholesterol Monohydrate Crystal Nucleation and Gallstone Formation in the Prairie Dog," *Surgery* 118 (1995): 517–23.

33. L.J. Schoenfield, J.M. Lachin, The Steering Committee, et al., "Chenodiol (Chenodeoxycholic Acid) for the Dissolution of Gallstones: The National Cooperative Gallstone Study: A Controlled Trial of Efficacy and Safety," *Ann Int Med* 95 (1981): 257.

34. H. Fromm, "Gallstone Dissolution and the Cholesterol-Bile Acid-Lipoprotein Axis: Propitious Effects of Ursodeoxycholic Acid (editorial)," *Gastroenterol* 87 (1984): 229.

35. M.L. Petroni et al., "Repeated Bile Acid Therapy for the Long-Term Management of Cholesterol Gallstones," *J Hepatol* 25 (1996): 719–24.

36. G.D. Bell and J. Doran, "Gallstone Dissolution in Man Using an Essential Oil Preparation," *Br Med J* 278 (1979): 24.

37. J. Doran, R.B. Keighley, and G.D. Bell, "Rowachol: A Possible Treatment for Cholesterol Gallstones," *Gut* 20 (1979): 312–7.

38. W.R. Ellis and G.D. Bell, "Treatment of Biliary Duct Stones with a Terpene Preparation," *Br Med J* 282 (1981): 611.

39. K.W. Somerville, W.R. Ellis, B.H. Whitten, et al., "Stones in the Common Bile Duct: Experience with Medical Dissolution Therapy," *Postgrad Med J* 61 (1985): 313–6.

40. W.R. Ellis, G.D. Bell, B. Middleton, and D.A. White, "Adjunct to Bile-Acid Treatment for Gallstone Dissolution: Low Dose Chenodeoxycholic Acid Combined with a Terpene Preparation," *Br Med J* 282 (1981): 611–2.

41. G.D. Bell, R.J. Clegg, W.R. Ellis, et al., "How Does Rowachol, A Mixture of Plant Monoterpenes, Enhance the Cholelithic Potential of Low and Medium Dose Chenodeoxycholic Acid?" *Br J Pharm* 13 (1982): 278–9.

42. W.R. Ellis, K.W. Somerville, B.H. Whitten, and G.D. Bell, "Pilot Study of Combination Treatment for Gall Stones with Medium Dose Chenodeoxycholic Acid and a Terpene Preparation," *Br Med J* 289 (1984): 153–6.

43. S. Pavel, "Sunbathing and Gallstones," *Lancet* 339 (1992): 241.

Glaucoma

1. L.M. Tierney, S.J. McPhee, and M.A. Papadakis, eds., *Current Medical Diagnosis and Treatment* (Los Altos, CA: Lange Medical Publications, 1997), 183–4.

2. B. Tengroth and T. Ammitzboll, "Changes in the Content and Composition of Collagen in the Glaucomatous Eye: Basis for a New Hypothesis for the Genesis of Chronic Open-Angle Glaucoma," *Acta Ophthamol* 62 (1984): 999–1008.

3. J. Weiss and M. Jayson, *Collagen in Health and Disease* (New York: Churchill Livingston, 1982), 388–403.

4. H. Quigley and E. Addicks, "Regional Differences in the Structure of the Lamina Cribosa and Their Relation to Glaucomatous Optic Nerve Damage," *Arch Ophthamol* 99 (1983): 137–43.

5. T. Krakau, B. Bengston, and C. Holmin, "The Glaucoma Theory Updated," *Acta Ophthamol* 61 (1983): 737–41.

6. J. Rohen, "Why Is Intraocular Pressure Elevated in Chronic Simple Glaucoma?" *Ophthalmology* 90 (1983): 758–65.

7. G. Bietti, "Further Contributions on the Value of Osmotic Substances as Means to Reduce Intraocular Pressure," *Trans Ophthamol Soc U.K.* 86 (1966): 247–54.

8. S. Fishbein and S. Goodstein, "The Pressure Lowering Effect of Ascorbic Acid," *Annal Ophthamol* 4 (1972): 487–91.

9. E. Linner, "The Pressure Lowering Effect of Ascorbic Acid in Ocular Hypertension," *Acta Ophthamol* 47 (1969): 685–9.

10. T. Shen and M. Yu, "Clinical Evaluation of Glycerin-Sodium Ascorbate Solution in Lowering Intraocular Pressure," *Chinese Med J* 1 (1975): 64–8.

11. M. Virno, M. Bucci, J. Pecori-Giraldi, and A. Missiroli, "Oral Treatment of Glaucoma with Vitamin C," *Eye Ear Nose Throat Monthly* 46 (1967): 1502–8.

12. M. Gabor, "Pharmacologic Effects of Flavonoids on Blood Vessels," *Angiologica* 9 (1972): 355–374.

13. J. Monboisse, P. Braquet, and J. Borel, "Oxygen-Free Radicals as Mediators of Collagen Breakage," *Agents Actions* 15 (1984): 49–50.

14. A. Hagerman and L. Butler, "The Specificity of Proanthocyanidin-Protein Interactions," *J Biol Chem* 256 (1981): 4494–7.

15. L. Caselli, "Clinical and Electroretinographic Study on Activity of Anthocyanosides," *Arch Med Int* 37 (1985): 29–35.

16. F. Stocker, "New Ways of Influencing the Intraocular Pressure," *NY St J Med* 49 (1949): 58–63.

17. L.F. Raymond, "Allergy and Chronic Simple Glaucoma," *Ann Allergy* 22 (1964): 146–50.

18. A.Z. Gaspar, P. Gasser, and J. Flammer, "The Influence of Magnesium on Visual Field and Peripheral Vasospasm in Glaucoma," *Ophthalmologica* 209 (1995): 11–3.

19. B.C. Lane, "Diet and Glaucomas," *J Am Coll Nutr* 10/Abstract 11 (1991): 536.

20. R. McGuire, "Fish Oil Cuts Lower Ocular Pressure," *Medical Tribune* August 19, 1991: 25.

21. H.J. Merte and W. Merkle, "Long-Term Treatment with *Ginkgo biloba* Extract of Circulatory Disturbances of the Retina and Optic Nerve," *Klin Monatsbl Augenheilkd* 177(5) (1980): 577–83.

Gout

1. R. Petersdorf et al., eds., *Harrison's Principles of Internal Medicine* (New York: McGraw-Hill, 1983).

2. M.V. Krause and L.K. Mahan, *Food, Nutrition, and Diet Therapy*, 7th ed. (Philadelphia: W.B. Saunders, 1984), 677–9.

3. Nutrition Foundation, *Present Knowledge in Nutrition*, 5th ed. (Washington, DC: Nutrition Foundation, 1984), 740–56.

4. J. Faller and I.H. Fox, "Ethanol-Induced Hyperuricemia," *NEJM* 307 (1982): 1598–602.

5. F.X. Pi-Sunyer, "The Fattening of America," *JAMA* 272 (1994): 238.

6. J.T. Scott, "Obesity and Hyperuricaemia," *Clin Rheum Dis* 3 (1977): 25–35.

7. B.T. Emmerson, "Effect of Oral Fructose on Urate Production," *Ann Rheum Dis* 33 (1974): 276–9.

8. T. Terano et al., "Eicosapentaenoic Acid as a Modulator of Inflammation, Effect on Prostaglandin and Leukotriene Synthesis," *Biochem Pharmacol* 35 (1986): 779–85.

9. A.W. Ford-Hutchinson, "Leukotrienes: Their Formation and Role as Inflammatory Mediators," *Fed Proc* 44 (1985): 25–9.

10. R.V. Panganamala and D.G. Cornwell, "The Effects of Vitamin E on Arachidonic Acid Metabolism," *Ann NY Acad Sci* 393 (1982): 376–91.

11. A.S. Lewis, L. Murphy, C. McCalla, et al., "Inhibition of Mammalian Xanthine Oxidase by Folate Compounds and Amethopterin. *J Biol Chem* 259:12-5, 1984

12. T. Spector and R. Ferone, "Folic Acid Does Not Activate Xanthine Oxidase," *J Biol Chem* 259 (1984): 10784–6.

13. K.A. Oster, "Xanthine Oxidase and Folic Acid," *Ann Int Med* 87 (1977): 252.

14. S. Taussig, M. Yokoyama, A. Chinen, et al., "Bromelain: A Proteolytic Enzyme and Its Clinical Application: A Review," *Hiroshima J Med Sci* 24 (1975): 185–93.

15. A. Bindoli, M. Valente, and L. Cavallini, "Inhibitory Action of Quercetin on Xanthine Oxidase and Xanthine Dehydrogenase Activity," *Pharm Res Comm* 17 (1985): 831–9.

16. W.W. Busse, D.E. Kopp, and E. Middleton, "Flavonoid Modulation of Human Neutrophil Function," *J Allergy Clin Immunol* 73 (1984): 801–9.

17. T. Yoshimoto, M. Furukawa, S. Yamamoto, et al., "Flavonoids: Potent Inhibitors of Arachidonate 5-Lipoxygenase," *Biochem Biophys Res Comm* 116 (1983): 612–8.

18. H.B. Stein, A. Hasan, and I.H. Fox, "Ascorbic Acid-Induced Uricosuria: A Consequence of Megavitamin Therapy," *Ann Int Med* 84 (1976): 385–8.

19. S.L. Gershon and I.H. Fox, "Pharmacological Effects of Nicotinic Acid on Human Purine Metabolism," *J Lab Clin Med* 84 (1974): 179–86.

20. L.W. Blau, "Cherry Diet Control for Gout and Arthritis," *Texas Rep Biol Med* 8 (1950): 309–11.

21. M. Gabor, "Pharmacologic Effects of Flavonoids on Blood Vessels," *Angiologica* 9 (1972): 355–74.

22. J. Kuhnau, "The Flavonoids: A Class of Semi-Essential Food Components: Their Role in Human Nutrition," *World Rev Nutr Diet* 24 (1976): 117–91.

23. B. Havsteen, "Flavonoids: A Class of Natural Products Of High Pharmacological Potency," *Biochem Pharm* 32 (1983): 1141–8.

24. E. Middleton, "The Flavonoids," *Trends Pharm Sci* 5 (1984): 335–8.

25. J.A. Duke, *Handbook of Medicinal Herbs* (Boca Raton, FL: CRC Press, 1985), 222.

26. D.W. McLeod, P. Revell, and B.V. Robinson, "Investigations of *Harpagophytum procumbens* (Devil's Claw) in the Treatment of Experimental Inflammation and Arthritis in the Rat," *Br J Pharmacol* 66 (1979): 140P–1P.

27. L.W. Whitehouse, M. Znamirowski, and C.J. Paul, "Devil's Claw (*Harpagophytum procumbens*): No Evidence for Anti-Inflammatory Activity in the Treatment of Arthritic Disease," *Can Med Assoc J* 129 (1983): 249–51.

28. G.V. Ball and L.B. Sorensen, "Pathogenesis of Hyperuricemia in Saturnine Gout," *NEJM* 280 (1969): 1199–202.

29. T. Appelboom and J.C. Bennett, "Gout of the Rich and Famous," *J Rheumatol* 13 (1986): 618–22.

30. J.H. Graziano and C. Blum, "Lead Exposure from Lead Crystal," *Lancet* 337 (1991): 141–2.

Headache

1. E.L. Hurwitz et al., "Manipulation and Mobilization of the Cervical Spine: A Systematic Review of the Literature," *Spine* 21 (1996): 1746–59.

2. K.A. Holroyd et al., "A Comparison of Pharmacological and Nonpharmacological Therapies for Chronic Tension Headaches," *J Consult Clin Psychol* 59 (1991): 387–93.

3. B. Larsson and J. Carlsson, "A School-Based, Nurse-Administered Relaxation Training for Children with Chronic Tension-Type Headache," *J Pediatr Psychol* 21 (1996): 603–14.

4. J.M. Hammill, T.M. Cook, and J.C. Rosecrance, "Effectiveness of a Physical Therapy Regimen in the Treatment of Tension-Type Headache," *Headache* 36 (1996): 149–53.

Heart Disease

1. M.F. Chen et al., "Plasma and erythrocyte thiamin concentration in geriatric outpatients," *J Am Coll Nutr* 15 (1996): 231–6.

2. D. Leslie and M. Gheorghiade, "Is there a role for thiamine supplementation in the management of heart failure?" *Am Heart J* 131 (1996): 1248–50. ·(1994): 125–30.

3. S.S. Gottlieb et al., "Prognostic importance of serum magnesium concentration in patients with congestive heart failure," *J Am Coll Cardiol* 16 (1990): 827–31.

4. S.S. Gottlieb, "Importance of magnesium in congestive heart failure," *Am J Cardiol* 63 (1989): 39G–42G.

5. R.M. McLean, "Magnesium and its therapeutic uses: A review," *Am J Med* 96 (1994): 63–76.

6. B.M. Altura, "Basic biochemistry and physiology of magnesium: A brief review," *Magnes Trace Elem* 10 (1991): 167–71.

7. J.R. Purvis and A. Movahed, "Magnesium disorders and cardiovascular disease," *Clin Cardiol* 15 (1992): 556–68.

8. B.M. Altura, "Ischemic heart disease and magnesium," *Magnesium* 7 (1988): 57–67.

9. M.A. Brodsky et al., "Magnesium therapy in new-onset atrial fibrillation," *Am J Cardiol* 73 (1994): 1227–9.

10. L.D. Galland, S.M. Baker, and R.K. McLellan, "Magnesium deficiency in the pathogenesis of mitral valve prolapse," *Magnesium* 5 (1986): 165–74.

11. J.S. Fernandes et al., "Therapeutic effect of a magnesium salt in patients suffering from mitral valvular prolapse and latent tetany," *Magnesium* 4 (1985): 283–9.

12. T. Ishiyama et al., "A clinical study of the effect of coenzyme Q on congestive heart failure," *Jpn Heart J* 17 (1976): 32.

13. T. Tsuyusaki, C. Noro, and R. Kikawada, "Mechanocardiography of ischemic or hypertensive heart failure," in Y. Yamamura, K. Folkers, Y. Ito, eds., *Biomedical and Clinical Aspects of Coenzyme Q*, Vol 2 (Amsterdam: Elsevier/North-Holland Biomedical Press, 1980), 273–88.

14. W.V. Judy et al., "Myocardial effects of co-enzyme Q10 in primary heart failure," in K. Folkers and Y. Yamamura, eds., *Biomedical and Clinical Aspects of Coenzyme Q*, Vol 4 (Amsterdam: Elsevier Science Publ, 1984), 353–67.

15. J.H.P. Vanfraechem, C. Picalausa, and K. Folkers, "Coenzyme Q10 and physical performance in myocardial failure," in K. Folkers and Y. Yamamura, eds., *Biomedical and Clinical Aspects of Coenzyme Q*, Vol 4 (Amsterdam: Elsevier Science Publ, 1984), 281–90.

16. C. Hofman-Bang, N. Rehnquist, and K. Swedberg, "Coenzyme Q10 as an adjunctive treatment of congestive heart failure," *J Am Coll Cardiol* 19 (1992): 216A.

17. C. Morisco, B. Trimarco, and M. Condorelli, "Effect of coenzyme Q10 therapy in patients with congestive heart failure: A long-term multicenter randomized study," *Clin Investig* 71(Suppl.8) (1993): S134–6.

18. E. Baggio et al., "Italian multicenter study on the safety and efficacy of coenzyme Q10 as adjunctive therapy in heart failure," CoQ10 Drug Surveillance Investigators *Mol Aspects Med* 15(Suppl.) (1994): S287–94.

19. T. Oda and K. Hamamoto, "Effect of coenzyme Q10 on the stress-induced decrease of cardiac performance in pediatric patients with mitral valve prolapse," *Jap Circ J* 48 (1984): 1387.

20. K. Folkers, S. Vadhanavikit, and S.A. Mortensen, "Biochemical rationale and myocardial tissue data on the effective therapy of cardiomyopathy with coenzyme Q10," *Proc Natl Acad Sci* 82 (1985): 901.

21. P.H. Langsjoen, S. Vadhanavikit, and K. Folkers, "Response of patients in classes III and IV of cardiomyopathy to therapy in a blind and crossover trial with coenzyme Q10," *Proc Natl Acad Sci* 82 (1985): 4240.

22. K.L. Goa and R.N. Brogden, "L-carnitine—A preliminary review of its pharmacokinetics, and its therapeutic use in ischemic cardiac disease and primary and secondary carnitine deficiencies in relationship to its role in fatty acid metabolism," *Drugs* 34 (1987): 1–24.

23. M. Mancini et al., "Controlled study on the therapeutic efficacy of propionyl-L-carnitine in patients with congestive heart failure," *Arzneim Forsch* 42 (1992): 1101–4.

24. G. Pucciarelli et al., "The clinical and hemodynamic effects of propionyl-L-carnitine in the treatment of congestive heart failure," *Clin Ter* 141 (1992): 379–84.

25. V.M. O'Conolly et al., "Treatment of cardiac performance (NYHA stages I to II) in advanced age with standardized crataegus extract," *Fortschr Med* 104 (1986): 805–8.

26. V.M. O'Conolly et al., "Treatment of cardiac performance (NYHA stages I to II) in advanced age with standardized crataegus extract," *Fortschr Med* 104 (1986): 805–8.

27. H. Leuchtgens, "Crataegus Special Extract WS 1442 in NYHA II heart failure: A placebo controlled randomized double-blind study," *Fortschr Med* 111 (1993): 352–4.

Hemorrhoids

1. H. Trowell, D. Burkitt, and K. Heaton, *Dietary Fibre, Fibre-Depleted Foods and Disease* (London, UK: Academic Press, 1985).

2. F. Moesgaard, M.L. Nielsen, J.B. Hansen, and J.T. Knudsen, "High-Fiber Diet Reduces Bleeding and Pain in Patients with Hemorrhoids," *Dis Colon Rectum* 25 (1982): 454–56.

3. D.J. Webster, D.C. Gough, and J.L. Craven, "The Use of Bulk Evacuation in Patients with Hemorrhoids," *Br J Surg* 65 (1978): 291–92.

4. A.N. Wadworth and D. Faulds, "Hydroxyethylrutosides: A Review of Its Pharmacology, and Therapeutic Efficacy in Venous Insufficiency and Related Disorders," *Drugs* 44 (1992): 1013–32.

5. T. Poynard and C. Valterio, "Meta-Analysis of Hydroxyethylrutosides in the Treatment of Chronic Venous Insufficiency," *Vasa* 23 (1994): 244–50.

6. M.R. Boisseau et al., "Fibrinolysis and Hemorheology in Chronic Venous Insufficiency: A Double Blind Study of Troxerutin Efficiency," *J Cardiovasc Surg* 36 (1995): 369–74.

7. H.A. Neumann and M.J. van den Broek, "A Comparative Clinical Trial of Graduated Compression Stockings and O-(Beta-Hydroxyethyl)-Rutosides (HR) in the Treatment of Patients with Chronic Venous Insufficiency," *Z Lymphol* 19 (1995): 8–11.

8. S. Renton et al., "The Effect of Hydroxyethylrutosides on Capillary Filtration in Moderate Venous Hypertension: A Double Blind Study," *Int Angiol* 13 (1994): 259–62.

9. W.J. MacLennan et al., "Hydroxyethylrutosides in Elderly Patients with Chronic Venous Insufficiency: Its Efficacy and Tolerability," *Gerontology* 40 (1994): 45–52.

10. N.A.M. Bergstein, "Clinical Study on the Efficacy of O-(Beta-Hydroxyethyl)-Rutoside (HR) in Varicosis of Pregnancy," *J Int Med Res* 3 (1975): 189–93.

11. H. Wijayanegara et al., "A Clinical Trial of Hydroxyethylrutosides in the Treatment of Hemorrhoids of Pregnancy," *J Int Med Res* 20 (1992): 54–60.

12. F. Annoni et al., "Treatment of Actue Symptoms of Hemorrhoidal Disease with High Dose O-(Beta-Hydroxyethyl)-Rutoside," *Minerva Medica* 77 (1986): 1663–68.

13. A. Saggloro et al., "Treatment of Hemorrhoidal Syndrome with Mesoglycan," *Min Diet Gastr* 31 (1985): 311–15

Hepatitis

1. W.T. Branch, *Office Practice of Medicine* (Philadelphia: WB Saunders, 1982), 679–85.

2. R.F. Cathcart, "The Third Face of Vitamin C," *J Orthomol Med* 7 (1992): 197–200.

3. R.F. Cathcart, "The Method of Determining Proper Doses of Vitamin C for the Treatment of Disease by Titrating to Bowel Tolerance," *J Orthomol Psychiat* 10 (1981): 125–32.

4. F.R. Klenner, "Observations on the Dose of Administration of Ascorbic Acid When Employed Beyond the Range of a Vitamin in Human Pathology," *J Applied Nutr* 23 (1971): 61–88.

5. D. Baetgen, "Results of the Treatment of Epidemic Hepatitis in Children with High Doses of Ascorbic Acid for the Years 1957-1958," *Medizinische Monatchrift* 15 (1961): 30–6.

6. H. Baur and H. Staub, "Treatment of Hepatitis with Infusions of Ascorbic Acid: Comparison with Other Therapies," *JAMA* 156 (1954): 565.

7. A. Murata, "Viricidal Activity of Vitamin C: Vitamin C for Prevention and Treatment of Viral Diseases," in T. Hasegawa, *Proc First Intersectional Cong Int Assoc Microbiol Soc*, Vol 3. (Tokyo: Tokyo Univ. Press, 1975), 432–42.

8. A. Ohbayashi, T. Akioka, and H. Tasaki, "A Study of Effects of Liver Hydrolysate on Hepatic Circulation," *J Therapy* 54 (1972): 1582–5.

9. K. Sanbe et al., "Treatment of Liver Disease—with Particular Reference to Liver Hydrolysates," *Jap J Clin Exp Med* 50 (1973): 2665–76.

10. K. Fujisawa et al., "Therapeutic Effects of Liver Hydrolysate Preparation on Chronic Hepatitis: A Double Blind, Controlled Study," *Asian Med J* 26 (1984): 497–526.

11. M. Galli et al., "Attempt to Treat Acute Type B Hepatitis with an Orally Administered Thymic Extract (Thymomodulin): Preliminary Results," *Drugs Exptl Clin Res* 11 (1985): 665–9.

12. F. Bortolotti et al., "Effect of an Orally Administered Thymic Derivative, Thymodulin, in Chronic Type B Hepatitis in Children," *Curr Ther Res* 43 (1988): 67–72.

13. H. Suzuki et al., "Effects of Glycyrrhizin on Biochemical Tests in Patients with Chronic Hepatitis: Double Blind Trial," *Asian Med J* 26 (1984): 423–38.

14. K. Mori et al., "Effects of Glycyrrhizin (SNMC: Stronger Neo-Minophagen C) in Hemophilia Patients with HIV-1 Infection," *Tohoku J Exp Med* 162(2) (1990): 183–93.

15. J. Eisenburg, "Treatment of Chronic Hepatitis B. Part 2: Effect of Glycyrrhizinic Acid on the Course of Illness," *Fortschr Med* 110 (1992): 395–8.

16. S.K. Acharya et al., "A Preliminary Open Trial on Interferon Stimulator (SNMC) Derived from Glycyrrhiza Glabra in the Treatment of Subacute Hepatic Failure," *Ind J Med Res* 98 (1993): 75–8.

17. Y. Arase et al., "The Long Term Efficacy of Glycyrrhizin in Chronic Hepatitis C Patients," *Cancer* 79 (1997): 1494–500.

18. Y. Arase et al., "The Superiority of Laparoscopic Examination in Predicting Hepatocellular Carcinoma After Interferon Therapy for Chronic Type C Hepatitis," *Dig Endosc J Pharmacol* 10 (1997): 613–20.

19. R.V. Farese et al., "Licorice-Induced Hypermineralocorticoidism," *N Engl J Med* 325 (1991): 1223–7.

20. F.C. Stormer, R. Reistad, and J. Alexander, "Glycyrrhizic Acid in Liquorice: Evaluation of Health Hazard," *Fd Chem Toxicol* 31 (1993): 303–12.

21. G. Deak et al., "Immunomodulator Effect of Silymarin Therapy in Chronic Alcoholic Liver Diseases," *Orv Hetil* 131 (1990): 1291–2, 1295–6.

22. E. Magliulo, B. Gagliardi, and G.P. Fiori, "Results of a Double Blind Study on the Effect of Silymarin in the Treatment of Acute Viral Hepatitis, Carried Out at Two Medical Centres," *Med Klin* 73 (1978): 1060–5.

23. R. Schandalik, G. Gatti, and E. Perucca, "Pharmacokinetics of Silybin in Bile Following Administration of Silipide and Silymarin in Cholecystectomy Patients," *Arzneim Forsch* 42 (1992): 964–8.

24. N. Barzaghi et al., "Pharmacokinetic Studies on IdB 1016, a Silybin-Phosphatidylcholine Complex, in Healthy Human Subjects," *Eur J Drug Metab Pharmacokinet* 15 (1990): 333–8.

25. A. Vailati et al., "Randomized open study of the dose-effect relationship of a short course of IdB 1016 in patients with viral or alcoholic hepatitis," *Fitoterapia* 44(3) (1993): 219–28.

26. S. Mascarella et al., "Therapeutic and antilipoperoxidant effects of silybin-phosphatidylcholine complex in chronic liver disease: Preliminary results," *Curr Ther Res* 53(1) (1993): 98–102.

27. G. Buzzelli et al., "A pilot study on the liver protective effect of silybin-phosphatidylcholine complex (IdB1016) in chronic active hepatitis," *Int J Clin Pharmacol Ther Toxicol* 31 (1993): 456–60.

28. C. Marena and P. Lampertico, "Preliminary clinical development of silipide: A new complex of silybin in toxic liver disorders," *Planta Medical* 57(S2) (1991): A124–5.

29. S.P. Thyagarajan et al., "Effect of Phyllanthus amarus on chronic carriers of hepatitis B virus," *Lancet* II (1988): 764–6.

30. A. Leelarasamee et al., "Failure of Phyllanthus amarus to eradicate hepatitis B surface antigen from symptomless carriers," *Lancet* 335 (1990): 1600–1.

31. B.S. Blumberg et al., "Hepatitis B virus and primary hepatocellular carcinoma: Treatment of HBV carriers with Phyllanthus amarus," *Vaccine* 8 (1990): S86-92; L. Berk et al., "Beneficial effects of Phyllanthus amarus for chronic hepatitis B, not confirmed," *J Hepatol* 12(3) (1991): 405–6.

32. A. Milne et al., "Failure of New Zealand hepatitis B carriers to respond to Phyllanthus amarus," *New Zealand Med J* 107 (1994): 243.

Herpes

1. R. Steele, M. Vincent, S. Hensen, et al., "Cellular Immune Response to Herpes Simplex Type 1 Virus in Recurrent Herpes Labialis: In Vitro Blastogenesis and Cytotoxicity to Infected Cell Lines," *J Inf Dis* 131 (1984): 528–34.

2. F. Aiuti, M. Sirianni, A. Stella, et al., "A Placebo-Controlled Trial of

Thymic Hormone Treatment of Recurrent Herpes Simplex Labialis Infection in Immunodeficient Hosts," *Int J Clin Pharm Ther Tox* 21 (1983): 81–6.

3. J. Fitzherbert, "Genital Herpes and Zinc," *Med J Aust* 1 (1979): 399.

4. I. Brody, "Topical Treatment of Recurrent Herpes Simplex and Post-Herpetic Erythema Multiforme with Low Concentrations of Zinc Sulphate Solution," *Br J Dermatol* 104 (1981): 191–213.

5. T. Hovi et al., "Topical Treatment of Recurrent Mucocutaneous Herpes with Ascorbic Acid-Containing Solution," *Antiviral Research* 27 (1995): 263–270.

6. R. Griffith, D. DeLong, and J. Nelson, "Relation of Arginine-Lysine Antagonism to Herpes Simplex Growth in Tissue Culture," *Chemotherapy* 27 (1981): 209–13.

7. J. DiGiovanna and H. Blank, "Failure of Lysine in Frequently Recurrent Herpes Simplex Infection," *Arch Dermatol* 120 (1984): 48–51.

8. R. Griffith, A. Norins, and C. Kagan, "A Multicentered Study of Lysine Therapy in Herpes Simplex Infection," *Dermatol* 156 (1978): 257–67.

9. M.A. McCune et al., "Treatment of Recurrent Herpes Simplex Infections with L-Lysine Monohydrochlorite," *Cutis* 34 (1984): 366–73.

10. R.S. Griffith et al., "Success of L-Lysine Therapy in Frequently Recurrent Herpes Simplex Infection," *Dermatologica* 175 (1987): 183–90.

11. R.H. Wolbling and K. Leonhardt, "Local Therapy of Herpes Simplex with Dried Extract from *Melissa officinalis*," *Phytomed* 1 (1994): 25–31.

12. R. Pompei, A. Pani, O. Flore, et al., "Antiviral Activity of Glycyrrhizic Acid," *Experientia* 36 (1980): 304.

13. M. Partridge and D. Poswillo, "Topical Carbonoxolone Sodium in the Management of Herpes Simplex Infection," *Br J Oral Maxillofac Surg* 22 (1984): 138–45.

14. G. Csonka and D. Tyrrell, "Treatment of Herpes Genitalis with Carbonoxolone and Cicloxolone Creams: A Double-Blind Placebo-Controlled Trial," *Br J Ven Dis* 60 (1984): 178–81.

High Blood Pressure

1. Medical Research Council Working Party on Mild Hypertension, "MRC Trial of Treatment of Mild Hypertension: Principal Results," *Br Med J* 291 (1980): 97–104.

2. Report by the Management Committee, "The Australian Therapeutic Trial in Mild Hypertension," *Lancet* 1 (1980): 1261–7.

3. Veterans Administration Cooperative Study Group on Antihypertensive Agents, "Effects of Treatment on Morbidity in Hypertension, II: Results of Patients with Diastolic Blood Pressure Averaging 90 through 114 mm Hg," *JAMA* 213 (1970): 1143–51.

4. U.S. Public Health Service Hospitals Cooperative Study Group, "Treatment of Mild Hypertension: Results of a Ten-Year Intervention Trial," *Circ Res* 40(suppl. 1) (1977): I98–I105.

5. A. Helgeland, "Treatment of Mild Hypertension: A Five-Year Controlled Drug Trial: The Oslo Study," *Am J Med* 69 (1980): 725–32.

6. Multiple Risk Factor Intervention Trial Research Group, "Baseline Rest Electrocardiographic Abnormalities, Antihypertensive Treatment, and Mortality in the Multiple Risk Factor Intervention Trial," *Am J Cardiol* 55 (1985): 1–15.

7. T.A. Miettinen, "Multifactorial Primary Prevention of Cardiovascular Diseases in Middle-Aged Men: Risk Factor Changes, Incidence, and Mortality," *JAMA* 254 (1985): 2097–2102.

8. A. Amery, W. Birkenhager, P. Brixko et al., "Mortality and Morbidity Results from European Working Party on High Blood Pressure in the Elderly Trial," *Lancet* 1 (1985): 1349–54.

9. Hypertension Detection and Follow-up Program Cooperative Group, "Five Year Findings of the Hypertension Detection and Follow-up Program, I.: Reduction in Mortality in Persons with High Blood Pressure, Including Mild Hypertension," *JAMA* 242 (1979): 2562–71.

10. E.D. Freis, "Rationale against the Drug Treatment of Marginal Dias-

tolic Systemic Hypertension," *Am J Cardiol* 66 (1990): 368–71.

11. M.H. Alderman, "Which Antihypertensive Drugs First—and Why!" *JAMA* 267 (1992): 2786–7.

12. I.L. Rouse, L.J. Beilin, D.P. Mahoney et al, "Vegetarian Diet and Blood Pressure," *Lancet* 2 (1983): 742–3.

13. C.A. Silagy and H.A. Neil, "A Meta-Analysis of the Effect of Garlic on Blood Pressure," *J Hypertens* 12(4) (1994): 463–8.

14. B. Jansson, "Dietary, Total Body, and Intracellular Potassium-to-Sodium Ratios and Their Influence on Cancer," *Cancer Detect Prevent* 14 (1991): 563–5.

15. K.T. Khaw and E. Barrett-Connor, "Dietary Potassium and Stroke-Associated Mortality," *N Engl J Med* 316 (1987): 235–40.

16. F. Skrabal, J. Aubock, and H. Hortnagl, "Low Sodium/High Potassium Diet for Prevention of Hypertension: Probable Mechanisms of Action," *Lancet* 2 (1981): 895–900.

17. O. Iimura et al., "Studies on the Hypotensive Effect of High Potassium Intake in Patients with Essential Hypertension," *Clin Sci* 61(Supplement 7) (1981): 77S–80S.

18. H.G. Langford, "Dietary Potassium and Hypertension: Epidemiological Data," *Ann Intern Med* 98 (1990): 770–2.

19. S.A. MacGregor et al., "Moderate Potassium Supplementation in Essential Hypertension," *Lancet* 2 (1982): 567–70.

20. N.M. Kaplan, "Potassium Supplementation in Hypertensive Patients with Diuretic-Induced Hypokalemia," *New Engl J Med* 312 (1985): 746–9.

21. S.M. Matlou et al., "Potassium Supplementation in Blacks with Mild to Moderate Essential Hypertension," *J Hypertension* 4 (1986): 61–4.

22. A.O. Oble, "Placebo Controlled Trial of Potassium Supplements in Black Patients with Mild Essential Hypertension," *J Cardiovasc Pharmacol* 14 (1989): 294–6.

23. P.S. Patki et al., "Efficacy of Potassium and Magnesium in Essential Hypertension: A Double-Blind, Placebo-Controlled, Cross-

over Study," *Br J Med* 301 (1990): 521–3.

24. M.D. Fotherby and J.F. Potter, "Potassium Supplementation Reduces Clinic and Ambulatory Blood Pressure in Elderly Hypertensive Patients," *J Hypertension* 10 (1992): 1403–8.

25. L. Thijs et al., "Age-Related Effects of Placebo and Active Treatment in Patients Beyond the Age of 60 Years: The Need for a Proper Control Group," *J Hypertension* 8 (1990): 997–1002.

26. T. Motoyama, H. Sano, and H. Fukuzaki, "Oral Magnesium Supplementation in Patients with Essential Hypertension," *Hypertension* 13 (1989): 227–32.

27. P.K. Whelton and M.J. Klag, "Magnesium and Blood Pressure: Review of the Epidemiologic and Clinical Trial Experience," *Am J Cardiol* 63 (1989): 26G–30G.

28. M.R. Joffres, D.M. Reed, and K. Yano, "Relationship of Magnesium Intake and Other Dietary Factors to Blood Pressure: The Honolulu Heart Study," *Am J Clin Nutr* 45 (1987): 469–75.

29. J.S. Lindberg et al., "Magnesium Bioavailability from Magnesium Citrate and Magnesium Oxide," *J Am Coll Nutr* 9 (1990): 48–55.

30. T. Bohmer et al., "Bioavailability of Oral Magnesium Supplementation in Female Students Evaluated from Elimination of Magnesium in 24-Hour Urine," *Magnesium Trace Elem* 9 (1990): 272–8.

31. N.M. Kaplan, "Non-Drug Treatment of Hypertension," *Annals of Internal Medicine* 102 (1985): 359–73.

32. D.E. Anderson, A.Y. Bagrov, and J.L. Austin, "Inhibited Breathing Decreases Renal Sodium Excretion," *Psychosomatic Med* 57 (1995): 373–80.

33. J.A. Simon, "Vitamin C and Cardiovascular Disease: A Review," *J Am Coll Nutr* 11 (1992): 107–25.

34. J.L. Pierkle, J. Schwartz, J.R. Landis, and W.R. Harlan, "The Relationship between Blood Lead Levels and Blood Pressure and Its Cardiovascular Risk Implications," *Am J Epid* 121 (1985): 246–58.

35. M. Ayback et al., "Effect of Oral Pyridoxine Hydrochloride Supplementation on Arterial Blood Pressure in Patients with Essential Hypertension," *Arzneim Forsch* 45 (1995): 1271–3.

36. F.P. Cappuccio et al., "Epidemiologic Association between Dietary Calcium Intake and Blood Pressure: A Meta-Analysis of Published Data," *Am J Epidemiol* 142 (1995): 935–45.

37. R.B. Meese et al., "The Inconsistent Effects of Calcium Supplements upon Blood Pressure in Primary Hypertension," *Am J Med Sci* 29 (1987): 4219–24.

38. J.R. Sowers et al., "Calcium and Hypertension," *J Lab Clin Med* 114 (1989): 338–48.

39. Y. Takagi et al., "Calcium Treatment of Essential Hypertension in Elderly Patients Evaluated by 24 H Monitoring," *Am J Hypertens* 4 (1991): 836–9.

40. V. Digiesi et al., "Mechanism of Action of Coenzyme Q10 in Essential Hypertension," *Curr Ther Res* 51 (1992): 668–72.

41. P. Langsjoen et al., "Treatment of Essential Hypertension with Coenzyme Q10," *Mol Aspects Med* 15(Suppl.) (1994): S265-72.

42. V. Digiesi et al., "Coenzyme Q10 in Essential Hypertension," *Mol Aspects Med* 15(Suppl.) (1994): S257–63.

43. E.B. Schmidt and J. Dyerberg, "Omega-3 Fatty Acids: Current Status in Cardiovascular Medicine," *Drugs* 47 (1994): 405–24.

44. L.J. Appel et al., "Does Supplementation of Diet with 'Fish Oil' Reduce Blood Pressure? A Meta-Analysis of Controlled Clinical Trials," *Arch Intern Med* 153 (1993): 1429–38.

45. P. Singer, "Alpha-Linolenic Acid vs. Long-Chain Fatty Acids in Hypertension and Hyperlipidemia," *Nutr* 8 (1992): 133–5.

46. E.M. Berry and J. Hirsch, "Does Dietary Linolenic Acid Influence Blood Pressure," *Am J Clin Nutr* 44 (1986): 336–40.

47. V. Petkov, "Plants with Hypotensive, Antiatheromatous and Coronarodilating Action," *Am J Chin Med* 7 (1979): 197–236.

48. H.P.T. Ammon and M. Handel, "Crataegus, Toxicology and Pharmacology, Part I: Toxicity," *Planta Med* 43 (1981): 105–20; "Part II: Pharmacodynamics," *Planta Med* 43 (1981): 209–39; "Part III: Pharmacodynamics and Pharmacokinetics," *Planta Med* 43(4) (1981): 313–22.

Hives

1. B.M. Czarnetzki. *Urticaria* (New York: Springer-Verlag, 1986).

2. K.P. Mathews. "A Current View of Urticaria," *Med Clin North Am* 58 (1974): 185–205.

3. T.M. Keahey. "The Pathogenesis of Urticaria," *Derm Clin* 3 (1985): 13–28.

4. R.K. Winkelmann. "Food Sensitivity and Urticaria or Vasculitis," in: J. Brostoff and S.J. Challacombe, eds., *Food Allergy and Intolerance* (Philadelphia: WB Saunders, 1987), 602–17.

5. A.D. Ormerod, T.M.S. Reid, and R.A. Main. "Penicillin in Milk—Its Importance in Urticaria," *Clin Allergy* 17 (1987): 229–34.

6. K. Wicher and R.E. Reisman. "Anaphylactic Reaction to Penicillin in a Soft Drink," *J Allergy Clin Immunol* 66 (1980): 155–7.

7. H.J. Schwartz and T.H. Sher. "Anaphylaxis to Penicillin in a Frozen Dinner," *Ann Allergy* 52 (1984): 342–3.

8. W.J. Boonk and W.G. Van Ketel. "The Role of Penicillin in the Pathogenesis of Chronic Urticaria," *Br J Derm* 106 (1982): 183–90.

9. H. Lindemayr, R. Knobler, D. Kraft, and G. Baumgartner. "Challenge of Penicillin Allergic Volunteers with Penicillin Contaminated Meat," *Allergy* 36 (1981): 471–8.

10. R.A. Settipane, H.P. Constatine, and G.A. Settipane. "Aspirin Intolerance and Recurrent Urticaria in Adults," *Allergy* 35 (1980): 149–54.

11. R.P. Warin. "The Effect of Aspirin in Chronic Urticaria," *Br J Derm* 72 (1960): 350–1.

12. M. Moore-Robinson and R.P. Warin. "Effects of Salicylates in Urticaria," *Br Med J* 4 (1967): 262–4.

13. R.H. Champion, S.O.B. Roberts, R.G. Carpenter, and J.H. Roger. "Urticaria and Angioedema. A Review of 554 Patients," *Br J Derm* 81 (1969): 588–97.

14. J. James and R.P. Warin. "Chronic Urticaria: The Effect of Aspirin," *Br J Derm* 82 (1970): 204–5.

15. C. Genton, P.C. Frei, and, A. Pecoud: "Value of Oral Provocation Tests to Aspirin and Food Additives in the Routine Investigation of Asthma and Chronic Urticaria," *J Allergy Clin Immunol* 76 (1985): 40–5.

16. I. Bjarnason, P. Williams, P. Smethurst, et al. "Effect of Non-Steroidal Anti-Inflammatory Drugs and Prostaglandins on the Permeability of the Human Small Intestine," *Gut* 27 (1986): 1292–7.

17. P.J. August. "Successful Treatment of Urticaria Due to Food Additive with Sodium Cromoglycate and an Exclusion Diet," in: Pepys and Edwards (eds)., *The Mast Cell, Its Role in Health and Disease* (Turnbridge Wells: Pitman Medical, 1979).

18. H.M.G. Doeglas. "Reactions to Aspirin and Food Additives in Patients with Chronic Urticaria, Including the Physical Urticaria," *Br J Derm* 93 (1975): 135–44.

19. K. Egyedi and L. Torok. "Nachweis ·Einer Intoleranz von Lebensmittel-Additvstoffen Durch Proben mit Salizylaten bei Chronischer Urticaria," *Allergologie* 5.

20. M. Fujita, T. Yakimoto, T. Aoki, et al. "Provocation Tests with Aspirin and Sodium Benzoate in Urticaria," *Japan J Derm* 88 (1978): 709–13.

21. C. Genton, P.C. Frei, and A. Pecoud. "Value of Oral Provocation Tests to Aspirin and Food Additives in the Routine Investigation of Asthma and Chronic Urticaria," *J Allergy Clin Immunol* 76 (1985): 40–5.

22. A. Gibson and R. Clancy. "Management of Chronic Idiopathic Urticaria by the Identification and Exclusion of Dietary Factors," *Clin Allergy* 10 (1980): 699–704.

23. M. Hannuksela. "Food Allergy and Skin Diseases," *Ann Allergy* 51 (1983): 269–71.

24. L. Juhlin. "Recurrent Urticaria: Clinical Investigation of 330 Patients," *Br J Derm* 104 (1981): 369–81.

25. K. Kaaber. "Colouring and Preservative Agents and Chronic Urticaria. Value of a Provocative Trial and Elimination Diet," *Ugeskr Laeger* 140 (1978): 1473–6.

26. A.S. Kemp and G. Schembri. "An Elimination Diet for Chronic Urticaria of Childhood," *Med J Aust* 143 (1985): 234–5.

27. B. Kirchoff, U.F. Haustein, and M. Rytter. "Azetylsalizylsaure-Addition-Intoleranzphanomene bei Chronich Rezidivierender Urtikaria," *Derm Msch* 168 (1982): 513.

28. H. Lindemayr and J. Schmidt. "Intolerance to Acetylsalicylic Acid and Food Additives in Patients Suffering from Chronic Urticaria," *Wien Klin Wochenschr* 91 (1979): 817–22.

29. G. Merk and G. Goerz. "Analgetika-Intoleranz," *Z Hautkr* 58 (1983): 535–54.

30. J. Meynadier, et al. "Chronic Urticaria," *Ann Derm Venereol* 106 (1979): 153–8.

31. G. Michaelsson and L. Juhlin. "Urticaria Induced by Preservatives and Dye Additives to Food and Drugs," *Br J Derm* 88 (1973): 525–34.

32. H. Mikkelsen, J.C. Larsen, and F. Tarding. "Hypersensitivity Reactions to Food Colours with Special Reference to the Natural Colour Annatto Extract (Butter Colour)," *Arch Toxicol* 1(suppl) (1978): 141–3.

33. I. Neuman, R. Elian, H. Nahum, et al. "The Danger of 'Yellow Dyes' (Tartrazine) to Allergic Subjects," *Clin Allergy* 8 (1978): 65–8.

34. C. Ortolani, E. Pastorello, M.T. Luraghi, et al. "Diagnosis of Intolerance to Food Additives," *Ann Allergy* 53 (1984): 587–91.

35. P.D. Pigatto, F. Riva, A. Cattaneo, et al. "Orticaria Cronica," *G Ital Derm Venereol* 120 (1985): 113–7.

36. M. Samter and R.F. Beers. "Concerning the Nature of Intolerance to Aspirin," *J Allergy* 40 (1967): 281–91.

37. G.A. Settipane, F.H. Chafee, H. Postman, et al. "Significance of Tartrazine Sensitivity in Chronic Urticaria of Unknown Etiology," *J Allergy Clin Immunol* 57 (1976): 541–9.

38. R.A. Simon. "Adverse Reactions to Drug Additives," *J Allergy Clin Immunol* 74 (1984): 623–30.

39. G. Supramaniam and J.O. Warner. "Artificial Food Additive Intolerance in Patients with Angio-Oedema and Urticaria," *Lancet* ii (1986): 907–9.

40. P. Thune and A. Granhold. "Provocation Tests with Anti-Phlogistic and Food Additives in Recurrent Urticaria," *Dermatologica* 151 (1975): 360–72.

41. R.P. Warin and R.J. Smith. "Challenge Test Battery in Chronic Urticaria," *Br J Derm* 94 (1976): 401–10.

42. B. Wutrich and L. Fabro. "Acetylsalicylsaure unc Lebensmittel-Additiva-Intleranz bei Urticaria, Asthma Bronchiale and Chronischer Rhinopathie," *Schweiz Med Wochenschr* 111 (1981): 1445–50.

43. B. Ziegler and U.F. Haustein. "Intoleranzreaktionen anf Nicht-Steroidale Antiphogistika and Analgetika bei Chronisch Recidivierendes Urtikaria," *Derm Mschr* 172 (1986): 313–7.

44. S.I. Asad, L.J.F. Youlten, and M.H. Lessof. "Specific Desensitization in Aspirin Sensitive Urticaria," *Clin Allergy* 13 (1983): 459–66.

45. M.L. Kowalski, I. Grzelewski-Ryzmowski, J. Roznieki, and M. Szmidt. "Aspirin-Induced Tolerance in Aspirin Sensitive Asthmatics," *Allergy* 39 (1984): 171–8.

46. F.M. Atkins. "The Basis of Immediate Hypersensitivity Reactions to Foods. Nutrition," *Rev* 41 (1983): 229–34.

47. D.G. Wraith, J. Merrett, A. Roth, et al. "Recognition of Food Allergic Patients and Their Allergens by the RAST Technique and Clinical Investigation," *Clin Allergy* 9 (1975): 25–36.

48. T.M. Golbert, R. Patterson, and J.J. Pruzansky. "Systemic Reactions to Ingested Antigens," *J Allergy* 44 (1969): 96–107.

49. S.P. Galant, J. Bullock, and O.L. Frick. "An Immunological Approach to the Diagnosis of Food Sensitivity," *Clin Allergy* 3 (1973): 363–72.

50. M.L. Pachor, L. Andri, F. Nicolis, et al. "Elimination Diet and Challenge Test in Diagnosis of Food Intolerance," *Italian J Med* 2 (1986): 1–6.

51. W.B. Rawls and V.C. Ancona, "Chronic Urticaria Associated with Hypochlorhydria or Achlorhydria," *Rev Gastroenterol* 18 (1951): 267–71.

52. P.C. Baird. "Etiology and Treatment of Urticaria: Diagnosis, Prevention and Treatment of Poison-Ivy Dermatitis," *NEJM* 224 (1941): 649–58.

53. J.R. Allison. "The Relation of Hydrochloric Acid and Vitamin B Complex Deficiency in Certain Skin Diseases," *Southern Med J* 38 (1945): 235–41.

54. M. Gloor, K. Henkel, and U. Schulz. "Zur Pathogenetischen Bedeutung von Magenfunktionsstoringen bie Allergish Bedingter Chronischer Urtikaria," *Derm Msch* 158 (1972): 96–102.

55. S. Husz, G. Berko, R. Szabo, and N. Simon. "Immunoelectrophoresis in the Dermatologic Practice. III. Dysproteinemias (Chronic Urticaria, Drug Allergy)," *Derm Msch* 160 (1974): 93–100.

56. J.R. Allison. "The Relation of Hydrochloric Acid and Vitamin B Complex Deficiency in Certain Skin Diseases," *Southern Med J* 38 (1945): 235–41.

57. L. Juhlin. "Additives and Chronic Urticaria," *Ann Allergy* 59 (1987): 119–23.

58. T. Zuberbier, et al. "Pseudoallergen-Free Diet in the Treatment of Chronic Urticaria," *ACTA Dermatologica Venerol* (Stockh) 75 (1995): 484–7.

59. S.D. Lockey. "Allergic Reactions to F D & C Yellow No. 5, Tartrazine, an Aniline Dye Used as a Coloring and Identifying Agent in Various Steroids," *Ann Allergy* 17 (1959): 719–21.

60. C. Collins-Williams. "Clinical Spectrum of Adverse Reactions to Tartrazine," *J Asthma* 22 (1985): 139–43.

61. M.H. Lessof, et al. "Reactions to Food Additives," *Clin Exp Allergy* 25(Suppl 1) (1995): 27–8.

62. R.J. Warrington, P.J. Sauder, and S. McPhillips. "Cell-Mediated Immune Responses to Artificial Food Additives in Chronic Urticaria," *Clin Allergy* 16 (1986): 527–33.

63. S.F. Natbony, M.E. Phillips, J.M. Elias, et al. "Histologic Studies of Chronic Idiopathic Urticaria," *J Allergy Clin Immunol* 71 (1983): 177–83.

64. H.M.G. Doeglas. "Dietary Treatment of Patients with Chronic Urticaria and Intolerance to Aspirin and Food Additives," *Dermatologica* 154 (1977): 308–10.

65. A.M. Ros, L. Juhlin, and G. Michaelsson. "A Follow-Up Study of Patients with Recurrent Urticaria and Hypersensitivity to Aspirin, Benzoates and Azo Dyes," *Br J Derm* 95 (1976): 19–24.

66. E. Valverde, J.M. Vich, J.V. Garcia-Calderon, et al. "In Vitro Stimulation of Lymphocytes in Patients with Chronic Urticaria Induced by Additives and Food," *Clin Allergy* 10 (1980): 691–8.

67. A. Verschave, E. Stevens, and H. Degreef. "Pseudo-Allergen Free Diet in Chronic Urticaria," *Dermatologica* 167 (1983): 256–9.

68. A.R. Swain, S.P. Dutton, and A.S. Truswell. "Salicylates in Foods," *J Am Diet Assoc* 85 (1985): 950–60.

69. A. Kulczycki. Aspartame-Induced Urticaria," *Annals Int Med* 104 (1986): 207–8.

70. D.A. Moneret-Vautrin, G. Faure, and M.C. Bene. "Chewing-Gum Preservative Induced Toxidermic Vasculitis," *Allergy* 41 (1986): 546–8.

71. J.G.D. Birkmayer and W. Beyer. "Biological and Clinical Relevance of Trace Elements," *Arztl Lab* 36 (1990): 284–7.

72. G.A. Vaida, M.A. Goldman, and K.J. Bloch. "Testing for Hepatitis B Virus in Patients with Chronic Urticaria and Angioedema," *J Allergy Clin Immunol* 72 (1983): 193–8.

73. C. Schade, U. Kuben, and H.J. Westphal. "Incidence of Yeasts and Therapeutic Results in Chronic Urticaria," *Derm Msch* 161 (1975): 187–95.

74. H. Serrano. "Hypersensitivity to Candida Albicans and Other Yeasts in Patients with Chronic Urticaria," *Allergol Immunopathol* 3 (1975): 289–98.

75. J. James and R.P. Warin. "An Assessment of the Role of Candida Albicans and Food Yeast in Chronic Urticaria," *Br J Derm* 84 (1971): 227–37.

76. G. Green, G. Koelsche, and R. Kierland: "Etiology and Pathogenesis of Chronic Urticaria," *Ann Allergy* 23 (1965): 30–6.

77. C.L. Shertzer and D.P. Lookingbill. "Effects of Relaxation Therapy and Hypnotizability in Chronic Urticaria," *Arch Derm* 123 (1987): 913–6.

78. M. Hannuksela and E.L. Kokkonen. "Ultraviolet Light Therapy in Chronic Urticaria," *Acta Derm Venereol* 65 (1985): 449–50.

79. J.H. Olafsson, O. Larko, G. Roupe et al: "Treatment of Chronic Urticaria with PUVA or UVA Plus Placebo: a Double-Blind Study," *Arch Derm Res* 278 (1986): 228–31.

80. C.S. Johnston, L.J. Martin, and X. Cai. "Antihistamine effect of supplemental ascorbic acid and neutrophil chemotaxis," *J Am Coll Nutr* 11 (1992): 172–6.

81. S.W. Simon. "Vitamin B_{12} Therapy in Allergy and Chronic Dermatoses," *J Allergy* 22 (1951): 183–5.

82. S.W. Simon and P. Edmonds. "Cyanocobalamin (B12): Comparison of Aqueous and Repository Preparations in Urticaria; Possible Mode of Action," *J Am Geriatr Soc* 12 (1964): 79–85.

83. E. Middleton and G. Drzewieki. "Naturally Occurring Flavonoids and Human Basophil Histamine Release," *Int Arch Allergy Appl Immunol* 77 (1985): 155–7.

84. M. Amella, C. Bronner, F. Briancon, et al. "Inhibition of Mast Cell Histamine Release by Flavonoids and Bioflavonoids," *Planta Medica* 51 (1985): 16–20.

85. G.W. Canonica, G. Ciprandi, M. Bagnasco, and A. Scordamaglia: "Oral Cromolyn in Food Allergy: In Vivo and In Vitro Effects," *Clinical Immunol Immunopathol* 41 (1986): 154–8.

86. J. Rumbyrt, J.L. Katz and A.L. Schocket. "Resolution of chronic urticaria in patients with thyroid autoimmunity," *J Allergy Clin Immunol* 96 (1995): 901–5.

Hypoglycemia

1. J.B. Wyngaarden, L.H. Smith, and J.C. Bennett, eds., *Cecil Textbook of Medicine* (Philadelphia, PA: W.B. Saunders), 1992.

2. S.A. Chalew et al., "Diagnosis of Reactive Hypoglycemia: Pitfalls in the Use of the Oral Glucose Tolerance Test," *Southern Medical J* 79 (1986): 285–7.

3. S.A. Chalew et al., "The Use of the Plasma Epinephrine Response in the Diagnosis of Idiopathic Postprandial Syndrome," *JAMA* 251 (1984): 612–5.

4. A. Hadji-Georgopoulus et al., "Elevated Hypoglycemic Index and Late Hyperinsulinism in Symptomatic Postprandial Hypoglycemia," *J Clin Endocrinol Metabl* 50 (1980): 371–6.

5. M. Fabrykant, "The Problem of Functional Hyperinsulinism on Functional Hypoglycemia Attributed to Nervous Causes, 1: Laboratory and Clinical Correlations," *Metabolism* 4 (1955): 469–79.

6. Editorial: "Statement on Hypoglycemia," *JAMA* 223 (1972): 682.

7. G.F. Cahill and J.S. Soelder, "A Non-Editorial on Non-Hypoglycemia," *N Engl J Med* 291 (1974): 905–6.

8. F.D. Hofeldt, "Patients with Bona Fide Meal-Related Hypoglycemia Should Be Treated Primarily with Dietary Restriction of Refined Carbohydrate," *Endocrinol Metab Clin North Am* 18 (1989): 185–201.

9. L.R. Sanders et al., "Refined Carbohydrate as a Contributing Factor in Reactive Hypoglycemia," *Southern Medical Journal* 75 (1982): 1072–5.

10. National Research Council, *Diet and Health: Implications for Reducing Chronic Disease Risk* (Washington, DC: National Academy Press, 1989).

11. A. Winokur, G. Maislin, J.L. Phillips, and J.D. Amsterdam, "Insulin Resistance after Glucose Tolerance Testing in Patients with Major Depression," *Am J Psychiatry* 145 (1988): 325–30.

12. J.H. Wright, J.J. Jacisin, N.S. Radin, et al., Glucose Metabolism in Unipolar Depression," *Br J Psychiatry* 132 (1978): 386–93.

13. A.G. Schauss, "Nutrition and Behavior: Complex Interdisciplinary Research," *Nutr Health* 3 (1984): 9–37.

14. D. Benton, "Hypoglycemia and Aggression: A Review," *Int J Neurosci* 41 (1988): 163–8.

15. M. Virkkunen, "Reactive Hypoglycemic Tendency among Arsonists," *Acta Psychiatr Scan* 69 (1984): 445–52.

16. S.J. Schoenthaler, "Diet and Crime: An Empirical Examination of the Value of Nutrition in the Control and Treatment of Incarcerated Juvenile Offenders," *Int J Biosocial Research* 4 (1983): 25–39.

17. S.J. Schoenthaler, "The Northern California Diet-Behavior Program: An Empirical Evaluation of 3,000 Incarcerated Juveniles in Stanslaus County Juvenile Hall," *Int J Biosocial Res* 5 (1983): 99–106.

18. G.E. Abraham, "Nutritional Factors in the Etiology of the Premenstrual Tension Syndromes," *J Repro Med* 28 (1983): 446–64.

19. C.H. Walsh and D.J. O'Sullivan, "Studies of Glucose Tolerance, Insulin and Growth Hormone Secretion during the Menstrual Cycle in Healthy Women," *Irish J Med Sci* 144 (1975): 18–24.

20. M. Critchley, "Migraine," *Lancet* 1 (1933): 123–6.

21. J.D. Dexter, J. Roberts, and J.A. Byer, "The Five Hour Glucose Tolerance Test and Effect of Low Sucrose Diet in Migraine," *Headache* 18 (1978): 91–4.

22. L. Mykkanen, L. Markku, and K. Pyorala, "High Plasma Insulin Levels Associated with Coronary Heart Disease in the Elderly," *Am J Epidem* 137 (1993): 1190–1202.

23. J. Yudkin, "Metabolic Changes Induced by Sugar in Relation to Coronary Heart Disease and Diabetes," *Nutr Health* 5 (1987): 5–8.

24. K. Pyorala, "Relationship of Glucose Tolerance and Plasma Insulin to the Incidence of Coronary Heart Disease: Results from Two Population Studies in Finland," *Diabetes Care* 2 (1979): 131–41.

25. S. Bansal, S.H. Toh, and K.A. LaBresh, "Chest Pain as a Presentation of Reactive Hypoglycemia," *Chest* 84 (1983): 641–2.

26. M. Hanson et al., "The Oral Glucose Tolerance Test in Men Under 55 Years of Age with Intermittent Claudication," *Angiology* June (1987): 469–73.

27. I. Hjermann, "The Metabolic Cardiovascular Syndrome: Syndrome X, Reaven's Syndrome, Insulin Resistance Syndrome, Atherothrombogenic Syndrome," *J Cardiovascular Pharm* 20(Suppl.8) (1992): S5–S10.

28. A. Maseri, "Syndrome X: Still an Appropriate Name," *J Am Coll Cardiol* 17 (1991): 1471–2.

29. J. Anderson, "Nutrition Management of Diabetes Mellitus," in R. Goodhart and V.R. Young, eds., *Modern Nutrition in Health and Disease* (Philadelphia, PA: Lea and Febiger, 1988), 1201–29.

30. S. Gregersen, O. Rasmussen, S. Larsen, and K. Hermansen, "Glycaemic and Insulinaemic Responses to Orange and Apple Compared with White Bread in Non-Insulin Dependent Diabetic Subjects," *Eur J Clin Nutr* 46 (1992): 301–3.

31. V.A. Koivisto and H. Yki-Jarvinen, "Fructose and Insulin Sensitivity in Patients with Type 2 Diabetes," *Journal of Internal Medicine* 233 (1993): 145–53.

32. J. Rodin, "Effects of Pure Sugar vs. Mixed Starch Fructose Loads on Food Intake," *Appetite* 17 (1991): 213–9.

33. J. Rodin, "Comparative Effects of Fructose, Aspartame, Glucose, and Water Preloads on Calorie and Macronutrient Intake," *AJCN* 51 (1990): 428–35.

34. L. Spitzer and J. Rodin, "Effects of Fructose and Glucose Preloads on Subsequent Food Intake," *Appetite* 8 (1987): 135–45.

35. D.J.A. Jenkins et al., "Glycemic Index of Foods: A Physiological Basis for Carbohydrate Exchange," *AJCN* 24 (1981): 362–6.

36. A.S. Truswell, "Glycemic Index of Foods," *Eur J Clin Nutr* 46(Suppl 2) (1992): S91–101.

37. D. Burkitt and H. Trowell, *Western Diseases: Their Emergence and Prevention* (Cambridge, MA: Harvard University Press, 1981).

38. R.A. Anderson, "Chromium, Glucose Tolerance, and Diabetes," *Biological Trace Element Research* 32 (1992): 19–24.

39. R.A. Anderson, M.M. Polansky, N.A. Bryden, et al., "Effects of Supplemental Chromium on Patients with Symptoms of Reactive Hypoglycemia," *Metabolism* 36 (1987): 351–5.

40. Y. Hirata, "Diabetes and Alcohol," *Asian Med J* 31 (1988): 564–9.

41. J.V. Selby, B. Newman, M.C. King, et al., "Environmental and Behavioral Determinants of Fasting Plasma Glucose in Women. A Matched Co-Twin Analysis," *Am J Epidem* 125 (1987): 979–88.

42. A.L. Vallerand, J.P. Cuerrier, D. Shapcott, et al., "Influence of Exercise Training on Tissue Chromium Concentrations in the Rat," *AJCN* 39 (1984): 402–9.

Hypothyroidism

1. J.C. Bennet and F. Plum (eds.). *Cecil Textbook of Medicine, 20th*

Edition (Philadelphia: WB Saunders, 1996), pp.1227–1245.

2. C. Wang and L.M. Crapo. "The Epidemiology of Thyroid Disease and Implications for Screening," *Endocrinol Metab Clin North Am* 26 (1997): 189–218.

3. A.P. Weetman. "Hypothyroidism: Screening and Subclinical Disease," *BMJ* 314 (1977): 1175–8.

4. P.J. Drinka and W.E. Nolten. "Review: Subclinical Hypothyroidism in the Elderly: To Treat or Not to Treat?" *Am J Med Sci* 295 (1988): 125–8.

5. K. Banovac, M. Zakarija, and J.M. McKenzie. "Experience with Routine Thyroid Function Testing: Abnormal Results in "Normal" Populations," *J Florida Med Assoc* 72 (1985): 835–9.

6. M.J. Rosenthal, W.C. Hunt, P.J. Garry, and J.S. Goodwin. "Thyroid Failure in the Elderly: Microsomal Antibodies as Discriminate for Therapy," *JAMA* 258(1987): 209–13.

7. R. Arem and D. Escalante. "Subclinical Hypothyroidism: Epidemiology, Diagnosis, and Significance," *Adv Intern Med* 41 (1996): 213–50.

8. B.O. Barnes and L. Galton. *Hypothyroidism: The Unsuspected Illness* (New York: Thomas Crowell, 1976).

9. S.E. Langer and J.F. Scheer. *Solved: The Riddle of Illness* (New Canaan: Keats, 1984).

10. U. Althaus, J.J. Staub, A. Ryff-De Leche, et al. "LDL/HDL-Changes in Subclinial Hypothyroidism: Possible Risk Factors for Coronary Heart Disease," *Clinical Endocrinology* 28 (1988): 157–63.

12. J.W. Dean and P.B.S. Fowler. "Exaggerated Responsiveness to Thyrotrophin Releasing Hormone: A Risk Factor in Women with Artery Disease," *Brit Med J* 290 (1985): 1555–61.

13. W.M.G. Turnbridge, D.C. Evered, and R. Hall, "Lipid Profiles and Cardiovascular Disease in the Wickham Area with Particular Reference to Thyroid Failure," *Clin Endocrinol* 7 (1977): 495–508.

14. M. Gold, A. Pottash, and I. Extein, "Hypothyroidism and Depression, Evidence from Complete Thyroid Function Evaluation," *JAMA* 245 (1981): 1919–22.

15. S. Esposito, A.J. Prange, and R. Golden, "The Thyroid Axis and Mood Disorders: Overview and Future Prospects," *Psychopharmacol Bull* 33 (1997): 205–17.

16. M. Krupsky et al., "Musculoskeletal Symptoms As a Presenting Sign of Long-Standing Hypothyroidism," *Isr J Med Sci* 23 (1987): 1110–3.

17. M.C. Hochberg et al., "Hypothyroidism Presenting As a Polymyositis-Like Syndrome," *Arthr Rheum* 19 (1976): 1363–6.

18. A. Prasad, "Clinical, Biochemical and Nutritional Spectrum of Zinc Deficiency in Human Subjects: An Update," *Ntr Rev* 41 (1983): 197–208.

19. D. Lennon, F. Nagle, F. Stratman et al., "Diet and Exercise Training Effects on Resting Metabolic Rate," *Int J Obesity* 9 (1985): 39–47.

Impotence

1. NIH Consensus Conference Panel on Impotence. "Impotence," *JAMA* 270 (1993): 83–90.

2. S.E. Lerner, A. Melman, and G.J. Christ. "A Review of Erectile Dysfunction: New Insights and More Questions," *Journal of Urology* 149 (1993): 1246–55.

3. J.E. Morley. "Management of Impotence," *Postgraduate Medicine* 93 (1993): 65–72.

4. D. Ornish, et al. "Can Lifestyle Changes Reverse Coronary Heart Disease?" *Lancet* 336 (1990): 129–33.

5. The Expert Panel. "Report of the National Cholesterol Education Program Expert Panel on Detection, Evaluation, and Treatment of High Cholesterol in Adults," *Arch Intern Med* 148 (1988): 136–69.

6. P.L. Canner and the Coronary Drug Project Group. "Mortality in Coronary Drug Project Patients During a Nine-Year Post-Treatment Period," *J Am Coll Cardiol* 8 (1986): 1245–55.

7. A.L. Welsh and M. Ede. "Inositol Hexanicotinate for Improved Nicotinic Acid Therapy," *Int Record Med* 174 (1961): 9–15.

8. A.M.A. El-Enein, Y.S. Hafez, H. Salem, and M. Abdel. "The Role of Nicotinic Acid and Inositol Hexaniacinate as Anticholesterolemic and Antilipemic Agents," *Nutr Rep Intl* 28 (1983): 899–911.

9. G.T. Sunderland, J.J.F. Belch, R.D. Sturrock, et al. "A Double Blind Randomised Placebo Controlled Trial of Hexopal in Primary Raynaud's Disease," *Clin Rheumatol* 7 (1988): 46–9.

10. R. Witherington. "Mechanical Devices for the Treatment of Erectile Dysfunction," *Am Fam Pract* 43 (1991): 1611–20.

11. J.R. White, et al. "Enhanced Sexual Behavior in Exercising Men," *Arch Sex Behav* 19 (1990): 193–209.

12. J.G. Susset, et al. "Effect of Yohimbine Hydrochloride on Erectile Impotence: A Double-Blind Study," *J Urology* 141 (1989): 1360–3.

13. A. Morales, et al. "Is Yohimbine Effective in the Treatment of Organic Impotence? Results of a Controlled Trial," *J Urology* 137 (1987): 1168–72.

14. J. Betz, K.D. White, and A.H. der Marderosian. "Chemical Analysis of 26 Commercial Yohimbe Products," *J Am Chem Soc* 78 (1995): 1189–94.

15. J.A. Duke. *Handbook of Medicinal Herbs* (Boca Raton: CRC Press, 1985).

16. J. Waynberg. "Aphrodisiacs: Contribution to the Clinical Validation of the Traditional Use of Ptychopetalum Guyanna," Presented at The First International Congress on Ethnopharmacology, Strasbourg, France, June 5–9, 1990.

17. R. Sikora, et al. "Ginkgo Biloba Extract in the Therapy of Erectile Dysfunction," *Journal of Urology* 141 (1989): 188A.

18. M. Sohn and R. Sikora. "Ginkgo Biloba Extract in the Therapy of Erectile Dysfunction," *J Sex Educ Ther* 17 (1991): 53–61.

19. S. Shibata, O. Tanaka, J. Shoji, and H. Saito. "Chemistry and Pharmacology of Panax," *Economic and Medicinal Plant Research* 1 (1985): 217–84.

20. C. Kim, H. Choi, C.C. Kim, et al. "Influence of Ginseng on Mating Behavior of Male Rats," *Am J Chinese Med* 4 (1976): 163–8.

21. W.S. Fahim, J.M. Harman, T.E. Clevenger, et al. "Effect of Panax Ginseng on Testosterone Level and

Prostate in Male Rats," *Arch Androl* 8 (1982): 261–3.

22. P.G. Merz, et al. "The Effects of a Special Agnus Castus Extract (BP1095E1) on Prolactin Secretion in Healthy Male Subjects," *Exp Clin Endocrinol Diabetes* 104 (1996): 447–53.

Infertility

1. K. Purvis and E. Christiansen, "Male Infertility: Current Concepts," *Annals Med* 24 (1992): 259–72.

2. J.B. Wyngaarden, L.H. Smith, and J.C. Bennett, eds., *Cecil Textbook of Medicine,* 19th ed. (Philadelphia, PA: W.B. Saunders, 1992).

3. E. Carlsen et al., "Evidence for Decreasing Quality of Semen During Past 50 Years," *British Med J* 305 (1992): 609–13.

4. N.H. Lauersen and C. Bouchez, *Getting Pregnant: What Couples Need to Know Right Now* (New York: Fawcett Columbine, 1991).

5. K. Purvis and E. Christiansen, "Review: Infection in the Male Reproductive Tract; Impact, Diagnosis and Treatment in Relation to Male Infertility," *Int J Androl* 16 (1993): 1–13.

6. R.M. Sharpe and N.E. Skakkebaek, "Are Oestrogens Involved in Falling Sperm Counts and Disorders of the Male Reproduction Tract?" *Lancet* 341 (1993): 1392–5.

7. B. Field, M. Selub, and C.L. Hughes, "Reproductive Effects of Environmental Agents," *Semen Reprod Endocrinol* 8 (1990): 44–54.

8. M. Messina and V. Messina, "Increasing the Use of Soyfoods and Their Potential Role in Cancer Prevention," *J Am Diet Assoc* 91 (1991): 836–40.

9. R.J. Aitken, "The Role of Free Oxygen Radicals and Sperm Function," *Int J Androl* 12 (1989): 95–7.

10. S. Kaur, "Effect of Environmental Pollutants on Human Semen," *Bull Environ Contam Toxicol* 40 (1988): 102–4.

11. O.P. Steeno and A. Pangkahila, "Occupational Influences on Male Fertility and Sexuality," *Andrologia* 16 (1984): 5–22.

12. V.D. Kulikauskas, D. Blaustein, and D. Ablin, "Cigarette Smoking and Its Possible Effects on Sperm," *Fertil Steril* 44 (1985): 526–8.

13. A. Zini, E. De Lamirande, and C. Gagnon, "Reactive Oxygen Species in Semen of Infertile Patients: Levels of Superoxide Dismutase- and Catalase-Like Activities in Seminal Plasma and Spermatozoa," *Int J Androl* 16 (1993): 183–8.

14. C. Fraga et al., "Ascorbic Acid Protects Against Endogenous Oxidative DNA Damage in Human Sperm," *Proc Natl Acad Sci* 88 (1991): 11003–6.

15. National Research Council, "Recommended Dietary Allowances," 10th ed. (Washington, D.C.: National Academy Press, 1989).

16. E. Dawson, W. Harris, and L. Powell, "Effect of Vitamin C Supplementation on Sperm Quality of Heavy Smokers," *FASEB J* 5 (1991): A915.

17. E.B. Dawson et al., "Effect of Ascorbic Acid on Male Fertility," *Ann NY Acad Sci* 498 (1987): 312–23.

18. R.J. Aitkin et al., "Analysis of the Relationship between Defective Sperm Function and the Generation of Reactive Oxygen Species in Cases of Oligospermia," *J Androl* 10 (1989): 214–20.

19. S.A. Suleiman, M.E. Ali, Z.M. Zaki, et al., "Lipid Peroxidation and Human Sperm Mobility: Protective Role of Vitamin E," *J Androl* 17 (1996): 530–7.

20. D.P. Weller, J.D. Zaneveld, and N.R. Farnsworth, "Gossypol: Pharmacology and Current Status as a Male Contraceptive," *Econ Med Plant Res* 1 (1985): 87–112.

21. A.S. Prasad, "Zinc in Growth and Development and Spectrum of Human Zinc Deficiency," *J Am Coll Nutr* 7 (1988): 377–84.

22. M. Tikkiwal et al., "Effect of Zinc Administration on Seminal Zinc and Fertility of Oligospermic Males," *Ind J Physiol Pharmacol* 31 (1987): 30–4.

23. H. Takihara et al., "Zinc Sulfate Therapy for Infertile Males with or without Varicocelectomy," *Urology* 29 (1987): 638–41.

24. A. Netter et al., "Effect of Zinc Administration on Plasma Testosterone, Dihydrotestosterone, and Sperm Count," *Arch Androl* 7 (1981): 69–73.

25. B. Sandler and B. Faragher, "Treatment of Oligospermia with Vitamin B12," *Infertility* 7 (1984): 133–8.

26. Y. Kumamoto et al., "Clinical Efficacy of Mecobalamin in Treatment of Oligospermia: Results of a Double-Blind Comparative Clinical Study," *Acta Urol Japan* 34 (1988): 1109–32.

27. A. Schacter, J.A. Goldman, and Z. Zukerman, "Treatment of Oligospermia with the Amino Acid Arginine," *J Urol* 110 (1973): 311–3.

28. G. Vitali, R. Parente, and C. Melotti, "Carnitine Supplementation in Human Idiopathic Asthenospermia: Clinical Results," *Drugs Exp Clin Res* 21 (1995): 157–9.

29. S. Shibata, O. Tanaka, J. Shoji, and H. Saito, "Chemistry and Pharmacology of Panax," *Economic and Medicinal Plant Research* 1 (1985): 217–84.

30. M. Yamamoto and T. Uemura, "Endocrinological and Metabolic Actions of P. Ginseng Principles," Proceedings 3rd International Ginseng Symposium, 1980: 115–9.

31. C. Kim, H. Choi, C.C. Kim, et al., "Influence of Ginseng on Mating Behavior of Male Rats," *Am J Chinese Med* 4 (1976): 163–8.

32. W.S. Fahim, J.M. Harman, T.E. Clevenger, et al., Effect of *Panax ginseng* on Testosterone Level and Prostate in Male Rats," *Arch Androl* 8 (1982): 261–3.

33. N.R. Farnsworth et al., "Siberian Ginseng (*Eleutherococcus senticosus*): Current Status as an Adaptogen," *Economic and Medicinal Plant Research* 1 (1985): 156–215.

34. G. Lucchetta, A. Weill, N. Becker, et al., "Reactivation from the Prostatic Gland in Cases of Reduced Fertility," *Urol Int* 39 (1984): 222–4.

35. G.F. Menchini-Fabris, P. Giorgi, F. Andreini, et al., "New Perspectives of Treatment of Prostato-Vesicular Pathologies with *Pygeum africanum*," *Arch Int Urol* 60 (1988): 313–22.

36. A. Clavert, C. Cranz, J.P. Riffaud, et al., "Effects of an Extract of the Bark of *Pygeum africanum* on Prostatic Secretions in the Rat and Man," *Ann Urol* 20 (1986): 341–3.

37. C. Carani, C. Salvioli, A. Scuteri, et al., "Urological and Sexual Evaluation of Treatment of Benign Prostatic Disease Using *Pygeum africanum* at High Dose," *Arch Ital Urol Nefrol Androl* 63 (1991): 341–5.

Inflammatory Bowel Disease

1. L. Demling, "Is Crohn's Disease Caused by Antibiotics?" *Hepato-Gastroenterol* 41 (1994): 549–51.

2. A.J. Levi, "Diet in the Management of Crohn's Disease," *Gut* 26 (1985): 985–8.

3. J. Jarnerot, I. Jarnmark, and K. Nilsson, "Consumption of Refined Sugar by Patients with Crohn's Disease, Ulcerative Colitis, or Irritable Bowel Syndrome," *Scand J Gastroenterol* 18 (1983): 999–1002.

4. J.F. Mayberry, J. Rhodes, and R.G. Newcombe, "Increased Sugar Consumption in Crohn's Disease," *Digestion* 20 (1980): 323–6.

5. D.S. Grimes, "Refined Carbohydrate, Smooth-Muscle Spasm, and Diseases of the Colon," *Lancet* i (1976): 395–7.

6. J.R. Thornton, P.M. Emmett, and K.W. Heaton, "Diet and Crohn's Disease: Characteristics of the Pre-Illness Diet," *Br Med J* 279 (1979): 762–4.

7. K.W. Heaton, J.R. Thornton, and P.M. Emmett, "Treatment of Crohn's Disease with an Unrefined-Carbohydrate, Fiber-Rich Diet," *Br Med J* 279 (1979): 764–6.

8. C.O. Morain, A.W. Segal, and A.J. Levi, "Elemental Diet as Primary Treatment of Acute Crohn's Disease: A Controlled Trial," *Br Med J* 288 (1984): 1859–62.

9. A.D. Harries, V. Danis, R.V. Heatley, et al., "Controlled Trial of Supplemented Oral Nutrition in Crohn's Disease," *Lancet* i (1983): 887–90.

10. C. Axelsson and S. Jarnum, "Assessment of the Therapeutic Value of an Elemental Diet in Chronic Inflammatory Bowel Disease," *Scand J Gastroenterol* 12 (1977): 89–95.

11. A.J. Voitk et al., "Experience with Elemental Diet in the Treatment of Inflammatory Bowel Disease," *Arch Surg* 107 (1973): 329–33.

12. E. Workman, A. Jonmes, A.J. Wilson, and J.O. Hunter, "Diet in the Management of Crohn's Disease," *Human Nutr: Applied Nutr* 38A (1984): 469–73.

13. V.A. Jones, E. Workman, A.H. Freeman, et al., "Crohn's Disease: Maintenance of Remission by Diet," *Lancet* ii (1985): 177–80.

14. A.H. James, "Breakfast and Crohn's Disease," *Br Med J* 276 (1977): 943–5.

15. J.R. Thornton, P.M. Emmett, and K.W. Heaton, "Diet and Ulcerative Colitis," *Br Med J* 280 (1980): 293–4.

16. S. Meyers and H.D. Janowitz, "Natural History of Crohn's Disease: An Analytical Review of the Placebo Lesson," *Gastroenterol* 87 (1984): 1189–92.

17. H.S. Mekhjian et al., "Clinical Features and Natural History of Crohn's Disease," *Gastroenterol* 77 (1979): 898–906.

18. H. Malchow et al., "European Cooperative Crohn's Disease Study (ECCDS): Results of Drug Treatment," *Gastroenterol* 86 (1984): 249–66.

19. M. Donowitz, "Arachidonic Acid Metabolites and Their role in Inflammatory Bowel Disease," *Gastroenterol* 88 (1985): 580–7.

20. A.W. Ford-Hutchinson, "Leukotrienes: Their Formation and Role as Inflammatory Mediators," *Fed Proc* 44 (1985): 25–9.

21. P. Sharon and W.F. Stenson, "Enhanced Synthesis of Leukotriene B4 by Colonic Mucosa in Inflammatory Bowel Disease," *Gastroenterol* 86 (1984): 453–60.

22. M.W. Musch, R.J. Miller, M. Field, and M.I. Siegel, "Stimulation of Colonic Secretion by Lipoxygenase Metabolites of Arachidonic Acid," *Science* 217 (1982): 1255–6.

23. D.K. Podolsky and K.J. Isselbacher, "Glycoprotein Composition of Colonic Mucosa," *Gastroenterol* 87 (1984): 991–8.

24. Y.S. Kim and J.C. Byrd, "Ulcerative Colitis: A Specific Mucin Defect?" *Gastroenterol* 87 (1984): 1193–5.

25. C.R. Boland, P. Lance, B. Levin, et al., "Abnormal Goblet Cell Glycoconjugates in Rectal Biopsies Associated with an Increased Risk of Neoplasia in Patients with Ulcerative Colitis: Early Results of a Prospective Study," *Gut* 25 (1984): 1364–71.

26. D.J. Hentges, *Human Intestinal Microflora in Health and Disease* (New York: Academic Press, 1983).

27. R. Marcus and J. Watt, "Seaweeds and Ulcerative Colitis in Laboratory Animals," *Lancet* ii (1969): 489–90.

28. P. Grasso et al., "Studies on Carrageenan and Large Bowel Ulceration in Mammals," *Food Cosmet Toxicol* 11 (1973): 555–64.

29. N.K. Motet, "Editorial: On Animal Models for Inflammatory Bowel Disease," *Gastroenterology* 62 (1972): 1269–71.

30. K.R. Bentiz, L. Goldberg, and F. Coulston, "Intestinal Effect of Carrageenans in the Rhesus Monkey," *Food Cosmet Toxicol* 11 (1973): 565–75.

31. S. Bonfils, "Carrageenan and the Human Gut," *Lancet* ii (1970): 414.

32. J.B. Levine and D. Lukawski-Trubish, "Extraintestinal Considerations in Inflammatory Bowel Disease," *Gastroenterol Clin North Am* 24 (1995): 633–46.

33. M.T. Murray, "The Healing Power of Herbs," (Rocklin, CA: Prima Publishing, 1995), 243–52.

34. I.H. Rosenberg, J.M. Bengoa, and M.D. Sitrin, "Nutritional Aspects of Inflammatory Bowel Disease," *Ann Rev Nutr* 5 (1985): 463–84.

35. H.V. Heatley, "Review: Nutritional Implications of Inflammatory Bowel Disease," *Scand J Gastroenterol* 19 (1984): 995–8.

36. K.J. Motil and R.J. Grand, "Nutritional Management of Inflammatory Bowel Disease," *Ped Clinics North Amer* 32 (1985): 447–69.

37. A.A. Salyers, A.P. Kurtitza, and R.E. McCarthy, "Influence of Dietary Fiber on the Intestinal Environment," *Proc Soc Exp Biol Med* 180 (1985): 415–21.

38. C.R. Fleming et al., "Zinc Nutrition in Crohn's Disease," *Dig Dis Sci* 26 (1981): 865–70.

39. A.N.H. Main, R.I. Russell, G.S. Fell, et al., "Clinical Experience of Zinc Supplementation During Intravenous Nutrition in Crohn's Disease: Value of Serum and Urine Zinc Measurements," *Gut* 23 (1982): 984–91.

40. L. Elsborg and L. Larsen, "Folate Deficiency in Chronic Inflammatory

Bowel Diseases," *Scand J Gastroenterol* 14 (1979): 1019–24.

41. R. Hellberg, L. Hulten, and E. Bjorn-Rasmussen, "The Nutritional and Haematological Status Before and After Primary and Subsequent Resectional Procedures for Classical Crohn's Disease and Crohn's Colitis," *Acta Chir Scand* 148 (1982): 453–60.

42. J.L. Franklin and I.H. Rosenberg, "Impaired Folic Acid Absorption in Inflammatory Bowel Disease: Effects of Salicylasosulfapyridine (Azulfidine)," *Gastroenterol* 64 (1973): 517–25.

43. L.B. Carruthers, "Chronic Diarrhea Treated with Folic Acid," *Lancet* i (1946): 849–50.

44. S. Filipsson, L. Hulten, and G. Lindstedt, "Malabsorption of Fat and Vitamin B12 Before and After Intestinal Resection for Crohn's Disease," *Scand J Gastroenterol* 13 (1978): 529–36.

45. W.R. Best et al., "Development of a Crohn's Disease Activity Index," *Gastroenterology* 70 (1976): 439–444.

46. J. Lloyd-Still and O.C. Green, "A Clinical Scoring System for Chronic Inflammatory Bowel Disease in Children," *Dig Dis Sci* 24 (1979): 620–4.

Insomnia

1. H. Spiro, *Clinical Gastroenterology*, 3rd ed. (New York: Macmillan Publishing, 1983), 713–35.

2. G.F. Longstreth, "Irritable Bowel Syndrome: A Multibillion-Dollar Problem," *Gastroenterol* 109 (1995): 2029–42.

3. J. Fielding, "Detailed History and Examination Assist Positive Clinical Diagnosis of the Irritable Bowel Syndrome," *J Clin Gastroenterol* 5 (1983): 495–7.

4. P. Cann, N. Read, and C. Holdsworth, "What Is the Benefit of Coarse Wheat Bran in Patients with Irritable Bowel Syndrome?" *Gut* 25 (1984): 168–73.

5. J. Fielding and M. Kehoe, "Different Dietary Fibre Formulations and the Irritable Bowel Syndrome," *Irish J Med Sci* 153 (1984): 178–80.

6. E. Hollander, "Mucous Colitis Due to Food Allergy," *Am J Med Sci* 174 (1927): 495–500.

7. L. Gay, "Mucous Colitis, Complicated by Colonic Polyposis, Relieved by Allergic Management," *Am J Dig Dis* 3 (1937): 326–9.

8. V. Jones, P. McLaughlin, M. Shorthouse, et al., "Food Intolerance: A Major Factor in the Pathogenesis of Irritable Bowel Syndrome," *Lancet* ii (1982): 1115–8.

9. M. Petitpierre, P. Gumowski, and J. Girard, "Irritable Bowel Syndrome and Hypersensitivity to Food," *Annals Allergy* 54 (1985): 538–40.

10. R. Nanda et al., "Food Intolerance and the Irritable Bowel Syndrome," *Gut* 30 (1989): 1099–1104.

11. D. Gertner and J. Powell-Tuck, "Irritable Bowel Syndrome and Food Intolerance," *Practitioner* 238 (1994): 499–504.

12. J. Zwetchkenbaum and R. Burakoff, "The Irritable Bowel Syndrome and Food Hypersensitivity," *Annals Allergy* 61 (1988): 47–9.

13. A. Russo, R. Fraser, and M. Horowitz, "The Effect of Acute Hyperglycemia on Small Intestinal Motility in Normal Subjects," *Diabetologia* 39 (1996): 984–9.

14. J.M. Hills and P.I. Aaronson, "The Mechanism of Action of Peppermint Oil in Gastrointestinal Smooth Muscle," *Gastroenterol* 101 (1991): 55–65.

15. K. Somerville, C. Richmond, and G. Bell, "Delayed Release Peppermint Oil Capsules (Colpermin) for the Spastic Colon Syndrome: A Pharmacokinetic Study," *Br J Clin Pharmacol* 18 (1984): 638–40.

16. R. Leicester and R. Hunt, "Peppermint Oil to Reduce Colonic Spasm during Endoscopy," *Lancet* ii (1982): 989.

17. W. Rees, B. Evans, and J. Rhodes, "Treating Irritable Bowel Syndrome with Peppermint Oil," *Br Med J* ii (1979): 835–6.

18. B. May et al., "Efficacy of a Fixed Peppermint Oil/Caraway Oil Combination in Non-Ulcer Dyspepsia," *Arzneim Forsch* 46 (1996): 1149–53.

19. J.C. Stiles et al., "The Inhibition of *Candida albicans* by Oregano," *J Applied Nutr* 47 (1995): 96–102.

20. J. Svedlund, I. Sjodin, G. Doteval, and R. Gillberg, "Upper Gastroin-

testinal and Mental Symptoms in the Irritable Bowel Syndrome," *Scand J Gastroenterol* 20 (1985): 595–601.

21. G. Goldsmith and J.S. Levin, "Effect of Sleep Quality on Symptoms of Irritable Bowel Syndrome," *Dig Dis Sci* 38 (1993): 1809–14.

22. W. Ryan, M. Kelly, and J. Fielding, "The Normal Personality Profile of Irritable Bowel Syndrome Patients," *Irish J Med Sci* 153 (1984): 127–9.

23. F. Narducci, W. Snape, W. Battle, R. Lodon, and S. Cohen, "Increased Colonic Motility during Exposure to a Stressful Situation," *Dig Dis Sci* 30 (1985): 40–4.

24. E.B. Blanchard et al., "Relaxation Training as a Treatment for Irritable Bowel Syndrome," *Biofeedback Self-Regulation* 18 (1993): 125–32.

25. G. Goldsmith and M. Patterson, "Irritable Bowel Syndrome: Treatment Update," *Am Fam Phys* 31 (1985): 191–5.

26. S.P. Schwarz et al., "A Four-Year Follow-Up of Behaviorally Treated Irritable Bowel Syndrome Patients," *Behavior Res Ther* 28 (1990): 331–5.

27. G. Shaw et al., "Stress Management for Irritable Bowel Syndrome: A Controlled Trial," *Digestion* 50 (1991): 36–42.

Irritable Bowel Syndrome

1. H. Spiro, *Clinical Gastroenterology*, 3rd ed. (New York: Macmillan Publishing, 1983), 713–35.

2. G.F. Longstreth, "Irritable Bowel Syndrome: A Multibillion-Dollar Problem," *Gastroenterol* 109 (1995): 2029–42.

3. J. Fielding, "Detailed History and Examination Assist Positive Clinical Diagnosis of the Irritable Bowel Syndrome," *J Clin Gastroenterol* 5 (1983): 495–97.

4. P. Cann, N. Read, and C. Holdsworth, "What is the Benefit of Coarse Wheat Bran in Patients with Irritable Bowel Syndrome?" *Gut* 25 (1984): 168–73.

5. J. Fielding and M. Kehoe, "Different Dietary Fibre Formulations and the Irritable Bowel Syndrome," *Irish J Med Sci* 153 (1984): 178–80.

6. E. Hollander, "Mucous Colitis Due to Food Allergy," *Am J Med Sci* 174 (1927): 495–500.

7. L. Gay, "Mucous Colitis, Complicated by Colonic Polyposis, Relieved by Allergic Management," *Am J Dig Dis* 3 (1937): 326–29.

8. V. Jones, P. McLaughlin, M. Shorthouse, et al., "Food Intolerance: A Major Factor in the Pathogenesis of Irritable Bowel Syndrome," *Lancet* ii (1982): 1115–18.

9. M. Petitpierre, P. Gumowski, and J. Girard, "Irritable Bowel Syndrome and Hypersensitivity to Food," *Annals Allergy* 54 (1985): 538–40.

10. R. Nanda et al., "Food Intolerance and the Irritable Bowel Syndrome," *Gut* 30 (1989): 1099–1104.

11. D. Gertner and J. Powell-Tuck, "Irritable Bowel Syndrome and Food Intolerance," *Practitioner* 238 (1994): 499–504.

12. J. Zwetchkenbaum and R. Burakoff, "The Irritable Bowel Syndrome and Food Hypersensitivity," *Annals Allergy* 61 (1988): 47–49.

13. A. Russo, R. Fraser, and M. Horowitz, "The Effect of Acute Hyperglycemia on Small Intestinal Motility in Normal Subjects," *Diabetologia* 39 (1996): 984–89.

14. J.M. Hills and P.I. Aaronson, "The Mechanism of Action of Peppermint Oil in Gastrointestinal Smooth Muscle," *Gastroenterol* 101 (1991): 55–65.

15. K. Somerville, C. Richmond, and G. Bell, "Delayed Release Peppermint Oil Capsules (Colpermin) for the Spastic Colon Syndrome: A Pharmacokinetic Study," *Br J Clin Pharmacol* 18 (1984): 638–40.

16. R. Leicester and R. Hunt, "Peppermint Oil to Reduce Colonic Spasm during Endoscopy," *Lancet* ii (1982): 989.

17. W. Rees, B. Evans, and J. Rhodes, "Treating Irritable Bowel Syndrome with Peppermint Oil," *Br Med J* ii (1979): 835–36.

18. B. May et al., "Efficacy of a Fixed Peppermint Oil/Caraway Oil Combination in Non-Ulcer Dyspepsia," *Arzneim Forsch* 46 (1996): 1149–53.

19. J.C. Stiles et al., "The Inhibition of *Candida Albicans* by Oregano," *J Applied Nutr* 47 (1995): 96–102.

20. J. Svedlund, I. Sjodin, G. Doteval, and R. Gillberg, "Upper Gastrointestinal and Mental Symptoms in the Irritable Bowel Syndrome," *Scand J Gastroenterol* 20 (1985): 595–601.

21. G. Goldsmith and J.S. Levin, "Effect of Sleep Quality on Symptoms of Irritable Bowel Syndrome," *Di Dis Sci* 38 (1993): 1809–14.

22. W. Ryan, M. Kelly, and J. Fielding, "The Normal Personality Profile of Irritable Bowel Syndrome Patients," *Irish J Med Sci* 153 (1984): 127–29.

23. F. Narducci, W. Snape, W. Battle, R. Lodon, and S. Cohen, "Increased Colonic Motility during Exposure to a Stressful Situation," *Dig Dis Sci* 30 (1985): 40–44.

24. E.B. Blanchard et al., "Relaxation Training as a Treatment for Irritable Bowel Syndrome," *Biofeedback Self-Regulation* 18 (1993): 125–32.

25. G. Goldsmith and M. Patterson, "Irritable Bowel Syndrome: Treatment Update," *Am Fam Phys* 31 (1985): 191–95.

26. S.P. Schwarz et al., "A Four-Year Follow-Up of Behaviorally Treated Irritable Bowel Syndrome Patients," *Behavior Res Ther* 28 (1990): 331–35.

27. G. Shaw et al., "Stress Management for Irritable Bowel Syndrome: A Controlled Trial," *Digestion* 50 (1991): 36–42.

Kidney Stones

1. P. Shaw, et al., "Idiopathic Hypercalciuria: Its Control with Unprocessed Bran," *Br J Urol* 52 (1980): 426–9.

2. J. Thom, et al:, "The Influence of Refined Carbohydrate on Urinary Calcium Excretion," *Br J Urol* 50 (1978): 459–64.

3. J. Lemann, et al., "Possible Role of Carbohydrate-Induced Hypercalciuria in Calcium Oxalate Kidney-Stone Formation," *N Eng J Med* 280 (1969): 232–7.

4. O. Zechner, et al., "Nutritional Risk Factors in Urinary Stone Disease," *J Urol* 125 (1981): 51–5.

5. W. Robertson, et al., "Prevalence of Urinary Stone Disease in Vegetarians," *Eur Urol* 8 (1982): 334–9.

6. H. Griffith, et al., "A Control Study of Dietary Factors in Renal Stone Formation," *Br J Urol* 53 (1981): 416–20.

7. G. Rose and E. Westbury, "The Influence of Calcium Content of Water, Intake of Vegetables and Fruit and of Other Food Factors upon the Incidence of Renal Calculi," *Urol Res* 3 (1975): 61–66.

8. A. Ulmann, et al., "Effects of Weight and Glucose Ingestion on Urinary Calcium and Phosphate Excretion: Implications for Calcium Urolithiasis," *J Clin Endo Metab* 54 (1982): 1063–7.

9. N. Rao, et al., "Are Stone Formers Maladaptive to Refined Carbohydrates?" *Br J Urol* 54 (1982): 575–7.

10. N.J. Blacklock, "Sucrose and Idiopathic Renal Stone," *Nutr Health* 5 (1987): 9–17.

11. G. Johansson, et al., "Biochemical and Clinical Effects of the Prophylactic Treatment of Renal Calcium Stones with Magnesium Hydroxide," *J Urol* 124 (1980): 770–4.

12. W. Wunderlich, "Aspects of the Influence of Magnesium Ions on the Formation of Calcium Oxalate," *Urol Res* 9 (1981): 157–60.

13. P. Hallson, G. Rose, and M. Sulaiman, "Magnesium Reduces Calcium Oxalate Crystal Formation in Human Whole Urine," *Clin Sci* 62 (1982): 17–9.

14. G. Johansson, U. Backman, B. Danielson, et al., "Magnesium Metabolism in Renal Stone Formers. Effects of Therapy with Magnesium Hydroxide," *Scand J Urol Nephrol* 53 (1980): 125–30.

15. E. Prien and S. Gershoff, "Magnesium Oxide-Pyridoxine Therapy for Recurrent Calcium Oxalate Calculi," *J Urol* 112 (1974): 509–12.

16. S. Gershoff and E. Prien, "Effect of Daily MgO and Vitamin B6 Administration to Patients with Recurring Calcium Oxalate Stones," *Am J Clin Nutr* 20 (1967): 393–9.

17. E. Will and L. Bijvoet, "Primary Oxalosis: Clinical and Biochemical Response to High-Dose Pyridoxine Therapy," *Metab* 28 (1979): 542–8.

18. E. Lyon, et al.:, "Calcium Oxalate Lithiasis Produced by Pyridoxine Deficiency and Inhibition with High-Magnesium Diets," *Invest Urol* 4 (1966): 133–42.

19. M. Murthy et al., "Effect of Pyridoxine Supplementation on Recurrent Stone Formers," *Int J Clin Pharm Ther Tox* 20 (1982): 434–7.

20. L. Azowry, et al., "May Enzyme Activity in Urine Play a Role in Kidney Stone Formation?" *Urol Res* 10 (1982): 185–9.

21. M. Liebman and W. Chai, "Effect of Dietary Calcium on Urinary Oxalate Excretion after Oxalate Loads," *Am J Clin Nutr* 65 (1997): 1453–9.

22. C.Y.C. Pak and C. Fuller, "Idiopathic Hypocitraturic Calcium-Oxalate Nephrolithiasis Successfully Treated with Potassium Citrate," *Ann Int Med* 104 (1986): 33–7.

23. N.A. Whalley et al., "Long-Term Effects of Potassium Citrate Therapy on the Formation of New Stones in Groups of Recurrent Stone Formers With Hypocitraturia," *Br J Urology* 78 (1996): 10–14.

24. Y. Nakagawa, et al., "Purification and Characterization of a Calcium Oxalate Monohydrate Crystal Growth Inhibitor from Human Kidney Tissue Culture Medium," *J Biol Chem* 256 (1981): 3936–44.

25. K. Dharmsathaphorn, et al., "Increased Risk of Nephrolithiasis in Patients with Steatorrhea," *Dig Dis Sci* 27 (1982): 401–5.

26. F. Coe, E. Moran, and A. Kavalich, "The Contribution of Dietary Purine Over-Consumption to Hyperuricosuria in Calcium Oxalate Stone Formers," *J Chron Dis* 29 (1976): 793–800.

27. R. Anton and M. Haag-Berrurier, "Therapeutic Use of Natural Anthraquinone for Other Than Laxative Actions," *Pharmacology* 20 (1980): 104–12.

28. W. Berg, et al., "Influence of Anthraquinones on the Formation of Urinary Calculi in Experimental Animals," *Urologe A* 15 (1976): 188–91.

29. I. Light, E. Gursel, and H.H. Zinnser, "Urinary Ionized Calcium in Urolithiasis: Effect of Cranberry Juice," *Urology* 1 (1973): 67–70.

30. K. Samaan, "The Pharmacological Basis of Drug Treatment of Spasm of the Ureter or Bladder and of Ureteral Stone," *Br J Urol* 5 (1933): 213–24.

31. R. Scott, et al., "The Importance of Cadmium as a Factor in Calcified Upper Urinary Tract Stone Disease: A Prospective 7-Year Study," *Br J Urol* 54 (1982): 584–9.

32. J.M. Rivers, "Safety of High-Level Vitamin C Ingestion," *Int J Vitamin Nutr Res* 30(suppl.) (1989): 95–102.

33. T.R. Wanzilak et al., "Effect of High Dose Vitamin C on Urinary Oxalate Levels," *J Urol* 151 (1994): 834–7.

34. L.K. Massey, "Dietary Salt, Urinary Calcium, and Kidney Stone Risk," *Nutr Rev* 53 (1995): 131–9.

Leukoplakia

1. A.A. Abel and E.M. Farber, "Disorders of Pigmentation, Hair, Nails, and Oral Mucosa," in: D.C. Dale and D.D. Fedeman, eds. *Scientific American Medicine* (New York: Scientific American Inc., 1997), 12–13.

2. M. Krupp and M. Chatton, *Current Medical Diagnosis and Treatment* (Los Altos, CA: Lange Medical Publications, 1982), 346.

3. J. Johnson, W. Ringsdorf, and E. Cheraskin, "Relationship of Vitamin A and Oral Leukoplakia," *Arch Derm* 88 (1963): 607–612.

4. D. Mulay and F. Urbach, "Local Therapy of Oral Leukoplakia with Vitamin A," *Arch Derm Syph* 78 (1958): 637–8.

5. J. Smith, "Clinical Evaluation of Massive Buccal Vitamin A Dosage in Oral Hyperkeratosis," *Oral Surg Med Path* 15 (1962): 282–92.

6. E. Zegarelli, A. Kutscher, and H. Stevers, "Keratotic Lesions of the Oral Mucosa Membranes Treated with High Dosage Topical and Systemic Vitamin A," *NY State Dent J* 25 (1959): 244–52.

7. H. Stich, M. Rosin, and M. Vallejera, "Reduction with Vitamin A and Beta-Carotene Administration of Proportion of Micronucleated Buccal Mucosal Cells in Asian Betel Nut and Tobacco Chewers," *Lancet* i (1984): 1204–6.

8. H. Stich, W. Stich, M. Rosin, and M. Vallejera, "Use of the Micronucleus Test to Monitor the Effect of Vitamin A, Beta-Carotene and Canthaxanthin on the Buccal Mucosa of Betel Nut/Tobacco Chewers," *Int J Cancer* 34 (1984): 745–50.

9. H.S. Garewal and S. Schantz, "Emerging Role of Beta-Carotene and Antioxidant Nutrients in Prevention of Oral Cancer," *Arch Oto-laryngol Head Neck Surg* 121 (1995): 141–5.

10. K. Ibraham, N. Zafarey, and S. Zuberi, "Plasma Vitamin 'A' and Carotene Levels in Squamous Cell Carcinoma of Oral Cavity and Oro-Pharynx," *Clin Oncol* 3 (1977): 203–7.

11. M. Hyams and P. Gallagher, "Vitamin A Therapy in the Treatment of Vulvar Leukoplakia," *Am J Obstet Gynecol* 59 (1950): 1346–54.

12. E. Hunt, "Vitamin A in Leukoplakia," *Lancet* ii (1947): 141.

13. H.S. Garewal, F.L. Meyskens, and D. Killen, "Response of Oral Leukoplakia to Beta-Carotene," *J Clin Oncol* 8 (1990): 1715–20.

14. R. Brandt et al., "Response of Oral Lesions with the Use of Antioxidant Vitamins and Beta-Carotene Supplements," in: G.A. Bray and D.H. Ryan, eds. *Vitamins and Cancer Prevention* vol. 2 (Baton Rouge, LA: Louisiana State Press, 1991), 220–221.

15. S. Toma et al., "Treatment of Oral Leukoplakia with Beta-Carotene," *Oncology* 49 (1992): 77–81.

16. K. Malaker et al., "Management of Oral Leukoplakia with Beta-Carotene and Retinoic Acid: A Pilot Crossover Study," *Cancer Detect Prev* 15 (1991): 335–40.

17. H.S. Garewal et al., "Beta-Carotene in Oral Leukoplakia," *Proc Am Soc Clin Oncol* 11 (1992): 141.

18. S.E. Benner et al., "Regression of Oral Leukoplakia with Alpha-Tocopherol," *J Natl Cancer Inst* 85 (1993): 44–7.

19. G.E. Kaugars et al., "Use of Antioxidant Supplements in the Treatment of Human Oral Leukoplakia," *Oral Surg Oral Med Oral Pathol* 81 (1996): 5–14.

Macular Degeneration

1. R.W. Young, "Pathophysiology of Age-Related Macular Degeneration," *Survey Ophthalmol* 31 (1987): 291–306.

2. D.A. Newsome, "Medical Treatment of Macular Diseases," *Ophthalmol Clinics North Amer* 6 (1993): 307–14.

3. J.R. Vinderling et al., "Age-Related Macular Degeneration Is Associated

with Atherosclerosis," *Am J Epidemiol* 142 (1995): 404–9.

4. Eye Disease Case-Control Study Group, "Antioxidant Status and Neovascular Age-Related Macular Degeneration," *Arch Ophthalmol* 111 (1993): 104–9.

5. D.M. Snoddorly, "Evidence for Protection Against Age-Related Macular Degeneration by Carotenoids and Antioxidant Vitamins," *Am J Clin Nutr* 62(6 Suppl) (1995): 1448S–1461S.

6. J.A. Mares-Perlman et al., "Serum Antioxidants and Age-Related Macular Degeneration in a Population-Based Case-Control Study," *Arch Ophthalmol* 113 (1995): 1518–23.

7. J.T. Landrum, R.A. Bone, and M.D. Kilburn, "The Macular Pigment: A Possible Role in Protection from Age-Related Macular Degeneration," *Adv Pharmacol* 38 (1997): 537–56.

8. A. Ben-Amotz et al., "Bioavailability of a Natural Isomer Mixture as Compared with Synthetic All-Trans-Beta-Carotene in Rats and Chicks," *J Nutr* 119 (1989): 1013–9.

9. S. Mokady, M. Avron, and A. Ben-Amotz, "Accumulation in Chick Livers of 9-Cis Versus All-Trans Beta-Carotene," *J Nutr* 120 (1990): 889–92.

10. A. Carughi and F.G. Hooper, "Plasma Carotenoid Concentrations Before and After Supplementation with a Carotenoid Mixture," *Am J Clin Nutr* 59 (1994): 896–9.

11. T. Morinobu et al., "Changes in Beta-Carotene Levels by Long-Term Administration of Natural Beta-Carotene Derived from *Dunaliella bardawil* in Humans," *J Nutr Sci Vitaminol* 40 (1994): 421–30.

12. S. Richer, "Multicenter Ophthalmic and Nutritional Age-Related Macular Degeneration Study, Part 1: Design, Subjects, and Procedures," *J Am Optom Assoc* 67 (1996): 12–29.

13. S. Richer, "Multicenter Ophthalmic and Nutritional Age-Related Macular Degeneration Study, Part 2: Antioxidant Intervention and Conclusions," *J Am Optom Assoc* 67(1) (1996): 30–49.

14. J.M. Seddon et al., "A Prospective Study of Cigarette Smoking and Age-Related Macular Degeneration in Women," *JAMA* 276 (1996): 1141–6.

15. D.A. Newsome et al., "Oral Zinc in Macular Degeneration," *Arch Ophthalmol* 106 (1988): 192–8.

16. M. Stur et al., "Oral Zinc and the Second Eye in Age-Related Macular Degeneration," *Invest Ophthalmol Vis Sci* 37 (1996): 1225–35.

17. A. Scharrer and M. Ober, "Anthocyanosides in the Treatment of Retinopathies," *Klin Monatsbl Augenheilkd* 178 (1981): 386–9.

18. L. Caselli, "Clinical and Electroretinographic Study on the Activity of Anthocyanosides," *Arch Med Int* 37 (1985): 29–35.

19. D.A. Lebuisson, L. Leroy, and G. Rigal, "Treatment of Senile Macular Degeneration with *Ginkgo biloba* Extract: A Preliminary Double-Blind, Drug Versus Placebo Study," *Presse Med* 15 (1986): 1556–8.

20. C. Corbe, J.P. Boisin, and A. Siou, "Light Vision and Chorioretinal Circulation: Study of the Effect of Procyanidolic Oligomers (Endotelon)," *J Fr Ophtalmol* 11 (1988): 453–60.

21. R.J. Olson, "Supplemental Antioxidant Vitamins and Minerals in Patients with Macular Degeneration," *J Am Coll Nutr* 10 (1991): 550/Abstract 52.

22. W.G. Christen et al., "A Prospective Study of Cigarette Smoking and Risk of Age-Related Macular Degeneration in Men," *JAMA* 276 (1996): 1147–51.

Menopause

1. S.C. Theisen and P.K. Mansfield, "Menopause: Social Construction or Biological Destiny?" *J Health Educ* 24 (1993): 209–13.

2. M.C. Martin, J.E. Block, S.D. Sanchez, et al., "Menopause without Symptoms: The Endocrinology of Menopause among Rural Mayan Indians," *Am J Obstet Gynecol* 168 (1993): 1839–45.

3. R.A. Wilson, *Feminine Forever* (New York: Evans, 1966).

4. G.L. Rubin, H.B. Peterson, N.C. Lee, et al., "Estrogen Replacement Therapy and the Risk of Endometrial Cancer: Remaining Controversies," *Am J Obstet Gynecol* 162 (1990): 148–54.

5. M.I. Whitehead, P.T. Townsend, J. Davies-Pryse, et al., "Effects of Estrogens and Progestins on the Biochemistry and Morphology of the Postmenopausal Endometrium," *N Engl J Med* 305 (1981): 1599–685.

6. D.R. Session, A.C. Kelly, and R. Jewelewicz, "Current Concepts in Estrogen Replacement Therapy in the Menopause," *Fertil Steril* 59 (1993): 277–84.

7. A. Birkenfeld and N.G. Kase, "Menopause Medicine: Current Treatment Options and Trends," *Comprehen Ther* 17 (1991): 36–45.

8. J.B. Henrich, "The Postmenopausal Estrogen/Breast Cancer Controversy," *JAMA* 268 (1992): 1900–2.

9. A. Tavani, C. Braga, C. LaVecchia, et al., "Hormone Replacement Treatment and Breast Cancer Risk: An Age-Specific Analysis," *Canc Epidem Biomark Prev* 6 (1997): 11–4.

10. L. Bergkvist, I. Persson, "Hormone Replacement Therapy and Breast Cancer. A Review of Current Knowledge," *Drug Saf* 15 (1996): 360–70.

11. K.K. Steinberg, S.B. Thacker, S.J. Smith, et al., "A Meta-Analysis of the Effect of Estrogen Replacement Therapy on the Risk of Breast Cancer," *JAMA* 265 (1991): 1985–90.

12. R.J. Toisi, F.E. Speizer, W.C. Willett, et al., "Menopause, Postmenopausal Estrogen Preparations, and the Risk of Adult-Onset Asthma: A Prospective Cohort Study," *Am J Respir Crit Care Med* 152 (1995): 1183–8.

13. H. Aldercreutz, W. Mazur, "Phyto-Estrogens and Western Diseases," *Ann Med* 29 (1997): 95–120.

14. M. Messina and S. Barnes, "The Roles of Soy Products in Reducing Risk of Cancer," *J Natl Cancer Inst* 83 (1991): 541–6.

15. M. Messina and V. Messina, "Increasing the Use of Soyfoods and Their Potential Role in Cancer Prevention," *J Am Diet Assoc* 91 (1991): 836–40.

16. G.R. Howe et al., "Dietary Factors and the Risk of Breast Cancer: Combined Analysis of 12 Case-Controlled Studies," *J Natl Cancer Inst* 82 (1990): 561–9.

17. C.J. Christy, "Vitamin E in Menopause," *Am J Ob Gyn* 50 (1945): 84–7.

18. H.C. McLaren, "Vitamin E in the Menopause," *Br Med J* ii (1949): 1378–81.

19. R.S. Finkler, "The Effect of Vitamin E in the Menopause," *J Clin Endocrinol Metab* 9 (1949): 89–94.

20. C.J. Smith, "Non-Hormonal Control of Vasomotor Flushing in Menopausal Patients," *Chic Med* 67 (1964): 193–5.

21. Y. Murase and H. Iishima, "Clinical Studies of Oral Administration of Gamma-Oryzanol on Climacteric Complaints and Its Syndrome," *Obstet Gynecol Prac* 12 (1963): 147–9.

22. M. Ishihara, "Effect of Gamma-Oryzanol on Serum Lipid Peroxide Levels and Climacteric Disturbances," *Asia Oceania J Obstet Gynecol* 10 (1984): 317.

23. G. Yoshino, T. Kazumi, M. Amano, et al., "Effects of Gamma-Oryzanol on Hyperlipidemic Subjects," *Current Ther Res* 45 (1989): 543–52.

24. M. Harada, M. Suzuki, and Y. Ozaki, "Effect of Japanese Angelica Root and Peony Root on Uterine Contraction in the Rabbit in Situ," *J Pharm Dyn* 7 (1984): 304–11.

25. K. Yoshiro, "The Physiological Actions of Tang-Kuei and Cnidium," *Bull Oriental Healing Arts Inst USA* 10 (1985): 269–78.

26. O. Thastrup, B. Fjalland, and J. Lemmich, "Coronary Vasodilatory, Spasmolytic and cAMP-phosphodiesterase Inhibitory Properties of Dihydropyranocoumarins and Dihydrofuranocoumarins," *Acta Pharmacol et Toxicol* 52 (1983): 246–53.

27. C.H. Costello and E.V. Lynn, "Estrogenic Substances from Plants: I. Glycyrrhiza," *J Am Pharm Soc* 39 (1950): 177–80.

28. A. Kumagai, K. Nishino, A. Shimomura, T. Kin, and Y. Yamamura, "Effect of Glycyrrhizin on Estrogen Action," *Endocrinol Japan* 14 (1967): 34–8.

29. J. Haller, "Animal Experimentation with the Lipshutz Technique on the Activity of a Phytohormone on Gonadotropin Function," *Geburt Frauen* 18 (1958): 1347.

30. H. Stolze, "An Alternative to Treat Menopausal Complaints," *Gyne* 3 (1982): 14–6.

31. G. Warnecke, "Influencing Menopausal Symptoms with a Phytotherapeutic Agent," *Med Welt* 36 (1985): 871–4.

32. W. Stoll, "Phytopharmacon Influences Atrophic Vaginal Epithelium. Double-Blind Study: Cimicifuga vs. Estrogenic Substances," *Therapeuticum* 1 (1987): 23–31.

33. T. Nesselhut, S. Borth, and W. Kuhn, "Influence of Cimicifuga Racemosa Extracts with Estrogen-Like Activity on the in Vitro Proliferation of Mamma Carcinoma Cells," *Arch Gynecol Obstet* 254 (1993): 817–8.

34. W.D. Korn, *Six-Month Oral Toxicity Study with Remifemin-Granulate in Rats Followed by an 8-Week Recovery Period* (Hannover, Germany: International Bioresearch, 1991).

35. J. Kleijnen and P. Knipschild, "Drug Profiles: Ginkgo biloba," *Lancet* 340 (1993): 1136–9.

36. V.G. Rudofsky, "The Effect of Ginkgo biloba Extract in Cases of Arterial Occlusive Disease: A Randomized Placebo Controlled Double-Blind Cross-Over Study," *Fortschr Med* 105 (1987): 397–400.

37. I. Hindmarch and Z. Subhan, "The Psychopharmacological Effects of Ginkgo biloba Extract in Normal Healthy Volunteers," *Int J Clin Pharmacol Res* 4 (1984): 89–93.

38. M. Hammar, G. Berg, and R. Lindgren, "Does Physical Exercise Influence the Frequency of Postmenopausal Hot Flushes?" *Acta Obstet Gynecol Scand* 69 (1990): 409–12.

39. L. Slaven and C. Lee, "Mood and Symptom Reporting among Middle-Aged Women: The Relationship between Menopausal Status, Hormone Replacement Therapy, and Exercise Participation," *Health Psychol* 16 (1997): 203–8.

40. A.S. Midgette and J.A. Baron, "Cigarette Smoking and the Risk of Natural Menopause," *Epidemiology* 1 (1990): 474–80.

Menstrual Blood Loss, Excessive

1. P.J. Haynes, H. Hodgson, A.B.M. Anderson, and A.C. Turnbill, "Measurement of Menstrual Blood Loss in Patients Complaining of Menorrhagia," *Br J Ob Gyn* 84 (1977): 763–8.

2. I. Downing, D.J.R. Hutchon, and N.L. Poyser, "Uptake of [3H]-Arachidonic Acid by Human Endometrium: Differences between Normal and Menorrhagic Tissue," *Prostaglandins* 26 (1983): 55–69.

3. R.W. Kelly, M.A. Lumsden, M.H. Abel, and D.T. Baird, "The Relationship between Menstrual Blood Loss and Prostaglandin Production in the Human: Evidence for Increased Availability of Arachidonic Acid in Women Suffering from Menorrhagia," *Prostaglandins Leukotrienes Med* 16 (1984): 69–78.

4. B. Arvidsson, G. Ekenved, G. Rybo, and L. Solvell, "Iron Prophylaxis in Menorrhagia," *Acta Ob Gyn Scand* 60 (1981): 157–60.

5. M.L. Taymor, S.H. Sturgis, and C. Yahia, "The Etiological Role of Chronic Iron Deficiency in Production of Menorrhagia," *JAMA* 187 (1964): 323–7.

6. D. Lithgow and W. Politzer, "Vitamin A in the Treatment of Menorrhagia," *S Afr Med J* 51 (1977): 191–3.

7. J.D. Cohen and H.W. Rubin, "Functional Menorrhagia: Treatment with Bioflavonoids and Vitamin C," *Curr Ther Res* 2 (1960): 539–42.

8. P.R. Dasgupta, S. Dutta, P. Banerjee, and S. Majumdar, "Vitamin E (Alpha Tocopherol) in the Management of Menorrhagia Associated with the Use of Intrauterine Contraceptive Devices (IUCD)," *Int J Fertil* 28 (1983): 55–6.

9. R. Gubner and H.E. Ungerleider, "Vitamin K Therapy in Menorrhagia," *South Med J* 37 (1944): 556–8.

10. C.S. Stoffer, "Menstrual Disorders and Mild Thyroid Insufficiency," *Postgraduate Med* 72 (1982): 75–82.

11. E. Schumann, "Newer Concepts of Blood Coagulation and Control of Hemorrhage," *Am J Ob Gyn* 38 (1939): 1002–7.

12. A. Steinberg, H.I. Segal, and H.M. Parris, "Role of Oxalic Acid and Certain Related Dicarboxylic Acids in the Control of Hemorrhage," *Annals Oto Rhino Laryngo* 49 (1940): 1008–21.

Migraine Headache

1. E. Rubenstein and D.D. Federman, *Scientific American Medicine* (New

York: Scientific American, 1987), 11:XI:1–3.

2. F.C. Rose, "The Pathogenesis of a Migraine Attack," *TINS* 6 (1983): 247.

3. E. Shinhoj, "Hemodynamic Studies within the Brain during Migraine," *Arch Neurol* 29 (1979): 257–66.

4. R.S. Blacklow, *MacBrydes Signs and Symptoms,* 6th ed. (New York: J.B. Lippincott, 1983), 64–8.

5. J. Olesen, "The Ischemic Hypothesis of Migraine," *Arch Neurol* 44 (1987): 321–2.

6. E. Hanington, "The Platelet and Migraine," *Headache* 26 (1986): 411–5.

7. J.D. Spence, D.G. Wong, L.J. Melendez, et al., "Increased Incidence of Mitral Valve Prolapse in Patients with Migraine," *Can Med Assoc J* 131 (1984): 1457–60.

8. G. Gamberini, R. D'Alessandro, E. Labriola, et al., "Further Evidence on the Association of Mitral Valve Prolapse and Migraine," *Headache* 24 (1984): 39–40.

9. G. Lanzi, A.M. Grandi, G. Gamba, et al., "Migraine, Mitral Valve Prolapse, and Platelet Function in the Pediatric Age Group," *Headache* 26 (1986): 142–5.

10. K.M.A. Welch, "Migraine: A Biobehavioral Disorder," *Arch Neurol* 44 (1987): 323–7.

11. M.D. Ferrari et al., "Serotonin Metabolism in Migraine," *Neurology* 33 (1989): 1239–42.

12. L. Fioroni et al., "Platelet Serotonin Pathway in Menstrual Migraine," *Cephalgia* 16 (1996): 427–30.

13. J.W. Lance et al., "5-hydroxytryptamine and Its Putative Aetological Involvement in Migraine," *Cephalgia* 9 (Suppl.9) (1989): 7–13.

14. F. Sicuteri, "Migraine, a Central Biochemical Dysnociception," *Headache* 16 (1986): 145–9.

15. J.R. Fozard and J.A. Gray, "5-HT$_{1c}$ Receptor Activation: A Key Step in the Initiation of Migraine?" *Trends Pharmacol Sci* 10 (1989): 307–9.

16. M.D. Ferrari et al., "Treatment of Migraine with Sumatriptan," *N Engl J Med* 325 (1991): 316–21.

17. A. Kagaya et al., "Serotonin-Induced Desensitization of Serotonin$_2$ Receptors in Human Platelets via Mechanism Involving Protein Kinase C," *J Pharmacol Exp Ther* 255 (1990): 305–11.

18. N.T. Mathew, "Chronic Refractory Headache," *Neurology* 43(suppl.3) (1993): S26–S33.

19. N.T. Mathew, "Transformed Migraine," *Cephalgia* 13(suppl.12) (1993): 78–83.

20. H. Isler, "Migraine Treatment as a Cause of Chronic Migraine," in F.C. Rose, ed., *Advances in Migraine Research and Therapy* (New York: Raven Press, 1982), 159–64.

21. L.E. Mansfield, T.R. Vaughan, S.T. Waller, et al., "Food Allergy and Adult Migraine: Double-Blind and Mediator Confirmation of an Allergic Etiology," *Ann Allergy* 55 (1985): 126–9.

22. C.M. Carter, J. Egger, and J.F. Soothill, "A Dietary Management of Severe Childhood Migraine," *Hum Nutr: Appl Nutr* 39A (1985): 294–303.

23. E.C. Hughes, P.S. Gott, R.C. Weinstein, and R. Binggeli, "Migraine: A Diagnostic Test for Etiology of Food Sensitivity by a Nutritionally Supported Fast and Confirmed by Long-Term Report," *Ann Allergy* 55 (1985): 28–32.

24. J. Egger, C.M. Carter, J. Wilson et al., "Is Migraine Food Allergy?" *Lancet* ii (1983): 865–9.

25. J. Monro, J. Brostoff, C. Carini, and K. Zilkha, "Food Allergy in Migraine," *Lancet* ii (1980): 1–4.

26. E.C.G. Grant, "Food Allergies and Migraine," *Lancet* i (1979): 966–9.

27. C.H. Little, A.G. Stewart, and M.R. Fennessy, "Platelet Serotonin Release in Rheumatoid Arthritis as Studied in Food Intolerant Patients," *Lancet* ii (1983): 297–9.

28. R.C. Peatfield, "Relationship Between Food, Wine, and Beer-Precipitated Headaches," *Headache* 35 (1995): 355–7.

29. R. Jarisch and F. Wantke, "Wine and Headache," *Int Arch Allergy Immunol* 110 (1996): 7–12.

30. F. Wantke, M. Gotz, and R. Jarisch, "Histamine-Free Diet: Treatment of Choice for Histamine-Induced Food Intolerance and Supporting Treatment for Chronic Headaches," *Clin Exp Allergy* 23 (1993): 982–5.

31. C. Ortolani, "Atlas on Mechanisms in Adverse Reaction to Foods," *Allergy* (50 Suppl.20) (1995): 5–81.

32. T.R. Vaughn, "The Role of Food in the Pathogenesis of Migraine

Headache," *Clin Rev Allergy* 12 (1994): 167–80.

33. J. Jarman, V. Glover, and M. Sandler, "Release of (^{14}C)5-Hydroxytryptamine from Human Platelets by Red Wine," *Life Sci* 48 (1991): 2297–2300.

34. P.M. Martner Hewes et al., "Vitamin B6 Nutriture and Plasma Diamine Oxidase Activity in Pregnant Hispanic Teenagers," *Am J Clin Nutr* 44 (1988): 907–13.

35. A. Sabbah et al., "Antihistaminic or Anti-Degranulating Activity of Pregnancy Serum," *Allergy Immunol Paris* 20 (1988): 236–40.

36. S. Lindberg, "14C-Histamine Elimination from Blood of Pregnant and Non-Pregnant Women with Special Reference to the Uterus," *Acta Obst Gynecol Scand* 62 (1963): 1–25.

37. I. Fettes et al., "Endorphin Levels in Headache Syndromes," *Headache* 25 (1984): 37–9.

38. M. Leone et al., "Beta-Endorphin Level in Lymphocytes of Primary Headache Patients," *Cephalgia* 11(Suppl.11) (1991): 188–9.

39. P.A. Battistella et al., "Beta-Endorphin in Plasma and Monocytes in Juvenile Headache," *Headache* 36 (1996): 91–4.

40. F. Titus et al., "5-Hydroxytryptophan Versus Methysergide in the Prophylaxis of Migraine: Randomized Clinical Trial," *Eur Neurol* 25 (1986): 327–9.

41. G. Bono et al., "Serotonin Precursors in Migraine Prophylaxis," *Adv Neurol* 33 (1982): 357–63.

42. C.P. Maissen and H.P. Ludin, "Comparison of the Effect of 5-hydroxytryptophan and Propranolol in the Interval Treatment of Migraine," *Med Wochenschr* 121 (1991): 1585–90.

43. G. De Giorgis et al., "Headache in Association with Sleep Disorders in Children: A Psychodiagnostic Evaluation and Controlled Clinical Study—L-5-HTP versus Placebo," *Drugs Exp Clin Res* 13 (1987): 425–33.

44. M. Santucci et al., "L-5-hydroxytryptophan versus Placebo in Childhood Migraine Prophylaxis: A Double-Blind Crossover Study," *Cephalgia* 6 (1986): 155–7.

45. G. Longo et al., "Treatment of Essential Headache in Develop-

mental Age with L-5-HTP (Cross-Over Double-Blind Study versus Placebo)," *Pediatr Med Chir* 6 (1984): 241–5.

46. J.M. Gerrard, J.G. White, and W. Krivit, "Labile Aggregation Stimulating Substance, Free Fatty Acids and Platelet Aggregation," *J Lab Clin Med* 87 (1976): 73–82.

47. T.A.B. Sanders and F. Roshanai, "The Influence of Different Types of Omega-3 Polyunsaturated Fatty Acids on Blood Lipids and Platelet Function in Healthy Volunteers," *Clin Sci* 64 (198): 91–9.

48. B.E. Woodcock, E. Smith, W.H. Lambert, et al., "Beneficial Effect of Fish Oil on Blood Viscosity in Peripheral Vascular Disease," *Br Med J* 288 (1984): 592–4.

49. J. Schoenen, M. Lenaerts, and E. Bastings, "High-Dose Riboflavin as a Prophylactic Treatment of Migraine: Results of an Open Pilot Study," *Cephalagia* 14 (1994): 328–9.

50. G. Mazzotta et al., "Electro-myographical Ischemic Test and Intracellular and Extracellular Mag-nesium Concentration in Migraine and Tension-Type Headache Patients," *Headache* 36 (1996): 357–61.

51. D.R. Swanson, "Migraine and Magnesium: Eleven Neglected Connections," *Perspect Biol Med* 31 (1988): 526–57.

52. N.M. Ramadan et al., "Low Brain Magnesium in Migraine," *Headache* 29 (1989): 590–3.

53. V. Gallai et al., "Magnesium Content of Mononuclear Blood Cells in Migraine Patients," *Headache* 34 (1994): 160–5.

54. V. Pfaffenrath et al., "Magnesium in the Prophylaxis of Migraine: A Double-Blind Placebo-Controlled Study," *Cephalagia* 16 (1996): 436–40.

55. A. Peikert et al., "Prophylaxis of Migraine with Oral Magnesium: Results from a Prospective, Multi-Center, Placebo-Controlled and Double-Blind Randomized Study," *Cephalagia* 16 (1996): 257–63.

56. L.D. Galland, S.M. Baker, and R.K. McLellan, "Magnesium Deficiency in the Pathogenesis of Mitral Valve Prolapse," *Magnesium* 5 (1986): 165–74.

57. J.S. Lindberg et al., "Magnesium Bioavailability from Magnesium Citrate and Magnesium Oxide," *J Am Coll Nutr* 9 (1990): 48–55.

58. P. Majumdar and M. Boylan, "Alteration of Tissue Magnesium Levels in Rats by Dietary Vitamin B6 Supplementation," *Int J Vitamin Nutr Res* 59 (1989): 300–3.

59. A. Mauskop et al., "Intravenous Magnesium Sulfate Rapidly Alleviates Headaches of Various Types," *Headache* 36 (1996): 154–60.

60. A. Mauskop et al., "Intravenous Magnesium Sulphate Relieves Migraine Attacks in Patients with Low Serum Ionized Magnesium Levels: A Pilot Study," *Clin Sci* 89 (1995): 633–6.

61. A. Mauskop et al., "Intravenous Magnesium Sulfate Relieves Cluster Headaches in Patients with Low Serum Ionized Magnesium Levels," *Headache* 35 (1995): 597–600.

62. G.B. Parker, H. Tupling, and D.S. Pryor, "A Controlled Trial of Cervical Manipulation for Migraine," *Aust NZ J Med* 8 (1978): 589–93.

63. P.G. Watts, K.M.S. Peet and R.P. Juniper, "Migraine and the Temporomandibular Joint: The Final Answer?" *Br Dent J* 161 (1986): 170–3.

64. S. Solomon and K.M. Guglielmo, "Treatment of Headache by Transcutaneous Electrical Stimulation," *Headache* 25 (1985): 12–5.

65. H. Doeer-Proske and H.U. Wittchen, "A Muscle and Vascular Oriented Program for the Treatment of Chronic Migraine Patients: A Randomized Clinical Comparative Study," *Z Psychosom Med Psychoanal* 31 (1985): 247–66.

66. V.A. Vesnina, "Current Methods of Migraine Reflexotherapy (Acupuncture, Electropuncture, and Electroacupuncture)," *Zh Nevropatol Psikhiatr* 80 (1980): 703–9.

67. H.D. Kurkland, "Treatment of Headache Pain with Auto-Acupressure," *Dis Nerv Sys* 37 (1976): 127–9.

68. L. Lenhard and P.M. Waite, "Acupuncture in the Prophylactic Treatment of Migraine Headache: Pilot Study," *NZ Med J* 96 (1983): 663–6.

69. F. Facchinetti, G. Nappi, F. Savoldi, and A.R. Genazzani, "Primary Headaches: Reduced Circulating Beta-Lipotropin and Beta-Endorphin Levels with Impaired Reactivity to Acupuncture," *Cephalgia* 1 (1980): 195–201.

70. V.F. Markelova, V.A. Vesnina, S.I. Malygina, and L.A. Dubovskaia, "Changes in Blood Serotonin Levels in Patients with Migraine Headaches Before and After a Course of Reflexotherapy," *Zh Nevropatol Psikhiatr* 84 (1984): 1313–6.

71. J. Laiten, "Acupuncture for Migraine Prophylaxis: A Prospective Clinical Study with Six Months' Follow-Up," *Am J Chin Med* 3 (1975): 271–4.

72. K.A. Holroyd and D.B. Penzien, "Pharmacological versus Non-Pharmacological Prophylaxis of Recurrent Migraine Headache: A Meta-Analytic Review of Clinical Trials," *Pain* 42 (1990): 1–13.

73. E.S. Johnson et al., "Efficacy of Feverfew as Prophylactic Treatment of Migraine," *Br Med J* 291 (1985): 569–73.

74. J.J. Murphy, S. Heptinstall, and J.R.A. Mitchell, "Randomized Double-Blind Placebo-Controlled Trial of Feverfew in Migraine Prevention," *Lancet* ii (1988): 189–92.

75. R.W.J. Barsby, U. Salan, B.W. Knight, and J.R.S. Hoult, "Feverfew and Vascular Smooth Muscle: Extracts From Fresh and Dried Plants Show Opposing Pharmacological Profiles, Dependent upon Sesquiterpene Lactone Content," *Planta Medica* 59 (1993): 20–5.

76. S. Heptinstall et al., "Parthenolide Content and Bioactivity of Feverfew (*Tanacetum parthenium* (L.) Schultz-Bip.). Estimation of Commercial and Authenticated Feverfew Products," *J Pharm Pharmacol* 44 (1992): 391–5.

77. F. Kiuchi et al., "Inhibition of Prostaglandin and Leukotriene Biosynthesis by Gingerols and Diarylheptanoids," *Chem Pharm Bull* 40 (1992): 387–91.

78. K.C. Srivastava, "Isolation and Effects of Some Ginger Components on Platelet Aggregation and Eicosanoid Biosynthesis," *Prosta-glandins Leurotri Med* 25 (1986): 187–98.

79. T. Mustafa and K.C. Srivastava, "Ginger (*Zingiber officinale*) in

Migraine Headaches," *J Ethnopharmacol* 29 (1990): 267–73.

Multiple Sclerosis

1. G.W. Ellison, B.R. Visscher, M.C. Graves, and J.L. Fahey, "Multiple Sclerosis," *Annals Int Med* 101 (1984): 514–26.

2. R.W.P. Cutler, "Demyelinating Disease," in C.D. Dale and D.D. Federman, *Scientific American Medicine* (1997): 11:IX:1–5.

3. R.G. Petersdorf, *Harrison's Principles of Internal Medicine* (New York: McGraw-Hill, 1983), 2098–103.

4. D.C. Hewson, "Is There a Role for Gluten-Free Diets in Multiple Sclerosis?" *Human Nutr Appl Nutr* 38A (1984): 417–20.

5. P.J. Butcher, "Milk Consumption and Multiple Sclerosis—an Etiological Hypothesis," *Medical Hypothesis* 19 (1986): 169–78.

6. B.A. Agranoff and D. Goldberg, "Diet and the Geographical Distribution of Multiple Sclerosis," *Lancet* 2 (1974): 1061–6.

7. R.L. Swank, "Multiple Sclerosis: A Correlation of Its Incidence with Dietary Fat," *Am J Med Sci* 220 (1950): 421–30.

8. M.L. Esparza et al., "Nutrition, Latitude, and Multiple Sclerosis Mortality: An Ecologic Study," *Am J Epidem* 142 (1995): 733–7.

9. R.L. Swank, "Multiple Sclerosis: Twenty Years on Low Fat Diet," *Arch Neurol* 23 (1970): 460–74.

10. R.L. Swank, O. Lerstad, A. Strom et al., "Multiple Sclerosis in Rural Norway: Its Geographic Distribution and Occupational Incidence in Relation to Nutrition," *NEJM* 246 (1952): 721–8.

11. J. Bernsohn and L.M. Stephanides, "Aetiology of Multiple Sclerosis," *Nature* 10 (1963): 523–30.

12. V.K.S. Shukla, G.E. Jensen, and J. Clausen, "Erythrocyte Glutathione Peroxidase Deficiency in Multiple Sclerosis," *Acta Neurol Scand* 56 (1977): 542–50.

13. A. Szeinberg, R. Golan, B. Ezzer et al., "Decreased Erythrocyte Glutathione Peroxidase Activity in Multiple Sclerosis," *Acta Neurol Scand* 60 (1979): 265–71.

14. G.E. Jensen, G. Gissel-Nielsen, and J. Clausen, "Leukocyte Glutathione Peroxidase Activity and Selenium Level in Multiple Sclerosis," *J Neurol Sci* 48 (1980): 61–7.

15. G.L. Mazzella, E. Sinfoiani, F. Savoldi et al., "Blood Cells Glutathione Peroxidase Activity and Selenium in Multiple Sclerosis," *Eur Neurol* 22 (1983): 442–6.

16. J. Wikstrom, T. Westermarck, and J. Palo, "Selenium, Vitamin E and Copper in Multiple Sclerosis," *Acta Neurol Scand* 54 (1976): 287–90.

17. R.L. Swank and M.H. Pullen, *The Multiple Sclerosis Diet Book* (Garden City, NY: Doubleday, 1977).

18. I.S. Neu, "Essential Fatty Acids in the Serum and Cerebrospinal Fluid of Multiple Sclerosis Patients," in R.E. Gonsette and P. Delmotte, eds., *Immunological and Clinical Aspects of Multiple Sclerosis* (Boston: MTP Press, 1984).

19. S.T. Homa, J. Belin, A.D. Smith et al., "Levels of Linolenate and Arachidonate in Red Blood Cells of Healthy Individuals and Patients with Multiple Sclerosis," *J Neurol Neurosurg Psychiat* 43 (1980): 106–10.

20. H.P. Wright, R.H.S. Thompson, and K.J. Zilkha, "Platelet Adhesiveness in Multiple Sclerosis," *Lancet* 2 (1965): 1109–10.

21. C.F. Cullen and R.L. Swank, "Intravascular Aggregation and Adhesiveness of the Blood Elements Associated with Alimentary Lipemia and Injection of Large Molecular Substances: Effect on Blood-Brain Barrier," *Circulation* 9 (1954): 335–46.

22. A.F. Haeren, W.W. Tourtellotte, K.A. Richard et al., "A Study of the Blood Cerebrospinal Fluid-Brain Barrier in Multiple Sclerosis," *Neurology* 14 (1964): 345–51.

23. R.L. Swank and H. Nakamura, "Oxygen Availability in Brain Tissues after Lipid Meals," *Am J Physiol* 198 (1960): 217–20.

24. R.W. Soll and P.B. Grenoble, *MS: Something Can Be Done and You Can Do It* (Chicago: Contemporary Books, 1984).

25. L.S. Lange and M. Shiner, "Small-Bowel Abnormalities in Multiple Sclerosis," *Lancet* 2 (1976): 1319–22.

26. L.A. Liversedge, "Treatment and Management of MS," *Br Med Bull* 33 (1976): 78–83.

27. L.A. Hunter, B.W.G. Rees, and L.T. Jones, "Gluten Antibodies in Patients with Multiple Sclerosis," *Hum Nutr Clin Nutr* 38A (1984): 142–3.

28. Z.H.D. Millar, K.J. Zilkha, M.J.S. Langman et al., "Double-Blind Trial of Linolate Supplementation of the Diet in Multiple Sclerosis," *Br Med J* 1 (1973): 765–8.

29. D. Bates, P.R.W. Fawcett, D.A. Shaw, and D. Weightman, "Polyunsaturated Fatty Acids in Treatment of Acute Remitting Multiple Sclerosis," *Br Med J* 2 (1978): 1390–1.

30. D.W. Paty, H.K. Cousin, S. Read, and K. Adlakkha, "Linoleic Acid in Multiple Sclerosis: Failure to Show Any Therapeutic Benefit," *Acta Neurol Scand* 58 (1978): 53–8.

31. R.H. Dworkin, D. Bates, J.H.D. Millar, and D.W. Paty, "Linoleic Acid and Multiple Sclerosis: A Reanalysis of Three Double-Blind Trials," *Neurology* 34 (1984): 1441–5.

32. R.H. Dworkin, D. Bates, J.H.D. Millar, D.A. Shaw, and D.W. Paty, "Chapter 3. Dietary Supplementation with Polyunsaturated Fatty Acids in Acute Remitting Multiple Sclerosis," in R.E. Gonsette and P. Delmotte, eds., *Immunological and Clinical Aspects of Multiple Sclerosis* (Boston: MTP Press, 1984).

33. E.J. Field and G. Joyce, "Multiple Sclerosis: Effect of Gamma Linolenate Administration upon Membranes and the Need for Extended Clinical Trials of Unsaturated Fatty Acids," *Eur Neurol* 22 (1983): 78–83.

34. C.J. Meade, J. Mertin, J. Sheena, and R. Hunt, "Reduction by Linoleic Acid of the Severity of Experimental Allergic Encephalomyelitis in the Guinea Pig," *J Neurol Sci* 35 (1978): 291–308.

35. D. Hughes, A.B. Kieth, J. Mertin, and E.A. Caspary, "Linoleic Acid Therapy in Severe Experimental Allergic Encephalomyelitis in the Guinea Pig: Suppression by Continuous Treatment," *Clin Exp Immunol* 41 (1980): 523–31.

36. D.V. Johnston and L.A. Mashall, "Dietary Fat, Prostaglandins and the

Immune Response," *Progress Food Nutr Sci* 8 (1984): 3–25.

37. G.J. Meade and J. Mertin, "Fatty Acids and Immunity," *Adv Lipid Res* 16 (1978): 127–65.

38. J. Mertin and A. Stackpoole, "The Spleen Is Required for Suppression of Experimental Allergic Encephalomyelitis by Prostaglandin Precursors," *Clin Exp Immunol* 36 (1979): 449–55.

39. J. Mertin and A. Stackpoole, "Suppression by Essential Fatty Acids of Experimental Allergic Encephalomyelitis Is Abolished by Indomethacin," *Prostaglandins Med* 1 (1978): 283–91.

40. S. Renaud and A. Norday, "Small Is Beautiful: Alpha-Linolenic Acid and Eicosapentaenoic Acid in Man," *Lancet* 1 (1983): 1169.

41. R.T. Holman, S.B. Johnson, and T.F. Hatch, "A Case of Human Linolenic Acid Deficiency Involving Neurological Abnormalities," *Am J Clin Nutr* 65 (1982): 617–23.

42. J. Mai, P.S. Sorenson, and J.C. Hansen, "High Dose Antioxidant Supplementation to MS Patients: Effects on Glutathione Peroxidase, Clinical Safety, and Absorption," *Biol Trace Elem Res* 24 (1990): 109–17.

43. J. Dyerberg, "Linolenate-Derived Polyunsaturated Fatty Acids and Prevention of Atherosclerosis," *Nutr Rev* 44 (1986): 125–34.

44. D.F. Horrobin, "Multiple Sclerosis: The Rational Basis for Treatment with Colchicine and Evening Primrose Oil," *Med Hypothesis* 5 (1979): 365–78.

45. R. Sandyk and G. Awerbuch, "Vitamin B12 and Its Relationship to Age of Onset of Multiple Sclerosis," *Int J Neurosci* 71 (1993): 93–9.

46. E. Reynolds, "Multiple Sclerosis and Vitamin B12 Metabolism," *J Neuroimmunol* 40 (1992): 225–30.

47. E.H. Reynolds et al., "Vitamin B12 Metabolism in Multiple Sclerosis," *Arch Neurol* 49 (1992): 649–52.

48. J. Kira, S. Tobimatsu, and I. Goto, "Vitamin B12 Metabolism and Massive-Dose Methyl Vitamin B12 Therapy in Japanese Patients with Multiple Sclerosis," *Int Med* 33 (1994): 82–6.

49. C.A. Simpson, D.J. Newell, and H. Miller, "The Treatment of Multiple

Sclerosis with Massive Doses of Hydroxocobalamin," *Neurology* 15 (1965): 599–602.

50. S.M. Baig and G.A. Qureshi, "Homocysteine and Vitamin B12 in Multiple Sclerosis," *Biogenic Amines* 11 (1995): 479–85.

51. J. Rio et al., "Serum Homocysteine Levels and Multiple Sclerosis," *Arch Neurol* 51 (1994): 1181.

52. K. Ransberger and W. van Schaik, "Enzyme Therapy in Multiple Sclerosis," *Der Kassenarzt* 41 (1986): 42–5.

53. J.K. Gupta, A.P. Ingegno, A.W. Cook and L.P. Pertschuk, "Multiple Sclerosis and Malabsorption," *Am J Gastroenterol* 68 (1977): 560–6.

54. K. Ransberger, "Enzyme Treatment of Immune Complex Diseases," *Arthritis Rheuma* 8 (1986): 16–9.

55. D. Squillacote, M. Martinez, and W. Sheremata, "Natural Alpha Interferon in Multiple Sclerosis: Results of Three Preliminary Series," *J Int Med Res* 24 (1996): 246–57.

56. V. Calabrese et al., "Changes in Cerebrospinal Fluid Levels of Malondialdehyde and Glutathione Reductase Activity in Multiple Sclerosis," *Int J Clin Pharmacol Res* 14 (1994): 119–23.

57. B. Brochet et al., "Double-Blind, Placebo-Controlled Multi-Center Study of Ginkgolide B in the Treatment of Acute Exacerbations of Multiple Sclerosis," *Journal of Neurology, Neurosurgery Psych* 58 (1995): 360–2.

58. V. Boschetty and j. Cernoch, "Aplikace kysliku za pretlaku u nekterych neurologickych onemocneni," *Bratisl Lek Listy* 53 (1970): 298–302.

59. J.H. Baixe, "Bilan de onze annees d'activite en medicine hyperbare," *Med Aer Spatiale Med Subaquatique Hyperbare* 17 (1978): 90–2.

60. R.A. Neubauer, "Treatment of Multiple Sclerosis with Monoplace Hyperbaric Oxygenation," *J Fl Med Assoc* 65 (1978): 101.

61. B.H. Fischler, M. Marks, and T. Reich, "Hyperbaric-Oxygen Treatment of Multiple Sclerosis," *N Engl J Med* 308 (1983): 181–6.

62. M.P. Barnes, D. Bates, N.E.F. Cartlidge et al., "Hyperbaric Oxygen and Multiple Sclerosis: Short Term

Results of a Placebo-Controlled, Double Blind Trial," *Lancet* 1 (1985): 297–300.

63. C.M. Wiles, C.R.A. Clarke, H.P. Irwin et al., "Hyperbaric Oxygen in Multiple Sclerosis: A Double Blind Trial," *Br Med J* 292 (1986): 367–71.

64. J. Kleijnen and P. Knipschild, "Hyperbaric Oxygen for Multiple Sclerosis: Review of Controlled Trials," *Acta Neurol Scand* 91 (1995): 330–4.

65. C.C. Whitacre et al., "Treatment of Autoimmune Disease by Oral Tolerance to Autoantigens," *Clin Immunol Immunopathol* 80 (1996): S31–9.

66. H. Fukaura et al., "Induction of Circulating Myelin Basic Protein and Proteolipid Protein-Specific Transforming Growth Factor-Beta1-Secreting Th3 T Cells by Oral Administration of Myelin in Multiple Sclerosis Patients," *J Clin Invest* 98 (1996): 70–7.

67. J.H. Petajan et al., "Impact of Aerobic Training on Fitness and Quality of Life in Multiple Sclerosis," *Ann Neurol* 39 (1996): 432–41.

Nausea and Vomiting of Pregnancy

1. A. Gaby, *The Doctor's Guide to B6* (Emmaus, PA: Rodale Press, 1984).

2. B. Weinstein et al., "Oral Administration of Pyridoxine Hydrochloride in the Treatment of Nausea and Vomiting of Pregnancy," *Am J Ob Gyn* 47 (1944): 389–94.

3. V. Sahakian et al., "Vitamin B6 Is Effective for Nausea and Vomiting of Pregnancy: A Randomized, Double-Blind Placebo-Controlled Study," *Obstet Gynecol* 78 (1991): 33–6.

4. T. Vutyananich, S. Wongtrangan, and R. Rungaroon "Pyridoxine for Nausea and Vomiting of Pregnancy: A Randomized, Double-Blind, Placebo-Controlled Trial," *Am J Obstet Gynecol* 173 (1995): 881–4.

5. R. Merkel, "The Use of Menadione Bisulfite and Ascorbic Acid in the Treatment of Nausea and Vomiting of Pregnancy," *Am J Ob Gyn* 64 (1952): 416–8.

6. D. Mowrey and D. Clayson, "Motion Sickness, Ginger, and Psychophysics," *Lancet* 1 (1982): 655–7.

7. W. Fischer-Rasmussen, S.K. Kjaer, C. Dahl and U. Asping, "Ginger Treatment of Hyperemesis Gravidarum," *Eur J Obstet Gynecol Reprod Biol* 38 (1990): 19–24.

8. S. Wolkind and E. Zajicek, "Psycho-Social Correlates of Nausea and Vomiting in Pregnancy," *H Psychosom Res* 22 (1978): 1–5.

9. C.M. FitzGerald, "Nausea and Vomiting in Pregnancy," *Br J Med Psycho* 57 (1984): 159–65.

10. E. Hyde, "Acupressure Therapy for Morning Sickness: A Controlled Clinical Trial," *J Nurse Midwifery* 34 (1989): 171–8.

Obesity

1. R. Kuczmarski et al., "Increasing Prevalence of Overweight among US Adults," *JAMA* 272 (1994): 205–11.

2. Centers for Disease Control and Prevention, "Prevalence of Overweight Among Adolescents—United States, 1988-91," *MMWR Morb Mortal Wkly Rep* 43(44) (1994): 818–21.

3. R.F. Gillum, "The Association of Body Fat Distribution with Hypertension, Hypertensive Heart Disease, Coronary Heart Disease, Diabetes and Cardiovascular Risk Factors in Men and Women Age 18-79 Years," *J Chron Dis* 40 (1987): 421–28.

4. W.H. Dietz and S.L. Gortmaker, "Do We Fatten Our Children at the Television Set?" *Pediatrics* 75 (1985): 807–12.

5. L.A. Tucker and M. Bagwell, "Television Viewing and Obesity in Adult Females," *Am J Public Health* 81 (1991): 908–11.

6. G. Kolata, "Why Do People Get Fat?" *Science* 227 (1985): 1327–28.

7. R.J. Wurtman and J.J. Wurtman, "Brain Serotonin, Carbohydrate-Craving, Obesity and Depression," *Adv Exp Med Biol* 398 (1996): 35–41.

8. J. Wurtman and S. Suffes, *The Serotonin Solution* (New York: Fawcett Columbine, 1997).

9. G.M. Goodwin et al., "Plasma Concentrations of Tryptophan and Dieting," *Br Med J* 300 (1990): 1499-1500.

10. M. Laville et al., "Decreased Glucose-Induced Thermogenesis at the Onset of Obesity," *Am J Clin Nutr* 57 (1993): 851–56.

11. E. Ravussin et al., "Evidence that Insulin Resistance is Responsible for the Decreased Thermic Effect of Glucose in Human Obesity," *J Clin Invest* 76 (1985): 1268–73.

12. A. Astrup, N.J. Christensen, and L. Breum, "Reduced Plasma Noradrenaline Concentrations in Simple-Obese and Diabetic Obese Patients," *Clin Sci* 80 (1991): 53–58.

13. K.M. Nelson et al., "Effect of Weight Reduction on Resting Energy Expenditure, Substrate Utilization, and the Thermic Effect of Food in Moderately Obese Women," *Am J Clin Nutr* 55 (1992): 924–33.

14. L.O. Schulz, "Brown Adipose Tissue: Regulation of Thermogenesis and Implications for Obesity," *J Am Diet Assoc* 87 (1987): 761–64.

15. E.A. Sims et al., "Endocrine and Metabolic Effects of Experimental Obesity in Man," *Rec Prog Hor Res* 29 (1973): 457–96.

16. R.L. Leibel and J. Hirsch, "Diminished Energy Requirements in Reduced Obese Patients," *Metabolism* 33 (1984): 164–70.

17. L.H. Eck, "Children at Familial Risk for Obesity: An Examination of Dietary Intake, Physical Activity, and Weight Status," *Int J Obes* 16 (1992): 71–78.

18. F. Ceci et al., "The Effects of Oral 5-Hydroxytryptophan Administration on Feeding Behavior in Obese Adult Female Subjects," *J Neural Transm* 76 (1989): 109–17.

19. C. Cangiano et al., "Effects of 5-Hydroxytryptophan on Eating Behavior and Adherence to Dietary Prescriptions in Obese Adult Subjects," *Adv Exp Med Biol* 294 (1991): 591–93.

20. C. Cangiano et al., "Eating Behavior and Adherence to Dietary Prescriptions in Obese Adult Subjects Treated with 5-Hydroxytryptophan," *Am J Clin Nutr* 56 (1992): 863–67.

21. A. Astrup et al., "The Effect of Chronic Ephedrine Treatment on Substrate Utilization, the Sympathoadrenal Activity, and Expenditure During Glucose-Induced Thermogenesis in Man," *Metabolism* 35 (1986): 260–65.

22. A. Astrup et al., "Pharmacology of Thermogenic Drugs," *Am J Clin Nutr* 55(1 Suppl.) (1992): 246S–248S.

23. A.G. Dulloo and D.S. Miller, "The Thermogenic Properties of Ephedrine/Methylxanthine Mixtures: Animal Studies," *Am J Clin Nutr* 43(1986): 388–94.

24. R. Pasquali, "A Controlled Trial Using Ephedrine in the Treatment of Obesity," *Int J Obes* 9 (1985): 93–98.

25. S. Toubro et al., "Safety and Efficacy of Long-Term Treatment with Ephedrine, Caffeine and an Ephedrine/Caffeine Mixture," *Int J Obes* 17(Suppl.1) (1993): S69–72.

26. A. Astrup et al., "The Effect and Safety of an Ephedrine/Caffeine Compound Compared to Ephedrine, Caffeine and Placebo in Obese Subjects on an Energy Restricted Diet. A Double Blind Trial," *Int J Obes* 16 (1992): 269–77.

27. A.G. Dulloo and D.S. Miller, "The Thermogenic Properties of Ephedrine/Methylxanthine Mixtures: Human Studies," *Int J Obes* 10 (1986): 467–81.

28. A. Astrup et al., "The Effect of Ephedrine/Caffeine Mixture on Energy Expenditure and Body Composition in Obese Women," *Metabolism* 41 (1992): 686–88.

29. G.A. Spiller, *Dietary Fiber in Health and Nutrition* (Boca Raton, FL: CRC Press, 1994).

30. M. Krotkiewski, "Effect of Guar on Body Weight, Hunger Ratings and Metabolism in Obese Subjects," *Clinical Science* 66 (1984): 329–36.

31. M. Krotkiewski and U. Smith, "Dietary Fibre in Obesity," in *Dietary Fiber Perspectives. Reviews and Bibliography*, eds. A.R. Leeds and A. Avenell (London: John Libbey, 1985), p.61.

32. M. Krotkiewski, "Effect of Guar Gum on Body-Weight, Hunger Ratings and Metabolism in Obese Subjects," *Br J Nutr* 52 (1984): 97–105.

33. Anonymous, "Better Than Oat Bran," *Science News* 145 (1994): 28.

34. D.E. Walsh, V. Yaghoubian and A. Behforooz, "Effect of Glucomannan on Obese Patients: A Clinical Study," *Int J Obesity* 8 (1984): 289–93.

35. G. Biancardi, L. Palmiero, and P.E. Ghirardi, "Glucomannan in the Treatment of Overweight Patients with Osteoarthrosis," *Curr Ther Res* 46 (1989): 908–12.

36. S.M. El-Shebini et al., "The Role of Pectin as a Slimming Agent," *J Clini Biochem Nutr* 4 (1988): 255–62.

37. T.T. Solum et al., "The Influence of a High-Fibre Diet on Body Weight, Serum Lipids and Blood Pressure in Slightly Overweight Persons. A Randomized, Double-Blind, Placebo-Controlled Investigation with Diet and Fibre Tablets (DumoVital)," *Int J Obesity* 11(Suppl.1) (1987): 67–71.

38. K.R. Ryttig, S. Larsen, and L. Haegh, "Treatment of Slightly to Moderately Overweight Persons: A Double-Blind Placebo-Controlled Investigation with Diet and Fibre Tablets (DumoVital)," *Tidsskr Nor Laegeforen* 104 (1984): 989–91.

39. S. Rossner et al., "Weight Reduction with Dietary Fibre Supplements. Results of Two Double-Blind Studies," *Acta Med Scand* 222 (1987): 83–88.

40. K.R. Ryttig et al., "A Dietary Fibre Supplement and Weight Maintenance After Weight Reduction: A Randomized, Double-Blind, Placebo-Controlled Long-Term Trial," *Int J Obesity* 14 (1989): 763–69.

41. D. Rigaud et al., "Mild Overweight Treated with Energy Restriction and a Dietary Fiber Supplement: A 6-Month Randomized, Double-Blind, Placebo-Controlled Trial," *Int J Obesity* 14 (1990): 763–69.

42. W. Mertz, "Chromium in Human Nutritiona: A Review," *J Nutr* 123 (1993): 626–33.

43. R.A. Anderson, "Chromium, Glucose Tolerance, and Diabetes," *Biological Trace Element Research* 32 (1992): 19–24.

44. R.A. Anderson, M.M. Polansky, N.A. Bryden et al., "Effects of Supplemental Chromium on Patients with Symptoms of Reactive Hypoglycemia," *Metabolism* 36 (1987): 351–55.

45. M.F. McCarthy, "Hypothesis: Sensitization of Insulin-Dependent Hypothalamic Glucoreceptors May Account for the Fat-Reducing Effects of Chromium Picolinate," *J Optimal Nutr* 21 (1993): 36–53.

46. G.W. Evans and D.J. Pouchnik, "Composition and Biological Activity of Chromium-Pyridine Carbosylate Complexes," *J Inorgranic Biochemistry* 49 (1993): 177–87.

47. G.W. Evans, "Chromium Picolinate is an Efficacious and Safe Supplement," *Int J Sport Nutr* 3 (1993): 117–22.

48. R.I. Press, J. Geller, and G.W. Evans, "The Effect of Chromium Picolinate on Serum Cholesterol and Apolipoprotein Fractions in Human Subjects," *Western J Med* 152 (1993): 41–45.

49. N. Baba, E.F. Bracco, and S.A. Hashim, "Enhanced Thermogenesis and Diminished Deposition of Fat in Response to Overfeeding with Diet Containing Medium Chain Triglyceride," *Am J Clin Nutr* 35 (1982): 678–82.

50. J.O. Hill et al., "Thermogenesis in Humans During Overfeeding with Medium-Chain Triglycerides in Man," *Amer J Clin Nutr* 44 (1986): 630–34.

51. J.O. Hill et al., "Thermogenesis in Man During Overfeeding with Medium Chain Triglycerides," *Metabolism* 38 (1989): 641–48.

52. H. Chee, D.R. Romsos, and G.A. Leveille, "Influence of (-)-Hydroxycitrate on Lipigenesis in Chickens and Rats," *J Nutr* 107 (1977): 112–19.

53. A.C. Sullivan et al., "Effect of (-)-Hydroxycitrate upon the Accumulation of Lipid in the Rat. I. Lipogenesis," *Lipids* 9 (1974): 121–28.

54. R.N. Rao and K.K. Sakariah, "Lipid-Lowering and Antiobesity Effect of (-)-Hydroxycitric Acid," *Nutr Res* 8 (1988): 209–12.

55. L. van Gaal et al., "Exploratory Study of Coenzyme Q10 in Obesity," in *Biomedical and Clinical Aspects of Coenzyme Q, Vol. 4.* K. Folkers and Y. Yamamura (eds.) (Amsterdam: Elsevier Science Publ, 1984), pp369-73.

Osteoarthritis

1. R. Petersdorf et al., eds., *Harrison's Principles of Internal Medicine* (New York: McGraw-Hill, 1983), 517–24.

2. J.H. Bland and S.M. Cooper, "Osteoarthritis: A Review of the Cell Biology Involved and Evidence for Reversibility: Management Rationally Related to Known Genesis and Pathophysiology," *Sem Arthr Rheum* 14 (1984): 106–33.

3. M.N. Summers et al., "Radiographic Assessment and Psychologic Variables As Predictors of Pain and Functional Impairment in Osteoarthritis of the Knee or Hip," *Arthritis Rheum* 31 (1988): 204–9.

4. G.H. Perry, M.J.G. Smith, and C.G. Whiteside, "Spontaneous Recovery of the Hip Joint Space in Degenerative Hip Disease," *Ann Rheum Dis* 31 (1972): 440–8.

5. M.J. Shield, "Anti-Inflammatory Drugs and Their Effects on Cartilage Synthesis and Renal Function," *Eur J Rheumatol Inflam* 13 (1993): 7–16.

6. P.M. Brooks, S.R. Potter, and W.W. Buchanan, "NSAID and Osteoarthritis—Help or Hindrance," *J Rheumatol* 9 (1982): 3–5.

7. N.M. Newman and R.S.M. Ling, "Acetabular Bone Destruction Related to Non-Steroidal Anti-Inflammatory Drugs," *Lancet* 2 (1985): 11–13.

8. L. Solomon, "Drug Induced Arthropathy and Necrosis of the Femoral Head," *J Bone Joint Surg* 55B (1973): 246–51.

9. H. Ronningen and N. Langeland, "Indomethacin Treatment in Osteoarthritis of the Hip Joint," *Acta Orthop Scand* 50 (1979): 169–74.

10. J. Dequeker, A. Burssens, and R. Bouillon, "Dynamics of Growth Hormone Secretion in Patients with Osteoporosis and in Patients with Osteoarthrosis," *Hormone Res* 16 (1982): 353–6.

11. A.J. Hartz, M.E. Fischer, G. Bril et al., "The Association of Obesity with Joint Pain and Osteoarthritis in the Hanes Data," *J Chron Dis* 39 (1986): 311–9.

12. D.T. Felson et al., "Weight Loss Reduces the Risk for Symptomatic Knee Osteoarthritis in Women," *Ann Intern Med* 116 (1992): 535–9.

13. N.F. Childers and G.M. Russo, *The Nightshades and Health* (Somer-

ville, NJ: Horticulture Publications, 1973).

14. T.E. McAlindon et al., "Do Antioxidant Micronutrients Protect against the Development and Progression of Knee Osteoarthritis?" *Arthritis Rheumatism* 39 (1996): 648–56.

15. K. Karzel and R. Domenjoz, "Effect of Hexosamine Derivatives and Uronic Acid Derivatives on Glycosaminoglycan Metabolism of Fibroblast Cultures," *Pharmacology* 5 (1971): 337–45.

16 R.R. Vidal y Plana et al., "Articular Cartilage Pharmacology: I. In Vitro Studies on Glucosamine and Non-Steroidal Antininflammatory Drugs," *Pharmacol Res Comm* 10 (1978): 557–69.

17. W. Noack et al., "Glucosamine Sulfate in Osteoarthritis of the Knee," *Osteoarthritis Cartilage* 2 (1994): 51–9.

18. G. Crolle and E. D'este, "Glucosamine Sulfate for the Management of Arthrosis: A Controlled Clinical Investigation," *Curr Med Res Opin* 7 (1980): 104–9.

19. J.M. Pujalte et al., "Double-Blind Clinical Evaluation of Oral Glucosamine Sulphate in the Basic Treatment of Osteoarthrosis," *Curr Med Res Opin* 7 (1980): 110–4.

20. A. Drovanti et al., "Therapeutic Activity of Oral Glucosamine Sulfate in Osteoarthrosis: A Placebo-Controlled Double-Blind Investigation," *Clin Ther* 3 (1980): 260–72.

21. Y. Vajaradul, "Double-Blind Clinical Evaluation of Intra-Articular Glucosamine in Outpatients with Gonarthrosis," *Clin Ther* 3 (1981): 336–43.

22. E.D. D'Ambrosia et al., "Glucosamine Sulphate: A Controlled Clinical Investigation in Arthrosis," *Pharmatherapeutica* 2 (1982): 504–8.

23. A.L. Vaz, "Double-Blind Clinical Evaluation of the Relative Efficacy of Ibuprofen and Glucosamine Sulfate in the Management of Osteoarthrosis of the Knee in Out-Patients," *Curr Med Res Opin* 8 (1982): 145–9.

24. H. Muller-Fassbender et al., "Glucosamine Sulfate Compared to Ibuprofen in Osteoarthritis of the Knee," *Osteoarthritis Cartilage* 2 (1994): 61–9.

25. L.C. Rovati et al., "A Large, Randomized, Placebo Controlled, Double-Blind Study of Glucosamine Sulfate vs Piroxicam and vs Their Association, on the Kinetics of the Symptomatic Effect in Knee Osteoarthritis," *Osteoarthritis Cartilage* 2(Suppl.1) (1994): 56.

26. M.J. Tapadinhas et al., "Oral Glucosamine Sulfate in the Management of Arthrosis: Report on a Multi-Centre Open Investigation in Portugal," *Pharmatherapeutica* 3 (1982): 157–68.

27. I. Setnikar et al., "Pharmacokinetics of Glucosamine in Man," *Arzneim Forsch* 43(10) (1993): 1109–13.

28. A. Baici et al., "Analysis of Glycosaminoglycans in Human Sera after Oral Administration of Chondroitin Sulfate," *Rheumatol Int* 12 (1992): 81–8.

29. A. Conte et al., "Biochemical and Pharmacokinetic Aspects of Oral Treatment with Chondroitin Sulfate," *Arzneim Forsch* 45 (1995): 918–25.

30. M. Shinmei et al., "Significance of the Levels of Carboxy Terminal Type II Procollagen Peptide, Chondroitin Sulfate Isomers, Tissue Inhibitor of Metalloproteinases, and Metalloproteinases in Osteoarthritis Joint Fluid," *J Rheumatol* 43(Suppl.) (1995): 78–81.

31. A. Baici and F.J. Wagenhauser, "Bioavailability of Oral Chondroitin Sulfate," *Rheumatology Int* 13 (1993): 41–43.

32. V.R. Pipitone, "Chondroprotection with Chondroitin Sulfate," *Drugs Exptl Clin Res* 18 (1991): 3–7.

33. J.L. L'Hirondel, "Double-Blind Clinical Study with Oral Administration of Chondroitin Sulfate versus Placebo in Tibiofemoral Gonarthrosis," *Litera Rheumatologica* 14 (1992): 77–82.

34. T. Conrozier and E. Vignon, "The Effect of Chondroitin Sulfate Treatment in Coxarthritis: A Double-Blind Placebo Study," *Litera Rheumatologica* 14 (1992): 69–75.

35. P. Morreale et al., "Comparison of the Antiinflammatory Efficacy of Chondroitin Sulfate and Diclofenac Sodium in Patients with Knee Osteoarthritis," *J Rheumatol* 23 (1996): 1385–91.

36. W. Kaufman, *The Common Form of Joint Dysfunction: Its Incidence and Treatment* (Brattleboro, VT: EL Hildreth Co., 1949).

37. A. Hoffer, "Treatment of Arthritis by Nicotinic Acid and Nicotinamide," *Can Med Assoc J* 81 (1959): 235–9.

38. W.B. Jonas, C.P. Rapoza, and W.F. Blair, "The Effect of Niacinamide on Osteoarthritis: A Pilot Study," *Inflamm Res* 45 (1996): 330–4.

39. M.F. Harmand et al., "Effects of S-Adenosylmethionine on Human Articular Chondrocyte Differentiation: An In Vitro Study," *Am J Med* 83(Suppl.5A) (1987): 48–54.

40. H. Konig et al., "Magnetic Resonance Tomography of Finger Polyarthritis: Morphology and Cartilage Signals after Ademetionine Therapy," *Aktuelle Radiol* 5 (19950: 36–40.

41. H. Muller-Fassbender, "Double-Blind Clinical Trial of S-Adenosylmethionine versus Ibuprofen in the Treatment of Osteoarthritis," *Am J Med* 83(Suppl.5A) (1987): 81–3.

42. S. Glorioso et al., "Double-Blind Multicentre Study of the Activity of S-adenosylmethionine in Hip and Knee Osteoarthritis," *Int J Clin Pharmacol Res* 5 (1985): 39–49.

43. R. Marcolongo et al., "Double-Blind Multicentre Study of the Activity of S-Adenosyl-Methionine in Hip and Knee Osteoarthritis," *Curr Ther Res* 37 (1985): 82–94.

44. Z. Domljan et al., "A Double-Blind Trial of Ademetionine vs Naproxen in Activated Gonarthrosis," *Int J Clin Pharmacol Ther Toxicol* 27 (1989): 329–33.

45. I. Caruso and V. Pietrogrande, "Italian Double-Blind Multicenter Study Comparing S-Adenosylmethionine, Naproxen, and Placebo in the Treatment of Degenerative Joint Disease," *Am J Med* 83(Suppl.5A) (1987): 66–71.

46. G. Vetter, "Double-Blind Comparative Clinical Trial with S-Adenosylmethionine and Indomethacin in the Treatment of Osteoarthritis," *Am J Med* 83(Suppl.5A) (1987): 78–80.

47. A. Maccagno, "Double-Blind Controlled Clinical Trial of Oral S-Adenosylmethionine versus Piroxicam in Knee Osteoarthritis,"

Am J Med 83(Suppl.5A) (1987): 72–7.

48. B. Konig, "A Long-Term (Two Years) Clinical Trial with S-Adeno-sylmethionine for the Treatment of Osteoarthritis," *Am J Med* 83 (Suppl.5A) (1987): 89–94.

49. R. Berger and H. Nowak, "A New Medical Approach to the Treatment of Osteoarthritis: Report of an Open Phase IV Study with Ademetionine (Gumbaral)," *Am J Med* 83 (Suppl.5A) (1987): 84–8.

50. K. Lund-Olesen and K.B. Menander, "Orgotein: A New Anti-Inflammatory Metalloprotein Drug: Preliminary Evaluation of Clinical Efficacy and Safety in Degenerative Joint Disease," *Curr Ther Res* 16 (1974): 706–17.

51. E.C. Huskisson and J. Scott, "Orgotein in Osteoarthritis of the Knee Joint," *Eur J Rheumatol Inflam* 4 (1981): 212.

52. S. Zidenberg-Cherr, C.L. Keen, B. Lonnerdal, and L.S. Hurley, "Dietary Superoxide Dismutase Does Not Affect Tissue Levels," *Am J Clin Nutr* 37 (1983): 5–7.

53. I. Machtey and L. Ouaknine, "Tocopherol in Osteoarthritis: A Controlled Pilot Study," *J Am Ger Soc* 26 (1978): 328–30.

54. E.R. Schwartz, "The Modulation of Osteoarthritic Development by Vitamins C and E," *Int J Vit Nutr Res Suppl* 26 (1984): 141–6.

55. C.J. Bates, "Proline and Hydroxyproline Excretion and Vitamin C Status in Elderly Human Subjects," *Clin Sci Mol Med* 52 (1977): 535–43.

56. A.P. Prins, J.M. Lipman, C.A. McDevitt, and L. Sokoloff, "Effect of Purified Growth Factors on Rabbit Articular Chondrocytes in Monolayer Culture," *Arthr Rheum* 25 (1982): 1228–32.

57. G. Krystal, G.M. Morris, and L. Sokoloff, "Stimulation of DNA Synthesis by Ascorbate in Cultures of Articular Chondrocytes," *Arth Rheum* 25 (1982): 318–25.

58. J.C. Anand, "Osteoarthritis and Pantothenic Acid," *J Coll Gen Pract* 5 (1963): 136–7.

59. J.C. Anand, "Osteoarthritis and Pantothenic Acid," *Lancet* 2 (1963): 1168.

60. A report from the General Practitioner Research Group, "Calcium Pantothenate in Arthritis Conditions," *Pract* 224 (1980): 208–11.

61. R.L. Travers, G.C. Rennie, and R.E. Newnham, "Boron and Arthritis: The Results of a Double-Blind Pilot Study," *J Nutr Med* 1 (1990): 127–32.

62. R.E. Newnham, "Arthritis or Skeletal Fluorosis and Boron," *Int Clin Nutr Rev* 11 (1991): 68–70.

63. V. Wright, "Treatment of Osteo-Arthritis of the Knees," *Ann Rheum Dis* 23 (1964): 389–91.

64. G.R. Clarke, L.A. Willis, L. Stenner, and P.J.R. Nichols, "Evaluation of Physiotherapy in the Treatment of Osteoarthrosis of the Knee," *Rheum Rehab* 13 (1974): 190–7.

65. H. Vanharantha, "Effect of Short-Wave Diathermy on Mobility and Radiological Stage of the Knee in the Development of Experimental Osteoarthritis," *Am J Phys Med* 61 (1982): 59–65.

66. Falconer J., Hayes K.W. and Chang R.W.: "Effect of Ultrasound on Mobility in Osteoarthritis of the Knee, a Randomized Clinical Trial." *Arthritis Care Res* 5 (1992): 29–35.

67. J. Stehlian et al., "Improvement of Pain in Elderly Patients with Degenerative Osteoarthritis of the Knee Treated with Narrow-Band Light Therapy," *J Am Geriat Soc* 40 (1992): 23–6.

68. N.M. Fisher, D.R. Pendergast, and G.E. Gresham, "Muscle Rehabilitation: Its Effects on Muscular and Functional Performance of Patients with Knee Osteoarthritis," *Arch Phys Med Rehabil* 72 (1991): 367–74.

69. P.A. Kovar et al., "Supervised Fitness Walking in Patients with Osteoarthritis of the Knee: A Randomized Controlled Trial," *Ann Intern Med* 116 (1992): 529–34.

70. R. Bingham, B.A. Bellew, and J.G. Bellew, "Yucca Plant Saponin in the Management of Arthritis," *J Appl Nutr* 27 (1975): 45–50.

71. T.I. Morales, L.M. Wahl, and V.C. Hascall, "The Effect of Lipopolysaccharides on the Biosynthesis and Release of Proteoglycans from Calf

Articular Cartilage Cultures," *J Biol Chem* 259 (1984): 6720–9.

72. L.R. Brady, V.E. Tyler, and J.E. Robbers, *Pharmacognosy*, 8th ed., (Philadelphia: Lea & Febiger, 1981), 480.

73. L.W. Whitehouse, M. Znamirowski, and C.J. Paul, "Devil's Claw (*Harpagophytum procumbens*): No Evidence for Anti-Inflammatory Activity in the Treatment of Arthritic Disease," *Can Med Assoc J* 129 (1983): 249–51.

74. D.W. McLeod, P. Revell, and B.V. Robinson, "Investigations of *Harpagophytum procumbens* (Devil's Claw) in the Treatment of Experimental Inflammation and Arthritis in the Rat," *Br J Pharm* 66 (1979): 140P–141P.

75. G.B. Singh and C.K. Atal, "Pharmacology of an Extract of Salai Guggal Ex-*Bosewellia serrata*, a New Non-Steroidal Anti-Inflammatory Agent," *Agents Action* 18 (1986): 407–12.

76. C.K. Reddy, G. Chandrakasan, and S.C. Dhar, "Studies on the Metabolism of Glycosaminoglycans under the Influence of New Herbal Anti-Inflammatory Agents," *Biochemical Pharmacol* 20 (1989): 3527–34.

77. R.R. Kulkani, P.S. Patki, V.P. Jog et al., "Treatment of Osteoarthritis with a Herbomineral Formulation: A Double-Blind, Placebo-Controlled, Cross-Over Study," *J Ethnopharmacol* 33 (1991): 91–5.

78. G.M. McCarthy and D.J. McCarty, "Effect of Topical Capsaicin in the Therapy of Painful Osteoarthritis of the Hands," *J Rheumatol* 19 (1992): 604–7.

Osteoporosis

1. D.W. Dempster and R. Lindsay, "Pathogenesis of Osteoporosis," *Lancet* 341 (1993): 797–805.

2. R. Lindsay, "The Burden of Osteoporosis: Cost," *Am J Med* 98 (Suppl.2A) (1995): 9S–11S.

3. M. Grossman, J. Kirsner, and I. Gillespie, "Basal and Histalog-Stimulated Gastric Secretion in Control Subjects and in Patients with Peptic Ulcer or Gastric Cancer," *Gastroenterology* 45 (1963): 15–26.

4. R. Recker, "Calcium Absorption and Achlorhydria," *New England Journal of Medicine* 313 (1985): 70–73.

5. M.J. Nicar and C.Y.C. Pak, "Calcium Bioavailability from Calcium Carbonate and Calcium Citrate," *J Clin Endocrinol Metabol* 61 (1985): 391–93.

6. F. Lore, R. Nuti, A. Vattimo, and Caniggia, "Vitamin D Metabolites in Postmenopausal Osteoporosis," *Horm Metabol Res* 16 (1984): 58.

7. N. Brautbar, "Osteoporosis: Is 1,25-(OH)2D3 of Value in Treatment?" *Nephron* 44 (1986): 161–66.

8. J. Kanis, "Bone Density Measurements and Osteoporosis," *J Int Med* 241 (1997): 173–75.

9. C.H. Chestnut et al., "Hormone Replacement Therapy in Postmenopausal Women: Urinary N-Telopeptide of Type I Collagen Monitors Therapeutic Effect and Predicts Response of Bone Mineral Density," *Am J Med* 102 (1997): 29–37.

10. J.F. Aloia, S.H. Cohn, A. Vaswani, et al., "Risk Factors for Postmenopausal Osteoporosis," *Am J Med* 78 (1985): 95–100.

11. S.B. Jaglar, N. Kreiger, and G. Darlington, "Past and Recent Physical Activity and the Risk of Osteoporosis," *Am J Epidemiol* 138 (1993): 107–118.

12. J.C. Opriot et al., "Physical Activity As Therapy for Osteoporosis," *Can Med Assoc J* 155 (1996): 940–44.

13. R. Marcus et al., "Osteoporosis and Exercise in Women," *Med Sci Sports Exer* 24 (1992): S301–307.

14. N.A. Pocock et al., "Physical Fitness Is the Major Determinant of Femoral Neck and Lumbar Spine Density," *J Clin Invest* 78 (1986): 618–21.

15. B. Krolner, B. Toft, S. Nielsen,and E. Tondevold, "Physical Exercise As Prophylaxis against Involutional Vertebral Bone Loss: A Controlled Trial," *Clin Sci* 64 (1983): 541–46.

16. R. Yeater and R. Martin, "Senile Osteoporosis: The Effects of Exercise," *Postg Med* 75 (1984): 147–49.

17. C. Donaldson, S. Hulley, J. Vogel, et al., "Effect of Prolonged Bed Rest on Bone Mineral," *Metabolism* 19 (1970): 1071–84.

18. J. Eaton-Evans, "Osteoporosis and the Role of Diet," *Br J Biomedical Sci* 51 (1994): 358–70.

19. P.D. Saltman and L.G. Strause, "The Role of Trace Minerals in Osteoporosis," *J Am Coll Nutr* 4 (1993): 384–89.

20. F. Ellis, S. Holesh, and J. Ellis, "Incidence of Osteoporosis in Vegetarians and Omnivores," *Am J Clin Nutr* 25 (1972): 55–58.

21. A. Marsh et al., "Bone Mineral Mass in Adult Lactovegetarian and Omnivorous Adults," *Am J Clin Nutr* 37 (1983): 453–56.

22. A. Licata, E. Bou, F. Bartter, and F, West, "Acute Effects of Dietary Protein on Calcium Metabolism in Patients with Osteoporosis," *J Geron* 36 (1981): 14–19.

23. C. Cooper, "Dietary Protein Intake and Bone Mass in Women," *Calcif Tissue Int* 58 (1996): 320–25.

24. J. Thom, J. Morris, A. Bishop, and Blacklock, "The Influence of Refined Carbohydrate on Urinary Calcium Excretion," *Br J Urol* 50 (1978): 459–64.

25. E. Mazariegos-Ramos et al., "Consumption of Soft Drinks with Phosphoric Acid As a Risk Factor for the Development of Hypocalcemia in Children: A Case-Control Study," *J Pediatr* 126 (1995): 940–42.

26. G. Wyshak and R.E. Frisch, "Carbonated Beverages, Dietary Calcium, the Dietary Calcium/Phosphorus Ratio, and Bone Fractures in Girls and Boys," *J Adolesc Health* 15 (1994): 210–15.

27. C. Vermeer et al., "Effects of Vitamin K on Bone Mass and Bone Metabolism," *J Nutr* 126 (1996): 1187S–91S.

28. L. Bitensky, J.P. Hart, A. Catterall, et al., "Circulating Vitamin K Levels in Patients with Fractures," *J Bone Joint Surg* 70-B (1988): 663–64.

29. T. Kanai et al., "Serum Vitamin K Level and Bone Mineral Density in Post-Menopausal Women," *Int J Gynecol Obstet* 56 (1997): 25–30.

30. F.H. Neilsen, C.D. Hunt, L.M. Mullen, and J.R. Hunt, "Effect of Dietary Boron on Mineral, Estrogen, and Testosterone Metabolism in Postmenopausal Women," *FASEB J* 1 (1987): 394–97.

31. G. Block, "Dietary Guidelines and the Results of Food Consumption Surveys," *Am J Clin Nutr* 53 (1991): 356S–57S.

32. F.H. Nielsen, S.K. Gallagher, L.K. Johnson, and E.J. Nielsen, "Boron Enhances and Mimics Some of the Effects of Estrogen Therapy in Postmenopausal Women," *J Trace Elem Exp Med* 5 (1992): 237–46.

33. I.R. Reid et al., "Long-Term Effects of Calcium Supplementation on Bone Loss and Fractures in Postmenopausal Women: A Randomized Controlled Trial," *Am J Med* 98 (1995): 331–35.

34. I.R. Reid, "Therapy of Osteoporosis: Calcium, Vitamin D, and Exercise," *Am J Med Sci* 312 (1996): 278–86.

35. A. Devine et al., "A 4-Year Follow-Up Study of the Effects of Calcium Supplementation on Bone Density in Elderly Postmenopausal Women," *Osteoporos Int* 7 (1997): 23–28.

36. R.P. Heaney, "Calcium in the Prevention and Treatment of Osteoporosis," *J Int Med* 231 (1992): 169–80.

37. C.J. Lee, G.S. Lawler, and G.H. Johnson, "Effects of Supplementation of the Diets with Calcium and Calcium-Rich Foods on Bone Density of Elderly Females with Osteoporosis," *Am J Clin Nutr* 34 (1981): 819–23.

38. J.F. Aloia et al., "Calcium Supplementation with and without Hormone Replacement Therapy to Prevent Postmenopausal Bone Loss," *Annals Intern Med* 120 (1994): 97–103.

39. I.R. Reid et al., "Long-Term Effects of Calcium Supplementation on Bone Loss and Fractures in Postmenopausal Women: A Randomized Controlled Trial," *Am J Med* 98 (1995): 331–35.

40. P.J.M. Elders et al., "Long-Term Effect of Calcium Supplementation on Bone Loss in Perimenopausal Women," *J Bone Min Res* 9 (1994): 963–70.

41. B.P. Bourgoin, D.R. Evans, J.R. Cornett, et al., "Lead Content in 70 Brands of Dietary Calcium Supplements," *Am J Public Health* 83 (1993): 1155–60.

42. C.J. Carr and R.F. Shangraw, "Nutritional and Pharmaceutical Aspects of Calcium Supplementation," *Am Pharm* 27 (1987): 49–57.

43. B. Dawson-Hughes et al., "Rates of Bone Loss in Postmenopausal Women Randomly Assigned to One of Two Dosages of the Vitamin D," *Am J Clin Nutr* 61 (1995): 1140–45.

44. M.E. Ooms et al., "Prevention of Bone Loss by Vitamin D Supplementation in Elderly Women: A Randomized Double-Blind Study," *J Clin Endocrinol Metabol* 80 (1995): 1052–58.

45. M.C. Chapuy et al., "Effect of Calcium and Cholecalciferol Treatment for Three Years on Hip Fractures in Elderly Women," *BMJ* 308 (1994): 1081–82.

46. B. Dawson-Hughes et al., "Effect of Calcium and Vitamin D Supplementation on Bone Density in Men and Women 65 Years of Age or Older," *N Engl J Med* 337 (1997): 701–2.

47. L. Cohen and R. Kitzes, "Infrared Spectroscopy and Magnesium Content of Bone Mineral in Osteoporotic Women," *Isr J Med Sci* 17 (1981): 1123–25.

48. G. Stendig-Lindberg, R. Tepper, and I. Leichter, "Trabecular Bone Density in a Two-Year Controlled Trial of Peroral Magnesium in Osteoporosis," *Magnesium Res* 6 (1993): 155–63.

49. R.K. Rude, J.S. Adams, E. Ryzen et al., "Low Serum Concentration of 1,25-Dihydroxyvitamin D in Human Magnesium Deficiency," *J Clin Endo Metabol* 61 (1985): 933–40.

50. G. Stendig-Lindberg, R. Tepper, and I. Leichter, "Trabecular Bone Density in a Two-Year Controlled Trial of Peroral Magnesium in Osteoporosis," *Magnesium Res* 6 (1993): 155–63.

51. L.E. Brattstrom, B.L. Hultberg, and J.E. Hardebo, "Folic Acid Responsive Postmenopausal Homocysteinemia," *Metabolism* 34 (1985): 1073–77.

52. J.B. Ubbink, W.J. van der Merwe, and R. Delport, "Hyperhomocysteinemia and the Response to Vitamin Supplementation," *Clin Invest* 71 (1993): 993–98.

53. R.J. Fessenden and J.S. Fessenden, "The Biological Properties of Silicon Compounds," *Adv Drug Res* 4 (1987): 95.

54. B. Riggs, E. Seeman, S. Hodgson, et al., "Effect of the Fluoride/Calcium Regimen on Vertebral Fracture Occurrence in Postmenopausal Osteoporosis," *New Engl J Med* 306 (1982): 446–50.

55. T.M. Murray and L.G. Ste-Marie, "Flouride Therapy for Osteoporosis," *Can Med Assoc J* 155 (1996): 949–54.

56. M.L. Brandi, "New Treatment Strategies: Ipriflavone, Strontium, Vitamin D Metabolites and Analogs," *Am J Med* 95 (Suppl.5A) (1993): 69S–74S.

57. M. Moscarinie et al., "New Perspectives in the Treatment of Postmenopausal Osteoporosis—Ipriflavone," *Gynecol Endocrinol* 8 (1994): 203–7.

58. M. Passeri et al., "Effect of Ipriflavone on Bone Mass in Elderly Osteoporotic Women," *Bone Miner* 19(Suppl.1) (1992): S57-62.

59. D. Agnusdei et al., "A Double Blind, Placebo-Controlled Trial of Ipriflavone for Prevention of Postmenopausal Spinal Bone Loss," *Calcif Tissue Int* 61 (1997): 142–47.

60. S. Adami et al., "Ipriflavone Prevents Radial Bone Loss in Postmenopausal Women with Low Bone Mass over 2 Years," *Osteoporos Int* 7 (1997): 119–25.

61. G.B. Melis et al., "Lack of Any Estrogenic Effect of Ipriflavone in Postmenopausal Women," *J Endocrinol Invest* 15 (1992): 755–61.

62. U.A. Liberman et al., "Effect of Oral Endronate on Bone Mineral Density and the Incidence of Fractures in Postmenopausal Osteoporosis," *New Engl J Med* 333 (1995): 1437–43.

63. J.Y. Reginster, "Calcitonin for Prevention and Treatment of Osteoporosis," *Am J Med* 95(Suppl.5A) (1993): 44S–47.

Periodontal Disease

1. F. Carranza. *Glickman's Clinical Periodontology* (Philadelphia: WB Saunders, 1984).

2. S. Robbins and R. Cotran. *Pathologic Basis of Disease* (Philadelphia: WB Saunders, 1979), pp. 893–5.

3. R. Page and H. Schroeder. "Current Status of the Host Response in Chronic Marginal Periodontitis," *J Periodontal* 52 (1981): 477–91.

4. K. James. "Complement: Activation, Consequences, and Control," *Am J Med Tech* 48 (1982): 735–43.

5. T. Hyyppa. "Gingival IgE and Histamine Concentrations in Patients with Periodontitis," *J Clin Periodontal* 11 (1984): 132–7.

6. S. Addya, Chakravarti, A. Basu, et al. "Effects of Mercuric Chloride on Several Scavenging Enzymes in Rat Kidney and Influence of Vitamin E Supplementation," *Acta Vitaminol Enzymol* 6 (1984): 103–7.

7. P. Bartold, O. Wiebkin, and J. Thonard. "The Effect of Oxygen-Derived Free Radicals on Gingival Proteoglycans and Hyaluronic Acid," *J Periodontal Res* 19 (1984): 390–400.

8. H.A. Schenkein, et al. "Smoking and Its Effects on Early-Onset Periodontitis," *J Am Dental Assoc* 126 (1995): 1107–13.

9. W.B. Kaldahl, et al. "Levels of Cigarette Consumption and Response to Periodontal Therapy," *J Periodont* 67 (1996): 675–81.

10. O. Pelletier. "Smoking and Vitamin C Levels in Humans," *Am J Clin Nutr* 21 (1968): 1259–67.

11. I. Prerovsky and J. Hladovec. "Suppression of the Desquamating Effect of Smoking on the Human Endothelium by Hydroxyethylrutosides," *Blood Vessels* 16 (1979): 239–40.

12. G. Burton and K. Ingold. "Beta-Carotene: An Unusual Type of Lipid Antioxidant," *Science* 224 (1984): 569–73.

13. L. Junqueira and J. Carneiro. "Basic Histology," *Lange Med Publ*, Los Altos, Ca (1980): 312.

14. P. Bartold, O. Wiebkin, and J. Thonard. "The Active Role of Gingival Proteoglycans in Periodontal Disease," *Med Hypothesis* 12 (1983): 377–87.

15. P. Bartold, O. Wiebkin, and J. Thonard. "Proteoglycans of Human Gingival Epithelium and Connective Tissue," *Biochem J* 11 (1983): 119–27.

16. P. Bartold, O. Wiebkin, and J. Thonard. "Glycosaminoglycans of Human Gingival Epithelium and Connective Tissue," *Connective Tissue Research* 9 (1981): 99–106.

17. F. Abbas, U. van der Velden, and A. Hart. "Relation Between Wound

Healing After Surgery and Susceptibility to Periodontal Disease," *J Clin Periodontal* 11 (1984): 221–9.

18. O. Alvares. "Nutrition, Diet and Oral Health," Chapter 14 in *Contemporary Developments in Nutrition*. ed. B. Worthington-Roberts (St. Louis: Mosby, 1981).

19. O. Alvares, L. Altman, S. Springmeyer, et al. "The Effect of Subclinical Ascorbate Deficiency on Periodontal Disease in Nonhuman Primates," *J Periodontal Res* 16 (1984): 628–36.

20. S. Woolfe, W. Hume, and E. Kenney. "Ascorbic Acid and Periodontal Disease: A Review of the Literature," *J Western Soc Periodontal* 28 (1980): 44–60.

21. M. Alfano, S. Miller, and J. Drummond. "Effect of Ascorbic Acid Deficiency on the Permeability and Collagen Biosynthesis of Oral Mucosal Epithelium," *Ann NY Acad Sci* 258 (1975): 253–63.

22. O. Alvares and I. Siegel. "Permeability of Gingival Sulcular Epithelium in the Development of Scorbutic Gingivitis," *J Oral Path* 10 (1981): 40–8.

23. C. Stephens and R. Snyderman. "Cyclic Nucleotides Regulate the Morphologic Alterations Required for Chemotaxis in Monocytes," *J Immunol* 128 (1982): 1192–7.

24. G. Mann and P. Newton. "The Membrane Transport of Ascorbic Acid," *Ann NY Acad Sci* 258 (1975): 243–51.

25. W. Ringsdorf, E. Cheraskin, and R. Ramsay. "Sucrose, Neutrophil Phagocytosis and Resistance to Disease," *Dent Surv* 52 (1976): 46–8.

26. A. Sanchez, J. Reeser, H. Lau, et al. "Role of Sugars in Human Neutrophilic Phagocytosis," *Am J Clin Nutr* 26:1180–4, 1973

27. M. Krause and L. Mahan. *Food, Nutrition and Diet Therapy* (Philadelphia: WB Saunders, 1984).

28. A. Prasad. "Clinical, Biochemical and Nutritional Spectrum of Zinc Deficiency in Human Subjects: An Update," *Nutr Rev* 41 (1983): 197–208.

29. J. Freeland, R. Cousins, and R. Schwartz. "Relationship of Mineral Status and Intake to Periodontal Disease," *Am J Clin Nutr* 29 (1976): 745–9.

30. J. Nordstrom. "Trace Mineral Nutrition in the Elderly," *Am J Clin Nutr* 36 (1982): 788–95.

31. G. Harrap, C. Saxton, and J. Best. "Inhibition of Plaque Growth by Zinc Salts," *J Periodontal Res* 18 (1983): 634–42.

32. S. Hsieh, A. Hayali, and J. Navia. "Zinc," in *Trace Elements in Dental Disease*, eds. M. Curzon and T. Cutress (Boston: John Wright PSG Inc, 1983), chapter 9 pp 99–220.

33. S. Hazan and E. Cowan. *Diet, Nutrition and Periodontal Disease* (Chicago: Am Soc Prev Dent, 1975)

34. J. Kim and G. Shklar. "The Effect of Vitamin E on the Healing of Gingival Wounds in Rats," *J Periodontal* 54 (1983): 305–8.

35. K. Folkers and Y. Yamamura. *Biomedical and Clinical Aspects of Coenzyme Q, vol 1* (Amsterdam: Elsevier/North Holland Biomedical Press, 1977), 294–311.

36. K. Folkers and Y. Yamamura. *Biomedical and Clinical Aspects of Coenzyme Q, vol 3* (Amsterdam: Elsevier/North Holland Biomedical Press, 1981), 109–125.

37. J. Monboisse, P. Braquet, and J. Borel. "Oxygen-Free Radicals as Mediators of Collagen Breakage," *Agents Actions* 15 (1984): 49–50.

38. C. Rao, V. Rao, and B. Steinman. "Influence of Bioflavonoids on the Metabolism and Cross Linking of Collagen," *Ital J Biochem* 30 (1981): 259–70.

39. M. L. Ferrandiz and M. J. Alcaraz. "Anti-inflammatory Activity and Inhibition of Arachidonic Acid Metabolism by Flavonoids," *Agents Action* (1991) 32:283–7.

40. M. Ronziere, D. Herbage, R. Garrone, and Frey. "Influence of Some Flavonoids on Reticulation of Collagen Fibrils In Vitro," *Biochem Pharm* 30 (1981): 1771–6.

41. C. Jones, C. Cummings, J. Ball, and P. Beighton. "A Clinical and Ultrastructural Study of Osteogenesis Imperfecta after Flavonoid (Catergen) Therapy," *S Afr Med J* 66 (1984): 907–10.

42. F. Pearce, A. Befus, and J. Bienenstock. "Effect of Quercetin and Other Flavonoids on Antigen-Induced Histamine Secretion from Rat Intestinal Mast Cells," *J*

Allerg Clin Immunol 73 (1984): 819–23.

43. W. Busse, D. Kopp, and E. Middleston. "Flavonoid Modulation of Human Neutrophil Function," *J Allerg Clin Immunol* 73 (1984): 801–9.

44. M. Gineste, et al. "Influence of 3-Methoxy 5,7,3'4'-Tetrahydroxyflavan (ME) on Experimental Periodontitis in the Golden Hamster," *J Biol Buccale* 12 (1984): 259–65.

45. R. Vogel, R. Fink, L. Schneider, et al. "The Effect of Folic Acid on Gingival Health," *J Periodontal* 47 (1976): 667–8.

46. R. Vogel, R. Fink, L. Schneider, et al. "The Effect of Topical Application of Folic Acid on Gingival Health," *J Oral Med* 33 (1978): 20–2.

47. A. Pack and M. Thomson. "Effects of Topical and Systemic Folic Acid Supplementation on Gingivitis in Pregnancy," *J Clin Periodontal* 7 (1980): 402–4.

48. A. Pack and M. Thomson. "Effects of Extended Systemic and Topical Folate Supplementation on Gingivitis of Pregnancy," *J Clin Periodontal* 9 (1982): 275–80.

49. A. Pack. "Folate Mouthwash: Effects on Established Gingivitis in Periodontal Patients," *J Clin Periodontal* 11 (1984): 619–28.

50. M. da Costa and S. Rothenberg. "Appearance of Folate Binder in Leukocytes and Serum of Women Who Are Pregnant or Taking Oral Contraceptives," *J Lab Clin Med* 83 (1974): 207–14.

51. K.C. Godowski. "Antimicrobial Action of Sanguinarine," *J Clin Dent* 1 (1989): 96–101.

52. E. Grossman, et al. "A Clinical Comparison of Antibacterial Mouthrinses: Effects of Chlorhexidine, Phenolics, and Sanguinarine on Dental Plaque and Gingivitis," *J Periodontol* 60 (1989): 435–40.

53. A. Benedicenti, D. Galli and A. Merlini. "The Clinical Therapy of Periodontal Disease: The Use of Potassium Hydroxide and the Water-Alcohol Extract of Centella Asiatica in Combination with Laser Therapy in the Treatment of Severe Periodontal Disease," *Parodontol Stomatol* 24 (1985): 11–26.

Premenstrual Syndrome

1. K.T. Barnhart, E.W. Freeman, and S.J. Sondheimer. "A Clinician's Guide to the Premenstrual Syndrome," *Med Clin North Am* 79 (1995): 1457–72.

2. M. Steiner. "Premenstrual Dysphoric Disorder. An Update," *Gen Hosp Psychiatry* 18 (1996): 244–50.

3. J.T. Richardson. "The Premenstrual Syndrome: A Brief History," *Soc Sci Med* 41 (1995): 761–7.

4. J.F. Mortola. "A Risk-Benefit Appraisal of Drugs Used in the Management of Premenstrual Syndrome," *Drug Safety* 10 (1994): 160–9.

5. S. Nader. "Premenstrual Syndrome," *Postgraduate Med* 90 (1991): 173–80.

6. S. Smith. "The Premenstrual Syndrome—Diagnosis and Management," *Fertility Sterility* 53 (1989): 527–43.

7. D. Propping, T. Katzorke, and L. Belkien. Diagnosis and Therapy of Corpus Luteum Insufficiency in General Practice," *Therapiwoche* 38 (1988): 2992–3001.

8. S. Smith. "The Premenstrual Syndrome—Diagnosis and Management," *Fertility Sterility* 53 (1989): 527–43.

9. G.E. Abraham. "Nutritional Factors in the Etiology of the Premenstrual Tension Syndromes," *J Reprod Med* 28 (1983): 446–64.

10. M. Wang, et al. "Relationship between Symptom Severity and Steroid Variation in Women with Premenstrual Syndrome: Study on Serum Pregnenolone, Pregnenolone Sulfate, 5 Alpha-Pregnane-3,20-Dione and 3 Alpha-Hydroxy-5 Alpha-Pregnan-20-One," *J Clin Endocrinol* 81(1996): 1076–82.

11. F. Facchinetti, et al. "Oestradiol/Progesterone Imbalance and the Premenstrual Syndrome," *Lancet* 2 (1983): 1302.

12. M.R. Munday, M.G. Brush, and R.W. Taylor. "Correlations between Progesterone, Oestradiol and Aldosterone Levels in the Premenstrual Syndrome," *Clin Endocrinol* 14 (1981): 1–9.

13. T. Backstrom and B. Mattson. "Correlation of Symptoms in Pre-Menstrual Tension to Oestrogen and Progesterone Concentrations in Blood Plasma," *Neuropsychobiol* 1 (1975): 80–6.

14. R.L. Reid. "PMS Etiology: Medical Theories," in *Gynecology: Essentials of Clinical Practice*, ed. W.R. Keye Jr (Philadelphia: WB Saunders, 1988), 66–93.

15. M.S. Biskind and G.R. Biskind. "Diminution in Ability of the Liver to Inactivate Estrone in Vitamin B Complex Deficiency," *Science* 94 (1941): 462.

16. M.S. Biskind. "Nutritional Deficiency in the Etiology of Menorrhagia, Metrorrhagia, Cystic Mastitis and Premenstrual Tension; Treatment with Vitamin B Complex," 3 (1943): 227–34.

17. C.J. Chuong, B.P. Hsi, and W.E. Gibbons. "Periovulatory Beta-Endorphin Levels in Premenstrual Syndrome," *Obstet Gynecol* 83 (1995): 755–60.

18. V. Wynn, et al. "Tryptophan, Depression and Steroidal Contraception," *J Steroid Biochem* 6 (1975): 965–70.

19. P. Bermond. "Therapy of Side Effects of Oral Contraceptive Agents with Vitamin B6," *Acta Vitaminol-Enzymol* 4 (1982): 45–54.

20. U. Halbreich, et al. "Serum-Prolactin in Women with Premenstrual Syndrome," *Lancet* 2 (1976): 654–6.

21. P.M. O'Brien and E.M. Symonds. "Prolactin Levels in the Premenstrual Syndrome," *Br J Obst Gyn* 89 (1982): 306–8.

22. B. Goldin and S. Gorsbach. "The Effect of Milk and Lactobacillus Feeding on Human Intestinal Bacterial Enzyme Activity," *Am J Clin Nutr* 39 (1984): 756–61.

23. E. Freeman, et al. "Ineffectiveness of Progesterone Suppository Treatment for Premenstrual Syndrome," *JAMA* 264 (1990): 349–53.

24. S. Maddocks, et al. "A Double-Blind Placebo-Controlled Trial of Progesterone Vaginal Suppositories in the Treatment of Premenstrual Syndrome," *Am J Obstet Gynecol* 154 (1986): 573–81.

25. B. Andersch and L.J. Hahn. "Progesterone Treatment of Premenstrual Tension—A Double Blind Study," *Psychosom Res* 29 (1985): 489–93.

26. L. Dennerstein, et al. "Progesterone and the Premenstrual Syndrome: A Double Blind Crossover Trial," *Br Med J* 290 (1985): 1617–21.

27. E.R. Baker, et al. "Efficacy of Progesterone Vaginal Suppositories in Alleviation of Nervous Symptoms in Patients with Premenstrual Syndrome," *J Assist Reprod Genet* 12(3) (1995): 205–9.

28. P.J. Magill. "Investigation of the Efficacy of Progesterone Pessaries in the Relief of Symptoms of Premenstrual Syndrome. Progesterone Study Group," *Br J Gen Pract* 45(400) (1995): 589–93.

29. N.D. Brayshaw and D.D. Brayshaw. "Thyroid Hypofunction in Premenstrual Syndrome," *New Engl J Med* 315 (1986): 1486–7.

30. P.P. Roy-Byrne, et al. "TSH and Prolactin Responses to TRH in Patients with Premenstrual Syndrome," *Am J Psychiatry* 144 (1987): 480–4.

31. S.S. Girdler, C.A. Pedersen, and K.C. Light. "Thyroid Axis Function during the Menstrual Cycle in Women with Premenstrual Syndrome," *Psychoneuroendocrin* 20 (1995): 395–403.

32. P.J. Schmidt, et al. "Thyroid Function in Women with Premenstrual Syndrome," *J Clin Endocrinol Metab* 76 (1993): 671–74.

33. J.A. Aganoff and G.J. Boyle. "Aerobic Exercise, Mood States and Menstrual Cycle Symptoms," *J Psychosom Res* 38 (1994): 183–92.

34. P.Y. Choi and P. Salmon. "Symptom Changes across the Menstrual Cycle in Competitive Sportswomen, Exercisers and Sedentary Women," *Br J Clin Psychol* 34 (1995): 447–60.

35. J.F. Steege and J.A. Blumenthal. "The Effects of Aerobic Exercise on Premenstrual Symptoms in Middle-Aged Women: A Preliminary Study," *J Psychosom Res* 37(2) (1993): 127–33.

36. A.R. Kuczmierczyk, C.C. Johnson, and A.H. Labrum. "Coping Styles in Women with Premenstrual Syndrome," *Acta Psychiatr Scand* 89 (1994): 301–5.

37. D.B. Van Zak, et al. "Biofeedback Treatments for Premenstrual and Premenstrual Affective Syndromes," *Int J Psychosom* 41 (1994): 53–60.

38. R.J. Kirkby. "Changes in Premenstrual Symptoms and Irrational Thinking Following Cognitive-Behavioral Coping Skills Training," *J Consult Clin Psychol* 62 (1994): 1026–32.

39. K.T. Barnhart, E.W. Freeman and S.J. Sondheimer. "A Clinician's Guide to the Premenstrual Syndrome," *Med Clin North Am* 79 (1995): 1457–72.

40. E. Eriksson, et al. "Cerebrospinal Fluid Levels of Monoamine Metabolites. A Preliminary Study of Their Relation to Menstrual Cycle Phase, Sex Steroids, and Pituitary Hormones in Healthy Women and in Women with Premenstrual Syndrome," *Neuropsychopharmacology* 11 (1994): 201–13.

41. U. Halbreich, et al. "Low Plasma Gamma-Aminobutyric Acid Levels During the Late Luteal Phase of Women with Premenstrual Dysphoric Disorder," *Am J Psychiatry* 153(5) (1996): 718–20.

42. S.L. Gorbach and B.R. Goldin. "Diet and the Excretion and Enterohepatic Cycling of Estrogens," *Prev Med* 16 (1987): 525–31.

43. B.R. Goldin, et al. "Estrogen Patterns and Plasma Levels in Vegetarian and Omnivorous Women," *New Engl J Med* 307 (1982): 1542–7.

44. C. Longcope, et al. "The Effect of a Low Fat Diet on Oestrogen Metabolism," *J Clin Endocrinol Metab* 64 (1987): 1246–50.

45. M.N. Woods, et al. "Low-Fat, High-Fiber Diet and Serum Estrone Sulfate in Premenopausal Women," *Am J Clin Nutr* 49 (1989): 1179–83.

46. D.Y. Jones. "Influence of Dietary Fat on Self-Reported Menstrual Symptoms," *Physiol Behav* 40 (1987): 483–7.

47. A.M. Rossignol and H. Bonnlander. "Prevalence and Severity of the Premenstrual Syndrome. Effects of Foods and Beverages that Are Sweet or High in Sugar Content," *J Reprod Med* 36 (1991): 131–6.

48. J. Yudkin and O. Eisa. "Dietary Sucrose and Oestradiol Concentration in Young Men," *Ann Nutr Metabol* 32 (1988): 53–5.

49. F. Falck, et al. "Pesticides and Polychlorinated Biphenyl Residues in Human Breast Lipids and Their Relation to Breast Cancer," *Archives of Environmental Health* 47 (1992): 143–6.

50. R.M. Sharpe and N.E. Skakkebaek. "Are Oestrogens Involved in Falling Sperm Counts and Disorders of the Male Reproduction Tract," *Lancet* 341 (1993): 1392–5.

51. A.M. Rossignol and H. Bonnlander. "Caffeine-Containing Beverages, Total Fluid Consumption, and Premenstrual Syndrome," *Am J Public Health* 80 (1990): 1106–10.

52. M.K. Berman, et al. "Vitamin B6 in Premenstrual Syndrome," *J Am Diet Assoc* 90 (1990): 859–61.

53. J. Kliejnen, G. Ter Riet, and P. Knipschild. "Vitamin B6 in the Treatment of Premenstrual Syndrome—A Review," *Br J Obstet Gynaecol* 97 (1990): 847–52.

54. W. Barr. "Pyridoxine Supplements in the Premenstrual Syndrome," *Practitioner* 228 (1984): 425–7.

55. J. Zempleni. "Pharmacokinetics of Vitamin B6 Supplements in Humans," *J Am Coll Nutr* 14 (1995): 579–86.

56. M. Cohen and A. Bendich. "Safety of Pyridoxine—A Review of Human and Animal Studies," *Toxicol Letters* 34 (1986): 129–39.

57. G.J. Parry and D.E. Bredesen. "Sensory Neuropathy with Low-Dose Pyridoxine," *Neurol* 35 (1985): 1466–8.

58. J.A. Waterston and B.S. Gilligan. "Pyridoxine Neuropathy," *Med J Aust* 146 (1987): 640–2.

59. P. Majumdar and M. Boylan. "Alteration of Tissue Magnesium Levels in Rats by Dietary Vitamin B6 Supplementation," *Int J Vitamin Nutr Res* 59 (1989): 300–3.

60. C. Posacki, et al. "Plasma, Copper, Zinc, and Magnesium Levels in Patients with Premenstrual Tension Syndrome," *Acta Obstet Gynecol Scand* 73 (1994): 452–5.

61. J.W. Piesse. "Nutritional Factors in the Premenstrual Syndrome," *Int Clin Nutr Rev* 4 (1984): 54–81.

62. F. Facchinetti, et al. "Oral Magnesium Successfully Relieves Premenstrual Mood Changes," *Obstet Gynecol* 78 (1991): 177–81.

63. D.L. Rosenstein, et al. "Magnesium Measures across the Menstrual Cycle in Premenstrual Syndrome," *Biol Psychiatr* 35 (1994): 557–61.

64. R.S. London, R. Bradley, and N.Y. Chiamori. "Effect of a Nutritional Supplement on Premenstrual Symptomatology in Women with Premenstrual Syndrome: A Double-Blind Longitudinal Study," *J Am Coll Nutr* 10 (1991): 494–9.

65. A. Stewart. "Clinical and Biochemical Effects of Nutritional Supplementation on the Premenstrual Syndrome," *J Reprod Med* 32 (1987): 435–41.

66. J.S. Lindberg, et al. "Magnesium Bioavailability from Magnesium Citrate and Magnesium Oxide," *J Am Coll Nutr* 9 (1990): 48–55.

67. T. Bohmer, et al. "Bioavailability of Oral Magnesium Supplementation in Female Students Evaluated from Elimination of Magnesium in 24-hour Urine," *Magnesium Trace Elem* 9 (1990): 272–8.

68. J.G. Penland and P.E. Johnson. "Dietary Calcium and Manganese Effects on Menstrual Cycle Symptoms," *Am J Obstet Gynecol* 168 (1993): 1417–23.

69. S. Thys-Jacob, et al. "Calcium Supplementation in Premenstrual Syndrome: A Randomized Crossover Trial," *J Gen Intern Med* 4 (1989): 183–9.

70. S. Thys-Jacobs, et al. "Reduced Bone Mass in Women with Premenstrual Syndrome," *J Women Health* 4 (1995): 161–8.

71. C.J. Chuong and E.B. Dawson. "Zinc and Copper Levels in Premenstrual Syndrome," *Fertility Sterility* 62 (1994): 313–20.

72. A.M. Judd, R.M. Macleod, and I.S. Login "Zinc Acutely, Selectively and Reversibly Inhibits Pituitary Prolactin Secretion," *Brain Res* 294 (1984): 190–2.

73. R.S. London, et al. "The Effect of Alpha-Tocopherol on Premenstrual Symptomatology: A Double-Blind Study. II. Endocrine Correlates," *J Am Col Nutr* 3 (1984): 351–6.

74. D.F. Horrobin, et al. "Abnormalities in Plasma Essential Fatty Acid Levels in Women with Premenstrual Ssyndrome and with Non-Malignant Breast Disease," *J Nutr Med* 2 (1991): 259–64.

75. D. Budeiri, et al. "Is Evening Primrose Oil of Value in the Treatment of Premenstrual Syndrome?" *Control Clin Trials* 17 (1996): 60–8.

76. S.K. Khoo, C. Munro, and D. Battistutta. "Evening Primrose Oil and Treatment of Premenstrual Syndrome," *Med J Austral* 153 (1990): 189–92.

77. A. Cerin, et al. "Hormonal and Biochemical Profiles of Premenstrual Syndrome. Treatment with Essential Fatty Acids," *Acta Obstet Gynecol Scand* 72 (1993): 337–43.

78. A. Collins, et al. "Essential Fatty Acids in the Treatment of Premenstrual Syndrome," *Acta Obstet Gynecol* 81 (1993): 93–8.

79. M. Harada, M. Suzuki, and Y. Ozaki. "Effect of Japanese Angelica Root and Peony Root on Uterine Contraction in the Rabbit In Situ," *J Pharm Dyn* 7 (1984): 304–11.

80. K. Yoshiro. "The Physiological Actions of Tang-Kuei and Cnidium," *Bull Oriental Healing Arts Inst USA* 10 (1985): 269–78.

81. C.H. Costello and E.V. Lynn. "Estrogenic Substances from Plants: I. Glycyrrhiza," *J Am Pharm Soc* 39 (1950): 177–80.

82. A. Kumagai, K. Nishino, A. Shimomura, T. Kin, and Y. Yamamura. "Effect of Glycyrrhizin on Estrogen Action," *Endocrinol Japon* 14 (1967): 34–8.

83. R.V. Farese, et al. "Licorice-Induced Hypermineralocorticoidism," *N Engl J Med* 325 (1991): 1223–7.

84. F.C. Stormer, R. Reistad, and J. Alexander. "Glycyrrhizic Acid in Liquorice—Evaluation of Health Hazard," *Fd Chem Toxicol* 31 (1993): 303–12.

85. J. Baron, et al. "Metabolic Studies, Aldosterone Secretion Rate and Plasma Renin after Carbonoxolone Sodium as Biogastrone," *Br Med J* 2 (1969): 793–5.

86. E. Schildge. "Essay on the Treatment of Premenstrual and Menopausal Mood Swings and Depressive States," *Rigelh Biol Umsch* 19(2) (1964): 18–22.

87. F.W. Dittmar, et al. "Premenstrual Syndrome. Treatment with a Phytopharmaceutical," *Therapiewoche Gynakol* 5 (1992): 60–8.

88. C. Peteres-Welte and M. Albrecht. "Menstrual Abnormalities and PMS: Vitex Agnus-castus," *Therapiewoche Gynakol* 7 (1994): 49–52.

89. A. Milewicz, et al. "Vitex Agnus-castus in the Treatment of Luteal Phase Defects Due to Hyperprolactinemia," *Arzneim-Forsch* 43 (1993): 752–6.

Prostate Enlargement

1. J.E. Oesterling, "Benign Prostatic Hyperplasia: A Review of Its Histogenesis and Natural History," *Prostate* 6 (Suppl.) (1996): 67–73.

2. R. Horton, "Benign Prostatic Hyperplasia: A Disorder of Androgen Metabolism in the Male," *J Am Geri Soc* 32 (1984): 380–5.

3. A. Kappas, K.E. Anderson, A.H. Conney et al., "Nutrition-Endocrine Interactions: Induction of Reciprocal Changes in the Delta-5-Alpha-Reduction of Testosterone and the Cytochrome P-450-Dependent Oxidation of Estradiol by Dietary Macronutrients in Man," *Proc Natl Acad Sci USA* 80 (1983): 7646–9.

4. I.M. Bush et al., "Zinc and the Prostate," Presented at the annual meeting of the AMA, 1974.

5. M. Fahim, Z. Fahim, R. Der, and J. Harman, "Zinc Treatment for the Reduction of Hyperplasia of the Prostate," *Fed Proc* 35 (1976): 361.

6. A. Leake, G.D. Chrisholm, A. Busuttil, and F.K. Habib, "Subcellular Distribution of Zinc in the Benign and Malignant Human Prostate: Evidence for a Direct Zinc Androgen Interaction," *Acta Endocrinol* 105 (1984): 281–8.

7. V.Y. Zaichick et al., "Zinc Concentration in Human Prostatic Fluid: Normal, Chronic Prostatitis, Adenoma and Cancer," *Int Urol Nephrol* 28 (1996): 687–94.

8. A. Leake, G.D. Chisholm, and F.K. Habib, "The Effect of Zinc on the 5-Alpha-Reduction of Testosterone by the Hyperplastic Human Prostate Gland," *J Steroid Biochem* 20 (1984): 651–5.

9. A.M. Wallae and J.K. Grant, "Effect of Zinc on Androgen Metabolism in the Human Hyperplastic Prostate," *Biochem Soc Trans* 3 (1975): 540–2.

10. A.M. Judd, R.M. MacLeod, and I.S. Login, "Zinc Acutely, Selectively and Reversibly Inhibits Pituitary Prolactin Secretion," *Brain Res* 294 (1984): 190–2.

11. I.S. Login, M.O. Thorner, and R.M. MacLeod, "Zinc May Have a Physiological Role in Regulating Pituitary Prolactin Secretion," *Neuroendocrinology* 37 (1983): 317–20.

12. W.E. Farnsworth, W.R. Slaunwhite, M. Sharma et al., "Interaction of Prolactin and Testosterone in the Human Prostate," *Urol Res* 9 (1981): 79–88.

13. D.J. Farrar and J.S. Pryor, "The Effect of Bromocriptine in Patients with Benign Prostatic Hyperplasia," *Br J Urol* 48 (1976): 73–5.

14. G. DeRosa, S.M. Corsello, M.P. Ruffilli et al., "Prolactin Secretion After Beer," *Lancet* 2 (1981): 934.

15. B. Corenblum and M. Whitaker, "Inhibition of Stress-Induced Hyperprolactinaemia," *Br Med J* 275 (1977): 1328.

16. P.H. Chyou et al., "A Prospective Study of Alcohol, Diet, and Other Lifestyle Factors in Relation to Obstructive Uropathy," *Prostate* 22 (1993): 253–64.

17. J.P. Hart and W.L. Cooper, *Vitamin F in the Treatment of Prostatic Hyperplasia* Report Number 1 (Milwaukee, WI: Lee Foundation for Nutritional Research, 1941).

18. W.W. Scott, "The Lipids of the Prostatic Fluid, Seminal Plasma and Enlarged Prostate Gland of Man," *J Urol* 53 (1945): 712–8.

19. E.M. Boyd and N.E. Berry, "Prostatic Hypertrophy As Part of a Generalized Metabolic Disease: Evidence of the Presence of a Lipopenia," *J Urol* 41 (1939): 406–11.

20. F. Dumrau, "Benign Prostatic Hyperplasia: Amino Acid Therapy for Symptomatic Relief," *Am J Ger* 10 (1962): 426–30.

21. H.M. Feinblatt and J.C. Gant, "Palliative Treatment of Benign Prostatic Hypertrophy: Value of Glycine, Alanine, Glutamic Acid Combination," *J Maine Med Assoc* 49 (1958): 99–102.

22. F. Hinman, *Benign Prostatic Hyperplasia* (New York: Springer-Verlag, 1983).

23. R.S. Tilvis and T.A. Miettinen, "Serum Plant Sterols and Their Relation to Cholesterol Absorption," *Am J Clin Nutr* 43 (1986): 92–7.

24. R.R. Berges et al., "Randomized, Placebo-Controlled, Double-Blind Clinical Trial of Beta-Sitosterol

in Patients with Benign Prostatic Hyperplasia," *Lancet* 345 (1995): 1529–32.

25. M.S. Morton, K. Griffiths, and N. Blacklock, "The Preventive Role of Diet in Prostatic Disease," *Br J Urol* 77 (1996): 481–93.

26. M. Messina and S. Barnes, "The Roles of Soy Products in Reducing Risk of Cancer," *J Natl Cancer Inst* 83 (1991): 541–6.

27. R. Lahtonen, "Zinc and Cadmium Concentrations in Whole Tissue and in Separated Epithelium and Stroma from Human Benign Prostatic Hypertrophic Glands," *Prostate* 6 (1985): 177–83.

28. G. Sinquin et al., "Testosterone Metabolism by Homogenates of Human Prostates with Benign Hyperplasia: Effects of Zinc, Cadmium, and Other Bivalent Cations," *J Steroid Biochem* 20 (1984): 733–80.

29. A.C. Buck, "Phytotherapy for the Prostate," *Br J Urol* 78 (1996): 325–36.

30. F.C. Lowe and J.C. Ku, "Phytotherapy in Treatment of Benign Prostatic Hyperplasia: A Critical Review," *Urology* 48 (1996): 12–20.

31. D. Bach, M. Schmitt, and L. Ebeling, "Phytopharmaceutical and Synthetic Agents in the Treatment of Benign Prostatic Hyperplasia," *Phytomed* 3 (1996): 309–13.

32. S. Boccafoschi, and S. Annoscia, "Comparison of *Serenoa repens* Extract with Placebo by Controlled Clinical Trial in Patients with Prostatic Adenomatosis," *Urologia* 50 (1983): 1257–68.

33. E. Cirillo-Marucco, A. Pagliarulo, G. Tritto et al., "Extract of *Serenoa repens* (Permixon^R) in the Early Treatment of Prostatic Hypertrophy," *Urologia* 5 (1983): 1269–77.

34. V. Tripodi, M. Giancaspro, M. Pascarella et al., "Treatment of Prostatic Hypertrophy with *Serenoa repens* Extract," *Med Praxis* 4 (1983): 41–6.

35. E. Emili, M. Lo Cigno, and U. Petrone, "Clinical Trial of a New Drug for Treating Hypertrophy of the Prostate (Permixon)," *Urologia* 50 (1983): 1042–8.

36. P. Greca and R. Volpi, "Experience with a New Drug in the Medical Treatment of Prostatic Adenoma," *Urologia* 52 (1985): 532–5.

37. R. Duvia, G.P. Radice, and R. Galdini, "Advances in the Phytotherapy of Prostatic Hypertrophy," *Med Praxis* 4 (1983): 143–8.

38. A. Tasca, M. Barulli, A. Cavazzana et al., "Treatment of Obstructive Symptomatology Caused by Prostatic Adenoma with an Extract of *Serenoa repens*: Double-Blind Clinical Study vs. Placebo," *Minerva Urol Nefrol* 37 (1985): 87–91.

39. Cukier (Paris), Ducassou (Marseille), Le Guillou (Bordeaux) et al., "Permixon versus Placebo," *C R Ther Pharmacol Clin* 4/25 (1985): 15–21.

40. A. Crimi and A. Russo, "Extract of *Serenoa repens* for the Treatment of the Functional Disturbances of Prostate Hypertrophy," *Med Praxis* 4 (1983): 47–51.

41. G. Champlault, J.C. Patel, and A.M. Bonnard, "A Double-Blind Trial of an Extract of the Plant *Serenoa repens* in Benign Prostatic Hyperplasia," *Br J Clin Pharmacol* 18 (1984): 461–2.

42. G. Champlault, A.M. Bonnard, J. Cauquil, and J.C. Patel, "Medical Treatment of Prostatic Adenoma: Controlled Trial: PA 109 vs Placebo in 110 Patients," *Ann Urol* 18 (1984): 407–10.

43. F.M. Mattei, M. Capone, and A. Acconcia, "*Serenoa repens* Extract in the Medical Treatment of Benign Prostatic Hypertrophy," *Urologia* 55 (1988): 547–52.

44. J. Braeckman, "The Extract of *Serenoa repens* in the Treatment of Benign Prostatic Hyperplasia: A Multicenter Open Study," *Curr Ther Res* 55 (1994): 776–85.

45. D. Bach and L. Ebeling, "Long-Term Drug Treatment of Benign Prostatic Hyperplasia—Results of a Prospective 3-Year Multicenter Study Using Sabal Extract IDS89," *Phytomed* 3 (1996): 105–11.

46. R. Yasumoto et al., "Clinical Evaluation of Long-Term Treatment Using Cerniltin Pollen Extract in Patients with Benign Prostatic Hyperplasia," *Clinical Therapeutics* 17 (1995): 82–6.

47. A.C. Buck et al., "Treatment of Outflow Tract Obstruction Due to Benign Prostatic Hyperplasia with the Pollen Extract, Cernilton®: A Double-Blind, Placebo-Controlled Study," *Br J Urol* 66(4) 1990: 398–404.

48. H. Becker and L. Ebeling, "Conservative Therapy for Benign Prostatic Hyperplasia (BPH) with Cernilton," *Br J Urol* 66 (1988): 398–404.

49. K. Habib Fouad et al., "Identification of a Prostate Inhibitory Substance in a Pollen Extract," *Prostate* 26 (1995): 133–139.

50. M.C. Andro and J.P. Riffaud, "Pygeum Africanum Extract for the Treatment of Patients with Benign Prostatic Hyperplasia: A Review of 25 Years of Published Experience," *Curr Ther Res* 56 (1995): 796–817.

51. P. Guillemin, "Clinical Trials of V1326, or Tadenan, in Prostatic Adenoma," *Med Prat* 386 (1970): 75–6.

52. J. Lange and P. Muret," "Clinical Trial of V1326 in Prostatic Disease," *Med* 11 (1970): 2807–11.

53. L. Wemeau, J. Delmay, and J. Blankaert, "Tadenan in Prostatic Adenoma," *Vie Medicale* (January 1970): 585–8.

54. G. Viollet, "Clinical Experimentation of a New Drug from Prostatic Adenoma," *Vie Medicale* (June 1970): 3457–8.

55. A. Lhez and G. Leguevague, "Clinical Trials of a New Lipid-Sterolic Complex of Vegetal Origin in the Treatment of Prostatic Adenoma," *Vie Medicale* (December 1970): 5399–5404.

56. J.P. Thomas and F. Rouffilange, "The Action of Tadenan in Prostatic Adenoma," *Rev Int Serv* 43 (1970): 43–5.

57. J.A. Huet, "Prostatic Disease in Old Age," *Med Intern* 5 (1970): 405–8.

58. A. Rometti, "Medical Treatment of Prostatic Adenoma," *La Provence Medicale* 38 (1970): 49–51.

59. F. Gallizia and G. Gallizia, "Medical Treatment of Benign Prostatic Hypertrophy with a New Phytotherapeutic Principle," *Recent Med* 9 (1972): 461–8.

60. A. Durval, "The Use of a New Drug in the Treatment of Prostatic Disorders," *Minerva Urol* 22 (1970): 106–11.

61. V. Pansadoro and A. Benincasa, "Prostatic Hypertrophy: Results Obtained with *Pygeum africanum* Extract," *Minerva Med* 11 (1972): 119–44.

62. A. Maver, "Medical Therapy of the Fibrous-Adematose Hypertrophy of the Prostate with a New Vegetal Substance," *Minerva Med* 63 (1972): 2126–36.

63. G. Bongi, "Tadenan in the Treatment of Prostatic Adenoma," *Minerva Urol* 24 (1972): 129–39.

64. J. Doremieux, J.C. Masson, and C. Bollack, "Prostatic Hypertrophy, Clinical Effects and Histological Changes Produced by a Lipid Complex Extracted from *Pygeum africanum*," *J Med Strasbourg* 4 (1973): 253–7.

65. B. Del Valio, "The Use of a New Drug in the Treatment of Chronic Prostatitis," *Minerva Urol* 26 (1974): 81–94.

66. G. Colpi and U. Farina, "Study of the Activity of Chloroformic Extract of *Pygeum africanum* Bark in the Treatment of Urethral Obstructive Syndrome Caused by Non-Cancerous Prostapathy," *Urologia* 43 (1976): 441–8.

67. T. Donkervoort, J. Sterling, J. van Ness, and P.J. Donker, "A Clinical and Urodynamic Study of Tadenan in the Treatment of Benign Prostatic Hypertrophy," *Urol* 8 (1977): 218–25.

68. B. Dufour and C. Choquenet, "Trial Controlling the Effects of *Pygeum africanum* Extract on the Functional Symptoms of Prostatic Adenoma," *Ann Urol* 18 (1984): 193–5.

69. C. Legramandi, V. Ricci-Barbini, and A. Fonte, "The Importance of *Pygeum africanum* in the Treatment of Chronic Prostatitis Void of Bacteria," *Gazz Medica Ital* 143 (1984): 73–6.

70. S. Ranno et al., "Efficacy and Tolerability in the Treatment of Prostatic Adenoma with Tadenan 50," *Progresso Medico* 42 (1986): 165–9.

71. G. Frasseto et al., "Study of the Efficacy and Tolerability of Tadenan 50 in Patients with Prostatic Hypertrophy," *Progresso Medico* 42 (1986): 49–52.

72. P. Bassi et al., "Standardized Extract of *Pygeum africanum* in the Treatment of Benign Prostatic Hypertrophy," *Minerva Urol* 39 (1987): 45–50.

73. R. Duvia, G.P. Radice, and R. Galdini, "Advances in the Phytotherapy of Prostatic Hypertrophy," *Med Praxis* 4 (1983): 143–8.

74. P. Belaiche and O. Lievoux, "Clinical Studies on the Palliative Treatment of Prostatic Adenoma with Extract of Urtica Root," *Phytother Res* 5 (1991): 267–9.

75. I. Romics, "Observations with Bazoton in the Management of Prostatic Hyperplasia," *Int Urol Nephrol* 19(3) (1987): 293–7.

76. H. Wagner et al., "Search for the Antiprostatic Principle of Stinging Nettle (*Urtica dioica*) Roots," *Phytomedicine* 1 (1994): 213–24.

Psoriasis

1. J. Voorhees and E. Duell. "Imbalanced Cyclic AMP-Cyclic GMP Levels in Psoriasis," *Adv Cyc Nucl Res* 5 (1975): 755–7.

2. S. Robbins and R. Cotran. *Pathological Basis of Disease* (Philadelphia: W B Saunders, 1979), p1449.

3. M. Proctor, et al. "Lowered Cutaneous and Urinary Levels of Polyamines with Clinical Improvement in Treated Psoriasis," *Arch Dermatol* 115 (1979): 945–9.

4. Editorial. "Polyamines and Psoriasis," *Arch Dermatol* 115 (1979): 943–4.

5. Editorial. "Polyamines in Psoriasis," *J Invest Dermatol* 81 (1983): 385–7.

6. M. Haddox, K. Frassir, and D. Russel. "Retinol Inhibition of Ornithine Decarboxylase Induction and G1 Progression in CHD Cells," *Cancer Res* 39 (1979): 4930–8.

7. S. Kuwano and K. Yamauchi. "Effect of Berberine on Tyrosine Decarboxylase Activity of Streptococcus Faecalis," *Chem Pharm Bull* 8 (1960): 491–6.

8. E. Rosenberg and P. Belew. "Microbial Factors in Psoriasis," *Arch Dermatol* 118 (1982): 1434–44.

9. M. Rao and M. Field. "Enterotoxins and Anti-Oxidants," 12 (1984): 177–80.

10. L. Juhlin and C. Vahlquist. "The Influence of Treatment and Fibrin Microclot Generation in Psoriasis," *Br J Dermatol* 108 (1983): 33–7.

11. F.M. Thurmon. "The Treatment of Psoriasis with Sarsaparilla Compound," *NEJM* 227 (1942): 128–33.

12. G. Weber and K. Galle. "The Liver, a Therapeutic Target in Dermatoses," *Med Welt* 34 (1983): 108–11.

13. B.E. Monk and S.M. Neill. "Alcohol Consumption and Psoriasis," *Dermatologica* 173 (1986): 57–60.

14. H. Hikino, et al. "Antihepatotoxic Actions of Flavanolignans from Silybum Marianum Fruits," *Planta Medica* 50 (1984): 248–50.

15. T. Adzet. "Polyphenolic Compounds with Biological and Pharmacological Activity," *Herbs Spices Medicinal Plants* 1 (1986): 167–84.

16. NB. Zlatkov, J.J. Ticholov, and A.L. Dourmishev. "Free Fatty Acids in the Blood Serum of Psoriatics," *Acta Derm Vener (Stockh)* 64 (1984): 22–5.

17. S.B. Bittiner, et al. "A Double-Blind, Randomized, Placebo-Controlled Trial of Fish Oil in Psoriasis," *Lancet* i (1988): 378–80.

18. F. Grimmunger, et al. "A Double-Blind, Randomized, Placebo-Controlled Trial of N-3 Fatty Acid Based Lipid Infusion in Acute, Extended Guttate Psoriasis," *Clin Invest* 71 (1993): 634–43.

19. P.D.L. Maurice, et al. "The Effects of Dietary Supplementation with Fish Oil in Patients with Psoriasis," *Br J Dermatol* 1117 (1987): 599–606.

20. Editorial. "Leukotrienes and Other Lipoxygenase Products in the Pathogenesis and Therapy of Psoriasis and Other Dermatoses," *Arch Dermatol* 119 (1983): 541–7.

21. K. Kragballe and M.D. Herlin. "Benoxaphren Improves Psoriasis," *Arch Deramatol* 119 (1983): 548–52.

22. H. Lithell, et al. "A Fasting and Vegetarian Diet Treatment Trial on Chronic Inflammatory Disorders," *Acta Derm Vener (StockH)* 63 (1983): 397–403.

23. A. Bazex. "Diet without Gluten and Psoriasis," *Ann Derm Symp* 103 (1976): 648.

24. J.M. Douglass. "Psoriasis and Diet," *Calif Med* 133 (1980): 450.

25. S. Majewski, et al. "Decreased Levels of Vitamin A in Serum of Patients with Psoriasis," *Arch Dermatol Res* 280 (1989): 499–501.

26. L.J. Hinks, et al. "Trace Element Status in Eczema and Psoriasis," *Clin Exp Dermatol* 12 (1987): 93–7.

27. A. Donadini, A. Dazzaglia, and G. Desirello. "Plasma Levels of Zn, Cu and Ni in Healthy Controls and in Psoriatic Patients," *Acta Vitamin Enzymol* 1 (1980): 9–16.

28. P. Fratino, C. Pelfini, A. Jucci, and R. Bellazi. "Glucose and Insulin in Psoriasis: The Role of Obesity and Genetic History," *Panminerva Medica* 21 (1979): 167.

29. L. Juhlin, L. Bedquist, G. Echman, et al. "Blood Glutathione-Peroxide Levels in Skin Diseases: Effect of Selenium and Vitamin E Treatment," *Acta Dermat Vener (StockH)* 62 (1982): 211–4.

30. S. Morimoto, S. Takamoto, T. Onishi, et al. "Therapeutic Effect of 1,25-Dihydroxyvitamin D3 for Psoriasis: Report of Five Cases," *Calcif Tissue Int* 38 (1986): 119–22.

31. S. Takamoto, T. Onishi, S. Morimoto, et al. "Effect of 1-Alpha-Hydroxycholecalciferol on Psoriasis Vulgaris: A Pilot Study," *Calcif Tissue Int* 39 (1986): 360–4.

32. B. Staberg, A. Oxholm, P. Klemp, and C. Christiansen. "Abnormal Vitamin D Metabolism in Patients with Psoriasis," *Acta Derm Venereol (Stockh)* 67 (1987): 65–8.

33. C. Nieboer, et al. "Systemic Therapy with Fumaric Acid Derivates: New Possibilities in the Treatment of Psoriasis," *J Am Acad Dermatol* 20 (1989): 601–8.

34. R.H. Seville. "Psoriasis and Stress," *Br J Dermatol* 97 (1977): 297.

35. S.A. Winchell and R.A. Watts. "Relaxation Therapies in the Treatment of Psoriasis and Possible Pathophysiologic Mechanisms," *J Am Acad Dermatol* 18 (1988): 101–4.

36. J. Parrish. "Phototherapy and Photochemotherapy of Skin Diseases," *J Incest Dermatol* 77:1 (1981): 167–71.

37. O. Larko and G. Swanbeck. "Is UVB Treatment of Psoriasis Safe?" *Acta Dermat Vener (StockH)* 62 (1982): 507–12.

38. J. Boer, J. Hermans, A. Schothorst, and D. Suurmond. "Comparison of Phototherapy (UV-B) and Photochemotherapy (PUVA) for Clearing and Maintenance Therapy of Psoriasis," *Arch Dermatol* 120 (1984): 52–7.

39. H. Katayama and H. Hori. "The Influence of UVB Irradiation on the Excretion of the Main Urinary Metabolite of Prostaglandin F1a and F2a in Psoriatic and Normal Subjects," *Acta Dermatol Vener (StockH)* 64 (1984): 1–4.

40. H. Urabe, K. Nishitani, and H. Kohda. "Hyperthermia in the Treatment of Psoriasis," *Arch Dermatol* 117 (1981): 770–4.

41. E. Orenberg, D. Deneau, and E. Farber. "Response of Chronic Psoriatic Plaques to Localized Heating Induced by Ultrasound," *Arch Dermatol* 116 (1980): 893–7.

42. F.Q. Evans. "The Rational Use of Glycyrrhetinic Acid in Dermatology," *Br J Clin Pract* 12 (1958): 269–79.

43. S. Teelucksingh, et al. "Potentiation of Hydrocortisone Activity in Skin by Glycyrrhetinic Acid," *Lancet* 335 (1990): 1060–3.

44. C. Mann and E.J. Staba. "The Chemistry, Pharmacology, and Commercial Formulations of Chamomile," *Herbs, Spices, and Medicinal Plants* 1 (1984): 235–80.

45. C.N. Ellis, et al. "A Double-Blind Evaluation of Topical Capsaicin in Pruritic Psoriasis," *J Am Acad Dermatol* 29 (1993): 438–42.

46. J.E. Bernstein, et al. "Effects of Topically Applied Capsaicin on Moderate and Severe Psoriasis Vulgaris," *J Am Acad Dermatol* 15 (1986): 504–7.

Rheumatoid Arthritis

1. J.C. Bennett and F. Plum, eds., *Cecil Textbook of Medicine* (Philadelphia: WB Saunders, 1996), 1459–66.

2. L.M. Tierney, S.J. McPhee, and M.A. Papadakis, eds., *Current Medical Diagnosis and Treatment* (Los Altos, CA: Lange Medical Publications, 1997), 161.

3. M.D. Smith, R.A. Gibson, and P.M. Brooks, "Abnormal Bowel Permeability in Ankylosing Spondylitis and Rheumatoid Arthritis," *J Rheum* 12 (1985): 299–305.

4. G.C. Zaphiropoulos, "Rheumatoid Arthritis and the Gut," *Br J Rheum* 25 (1986): 138–40.

5. A.W. Segal, D.A. Isenberg, V. Hajirousou et al., "Preliminary Evidence for Gut Involvement in the Pathogenesis of Rheumatoid Arthritis," *Br J Rheum* 25 (1986): 162–6.

6. A.E.K. Henriksson et al., "Small Intestinal Bacterial Overgrowth in Patients with Rheumatoid Arthritis," *Annals Rheumatic Dis* 52 (1993): 503–10.

7. P.E. Philips, "Seminars in Arthritis and Rheumatism: Infectious Agents in the Pathogenesis of Rheumatoid Arthritis," *Semin Arthr Rheum* 16 (1986): 1–100.

8. P. Venables, "Epstein-Barr Virus Infection and Autoimmunity in Rheumatoid Arthritis," *Ann Rheum Dis* 47 (1988): 265–9.

9. H.W. Clark, M.R. Coker-Vann, J.S. Bailey, and T.M. Browm, "Detection of Mycoplasmal Antigens in Immune Complexes from Rheumatoid Arthritis Synovial Fluids," *Ann Allergy* 60 (1988): 394–8.

12. G.M. Hall and T.D. Spector, "Depressed Levels of Dehydroepiandrosterone Sulphate in Postmenopausal Women with Rheumatoid Arthritis but No Relation with Axial Bone Density," *Annals Rheum Dis* 52 (1993): 211–4.

13. R.F. van Vollenhoven et al., "An Open Study of Dehydroepiandrosterone in Systemic Lupus Erythematosus," *Arthritis Rheum* 37(9) (1994): 1305–10.

14. R. van Vollenhoven, E.G. Engleman, and J.L. McGuire, "Dehydroepiandrosterone in Systemic Lupus Erythematosus: Results of a Double-Blind, Placebo-Controlled, Randomized Clinical Trial," *Arthr Rheum* 38 (1995): 1826–31.

15. R. Jenkins, P. Rooney, D. Jones et al., "Increased Intestinal Permeability in Patients with Rheumatoid Arthritis: A Side Effect of Oral Nonsteroidal Anti-Inflammatory Drug Therapy?" *Br J Rheum* 26 (1987): 103–7.

16. J.F. Fries et al., "Toward an Epidemiology of Gastropathy Associated with Nonsteroidal Anti-inflammatory Drug Use," *Gastroenterol* 96 (1989): 647–55.

17. D.L. Scott et al., "Long-Term Outcome of Treating Rheumatoid

Arthritis: Results after 20 Years," *Lancet* 1 (1989): 1108–11.

18. H. Trowell and D. Burkitt, *Western Diseases: Their Emergence and Prevention* (Cambridge, MA: Harvard University Press, 1981).

19. L.G. Darlington and N.W. Ramsey, "Clinical Review: Review of Dietary Therapy for Rheumatoid Arthritis," *Br J Rheumatol* 32 (1993): 507–14.

20. H.M. Buchanan, S.J. Preston, P.M. Brooks et al., "Is Diet Important in Rheumatoid Arthritis," *Br J Rheumatol* 30 (1991): 125–34.

21. F. McCrae, K. Veerapen, and P. Dieppe, "Diet and Arthritis," *Practitioner* 230 (1986): 359–61.

22. L.G. Darlington, N.W. Ramsey, and J.R. Mansfield, "Placebo-Controlled, Blind Study of Dietary Manipulation Therapy in Rheumatoid Arthritis," *Lancet* 1 (1986): 236–8.

23. J.A. Hicklin, L.M. McEwen, and J.E. Morgan, "The Effect of Diet in Rheumatoid Arthritis," *Clinical Allergy* 10 (1980): 463–7.

24. R.S. Panush, "Delayed Reactions to Foods: Food Allergy and Rheumatic Disease," *Annals of Allergy* 56 (1986): 500–3.

25. M.A.F.J. Van de Laar and J.K. Ander Korst, "Food Intolerance in Rheumatoid Arthritis, I. A Double-Blind, Controlled Trial of the Clinical Effects of Elimination of Milk Allergens and Azo Dyes," *Annals Rheum Dis* 51 (1992): 298–302.

26. J. Kjeldsen-Kragh et al., "Controlled Trial of Fasting and One-Year Vegetarian Diet in Rheumatoid Arthritis," *Lancet* 338 (1991): 899–902.

27. L. Skoldstam, L. Larsson and F.D. Lindstrom, "Effects of Fasting and Lactovegetarian Diet on Rheumatoid Arthritis," *Scand J Rheumatol* 8 (1979): 249–55.

28. G.P. Kroker et al., "Fasting and Rheumatoid Arthritis: A Multicenter Study," *Clinical Ecology* 2 (1984): 137–44.

29. I. Hafstrom et al., "Effects of Fasting on Disease Activity, Neutrophil Function, Fatty Acid Composition, and Leukotriene Biosynthesis in Patients with Rheumatoid Arthritis," *Arthr Rheum* 31 (1988): 585–92.

30. J. Kjeldsen-Kragh et al., "Vegetarian Diet for Patients with Rheumatoid Arthritis—Status: Two Years After

Introduction of the Diet," *Clin Rheumatol* 13 (1994): 475–82.

31. R. Peltonen et al., "Changes in Faecal Flora in Rheumatoid Arthritis during Fasting and One-Year Vegetarian Diet," *Br J Rheumatol* 33 (1994): 638–43.

32. R. Peltonen et al., "Faecal Microbial Flora and Disease Activity in Rheumatoid Arthritis during a Vegan Diet," *Br. J Rheumatol* 36 (1997): 64–8.

33. T.J. De Witte et al., "Hypochlorhydria and Hypergastrinemia in Rheumatoid Arthritis," *Ann Rheumatic Dis* 38 (1979): 14–17

34. K. Henriksson et al., "Gastrin, Gastric Acid Secretion, and Gastric Microflora in Patients with Rheumatoid Arthritis," *Ann Rheumatic Dis* 45 (1986): 475–83.

35. I. Horger, "Enzyme Therapy in Multiple Rheumatic Diseases," *Therapiewoche* 33 (1983): 3948–57.

36. K. Ransberger, "Enzyme Treatment of Immune Complex Diseases," *Arthritis Rheuma* 8 (1986): 16–19.

37. J.A. Shapiro et al., "Diet and Rheumatoid Arthritis in Women: A Possible Protective Effect of Fish Consumption," *Epidemiology* 7 (1996): 256–63.

38. J. Jantti et al., "Evening Primrose Oil in Rheumatoid Arthritis: Changes in Serum Lipids and Fatty Acids," *Ann Rheum Dis* 48 (1989): 124–7.

39. M. Brzeski, R. Madhok, and H.A. Capell, "Evening Primrose Oil in Patients with Rheumatoid Arthritis and Side Effects of Non-Steroidal Anti-Inflammatory Drugs," *Br J Rheumatol* 30 (1991): 371–2.

40. J.F. Belch et al., "Effects of Altering Dietary Essential Fatty Acids on Requirements for Non-Steroidal Anti-Inflammatory Drugs in Patients with Rheumatoid Arthritis: A Double Blind Placebo Controlled Study," *Ann Rheum Dis* 47 (1988): 96–104.

41. L.J. Levanthal et al., "Treatment of Rheumatoid Arthritis with Gammalinoleic Acid," *Annals Int Med* 119 (1993): 867–73.

42. J. Kremer et al., "Effects of Manipulation of Dietary Fatty Acids on Clinical Manifestation of Rheumatoid Arthritis," *Lancet* 1 (1985): 184–7.

43. J. Kremer et al., "Fish-Oil Supplementation in Active Rheumatoid Arthritis: A Double-Blinded, Controlled Cross-Over Study," *Ann Intern Med* 106 (1987): 497–502.

44. R. Sperling et al., "Effects of Dietary Supplementation with Marine Fish Oil on Leukocyte Lipid Mediator Generation and Function in Rheumatoid Arthritis," *Arthritis Rheum* 30 (1987): 988–97.

45. L.G. Cleland et al., "Clinical and Biochemical Effects of Dietary Fish Oil Supplements in Rheumatoid Arthritis," *J Rheumatol* 15 (1988): 1471–5.

46. M. Magaro et al., "Influence of Diet with Different Lipid Composition on Neutrophil Composition on Neutrophil Chemiluminescence and Disease Activity in Patients with Rheumatoid Arthritis," *Ann Rheum Dis* 47 (1988): 793–6.

47. H. van der Temple et al., "Effects of Fish Oil Supplementation in Rheumatoid Arthritis," *Ann Rheum Dis* 49 (1990): 76–80.

48. J.M. Kremer et al., "Dietary Fish Oil and Olive Oil Supplementation in Patients with Rheumatoid Arthritis," *Arth Rheum* 33 (1990): 810–20.

49. C.S. Lau et al., "Maxepa on Nonsteroidal Anti-Inflammatory Drug Usage in Patients with Mild Rheumatoid Arthritis," *Br J Rheumatol* 30 (1991): 137.

50. G.L. Nielsen et al., "The Effects of Dietary Supplementation with N-3 Polyunsaturated Fatty Acids in Patients with Rheumatoid Arthritis: A Randomized, Double-Blind Trial," *Eur J Clin Invest* 22 (1992): 687–91.

51. V.K.S. Shukla and E.G. Perkins, "The Presence of Oxidative Polymeric Materials in Encapsulated Fish Oils," *Lipids* 26 (1991): 23–6.

52. K.L. Fritshe and P.V. Johnston, "Rapid Autoxidation of Fish Oil in Diets without Added Antioxidants," *J Nutr* 118 (1988): 425–6.

53. D. Harats et al., "Fish Oil Ingestion in Smokers and Nonsmokers Enhances Peroxidation of Plasma Lipoproteins," *Atherosclerosis* 90 (1991): 127–39.

54. J.A. Nettleton, "Omega-3 Fatty Acids: Comparison of Plant and Seafood Sources in Human

Nutrition," *J Am Diet Assoc* 91 (1991): 331–7.

55. S.C. Cunnane et al., "Alpha-Linolenic Acid in Humans: Direct Functional Role or Dietary Precursor," *Nutrition* 7 (1991): 437–9.

56. E. Mantzioris et al., "Dietary Substitution with Alpha-Linolenic Acid-Rich Vegetable Oil Increases Eicosapentaenoic Acid Concentrations in Tissues," *Am J Clin Nutr* 59 (1994): 1304–9.

57. D.S. Kelley, "Alpha-Linolenic Acid and Immune Response," *Nutrition* 8 (1992): 215–7.

58. D.C.E. Nordstrom et al., "Alpha-Linolenic Acid in the Treatment of Rheumatoid Arthritis: A Double-Blind Placebo-Controlled and Randomized Study: Flaxseed vs. Safflower Oil," *Rheumatol Int* 14 (1995): 231–4.

59. V. Cody, E. Middleton, and J.B. Harborne, *Plant Flavonoids in Biology and Medicine—Biochemical, Pharmacological, and Structure-Activity Relationships* (New York: Alan R Liss, 1986); V. Cody, E. Middleton, J.B. Harborne, and A. Beretz, *Plant Flavonoids in Biology and Medicine II—Biochemical, Pharmacological, and Structureactivity Relationships* (New York: Alan R. Liss, 1988).

60. G.W. Comstock et al., "Serum Concentrations of Alpha Tocopherol, Beta Carotene, and Retinol Preceding the Diagnosis of Rheumatoid Arthritis and Systemic Lupus Erythematosus," *Ann Rheum Dis* 56 (1997): 323–5.

61. U. Tarp et al., "Low Selenium Level in Severe Rheumatoid Arthritis," *Scandinavian Journal of Rheumatology* 14 (1985): 97–101.

62. U. Tarp et al., "Selenium Treatment in Rheumatoid Arthritis," *Scandinavian Journal of Rheumatology* 14 (1985): 364–8.

63. E. Munthe and J. Aseth, "Treatment of Rheumatoid Arthritis with Selenium and Vitamin E," *Scandinavian Journal of Rheumatology* 53 (suppl.) 1984: 103.

64. S.P. Pandley, S.K. Bhattacharya, and S. Sundar, "Zinc in Rheumatoid Arthritis," *Indian Journal of Medical Research* 81 (1985): 618–20.

65. P.A. Simkin, "Treatment of Rheumatoid Arthritis with Oral Zinc Sulfate," *Agents and Actions* (suppl.) 8 (1981): 587–95.

66. P.C. Mattingly and A.G. Mowat, "Zinc Sulphate in Rheumatoid Arthritis," *Annals of the Rheumatic Diseases* 41 (1982): 456–7.

67. C. Pasquier et al., "Manganese-Containing Superoxide-Dismutase Deficiency in Polymorphonuclear Leukocytes of Adults with Rheumatoid Arthritis," *Inflammation* 8 (1984): 27–32.

68. K.B. Menander-Huber, "Orgotein in the Treatment of Rheumatoid Arthritis," *Europ J Rheum Inflammation* 4 (1981): 201–11.

69. S. Zidenberg-Cherr et al., "Dietary Superoxide Dismutase Does Not Affect Tissue Levels," *Am J Clin Nutr* 37 (1983): 5–7.

70. G.D. Rosa et al., "Regulation of Superoxide Dismutase Activity by Dietary Manganese," *J Nutr* 110 (1980): 795–804.

71. A. Mullen and C.W.M. Wilson, "The Metabolism of Ascorbic Acid in Rheumatoid Arthritis," *Proc Nutr Sci* 35 (1976): 8A–9A.

72. N. Subramanian, "Histamine Degradation Potential of Ascorbic Acid," *Agents and Actions* 8 (1978): 484–7.

73. M. Levine, "New Concepts in the Biology and Biochemistry of Ascorbic Acid," *New Engl J Med* 314 (1986): 892–902.

74. E.C. Barton-Wright and W.A. Elliott, "The Pantothenic Acid Metabolism of Rheumatoid Arthritis," *Lancet* 2 (1963): 862–3.

75. General Practitioner Research Group, "Pantothenic Acid in Rheumatoid Arthritis," *Practitioner* 224 (1980): 208–11.

76. J.R.J. Sorenson and W. Hangarter, "Treatment of Rheumatoid and Degenerative Disease with Copper Complexes: A Review with Emphasis on Copper Salicylate," *Inflammation* 2 (1977): 217–38.

77. A.J. Lewis, "The Role of Copper in Inflammatory Disorders," *Agents Actions* (1984): 513–9.

78. W.R. Walker and D.M. Keats, "An Investigation of the Therapeutic Value of the "Copper Bracelet"—Dermal Assimilation of Copper in Arthritic/Rheumatoid Conditions," *Agents Actions* 6 (1976): 454–8.

79. M.H. Chung, L. Kessner, and P.C. Chan, "Degradation of Articular Cartilage by Copper and Hydrogen Peroxide," *Agents Actions* 15 (1984): 328–35.

80. M.X. Sullivan and W.C. Hess, "Cystine Content of Fingernails in Arthritis," *J Bone Joint Surg* 16 (1935): 185–8.

81. B.D. Senturia, "Results of Treatment of Chronic Arthritis and Rheumatoid Conditions with Colloidal Sulphur," *J Bone Joint Surg* 16 (1934): 119–25.

82. K. Wheeldon, "The Use of Colloidal Sulphur in the Treatment of Arthritis," *J Bone Joint Surg* 17 (1935): 693–726.

83. W. Kaufman, *The Common Form of Joint Dysfunction: Its Incidence and Treatment* (Brattleboro, VT: E.L. Hildreth Company, 1949).

84. A. Hoffer, "Treatment of Arthritis by Nicotinic Acid and Nicotinamide," *Canadian Medical Association Journal* 81 (1959): 235–9.

85. H.P.T. Ammon and M.A. Wahl, "Pharmacology of Curcuma Longa," *Planta Medica* 57 (1991): 1–7.

86. O.P. Sharma, "Antioxidant Properties of Curcumin and Related Compounds," *Biochem Pharmacol* 25 (1976): 1811–25.

87. S. Toda, T. Miyase, H. Arich et al., "Natural Antioxidants: Antioxidative Compounds Isolated from Rhizome of Curcuma Longa L," *Chem Pharmacol Bull* 33 (1985): 1725–8.

88. R. Srimal and B. Dhawan, "Pharmacology of Diferuloyl Methane (Curcumin), a Non-Steroidal Anti-Inflammatory Agent," *J Pharm Pharmac* 25 (1973): 447–52.

89. R. Srivastava, "Inhibition of Neutrophil Response by Curcumin," *Agents Actions* 28 (1989): 298–303.

90. D.L. Flynn and M.F. Rafferty, "Inhibition of 5-Hydroxy-Eicosatetraenoic Acid (5-HETE) Formation in Intact Human Neutraphils by Naturally-Occurring Diarylheptanoids: Inhibitory Activities of Curcuminoids and Yakuchinones," *Prost Leukotri Med* 22 (1986): 357–60.

91. S.D. Deodhar, R. Sethi, and R.C. Srimal, "Preliminary Studies on Antirheumatic Activity of Curcumin

(Diferuloyl Methane)," *Ind J Med Res* 71 (1980): 632–4.

92. R.R. Satoskar, S.J. Shah, and S.G. Shenoy, "Evaluation of Anti-Inflammatory Property of Curcumin (Diferuloyl Methane) in Patients with Postoperative Inflammation," *Int J Clin Pharmacol Ther Toxicol* 24 (1986): 651–4.

93. T.N.B. Shankar, N.V. Shantha, H.P. Ramesh et al., "Toxicity Studies on Turmeric (Curcuma longa): Acute Toxicity Studies in Rats, Guinea Pigs & Monkeys," *Indian J Exp Biol* 18 (1980): 73–5.

94. S. Taussig and S. Batkin, "Bromelain, the Enzyme Complex of Pineapple (Ananas comosus) and Its Clinical Application: An Update," *J Ethnopharmacol* 22 (1988): 191–203.

95. A. Cohen and J. Goldman, "Bromelain Therapy in Rheumatoid Arthritis," *Penn Med J* 67 (1964): 27–30.

96. A. Leung, *Encyclopedia of Common Natural Ingredients Used in Food, Drugs, and Cosmetics* (New York: John Wiley & Sons, 1980).

97. F. Kiuchi et al., "Inhibition of Prostaglandin and Leukotriene Biosynthesis by Gingerols and Diarylheptanoids," *Chem Pharm Bull* 40 (1992): 387–91.

98. K.C. Srivastava and T. Mustafa, "Ginger (Zingiber officinale) and Rheumatic Disorders," *Med Hypothesis* 29 (1989): 25–28.

99. K.C. Srivastava and T. Mustafa, "Ginger (Zingiber officinale) in Rheumatism and Musculoskeletal Disorders," *Med Hypothesis* 39 (1992): 342–8.

100. K. Shimizu, S. Amagaya, and Y. Ogihara, "Combination of Shosaikoto (Chinese Traditional Medicine) and Prednisolone on the Anti-Inflammatory Action," *J Pharmaco Dyn* 7 (1984): 891–9.

101. M. Yamamoto, A. Kumagai, and Y. Yokoyama, "Structure and Actions of Saikosaponins Isolated from Bupleurum Falcatum L," *Arzniem Forsch.* 25 (1975): 1021–40.

102. S. Hiai et al., "Stimulation of the Pituitary-Adrenocortical Axis by Saikosaponin of Bupleuri Radix," *Chem Pharm Bull* 29 (1981): 495–9.

103. H. Hikino, "Recent Research on Oriental Medicinal Plants," *Economic and Medicinal Plant Research* 1 (1985): 53–85.

104. S. Sukenik et al., "Balneotherapy for Rheumatoid Arthritis at the Dead Sea," *Isr Med J* 31 (1995): 210–4.

105. A. Ebringer, S. Khalpfour, and C. Wilson, "Rheumatoid Arthritis and Proteus: A possible Aetiological Association," *Rheumatol Int* 9 (1989): 223–228.

106. A. Ebringer, N. Cox, A.I. Abuljadayel et al., "Klebsiella Antibodies in Ankylosing Spondylitis and Proteus Antibodies in Rheumatoid Arthritis," *Bri J of Rheu* (1988): 2772–85.

Rosacea

1. J. Ryle and H. Barber, "Gastric Analysis in Acne Rosacea,". *Lancet* 2 (1920): 1195–96.

2. A. Barba, B. Rosa, G. Angelini, et al., "Pancreatic Exocrine Function in Rosacea," *Dermatologica* 165 (1982): 601–6.

3. W. Poole, "Effect of Vitamin B Complex and S-Factor on Acne Rosacea," *S Med J* 50 (1957): 207–10.

4. L. Tulipan, "Acne Rosacea: A Vitamin B Complex Deficiency," *NY State J Med* 29 (1929): 1063–64.

5. L. Johnson and R. Eckardt, "Rosacea Keratitis and Conditions with Vascularization of the Cornea Treated with Riboflavin," *Arch Ophth* 23 (1940): 899.

Seasonal Affective Disorder

1. H.S. Yu and R.J. Reiter eds., *Melatonin Biosynthesis, Physiological Effects and Clinical Applications* (Boca Raton, USA: CRC Press, 1993).

2. A. Miles and D.R.S. Philbrick, "Melatonin and Psychiatry," *Biol Psychiatry* 23 (1988): 405–25.

3. N. Rosenthal et al., "Antidepressant Effects of Light in Seasonal Affective Disorders," *Am J Psychiat* 142 (1985): 163–70.

4. N. Rosenthal et al., "Seasonal Affective Disorder: A Description of the Syndrome and Preliminary Findings with Light Treatment," *Arch Gen Psychiat* 41 (1984): 72–80.

5. D. Kripke, S. Risch, and D. Janowsky, "Bright White Light Alleviates Depression," *Psychiat Res* 10 (1983): 105–12.

6. B. Martinez et al., "Hypericum in the Treatment of Seasonal Affective Disorders," *J Geriatr Psychiatry Neurol* 7 (Suppl. 1) (1994): S29–33.

Seborrheic Dermatitis

1. J. Eppic, "Seborrhea Capitis in Infants: A Clinical Experience in Allergy Therapy," *Ann Allergy* 29 (1971): 323–4.

2. A. Nisenson, "Seborrheic Dermatitis of Infants and Leiner's Disease: A Biotin Deficiency," *J Ped* 51 (1957): 537–49.

3. A. Nisenson, "Treatment of Seborrheic Dermatitis with Biotin and Vitamin B Complex," *J Ped* 81 (1972): 630–1.

4. A. Schreiner, W. Slinger, V. Hawkins, et al., "Seborrheic Dermatitis: A Local Metabolic Defect Involving Pyridoxine," *J Lab Clin Med* 40 (1952): 121–30.

5. A. Schreiner, E. Rockwell, and R. Vilter, "A Local Defect in the Metabolism of Pyridoxine in the Skin of Persons with Seborrheic Dermatitis of the 'Sicca' Type," *J invest Dermatol* 19 (1952): 95–6.

6. H. Effersoe, "The Effect of Topical Application of Pyridoxine Ointment on the Rate of Sebaceous Secretion in Patients with Seborrheic Dermatitis," *Acta Dermatol* 3 (1954): 272–7.

7. D.A. Roe, *Drug-Induced Nutritional Deficiencies* (Westport, CT: AVI Publishing, 1976), 168–77.

8. T. Callaghan, "The Effect of Folic Acid on Seborrheic Dermatitis," *Cutis* 3 (1967): 584–8.

9. G. Andrews, C. Post, and A. Domonkos, "Seborrheic Dermatitis: Supplemental Treatment with

Vitamin B12," *NY State J M* (1950): 1921–5.

Sinusitis (Bacterial)

1. W. Stalman, et al., "Maxillary Sinusitis in Adults: An Evaluation of Placebo-Controlled Double-Blind Trials," *Fam Pract* 14 (1997): 124–9.
2. M.D. Poole, "Antimicrobial Therapy for Sinusitis," *Otolaryngol Clin North Am* 30 (1997): 331–9.
3. R. Cohen, "The Antibiotic Treatment of Acute Otitis Media and Sinusitis in Children," *Diagn Microbiol Infect Dis* 27 (1997): 35–9.
4. A.W. Dohlman, M.P.B. Hamstreet, G.T. Odrezin, and A.A. Bartolucci, "Subacute Sinusitis: Are Antimicrobials Necessary?" *J Allergy Clin Immunol* 91 (1993): 1015–23.
5. C. Bullock, "Chronic Infectious Sinusitis Linked to Allergies," *Med Trib* December 7 (1995): 1.
6. R. Evans, "Environmental Control and Immunotherapy for Allergic Disease," *J Allergy Clin Immunol* 90 (1992): 462–8.
7. A. C. Chester, "Sick Building Syndrome and Sinusitis," *Lancet* 339 (1992): 249–50.
8. C. Laino, "*H. pylori* Implicated in Allergies," *Med Trib* March 24 (1994): 1.
9. R. Ryan, "A Double-Blind Clinical Evaluation of Bromelains in the Treatment of Acute Sinusitis," *Headache* 7 (1967): 13–7.
10. A. Yerushalmi, S. Karman, and A. Lwoff, "Treatment of Perennial Allergic Rhinitis by Local Hyperthermia," *Proc Natl Acad Sci USA* 79 (1982): 4766–9.

Sore Throat

1. J.T. Badgett and L.K. Hesterberg, "Management of Group A Streptococcus Pharyngitis with a Second-Generation Rapid Strep Screen: Strep A OIA," *Microb Drug Resist* 2 (1996): 371–6.
2. C.F. Dagnelie, Y. van der Graaf, and R.A. De Melker, "Do Patients with Sore Throat Benefit from Penicillin? A Randomized Double-Blind Placebo-Controlled Clinical Trial with Penicillin V in General Practice," *Br J Gen Pract* 46 (1996): 589–93.
3. W.J. McIsaac et al., "Reconsidering Sore Throats, Part I: Problems with Current Clinical Practice," *Can Fam Physician* 43 (1997): 485–93.
4. W.J. McIsaac et al., "Reconsidering Sore Throats, Part 2: Alternative Approach and Practical Office Tool," *Can Fam Physician* 43 (1997): 495–500.
5. I. Brook, "Treatment of Group A Streptococcal Pharyngotonsillitis," *JAMA* 247 (1982): 2496.
6. T. McKowen, *The Role of Medicine: Dream, Mirage, or Nemesis?* (London: Nuffield Provincial Hospitals Trust, 1975).
7. J.F. Rinehart, "Studies Relating Vitamin C Deficiency to Rheumatic Fever and Rheumatoid Arthritis: Experimental, Clinical, and General Considerations, I.: Rheumatic Fever," *Ann Int Med* 9 (1935): 586–99.
8. J.F. Rinehart, "Studies Relating Vitamin C Deficiency to Rheumatic Fever and Rheumatoid Arthritis: Experimental, Clinical, and General Considerations, II. Rheumatoid (Atrophic) Arthritis," *Ann Int Med* 9 (1935): 671–89.
9. D. Sun, H.S. Courtney, and E.H. Beachey, "Berberine Sulfate Blocks Adherence of Streptococcus Pyogenes to Epithelial Cells, Fibronectin, and Hexadecane," *Antimicrobial Agents and Chemotherapy* 32 (1988): 1370–4.
10. M.G. Barros, "Soothing Sore Throats Gingerly," *Cortlandt Forum* 67 (1995): 86–16.
11. D.W. Asher, "Chronic Sore Throat: The Toothbrush Connection," *Cortlandt Forum* 57 (1990): 17–28.
12. W.P. King, "Food Hypersensitivity in Otolaryngology: Manifestations, Diagnosis and Treatment," *Otolaryngol Clin North Am* 25 (1992): 163–79.
13. G. Zoppi, A. Deganello, G.G. Benoni, and F. Saccomani, "Oral Bacteriotherapy in Clinical Practice, I. The Use of Different Preparations in Infants Treated with Antibiotics," *Eur J Ped* 139 (1982): 18–21.
14. V.P. Gotz, J.A. Romankiewics, J. Moss, and H.W. Murray, "Prophylaxis against Ampicillin-Induced Diarrhea with a Lactobacillus Preparation," *Am J Hosp Pharm* 36 (1979): 754–7.

Sports Injuries, Tendinitis, and Bursitis

1. B. Havsteen, "Flavonoids, a Class of Natural Products of High Pharmacological Potency," *Biochem Pharmacol* 32 (1983): 1141–8.
2. T. Yoshimoto, M. Furukawa, S. Yamamoto, et al., "Flavonoids: Potent Inhibitors of Arachidonate 5-Lipoxygenase," *Biochem Biophys Res Common* 116 (1983): 612–8.
3. M. Amella, C. Bronner, F. Briancon, et al., "Inhibition of Mast Cell Histamine Release by Flavonoids and Bioflavonoids," *Planta Medica* 51 (1985): 16–20.
4. M.J. Miller, "Injuries to Athletes," *Med Times* 88 (1960): 313–4.
5. R.B. Cragin, "The Use of Bioflavonoids in the Prevention and Treatment of Athletic Injuries," *Med Times* 90 (1962): 529–30.
6. I.S. Klemes, "Vitamin B12 in Acute Subdeltoid Bursitis," *Indust Med Surg* 26 (1957): 290–2.
7. S. Taussigand and S. Batkin, "Bromelain, the Enzyme Complex of Pineapple (Ananas comosus) and Its Clinical Application. An Update," *J Ethnopharmacol* 22 (1988): 191–203.
8. J. Blonstein, "Control of Swelling in Boxing Injuries," *Practitioner* 203 (1960): 206.
9. G. Saveriano, P. Lioretti, F. Maiolo, and E. Battista, "Our Experience in the Use of a New Objective Pain Measuring System in Rheumarthropatic Subjects Treated with Transcutaneous Electroanalgesia and Ultrasound," *Minerva Med* 77 (1986): 745–52.
10. F.H. Krusen, F.J. Kottke and P.M. Ellwood, *Handbook of Physical Medicine and Rehabilitation* (Philadelphia: W.B. Saunders, 1971), 297–321.

Ulcers (Duodenal and Gastric)

1. K. Berstad and A. Berstad, "*Helicobacter pylori* Infection in Peptic Ulcer Disease," *Scand J Gastroenterol* 28 (1993): 561–7.

2. S. A. Sarker and K. Gyr, "Non-Immunological Defense Mechanisms of the Gut," *Gut* 33 (1992): 987–93.

3. J. Weil, et al., "Prophylactic Aspirin and Risk of Peptic Ulcer Bleeding," *BMJ* 310 (1995): 827–30.

4. G.M. Gray. "Peptic Ulcer Diseases," In, D.C. Dale, D.D. Federman, *Scientific American Medicine* (New York, NY: Sci Am, 1995).

5. E.J. Feldman and K.A. Sabovich, "Stress and Peptic Ulcer Disease," *Gastroenterol* 78 (1980): 1087–9.

6. R.F. Anda, D.F. Williamson, L. Escobedo, et al., "Self-Perceived Stress and the Risk of Peptic Ulcer Disease," *Arch Int Med* 152 (1992): 829.

7. J. Siegel, "Gastrointestinal Ulcer—Arthus Reaction!" *Ann Allergy* 32 (1974): 127–30.

8. C. Andre, B. Moulinier, F. Andre, and S. Daniere, "Evidence for Anaphylactic Reactions in Peptic Ulcer and Varioliform Gastritis," *Ann Allergy* 51 (1983): 325–8.

9. J. Siegel, "Immunologic Approach to the Treatment and Prevention of Gastrointestinal Ulcers," *Ann Allergy* 38 (1977): 27–9.

10. J. Rebhun, "Duodenal Ulceration in Allergic Children," *Ann Allergy* 34 (1975): 145–9.

11. N. Kumar, A. Kumar, S.L. Broor, et al., "Effect of Milk on Patients with Duodenal Ulcers," *Brit Med J* 293 (1986): 666.

12. A. Rydning, A. Berstad, E. Aadland, and B. Odegaard, "Prophylactic Effects of Dietary Fiber in Duodenal Ulcer Disease," *Lancet* 2 (1982): 736–9.

13. J.Y. Kang, et al., "Dietary Supplementation with Pectin in the Maintenance Treatment of Duodenal Ulcer," *Scand J Gastroenterol* 23 (1988): 95–9.

14. E. Harju and T.K. Larme, "Effect of Guar Gum Added to the Diet of Patients with Duodenal Ulcers," *J Parenteral Enteral Nutr* 9 (1985): 496–500.

15. G. Cheney, "Rapid Healing of Peptic Ulcers in Patients Receiving Fresh Cabbage Juice," *Cal Med* 70 (1949): 10–14.

16. G. Cheney, "Anti-Peptic Ulcer Dietary Factor," *J Am Diet Assoc* 26 (1950): 668–72.

17. W. Shive, R.N. Snider, B. DuBiler, et al., "Glutamine in Treatment of Peptic Ulcer," *Tex J Med* 53 (1957): 840–3.

18. J.Y. Kang, et al., "Effect of Colloidal Bismuth Subcitrate on Symptoms and Gastric Histology in Non-Ulcer Dyspepsia. A Double Blind Placebo Controlled Study," *Gut* 31 (1990): 476–80.

19. B.J. Marshall, et al., "Bismuth Subsalicylate Suppression of *Helicobacteria pylori* in Non-Ulcer Dyspepsia: A Double-Blind Placebo-Controlled Trial," *Dig Dis Scie* 38 (1993): 1674–80.

20. N. Parmar and M. Ghosh, "Gastric Anti-Ulcer Activity of (+)-Cyanidanol-3, a Histidine Decarboxylase Inhibitor," *Eur J Pharmacol* 69 (1981): 25–32.

21. P. Wendt, H. Reiman, K. Swoboda, G. Hennings, and G. Blumel, "The Use of Flavonoids as Inhibitors of Histidine Decarboxylase in Gastric Diseases, Experimental and Clinical Studies," *Naunyn-Schmiedeberg's Arch Pharma* (Suppl.) 313 (1980): 238.

22. W. Beil, Birkholz, and K.F. Sewing, "Effects of Flavonoids on Parietal Cell Acid Secretion, Gastric Mucosal Prostaglandin Production and *Helicobacter pylori* Growth," *Arzneim Forsch* 45 (1995): 697–700.

23. V.V. Schumpelik and E. Farthmann, "Untersuchung Zur Protektiven Wirkung Von Vitamin A Beim Stressulkus Der Ratte," *Arz For (Drug Res)* 26 (1976): 386.

24. P.L. Harris, et al., "Dietary Production of Gastric Ulcers in Rats and Prevention by Tocopherol Administration," *Proc Soc Exp Biol Med* 4 (1947): 273–7.

25. G. Oner, N.M. Bor, E. Onuk, and Z.N. Oner, "The Role of Zinc Ion in the Development of Gastric Ulcers in Rats," *Eur J Pharmacol* 70 (1981): 241–3.

26. D.J. Formmer, "The Healing of Gastric Ulcers by Zinc Sulphate," *Med J Austr* 2 (1975): 793.

27. J. Marle, et al., "Deglycyrrhizinised Liquorice (DGL) and the Renewal of Rat Stomach Epithelium," *Eur J Pharm* 72 (1981): 219.

28. Ag. Morgan et al., "Comparison Between Cimetidine and Caved-S in the Treatment of Gastric Ulceration, and Subsequent Maintenance Therapy," *Gut* 23 (1982): 545–51.

29. Z.A. Kassir, "Endoscopic Controlled Trial of Four Drug Regimens in the Treatment of Chronic Duodenal Ulceration," *Irish Med J* 78 (1985): 153–6.

30. A.G. Turpie, J. Runcie and T.J. Thomson, "Clinical Trial of Deglycyrrhizinate Liquorice in Gastric Ulcer," *Gut* 10 (1969): 299–303.

31. W.D.W. Rees, et al., "Effect of Deglycyrrhizinated Liquorice on Gastric Mucosal Damage by Aspirin," *Scand J Gastroent* 14 (1979): 605–7.

32. S.N. Tewari and A.K. Wilson, "Deglycyrrhizinated Liquorice in Duodenal Ulcer," *Practitioner* 210 (1972): 820–5.

33. H. Zhou and D. Jiao, "312 Cases of Gastric and Duodenal Ulcer Bleeding Treated with 3 Kinds of Alcoholic Extract Rhubarb Tablets," *Chung Hsi I Chieh Ho Tsa Chih* 10 (1990): 150–1.

Vaginitis

1. D. Eschenbach, "Vaginal Infection," *Clin Ob Gyn* 26 (1986): 186–202.

2. B. Woo and W.T. Branch, "Vaginitis," in *Office Practice of Medicine* (Philadelphia: WB Saunders, 1982), 461–70.

3. J. McCue, A. Kamanoff, T. Pass, and G. Friedland, "Strategies for Diagnosing Vaginitis," *J Fam Prac* 9 (1979): 395–402.

4. T. Stamey, "The Role of Introital Enterobacteria in Recurrent Urinary Infections," *J Urol* 109 (1973): 467–72.

5. N.R. Netto, P. Rangel, R. DaSilva, et al., "The Importance of Vaginal Infection on Recurrent Cystitis in Women," *Int Surg* 64 (1979): 79–82.

6. B. Larsen and R. Galask, "Vaginal Microbial Flora: Practical and Theoretic Relevance," *Ob Gyn* 55 (Suppl.) (1980): 100S–113S.

7. C.I. Meeker, "Candidiasis—an Obstinate Problem," *Med Times* 106 (1978): 26–32.

8. F. Heidrich, A. Berg, F. Gergman, et al., "Clothing Factors and Vaginitis," *J Fam Prac* 19 (1984): 491–94.

9. H. Gardner, "Vulvovaginitis: Prevalence and Diagnosis," *Med Times* 106 (1978): 21–25.

10. R.J. Hildebrandt, "Trichomoniasis: Always with Us—but Controllable," *Med Times* 106 (1978): 44–48.

11. K. Holmes and H. Handsfield, "Sexually Transmitted Diseases," in *Harrison's Principles of Internal Medicine* (New York: McGraw Hill, 1983), 889–902.

12. M.R. Miles, L. Olsen, A. Rogers, et al., "Recurrent Vaginal Candidiasis—Importance of an Intestinal Reservoir," *JAMA* 238 (1977): 1836–37.

13. N. Kudelco, "Allergy in Chronic Monilial Vaginitis," *Ann Allergy* 29 (1971): 266–67.

14. F.J. Fleury, "Is There a 'Non-Specific' Vaginitis?" *Med Times* 106 (1978): 37–43.

15. L. Vontver and D. Eschenbach, "The Role of Gardnerella Vaginalis in Nonspecific Vaginitis," *Clin Ob Gyn* 24 (1981): 439–60.

16. M. Balsdon, L. Pead, G. Taylor, and R. Maskell, "Corynebacterium Vaginale and Vaginitis: A Controlled Trial of Treatment," *Lancet* 1 (1980): 501–3.

17. C. Spiegel, R. Amsel, D. Eshenbach, et al., "Anaerobic Bacteria in Nonspecific Vaginitis," *NEJM* 303 (1980): 601–7.

18. K.K. Holmes, "The Chlamydia Epidemic," *JAMA* 245 (1981): 1718–23.

19. M. Khatamee, "Chlamydia Mycoplasma: What Are the Hidden Risks of These STDs?" *Mod Med* 52 (1984): 156–74.

20. S. Maneksha, "Comparison of Povidone Iodine (Betadine) Vaginal Pessaries and Lactic Acid Pessaries in the Treatment of Vaginitis," *J Int Med Res* 2 (1974): 236–39.

21. P. Reeve, "The Inactivation of Chlamydia Trachomatis by Povidone Iodine," *J Antimicrob Chemo* 2 (1976): 77–80.

22. J. Ratzen, "Monilial and Trichomonal Vaginitis—Topical Treatment with Povidone Iodine Treatments," *Cal Med* 110 (1969): 24–27.

23. S. Mayhew, "Vaginitis: A Study of the Efficacy of Povidone Iodine in Unselected Cases," *J Int Med Res* 9 (1981): 157–59.

24. T. Swate and J. Weed, "Boric Acid Treatment of Vulvovaginal Candidiasis," *Ob Gyn* 43 (1974): 894–95.

25. K. Keller Van Slyke, "Treatment of Vulvovaginal Candidiasis with Boric Acid Powder," *Am J Ob Gyn* 141 (1981): 145–48.

26. C.I. Meeker, "Candidiasis—an Obstinate Problem," *Med Times* 106 (1978): 26–32.

Varicose Veins

1. S. Rose, "What Causes Varicose Veins?" *Lancet* 1 (1986): 320–1.

2. R. Berkow, ed., *The Merck Manual of Diagnosis and Therapy*, 14th ed. (Rahway, NJ: Merck & Co, 1982), 560–6.

3. H. Trowell, D. Burkitt and K. Heaton, *Dietary Fibre, Fibre-Depleted Foods and Disease* (London: Academic Press, 1985).

4. G. Vahouny and D. Kritchevsky, *Dietary Fiber in Health and Disease* (New York: Plenum Press, 1982).

5. C. Latto, R.W. Wilkinson, and O.J.A. Gilmore, "Diverticular Disease and Varicose Veins," *Lancet* 1 (1973): 1089–90.

6. C. Allegra, G. Pollari, A. Criscuolo et al., "*Centella asiatica* Extract in Venous Disorders of the Lower Limbs: Comparative Clinico-Instrumental Studies with a Placebo," *Clin Terap* 99 (1981): 507–13.

7. Monograph: *Centella asiatica* (Milan, Italy: Indena S.p.A., 1987).

8. C. Allegra, "Comparative Capillaroscopic Study of Certain Bioflavonoids and Total Triterpenic Fractions of *Centella asiatica* in Venous Insufficiency," *Clin Terap* 110 (1984): 550.

9. J.P. Pointel, H. Boccalon, M. Cloarec et al., "Titrated Extract of *Centella asiatica* (TECA) in the Treatment of Venous Insufficiency of the Lower Limbs," *Angiology* 38 (1987): 46–50.

10. F. Marastoni, A. Baldo, G. Redaelli, and L. Ghiringhelli, "*Centella asiatica* Extract in Venous Pathology of the Lower Limbs and Its Evaluation As Compared with Tribenoside," *Minerva-Cardioangiol* 30 (1982): 201–7.

11. C. Diehm et al., "Comparison of Leg Compression Stocking and Oral Horse-Chestnut Seed Extract Therapy in Patients with Chronic Venous Insufficiency," *Lancet* 347 (1996): 292–4.

12. F. Annoni, A. Mauri, F. Marincola, and L.F. Resele, "Venotonic Activity of Escin on the Human Saphenous Vein," *Arzneim-Forsch.* 29 (1979): 672–5.

13. G. Hitzenberger, "The Therapeutic Effectiveness of Chestnut Extract," *Wien Med Wochenschr* 139 (17) (1989): 385–9.

14. J. Lucas, "Erfahrungen mit Aescin in der internen therapie," *Med Wel* 14 (1963): 913.

15. G. Marcelon, T.J. Verbeuren, H. Lauressergues, and P.M. Vanhoutte, "Effect of *Ruscus aculeatus* on Isolated Canine Cutaneous Veins," *Gen Pharmacol* 14 (1983): 103.

16. G. Rudofsky, "Improving Venous Tone and Capillary Sealing: Effect of a Combination of Ruscus Extract and Hesperidine Methyl Chalcone in Healthy Probands in Heat Stress," *Fortschr Med* 107(19) (1989): 52, 55–8.

17. R. Cappelli, M. Nicora, T. Di Perri, "Use of Extract of Ruscus Aculeatus in Venous Disease in the Lower Limbs," *Drugs Exp Clin Res* 14(4) (1988): 277–83.

18. M. Gabor, "Pharmacologic Effects of Flavonoids on Blood Vessels," *Angiologica* 9 (1972): 355–74.

19. J. Kuhnau, "The Flavonoids: A Class of Semi-Essential Food Components: Their Role in Human Nutrition," *World Review Nutrition and Dietetics* 24 (1976): 117–91.

20. H. Pourrat, "Anthocyanidin Drugs in Vascular Disease," *Plant Med Phytothera* 11 (1977): 143–51.

21. J.P. Henriet, "Veno-Lymphatic Insufficiency: 4,729 Pts: Undergoing Hormonal and Procyanidol Oligomer

Therapy," *Phlebologie* 46(2) (1993): 313–25.

22. N. Ihme et al., "Leg Edema Protection from Buckwheat Herb Tea in Patients with Chronic Venous Insufficiency: A Single-Center, Randomized, Double-Blind, Placebo-Controlled Clinical Trial," *Eur J Clin Pharmacol* 50 (1995): 443–7.

23. H.W. Kreysel, H.P. Nissen, and E. Enghoffer, "A Possible Role of Lysosomal Enzymes in the Pathogenesis of Varicosis and the Reduction in Their Serum Activity by Venostasin," *VASA* 12 (1983): 377–82.

24. S. Visudhiphan et al., "The Relationship between High Fibrinolytic Activity and Daily Capsicum Ingestion in Thais," *Am J Clin Nutr* 35 (1982): 1452–8.

25. A.K. Bordia, H.K. Josh, and Y.K. Sanadhya, "Effect of Garlic Oil on Fibrinolytic Activity in Patients with CHD," *Atherosclerosis* 28 (1977): 155–9.

26. K.I. Baghurst, M.J. Raj, and A.S. Truswell, "Onions and Platelet Aggregation," *Lancet* 1 (1977): 101.

27. K. Srivastava, "Effects of Aqueous Extracts of Onion, Garlic and Ginger on the Platelet Aggregation and Metabolism of Arachidonic Acid in the Blood Vascular System: In Vitro Study," *Prost Leukotri Med* 13 (1984): 227–35.

28. H. Ako, A. Cheung, and P. Matsura, "Isolation of a Fibrinolysis Enzyme Activator from Commercial Bromelain," *Arch Int Pharmacodyn* 254 (1981): 157–67.

INDEX

A

AA, *see* Alcoholics Anonymous
Abbott Laboratories, 250
Abraham, Guy, 552
Absorptiometry, 710–711
Acceptance, 21
Acetic acid, 266
Acetylation, 119
L-Acetylcarnitine, 230
Acetylcholine
memory and, 227
phosphatidylcholine and, 229
N-Acetylcysteine
AIDS and, 203–204
glutathione and, 117–118
Achilles reflex time, 561
Acne
azelaic acid for, 197
benzoyl peroxide for, 193
causes, 191–193
chromium for, 194
forms, 191
hypothyroidism and, 196
insulin for, 194
like-legions, causes, 193
pantothenic acid for, 196
pyridoxine for, 196
retin-A for, 193–194
selenium for, 195–196
sulfur for, 197
treatment summary, 198
tropical treatments, 196–197
vitamin A for, 194–195
vitamin E for, 195–196
zinc for, 195
Acne conglobata, 191
Acne rosacea, 191
Acne vulgaris, 191
ACP, *see* Alternate complement
pathway
Acquired immunodeficiency syndrome,
see AIDS
Acrodermatitis enteropathica, 156–157
ACTH, *see* Adrenocorticotropic
hormone
Active listening, 183–184
Acupressure, 679

Acupuncture
CTS and, 317
description, 5
migraines and, 662
smoking cessation by, 34
ADA, *see* American Diabetes Association
Adaptogen, 186–187
ADD, *see* Attention deficit disorders
Adenosine monophosphate, 763–764
Adenosylcobalamin
availability, 238
description, 228
S-Adenosylmethionine, *see also*
Methionine
bile flow and, 122
depression and, 386–387, 394–396
lipotropic formulas and, 123
osteoarthritis and, 701–702
synthesis, 118
Adrenal gland
abnormal response by, 185–187
asthma and, 262
CFS and, 366–367
depression and, 383
description, 175–176
Adrenaline, 175–176
Adrenocorticotropic hormone, 176
Adventist Battle Creek Sanitarium, 3
AE, *see* Acrodermatitis enteropathica
Aerobics Center Longitudinal Study,
37–38
Aesculus hippocastanum, see Horse
chestnut
AF, *see* Atrial fibrillation
Affirmations, 29
Age spots, 166
Aggression
hypoglycemia and, 551–552
turned-inward model, 378
Aging, *see also* Longevity
Alzheimer's disease and, 221
blood-pressure and, 527
causes, 164–165
cellular, 166
free-radical theory, 167–168
gallstones and, 478
glycosylation, 168

Hayflick limit, 164–166
oldest people list, 165
telomere-shortening theory, 166–167
varicose veins and, 826
Agoraphobia, 255
AIDS
antioxidants for, 203–205
botanical treatment, 207–209
description, 199–200
glutathione for, 116
nutrition, 202–203
T cells and, 147
treatment summary, 209–210
vitamin B6 for, 206
vitamin B12 for, 206
zinc for, 206
Alarm reaction, *see* Fight-or-flight
response
Alcohol
BPH and, 756
gout and, 491–492
hypoglycemia and, 556–557
immune system and, 152–153
impotence and, 567
intestinal flora, 215
liver and, 122
psoriasis and, 765
stress and, 184–185
use disorder inventory test, 214
Alcoholics Anonymous, 213
Alcoholism
amino acid levels, 216–217
antioxidants and, 216
carnitine for, 216
causes, 212
consequences, 211–212
depression and, 215, 384
description, 211
EFA for, 217
exercise for, 217–218
folic acid levels and, 236
glutamine for, 217
hypoglycemia and, 214–215
magnesium for, 217
milk thistle for, 218
psychosocial aspects, 213
pyridoxine for, 217

Alcoholism, *continued*
  test for, 214
  thiamin for, 217
  treatment summary, 219–220
  vitamin A for, 215–216
  vitamin C for, 217
  zinc for, 215
Alder, Alfred, 41–42
Aldicarb, 55
Aldose reductase, 411
Aldosterone, 738
Alexander technique, 79–80
Allergens, airborne, 264
Allergic tension-fatigue syndrome, 185
Allergic toxemia, 388
Allergies
  colds and, 371
  food, *see* Food allergies
  food coloring, 57
  preservatives, 58
  sinusitis and, 798
Allicin, *see* Garlic
Allium cepa, see Onions
Allium sativum, see Garlic
Allopathy, *see* Conventional medicine
Allopurinol, 493
Allyl propyl disulphide, 425
Aloe vera
  kidney stones and, 618
  ulcers and, 816
Alternate complement pathway, 448
Alternative complement pathway, 160
Aluminum, 222, 226–227
Alzheimer's disease
  aluminum and, 222, 226–227
  antioxidants for, 224–226
  causes, 221–222
  description, 221
  DHEA for, 230–231
  diagnosing, 222–224
  estrogen for, 226
  fingerprints and, 223–224
  ginkgo biloba for, 231–232
  LAC and, 230
  phosphatidylcholine for, 229
  treatment summary, 232
  vitamin B12 for, 227–228
  zinc for, 228–229
Amalgam restorations, 724
American Cancer Society, 49
American Celiac Society, 328
American College for the Advancement
  in Medicine, 250
American Diabetes Association, 415
American Digestive Disease Society, 328
American Heart Association, 49
American Journal of Cardiology, 525
American Journal of Epidemiology, 36
*American Journal of Industrial
  Medicine*, 124
Amino acids
  alcoholism and, 216–217
  BPH and, 756
  conjugation, 118

gout and, 494
  sulfur-containing, 172
γ-Amino-butyric acid, 389
Ammi visnaga, see Khella
AMP, *see* Adenosine monophosphate
Amylases, 127
Anaerobic metabolism, 253
Anatomy of an Illness, 149
Anderson, James, 415
Andy Griffith Show, 31
Anemia
  causes, 233–236
  chlorophyll and, 237
  description, 233
  folic acid and, 236, 240
  hydrochloric acid for, 237
  iron-deficiency, 234–235
    nutritional support, 237
  pernicious, 235, 239
  supplements, 237
  treatment summary, 241
  vitamin B12 and, 235–236, 238–240
Angelica sinensis, see Dong quai
Anger, *see* Type A personality
Angina
  carnitine for, 246–247
  causes, 242
  chelation therapy, 249–250
  CoQ_{10} for, 246
  description, 242
  hawthorn for, 248–249
  hypoglycemia and, 553
  khella for, 249
  pantethine for, 246–247
  pectoris, 248
  Prinzmetal's variant
    description, 242
    magnesium for, 242
  therapy goals, 246
  treatment summary, 251
Angioedema, 536
Angiograms
  description, 242–246
  supplements for, 245–246
Angiography, cerebral, 335–336
Angioplasty, 102, 242–246
Annals of the Rheumatic Diseases, 139
Antacids, 134
Anthocyanosides
  diabetes and, 427
  glaucoma and, 486
Antibiotics, *see also specific types*
  bronchitis and, 296
  candidiasis and, 301–302
  Crohn's diesese and, 589–590
  diarrhea and, 438
  ear infections and, 441–442
  hives and, 538
  role, 7–8
  sinusitis and, 797–798
  sore throat and, 801
Antibodies
  α-1-gliadin assay, 313–314
  B cells and, 147–148

RA and, 771–772
Antigen-antibody complexes, 110
Antioxidants
  AIDS, 202–207
  alcoholism and, 216
  Alzheimer's disease and, 226–228
  asthma and, 267–268
  cardiovasular disease and, 91
  leukoplakia and, 622
  longevity and, 168–169
  male infertility and, 581–583
  Parkinson's disease and, 224–225
  as preservative, 57–58
  RA and, 781
  recommended, 75
  thymus and, 158
  vitamin C as, 93–94
  vitamin E as, 77
Anxiety
  caffeine and, 255
  causes, 252–254
  Chinese ginseng for, 254
  description, 251
  ERPs, 257
  food allergies and, 255
  Hamilton scale, 256
  IBS and, 612
  kava for, 254, 255–258
  lactic acid for, 255
  treatment summary, 259
APDS, *see* Allyl propyl disulphide
Arachidonic acid
  asthma and, 265
  migraines and, 660
  source, 50–51
Arbutin, 289
Arctostaphylos uva ursi, see Uva ursi
Arginine
  herpes simplex and, 521–522
  male infertility and, 584
Arrhythmias
  description, 500–501
  magnesium for, 502–503
Artery, structure, 85–86
Artery bypass surgery, 242–246
Arthritis, *see* Osteoarthritis; Rheumatoid arthritis
Ascorbic acid, *see* Vitamin C
Asians, 325
Asparagus, 120
Aspartame, *see* NutraSweet
Aspartate, 368
Aspirin, see also Nonsteroidal anti-
  inflammatory drugs
  alternatives to, 101
  heart attacks and, 100–101
  hives and, 540
  safety, 100–101
Association for the Study of Dreams, 43
Asthma, *see also* Hayfever
  adrenal gland and, 262
  alliums and, 270
  antioxidants for, 267–268
  botanical and, 269–270

Candida albicans and, 265
carotenes for, 268
description, 260–261
DHEA for, 269
dietary factors, 265–266
flavonoids for, 268
food additives and, 266
ginkgo biloba for, 271
histamines and, 261
hypochlorhydria and, 264–265
Indian tobacco for, 270
leukotrienes and, 261
licorice for, 270
magnesium for, 269
mast cells and, 261
omega-3 for, 266
pyridoxine for, 266–267
salt and, 269
selenium for, 268
treatment summary, 271–272
tryptophan for, 266–267
Tylophora asthmatica and,
       270–271
types, 261
vitamin B12 for, 268–269
vitamin C for, 267–268
vitamin E for, 268
Astragalus membranaceus, see
       Astragalus root
Astragalus root, 160
Atherosclerosis
angina and, 242
description, 85–87
diabetes and, 412
free radicals and, 250
homocysteine levels and, 98
hypoglycemia and, 553
impotence and, 566–569
macular degeneration and,
       624–625
process, 83, 86
Atopic dermatitis, *see* Eczema
Atrial fibrillation, 503–504
Atriplex halimu, see Salt bush
Attention deficit disorders
description, 273–274
Feingold hypothesis, 274–276
food additives, 274–277
food allergies and, 277–278
heavy metals and, 279
with hyperactivity, 273–274
hyproglycemia and, 277
nutrient deficiency and, 279
sugar and, 277
treatment summary, 281
types, 273
without hyperactivity,
       278–279
Awaken the Giant Within, 28
Awareness, 28
Azelaic acid, 197
Azoospermia, 575
AZT, *see* Ziodvudine

B
Bacteria, *see also specific types*
ACP and, 448
beneficial
       CDSA, 131
bladder infection and, 285
hives and, 545
overgrowth, 139–141
pathogenic
       CDSA, 131–132
periodontal disease and, 723
Bacteroides vulgatus, 593
Balneotherapy, 786–787
Barberry, 310
Barnes, Broda, 549
Basics of Food Allergy, 480
Basophils, 147
Bastyr University, 13
B cells, 147–148
Behavior, *see* Lifestyles
Benadryl, 602
Benign prostatic hyperplasia, *see*
       Prostate enlargement
Benson, Herbert, 181
Benzoates
allergies and, 59
hives and, 544
Benzoic acid, 58
Benzoyl peroxide, 193
Berberine
diarrhea and, 437–438
poultices, 293
small-intestinal bacteria and, 140
Berberis aquifolium, see Grapes
Berberis vulgaris, see Barberry
Bereavement, 149
Bernard, Claude, 7
Beta-carotenes
AIDS and, 204–205
cataracts and, 322
cervical dysplasia and, 344
colds and, 374
description, 48
leukoplakia and, 621–622
BH$_4$, *see* Tetrahydrobiopterin
BHA, *see* Butylated hydroxyanisole
BHT, *see* Butylated hydroxytoluene
Bifidobacterium bifidum
candidiasis and, 309
dysbiosis and, 143
GI tract levels, 739
sore throat and, 803
Bilberry
cataracts, 322–323
diabetes and, 427
glaucoma and, 486
Bile
acids, 483
description, 476
detoxification by, 110–111
digestion and, 128
flow, importance, 121–122
salt, 812–813

Biodegradable cleansers, 56
Biofeedback, 662–663
Bioflavonoids, *see* Flavonoids
Biogenic amine model, 378–380
Biotin
diabetes and, 419
seborrheic dermatitis and, 794–795
Bipolar disorder
circadian rhythms, 284
description, 282
lecithin for, 283
SAM and, 394–396
treatment summary, 284
tryptophan for, 283
vanadium for, 283–284
Biskind, Morton, 736
Biskind's theory, 736–737
Bismuth sybsalicylate, *see*
       Pepto-Bismol
Bitter Melon, 425
Black cohosh
menopause and, 639–641
PMS and, 750
Bladder infection
cause, 285
chronic interstitial, 287
description, 285–286
goldenseal for, 289
menopausal, 634–635
therapy goals, 287
treatment summary, 290–291
uva ursi for, 289
Bladderwrack, 333
Blood
CDSA, 133
filtering, 110
flow, 245
lactic acid levels, 253
loss, excessive, 233
pressure, *see* High blood pressure
red cells
       deficient production, 233–234
       destruction, 233
stress and, 177
sugar, 214–215
test, allergy, 470–471
white cells, *see* Mast cells
Bloodroot
doctrine of signature, 171
periodontal disease and, 728
Blue cohosh signature, 171
Body
calming, 180–181
fats, types, 685
physical status, 77–80
weight, 61–62
Bodywork
about, 78–80
cellulite and, 332
CFS and, 368
headaches, 499
osteoarthritis and, 703
RA and, 785–786

Boils
  botanical medicines and, 292–293
  description, 292
  therapy goals, 292
  treatment summary, 294
Boric acid, 823–824
Boswellia serrata, 704
Botanical medicines, *see also specific types*
  description, 5
  immune function and, 159–160
Bowels
  abnormal permeability, 771
  inflamed, *see* Inflammatory bowel disease
  irritable, *see* Irritable bowel syndrome
  retraining, 142
  toxemia, 764–765
Boxer study, 807
BPH, *see* Prostate enlargement
Brain function, 227
Breast disease, 455–458
Breasts feeding
  eczema and, 449
  immune function and, 157–158
Breathing
  CFS and, 368
  diaphragmatic, 182
  proper, 77–78
Breneman, J. S., 480
Bromelain
  AIDS and, 208
  bronchitis and, 297–298
  bursitis and, 807
  CTS and, 318
  gout and, 493–494
  impotence and, 568
  RA and, 784
  sinusitis and, 798
  tendinitis and, 807
  varicose veins and, 829–830
Bronchitis
  botanical medicines, 298
  bromelain and, 297–298
  description, 294
  expectorants, 298
  naturopathic approach, 296–297
  postural draining, 299
Bulimia, 683
Bulking agents, 509, 827
Bupleuri falcatum, *see* Chinese thoroughwax
Bursitis
  bromelain for, 807
  cause, 805
  curcumin for, 807
  description, 805
  flavonoids for, 807
  nutrition and, 806–807
  physical therapy for, 807–808
  RICE for, 805–806
  treatment summary, 808–809
  vitamin B12 for, 807

Butcher's broom, 829
Butylated hydroxyanisole, 57–58, 544
Butylated hydroxytoluene, 57–58, 544
Butyrate, 132
  iso-Butyrate, 131
B vitamins
  canker sores and, 314
  heart disease and, 501
  immune function and, 156
  osteoporosis and, 719
  rosacea and, 791

C

Cabbage, 813–814
Cadmium, 757
Caffeine
  anxiety and, 255
  CFS and, 367
  depression and, 384–385
  FBD and, 455–456
  metabolic rate and, 688–689
  PMS and, 744
  stress and, 184
Caffeinism, 184, 384–385
Caffien
  gallstones and, 491
Calcium
  blood vessel influx, 249
  forms, 717–718
  hypertension and, 532–533
  kidney stones and, 616–617
  osteoporosis and, 707, 715–718
  PMS and, 747
Calcium citrate, 289
Calment, Jeanne Louise, 163–164
Calories
  needs, 61–62
  restriction
    gallstones, 480–481
    longevity, 168
Cancer
  detoxification and, 108–109
  food additives and, 58
  HRT and, 631–632
  pesticides and, 53
Candida albicans
  acne and, 193
  asthma and, 265
  bronchitis and, 295–296
  characteristics, 306–307
  description, 140–141
  dysbiosis and, 143–144
  echinacea and, 160
  eczema and, 450
  eradication, 304–305
  gentian violet and, 824–825
  habitat, 300
  hives and, 545
  IBS and, 612
  overgrowth factors, 301
  vaginitis and, 819, 823
Candid Camera, 149

Candidiasis
  causes, 301–302
  CFS and, 366
  description, 300
  detoxification, 307–308
  diagnosing, 302–304
  dietry factors, 305
  drugs for, 306
  elimination and, 308
  lipotropic factors, 308
  liver damage and, 307–308
  milk thistle for, 308–309
  natural agents, 309–311
  patient profile, 300–301
  questionnaire, 302–304
  related syndromes, 302
  therapy goals, 307
  treatment summary, 311–312
  triggers, 307
Canker sores
  B vitamins for, 314
  description, 313
  DGL for, 315
  gluten sensitivity and, 313–314
  nutrient deficiency and, 314
  quercetin for, 314–315
  stress and, 314
  treatment summary, 315
Caprylic acid, 310
Capsaicin, 768
Capsella bursa pastoris, *see* Shepherd's purse
Capsicum frutescens, *see* Cayenne pepper
Carbohydrates, *see also* Sugar
  complex, 67
  gout and, 493
  hypoglycemia, 554–555
  IBD and, 596
  refined
    stress and, 185
Cardiac risk factor ratios, 347
Cardiomyopathy
  coenzyme Q10, 505
  description, 500
  magnesium and, 504
Cardiovascular disease
  antioxidants for, 91
  cholesterol levels, 90–92
  diabetes and, 91
  dietry factors, 101–102
  earlobe crease and, 102–103
  EFA for, 95–96
  exercise for, 91
  fibrinogen formation, 97–98
  high blood pressure and, 91
  homocysteine levels and, 98
  hypothyroidism and, 560
  magnesium for, 96
  platelet aggregation and, 97
  potassium for, 96
  preventing, 88–90
  proanthocyanidins and, 94–95

risk factors, 87–88
risk scale, 89
smoking and, 88–90
vitamin E for, 91–93
worry and, 99–100
Cardiovascular system
atherosclerosis in, 85–87
description, 83–85
Carnitines, *see also specific types*
AIDS and, 206–207
alcoholism and, 216
angina and, 246–247
diabetes and, 424
heart disease and, 505–506
lipids and, 152
male infertility and, 584
Carob, 435
Carotenes, *see also specific types*
about, 46
asthma and, 268
beta, *see* Beta-carotene
description, 48
immune function and, 154–155
longevity and, 169
macular degeneration and, 625
Carpal tunnel syndrome
acupuncture and, 317
bromelain for, 318
B vitamins for, 316–317
description, 316
stretching for, 318–319
treatment summary, 318
water treatments, 317
Carrageenan, 593
Carrel, Alexis, 164–164
Carson, Rachel, 54
Cartilage, 8
Castille soap, 56
Cataracts
amino acids for, 322
antioxidants for, 322
botanical medicines,
322–323
description, 319
diabetes and, 411
dietary factors, 322
glutathione for, 320
heavy metals and, 322
hydrogen peroxide and, 321
melatonin for, 322
riboflavin for, 321–322
selenium for, 320–321
SOD for, 321
tetrahydrobiopterin for, 321
treatment summary, 324
vitamin C for, 319–320
vitamin E for, 320–321
Caulophyllum thalictroides, see
Blue cohosh
Cayenne pepper, 768
CDSA, see Comprehensive Digestive
Stool Analysis
Celery, 526–527

Celiac disease
associated conditions, 327–328
causes, 326
description, 325
diagnosing, 327
genetic factors, 325
pancreatic enzymes and, 327–328
societies for, 328
treatment summary, 328
Cell-mediated immunity, 146–147
Cellular aging, 166
Cellulite
botanical medicines, 332–333
description, 329–331
exercise for, 332
stages, 331–332
treatment summary, 334
weight loss and, 332
Centella asiatica, see Gotu kola
Centers for Disease Control
CFS criteria, 363–364
CFS definition, 359–360
tryptophan case, 389–390
Cerebral vascular insufficiency
carotid endarterectomy, 336–337
description, 335
diagnosing, 335–336
GAGs and, 337
GBE for, 337–339
treatment summary, 340
Cernilton, 759–760
Cervical dysplasia
beta-carotene for, 344
contraceptives and, 344
description, 340
folic acid for, 345
Pap smears and, 341–342
pyridoxine for, 345–346
risk factors, 342–343
selenium for, 346
sexual activity and, 343
smoking and, 343–344
treatment summary, 346
viruses and, 343
vitamin A for, 344
vitamin C for, 344–345
CFS, *see* Chronic fatigue syndrome
CGI scale, *see* Clinical global impressions
scale
Challenges, facing, 26
Chalmers, Thomas, 373
Chamomile, 767–768
Charantin, 425
Chasteberry
impotence, 572
menopause and, 639
PMS and, 739–740, 750–751
prolactins and, 738
Chediak-Higashi syndrome, 726
Chelation therapy, 249–250, 337
Chemotaxis, 268
Chenodeoxycholic acid, 483
Cherries, 494

CHF, *see* Congestive heart failure
Childers, Norman, 697–698
Children
early aging, 166
food additives and, 542–544
IBD in, 598–600
playing with, 31
vitamin A in, 153–154
Chinese ginseng
anxiety and, 254
impotence and, 572
RA and, 785
stress management by, 186–187
Chinese medicine, 5
Chinese thoroughwax, 785
Chiropractoric care, 498, 661–662
Chlamydia trachomatis
male infertility and, 579
vaginitis and, 822
Chlorophyll
anemia and, 237
menorrhagia and, 646
Cholera, 438
Cholestasis
causes, 122
PMS and, 737
SAM and, 118
Cholesterol, *see also*
Hypercholesterolemia
BPH and, 756
cardiovasular disease and, 90–91
CDSA, 131
description, 347–348
drug therapy, 350–351
elevations, *see* Hypercholesterolemia
gallstones and, 479
garlic for, 355–356
gugulipid and, 356–357
hypertension and, 533
niacin for, 351–354
oxidized, 91
pantethine for, 247, 354
treatment summary, 357–358
types, 52
vitamin C for, 354–355
vitamin E for, 91–93
Cholesterol Lowering Atherosclerosis
Study, 93
Cholinergic urticaria, 538–539
Chondroitin sulfate, 700–701
Chromium
acne and, 194
diabetes and, 407, 416–417
glaucoma and, 487
hypoglycemia and, 556
obesity and, 690–691
Chronic fatigue syndrome
adrenals and, 366–367
candidiasis and, 366
causes, 361–364
CFS and, 365, 365–366
criteria for, 360–361
depression and, 364

Chronic fatigue syndrome, *continued*
  description, 359–360
  dietary factors, 367
  emotions and, 367
  exercise, 368
  fibromyalgia *vs.*, 459–460
  food allergies and, 185, 366
  hypoglycemia and, 366
  hypothyroidism and, 366
  immune system and, 363–364
  licorice for, 368–369
  Siberian ginseng for, 368–369
  stress and, 364
  supplements for, 367–368
  treatment summary, 369–370
Chyme, 127
Chymotrypsin, 130
Cigarette smoking, *see* Smoking
Cimetidine, *see* Tagamet
Cimicifuga racemosa,
    see Black cohosh
Circadian rhythm, 173
Cirrhosis, 215, 218
Citrate, *see* Citric acid
Citric acid, 617
Clark, Norman, 250
Claudication, intermittent, 553
Clinical global impressions scale, 231
Clinical nutrition, 5
CoA, *see* Coenzyme A
Coca Cola, 276
Coenzyme A
  cholesterol and, 354
  pantethine and, 247
Coenzyme Q$_{10}$
  angina and, 246, 247–248
  angiograms and, 245–246
  heart disease and, 504–505
  hypertension and, 533
  obesity and, 693
  periodontal disease and, 727
Coenzymes, 72–73
Coffee, *see* Caffeine
Cognitive therapy, 382
Cola vera, 333
Colchicine, 491–492
Colds, *see* Common cold
Cold urticaria, 539
Colestipol, 93
Coleus forskolii, 451
Collagen
  glaucoma and, 485
  homocysteine levels and, 98
  matrix structure
    about, 725
    flavonoids and, 727
Colon
  characterization, 128–129
  description, 128–129
  FBD and, 457–458
  function, 141
Colony-stimulating factors, 159
Commission E, 355

Common cold, *see also* Sore throat
  beta-carotene for, 374
  description, 371
  echinacea for, 374–375
  liquids for, 372–373
  rest for, 372
  sugar and, 373
  treatment summary, 375–376
  vitamin A for, 374
  vitamin C for, 373
  zinc for, 157
Communication, 183–184
Complement system, 723–724
Comprehensive digestive stool analysis
  application, 129–130
  description, 129–130
  diarrhea, 432
Cone biopsy, 341
Congestive heart failure
  coenzyme Q10, 504–505
  description, 500
  magnesium for, 502–503
  thiamin for, 501
Conners, C. Keith, 275–277
Constipation, 141–142
Contraceptives, 344
Conventional medicine, *see also specific treatments*
  cholesterol regulation and, 350–351
  cost, 10–11
  diabetes and, 408–410
  ear treatment, 440–442
  natural substance use, 15–16
  naturopathy and, 9
  naturopathy *vs.*, 6–8
  paradigm shift, 1–2
Copper, 782
CoQ$_{10}$, *see* Coenzyme Q$_{10}$
Coronary artery bypass, 102
The Coronary drug project, 351–352
Corpus luteum insufficiency, 732
Corticosteroids, 186
Cortisol, 262
Corynebacterium acnes, 192
Counseling, 5–6
Cousin, Norman, 149
Cranberry juice
  bladder infections and, 287–288
  kidney stones and, 618
Crataegus sp., see Hawthorn
Creativity, 22
Crohn's disease
  activity index, 598
  antibiotics and, 589–590
  description, 587
  dietary factors, 590
  food allergies and, 590–591
  intestinal microflora, 593
  mucin defects, 592–594
  occurrence, 588
  placebo therapy, 591–592
  prostaglandins and, 592
Crook, William, 300

CTS, *see* Carpal tunnel syndrome
CT Scan, 223
Curcuma longa, see Curcumin
Curcumin
  AIDS and, 207–208
  bursitis and, 807
  detoxification by, 113–114
  RA and, 783–784
  smokers and, 114
  tendinitis and, 807
Curries, 113
Cyamopsis tetragonoloba, see Indian
    cluster bean
Cyanocobalamin
  absorption, 239
  availability, 238
Cyclo-oxygenase, 765–766
Cysteine
  cataracts and, 322
  detoxification and, 116
  longevity and, 172
Cystic fibrosis, 138
Cystitis, *see* Bladder infection
Cytochrome P450, 111–113
Cytokines, 202

D

Dairy products, *see also specific types*
  candidiasis and, 305
  cataracts and, 322
  diarrhea and, 434–435
  multiple sclerosis and, 667–668
Damiana, 572
DART, *see* Dietary and Reinfarction Trial
DDE, 54
DDT, 54, 108
Dead Sea baths, 786–787
Death
  causes, 163
  pneumonia-related, 294
Decarboxylases
  digestion and, 139
  small-intestinal bacteria and, 140
Deficiency, subclinical, 73–74
Deglycyrrhizinated licorice
  canker sores and, 315
  heartburn and, 135
  Helicobacter pylori and, 137
  indigestion and, 315
  ulcers and, 815–186
7-Dehydrocholesterol, 707–708
Dehydroepiandrosterone
  Alzheimer's disease and, 230–231
  asthma and, 269
  depression and, 383
  longevity and, 172–173
  RA and, 773–774
DeLeon, Ponce, 162
Dement, William C., 41
Dementia
  depression and, 223
  phosphatidylcholine and, 229
Demulcents, 593

Deoxycholic acid, 479–480
Deprenyl, 225
Depression
  alcohol and, 215, 384
  counseling for, 382
  CSF and, 364
  dementia and, 223
  description, 377
  dietary factors, 385–386
  drugs for, 381
  exercise and, 385
  folic acid for, 386–387
  food allergies and, 388
  GBE for, 398–399
  hormonal factors, 382–383
  5-HTP and, 391–392
  IBS and, 612
  kava for, 397–398
  lifestyle factors, 383–386
  manic, *see* Bipolar disorder
  monoamine metabolism and, 389
  omega-3 fatty acids for, 388
  PEA and, 393–394
  phosphatidylserine and, 229
  physical causes, 381–382
  PMS and, 742
  pyridoxine for, 387–388
  SAM and, 394–396
  serotonin and, 380–381
  smoking and, 384
  SSRI drugs for, 391–392
  St. John's wort, 396–397
  sugar and, 385–386
  theories on, 378–381
  thyroid and, 382–383
  toxins and, 383
  treatment summary, 400
  tryptophan and, 389–391
  tyrosine and, 393–394
Dermatitis
  atopic, *see* Eczema
  seborrheic, *see* Seborrheic dermatitis
Dermographism, 538
DES, *see* Diethylstilbestrol
δ-6-Desaturase, 450
Descartes, René, 1, 173
Desferrioxamine, 222
Detachment, 21
Detoxification, *see also* Toxins
  applications, 120
  candidiasis, 307–308
  CFS and, 365
  fasting, 124–125
  nutritional supplementation and,
    122–123
  overview, 103–104
  phase I
    inducers, 112–113
    inhibitors, 113–114
    process, 111–112
  phase II
    acetylation, 119
    amino acid conjugation, 118

    glucuronidation, 119–120
    glutathione conjugation, 113–118
    methylation, 118–119
    process, 113–114
    sulfation, 119
    sulfoxidation, 120
Detoxification system
  bile flow, importance, 121–122
    function, 110–111
  blood filtering, 110
  cancer and, 108–109
  liver as, 108–110
Devil's claw
  gout and, 494–495
  osteoarthritis, 704
DGL, *see* Deglycyrrhizinated licorice
DHA, *see* Docosahexanoic acid
DHEA, *see* Dehydroepiandrosterone
DHGLA, *see* Dihomogamma-linolenic
  acid
DHT, *see* Dihydrotestosterone
Diabetes mellitus
  alliums for, 424–425
  bilberry for, 427
  biotin for, 419
  bitter melon for, 425
  botanical medicines, 424
  B vitamins for, 419–420
  cardiovasular disease and, 91
  carnitine for, 424
  causes, 405–410
  chromium for, 407, 416–417
  complications, 410–413
  description, 401
  diagnosing, 404–405
  dietary factors, 413–416
  dietary fat and, 406
  EFA for, 422–424
  epicatechin plants, 427
  epidemiology, 403
  exercise for, 428
  fenugreek for, 426–427
  flavonoids for, 422
  GBE for, 427–428
  ginseng and, 422
  GLA and, 422
  glycemic index, 415
  Gymnema sylvestre and, 425–426
  hypoglycemia link, 403–404
  immune system and, 406
  impotence and, 567
  inositol for, 424
  magnesium for, 420–421
  manganese for, 421
  monitoring, 408
  obesity and, 406
  potassium for, 421
  prenatal factors, 407–408
  Pterocarpus marsupium and, 427
  salt bush for, 426–427
  treatment summary, 429–430
  types, 401–402
  virus and, 406

  vitamin C for, 417–418
  vitamin E for, 420
  zinc for, 421–422
Diamine oxidase, 658
Diaphragmatic breathing, 182
Diarrhea
  antibiotic-associated, 438
  berberine for, 437–438
  carob for, 435
  causes, 432
  dairy products and, 434–435
  description, 431
  diagnosing, 432
  food allergies and, 435
  general support for, 434–435
  kaolin for, 435
  Lactobacillus acidophilus for, 435, 438
  lactose and, 435–436
  parasites and, 436–437
  pectin for, 435
  treatment summary, 439
  types, 431
  water and, 434
Diazepam, *see* Valium
Dietary and Reinfarction Trial, 101–102
Dietary fats, *see also specific types*
  cellulite, 329–334
  description, 68
  diabetes and, 406
  fecal, 131
  food content, 50
  gout and, 493
  hydrogenation, 52
  intake, 49–53
  male infertility, 583
  meat content, 45
  PMS and, 743
  proteins and, 493
  RA and, 778–779
Dietary fiber
  candidiasis and, 308
  constipation and, 142
  description, 46
  diabetes and, 414–415
  digestion and, 129
  FBD and, 457
  food content, 47–48
  gallstones and, 479–480
  hemorrhoids and, 508–509
  hypoglycemia and, 555
  IBD and, 596
  IBS and, 610
  obesity and, 689–690
  psoriasis and, 765
  ulcers and, 813
  varicose veins and, 827
Diethylstilbestrol, 580
Diets, *see also* Foods
  acne care, 193–196
  ADA, 415
  anemia, 237
  arthritis, 776–777
  BPH and, 755

Diets, *continued*
    caloric need, 61–62
    candidiasis, 305
    cataracts and, 322
    cellulite, 332
    CFS, 367
    cholesterol levels and, 349–350
    Crohn's diesese and, 590
    depression, 385–386
    diabetes, 413–416
    EFA levels, 95–96
    elemination, *see* Elimination diet
    fat intake
        from meats, 45
        reducing, 49–53
    fiber intake
        constipation and, 142
        digestion, 129
        importance, 46
    French paradox, 92, 94
    gallstones, 479–480
    gastrointestinal tract and, 44–45
    glutathione in, 116–117
    gout, 492–493
    healthy exchange system, 62–70
    healthy heart, 85, 101, 245
    hemorrhoids and, 508–509
    herbicides in, 53–56
    hypertension and, 525–527
    hypoglycemia, 553–554
    immune function and, 150
    kidney stones and, 616–617
    liver and, 122
    low-purine, 492
    magnesium levels, 96
    menopause and, 636
    migraines, 656–657
    multiple sclerosis and, 667–668
    osteoarthritis, 697–698
    pesticides in, 53–56
    plant-based
        components, 45–46, 48–49
        importance, 44–45
    PMS, 742–743
    potassium intake
        heart disease and, 96
        sodium *vs.*, 58–60
    rotary diversified, 471–474
    salt intake, 58–60
    stress and, 184
    sugar intake, 53
    Swank, 670–671
    vaginitis, 822
    vegetarian, *see* Vegetarianism
    water in, 60
Digestion, see also Gastrointestinal tract;
    Indigestion
    bacterial overgrowth, 139–141
    biliary system, 128
    candidiasis and, 305–306
    evaluating, 129–133
    fiber and, 129
    liver, 128

    MS and, 674
    pancreas, 127–128
    pancreatic insufficiency, 137–138
    process, 126–127
    RA and, 778
    secretions, 177
    stress and, 133–134
Dihomogamma-linolenic acid, 51
Dihydrotestosterone, 192, 195
Diosgenin, 740
Diseases, chronic, 11–12
Disodium cromoglycate, 314
Diverticular disease, 142–143
DNA
    damage, 580
    HIV and, 200
    mutations, 167–168
    repair, 167–168
    telomere-shortening, 166–167
    zinc and, 228–229
Docosahexaenoic acid
    asthma and, 266
    eczema and, 450–451
Doctrine of signature, 171
Dong quai
    menopause, 639
    PMS and, 749
Dopamine, 259
Dowd, 277
Downs' syndrome, 223–224
Dreams
    importance, 41
    interpretation, 42
    recall techniques, 42–43
    resources, 43
    views of, 41–42
Drugs, *see also specific types*
    BPH and, 757
    cholesterol lowering, 350–352
    gallstones, 478
    hives and, 539–540, 542
    impotence and, 566–568
Duesberg, Peter, 199–200
Duffy, William, 549
Duodenum, 127
Dysbiosis
    description, 143–144
index, 133
Dysplasia, *see* Cervical dysplasia
Dysthymia, 377

E
Ear infections
    antibiotics for, 440–441
    bottle feeding and, 443
    causes, 442–443
    conventional treatment, 440–442
    description, 440
    food allergies and, 443–445
    humidifiers for, 445
    surgery for, 440–441
    thymus gland and, 445
    treatment summary, 446–447

Earlobe crease, 102–103
EBV, *see,*Epstein-Barr virus
Echinacea
    AIDS and, 202
    colds and, 374–375
    immune function and, 159–160
    sore throat and, 802–803
Echinacea angustifolia, *see* Echinacea
Echinacea purpurea, *see* Echinacea
Ecuador, Vilcabamba, 163
Eczema
    Candida albicans and, 450
    description, 448–449
    food allergies and, 449
    licorice for, 451–452
    treatment summary, 452–453
    zinc for, 451
Edison, Thomas, 16
EDTA, *see* Ethylenediaminetetraacetic
    acid
Education, *see* Training
EEG, *see* Electroencephalogram
EFA, *see* Essential Fatty Acids
Egger, 278
Eggs, 69
Eicosapentaenoic acid
    about, 51–52
    asthma and, 266
    eczema and, 450–451
    gout and, 493
Ein Gedi Spa, 786
Einstein, Albert, 1
Ejection fraction, 244, 501
Electroencephalogram, 223
Electrolytes, 434–435
Eleutherococus senticosus, see Siberian
    ginseng
Elimination
    bowel retraining, 142
    candidiasis, 308
    constipation, 141–142
    dysbiosis, 143–144
    IBS and, 143
    parasites and, 144
Elimination diet
    asthma and, 264
    food allergies, 469–470
    hives and, 546
    IBD, 595–596
Ellis, John, 316
Emotions, *see* Moods
Empathy, 21
EMS, *see* Eosinophilia-myalgia syndrome
Endarterectomy, 336–337
Endometrium, 645
Endorphins
    estrogen and, 737–738
    menopause and, 635
    mood and, 36
Endotoxins, 110
English, 235
Environmental Protection Agency,
    54–55

Enzymes, *see also specific types*
co-, 72–73
glycosylation and, 168
supplementation, 72–73
Eosinophilia-myalgia syndrome, 389–390
Eosinophils
function, 147
tryptophan and, 389
EPA, see Eicosapentaenoic acid; Environmental Protection Agency
Ephedrine, 688–689
Epinephrine, 262
Epstein-Barr virus
CFS and, 361–362
RA link, 772–773
Erectile dysfunction, *see* Impotence
Ergotamine, 655–656
ERP, *see* Event-related potentials
Escherichia coli, 285–286, 288
Essential fatty acids, *see also specific types*
alcoholism and, 217
BPH and, 756
Crohn's disease and, 592
diabetes and, 422
dietary levels, 95–96
eczema and, 450–451
menorrhagia and, 647
migraines and, 660
in plants, 49–51
prostaglandins in, 50
RA and, 778–81
supplements, 77
in wild meat, 45
Estrogen
aldosterone and, 738
Alzheimer's disease and, 226
endorphins and, 737–738
fibroids and, 738
in food, 743–744
liver and, 736–737
male infertility and, 579–580
neurotransmitters and, 737
PMS and, 736–741
–progesterone ratio, 738–741
prolactins and, 738
pyridoxine and, 738
Ethics, 22
Ethylenediaminetetraacetic acid, 249–250
Ethylenediaminetetra acetic acid, 383
European Cooperative Crohn's Disease Study, 592
Europeans, 325
Evening primrose, 672
Event-related potentials, 257
Exercise
alcoholics and, 217–218
cardiovasular disease and, 91
cellulite and, 332
CFS and, 368
CTS and, 318–319
depression and, 385

description, 36–37
diabetes and, 428, 430
fasting and, 125
hypoglycemia and, 557
hypothyroidism and, 562
IBS and, 612
importance, 35–36
impotence and, 570
insomnia and, 605
longevity and, 37–38, 168
menopause and, 642–643
mood and, 36–37
MS and, 675–676
osteoarthritis and, 703
osteoporosis, 711, 713
PMS and, 741
routine, creating, 38–40
stress and, 184
varicose veins and, 827
Exhaustion, 178
Expectorants, herbal, 298

F
Fasting
detoxification by, 124–125
exercise and, 125
immune function and, 152
psoriasis and, 766
RA and, 776–777
sleep in, 125
Fats, *see* Dietary fats
Fatty acid chains, 131–132
FBD, *see* Fibrocystic breast disease
FDA, *see* Food and Drug Administration
Feces, 131, 133
Feingold, Benjamin, 58, 274–276
Feingold hypothesis, 58, 274–276
Feldene, *see* Piroxicam
Feldenkrais Guild, 80
Feldenkrais technique, 80
Feminine Forever, 629
Fenclonine, 461
Fenugreek, 426–427
Ferritin, 607
Ferulic acid, 638
Feverfew, 663–664
Fiber, *see* Dietary fiber
Fibrinogen formation, 97–98
Fibroblasts, 164–166
Fibrocystic breast disease
B vitamins and, 457
caffeine and, 455–456
colon and, 457–458
description, 455
iodine, 456–457
liver and, 457
methylxanthines and, 455–456
thyroid and, 456–457
treatment summary, 458
vitamin A and, 456
vitamin E and, 456
Fibroids, uterine, 738

Fibromyalgia
CFS and, 363–364
CFS *vs.*, 459–460
description, 459
5-HTP and, 461–462
magnesium and, 462
sleep and, 460–461
St. John's wort and, 462
treatment summary, 463
Fibrosis, 457
Fight-or-flight response, 176–177
Fingerprints, 223–224
Fish oil
diabetes, 423–424
gallstones and, 482
MS and, 672
Flavonoids
asthma and, 268
bursitis and, 807
diabetes and, 422
dietary sources, 48–49
eczema and, 451
glaucoma and, 486–487
heart benefits, 94–95
longevity and, 170
macular degeneration and, 625–627
menorrhagia and, 646
periodontal disease and, 727–728
tendinitis and, 807
ulcers and, 814–815
varicose veins and, 829
Flaxseed oil
agoraphobia and, 255
benefits, 75, 77
diabetes and, 424
dressing with, 77
eczema and, 451
hypertension and, 533–534
MS and, 672
RA and, 780
Fluids, *see* Juices; Water
Fluoride, 720
FM, *see* Fibromyalgia
Folic acid
anemia and, 236
cervical dysplasia and, 345
–deficiency anemia, 240
depression and, 386–387
gout and, 493
IBD and, 597–598
immune function and, 156
osteoporosis and, 719
periodontal disease and, 728
restless-legs syndrome and, 607
seborrheic dermatitis and, 795
Folkers, Karl, 316
Follicle-stimulating hormone, 580, 628
Food additives
about, 56–58
ADD and, 274–277
asthma and, 266
Feingold hypothesis, 58
hypoglycema and, 542–544

Food allergies
ADD and, 277–278
anxiety and, 255
asthma and, 264
bladder infection and, 287
candidiasis and, 305
causes, 465–466
CFS and, 366
Crohn's diesese and, 590–591
depression and, 388
description, 464–465
diagnosing, 469–470
diarrhea and, 435
ear infections and, 443–445
eczema and, 449
elimination diets, 469–470
gallstones and, 480
glaucoma and, 487
hives and, 542
IBS and, 610
immune system and, 467–469
migraines and, 655–656
MS and, 671
pancreatin and, 138–139
psoriasis and, 766
RA and, 776–777
seborrheic dermatitis and, 794
sore throat and, 803
stress and, 185, 466–467
sugar, 53
testing for, 470–471
treatment summary, 475
types, 467–469
ulcers and, 813
Food and Drug Administration
additive approval, 57
cholesterol-lowering drugs, 350–351
folic acid, 607
food dyes, 275
pesticide monitoring, 54–55
potassium supplements, 530
preservatives, 58
sulfur approval, 197
thyroid extracts, 562
wax approval, 55
yohimbe classification, 571
Food challenge testing, 469
Foods, *see also* Diets; *specific types*
allergies, *see* Food allergies
dyes, 261, 274–277
estrogens in, 743–744
fat content, 50
fermented, 238
fiber content, 47–48
glutathione rich, 118
healthy exchange system, 65–70
junk, 234
mold containing, 305
organic, 56
pesticide residue, 54
phase I detoxification, 112–113
phyoesterogen containing, 636–637
potassium content, 59

prepared, 528
preservatives in
about, 58
hives and, 542
protein-rich, 118
salt content, 59
smoke meats, diabetes and, 406
solid, diarrhea and, 434
sugar content, 53
taxonomic list, 472–473
toxins in, 53–55
waxes, 55–56
yeast containing, 305
Foot ulcers, diabetic, 413
Frame size, 61–62
Framingham Osteoarthritis Cohort
Study, 698
France, Anatole, 30
Free radicals
aging theory
antioxidants role, 168
description, 167–168
alcohol and, 216
atherosclerosis and, 250
cytochrome P450 and, 111–112
description, 75
scavengers, *see* Antioxidants
French paradox, 92, 94
Freud, Sigmund, 41
Friendliness, 22
Fructose, *see* Fruits
Fruits
description, 66–67
diabetes and, 415–416
hypoglycemia and, 553–554
macular degeneration and, 625–626
taxonomic list, 472
FSH, *see* Follicle-stimulating hormone
Fucus vesiculosus, see Bladderwrack
Fumaric acid, 767
Furosemide, 501
Furuncles, *see* Boils
Futcher, Bruce, 166

G

GAGs, *see* Glycosaminoglycans
Gallstones
aging and, 478
bile acids and, 483
bile flow and, 121
caloric restriction, 480–481
causes, 476–477
chemical dissolution, 482–483
choleretics and, 482
coffee and, 481
description, 476
dietary factors, 479–480
drugs and, 478
fish oils and, 482
foods allergies and, 480
GI tract and, 478
lecithin and, 481

lipotropic factors and, 482
obesity and, 477–478
olive oil and, 481
risk factors, 477, 478–479
silent, 479
sugar and, 480
sunbathing and, 483
terpenes, 483
treatment summary, 483–484
types, 476
vitamin deficiency and, 481
Garcinia cambogia, see Malabar
Gardnerella vaginalis, 820
Garlic
asthma and, 270
candidiasis and, 310–311
cholesterol and, 355
commercial, 355–356
diabetes and, 424–425
hypertension and, 527, 534
platelet aggregation and, 97
Gastric acid, 810–811
Gastrointestinal tract, see also Bowels;
Digestion
aspirin and, 100
dietary factors, 44–45
diseases, 478
flora levels, maintaining, 739
intestinal motility, 540
microbial flora, 612
RA and, 777–778
microflora in, 593
stomach acid, 707
Gastrointestinal tract
microflora in, 215
small intestines, 139–140, 771
GBE, *see* Ginkgo biloba
Gemfibrozil, 353
Gender differences
gallstone development, 477
skin, 331
General adaption syndrome,
176–178, 187
General Foods, 276
General tonic effects, *see* Adaptogen
Genes
celiac disease and, 325
diabetes, 405
gallstones and, 477
IBD and, 589
long terminal repeat, 207
RA and, 770–771
Gentian violet
Candida albicans and, 824–825
vaginitis and, 824–825
Germ theory, 7
Gerontology, 164
Giardia, 437
Gilbert's syndrome, 119–120
Gilligan's Island, 31
Ginger
migraines and, 664
morning sickness and, 678

RA and, 784
sore throat and, 803
Gingival sulcus, 723
Ginkgo biloba
    Alzheimer's disease and, 231–232
    asthma and, 268, 271
    depression and, 398–399
    doctrine of signature, 171
    glaucoma and, 487–488
    impotence and, 572
    longevity and, 170–172
    menopause and, 641–642
    MS and, 674
    vascular insufficiency and, 337–339
Ginseng, *see also* Chinese ginseng;
        Siberian ginseng
    diabetes and, 422
    doctrine of signature, 171
    male infertility, 584–585
    stress and, 186–187
GLA, *see* Gamma-Linolenic acid
Glands, *see specific types*
Glaucoma
    chromium for, 487
    description, 485
    EFAs and, 487
    flavonoids and, 486–487
    food allergies and, 487
    Ginkgo biloba for, 487–488
    magnesium for, 487
    treatment summary, 488
    vitamin C for, 486
α-1-Gliadin antibody assay, 313–314
Gliadins, 325–326
Glucocorticoids, adrenal, 178
Glucokinase, 419
Glucosamine sulfate
    osteoarthritis and, 698–700
    as osteoarthritis treatment, 9
Glucose, *see also* Sugar
    anxiety and, 253–254
    insulin and, 548
    skin levels, 194
Glucose-insulin tolerance test, 404–405, 549
Glucose tolerance factor, 407, 556
Glucose tolerance test, 404, 549
β-Glucuronidase
    GI flora and, 739
β-Glucuronidase
    CDSA, 132
Glucuronidation, 119–120
Glutamic acid, 617
Glutamine, 217
Glutathione
    AIDS and, 203–204
    cataracts and, 320
    conjugation, 115–118
    detoxification by, 112
    liver function and, 123–124
    longevity and, 172
Glutathione peroxidase
    acne and, 196
    asthma and, 268

MS and, 668–669, 672–673
    selenium-dependent, 205
Gluten
    opioid activity, 326
    sensitivity, 313–314, 325
Gluten Tolerance Group of North
        America, 328
Glycemic index, 415, 555
Glycine, 374
Glycoasminoglycans,
    700–701
Glycogen, 528
Glycosaminoglycans
    aortic, 85–87, 337
    blood flow and, 246
    botanicals for, 510
    cardiovascular disease and, 102
    cellulite and, 333
    hemorrhoids and, 510
    NSAIDs and, 8–9
Glycosylation, 168
Glycyrrhetinic acid
    asthma, 270
    eczema and, 452
    psoriasis and, 767–768
Glycyrrhiza glabra, *see* Licorice
GMP, *see* Guanidine monophosphate
Goal setting, 29–30
Goblet cells, 592
Goiters, 559
Goldenseal
    bladder infection and, 289
    candidiasis and, 310
    doctrine of signature, 171
    poultices, 293
    sore throat and, 802–803
Gonorrhea, 820, 822
Gossypol, 583
Gotu kola
    bladder infection and, 287
    cellulite and, 333
    periodontal disease, 728
    varicose veins and, 828
Gout
    alcohol and, 491–492
    amino acids for, 494
    bromelain for, 493–494
    carbohydrates and, 493
    causes, 490–491
    cherries for, 494
    colchicine for, 491–492
    description, 489–490
    devil's claw for, 494–495
    EPA for, 493
    fats and, 493
    fluid intake, 493
    folic acid for, 493
    kidneys and, 491
    lead and, 495
    niacin for, 494
    obesity and, 491–492
    quercetin for, 494
    treatment summary, 496

vitamin C for, 494
vitamin E for, 493
Grains
    description, 67
    proteins, chemistry, 325–326
Grapes
    candidiasis and, 310
    seed extract
        about, 94–95
        cataracts and, 323
Gravel root, 618
Greider, Carol, 166
GSH, *see* Glutathione
Guanidine monophosphate, 763–764
Gugulipid, 356–357
Gymnema sylvestre
    diabetes and, 425–426

H
Habits, 3
Hachimijiogan, 323
Haemophilus vaginalis, *see* Gardnerella
        vaginalis
Hair
    analysis, 107
    hypothyroidism and, 560
Halogenated hydrocarbons, 54
Hamilton, William, 171
Hamilton anxiety scale, 256
Harley, Cal, 166
Harmine, 607
Harpagophytum procumbens, *see*
        Devil's claw
Harvard Alumni Health Study, 37–38
Harvard Medical School
    curcumin study, 207
    ginkgo biloba study, 231
Hawking, Stephen, 1
Hawthorn
    angina and, 248–249
    heart disease and, 506
    hypertension and, 534
Hayfever, *see also* Asthma
    causes, 261–262
    description, 260–261
Hayflick, Leonard, 165
Hayflick limit, 164–166
HDL, *see* High-density lipoproteins
Headaches, *see also* Migraines
    bodywork for, 499
    description, 497
    diagnosing, 497
    menopausal, 634
    treatment summary, 499
    triggers, 497
Healing force, 3
Health care cost, 10–11
Healthy exchange system
    cheese list, 69–70
    constructing, 62–63
    fats list, 68–69
    fruit list, 66–67
    grain list, 67–68

Healthy exchange system, *continued*
  legume list, 68
  meat list, 69–70
  menu planning, 65
  milk list, 69
  recommendations, 63–64
  seafood list, 69–70
  vegetable list, 65–66
Heart attacks
  aspirin and, 100–101
  description, 84, 96–96
  recurrent, 100
Heartburn, *see* Indigestion
Heart disease, *see also specific types*
  carnitine for, 505–506
  coenzyme Q and, 504–505
  description, 499
  diagnosing, 500
  hawthorn for, 506
  thiamin for, 501–502
  treatment summary, 506
  types, 499–500
Heavy metals
  ADD and, 279
  cataracts and, 322
  description, 105–106
  male infertility and, 581
Heidelberg gastric analysis, 135–136
  Helicobacter pylori
  hypochlorhydria and, 136–137
  Pepto-Bismol and, 814
  sinusitis and, 798
  ulcers and, 811, 814
Hellerwork, 79
Hemoglobin
  glycosylated, 408
  iron absorption, 237–238
Hemolysis, 468
Hemorrhoids
  bulking agents for, 509
  causes, 507
  description, 507
  diagnosing, 508
  fiber for, 508–509
  flavonoids for, 510
  GAGs for, 510–511
  hydrotherapy for, 509
  topical therapy, 509–510
  treatment summary, 510–511
  types, 507–508
HEPA filters, 798
Hepatitis
  description, 512
  diagnosing, 512–513
  dietary factors, 514–515
  licorice for, 516–517
  liver extracts for, 515–516
  milk thistle for, 517–518
  Phyllanthus amarus for, 518
  prevention, 514
  thymus extracts for, 516
  treatment summary, 519
  vitamin C for, 515

HER, *see* Hydroxyethylrutosides
Herbal detoxification, 113
Herbicides, 53–54
Herpes simplex
  arginine and, 521–522
  cervical dysplasia and, 343
  CFS and, 361–362
  creams for, 522
  description, 520
  licorice for, 522
  lysine for, 521–522
  treatment summary, 523
  vitamin C for, 521
  zinc for, 157, 521
Herxheimer reaction, 309–310
Hesperidin, 638
Hierarchy of needs, 20
High blood pressure
  alliums and, 527
  calcium for, 532–533
  coenzyme Q and, 533
  description, 524
  dietary factors, 525–528
  EFAs and, 533–534
  garlic for, 534
  hawthorn for, 534
  licorice for, 369
  lifestyle factors, 525–527
  potassium and, 527–530
  as risk factor, 91
  stress and, 531–532
  treatment summary, 534–535
  vitamin C for, 532
High-density lipoproteins
  atherosclerosis and, 86
  garlic and, 356
  gugulipid and, 357
  LDL *vs.*, 90–91
  levels, 349
  trans fatty acids and, 52
  vitamin C and, 354
  vitamin E and, 91–93
Hippocrates
  medicinal food, 44
  milk, 464
Hippuric acid, 287
Histamines
  asthma and, 261
  eczema and, 448
  inhibition, 451
  lesions and, 536
  ulcers and, 814–815
  vitamin C and, 268
HIV, *see* AIDS
Hives
  antibiotics and, 540
  aspirin and, 540
  bacterial factors, 545
  Candida albicans and, 545
  causes, 536–539
  clinical aspects, 537
  description, 536
  food additives and, 542–545

  hydrochloric acid for, 542
  infections and, 545
  quercetin for, 546–547
  stress and, 545–546
  thyroid gland and, 547
  treatment summary, 547
  types, 536–537
  UV therapy for, 546
  viruses and, 545
  vitamin B12 for, 546
  vitamin C for, 546
HIV integrase, 207
Hoffer, Abram, 782–783
Homeopathy, 5
Homocysteine
  cardiovascular disease and, 98
  osteoporosis and, 719
Honolulu heart study, 529–530
Hope for Hypoglycemia, 549
Hormone replacement therapy
  Alzheimer's disease and, 226
  benefits, 630–631
  cancer and, 631–632
  evaluation, 630
  osteoporosis and, 711
  side effects, 632
  types, 632–633
Hormones, *see also specific types*
  BPH and, 754–755
  depression and, 382–383
  menstrual cycle and, 731–733
  osteoarthritis and, 697
  osteoporosis and, 707, 709–710
Horse chestnut
  cellulite and, 333
  varicose veins and, 828
Hot flashes, 634–635
HPV, *see* Human papillomavirus
HRT, *see* Hormone replacement therapy
Human immunodeficiency virus,
  see HIV
Human papillomavirus, 343, 345
Humidifiers, 445
Humor, *see* Laughter
Hutchinsom-Gilford syndrome,
  166–167
Hyaluronidase, 160
Hydrastis canadensis, see Goldenseal
Hydrocarbons
  halogenated, 54
  polycyclic, 108
Hydrochloric acid
  anemia and, 237
  candidiasis and, 305–306
  digestion and, 136
  hives and, 542
Hydrogenation, 52
Hydrogen peroxide, 321
Hydrotherapy
  description, 5
  hemorrhoids and, 509
Hydroxycitrate, 692–693
Hydroxyethylrutosides, 510

5-Hydroxyindoleacetic acid
asthma and, 266
migraines and, 651–652
5-Hydroxytryptophan
bipolar disorder and, 282
depression and, 391–393
fibromyalgia and, 461–462
insomnia and, 605–606
migraines and, 659–660
obesity and, 686–688
Hyperactivity, 273–274, 278–279
Hypercholesterolemia, 348–349
Hypericum perforatum, see St. John's
wort
Hyperimmune globulin, 514
Hyperosmolar syndrome, non-
ketogenic, 411
Hyperplasia, prostatic, *see* Prostate
enlargement
Hypertension, *see* High blood pressure
Hypertension in the Elderly Trial, 525
Hypnosis, 34
Hypochlorhydria
asthma and, 264–265
cause, 136–137
description, 135–136
food allergies and, 138
supplements for, 136
Hypoglycemia
ADD and, 277
adrenal glucocorticoid and, 178
aggression and, 551–552
alcohol and, 556–557
alcoholism and, 214–215
cardiovascular disease and, 553
CFS and, 366
chromium for, 556
consequences, 550–551
description, 548
diabetes link, 403–404, 410–411
diagnosing, 548–549
dietary factors, 553–554
exercise for, 557
fiber for, 556
glycemic Index, 555
history, 549–550
insomnia and, 603–604
migraines and, 552–553
PMS and, 552
treatment summary, 557
types, 548
Hypothalamus, 635
Hypothyroidism
acne and, 196
causes, 559
depression and, 382–383
description, 558–559
diagnosing, 560–561
exercise for, 562
impotence and, 567
iodine for, 562
related conditions, 560
supplements for, 562

treatment summary, 563
types, 559–560
tyrosine for, 562

I

IBD, *see* Inflammatory bowel disease
IBS, *see* Irritable bowel syndrome
Idiopathic thrombocytic purpurea, 159
Ileum, 127
Immune system
alcohol and, 152–153
Astragalus membranaceus
and, 160
botanicals and, 159–160
breast-feeding and, 157–158
B vitamins and, 156
candidiasis and, 306–307
carotenes and, 154–155
CFS and, 363–364, 365–366
cholera and, 7
components, 145–148
diabetes and, 406–407
echinacea and, 159–160
emotions and, 149
fatty acids and, 671–672
folic acid and, 156
food allergies and, 467–469
functions, 145
IBD and, 590
iron and, 156
lifestyle factors, 150
lipids and, 152
microbial compounds and, 107
multiple sclerosis and, 667
obesity and, 152
proteins and, 151
RA and, 771–772
selenium and, 157
spleen extracts and, 159
stress and, 149–150
sugar and, 151–152
supporting, 148–149
thymus extracts and, 158–159
treatment summary, 161
vitamin A and, 153–154
vitamin C and, 155
vitamin E and, 155–156
zinc and, 156–157
Immunity, cell-mediated, 146–147
Immunizations, 260–261
Immunoglobulins
IgA
allergies and, 466–467
CDSA, 133
semen and, 585
small-intestinal bacteria and, 140
IgE
asthma and, 261, 264, 265
food allergies and, 464
periodontal disease and, 724
IgM
asthma and, 265
levels, testing, 470–471

Impotence
alcohol and, 567
atherosclerosis and, 566–568, 568–569
causes, 565–566
chasteberry for, 572
Chinese ginseng for, 572
damiana for, 572
description, 564
diagnosing, 566–568
drugs and, 567
exercise for, 570
Ginkgo biloba for, 572
penile prosthesis, 570
potency wood for, 571–572
psychotherapy for, 569
smoking and, 567
treatment summary, 573–574
vacuum constrictive devices, 569–570
yohimbe for, 571
Indian cluster bean, 689
Indian tobacco, 270
Indigestion, *see also* Digestion
description, 134
food allergies and, 138–139
hypochlorhydria, 135–137
treatments, 134–135
Indole-3-carbinol, 113
Infants, 443, 449
Infection equation, 7
Infections
hives and, 545
IBD and, 587
infertility and, 579
Infertility, *see* Male infertility
Inflammatory bowel disease, *see also*
Crohn's disease; Ulcerative colitis
carbohydrates and, 596
complications, 594
elementation diet, 595–596
emergency status, 600
fiber and, 596
folic acid for, 597–598
genetic link, 589
infections and, 587
monitoring, 598–600
nutritional impact, 594–595
pancreatic extracts for, 598
Robert's formula, 598
supplements for, 596–597
treatment summary, 600
vitamin B12 for, 597–598
vitamin C for, 597
vitamin E for, 597
zinc for, 597–598
Inositol hexaniacinate
cholesterol and, 569
diabetes and, 419, 424
Insomnia, *see also* Sleep
description, 602
dietary factors, 603
exercise for, 605
hypoglycemia and, 603–604
melatonin for, 606

Insomnia, *continued*
  myoclonus and, 606–607
  passionflower for, 607
  progressive relaxation for, 604–605
  restless-legs syndrome and,
    606–607
  sedatives for, 605
  serotonin therapy, 605–606
  sleeping pills for, 602
  stimulants and, 603
  treatment summary, 608
  types, 602–603
  valerian and, 607–608
Institute of Sexology, 571
Insulin
  acne and, 194
  chromium and, 691
  diabetes and, 408–409
  diabetes mellitus, 401–402
  fat burning and, 685
  glucose levels and, 548
  obesity and, 684
α-Interferon, 674
Interpersonal relationship
model, 378
Intrinsic factor, 235
Iodine
  FBD and, 456–457
  hypothyroidism and, 562
  vaginitis and, 823
Ipriflavone, 720
Irish
  anemia and, 235
  celiac diesase and, 325
Iron
  deficiency
    ADD and, 279
    diet and, 234–235
    nutritional support, 237
  forms, 237–238
  immune function and, 156
  menorrhagia and,
    645–446
Irritable bowel syndrome
  description, 143, 609
  diagnosing, 609–610
  digestion and, 143
  fiber and, 610
  food allergies and, 610
  psychological factors, 612
  sugar and, 611
  treatment summary, 613
  volatile oils and, 611–612
ITP, *see* Idiopathic thrombocytic
    purpurea
Ivory soap, 56

J
JAMA, *see Journal of the American
    Medical Association*
Japanese, 668
Jejunum, 127

Jenkins, David, 415
Joint Food and Agriculture
    Organization, 58
*Journal of the American College of
    Nutrition*, 373
*Journal of the American Medical
    Association*
  cholesterol-lowering drugs, 350
  CTS reports, 317
  hypertension, 525
  hypoglycemia, 549
  myringotomy, 441
  niacin toxicity, 353
  vitamin B12 administration, 239
Juices
  common cold and, 372–373
  cranberry, 287–288, 618
  fast, 124
  gout and, 493
  urine flow and, 287
Jung, Carl, 41–42

K
Kani, 257–258
Kaolin, 435
Kaufman, William, 782–783
Kava
  anxiety and, 254, 255–258
  benefits, 256–257
  depression and, 397–398
  side effects, 259–260
Kavain, 255–257
Kellogg, John, 3
Kellogg, William, 3
Keratin, 191–192
Ketoacidosis, diabetic, 411
Khella
  angina and, 249
  kidney stones, 618
Kidneys
  failure, EDTA and, 250
  gout and, 491
Kidney stones
  Aloe vera and, 618
  calcium and, 616
  citric acid and, 617
  description, 614
  diagnosing, 614, 616
  dietary factors, 616–617
  glutamic acid and, 617
  khella for, 618
  magnesium for, 617
  pyridoxine for, 617
  senna for, 618
  sodium and, 618
  treatment summary, 619–620
  uric acid and, 618
  vitamin C for, 618
  vitamin K for, 617
Kindness, 22
Kinsbourne, 275–276
Kneipp, Father Sebastian, 2
Kool-Aid study, 384–385

Krebs cycle
  aspartate in, 368
  magnesium in, 531
  osteoporosis and, 718
Kupperman menopausal index, 640

L
LAC, *see* L-Acetylcarnitine
Lactase, 434
Lactate, *see* Lactic acid
Lactic acid
  anxiety and, 253–254
  level reduction, 255
  pyruvic acid and, 255
Lactobacillus acidophilus
  bladder infection and, 286–287
  candidiasis and, 309
  diarrhea and, 435, 438
  dysbiosis and, 143
  GI tract levels, 739
  IBS and, 612
  sore throat and, 803
  vaginitis and, 822–823
Lactose intolerance, 435–436
The Lancet, 279–280
Langseth, 277
Laughter, 30–31
Laxatives, 142
LDL, *see* Low-density lipoproteins
Lead, 495
Leaky gut syndrome
  asthma, 264–265
  bacterial overgrowth, 139
  eczema and, 449
Learned helplessness model, 378–380
Learning disabilities, 278–279
Lecithin
  Alzheimer's disease and, 229
  bipolar disorder and, 283
  gallstones and, 481
Legumes, 68
Lemon balm, 522
Lequesne index, 699
Lesions, 536
Leukoplakia
  antioxidants for, 622
  beta-carotenes and, 621–622
  description, 621
  treatment summary, 622
  vitamin A for, 621–622
Leukotrienes
  asthma and, 261, 265, 266
  psoriasis and, 765–766
LH, *see* Luteinizing hormone
Licorice
  AIDS and, 208–209
  anti-allergy properties, 451
  asthma and, 270
  CFS and, 368–369
  Chinese herbal formula with, 452
  DGL, *see* Deglycyrrhizinated licorice
  eczema and, 451–452
  hepatitis and, 516–517

herpes simplex and, 522
menopause and, 639
PMS and, 749–750
thoroughwax and, 785
ulcers and, 815
Life-expectancy, 163
Life-extension, *see* Longevity
Life span, 163
Lifestyle Heart Trial, 101
Lifestyles, *see also* Diets; Exercise
 AIDS prevention, 210
 Alzheimer's disease and, 232
 anxiety reducing, 259
 behavior, *see* Self-actualization
 cholesterol levels and, 350
 depression and, 383–386
 exercise and, 35–40
 farmer's, 53
 gallstones and, 483
 heart healthy, 85
 hypertension and, 525–527
 IgE levels and, 264
 immune function and, 150
 insomnia and, 603
 macular degeneration and, 627
 mealtime atmosphere, 185
 menopause and, 642–643
 modification, 5–6
 sleep and, 40–43
 smoking and, 33–35
 stress factors, 182–185
 type A behavior, 98–99
 ulcers and, 812–813
Light therapy, 792–793
Limonene, 113
Linoleic acid
 description, 49–51
 eczema and, 450
 MS and, 671–672
 supplements, 77
Linolenic acid
 description, 49
 supplements, 77
α-Linolenic acid
 dietary levels, 95
γ-Linolenic acid
 PMS and, 748
 RA and, 779
γ-Linolenic acid
 diabetes and, 422
Lipases, 127
Lipid peroxides, 91
Lipids
 immune function and, 153
 MS and, 668–669
Lipofuscin
 longevity and, 166
 macular degeneration and, 623
Lipoic acid, 205
Lipoproteins, 347
Lipotropic factors, *see also specific types*
 detoxification and, 123
 gallstones and, 482

Liquids, *see* Juices; Water
Listening techniques, 183–184
Liver
 candidiasis and, 307–308
 cirrhosis, 215, 218
 detoxification, 108–110, 739
 detoxification by, 457
 diet and, 122
 digestion and, 128
 estrogen and, 736–737
 extracts, 515–516
 fatty, alcohol and, 213–214
 flush, 481
 IBD and, 594
 niacin for, 353
 plant-based medicines for, 123–124
 psoriasis and, 765
 toxicants, 106
 vitamin A for, 216
Lobelia inflata, see Indian tobacco;
  Lobelia signature
Lobelia signature, 171
Lobstein, Dennis Ph.D., 36
London Migraine Clinic, 663
Longevity, *see also* Aging
 amino acids for, 172
 antioxidants for, 168–169
 caloric restriction, 168
 DHEA for, 172–173
 exercise for, 37–38, 168
 flavonoids for, 170
 Ginkgo biloba for, 170–172
 melatonin for, 173–174
 myths, 163–164
 overview, 162
Loss model, 378
Lovastatin, 352–353
Low-density lipoproteins
 atherosclerosis and, 86
 description, 52
 garlic and, 356
 gugulipid and, 357
 HDL *vs.*, 90–91
 levels, 348
 niacin and, 351
 smoking and, 88–89
 vitamin E and, 91–93
Low sperm count, *see* Male infertility
LTR gene, 207
Lust, Benedict, 2–3
Luteinizing hormone, 628
Lymphocytes, *see* B cells; T cells
Lymph system, 144–146
Lysine, 521–522

M

Macrophages
 function, 148
 tuftsin and, 159
Macular degeneration
 atherosclerosis and, 624–625
 description, 623
 dietary factors, 625–626

flavonoids for, 625–627
 lifestyle factors, 627
 supplements for, 626
 treatment summary, 627
 types, 623–624
 zinc for, 626
Magnesium
 alcoholism and, 217
 angina and, 242
 asthma and, 269
 CFS and, 367–368
 diabetes and, 420–421
 dietary levels, 96
 dietary sources, 96
 dosage, 530–531, 746–747
 fibromyalgia and, 462
 glaucoma and, 487
 heart attacks and, 96–97
 heart disease and, 502–504
 kidney stones and, 617
 migraines and, 660–661
 osteoporosis and, 719
 PMS and, 746–747
 –potassium
  interaction, 529–530
  risks, 531
Malabar, 692–693
Male infertility
 antioxidants and, 581–583
 arginine and, 584
 carnitine and, 584
 causes, 575
 description, 575
 diagnosing, 576
 fats and, 583
 ginseng and, 584–585
 glandular therapy, 585
 heavy metals and, 581
 hormonal factors, 579–581
 infections and, 579
 Pygeum africanum and, 585
 soy products and, 581
 sperm-damaging factors, 578
 treatment summary, 585–586
 vitamin B12 and, 584
 vitamin C and, 581–583
 vitamin E and, 582–583
 zinc and, 583
Manganese
 diabetes and, 421
 RA and, 781–782
Manic depression, *see* Bipolar disorder
Marcus, 593
Marx Brothers, 149
Mary Tyler Moore, 31
Maslow, Abraham, 19–20
Massachusetts Institute of
  Technology, 682
Massage, *see* Bodywork
Mast cells
 allergies and, 57
 asthma and, 261
 carnitine and, 206–207

Mast cells, *continued*
  ear infections and, 445
  eczema and, 448
  function, 147–148, 148
  periodontal disease and, 724
  skill allergies and, 536
  sugar and, 151
  tuftsin and, 159
Matricaria chamomilla, see Chamomile
Mayans, 629
McMaster University, 166
MCS, *see* Multiple chemical sensitivities
Mealtime atmosphere, 185
Measles, 667
Meats
  description, 69
  fibers, CDSA, 130–131
  taxonomic list, 473
  wild, 45
Medicines
  botanical, 5
  Chinese, 5
  conventional, *see* Conventional
    medicine
  natural, *see* Naturopathic medicine
  physical, 5
Melaleuca alternifolia, see Tea tree oil
Melanin, 173
Melatonin
  cataracts and, 322
  insomnia and, 606
  longevity and, 173–174
Melissa officinalis, see Lemon balm
Memory
  acetylcholine and, 227
  DHEA for, 230–231
  dream, 42–43
  Ginkgo biloba for, 231–232
  LAC and, 230
  menopause and, 635, 642
  phosphatidylcholine for, 229
Menopause
  black cohosh for, 639–641
  bladder infections and, 634–635
  causes, 628–629
  chasteberry for, 639
  cold extremities in, 635
  description, 628
  DHEA and, 173
  dietary factors, 636
  endorphins in, 635
  exercise and, 642–643
  ferulic acid and, 638
  Ginkgo biloba for, 641–642
  headaches with, 634
  hesperidin and, 638
  hot flashes with, 634–635
  HRT for, 630–634
  hypothalamus in, 635
  hypothyroidism and, 635
  licorice for, 639
  medical test during, 635–636
  memory and, 635, 642

osteoporosis and, 711
phytoestrogens for, 636–637
smoking and, 643
as social construct, 629–630
soy for, 637
treatment summary, 643–644
uterine tonics and, 638–639
vaginitis and, 634
vitamin C for, 638
vitamin E for, 637–638
Menorrhagia
  chlorophyll for, 646
  description, 645
  EFAs for, 647
  flavonoids for, 646
  iron balance and, 645–446
  shepherd's purse for, 647
  thyroid gland and, 646–647
  treatment summary, 647
  vitamin A for, 646
  vitamin E for, 646
  vitamin K for, 646
Men's Fitness, 40
Mental attitudes, *see* Moods; Self-
  actualization
Mental illness, *see specific types*
Mentastics, 79
Menthol, 611–612
Merck, 390
Metchnikoff, Elie, 7
Methionine, *see also*
    S-Adenosylmethionine
  cataracts and, 322
  glutathione and, 116
  longevity and, 172
Methylation, 118–119
Methylcobalamin
  availability, 238
  description, 228
Microbial compounds, 106
Migraines, *see also* Headaches
  acupuncture for, 662
  analgesic-induced, 654–655
  arachidonic acid for, 660
  biofeedback for, 662–663
  causes, 649–653
  chiropractoric care for, 661–662
  description, 648
  drug reactions, 653–656
  EFAs for, 660
  ergotamine-induced, 655–656
  feverfew for, 663–664
  food allergy-induced, 656–657
  ginger root for, 664
  histimine-induced, 657–659
  5-HTP for, 659–660
  hypoglycemia and, 552–553
  magnesium for, 660–661
  mechanism, 652
  nerve disorder and, 651
  platelet disorder and, 650–651
  pyridoxine for, 658–659
  relaxation for, 662–663

riboflavin for, 660
serotonin deficiency and, 651–652
TENS for, 662
TMJ and, 662
treatment summary, 664–665
types, 648–649
vascular instability and, 650
Milk
  allergies, 464
  description, 69
Milk thistle
  alcoholism and, 218
  candidiasis and, 308–309
  hepatitis and, 517–518
  liver function and, 123–124
Mind, *see* Moods
Minerals, *see also specific types*
  absorption, 127
  multiple, taking, 74–75
  optimal ranges, 76
  PMS and, 748–749
  subclinical deficiency, 73–74
The Mission Diagnosis, 300
Mitochondria, 115, 246
Mitral valve prolapse
  coenzyme Q_{10}, 505
  description, 500
  magnesium and, 504
  migraines, 651
Molds, 305
Molybdenum, 120
Momordica, 425
Momordica charantia, see Bitter Melon
Monamine hypothesis, 378–380
Monocytes, 148
Moods
  calming, 180–181
  CFS and, 367
  disorders, *see specific types*
  exercise and, 36–37
  hypothyroidism and, 560
  immune function and, 149
  sleep and, 40
  ulcers and, 812
Morality, 22
Morning sickness, *see* Pregnancy
Mozart, Wolfgang Amadeus, 22
MS, *see* Multiple sclerosis
Mucin, 592–594
Mucus, 133
Muira puama, see Potency wood
Multiple chemical sensitivities, 363–364
Multiple Risk Factor Intervention
  Trial, 525
Multiple sclerosis
  autoimmune reaction, 667
  causes, 666–669
  description, 666
  diagnosing, 669
  dietary factors, 667–668, 670–671
  evening primrose for, 672
  exercise for, 675–676
  fish oils and, 672

flaxseed for, 672
food allergies and, 671
Ginkgo biloba for, 674
hyperbaric oxygen for, 674–675
interferon for, 674
linoleic acid for, 671–672
lipid peroxidation and, 668–669
oral antigen therapy, 675
pancreatic enzymes for, 673–674
selenium for, 672–673
treatment summary, 676
viral infections and, 666–667
vitamin B12 for, 673
vitamin E for, 672–673
Muscle & Fitness, 40
Muscular Development, 40
Mustard, 297
Mutations, 167–168
Mycology, 132
Mycoplasmas, 773
Myocardial infarction,
   see Heart attacks
Myoclonus, 606–607
Myoglobin, 237–238
Myringotomy, 440–441
Mystical experiences, 21

N

Nabisco, 276
NAC, *see* N-Acetylcysteine
National Diabetes Data Group, 404
National Digestive Disease Education
   and Information Clearing House,
   328
National Resources Defense Council
   DDT levels, 54
   pesticide monitoring, 55
Native Americans, 477
Natural killer cells
   function, 148
   lifestyle and, 150
Naturopathic medicine
   allopathy and, 9
   allopathy vs., 6–8
   definition, 1
   future, 15–16
   goals, 4
   history, 2–4
   licensing, 14–15
   need for, 10–12
   patient satisfaction, 12–13
   philosophy, 4
   practice, 6
   prescription privileges, 5
   prevention and, 9–10
   principles, 1
   professional organizations, 15
   program, 3
   therapies, 4–6
   training, 13–14
   treatment with, 8–9
Naturopathic physicians licensing
   exam, 15

Naturopathy, see Naturopathic
   medicine
Naylor, G., 283–284
Needs, hierarchy of, 20
Neisseria gonorrhea, see Gonorrhea
Nerve disorders, 651
Nervous system
   description, 150
   diet-induced thermogenesis, 685
   male sex act and, 564–565
   MS and, 673
   stress and, 181
Neurofibrillary tangles, 221
Neuropathy, diabetic
   about, 412–413
   pyridoxine and, 419–420
Neurotransmitters, 737
Neutrophils
   function, 147
   periodontal disease and, 723
New England Journal of Medicine
   Alzheimer's disease, 226
   carotid endarterectomy, 337
   hypoglycemia, 549
   khella, 249
   psoriasis, 765
   vitamin A, 154
   vitamin D, 718
Newton, Sir Isaac, 1
New York Institute for Medical
   Research, 231
Niacin
   cholesterol and, 351–353, 569
   colestipol and, 93
   gout and, 494
   liver and, 353
   niacinamide and, 418–419
Niacinamide
   kani and, 258
   niacin and, 418–419
   osteoarthritis and, 701
   RA and, 782–783
Night blindness, 73
Nitrosamines, 69
NK, *see* Natural killer cells
Nonsteroidal anti-inflammatory drugs,
   see also Aspirin
   asthma and, 261
   osteoarthritis and, 8–9, 697, 698–700
   RA and, 774–776
   safety, 100–101
   ulcers and, 811–812
North American Society of Teachers of
   the Alexander Technique, 80
Northwick Park Heart Study, 98
NPLEX, *see* Naturopathic Physicians
   Licensing Exam
NSAIDS, *see* Nonsteroidal anti-
   inflammatory drugs
Nurses health study, 632
NutraSweet, 555
Nutrients
   accessory, 74

essential, 73–74
immune function and, 150–151
phase I detoxification, 113
*Nutritional Influences of Mental
   Illness,* 255
Nutritional supplementation, *see also
   specific types*
   about, 72–77
   angiograms, 245–246
   clinical, 5
   description, 72–73
   detoxification and, 122–123
   heavy-metals and, 105–106
   hypochlorhydria, 136
   popularity, 73–74
   program, recommendations, 74–75, 77
   RDA and, 73–74
Nutrition Foundation, 276
Nystatin, 545
Nytol, 602

O

Obesity
   causes, 681–686
   chromium for, 690–691
   coenzyme Q_{10} for, 693
   description, 680
   diabetes and, 406
   diet-induced thermogenesis,
      684–686
   exercise for, 35–36
   fiber and, 689–690
   gallstones and, 477–478
   gout, 491–492
   5-HTP, 686–688
   hydroxycitrate for, 692–693
   immune function and, 152
   medium-chain triglycerides, 691–692
   physiological factors, 681–686
   psychological factors, 681
   serotonin and, 682–683
   set-point theory, 683–684
   thermogenic formulas for, 688–689
   treatment summary, 693–694
   types, 680–681
   weight-loss and, 686
Oils, *see specific types*
Ointments, 334
Oleic acid
   dietary levels, 95
   gallstones and, 481
Oligomers, procyanidolic, 95
Oligospermia, 575
Olive oil, 481
Olovnikov, Alexaie, 166
Omega-3 fatty acids
   agoraphobia and, 255
   asthma and, 266
   depression and, 388
   diabetes and, 422–424
   in diet, 95
   eczema and, 451
   glaucoma and, 487

Omega-3 fatty acids, (continued)
heart disease and, 101
hypertension and, 533–534
metabolism, 51
platelet aggregation and, 97
psoriasis and, 765–766
RA and, 779–781
in wild meat, 45
Omega-6 fatty acids
metabolism, 51
prostaglandins in, 50
Onions
asthma and, 270
diabetes and, 424–425
hypertension and, 527
Optimism
depression and, 380
importance, 22–23
learning, 27–31
pessimism vs., 26–27
quiz for, 23–25
reading list, 31–32
Oral antigen therapy, 675
Ornish, Dean, 101
γ-Oryzanol, see Ferulic acid
O'Shea, 278
Osteoarthritis
antioxidants for, 698
Boswellia serrata for, 704
chondroitin sulfate and, 700–701
conventional treatment, 8–9
description, 695
devil's claw and, 704
dietary factors, 697–698
exercise and, 703
GAGs and, 700–701
glucosamine sulfate for, 698–700
hormonal factors, 697
methionine for, 701–702
minerals for, 702
natural course, 696–697
niacinamide for, 701
NSAIDs and, 697, 698–700
physical therapy for, 703
SOD for, 702
supplements for, 702
topical treatments, 704
treatment summary, 704–705
vitamin C and, 698
yucca for, 703
Osteocalcin, 714–715
Osteomark-NTX, 711
Osteoporosis
B vitamins for, 719
calcium for, 715–718
best form, 717–718
as preventive, 716–717
causes, 706–707
description, 706
diagnosing, 710–711
dietary factors, 713–715
fluoride for, 720
folic acid for, 719

hormonal factors, 707
HRT and, 711
lifestyle factors, 711, 713
magnesium for, 719
phytoestrogens for, 720
self-test, 712–713
silicon for, 720
soft drinks and, 714
stomach acid and, 707
treatment summary, 721
vitamin D for, 707–709, 718
vitamin K for, 714–715
Otitis media, 278–279, see Ear infections
Oxazepam, 256–257
Oxidized cholesterol, 91
Oxygen
hyperbaric, 674–675
molecules, 167

P

PAF, see Platelet activating factor
Palm oil, 625–626
Panax ginseng, see Chinese ginseng
Pancreas
extracts, 598
function, 127–128
insufficiency, 137–138
Pancreatic enzymes
candidiasis and, 306
celiac disease, 327–328
MS and, 673–674
Pancreatin, 138
Panic attacks, see Anxiety
Pantethine
angina and, 246–247
cholesterol and, 354
CoA and, 247
Pantothenic acid
acne and, 196
osteoarthritis and, 702
RA and, 782
stress management by, 186
Pantyhose, 818–819
Pap smears, 341–342
Parasites
diarrhea and, 436–437
infection, 144
Parietal cells, 810–811
Parkinson's disease
antioxidants and, 224–225
kava for, 257
Passiflora incarnata, see Passionflower
Passionflower, 607
Pasture, Louis, 7
Pauling, Linus, 373
PCB, 54
PCO, see Procyanidolic oligomers
PCP, 54
PEA, see Phenylethylamine
Peak experiences, 21
Pectin, 435
Penicillin, 538
Penile prosthesis, 570

Peppermint oil, 611–612
Pepsin, 127
Pepto-Bismol
Helicobacter pylori inhibition, 137
ulcers and, 814
Perceptions, 21
Periodontal disease
amalgam restorations, 724
bloodroot for, 728
coenzyme Q₁₀, 727
collagen matrix and, 725
complement system and,
723–724
description, 722
disease process, 722–723
flavonoids for, 727–728
folic acid for, 728
gingival sulcus, 723
guto kola for, 728
local factors, 724
mast cells, 724
smoking and, 725
sugar and, 276
treatment goals, 725–726
treatment summary, 729
vitamin A for, 276
vitamin C for, 726
vitamin E for, 727
zinc for, 276–727
Pertussis, 260–261
Pessimism, 26–27
Pesticides, see also specific types
BPH and, 757
current use, 54–55
exposure, reducing, 53–56
history, 54
monitoring, 54–55
in water, 60
wax and, 56
Peyronie's disease, 567–568
pH
CDSA, 132
hypochlorhydria, 135–136
indigestion and, 134
Phalen, George, 316
Phenolsulphotransferase, 658
Phenylalanine, 393–394
Phenylbutazone, 783
Phenylethylamine, 393–394
Phlethysmorgraph, 828
Phosphatidylcholine, see Lecithin
Phosphatidylserine, 229–230
2-n-butyl Phthalide, 527
Phyllanthus amarus, 518
Physical fitness, see Exercise
Physical medicine, see also specific
types
acne, 198
cellulite, 334
CTS, 318
description, 5
Physical therapy, see Bodywork
Physician's Desk Reference, 567

Phytoestrogens
  menopause and, 636–637
  osteoporosis and, 720
Pimples, 173
Pineal gland, 173
Pine bark
  about, 94–95
  cataracts and, 323
Pinus maritima, see Pine bark
Piper mythisticum, see Kava
Piroxicam, 9
Plants, *see also specific types*
  berberine-containing, 310
  epicatechin-containing, 427
Plaques, 221
Platelet activating factor, 271
Platelets
  aggregation, 97
  disorder, 650–651
Pleasure, 21
PMS, *see* Premenstrual syndrome
Pneumonia
  description, 294
  naturopathic approach,
    296–297
  vitamin C for, 297
Polycyclic hydrocarbons, 108
Post, C. W., 3
Postural draining, 297
Posture, 78
Potassium
  bladder infection and, 288
  CFS and, 368
  diabetes and, 421
  dietary levels, 96
  dosage, 530
  hypertension and, 527–530
  intake, 58–60
  –magnesium
    interaction, 529–530
    risks, 531
  –sodium ratio, 528
Potency wood, 571–572
Poultices
  berberine, 293
  boils, 293
  goldenseal, 293
  mustard, 297
Praag, Herman van, 393–394
Prednisone, *see* Corticosteroids
Pregnancy
  anemia and, 234
  diabetes and, 407–408
  folic acid and, 236
  goldenseal during, 290
  as infertility test, 577–578
  morning sickness
    acupressure for, 679
    description, 677
    ginger for, 678
    psychological aspects, 678–679
    treatment summary, 679
    vitamin C for, 677–678

  vitamin K for, 677–678
  uva ursi during, 290
Premenstrual syndrome
  black cohosh for, 750
  calcium for, 747
  chasteberry for, 750–751
  corpus luteum and, 732
  description, 730
  diagnosing, 733
  dietary factors, 742–744
  dong quai for, 749
  EFAs for, 748
  estrogen and, 736–741
  exercise for, 741
  hypoglycemia and, 552
  licorice for, 749–750
  magnesium for, 746–747
  menstrual cycle and, 731–732
  progesterone for, 740–741
  psychotherapy, 742
  pyridoxine for, 745
  questionnaire, 734
  stress and, 741–742
  supplements for, 748–749
  thyroid and, 741
  treatment summary, 751–752
  types, 733, 735–736
  vitamin E for, 747–748
  zinc for, 747
Prescriptions, 5
Preservatives, 58
Prevention
  cardiovascular disease, 88–90
  cellulite, 332
  naturopathy and, 9–10
*The Principles, Aim, and Program of
  the Nature Cure*, 3
Principles of living, 3
Prinzmetal's variant angina
  description, 242
  magnesium for, 242
Privacy, 21
Proanthocyanidins, 94–95
Probiotics dysbiosis treatment, 143
Problem solving, 21
Procyanidins, *see* Proanthocyanidins
Procyanidolic oligomers, 95
Professional licensing, 14–15
Professional organizations, 15
Progeria, *see* Hutchinsom-Gilford
    syndrome
Progesterone
  –estrogen ratio, 738–741
  therapy, 740–741
Progressive relaxation, 182
Proiotics, *see specific types*
Prolactins
  estrogen and, 738
  FBD and, 455
Proline hydroxylase, 73
Propionibacterium acnes, 192
Prostaglandins
  asthma and, 265

  Crohn's disease and, 592
  EFAs and, 49–52
  fatty acids and, 672
  synthesis, 645
Prostate enlargement
  amino acids for, 756
  botanical use, 757–758
  cernilton for, 759–760
  cholesterol and, 756
  description, 753
  diagnosing, 753–754
  dietary factors, 755
  EFAs for, 756
  hormonal factors, 754–755
  Pygeum africanum for, 760–761
  saw palmetto for, 758–759
  soy for, 757
  stinging nettle for, 761–762
  treatment summary, 762
  TURP and, 755
  zinc for, 755–756
Proteases
  candidiasis and, 306
  digestion and, 127–128
  small-intestinal bacteria and, 140
Proteins, *see also specific types*
  acne and, 194
  complement system, 723–724
  digestion, 764
  fats and, 493
  glycosylated, diabetes and, 411
  grain, chemistry, 325–326
  immune system and, 151
  metabolism byproducts, 107
Provitamin A, *see* Carotenes
Prozac
  depression and, 386
  PMS and, 737, 742
Psoriasis
  alcohol and, 765
  bowel toxemia and, 764–765
  capsaicin for, 768
  causes, 763–765
  cayenne pepper for, *see* Cayenne
    pepper
  chamomile for, 767–768
  description, 763
  EFAs and, 765–766
  fasting for, 766
  food allergies and, 766
  fumaric acid for, 767
  glycyrrhetinic acid for, 767–768
  liver and, 765
  protein digestion and, 764
  stress and, 767
  supplements for, 766
  treatment summary, 768–769
  tropical treatments, 767–768
  UV light for, 767
Psychotherapy
  impotence, 569
  PMS, 742
Pterocarpus marsupium, 427

Purine deficient diet, 492
Pygeum africanum
　BPH and, 760–761
　male infertility and, 585
Pyridoxine
　acne and, 196
　AIDS and, 206
　alcoholism and, 217
　asthma and, 266–267
　cervical dysplasia and, 345–346
　CTS and, 316–317
　depression and, 387–388
　diabetes and, 419–420
　dosage, 745
　estrogen and, 738
　homocysteine levels and, 98
　immune function and, 156
　kidney stones and, 617
　magnesium and, 745
　migraines and, 658–659
　morning sickness and, 677
　platelet aggregation and, 97
　PMS and, 745
　safety, 745
　seborrheic dermatitis and, 795
Pyruvic acid
　anxiety and, 253
　lactic acid and, 255

Q

Quercetin
　asthma and, 268
　canker sores and, 314–315
　eczema and, 451
　gout and, 494
　hives and, 546–547
Questions, asking, 28–29

R

Radical loops, 224
Raffray, Andre-François, 164
Ragweed, 261
Rand Corporation, 498
Ranitidine, *see* Zantac
Rapid eye movement, 41, 460
Rash, *see* Hives
RDA, *see* Recommend daily allowance
Recall, *see* Memory
Recommend daily allowance, 73–74
Red blood cells, 233–234
5-α-Reductase, 192
Red wine
　benefits, 94
　headaches and, 658
Reflective listening, 183–184
Reflux esophagitis, *see* Indigestion
Relationships
　self-actualized, 21–22
　stress in, 183–184
Relaxation
　migraines and, 662–663
　progressive, 182, 604–605
　response, 180–181

REM, *see* Rapid eye movement
REP, *see* Retinal pigmented epithelium
Resistance reaction, 177
Respiratory syncytial virus, 153–154
Restless-legs syndrome, 606–607
Retin-A, 193–194
Retinal pigmented epithelium, 623, 626
Retinopathy, diabetic, 413
Rheumatoid arthritis
　antibodies and, 771–772
　antioxidants for, 781
　bacterial factors, 139
　bromelain for, 784
　causes, 770–774
　conventional treatment, 774–776
　copper for, 782
　curcumin for, 783–784
　description, 770
　DHEA for, 773–774
　diagnosing, 774–775
　dietary factors, 776–777
　digestion and, 778
　EBV link, 772–773
　fecal flora and, 777–778
　ginger for, 784
　GI tract and, 771
　GLA and, 779
　immune system and, 771–772
　manganese for, 781–782
　microbial hypotheses, 772–773
　niacinamide for, 782–783
　NSAIDs, 774–776
　pantothenic acid for, 782
　physical therapy for, 785–786
　related diseases, 770–771
　selenium for, 781
　SOD for, 781–782
　sulfur for, 782
　treatment summary, 787–789
　vitamin C for, 782
　zinc for, 780–781
Rheum species, see Rhubarb
Rhubarb, 816
Riboflavin
　cataracts and, 321–322
　migraines and, 660
RICE therapy, 805–806
Rinkel, Herbert J., 471
Rippere, 275
Ritchie articular index, 786
RNA, 200
RNA-reverse transcriptase
　description, 200
　lipoic acid and, 205
Robbins, Anthony, 28
Robert's formula, 598
Rockefeller Institute, 164
Rolfing, 79
Roots, *see specific types*
Rosacea
　B vitamins for, 791
　description, 790

hypochlorhydria and, 790–791
　treatment summary, 791
Rotary diversified diet, 471–474
Rowe, Albert, 185, 366, 388
Royal Liverpool University, 607
RSV, *see* Respiratory syncytial virus
Ruscus aculeatus, see Butcher's broom
Russia, Georgia region, 163
Ruta graveolens, see Gravel root
Rutin, 487

S

SAD, *see* Seasonal affective disorder
Salicylates, 543–544
Salivary amylase, 127
Salivary glands, 127–128
Salt, *see* Sodium
Salt bush, 426–427
SAM, *see* S-Adenosylmethionine
Sanguinaria canadensis, see Bloodroot
Sanguinarine, 728
SAOX, see Serum antioxidant capacity
Saw palmetto, 758–759
Scandinavians, 235
Schauss, 275
Schizophrenia, 383
Seafood, 69
Seasonal affective disorder
　description, 792
　light therapy, 792–793
　St. John's wort for, 793
　treatment summary, 793
Sebaceous glands, 191–192
Seborrheic dermatitis
　biotin and, 794–795
　description, 794
　folic acid for, 795
　food allergies and, 794
　pyridoxine for, 795
　treatment summary, 795–796
　vitamin B12 for, 795
Sebum, 191
Second-hand smoke, 89–90
Sedatives
　chemical, 602
　natural, 605
Selenium
　acne and, 195–196
　AIDS and, 205
　asthma and, 268
　cataracts and, 320–321
　cervical dysplasia and, 346
　immune function and, 157
　MS and, 672
　RA and, 781
Self-actualization
　achieving, 22–31
　characteristics, 21–22
　importance, 19–21
Self-talk, 28
Seligman, Martin, 379–380
Selye, Hans, 178, 184

Semen analysis, 576
Senna, 618
Serenoa repens, see Saw palmetto
Serotonin
  deficiency syndrome, 651–652
  depression and, 380–381
  obesity and, 682–683
  platelet disorder and, 650–651
  sleep therapy, 605–606
Sertoli cells, 580
Serum
  factors, function, 148
  ferritin, 234
Serum antioxidant capacity, 94
Set-point theory, 683–684
Sex act, male, 564–565
Sex organs, male, 567–568
Shape, 40
Shepherd's purse, 647
Showa Denko, 389–390
Shute, Evan, 93
Shute, Wilfred, 93
Shute Institute and Medical Clinic, 93
Siberian ginseng
  CFS and, 368–369
  stress management by, 186–187
Sicuteri, Federigo, 461
Silicon, 720
Silybum marianum, see Milk thistle
Sinusitis
  allergies and, 798
  antibiotics for, 797–798
  bromelain for, 798
  description, 797
  Helicobacter pylori and, 798
  treatment summary, 799–800
Skin
  cellulite, 329–334
  eczema, 448–454
  gender differences, 331
  hypothyroidism and, 560
  kava and, 257–258
  lesions, IBD and, 594
  prick test, 470
  rosacea, 790–791
  seborrheic dermatitis, 794–796
Sleep, *see also* Insomnia
  BPH and, 759
  dreams, 41–43
  fasting and, 125
  fibromyalgia, 460–461
  importance, 40
  pills for, *see* Sedatives
  requirements, 40
Smoking
  aging and, 167
  cardiovascular disease and, 88–89
  cervical dysplasia and, 343–344
  cessation techniques, 34–35
  cytochrome P450 and, 111
  depression and, 384
  glutathione and, 116
  health hazards, 33–34

impotence and, 567
male infertility and, 581–582
menopause and, 643
passive, 89–90
periodontal disease and, 725
turmeric and, 114
ulcers and, 812–813
Social readjustment rating scale, 178–180
SOD, *see* Superoxide dismutase
Sodium
  asthma and, 269
  bladder infection and, 288
  intake, 58–60
  kidney stones and, 618
  PMS and, 744
  –potassium ratio, 528
  in prepared foods, 528
  stress and, 185
Sodium cromoglycate, 546–547
Soft drinks, 714
Sorbitol, 411–412, 418
Sore throat
  antibiotics and, 801
  description, 800
  herbal treatments, 802–803
  immune system and, 801–802
  treatment summary, 803–804
  vitamin C for, 802
Soy products
  BPH and, 757
  male infertility and, 581
  menopause and, 637
  osteoporosis and, 720
  PMS and, 744
Special tissue cells, 148
Sperm
  agglutinated, 583
  –damaging factors, 578
Spleen
  extracts, 159
  function, 147
Splenectomy, 159
Splenopentin, 159
Spontaneity, 21
Sport injuries, *see* Bursitis; Tendinitis
St. John's wort
  depression and, 396–397
  fibromyalgia and, 462
  SAD and, 793
Standing fat-cell chambers, 330
Staphylococcus aureus, 448–449
Stekel, William, 42
Steroids, *see specific types*
Stinging nettle, 761–762
Straphylococcus aureus, 293
Streptozotocin, 406
Stress
  adrenals and, 383
  alcohol and, 184–185
  caffeine and, 184
  canker sores and, 314
  carbohydrates and, 185
  conditions linked to, 178

CSF and, 364
digestion and, 133–134
food allergies and, 466–467
general adaption syndrome, 176–177
health view of, 178
hives and, 545–546
hypertension and, 531–532
immune function and, 149–150
levels, 178–180
PMS and, 741–742
potassium and, 185
psoriasis and, 767
recognizing, 175–176
response
  description, 175
  relaxation response *vs.,* 181
sodium and, 185
ulcers and, 812
Stress management
  body calming, 180–181
  diaphragmatic breathing, 182
  diets for, 184
  exercise for, 184
  ginseng for, 186–187
  herbal support, 185–187
  lifestyle factors, 182–185
  mind calming, 180–181
  negative coping patterns, 180
  nutritional support, 185–187
  overview, 175
  relaxation, progressive, 182
  techniques, general, 180
The Stress of Life, 178
Stroke, 102
Stronger neominophagen C, 516–517
Subclinical deficiency, 73–74
Subcutaneous tissue, 329–330
Sucrose, *see* Sugar
Sugar, *see also* Glucose; Hypoglycemia
  acne and, 194
  blood, 214–215
  candidiasis and, 305
  CFS and, 367
  common cold and, 373
  depression and, 385–386
  food dyes and, 277
  gallstones and, 480
  IBS and, 611
  immune system and, 151–152
  intake, 53
  kidney stones, 616–617
  periodontal disease, 276
  PMS and, 743
Sugar Blues, 549
Sulfation, 119
Sulfites
  about, 60
  hives and, 544
Sulfonylureas, *see* Sulfur
Sulfoxidation, 120

Sulfur
    acne and, 197
    diabetes, 409–410
    RA and, 782
Sunbathing, 483
Superoxide dismutase
    aging and, 168–169
    cataracts and, 321
    osteoarthritis and, 702
    RA and, 781–782
Supplementary measures
    overview, 71–72
    physical care, 77–80
Surgery, *see also specific types*
    increase in, 11, 440–441
Swank diet, 670–671
Swanson, 275–276
Sweet and Dangerous, 549
Sydenham, 489–490
Syndrome X, 550, 553

T

Tagamet, 306
Tai Chi, 368
The Talmud, 42
Tanacetum parthenium, see Feverfew
Tartrazine
    about, 57
    asthma and, 261
    CTS and, 316
    hives and, 542–544
T cells
    AIDS and, 200
    allergies and, 466
    carotenes and, 154
    counts, 200–202, 205
    description, 146
    function, 147
    licorice and, 208–209
    lipoic acid and, 205
    vitamin A and, 204–205
    vitamin E and, 155–156
Tea tree oil
    boils and, 292–293
    description, 196–197
Television, 681
Telomeres
    about, 166
    shortening theory, 166–167
Temperature, basal body, 560–561
Temporomandibular joint
    dysfunction, 662
Tendinitis
    bromelain for, 807
    cause, 805
    curcumin for, 807
    description, 805
    flavonoids for, 807
    nutrition and, 806–807
    physical therapy for, 807–808
    RICE for, 805–806
    treatment summary, 808–809
    vitamin B12 for, 807

TENS, Transcutaneous electrical
    stimulation
Terpenes, 483
Testicular hypothermia device, 578
Tetrahydrobiopterin
    cataracts and, 321
    depression and, 387
Thermogenesis, diet-induced, 684–686
Thiamin
    alcoholism and, 217
    brain function and, 227
    heart disease and, 501–502
Thoreau, Henry David, 1
Throats, *see* Sore throat
Thymus gland
    AIDS and, 207
    antioxidants, 158–159
    ear infections and, 445
    extracts, 158–159, 516
    function, 146–147, 157
    stress and, 149–150
Thymus index, 158
Thyroid gland
    CFS and, 366
    cholesterol levels and, 349
    deficient, *see* Hypothyroidism
    depression and, 382–383
    eczema and, 452–453
    FBD and, 456–457
    hives and, 547
    menorrhagia and, 646–647
    osteoporosis and, 709–710
    PMS and, 741
Thyroid-stimulating hormone, 558
TIA, *see* Transient ischemic attack
Time management, 182–183
Tissues, subcutaneous, 329–330
TMJ, *see* Temporomandibular joint
    dysfunction
TNF, *see* Tumor necrosis factor
α-Tocopherol, *see* Vitamin E
Tolbutamide, 410
Tonsillectomy, 440–441
Toxicity, diagnosing, 107–108
Toxins, *see also specific types*
    depression and, 383
    gout and, 495
    male infertility and, 580
    types, 105–107
Toynbee phenomenon, 444
Trager, Milton, 79
The Trager Institute, 80
Tragerwork, 79
Training
    naturopathy, 13–14
    in optimism, 27–31
Transcutaneous electrical stimulation,
    662, 808
Trans-fatty acids
    about, 52–53
    acne and, 194
Transient ischemic attack, 335
Tretinoin, *see* Retin-A

Trichomonas vaginalis, 819
Triglycerides
    CDSA, 130
    obesity and, 691–692
Trigonella foenumgraecum,
    see Fenugreek
Troendle, 351
Truss, Orion, 300
Trypsin, 235
Tryptophan
    asthma and, 266–267
    bipolar disorder and, 283
    catastrophe, 389–390
    depression and, 380, 390–391
    insomnia and, 605–606
    schizophrenia, 383
TSH, *see* Thyroid-stimulating hormone
Tuftsin, 159
Tumor necrosis factor, 208
Turmeric, *see* Curcumin
Turnera diffusa, see Damiana
Tylophora asthmatica, 270–271
Type A personality, 98–99
Tyrosine
    depression and, 393–394
    hypothyroidism, 562

U

Ubiquinone, *see* Coenzyme Q10
UDP-glucuronyl transferase, 119–120
UDPGT, *see* UDP-glucuronyl
    transferase
Ulcerative colitis, 593
Ulcers
    aloe vera for, 816
    cabbage for, 813–814
    description, 810–811
    DGL and, 815–186
    fiber for, 813
    flavonoids for, 814–815
    food allergies and, 813
    Helicobacter pylori and, 811
    licorice and, 815
    lifestyle factors, 812–813
    Pepto-Bismol and, 814
    psychological factors, 812
    rhubarb for, 816
    smoking and, 812–813
    supplements for, 814–815
    treatment summary, 816–817
    types, 810–811
Ulnar loops, 224
Ultraviolet therapy
    hives, 546
    psoriasis and, 767
Universal Group Diabetes Program, 415
University of California, Berkley, 199
University of Chicago, 526–527
University of Connecticut, 461
University of Nottingham, 663
University of Rome, 687
University of Surrey, 283
University of Texas, 316

Unlimited Power, 28
Uric acid
  gout and, 489, 491
  kidney stones and, 618
Urinary tract infection, *see* Bladder
    infection
Urine
  acidifying, 288–289
  alkalinizing, 288–289
  flow, increasing, 287
Ursodeoxycholic acid, 483
Urtica dioca, see Stinging nettle
Urticaria, *see* Hives
Uterine tonics, 638–639
Uva ursi, 289

V

Vaccinium macrocarpon, see
    Cranberry juice
Vacuum constrictive devices, 569–570
Vaginitis
  antiseptics for, 823–824
  bacterial factors, 819
  boric acid for, 823–824
  causes, 818–820, 822
  description, 818
  dietary factors, 822
  gentian violet, 824–825
  gonorrhea, 820, 822
  iodine for, 823
  Lactobacillus acidophilus, 822–823
  menopausal, 634
  treatment summary, 824–825
Valerate, 131
Valerian, 607–608
Valeriana officinalis, see Valerian
Valium, 187, 255
Vanadium, 283–284
Varicose veins
  bromelain for, 829–830
  butcher's broom for, 829
  causes, 826
  description, 826
  dietary fiber for, 827
  exercise for, 827
  flavonoids for, 829
  gotu cola for, 828
  horse chestnut for, 828
  supplements for, 827
  treatment summary, 830
Vascular instability, 650
Vasoactive amines, 139
Vegetables
  description, 65–66
  fibers, CDSA, 131
  green leafy, 714–715
  macular degeneration and, 625–626
  nightshade, 697–698
  taxonomic list, 472
Vegetarianism
  anemia and, 234, 235
  asthma and, 265–266
  biotin absorption, 419

description, 44–49
  estrogen and, 742–743
  gallstones and, 480
  hypertension and, 526
  osteoporosis and, 713
  RA and, 777–778
  vitamin B12 deficiency, 238
Venotonic activity, 828–829
Violet, *see* Gentian violet
Viruses, *see also specific types*
  diabetes and, 406
  hives and, 545
Visualization
  practicing, 30
  smoking cessation by, 34
Vitamin A
  acne and, 194–195
  AIDS and, 204
  alcoholism and, 215–216
  bladder infection and, 290
  cataracts and, 322
  cervical dysplasia and, 344
  colds and, 374
  FBD and, 456
  immune function and, 153–154
  leukoplakia and, 621–622
  menorrhagia and, 646
  periodontal disease and, 276
  ulcers and, 814
Vitamin B1, *see* Thiamin
Vitamin B2, 316
Vitamin B5, *see* Pantothenic acid
Vitamin B6, *see* Pyridoxine
Vitamin B12
  AIDS and, 206
  Alzheimer's disease and, 227–228
  anemia and, 235–236
  asthma and, 268–269
  deficiency, 238–240
  diabetes and, 419–420
  dosage, 240
  forms, 228, 238
  hives and, 546
  homocysteine levels and, 98
  IBD and, 597–598
  immune function and, 156
  injectable *vs.* oral, 238–240
  iron-deficiency anemia, 234
  male infertility, 584
  MS and, 673
  oral *vs.* injectable, 238–240
  seborrheic dermatitis and, 795
  tendinitis and, 807
Vitamin C
  AIDS and, 204
  alcoholism and, 217
  Alzheimer's disease and, 225–226
  angiograms, 245–246
  as antioxidant, 75, 93–94
  asthma and, 267–268
  bipolar disorder and, 283–284
  cataracts and, 319–320
  cervical dysplasia and, 344–345

cholesterol and, 354–355
  common cold and, 373
  diabetes and, 416–417
  enzyme interaction, 73
  gallstones, 491
  glaucoma and, 486–487
  glutathione and, 117–118
  gout and, 494
  hepatitis and, 515
  herpes simplex and, 521
  hives and, 546
  hypertension and, 532
  IBD and, 597
  immune function and, 155
  kidney stones and, 618
  leukoplakia and, 622
  male infertility and, 581–583
  menopause and, 638
  menorrhagia and, 646
  morning sickness and, 677–678
  osteoarthritis and, 698, 702
  PCO *vs.,* 95
  periodontal disease and, 726
  pneumonia and, 299
  RA and, 782
  red wine *vs.,* 94
  sore throat and, 802
  stress management by, 186
  sugar levels and, 151
*Vitamin C and the Common
    Cold,* 373
Vitamin D, 707–709, 718
Vitamin E
  for acne, 195–196
  acne and, 195–196
  AIDS and, 204
  Alzheimer's disease and,
    225–226
  as antioxidant, 75
  asthma and, 268
  cardiovasular disease and, 91–93
  cataracts and, 320–321
  diabetes and, 420
  FBD and, 456
  gallstones, 481
  gout and, 493
  IBD and, 597
  immune function and, 155–156
  leukoplakia and, 622
  male infertility and, 582–583
  menopause and, 637–638
  menorrhagia and, 646
  MS and, 672–673
  osteoarthritis and, 702
  PCO *vs.,* 95
  periodontal disease and, 727
  PMS and, 747–748
  ulcers and, 814
Vitamin K
  kidney stones and, 617
  menorrhagia and, 646
  morning sickness and, 677–678
  osteoporosis and, 714–715

Vitamins, *see also specific types*
  bursitis, 806–807
  hypothyroidism and, 562
  IBD and, 596–597
  multiple, taking, 74–75
  optimal ranges, 76
  PMS and, 748–749
  psoriasis and, 766
  subclinical deficiency, 73–74
  tendinitis and, 806–807
Vitex agnus castus, see Chasteberry
Vitis vinifera, see Grapes
Volatile oils, 311

W

Wasting syndrome, 202
Water
  blood pressure and, 529
  common cold and, 372–373
  consumption, 60
  diarrhea and, 434
  –filtration units, 60
  gout and, 493
  hot/cold treatments, 317
  urine flow and, 287
Water Quality Association, 60
Watson, James, 168
Watt, 593
Waxes, 55–56

Waynberg, Jacques, 571
Werbach, Melvin, 255, 386
Werner's syndrome, 166–167
White blood cells, *see* Mast cells
Whooping cough, *see* Pertussis
Williams, Roger, 74–75
Wilson, Robert A., 629–630
World Health Organization
  anitbiotic use, 301
  antibiotic use, 8, 441–442
  traditional medicines, 424
Worries scale, 99
Wright, Jonathan, 120, 136, 268–269
Wurtman, Judith, 682
Wurtman, Richard, 682

X

Xanthine oxidase, 493

Y

Yeast, 305
The Yeast Connection, 300
Yeast syndrome, *see* Candidiasis
Yellow #5, *see* Tartrazine
Yellow dye 5, 57
Yohimbe, 571
Yucca, 703
Yudkin, John, 549

Z

Zantac, 306
Zinc
  acne and, 195
  AIDS and, 206
  alcoholism and, 215
  Alzheimer's disease and,
    228–229
  BPH and, 755–756
  cataracts and, 322
  diabetes and, 421–422
  DNA and, 228–229
  eczema and, 451
  enzyme interaction, 73
  herpes simplex and, 521
  IBD and, 597–598
  immune function, 156–157
  lozenges, colds and, 373–374
  macular degeneration and, 626
  male infertility and, 583
  periodontal disease and, 276–727
  PMS and, 747
  RA and, 780–781
  ulcers and, 814
Zingiber officinale, see Ginger
Ziodvudine
  AIDS and, 200
  carnitine and, 207
  description, 200